GYNECOLOGY

Principles and Practice

GYNECOLOGY
PRINCIPLES AND PRACTICE

FOURTH EDITION

ROBERT W. KISTNER, M.D.

Associate Clinical Professor of Obstetrics and Gynecology
Harvard Medical School
Senior Gynecologist, Brigham and Women's Hospital
Formerly Associate Chief of Staff
Boston Hospital for Women
(formerly Free Hospital for Women and Boston Lying-In Hospital)
Boston, Massachusetts

YEAR BOOK MEDICAL PUBLISHERS, INC.

CHICAGO • LONDON

234567890K89888786

Library of Congress Cataloging in Publication Data
Main entry under title:

Gynecology: principles and practice.

   Rev. ed. of: Gynecology/Robert W. Kistner. 3d ed. c1979.
   Includes bibliographies and index.
   1. Gynecology.   I. Kistner, Robert W. (Robert
William), 1917–   . II. Kistner, Robert W. (Robert
William), 1917–   . Gynecology. [DNLM: 1. Genital
Diseases, Female.   2. Genital Neoplasms, Female.
WP 140 G9977]
RG101.G95   1986   618.1   85–14232
ISBN 0-8151-5082-2

Sponsoring Editor: James D. Ryan, Jr.
Manager, Copyediting Services: Frances M. Perveiler
Copyeditor: Deborah Thorp
Production Project Manager: R. Allen Reedtz
Proofroom Supervisor: Shirley E. Taylor

To my wife, JANET,
and my children,
DANA, SKIP, STEVE, *and* PETE

Contributors

Robert Barbieri, M.D.

Assistant Professor, Obstetrics and Gynecology
Harvard Medical School
Brigham and Women's Hospital
Boston, Massachusetts

Ross S. Berkowitz, M.D.

Associate Professor, Obstetrics and Gynecology
Harvard Medical School
Associate Director
New England Trophoblastic Disease Center
Brigham and Women's Hospital
Boston, Massachusetts

Richard W. Erbe, M.D.

Associate Professor, Genetics and Pediatrics
Harvard Medical School
Chief, Genetics Unit
Massachusetts General Hospital
Boston, Massachusetts

Stephen Evans, M.D.

Instructor, Obstetrics and Gynecology
Harvard Medical School
Fellow, Reproductive Endocrinology
Brigham and Women's Hospital
Boston, Massachusetts

Donald P. Goldstein, M.D.

Associate Professor, Obstetrics and Gynecology
Harvard Medical School
Director, New England Trophoblastic Disease Center
Brigham and Women's Hospital
Chief of Adolescent Gynecology
Children's Hospital
Boston, Massachusetts

Howard M. Goodman, M.D.

Instructor, Mount Sinai Medical Center
Attending, Mount Sinai Hospital
New York, New York

C. Thomas Griffiths, M.D.

Associate Professor, Gynecology
Harvard Medical School
Associate Chief, Gynecologic Oncology
Brigham and Women's Hospital
Dana Farber Cancer Institute
Boston, Massachusetts

Robert W. Kistner, M.D.

Associate Clinical Professor, Obstetrics and Gynecology
Harvard Medical School
Senior Gynecologist
Brigham and Women's Hospital
Formerly Associate Chief of Staff
Boston Hospital for Women (formerly Free Hospital for Women and Boston Lying-In Hospital)
Boston, Massachusetts

Robert C. Knapp, M.D.

William H. Baker Professor of Gynecology
Harvard Medical School
Director, Gynecology and Gynecologic
Oncology
Brigham and Women's Hospital
Dana Farber Cancer Institute
Boston, Massachusetts

Thomas Leavitt, Jr., M.D.

Associate Clinical Professor, Obstetrics
and Gynecology
Harvard Medical School
Obstetrician-Gynecologist
Brigham and Women's Hospital
Boston, Massachusetts

Wayne A. Miller, M.D.

Assistant Professor of Pediatrics (Genetics)
Harvard Medical School
Director, Prenatal Diagnostic Laboratory
Massachusetts General Hospital
Boston, Massachusetts

Veronica A. Ravnikar, M.D.

Instructor, Obstetrics and Gynecology
Harvard Medical School
Associate Director, Menopause Unit
Brigham and Women's Hospital
Boston, Massachusetts

Isaac Schiff, M.D.

Associate Professor, Obstetrics and
Gynecology
Harvard Medical School
Associate Director
Reproductive Endocrine Services
Brigham and Women's Hospital
Boston, Massachusetts

Robert L. Shirley, M.D.

Assistant Clinical Professor, Obstetrics and
Gynecology
Harvard Medical School
Brigham and Women's Hospital
Dana Farber Cancer Institute
Boston, Massachusetts

Phillip G. Stubblefield, M.D.

Associate Professor, Obstetrics and
Gynecology
Harvard Medical School
Chief, Department of Obstetrics and
Gynecology
Mount Auburn Hospital
Cambridge, Massachusetts

Ruth E. Toumala, M.D.

Instructor, Obstetrics and Gynecology
Harvard Medical School
Director, Infectious Diseases Service
Brigham and Women's Hospital
Boston, Massachusetts

Preface to First Edition

THIS WORK is designed both as a textbook and as a general reference book of gynecology to meet the needs of undergraduate medical students, young practitioners of gynecology, and specialists in this field. The format of each chapter is similar, the purpose being to provide a uniform and organized approach to the understanding of multiple disease processes of each organ of the female genital tract. Thus, in each chapter the embryology, anatomy, and histology are correlated with specific malformations. Morphologic variations are correlated with physiologic alterations. Recent advances in the diagnosis and therapy of infectious processes are described in detail. Particular emphasis has been given to the relationship of premalignant to malignant neoplasms, and methods for the prophylaxis of certain tumors are suggested. Because of the importance and increasing incidence of endometriosis a separate chapter on this disease is included. Particular emphasis has been placed on hormonal therapy, and details of management outlined.

Because of my interest in the practical endocrinologic aspects of gynecology, a chapter is devoted to steroid therapy. In this chapter an attempt is made to obviate many of the difficulties of administration associated with the new synthetic preparations. I have included (1) a brief résumé of basic steroid chemistry, (2) a summation of the pharmacology and physiology of androgens, estrogens, and progesterone, together with a similar discussion of the synthetic progestins, and (3) a discussion of proved and proposed indications for the use of these steroids, with specific contraindications and optimum dosage.

The observations and opinions expressed in this text summarize the sum and substance of the teaching and practice at the Free Hospital for Women during the past 15 years. This hospital was opened on November 2, 1875, and has been in continuous operation since that time. It is the only remaining specialty hospital in the United States whose primary objective is the diagnosis and treatment of medical and surgical diseases of the female.

The Free Hospital for Women became internationally known because of the *Textbook of Gynecology* written by Dr. William P. Graves, formerly Professor of Gynecology at Harvard Medical School. Although the fourth and last edition of Graves' textbook appeared in 1928, since that time a multiplicity of original and important contributions has been published by the members of the staff. Outstanding among these have been the innumerable works of Drs. George and Olive Smith concerning the measurement and metabolism of ovarian steroids and gonadotropic hormones during the menstrual cycle, the period of conception, and subsequent pregnancy. During the years 1938 through 1957 Drs. John Rock and Arthur T. Hertig accomplished their monumental studies on the earliest stages of human growth following fertilization. From 1928 through 1958 Dr. Rock directed intensive study and research projects relating to the etiologic factors in infertility. The pathogenesis of carcinoma in situ of the cervix and its relationship to invasive carcinoma have undergone thorough investigation and evaluation by Drs. Paul Younge, Arthur T. Hertig, and Donald G. MacKay. During the past seven years the synthetic progestational agents have been subjected to extensive clinical investigation in specific gynecologic disorders such as endometriosis and endometrial carcinoma.

In preparing a work of this type, material must be gathered not only from the author's personal experience, but to a still greater extent from the work of others. I have, therefore, attempted to include the important observations of numerous authors who have published data concerning the clinical material at the Free Hospital for Women. From the great number of publications consulted there have been several to which I have had frequent recourse, both for new material and for corroboration of personal observations. I must, therefore, express a general acknowledgment of indebtedness to Drs. George and Olive Smith, Arthur T. Hertig, Christopher J. Duncan, Paul A. Younge, Donald G. MacKay, and John Rock. I have also drawn on the writings of the late Joe V. Meigs and Langdon Parsons, both former residents at the Free Hospital for Women. In writing the sections on the relationship of endocrinology to gynecology I have received the greatest assistance from the excellent works, *Endocrine and Metabolic Aspects of Gynecology* by Joseph Rogers, *Human Endocrinology* by Herbert S. Kupperman, and *The Endocrinology of Reproduction*, edited by Joseph T. Velardo. The reader is referred to these publications for additional and specific details.

I am indebted to Mrs. Edith Tagrin for the excellent illustrations and to Mr. Leo Goodman and Dr. Robert Ehrmann for the photomicrographs. Dr. Arthur T. Hertig and Dr. Hazel M. Gore have also kindly given permission to reproduce many of their excellent photomicrographs previously published in *Tumors of the Female Sex Organs*, published by the Armed Forces Institute of Pathology. The student is advised to refer to these fascicles for a complete survey of the pathology of tumors of the female genital tract.

I also wish to acknowledge a deep indebtedness to the tireless fingers and indefatigable efforts of my secretaries, Mrs. Ann Gregory Metzger, Mrs. Constance M. Rakoske, Mrs. Linda Angelico, and Mrs. Rachel Markiewicz. Valuable assistance has been given to me by the Administrator of the Free Hospital for Women, Miss Lillian Grahn. Finally, the courtesies of the staff of Year Book Medical Publishers have made the final preparation of this manuscript a pleasant task.

ROBERT W. KISTNER

Preface to Fourth Edition

THE FIRST EDITION of this textbook, published in 1964, was designed to meet the needs of medical students, interns, and residents in obstetric and gynecologic training as well as established specialists in this field. The observations and opinions expressed in the first edition summarized the sum and substance of the teaching and practice at the former Free Hospital for Women, a teaching hospital of the Harvard Medical School. Subsequently, the Free Hospital for Women joined the Boston Lying-In Hospital to form the Boston Hospital for Women. In 1980, a new hospital was constructed, adjacent to the Harvard Medical School, which included the Boston Hospital for Women, the Peter Bent Brigham Hospital, and the Robert Breck Brigham Hospital. Despite this amalgamation, the Department of Obstetrics and Gynecology has retained its unique identity and the fourth edition of this textbook accurately reflects the principles and practice of gynecology in our new institution, The Brigham and Women's Hospital.

Twenty-five years ago I wrote the entire first edition, mostly from lectures given to junior and senior medical students. Mr. Fred Rogers, then Vice President of Year Book Medical Publishers, was responsible for the inception and development of this book since he indicated to me a need for an updated gynecologic textbook. Dr. William P. Graves, formerly Professor of Gynecology at Harvard Medical School, had published a textbook of gynecology but the fourth and last edition appeared in 1928. From 1930 until 1960 numerous original and important contributions had been published by the members of the staff of the Free Hospital for Women. The first edition included all of the important publications of George V. Smith, John Rock, Arthur Hertig, Paul A. Younge, and Donald G. McKay. My own contributions concerning the newly developed oral contraceptive, induction of ovulation, and hormonal therapy for endometriosis received full attention. A major criticism of the first edition was its rather parochial approach. In retrospect, the criticism was accurate.

Therefore, the second edition, published in 1971, was expanded to include advances in the rapidly advancing subspecialty areas of endocrinology and fertility, cytogenetics, conception control, and oncology. For the third edition, published in 1978, each chapter was either thoroughly updated and revised or completely rewritten. Dr. Donald P. Goldstein added new material to his already authoritative chapter on trophoblastic tumors and Dr. C. Thomas Griffiths revised the chapter on the ovary, with particular emphasis on changes in surgical and chemotherapeutic approaches.

The fourth edition of *Gynecology: Principles and Practice* introduces many new authors in an effort to provide the reader with the most authoritative and updated material in the various subspecialties of gynecology. Dr. Thomas Leavitt has revised and rewritten the chapter on diseases of the vulva and Drs. Ross Berkowitz and Donald Goldstein have updated the chapter on trophoblastic tumors. In addition, Dr. C. Thomas Griffiths and Dr. Berkowitz have combined to produce a completely new chapter on diseases of the ovary.

Dr. Phillip Stubblefield, an authority on conception control, has reviewed the vast amount of new investigation in this field and has written an excellent in-depth chapter providing the clinician with an overview of this controversial and perplexing subject. The chapter on infertility has been rewritten by Dr. Stephen Evans and the chapter on habitual abortion by Dr. Veronica Ravnikar. Both Dr. Evans and Dr. Ravnikar are members of the Section on Endocrinology and Infertility at the Brigham and Women's Hospital and both have contributed important research and clinical advances in this field. Dr. Ravnikar has also rewritten the chapter on endocrine aspects of gynecology.

I asked Dr. Robert Barbieri to write the chapter on endometriosis. Dr. Barbieri, also a member of the Section on Endocrinology and Infertility of the Brigham and Women's Hospital, has contributed important data concerning the hormonal management of this disease, specifically in regard to the physiologic action of Danocrine. He offers new insight into this disease particularly in the field of physiology and therapy. Dr. Barbieri has also revised the chapter on steroid therapy.

Drs. Howard Goodman and Robert Knapp have rewritten the chapter on the cervix, providing the reader with current data concerning diagnosis and treatment of premalignant and malignant diseases. Dr. Robert Shirley has updated his chapter on diseases of the breast in which he describes important diagnostic criteria and suggests methods for selection of appropriate therapy for both benign and malignant lesions.

Drs. Wayne A. Miller and Richard W. Erbe have accomplished the difficult task of placing in proper perspective the relationship of chromosomal abnormalities to gynecologic disorders. They have added significant data that has become available during the past decade to their excellent chapter.

Dr. Isaac Schiff, a member of the Section on Endocrinology and Fertility of the Brigham and Women's Hospital, has conducted extensive research in the pathophysiology of the menopause during the past decade and has initiated several ongoing studies to determine the effects of estrogen on osteoporosis and other degenerative diseases associated with this entity. I asked Dr. Schiff to revise and rewrite the chapter on menopause for the fourth edition.

The increase in the number and variety of venereal diseases during the past decade has necessitated the introduction of a new chapter on pelvic infections. Simultaneously, there has been a surge of new antibiotics and treatment regimens that have rendered previous therapy obsolete. This chapter provides the clinician with a therapeutic approach that is both timely and effective. It has been written by Dr. Ruth Tuomala, a recognized authority in the field of antibiotic therapy.

I wish to acknowledge the cooperation and assistance of the staff of Year Book Medical Publishers, in particular Mr. James Ryan. Finally, I am deeply indebted to my secretary, Mrs. Marlene Selig, for her assistance in the preparation of this edition.

ROBERT W. KISTNER, M.D.

Contents

CHAPTER ONE

Introduction

THE SPECIALTY OF gynecology has rapidly expanded during the past three decades to encompass disciplines of surgical, medical, endocrinologic, and obstetric endeavor. Prior to this time gynecology remained subservient to the field of general surgery—a stepchild with but limited possibilities in both clinical and laboratory investigation. The union of gynecology with obstetrics brought about an awareness of the all-inclusive problem of "femaleness," together with a reawakening of interest in basic scientific principles of human reproduction. It is now not sufficient for the physician to limit his scope to the surgical aspects of pelvic disorders since extirpation, although simple and expedient, may seriously alter the reproductive capacity and physiologic standards of the female.

A medical school gynecology lecture from only a decade and a half ago is already an antiquated exercise by today's standards and knowledge. Like it or not, the modern gynecologist is becoming more and more an endocrinologist.

The rapidly expanding field of reproductive biology and its clinical application to the problems of endocrinology, steroid chemistry, immunology, and gynecology can no longer be contained within the confines of a single subspecialty.

In addition to major advances within the factual foundations of gynecology, there are changes in the character of clinical practice. The modern gynecologist spends less and less time in the operating room and is rapidly becoming engulfed in a wave of relatively healthy patients whose major concerns are cancer prevention, conception control, hormonal replacement, and infertility.

Each of these entities is intrinsically related to, or dependent upon, endocrine homeostasis. Since endocrinologic maneuvers are an integral part of the day-to-day activities of the gynecologist, it is necessary that he be provided with the reasons for his therapeutic approach.

It is imperative, therefore, that medical students and residents appreciate the intimate relationships between metabolic disorders or aberrations of endocrine function and the genital tract. The importance of psychosomatic influences on the behavior of woman must be recognized and the intimate correlation of pregnancy, delivery, and the puerperium with both structure and function must be emphasized. An attempt will be made in this text to bring into clear focus the basic anatomic, physiologic, and pathologic facets of most gynecologic disorders, and, perhaps more important, each of these will be considered as alterations of "femaleness." Therapy to preserve, restore, or improve this desideratum will be outlined.

A word of caution regarding the intimacy of gynecology is perhaps in order for the beginner. Many of the problems that bring the patient to the physician concern subjects or body areas that she would rather forget than discuss. The patient who visits her physician frequently for respiratory or intestinal ailments is likely to neglect a vulvar lesion that may be, or develop into, cancer. The gynecologist must at the outset be both sympathetic and understanding but tactfully capable

1

of eliciting details that might be omitted purposely by the patient. He must be an attentive and interested listener and, in addition, should retain a reassuring and indulgent attitude. A brief explanation of the causes of symptoms together with logical reasons for the performance of diagnostic tests or surgery will help to diminish or dispel fears and misconceptions of most patients. Numerous visits are occasioned by cancerphobia and many more by episodes of vague, fleeting pain for which no explanation is evident. It is in such situations that much may be accomplished by reassurance and frank discussion.

THE HISTORY

Good history-taking is probably more closely related to the art than to the science of medicine. Yet it is important that a methodical approach be utilized so that important omissions may be avoided. A printed form, while sometimes cumbersome and at times inadequate, will serve this purpose in most instances and is essential for the student.

The chief complaint should be stated in the exact words of the patient, and its duration should be included. The present illness, which follows, is merely an expansion of the chief complaint. The account presents a chronologic sequence of events from the onset of illness up to the time of examination. It is not sufficient, however, merely to list such all-inclusive phrases as "irregular periods," "flowing on and off" or "trouble with periods." The clinician should determine the exact dates of the last normal menstrual period and the previous period. Bleeding intermenstrually should be described as to time of occurrence, duration, and the presence or absence of pain and/or clots. It will often be found that the abnormal bleeding complained of is simply staining due to endometrial breakdown at the time of ovulation. Similarly, the skips and delays in periods at the time of menopause may be easily explained on the basis of irregularities in ovulation. Bleeding

postcoitally or after a douche suggests a cervical polyp or malignancy. Postmenopausal bleeding is caused by malignancy of the cervix, uterine corpus, or ovary in about one half of all patients. Exacting detail in the description of bleeding is therefore most important.

Frequently a diagnosis is suggested by the first few sentences of the chief complaint. This may be misleading since "snap" diagnoses are likely to result. Subsequent complaints are glossed over, or a careful review of other systems is not completed. Should the physical and pelvic examination be equally sketchy, the gynecologist often becomes the victim of embarrassing "surprises" at the operating table. A common situation is the discovery of carcinoma or diverticulitis of the sigmoid colon when a fibroid or left ovarian mass was expected. The era of the master surgical technician has passed, and for the complete and successful treatment of the patient a combination of judgment, reason, skill, and humanity is desirable. An unnecessary operation by the most adept surgeon may still result in death from infection, pulmonary embolism, or unrecognized cardiac disease.

Previous hospitalizations are of interest, especially if pelvic surgery has been performed or radium and/or x-ray therapy has been administered. The location of the hospital, the name of the surgeon, and the date of surgery should be noted and a transcript of the patient's chart obtained. This will avoid misinterpretation of what the patient says was done or what was removed.

The past history merits consideration because of its bearing on the choice of anesthesia and on the advisability of certain surgical procedures. Obviously a patient with chronic bronchitis and a persistent cough should not be hurried to the hospital for an operation to cure stress incontinence until her pulmonary difficulties have improved. A simple checklist of serious infectious, pulmonary, cardiac, and renal diseases seems adequate in most cases, with elaboration when necessary.

The family history is recorded primarily to determine the incidence of diseases such as diabetes, cancer (especially breast), hypertension, or coronary occlusion. Occasionally, important entities such as a familial polyposis will be discovered in this fashion.

A history of the patient's social background is important. It should include her birthplace, national descent, religion, occupation, and previous marriages, if any. The age, occupation, religion, and health of the husband should also be obtained.

The systems review should include all pregnancies, listed in order by year, with the length of gestation, type of delivery, fetal weight, and complications, if any. Long periods of infertility, either primary or secondary, suggest endometriosis or pelvic inflammatory disease. In the patient who has been pregnant five or six times in the same number of years there may be a history of pelvic pain, sacral backache, dyspareunia, and vaginal discharge. This suggests a diagnosis of "married women's complaint" and is usually causally related to a uterine retroversion with pelvic vascular congestion and a diseased cervix.

The dates and normality of the last and previous menstrual periods should be accurately recorded. If this is neglected, intrauterine pregnancies, tubal pregnancies, and threatened or incomplete abortions will not be given serious consideration in the differential diagnosis. On occasion, the patient will deliberately falsify a recent period or neglect to describe its true length or character. A careful pelvic examination and visualization of the cervix will usually aid the examiner in recognizing these deceptions.

Pain associated with the menstrual flow should be classified as to site, duration, intensity, and nature. Midline, suprapubic, first day (or 24 hours before flow), dull, crampy pain is characteristic of primary (idiopathic) dysmenorrhea. The pain of endometriosis is, by contrast, sharp, aching, constant, lateral or deep in the pelvis around the rectum and seems to get progressively worse month after month. Pain on defecation or dyspareunia suggests cul-de-sac or rectosigmoid endometriosis or possibly blood or pus in the pelvic

cavity due to ectopic pregnancy or pelvic inflammation.

The review of systems is frequently of aid in establishing a gynecologic diagnosis or in the elimination of bowel or urinary tract disease. The proximity of bladder, uterus, and rectosigmoid and the inability of most patients to pinpoint their symptoms make this survey worthwhile.

The usual data regarding age of onset and interval and duration of menstrual periods are necessary requisites of every gynecologic history. The age of onset of the menses will vary, depending on climate and genetic background. In the United States the first period usually occurs between ages 11 and 16 years, the average about 13 years. The clinician should not become alarmed, however, if menses occur two years earlier or later than these extremes. Thus it has been noted that Jewish women menstruate sooner than Gentiles, and brunettes usually start about a year or so before blondes. Vaginal bleeding occurring in a child aged 6 or 8 years should, however, be investigated with the same thoroughness as amenorrhea in a woman of 20 years. An extensive endocrinologic survey is not indicated for primary amenorrhea before age 18 years.

An interval of 28 days between periods is time-honored but not exact, and in normal women the interval will vary between 26 and 32 days. The singular characteristic of menstrual (i.e., postovulatory) bleeding is rhythmicity. This distinguishes it from the marked irregular flowing of anovular origin. Patients who have maintained rhythmic cycles of 21 days, 35 days, or even 60 days should not be considered abnormal, although they cannot be called "average."

The average duration of menstruation is between three and four days with an average blood loss of 25 to 70 ml. A good deal of variation is noted in both of these variables since some normal women bleed for one or two days and others six to seven days, with extremes of blood loss from 10 to 200 ml. The presence of clots may mean the absence of a fibrinolysin (found normally in menstrual discharge), suggesting that the bleeding is anovular. Or it may mean that the vascular breakdown in the endometrium is so rapid that whatever fibrinolysin is present is unable to maintain the fluidity of blood, so that clotting occurs.

Vaginal discharge may be due to infection, malignancy, foreign bodies, or trauma. Therefore, inquiries should be made about its color, consistency, and the presence of blood. Pessaries and certain douche solutions may be irritating to the vaginal mucosa and should be thought of as possible etiologic factors. Bloody mucoid discharge occurring postmenopausally may be due to carcinoma of the endometrium or cervix. Occasionally, however, it will be due to prolonged use of estrogens, and cessation of this medication results in cure. A list of all medications the patient is presently taking or has received in the recent past should be noted. Broad-spectrum antibiotics frequently cause candidal (monilial) vaginitis, vaginal discharge, and pruritus, and their use should be determined.

The general health is investigated. Symptoms such as nausea, anorexia, lassitude, and low-grade temperature elevation may be due to pulmonary or genital tuberculosis. Weight loss, dizziness, and anemia with crampy right lower quadrant pain suggest cancer of the right colon or cecum. The finding of a large leiomyoma, while spectacular to the student, may be misleading. Generalized symptoms, such as those just noted, are not common with most gynecologic maladies, and one must not be content to explain all symptoms on the basis of one gross abnormality. The cardiorespiratory, gastrointestinal, urinary, and neuromuscular systems should be carefully investigated. Particular attention should be given to symptoms such as diminished appetite, change in bowel habits, alternating diarrhea and constipation, blood mixed with stool, tenesmus or pain with bowel movements, or change in the stool diameter. The gynecologist encounters sigmoid or rectal carcinoma all too often during surgery for a suspected ovarian cyst or myoma. Attention to

such symptoms will permit the correct diagnosis to be made before surgery.

Symptoms that arise from the urinary tract merit detailed discussion since there is frequently a correlation with the gynecologic complaint. Stress incontinence, or loss of urine while coughing, sneezing, laughing, etc., should be differentiated from urge incontinence since the stress incontinence may require surgical correction, whereas the urge incontinence may be treated by simple bladder irrigations or urinary antiseptics. Dysuria, frequency, and nocturia suggest bladder infections but may be secondary to radium or x-ray treatments. If urinary frequency occurs, it is important to know whether there is associated polyuria and polydipsia since these may be the first symptoms of early diabetes. If there is associated itching and vulvitis, diabetes should be strongly suspected. A common complaint of a bride is that of dysuria and frequency—"honeymoon cystitis." The details of the history are sufficient to make the diagnosis.

Further inquiry is also made regarding allergies or sensitivities to drugs, antibiotics, and anesthetic agents as well as previous thromboembolic disease.

THE PHYSICAL EXAMINATION

A complete physical examination is performed when the patient is seen for the first time. This includes gross inspection of head and neck and palpation of the thyroid gland, supraclavicular areas, and superficial lymph nodes. One should particularly note the patency of the nasal airway, irregularities or nodules in the thyroid, and the presence of supraclavicular nodes or masses.

The gynecologist should include a thorough examination of the breasts not only at the first visit but at subsequent visits (if the interval exceeds three months). Inspection of the breasts should be done first with the patient sitting erect with her arms at her sides and then with the arms raised. The maneuver will frequently outline asymmetry or fixation of the nipple or fixed masses under or adjacent to the areola. The supraclavicular areas and the axillae are then palpated with the patient sitting erect. An adequate examination of the axilla can be performed only if the pectoral muscles are relaxed. This is accomplished by supporting the patient's arm in slight abduction and palpating the axilla with the finger tips. Particular attention should be given to the apex of the axilla and the undersurface of the pectoralis major muscle. A systematic examination of the breasts is then performed in both the erect and supine positions. Masses in the breast are best determined by palpation with the flat surface rather than the tips of the fingers. The whole extent of the breast, as it lies relatively flattened out and balanced on the chest wall, should be systematically palpated. The medial portion is examined first with the patient's arm raised. This flattens the pectoral muscles under the breast, and the examiner's fingers trace a series of transverse lines across the breast from the nipple line to the sternum. Palpation of the lateral portion of the breast is then performed with the patient's arm at her side. The ducts and nipples should be compressed, and if bloody secretion is obtained it is submitted to cytologic examination. Cloudy fluid may be expressed from the nipples of parous women many years after pregnancy and is of no significance. A very common finding is thickening in the upper outer quadrant of the breast; if present, this is noted and repeated observations suggested. It should be borne in mind that the breast normally presents fine nodularity on palpation. During periods of engorgement (especially premenstrually), this nodularity may be accentuated almost to the point of simulating a dominant lump. Differentiation between tumor and such physiologic change is difficult. Usually, with care in palpation and reexamination at a different time in the menstrual cycle, a definite decision can be reached. About 65% of all cancers of the breast occur in this quadrant, and this area should therefore be given particular attention.

The use of a lubricant, glove powder, or soap and water provides a friction-free breast surface for optimum examination. When the patient is in the supine position with her arms above her head, lactiferous duct sinuses and previous biopsy sites are easily palpable, and any questionable areas become more distinct under the friction-free surface.

If a lump feels cystic, an attempt is made to aspirate the contents. If withdrawal of this fluid collapses the cyst and restores the breast to normal, nothing further is done except that repeated examination is advised every six months. If the fluid is clear and yellow, further examination of the aspirate is unnecessary. Nevertheless, if the fluid is discolored (brown, green) or cloudy, or if the cyst fills up again within six weeks to three months, an excisional biopsy is advised. Cytologic examination of areas of thickened, tender, or asymmetric breast tissue may be effective in detecting early carcinoma in a high percentage of patients. In the average clinic about 60% of patients who are seen because of breast symptomatology will have cystic disease or mastitis; 20% will have cancer; 15% fibroadenomas; and the remaining 5% fat necrosis, tuberculosis, or lipoma. The differential diagnosis of masses in the breast may be aided by the use of mammography, although the report of the radiologist should be tempered by clinical experience and judgment (see chapter 8, "The Breast"). All discrete masses or dominant lumps are excised in the operating room, a frozen section made, and appropriate therapy performed.

The examination of the abdomen is begun by inspection, noting the presence of scars, striae, distension, dilated veins, and umbilical eversion. The patient is then asked to lift her head and cough; this will delineate hernias or diastasis recti. Systematic palpation of the viscera is performed to determine abnormalities of liver, gallbladder, spleen, and kidneys. Palpation of the liver is best accomplished with the patient supine, her head and shoulders slightly elevated by pillows. The examiner should stand at the patient's right side, place his left hand under the patient's right flank, pressing gently upward with it, and then place the right hand gently but firmly on the abdominal wall. As the patient takes a deep breath the right hand is moved downward and as the diaphragm descends the liver is carried down and its margin and consistency may be noted. Hepatic enlargement, especially if irregular or nodular, suggests a primary bowel tumor rather than a cancer of the uterus or ovary. An enlarged or tense gallbladder may be similarly palpated. Hydrops of the gallbladder may be confused with acute appendicitis since the tip of the distended gallbladder may extend into the right lower quadrant and since symptoms of nausea and vomiting are frequently associated. The spleen is best palpated by placing the right hand flat with the abdominal wall just at the left costal margin; as the patient inspires, the spleen descends and is palpable if enlarged. The cecum, right colon, and sigmoid colon are similarly palpated. The first clue in the diagnosis of diverticulitis of the sigmoid may be obtained at this time if there is tenderness deep in the left lower quadrant. In symmetric midline tumors, regardless of consistency, consideration should be given to the possibility of an intrauterine pregnancy or a distended bladder. Catheterization will reveal the true nature of the latter, but early pregnancy, especially if coincident with other masses such as fibroids or ovarian cysts, is often difficult to diagnose unless constantly kept in mind. Ovarian cysts may usually be differentiated from ascites by percussion, since with large cysts one usually finds areas of dullness over the cyst with tympany in the flanks. With ascites, the small intestine usually floats anteriorly and is tympanitic, whereas the dullness is found laterally.

The costovertebral angles and flanks should also be carefully evaluated in the gynecologic patient since renal and ureteral lesions frequently cause symptoms which the patient interprets as "female trouble." Firm pressure exerted by the index finger in the angle between the spine and the twelfth rib will elicit inflammatory kidney processes, which otherwise might go undetected. The procedure for palpating the kidneys is similar to that for palpating the liver.

Both groins are inspected and palpated. Enlargement of the superficial inguinal nodes may be associated with venereal disease (syphilis, granuloma inguinale, chancroid, lymphopathia venereum), and varying degrees of ulceration, so-called buboes, may be revealed.

Cancer of the vulva or lower vagina, acute nongonorrheal vulvitis, tuberculosis, or, occasionally, superficial infections of the skin of the thigh may all cause inguinal lymphadenopathy. Other causes are plantar or lower extremity melanomas, thigh vaccination and acute bartholinitis. We have recently seen a patient whose chief complaint was a unilateral, firm, 4-cm inguinal mass. Review of the past history revealed that the right eye had been enucleated five years previously for a melanosarcoma; on excision the inguinal mass was found to be microscopically similar to the primary lesions in the eye. Hodgkin's disease and systemic illnesses characterized by generalized lymphadenopathy should also be considered. In many thin, asthenic females, firm, discrete, mobile inguinal nodes are palpable without apparent cause and need no further investigation. The patient should again be asked to raise her head and cough, and careful examination should be performed for detection of inguinal and femoral hernias. Frequently no cause can be found for a complaint of an "aching soreness" in the lower abdomen until the patient is asked to stand and cough or to exert intra-abdominal pressure. Examination below Poupart's ligament may often reveal a femoral hernia.

The extremities are examined for edema, ulceration, scars of previous surgery, and varicose veins. Bilateral edema may be caused by increased intrapelvic pressure from a pregnancy, an old phlebitis, or a lymphatic obstruction due to postpartum phlegmasia alba dolens as well as to excess intake of salt. It may, however, just as well be due to impaired nutrition associated with low serum albumin levels, carcinoma of the ovary with ascites, or to cardiac failure or chronic nephritis. Its cause bears investigation. Unilateral edema may follow postpartum or postoperative deep phlebothrombosis. Bilateral edema of the extremities is occasionally congenital and occurs without venous or lymphatic obstruction (Milroy's disease). Ulceration of the legs suggests peripheral vascular disease due to venous stasis or diabetes. Varicose veins or scars of previous vein ligation or stripping should be adequate warning to initiate prophylaxis against thromboembolic disease if surgery is contemplated.

It is well for the gynecologist, as well as the student, to stop at this point and consider the differential diagnosis suggested by the history and the general physical examination. In most gynecologic diseases the history, if accurately given and carefully taken, will narrow down the possibilities to three or four conditions. The general physical examination may further reduce this to two or three, or it may suggest that the original complaint may arise from another organ system. If this is so, appropriate x-rays, endoscopy, and laboratory procedures should be performed. This will avoid the embarrassment of operating on patients with unsuspected colonic or bladder carcinoma, diverticulitis, renal tumors, pelvic kidneys, and ulcerative colitis.

THE PELVIC EXAMINATION

The pelvic examination is the most important part of the armamentarium of the gynecologist—the ability to see, to palpate, and, most of all, to interpret abnormal findings of the female genitalia. Frequently these findings will adequately explain the symptoms of the patient. Often, however, they will bear no relationship, and one should not fall into the trap of *post hoc, ergo propter hoc* reasoning at this juncture. Occasionally the pelvic examination will be normal, but laboratory procedures such as cytologic examination will aid in diagnosis.

The pelvic examination should be carried out with the patient on an examining table with the legs supported and adequately abducted (Fig 1–1). The table should be

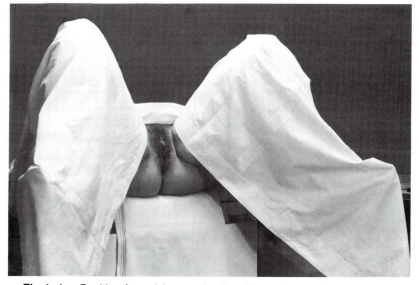

Fig 1–1.—Position for pelvic examination. The patient is placed so that the buttocks extend just beyond the edge of the table. The legs are supported in stirrups and are adequately abducted.

equipped with a movable backrest so that the head may be raised slightly, permitting better relaxation of abdominal muscles. Examinations in bed are difficult and may lead to erroneous interpretations. The buttocks should extend just beyond the end of the table. Good light is essential. The patient is instructed to urinate just before the examination, since a full bladder may be mistaken for a pregnant uterus or an ovarian cyst. If symptoms suggest urinary tract disease, the bladder is emptied by catheterization or a midstream "catch" specimen is obtained. Although routine enemas are not advised, a full rectum makes the pelvic examination difficult and inconclusive. A clean lower bowel is especially important if the examiner wishes to palpate the rectovaginal septum and uterosacral ligaments, since solid fecal particles may simulate masses and nodularity. If there is any doubt, an enema should be given and the patient reexamined.

A speculum is inserted without lubrication and a small amount of secretion is obtained from the cervix by aspiration or forceps technique and submitted to cytologic examination. Cervical scrapings are routinely performed since malignant cells are occasionally found in this specimen, but not in the aspirate. At the Brigham and Women's Hospital better correlation has been obtained between biopsies and cervical aspirations and scrapings than between biopsies and vaginal pool aspirations. This could conceivably be due to poor technique in aspirating the pool in the posterior vagina.

Some mention should be made of the technique of speculum examination. The gynecologist should attempt to use the speculum best adapted for a particular patient and he is aided in this by the variety of instruments available. The one used most commonly is the Graves speculum, which has a posterior blade approximately 4½ in. long and 1¼ in. wide at its tip. This speculum is available in lengths varying from 3½ to 5 in., and widths from ¾ to 1¼ in. The posterior blade of the Graves speculum is usually about ¼ in. longer than

the anterior blade so as to fit into the longer posterior vaginal wall. In some patients, however, when the cervix lies posteriorly or there is a large cystocele, it is advantageous to have a longer anterior blade. The ordinary speculum may then be rotated, or a modified Graves speculum with a longer anterior blade used. The Pederson speculum is narrower and flatter and may be used to advantage in nulliparous patients or when the vagina is contracted by senescence, scars, or radiation. In children, a Kelly cystoscope is an ideal instrument for visualization of the vagina.

Before insertion, the speculum should be warmed by holding it under warm water, and it should be adequately lubricated unless it is being used for cytologic aspiration. Slight pressure is then exerted on the posterior vaginal wall and perineum by the index and middle finger of the left hand, and care is taken to keep the blades away from the sensitive periurethral area. The speculum should be angled when inserted, so that its greatest width is in the anteroposterior diameter of the vagina (Fig 1–2). It is then rotated as it is passed along the posterior vaginal wall, and as the tip reaches the cervix the anterior blade is elevated by pressure on the lever under the lateral screw. When the proper exposure has been obtained the lateral set screw is adjusted. If increased vision in the anteroposterior field is desired, the central set screw may be loosened and the blades separated. When the speculum is removed only the lateral screw should be released, allowing the tips of the blades to fall together. The central screw should not be loosened since, in so doing, vaginal mucosa may be pinched between lateral aspects of the blades.

Before proceeding to the examination of the vagina and cervix the examiner should methodically inspect the external genitalia. The general features are illustrated in Figure 1–3. A good sequence is to start with the labia majora and minora, noting the size as well as the presence of edema, inflammation, ulceration, crusting, deformity, discoloration, or atrophy. Dilated veins, nevi, and melano-

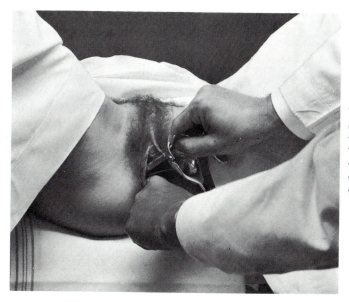

Fig 1–2.—Insertion of speculum. The posterior vaginal wall is depressed by slight pressure with the index finger of the left hand. The speculum is angled to conform to the anteroposterior diameter of the vagina. Care is taken to avoid the periurethral area.

mas are obvious. Evidence of recent trauma, as by rape, should be recorded. Secretions should be examined microscopically and by culture, if indicated. The labia minora should be followed to their junction in the prepuce over the clitoris and enlargement or adhesions noted. Enlargement of the clitoris should alert the examiner to search for other stigmata of virilism and the possibility of an adrenal tumor. At this point the mons veneris and pubic hair distribution are observed for pediculosis and dermatitis. The thumb and index finger of the right hand separate the labia minora as shown in Figure 1–4, exposing the vestibule with the vaginal and urethral openings as well as those of the periurethral (Skene's) and vulvovaginal (Bartholin's) glands. At this point the patient may be asked to strain down or cough. This will delineate pelvic floor relaxation and urinary incontinence. The index finger of the gloved (left) hand is then inserted gently under the urethra and it is compressed toward the external orifice. A purulent exudate suggests gonorrhea and should be stained and cultured. The urethral orifice should be observed also for polyps, prolapse of the mucosa, ulceration, or caruncle. The index finger may then be rotated and the ducts of the periurethral glands

stripped. The vulvovaginal glands should be sought for, placing the index finger in the vagina and the thumb on the perineal skin. Normally they are not palpable, but undue tenderness, swelling, or fluctuation suggests Bartholin's cyst or abscess. At this time the posterior commissure and perineal body may be inspected and palpated. The condition of previous episiotomies should be noted as should the presence of any small dimples, which indicate the presence of vaginoperineal or vaginorectal fistulas. The integrity of the levator ani muscle may be tested, but this is better done by a later combined rectovaginal examination.

Attention is next given to the condition of the hymen. In young adolescents one commonly finds the ring intact but with a small opening, which may admit the index finger. Occasionally the tissue is extremely fibrotic and even the smallest finger cannot be inserted. In parous women the hymen may be in excellent condition, depending on the rigors of delivery and the technique of the obstetrician. Usually, however, it is absent in its lower third, but remnants (the carunculae myrtiformes) are found anteriorly. In postmenopausal virgins the hymen is frequently tight and contracted so that even the passage

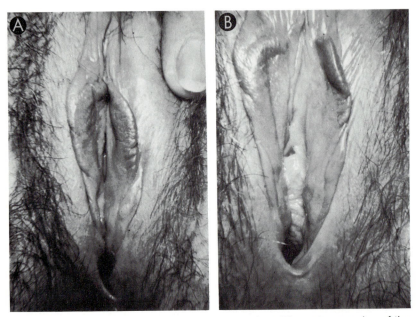

Fig 1–3.—A, normal vulva of multiparous patient. The outer margins of the labia majora are covered with hair, and a slight degree of gaping of the labia minora permits exposure of the introitus. **B,** labia majora are displaced laterally to show clitoris, which labia minora join anteriorly. The urethral orifice is seen just above a slight relaxation of the anterior vaginal wall. Vaginal orifice is at lowermost portion of labia minora.

Fig 1–4.—Method of beginning the internal examination. The labia majora and minora are held apart with the fingers of the right hand and first one and then two fingers of the left hand are gently inserted along the posterior vaginal wall.

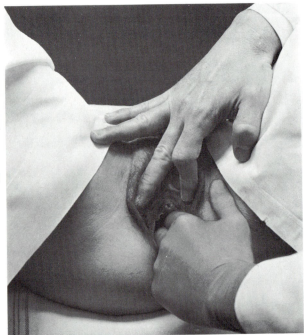

of a small glass tube is impossible. Hematomas and fresh lacerations may indicate recent attempts at rape.

The examination of the internal genitalia requires a minimum amount of equipment, which is both inexpensive and simple to use. Figure 1–5 illustrates a typical arrangement used in our clinic.

The internal examination is begun by introducing first one and then two fingers of the left hand along the posterior vaginal wall (Fig 1–4). The reason for a right-handed examiner to use his left hand for the internal examination is twofold: it allows freedom of the right hand for forceps, biopsy instruments, cautery, insufflator, etc., and it allows the more trained hand to palpate the pelvic viscera through the abdomen after they have been lifted into position by the left hand. Specifically then, the fingers elevate and support the uterus and adnexa while the external hand is used to determine the anatomic details of these structures. In addition, any abnormalities of the vagina are noted and the size, shape, and consistency of the cervix is determined, as is the patency of its external os.

The cervix may then be moved laterally; if pain results, it suggests the presence of an inflammatory process. A widely patulous, soft cervix is usually found in patients with an inevitable or incomplete abortion, whereas a widely patulous, firm cervix may be palpable around a protruding leiomyoma or pedunculated adenomyoma. Cervical polyps are easily palpable as movable, soft, fleshy projections, whereas stony hardness is characteristic of carcinoma.

The vaginal fingers may note at the outset a third-degree uterine retroversion as they advance toward the posterior cul-de-sac, or nodularity and scarring of the uterosacral ligaments may suggest the presence of endometriosis.

The normal position of the uterus is one of anteversion with some anteflexion of the corpus on the cervix. To palpate the uterus, the simplest method is to place the two vaginal fingers under the cervix and elevate it and the uterine corpus toward the abdominal wall (Fig 1–6). The external hand is gently placed on the abdomen with the fingers flat and is moved about from below the umbilicus to the

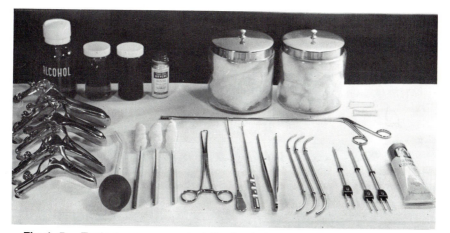

Fig 1–5.—Typical arrangement of the basic instruments and supplies for an adequate gynecologic examination. Bottles (left to right): alcohol, Alkalol, Schiller's solution, Oxycel. Jars contain gauze pledgets and cotton balls. Tampons are at right of jars. Three Graves and one Pederson specula are at far left. Then, in order, tube and aspiration bulb for cytology, cotton-tipped metal applicators, cervical tenaculum, uterine sound, endometrial curet, thumb forceps (long), three cervical dilators sizes 11 to 16, three nasal-tip cauteries, lubricating jelly. A cervical biopsy punch (extra long) is shown below the jars.

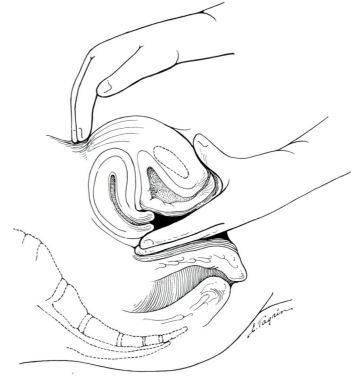

Fig 1–6.—Internal examination. The uterus is palpated by placing two fingers under the cervix, elevating it and the uterine corpus toward the abdominal wall. The external hand is gently placed on the abdomen with the fingers flat and moved about from below the umbilicus to the symphysis. The author prefers to stand at the left side of the patient, outside the abducted leg.

symphysis. Intermittent pressure on the uterus between the fingers of both hands will yield information as to size, shape, and consistency. Ballottement between the two hands yields important information regarding mobility.

The left adnexal area is usually examined next. This is accomplished by moving the vaginal fingers to the left of the cervix so that they occupy the lateral and uppermost part of the vagina (Fig 1–7). If the patient is cooperative, the vaginal fingers can actually be placed under the posterior portion of the broad ligament. On the left side the ovary is frequently underneath the sigmoid colon so that abdominal palpation must begin rather high. By a series of caudad displacements the hand is brought over the ovary, which can usually be palpated between the two hands. The vaginal fingers usually serve only to support the ovary while the external hand palpates for size, shape, and mobility. The oviduct is usually not palpable in its normal

state. The right ovary is palpated in the same fashion; however, if it is not easily felt, the examiner should change hands and place the right hand in the vagina. The natural curvature of the right hand sometimes makes it easier to outline the right adnexa.

In performing the internal examination it is important to bear in mind several points. (1) Always begin gently, usually with the insertion of one well-lubricated finger along the posterior vagina. (2) Gradually insinuate two fingers under the cervix. (3) Apply the abdominal hand easily, slowly, and keep it in motion. (4) Never apply force or use abrupt motion, since the initial reflex resistance will then actually increase and examination will become impossible. (5) Always examine the painful side last. (6) Employ reassuring discussion with the patient and have her breathe through her mouth during the examination to aid in securing relaxation.

Students are frequently discouraged about their inability to palpate the ovaries or masses in the sides of the pelvis, feeling that they cannot reach them. If the fingers are somewhat shorter than normal, or if a mass seems high up, additional length may be obtained by placing the left foot on a small stool, resting the left elbow against the knee and then invaginating the pelvic floor by firm pressure (Fig 1–8). Another method is to place the middle finger in the rectum and the index finger in the vagina (Fig 1–9). This will enable the examiner to reach almost 1 in. higher into the pelvis and is of inestimable value in differentiating left-sided ovarian cysts from diverticulitis or thickening of the sigmoid colon. Before withdrawal of the vaginal fingers an attempt should be made to palpate the ureters through the anterior vaginal wall. Unusual degrees of tenderness or thickening suggest inflammatory or neoplastic processes.

In describing the findings, it is important to bear in mind that all observers will not interpret the palpatory findings in the same way. Therefore, it is better to give accurate or estimated measurements in centimeters rather than in terms of fruit, eggs, or balls of various sizes. This need not be carried ad absurdum, however, and if both ovaries are normal in all respects, it is simpler to report "sides of the pelvis negative." Abnormal masses should be described as to size, shape, consistency, mobility, position, and whether or not they are tender.

The speculum examination is performed utilizing the technique previously described. The vaginal mucosa is inspected as the speculum is introduced, with observation made of the amount of rugation or the presence of discharge. Primary diseases of the vagina (excluding simple vaginitis) are not too common, but one should look for congenital abnormalities such as vaginal septa, double vaginas, double cervixes, and Gartner duct cysts. The cervix is then brought into view and the light adjusted so that the entire portio epithelium is visible. A cotton-tipped applicator is dipped in an alkaline, saline solution that dissolves mucus (Alkalol) or into tyloxapol (Alevaire), and the cervix is liberally swabbed. The entire area is then dried with a second applicator, and a third is used to apply Schiller's solution to the cervix and upper vagina. (Schiller's solution: 1 gm of iodine, 2 gm of potassium iodide, 300 ml of water.) The normal stratified squamous epithelium of the va-

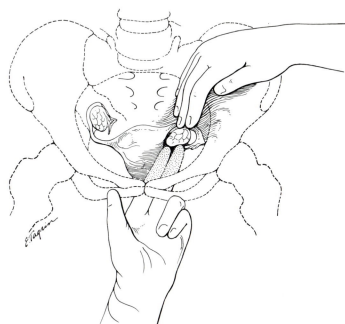

Fig 1–7.—Palpation of adnexal areas. The vaginal fingers are moved to the side of the cervix so that they occupy the lateral and uppermost part of the vagina. By a series of caudad displacements, the hand is brought over the ovary. The vaginal fingers serve only to *support* the ovary, while the external hand is used to determine size, shape, and mobility.

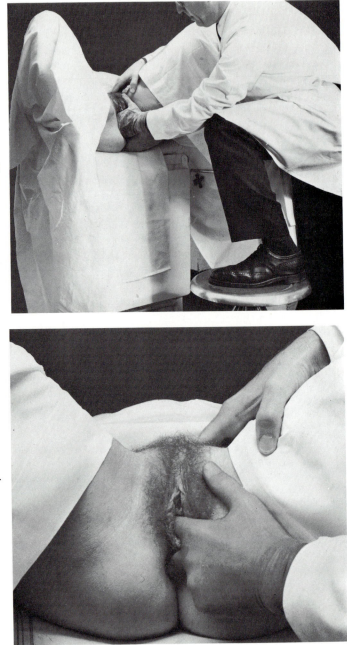

Fig 1–8.—Method of internal pelvic examination. To obtain additional length, the left foot may be placed on a small stool, the left elbow rested against the knee, and the pelvic floor then invaginated by firm pressure.

Fig 1–9.—Combined vaginorectal examination enables the examiner to reach almost 1 in. higher into the pelvis. Thickening of the rectovaginal septum, cul-de-sac nodules, fixed uterine retroversion, and involvement of the broad ligaments by tumor are more accurately outlined by this method.

gina and portio vaginalis of the cervix is rich in glycogen and stains dark brown with Schiller's solution. Abnormal squamous epithelium (whether it be acute inflammation, leukoplakia, parakeratosis, carcinoma in situ, or carcinoma) does not stain. The endocervical cells also do not stain, so that an obvious erosion (really an ectropion of endocervical cells) must be differentiated from a true "Schiller-positive" or nonstaining area of squamous epithelium. We routinely biopsy all Schiller-positive areas, preferably at the junction of the staining and nonstaining area. Biopsy is also done on all erosions prior to cauterization—reasons for which will be given in Chapter 4, "The Cervix."

After the cervix has been studied, a uterine sound is passed through the cervical os to determine the length of the uterine cavity. This is of particular value if the position and the size of the uterus are not definitely determined at the time of bimanual examination. The sound should be passed gently and not forced, since perforation may occur without undue pressure. In postmenopausal women it is especially important to know whether or not the cervical canal is patent. If it is closed, steps to open it should be taken, since endometrial carcinoma would not give the usual early symptom of bleeding in this instance.

The vaginorectal examination is performed as previously described. Its importance lies in the fact that, by gaining extra depth, lesions of the posterior cul-de-sac, uterosacral ligaments and rectovaginal septum will become obvious. Frequently a uterus in fixed third-degree retroversion can be outlined only by this method. This examination is followed by a thorough digital examination of the anus and rectum. The fact that about one half of the malignancies of the rectosigmoid may be palpated by careful digital exploration is adequate reason for making this part of the examination an integral step in the gynecologic survey. A guaiac test for blood in the stool should be routine in every rectal examination. If blood was noted in the examination of the vagina, the glove should be changed before the rectal examination is performed.

CHAPTER TWO

The Vulva

THOMAS LEAVITT, JR., M.D.

GENERAL CONSIDERATIONS

THE VULVA, or external female genitalia, includes the following structures: labia majora, labia minora, clitoris, vestibule, hymen, vestibular bulbs, mons veneris, urethral meatus, vulvovaginal glands, and periurethral gland ducts. The outer portion of the vulva is covered by somewhat altered skin, which contains hair follicles and sweat and sebaceous glands. This is modified on the inner surface so that the inner portions of the labia minora are moist and do not contain hair follicles. The vulva serves as the entrance to the vagina and, in the normal state, covers and protects the urethral orifice. The labia have specific importance in the process of urination since it has been found that, following vulvectomy, uncontrolled "spraying" is a common complaint.

The anatomic location of the vulva predisposes its structures to unusual and occasionally rare disorders. At the same time, systemic diseases such as diabetes, anemia, Addison's disease, and gout may manifest themselves first by vulvar changes and complaints therefrom. The importance of venereal diseases as a major cause of symptomatology from these structures is obvious, and each will be considered in this chapter. Since a good portion of the vulvar area may be properly classified as skin, it is at once evident that any specific cutaneous disease may occur here, but because of certain variations, diagnosis may be difficult or even impossible. Difficulty in diagnosis is aggravated by the tendency of the patient to procrastinate and to utilize self-medication when the lesion involves the genitalia. Patient delay is of extreme importance when the disease is malignant, since carcinoma involving these structures has a poor prognosis unless discovered early. Of equal importance in this problem is the responsibility of the physician. Numerous studies have shown that "physician delay" may actually exceed "patient delay" by many months.

Success in the diagnosis and treatment of lesions of the vulva will be forthcoming only if the physician investigates completely all possible etiologic factors and performs a meticulous examination. A thorough interview should determine the exact site and duration of specific complaints as well as generalized symptoms. Inquiry should be made about diarrhea or discharge, applications of lotions, medications or soaps, systemic medications, contraceptives, sexual habits, clothing changes, and, of major importance, events that might be causative in producing mental stress, worry, or anxiety. The examiner should scrutinize closely the oral mucosa, fingernails, scalp, and pubic hair as part of the gynecologic examination. It is not sufficient to allay symptoms, since recurrence is commonplace. Therefore, the cause of the disorder must be found and specific therapy instituted.

EMBRYOLOGY

In the female, as in the male, the external genitalia develop in connection with the genital tubercle, a conical prominence caudal to the umbilical cord. This tubercle appears in the 8-mm embryo (5 weeks)* as a simple protrusion (Fig 2–1) and later is noted to present a groove along its caudal surface—the urethral groove. The urethra is subsequently formed from this groove. The genital tubercle becomes clearly defined as a phallus in the 16- to 18-mm embryo (6 to 7 weeks), whereas the specific external genitalia of either male or female type are formed in the 40-mm embryo (10 weeks).

The cloacal membrane is an epithelial structure located in the ventral portion of the embryo caudal to the genital tubercle. This membrane consists of an inner (cephalic) layer of entodermal cells and an outer (caudal) layer of ectodermal cells. When the cloacal membrane perforates about the 12th week, the openings of the urethra, vagina, and anus are clearly visible. The rudimentary external genitalia appear about the sixth week of embryonic life as swellings on either side of the cloacal membrane. These swellings later project to form the genital folds, which extend cephalad to join the genital tubercle (Fig 2–2). The genital folds become the labia minora, and the clitoris is derived from the genital tubercle. The labia majora develop from swellings at the outer sides of the genital folds (lateral genital folds). These lateral genital folds join cephalad to form the genital eminence or mons veneris, whereas caudad they curve medially to form the posterior commissure. About the fifth or sixth month a secondary upgrowth of tissue around the clitoris forms a fold or hood about it, the preputium clitoridis or prepuce.

When the cloaca becomes divided into a dorsal and ventral segment by the downgrowth of a septum, which grows mainly from mesoderm, two compartments are formed. The ventral portion constitutes the urogenital sinus and is bounded at its lower end by the cloacal membrane. The wolffian ducts are embedded in this mesoderm of the down-

*Measurements correspond to values of F. P. Mall, and ages are "ovulation age," or two weeks less than menstrual age.

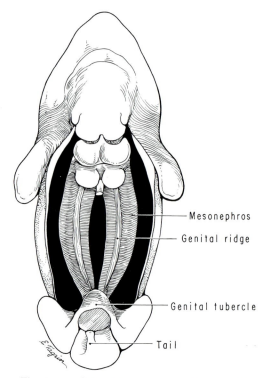

Fig 2–1.—Schematic representation of 9-mm human embryo in frontal section to show anatomic relations of the genital tubercle.

growing septum on either side and later become implanted in the septum. When division is complete they open into the urogenital sinus. Above the site of their implantation the urogenital sinus dilates to become the urinary bladder. The dorsal segment formed by the aforementioned downgrowth of mesoderm (sometimes called the urorectal fold) differentiates into the rectum. Thus, at this stage of development (12- to 14-mm embryo) both rectum and bladder are continuous with the urogenital sinus, which is closed at its lower end by the cloacal membrane (Fig 2–3). Bartholin's glands appear as outgrowths from the walls of the urogenital sinus.

At the site where the solid müllerian ducts join the sinus the hymen is ultimately formed. As these solid masses of cells at the termination of the müllerian ducts proliferate, vaginal bulbs form, which grow downward along the posterior wall of the sinus. They in-

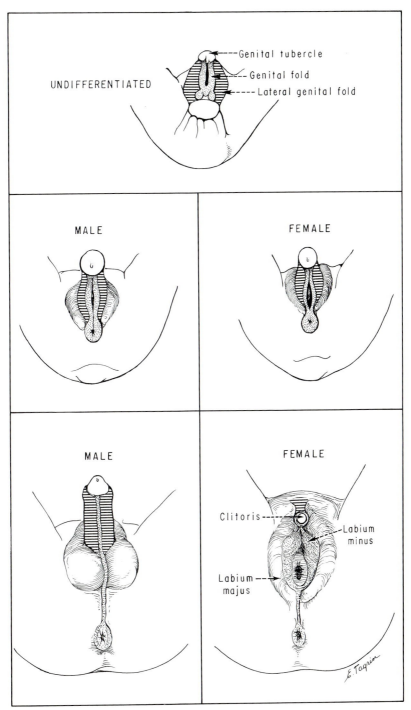

Fig 2–2.—Schematic drawing to show the homologous development of the external genitalia from the undifferentiated state.

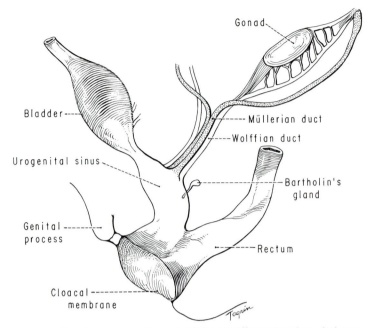

Fig 2–3.—Schematic drawing of the undifferentiated genital system of the 12- to 14-mm embryo.

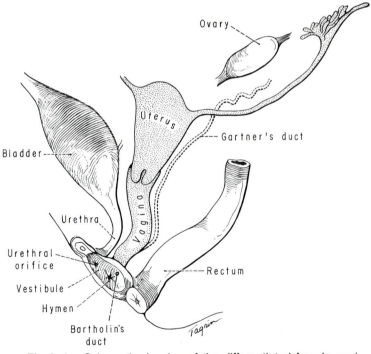

Fig 2–4.—Schematic drawing of the differentiated female genitalia.

crease in size and press against the walls of the sinus, invaginating it, so that the upper part of the sinus becomes gradually shortened. In this manner, the openings of the ducts of Bartholin's glands are brought close to the hymenal margin. Later, the solid vagina, thus formed, breaks down in the center and, at the site where its cavity opens into the sinus, the hymenal orifice is formed. The remainder of the urogenital sinus in front of the hymen forms the vestibule. Figure 2–4 illustrates the definitive female genital system.

ANATOMY AND HISTOLOGY

LABIA MAJORA.—The skin covering the labia majora is thick, contains many sebaceous and sweat glands and is covered by hair, except along the lower part of the inner aspect. The extent of the glandular development is pronounced and accounts for the frequency of sebaceous retention cysts and hair follicle infections in this region. On the inner aspect of the labia majora, the sebaceous glands empty directly on the skin surface and are less numerous. The skin is made up of typical stratified squamous epithelium with moderate keratosis and a well-vascularized dermis (Fig 2–5). Involuntary muscle fibers, or dartos, are present but are much less developed than in the corresponding tissue, the scrotum, of the male. A large amount of fatty tissue is usually present, situated in lobules separated by elastic and connective tissue fibers. This elastic connective tissue forms a well-defined sac with an inner opening pointing toward the inguinal region. It is at this point that the round ligament enters the labium from each side, its fibers dispersing and passing into the fibroelastic sac just described.

The labia majora form the lateral extent of the vulva. These folds continue cephalad to-

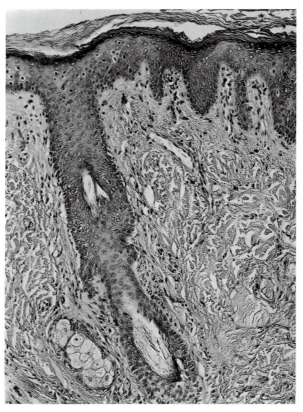

Fig 2–5.—Photomicrograph of labium majus, showing normal histology.

ward the lower abdomen and fuse in the midline as the anterior commissure or mons pubis. The union of the labia majora caudally is known as the posterior commissure and is the lowermost extent of the vulva (Fig 2–6).

The blood supply of the labia majora is derived from the internal pudendal artery through the posterior labial branch and also from a small branch of the obturator artery. The veins have approximately the same source but also communicate with the vesicovaginal plexus and the inferior hemorrhoidal veins. The nerve supply is from multiple sources. The pudendal nerve, derived from the second to fourth sacral nerves, gives off the perineal branch from which the posterior labial nerve arises. The latter innervates the labia majora and the lateral portion of the urethral triangle. In addition, adjunctive supply

is afforded by the ilioinguinal, internal branch of the genitocrural and the genital branch of the lesser sciatic (posterior femoral cutaneous). The nerve supply of the perineum and vulva is shown in Figure 2–7.

LABIA MINORA.—The labia minora consist of two cutaneous folds, which are usually concealed by the majora. In certain instances they may be greatly hypertrophied and project beyond the majora. They lie directly approximate to each other with a convex free border and extend caudad from the prepuce of the clitoris to join the labia majora as they terminate in the posterior fourchette. Between this fourchette and the hymenal ring is a curved depression, the fossa navicularis (see Fig 2–6). The labia minora are reduplications of skin and not mucosa, although some pathol-

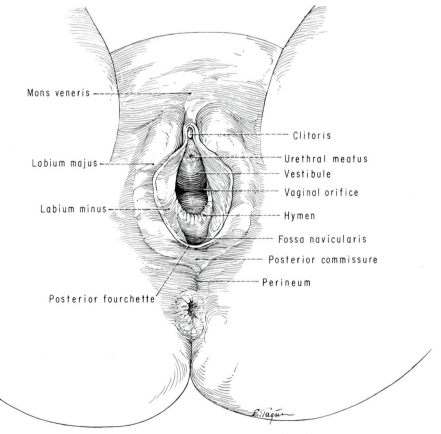

Fig 2–6.—External genitalia of the female.

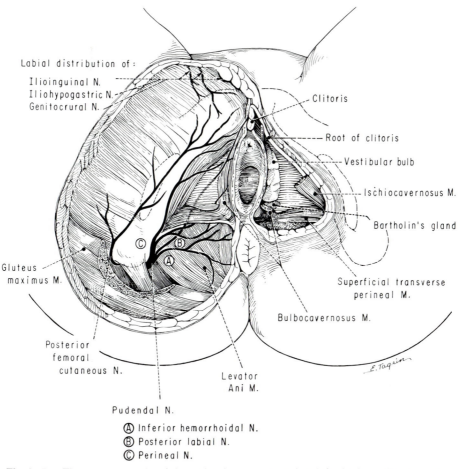

Labial distribution of:
Ilioinguinal N.
Iliohypogastric N.
Genitocrural N.

Clitoris

Root of clitoris

Vestibular bulb

Ischiocavernosus M.

Bartholin's gland

Gluteus maximus M.

Superficial transverse perineal M.

Bulbocavernosus M.

Posterior femoral cutaneous N.

Levator Ani M.

Pudendal N.
Ⓐ Inferior hemorrhoidal N.
Ⓑ Posterior labial N.
Ⓒ Perineal N.

Fig 2–7.—The nerve supply of the vulva is represented at left. At the right, the ischiocavernosus and bulbocavernosus muscles have been reflected to show the anatomy of the clitoris and vestibular bulbs.

ogists have classified the labia minora and vagina as "mucous membrane" and the labia majora as skin. Mucus, however, is not secreted from either the vagina or the labia minora.

The skin of the labia minora contains abundant pigment and blood vessels. Microscopically, the stratified squamous epithelium is characterized by minimal keratinization, but the rete ridges are numerous and prominent. The dermis is made up of connective tissue fibers with numerous bundles of elastic tissue and blood vessels but with minimal fatty tissue. Sweat glands and hair follicles are usually absent but sebaceous glands are abundant (Fig 2–8). As mentioned, the prepuce of the

clitoris is continuous with the labia minora and is histologically similar except for its extreme vascularity. The blood supply is derived from the labial vessels, as previously described, and from the dorsal artery to the clitoris, which is a terminal branch of the internal pudendal artery. The nerve supply is the same as that of the labia majora.

The labia minora may become enlarged following prolonged manipulation or masturbation so that, even in virginal women, they may project beyond the majora. Immediately preceding and during coitus they become moist and lubricated with secretions from the vulvovaginal and sebaceous glands.

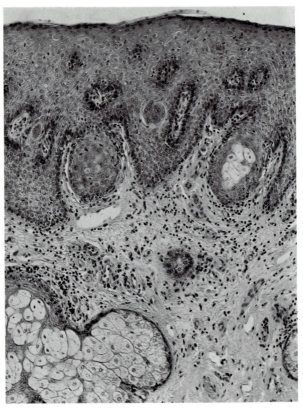

Fig 2–8.—Photomicrograph of labium minus, showing normal histology.

CLITORIS.—The clitoris is composed of two roots, which traverse the pubic rami to unite beneath the symphysis in the clitoridean body. The body terminates in the upper portion of the vestibule as the glans. The roots and body are covered by overlying muscle, but the glans is exposed. Figure 2–7 illustrates the relationship of the root of the clitoris to the overlying ischiocavernosus muscle. The roots, or crura, are 3 to 4 cm long in the flaccid state but in erection are 4.5 to 5.0 cm long. The body is 2.5 to 3.0 cm in length and is surrounded by a connective tissue capsule of fibroelastic tissue termed the clitoridean fascia. The covering of the glans is modified cutaneous tissue, not mucosa. Unlike the penis, the glans clitoridis contains no corpus spongiosum and does not possess as much erectile tissue.

The function of the clitoris seems to be that of a "nerve-center" for coitus. Prior to con-

tact, sexual stimulation causes vascular engorgement and enlargement, so that when the penis is inserted the clitoris becomes particularly sensitive to the to-and-fro motion of the shaft. Orgasm in the female may be brought about by this stimulation even in the absence of the vagina and consists of an interrelated reflex resulting in forceful contractions of both voluntary and involuntary musculature of the pelvis and pelvic viscera. After the process of orgasm has been experienced and a conditioned reflex established, the presence of the clitoris is not absolutely necessary. Women who have had simple or radical vulvectomy with excision of the clitoris are capable of experiencing orgasm.

The arteries of the clitoris arise from the internal pudendal artery. The veins correspond to the arteries, except for the large dorsal vein of the clitoris, which runs beneath the arcuate ligament of the symphysis through a small notch and communicates with the pelvic veins.

VESTIBULAR BULBS.—Vestibular bulbs correspond to the corpus spongiosum of the male and consist of truncated masses of erectile tissue placed on either side of the vaginal orifice. They are situated above the inferior fascia of the pelvic diaphragm and below the bulbocavernosus muscles (see Fig 2–7). The anterior ends taper to join the bulb of the opposite side in the pars intermedia, whereas the posterior surfaces are in contact with Bartholin's glands.

HYMEN.—The hymen is an irregular, membranous fold of varying thickness that partially occludes the vaginal orifice. It extends from the floor of the urethra to the fossa navicularis and may be complete (imperforate), totally absent, incomplete, or cribriform in type. The hymen may be avulsed by examination, trauma, surgery, or coitus. Usually irregular remnants persist, forming a fleshy fringe about the vaginal opening (the carunculae myrtiformes).

VESTIBULE.—The vestibule is an elliptical space that is situated just inside the labia minora and extends from the glans clitoridis to the posterior side of the hymenal ring. The orifices of the urethra, vagina, and vulvovaginal gland ducts open into the vestibule (see Fig 2–6).

MONS VENERIS.—The mons veneris is the most cephalad portion of the vulva (see Fig 2–6) and consists of an accumulation of subcutaneous fat in excess amount in a rounded pad overlying the symphysis pubis. It is covered by pubic hair and the skin is similar to that of the labia majora. The fat pad characteristically remains even after marked inanition and weight loss. The typical female escutcheon of hair over the mons is triangular in shape and usually does not extend upward along the abdomen although there is much variation in this respect, depending on racial and familial traits.

URETHRAL MEATUS.—The urethral meatus, the orifice of the urethra, is situated just caudad to the glans clitoridis and may be visualized by separating the labia minora. It has a cleftlike appearance with slightly raised lateral margins and is the uppermost structure of the vestibule (see Fig 2–6).

PERIURETHRAL GLAND DUCTS.—The periurethral gland ducts are the external orifices of the periurethral (Skene's) glands, which are situated beneath the urethral floor. The orifices are extremely small, yet are usually grossly visible crypts just lateral to and somewhat posterior to the urethral orifice. These glands arise, as do the mucous glands that empty into the distal urethra, from the urethral mucosa itself and are histologically similar. They are stated to be the rudimentary homologue of the prostate gland in the male and are commonly invaded by the gonococcus, in which case pus may be expressed from the openings.

VULVOVAGINAL GLANDS.—The vulvovaginal glands, known commonly as Bartholin's glands, are the homologue of the bulbourethral glands in the male. They are racemose in type and secrete mucus, particularly during sexual stimulation. Situated at each side of the vaginal orifice, below the hymen, the glands are normally small and can be palpated only in rather thin women or if enlarged by inflammation or tumor. The duct openings are in the posterior introitus. Rapid growth occurs at puberty and shrinkage occurs after menopause. Microscopically, the glands show a single layer of high columnar epithelium in the alveoli but the duct is lined by transitional epithelium except for a short invagination of stratified squamous epithelium at the orifice.

MALFORMATIONS

Congenital malformations of the vulva are rare but do occur in association with the stigmata of female hermaphroditism, hypospadias, or incomplete cloacal separations. Complete absence (aplasia) of the vulva occasionally accompanies rudimentary internal genitalia and resembles the secondary atrophy of senility. The labia majora may show some differentiation but are flattened and contain little fat and practically no hair follicles. The labia minora are present, the clitoris rudimentary, and the perineal body short.

Vulvar atresia may occur but is usually incomplete and consists of partial agglutination of the labia with stenosis of the introitus and occasionally an imperforate hymen. Vulvar duplication may occur along with duplication of the vagina, cervix, and uterus. Vulvar fusion has been described in the newborn following the administration of certain progestational agents to the mother during the first 12 weeks of gestation (see Chapter 11).

A comprehensive classification of abnormal

TABLE 2–1.—CLASSIFICATION OF
ABNORMAL SEXUAL DEVELOPMENT*†

Disorders with apparently normal sex chromosomes
    Female pseudohermaphroditism
        Adrenogenital syndrome
        Treatment of mother with progestins or
            androgens
        Maternal virilizing tumor
    Male pseudohermaphroditism
        Primary central nervous system (CNS) defect
            Abnormal gonadotropin secretion
            No gonadotropin secretion
        Primary gonadal defect
            Testicular regression syndrome (gonadal
                destruction)
            Leydig cell agenesis
            Defect in testosterone synthesis identifiable
            Defect in Müllerian Inhibiting System
        End-organ defect
            Androgen insensitivity syndrome (testicular
                feminization)
            5α-reductase deficiency
Disorders associated with obviously abnormal sex
    chromosomes
    Sexual ambiguity unusual
        Klinefelter's syndrome
        Turner's syndrome
    Sexual ambiguity frequent
        Mixed gonadal dysgenesis
        True hermaphroditism

*"Idiopathic" or "unclassified" conditions exist within each major category.
†From Welch W.R., Robboy S.J.: Abnormal sexual development: A classification with emphasis on pathology and neoplastic conditions, in Kogan S.J., Hafez E.S.E. (eds.): *Pediatric Andrology.* Hingham, Mass., Martinus Nijhoff, 1981, chap. 8.

sexual development has recently been devised by Welch and Robboy (Table 2–1). Such a classification depends on the basic criteria of genital anatomy, gonadal anatomy, chromosomal makeup, and specific genetic or metabolic defects (Table 2–1).

Normal development of the male or female genital tract begins with the influence of sex chromosomes on the indifferent gonad with a resulting ovary or testis, testicular differentiation preceding that of the ovary by five weeks. Testicular Sertoli's cells elaborate müllerian inhibiting substance (MIS). Absence of MIS permits development of fallopian tubes, uterus, and upper vagina. Production of MIS from both testes is mandatory since reduced unilateral output results in a streak or ovary with uterus and tube and vagina. Testosterone secretion in adequate amounts originates from Leydig's cells under the stimulus of human chorionic gonadotropin and is necessary for development of the epididymis, vas deferens, and seminal vesicles. On rare occasions, exogenous testosterone or testosterone derived from a maternal source may be responsible for the differentiation of female fetal organs into definitive male organs.

Absence of tissue ability to convert testosterone to dihydrotestosterone (DHT) results in failure of development of the prostate, penis, and scrotum. Therefore, absent development of female genitalia may be secondary to a lack of adequate secretion of testosterone or absent conversion in the end organ to DHT by 5α-reductase or 5α-reductase deficiency. End-organ insensitivity and mild deficiencies of 5α-reductase may result in hypospadias, persistent urogenital sinus, and defects in scrotal fusion.

Finally, internal and external female genitalia may develop and differentiate without any influence from hormones from the fetal ovary unless influenced by the effect of MIS. Elevated levels of androgen prior to 10 to 12 weeks of gestational age will result in ambiguous or normal-appearing external male genitalia with the urethra opening into the vagina. Elevation of androgen levels in the female fetus after 20 weeks' gestational age results only in clitoral hypertrophy. Drugs associated with female pseudohermaphroditism include 17α-ethinyltestosterone, 17α-ethinyl-19-nortestosterone, and, occasionally, diethylstilbestrol, androgens, and intramuscular progesterone. A variety of maternal ovarian tumors have been associated with virilization of the female infant, the most common being a persistent luteoma that manifests itself in mild degrees of fusion of the labia and clitoral enlargement.

Determination of such abnormalities early is important for gender identification in child-rearing, for alleviation of psychological problems attendant to a wrong gender being assigned, and for prevention of life-threatening situations (as in congenital adrenal hyperplasia) and possible malignancy (as in testicular feminization and mixed gonadal dysgenesis).

Correlation of sex chromosomes, external genital morphology, internal genital morphology, and gonadal histology is essential to the diagnosis of disorders of sexual development.

ADRENOGENITAL SYNDROME.—Clitoral hypertrophy may signal deficiency of 3β-hydroxysteroid dehydrogenase or 21-hydroxylase, the latter being the commonest finding in the adrenal-genital syndrome. If androgen excess was present prior to the 16th week of gestation, there may be a common urogenital sinus into which vagina and urethra open. More marked changes may result in a misdiagnosis of a cryptorchid male, with or without hypospadias. Associated deficiencies of other enzymes related to glucocorticoid and mineral-corticoid synthesis can be responsible for life-threatening metabolic problems.

The treatment of minor changes such as agglutination of labia can be accomplished in the early weeks of life by gentle massage and traction to separate the agglutination. If this fails, more vigorous efforts under anesthesia will be necessary. The use of estrogen cream is helpful in preparing these tissues and allowing them to remain apart once successful lysis of the fusion has been carried out.

HYMEN.—The hymen is often involved in developmental defects, the most common types being the (1) imperforate, (2) septate, (3) fenestrate, and (4) cribriform. An imperforate hymen is usually unnoticed until the menarche, at which time menstrual blood accumulates behind the membrane with resultant hematocolpos and hematometra. Blood may rarely be forced into the peritoneal cavity, giving rise to the signs and symptoms of peritonitis. The diagnosis is usually obvious by inspection, a bluish, bulging membrane presenting at the introitus (Fig 2–9). Rectal examination will reveal a distended vagina and an enlarged uterus (occasionally the size of a 12 to 14 week gestation). This condition should be treated in the operating room by a generous cruciate incision, or by excision of a portion of the hymen. Further surgery or exploration is not warranted at this time.

A rigid hymen is frequently seen as a cause for dyspareunia. This may be due to the presence of an excess amount of tough, fibrous tissue or to the presence of multiple small orifices, none of which is large enough to admit the penis. Although both of these types may be helped by gradual dilatation, surgical correction is preferable. A hymenectomy is a simple procedure, and the results are immediate and permanent.

CLITORIS.—The most common abnormality of the clitoris is not really a malformation but an enlargement seen in association with hermaphroditism. The latter condition may be due to adrenal hyperplasia or tumor, gonadal dysgenesis, or unknown causes. Arrhenoblastoma or hilus cell tumor of the ovary may also cause enlargement of the clitoris.

URETHRA.—Malformations of the urethra include stenosis, diverticula, and hypospadias. Mild degrees of stenosis are fairly common and usually cause no symptoms. In some patients there may be tenesmus and recurrent cystitis from urinary retention. Urethral dilatation and treatment of the cystitis are attended by marked relief. Diverticula may be regarded as an abnormality resulting from incomplete development of the urethrovaginal

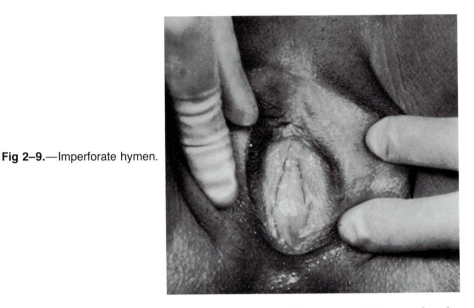

Fig 2–9.—Imperforate hymen.

septum. There may be single or multiple out-pouchings of the urethra along its caudal surface, but without connection with the vagina. The diagnosis is made by expressing urine or, occasionally, pus by firm pressure on the diverticulum. Treatment should be surgical excision. Hypospadias also results from an incomplete separation of the urethra from the vagina, with a resultant congenital urethrovaginal fistula. It may be looked on embryologically as an arrest in the normal development of the urethra in which the posterior (ventral) aspect is incomplete. Thus, in the female, an opening persists between the urethra and the vagina. (Epispadias is extremely rare and refers to the urethral orifice being anterior, i.e., ventral, to its normal position—e.g., clitoral, subsymphyseal, or complete, as in bladder exstrophy.) Treatment in hypospadias (or epispadias) is surgical.

PHYSIOLOGIC ALTERATIONS

The vulvar skin represents a surface area that is sensitive to many systemic alterations and diseases and may be the site of the first cutaneous manifestation of such conditions. The most commonly encountered diseases are diabetes, uremia, and blood dyscrasias.

DIABETES.—Diabetic vulvitis may be the first sign of previously undiagnosed diabetes and may present when known diabetes is out of control. There is marked acute erythema, often with some edema, and the patient will complain of external burning as urine crosses the vulva. Frequently there is an associated monilial vulvovaginitis. Hyperkeratosis ensues with the passage of time. Therefore, the clinical picture may be mixed, with patches appearing opaque and white interspersed with red areas on vulvar skin (Fig 2–10). Control of diabetes and the use of antifungal agents, both vaginally and topically on the vulva, when combined with the use of topical steroids provides marked improvement over a period varying from a week to ten days.

UREMIA.—Late-stage renal disease with uremia may result in "uremic frost" of the vulva as well as of the oral mucosa. Labial surfaces are covered with a gray-white-brown membrane containing urea and uric acid deposits. Treatment consists of local cleansing measures and correction of renal failure, if appropriate.

BLOOD DYSCRASIAS.—Leukemia, aplastic anemia, and agranulocytosis may cause rather typical vulvar ulceration. These ulcers are deep, well-demarcated oval lesions covered usually with a thin, gray membrane. Such lesions have been found following administration of drugs that result in depressed bone marrow function (e.g., methotrexate) and, if death does not ensue, they heal spontaneously following cessation of the drug. In pernicious anemia, vulvar ulceration and hyperpigmentation may be part of generalized tissue devitalization and hypovitaminosis so characteristic of that disease.

VITAMIN DEFICIENCY.—Pellagra may result in acute and, later, chronic hyperkeratotic vulvitis (white) without the presence of monilia. Sitz baths, topical corticosteroids, and vitamin B replacement will reverse this condition.

Apthous ulcers are nonspecific manifestations of such systemic diseases as immunodeficiency syndromes and will be dealt with elsewhere. Of interest, spider bite *(Loxosceles reclusa)* has been reported in patients with hypogammaglobulinemia to result in progressive, painful ulceration of the vulva.

CIRCULATORY DISTURBANCES.—Circulatory disturbances are most commonly evident as edema, varicose veins, and simple hypertrophy. Because of the loose connective tissue of the labia majora, marked edema may be found in generalized anasarca, portal obstruction, or pelvic tumors. A severe edema may be associated with inflammatory conditions such as a chancre or may follow prolonged scratching. The chronic edema of filariasis found especially in Oriental countries and due to an infection with *Acanthocheilonema (Dipetalonema) perstans* is considered to be due to blockage of lymphatic return, excessive intercourse, and a racial predisposition to skin hypertrophy. Varicose veins are especially prominent during the last trimester of pregnancy in association with hemorrhoids and leg varicosities. The patient may complain of burning, itching, and a feeling of heaviness in the vulva. Relief is accomplished by placing pressure against the vulva in the form of a sanitary napkin or foam rubber held in place by a girdle. Rest with the legs and hips elevated should be taken frequently during the day. Occasionally, surgical excision or injection with sclerosing solutions is necessary for relief. During the puerperium, the veins usually become smaller and asymptomatic.

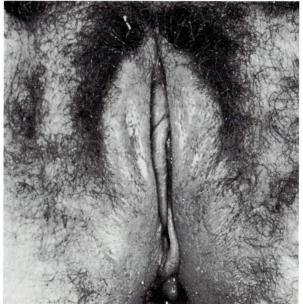

Fig 2–10.—Diabetic vulvitis.

Rarely a telangiectatic angioma may produce unilateral vulvar swelling.

Simple hypertrophy of the labia minora is said to occur when they project more than 4 to 5 cm from their attachment. Such an enlargement is usually symmetric and is thought to be due to masturbation or repeated sexual excitement with resultant chronic hyperemia. There is usually an associated hypersecretion of the sebaceous glands, giving the surface a moist and glistening appearance. It is found more often in blacks, in whom it may merely represent a racial tendency.

VULVAR INJURIES

ACCIDENTAL INJURIES.—The usual injury is a hematoma, brought about by a blow to the vulvar area, particularly if there are large varices, or by falling astride some object, with resultant damage to the vestibular bulbs or to the veins of the clitoris. Minor contusions may be treated by cold compresses and pressure. A large hematoma should be evacuated and packed, and antibiotics should be administered. Inspection should be done carefully to determine whether the urethra, bladder, or rectum has been injured. Fatal perforations into the peritoneal cavity, intestine, and bladder have been reported. The vascular trauma in vulvar injuries is usually venous, so that hemostasis may usually be secured by evacuation of the hematoma and firm packing. Individual ligation of small vessels is not necessary unless arterial bleeding is encountered. The venous pressure in the vulva may be reduced somewhat by elevating both hips on pillows, and the swelling may be reduced by application of cold compresses or ice.

Recreational pursuits such as waterskiing, use of snowmobiles, and riding of mechanical bucking bulls have been added to the list of conventional sources of vulvar trauma (accidental injuries). An indwelling catheter is indicated when dealing with suspected urethral or vesical trauma, or in the presence of large retroperitoneal hematomas or otherwise painful vulvar and perineal injuries, regardless of whether hematomas have been drained or packed or both.

COITAL INJURIES.—Most minor injuries about the hymen are so constantly associated with coitus that they may be termed *physiologic*. They are usually superficial lacerations at either side of the posterior commissure. Injuries following rape, however, may be extensive and occasionally fatal. Profuse hemorrhage may result from tears of the clitoris or posterior fourchette or from hymenal avulsion. If the hymen is thick and nonyielding, lacerations of the perineum into the rectum may occur.

Treatment consists of surgical repair and supportive measures. The clinician should make complete notes of his findings at the time of the first examination. Microscopic search for spermatozoa and smears and cultures for gonorrhea should be made and recorded, since such cases are frequently investigated in criminal court. Although bleeding may be severe enough to necessitate transfusion, treatment is simple and such lacerations usually heal without scarring. The possibility that syphilis and gonorrhea have been contracted at this time must be considered and prophylactic therapy given.

OBSTETRIC INJURIES.—Physiologic injuries occurring at the time of delivery include obliteration of the hymenal folds by the passage of the fetal head and abrasions and minor tears of the vestibule, periurethral area, and perineum. Occasionally, however, complete perineal lacerations with division of the anal sphincter occur. All such tears should be debrided and repaired by primary suture at the time of delivery.

Vulvar hematomas may occur following rapid spontaneous delivery or difficult forceps rotations. Large varicose veins seem to be a predisposing factor and should be ligated or excised just prior to delivery. If the hematoma is small and not extending, it may be treated by elevation of the hips and application of cold compresses. Large hematomas may extend retroperitoneally and be palpable above Poupart's ligament. These should be widely incised, packed, and a contralateral vaginal pack inserted. Blood transfusions and antibiotics are useful as adjunctive therapy. Only rarely can the bleeding vessel be found for ligation, and even if it is, the packing should be placed as described.

Massive vulvar edema following prolonged pushing during the second stage of labor while in the vertical position on the birthing chair may simulate or obscure hematomas of the vulva. Such edema contributes to extension of episiotomies, difficulty in repair, and subsequent poor healing.

X-RAY INJURIES.—The vulvar structures do not tolerate x-ray therapy well. In certain instances the reaction has been extreme, with marked erythema, edema, ulceration, and scarring. Although x-ray may be used occasionally as a palliative procedure for extensive vulvar carcinoma, its use for benign conditions such as neurodermatitis or lichen sclerosus is not without hazard.

PRURITUS VULVAE

Pruritus vulvae is a symptom and not a diagnosis, the word *pruritus* being derived from the Latin *prurire* ("to itch"). The cause for this distressing symptom is often obscure and difficult to determine. It has been estimated that in about 10% of patients seen in private gynecologic practice this is the chief complaint.

The neural mechanisms for the perception of itching are poorly understood, but it has been suggested that these impulses follow somatic pain fibers. The sensation of itching is therefore a subpain response mediated through the lateral spinothalamic tracts. This explains the absence of itching in patients who have had a chordotomy. Psychiatrists have pointed out that the central mediation of anger, resentment, and eroticism may be exhibited in certain areas of the skin, such as the vulva in the female or the perianal area in the male. The persistence of the

stimulus leads to scratching, trauma, and visible damage, thus setting up a vicious cycle. Pathologic changes in the skin, such as hyperkeratosis, rete ridge hyperplasia, and inflammatory changes in the dermis, may be produced experimentally in animals simply by scratching the same skin area repeatedly for a sufficiently long period.

The individual response and the choice of location are intimately allied with the patient's intrapsychic problem, leading to the complexity of the itch-scratch reflex. The intolerable, weak "pain" that is called "itch" is frequently so unpleasant that the patient tries to convert it to a strong pain by scratching. Itching disappears when strong pain is substituted, and such pain is often more endurable, at least temporarily, than the unpleasant sensation of itching. Examples of this are commonplace. Frequently women will, after years of vulvar scratching, resort to stiff brushes to convert itch to pain. Such trauma to the skin prevents natural healing and is followed by other effects, which prolong the dermatitis.

Thus it is often impossible for the clinician to determine whether the gross vulvar changes he sees are due to prolonged scratching or the itching is due to primary skin disease. Biopsy is the only method of making an accurate diagnosis.

Etiology.—Two general classifications of pruritus vulvae may be employed: (1) local genital tract causes and (2) systemic causes. In the first group may be included (*a*) trichomonas vulvovaginitis; (*b*) fungous vulvovaginitis; (*c*) nonspecific bacterial vulvovaginitis; (*d*) atrophic vulvovaginitis; (*e*) contact or atopic vulvovaginitis; (*f*) vulvar dystrophies; and (*g*) carcinoma. The second group includes (*a*) diabetes mellitus; (*b*) drug sensitivity and allergy; (*c*) chemical irritants; (*d*) skin diseases—herpes, intertrigo, lichen planus, psoriasis, and urticaria; (*e*) vitamin deficiencies, especially vitamin A and B complex vitamins; (*f*) diseases due to animal parasites—pediculosis and scabies; (*g*) systemic diseases—anemia, leukemia, hepatitis (with or without jaundice) and tuberculosis; and *(h)* neurogenic dermatitis.

Diagnosis.—Diagnosis will be aided by a meticulous history, careful examination and selected laboratory studies. The important features of the history are the intensity and duration of pruritus, the relationship to menses, associated leukorrhea or bleeding, and previous allergic or dermatologic episodes. Examination should include a careful survey of skin lesions elsewhere as well as inguinal lymphadenopathy. The local lesion should be examined in good light and its general and specific characteristics noted. Fissuring, ulceration, bleeding, scratch marks, thickening, and discoloration are important signs. In addition, inspection of the urethra, periurethral glands, vagina, cervix, anus, and Bartholin's glands should be made.

Selected laboratory tests of importance are: (1) a complete blood study for anemia or blood dyscrasia, (2) urinalysis for diabetes, (3) hanging-drop preparations of vaginal discharge for trichomoniasis and fungous diseases, (4) cultures for nonspecific bacterial infections, (5) cytologic studies for cancer, (6) serologic and antigen studies for venereal disease, (7) blood chemistry examinations for uremia and diabetes, and (8) biopsy for dystrophies or any derangement of skin not responding to short courses of local therapy.

Animal Parasites

SCABIES.—Scabies is caused by the female itch mite, *Sarcoptes (Acarus) scabiei.* Examination will reveal similar lesions in the sides and webs of the fingers, the palms, axillae, wrist flexures, and over the nipples. Pruritus may be intense but is usually nocturnal. The face is almost always uninvolved. Diagnosis is made by obtaining the acarus from a skin burrow with a needle and examining it under the microscope. Either γ-benzene hexachloride (Kwell) ointment or 25% benzyl benzoate in equal parts of tincture of green soap and water may be used to treat the infestation. A se-vere dermatitis should first be treated with soothing baths and lotions and topical use of an antibiotic if necessary. It is best to have the patient begin treatment with a prolonged soap-and-water bath, then rub the selected scabicide into the skin, bathe again only after 24 hours, and change the bed linen and clothing.

PEDICULOSIS PUBIS.—The pubic or crab louse *(Phthirus pubis)* pierces the skin and secretes a noxious substance, which produces severe pubic and vulvar pruritus. The disease is spread by coitus but possibly also by bedding or toilets. The lice may be found attached to the hairs about ½ in. above the skin or at the skin-hair junction. Diagnosis is made by removing the hair and examining it under the microscope. Kwell ointment or lotion are equally effective therapeutically.

OXYURIASIS.—The vulva of children may be affected by an intestinal focus of *Oxyuris vermicularis* (pinworms). Treatment includes oral administration of piperazine citrate (Antepar).

Gentian violet in enteric-coated tablets is an effective, inexpensive agent for the treatment of enterobiasis. Therapy for ten consecutive days is effective and relatively well tolerated, although nausea, vomiting, and abdominal pain are not uncommon.

SEXUALLY TRANSMITTED DISEASES

The major venereal diseases, such as syphilis, gonorrhea, and Herpesvirus hominis type 2 are dealt with in great detail in Chapter 18, and will therefore not be covered in this particular chapter. That is not to minimize their importance. It must be stressed that any lingering lesion of the vulva must be considered in the light of the major venereal diseases. The differential diagnosis of a multiplicity of vulvar diseases should include both syphilis and gonorrhea. Appropriate measures, including culture of the urethra, cervix, and anus, and serologic tests for syphilis should be undertaken quite routinely and, when in doubt, darkfield examination technique should be utilized. Culturing any vesicular eruption is extremely important, especially in an attempt to isolate herpes virus. Techniques are now available that allow for easy transport of culture material. Culture techniques themselves are now extremely reliable.

LYMPHOGRANULOMA VENEREUM.—Lymphogranuloma venereum is a venereal infection spread by coitus and now thought to be caused by an organism of the *Chlamydia* group. There is a latent period with prodromal symptoms and fever and malaise lasting from one to four weeks. Papules, pustules, or small ulcers are present for only a few days and may be relatively asymptomatic, with spontaneous healing. Suppurative inguinal adenitis may follow quickly, with subsequent necrosis, abscess formation, and, perhaps, ulceration. Fibrosis and scarring is a late manifestation, and obstruction of surrounding lymphatics may result in marked edema of the vulva. Lymphatic extension of the disease is responsible for involvement of other organs, such as rectum and lower colon, and may be productive of strictures of the urethra and rectum and eventual incontinence. The disfigurement and destruction of vulvar structures may raise a question of hidradinitis suppurativa. However, this entity will spare the labia minora, in contrast to lymphogranuloma venereum.

Diagnosis is made by complement fixation and the Frei test. In the absence of a positive Frei test result, a repeat complement-fixation study three or more weeks later should confirm the diagnosis. Treatment includes local cleansing and soothing measures. Buboes must be aspirated and never incised for relief of pain.

Treatment.—Tetracycline is very effective. Both penicillin and ampicillin have been reported to be beneficial as well. Therapy should be continued for three to four weeks in the face of early disease. In the chronic state, antibiotics will contribute nothing and vulvectomy for severe deformity and/or colostomy for rectal stricture will at times be necessary. In the presence of multiple, hard, enlarged lymph nodes it is extremely important to be careful to rule out the presence of carcinoma.

CHANCROID (SOFT CHANCRE).—Chancroid is a rare ulcerative vulvar lesion transmitted by coitus and caused by Ducrey's bacillus *(Hemophilus ducreyi)*. The lesion appears initially as a papule or ulcer. It is virtually the only sharply demarcated lesion with induration that is painful. The organisms may be cultured on blood agar plates.

Treatment consists of local measures, including sitz baths and intermittent washing of the vulva with povidone-iodine (Betadine). Erythromycin 500 mg p.o. four times a day or trimethoprim/sulfamethoxazole two single strengths or one double strength tablet p.o. twice daily for ten days is specific treatment.

GRANULOMA INGUINALE.—Granuloma inguinale is a chronic granulomatous disease found especially among blacks in the tropics or southern sections of the United States and is characterized by a severe ulcerative tendency. The etiologic agent is a large bacillus—*Donovania granulomatis (Calymmatobacterium)*. It is described in tissue stains as a Donovan body and it may be seen best using Wright's stain or Giemsa stain or ordinary hematoxylin-eosin preparations on scrapings or biopsies of the lesion. Treatment may be with tetracycline, 1 gm daily for ten days to two weeks. The disease initially begins as a small papular lesion on the labia minor or groin, later becoming serpiginous with pseudobubo or manifesting subcutaneous inguinal granulomas. Streptomycin has been extremely effective in the treatment of this disease but because of its ototoxicity should not be used, at least initially. Biopsies of the skin lesions are important to rule out the co-existence of carcinoma. Occasionally, late-stage manifestations with marked edema and distor-

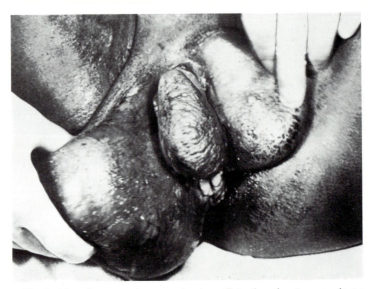

Fig 2–11.—Severe edema and vulvar distortion due to granuloma inguinale.

tion of the vulva may necessitate a vulvectomy (Fig 2–11).

CONDYLOMA ACUMINATA.—From 1966 to 1981, the number of consultations for complaints referable to condyloma acuminata have increased 459%, or more than three times the number of consultations required for genital herpes. More than 65% of these consultations were in the age group of 15 to 29 years. The highest risk group was 20 to 24 years of age, followed by the group aged 25 to 29 years. Although itch and vaginal discharge account for some of the presenting complaints, a large number of patients present with complaints of pain both in the genital and anal areas. The causative agent is a papillomavirus. The epidemiology and complications of these warts is relatively unknown. There is a marked propensity for prolongation of courses of treatment and recurrence. Treatment modalities consist of topical application of 25% podophyllin in tincture of benzoin, freezing, excision, laser, and desiccation. Treatment of vaginal lesions using topical podophyllin is contraindicated due to systemic absorption, which may be toxic. Transmission of the papillomavirus during birth ac-

counts for the presence of laryngeal warts in the newborn. There is early epidemiologic evidence relating the presence of condyloma to later appearance of cervical carcinoma.

MOLLUSCUM CONTAGIOSUM.—This is a sexually transmitted disease that is on the increase. The etiologic agent is a pox virus that has a long incubation period, resulting in the appearance of new warts two to three months after treatment of early lesions. This lesion is not thought to be premalignant. The typical wart is dome-shaped and papular, with a smooth surface varying from 2 to 6 mm in diameter. It may be skin-colored, white, red-purple, or even translucent. The older lesions have a central umbilication. However, only about a third of the lesions display this characteristic. The best treatment is incision and curettement to remove the molluscum body (Fig 2–12). Other therapies include the application of cantharidin, trichloracetic acid, or liquid nitrogen. Cantharidin must be used with care, since it will produce vesicles when applied to normal skin. Protection of skin adjacent to the lesion using Vaseline is recommended. Excision and electrodesiccation are not indicated, since they produce scarring.

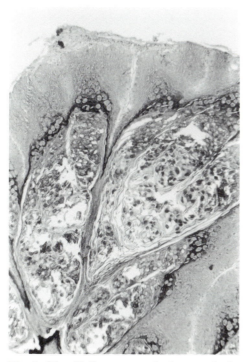

Fig 2–12.—Molluscum contagiosum. A demonstration of the molluscum body, which may be expressed or curetted after nicking the center of the lesion. Touching the cavity with silver nitrate or cryocautery gives good results.

TRICHOMONIASIS.—Trichomoniasis is usually evidenced as a vaginitis, but the thin, frothy, yellow-green discharge often may cause vulvar itching. The vagina is reddened and inflamed, with a granular or strawberry-like appearance. Diagnosis is made by placing a drop of the discharge on a warm slide to which warm normal saline is added, and noting motile *Trichomonas vaginalis*.

Treatment consists of the use of metronidazole (Flagyl), 250 mg three times a day. Although short courses from three to five days are now being utilized, many cases are refractory and will need retreatment for ten days at a time for two to three treatment schedules. Occasionally a patient is intolerant of the drug. Even after retreatment the disease may persist in some. An old-fashioned remedy consisting of hypertonic saline solution may be extremely beneficial in such instances. A formula for a douche consists of 1 cup of table salt stirred into 4 cups of water.

FUNGAL DISEASES

FUNGOUS VULVITIS.—The vulvar area harbors numerous fungi as saprophytes, and under conditions of lowered general resistance, increased heat, friction, or excessive perspiration these may become virulent pathogens. Predisposing causes to this transformation are pregnancy and diabetes, and the finding of a fungous vulvitis should be sufficient to alert the clinician to the possibility of the diabetic state. The most common forms are tinea cruris and candidiasis (moniliasis).

TINEA CRURIS.—Tinea cruris is characterized by superficial, pale pink to bright red lesions with well-defined scaly borders. By a process of coalescence the adjacent vulvar skin, thighs, and pubis may become involved. Following periods of scratching or maceration, the process may resemble a weeping type of eczema. Tinea cruris is caused by a specific fungus, *Epidermophyton inguinale*, and the diagnosis may be made by microscopic examination of the scales, by direct Gram stain, or by culture on Sabouraud's maltose agar. Direct mycologic examination of scales, hairs, and scrapings is facilitated by preparing the specimens without heating in an aqueous solution of 0.1% aminolipid and 0.2% basic fuchsin.

In office practice, scrapings planted on dermatophyte test medium (DTM) culture will result in colonies that change color from yellow to red, in contradistinction to *Candida* colonization, in which color change is rare. Examination with Wood's lamp will not demonstrate fluorescence.

Treatment.—Clotrimazole ointment (Lotrimin) used three times a day is as specific as it will be for *Candida*. Cool sitz baths relieve the itch. Intermittent use of topical corticosteroid cream and, in the severe case, an oral antihistamine-tranquilizer will provide faster relief of symptoms.

CANDIDIASIS.—Nine different yeasts have been identified in the etiology of mycotic vulvitis. Candidiasis (moniliasis) is caused by the most common saprophyte of the normal vagina and vulva, *Candida (Monilia) albicans.* The lesion begins as a reddish papule, which later becomes vesicular. After these rupture, a moist, red mucous membrane remains. Secondary infection is common, so that the vagina and vulva become markedly edematous and tender. The vulva may be covered with a tenacious, gray-white frosting (Fig 2–13), or there may be marked edema due to recurrent scratching. The most common symptoms of candidiasis (moniliasis) are intense itching, burning, and swelling. Itching is likely to persist or reappear unless the fungus is completely eliminated by treatment. A whitish, curdlike vaginal discharge, often with a yeasty or disagreeable odor, may develop as the infection becomes more severe. If chafing occurs, a secondary inflammation or dermatitis of the thighs may also be present. Sexual intercourse may be painful or impossible because of the swelling, abrasion, and inflammation. Walking may be uncomfortable because of chafing.

In some patients, these characteristic features of *Candida (Monilia)* infection are so obvious that diagnosis may be by inspection

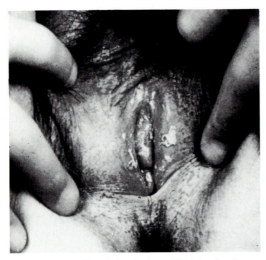

Fig 2–13.—Candidiasis (moniliasis) of vulva.

alone. In others, e.g., in older patients, in very early stages of infection, and when secondary bacterial infections are present, diagnosis is more difficult.

Diagnosis, as with tinea cruris, may be made by wet smear, Gram stain, or culture. Nickerson's medium has simplified culturing, since it is available in small vials that may be inoculated and kept in the office at room temperature. A dark brown or black growth occurs on the medium in about 48 hours if *Candida (Monilia)* organisms are present. Colonies growing on DTM culture will show no color. Specific treatment is available in the form of clotrimazole (Gyne-Lotrimin vaginal tablets and Lotrimin cream 1% and solution 1%), miconazole nitrate 2% (Monistat vaginal cream), nystatin (Mycostatin) vaginal tablets (100,000 units per tablet) and ointment (100,000 units of nystatin per gram) or chlordantoin with benzalkonium (Sporostacin) cream.

Mycolog cream applied locally three times daily is also helpful. In severe cases, especially those complicated by gastrointestinal tract candidiasis, treatment should include the oral administration of nystatin (500,000 units per tablet), two tablets three times a day for a total of ten days. Alternative therapeutic agents are 2% aqueous gentian violet (Genapax) suppositories for vaginal placement. Additionally, the vulva may be painted with 2% aqueous gentian violet.

Size 0 gelatin capsules containing 600 mg of boric acid powder provides an alternative regimen that is cheaper and less objectionable in terms of vaginal discharge, which is associated with other therapeutic creams and jellies. It may be especially helpful in retreatment of recurring or chronic cases of monilial vaginitis. It is important to utilize the powder form as opposed to crystals, which may be responsible for male dyspareunia in some cases. One capsule placed high in the vagina at bedtime over a period of 14 days is optimal treatment. However, in some cases it may be necessary to continue to use the capsule on a twice-a-week basis for as long as two to three months, especially in stubborn cases of mixed vaginal infections. Five percent boric acid ointment (Borofax) applied to the vulva is also extremely efficacious. Its effectiveness is unrelated to pH.

Discontinuation of oral contraceptives may be necessary when infection occurs frequently. Dilantin may relieve persistent symptoms (i.e., burning, soreness) in patients with neuritis after the skin clears.

OTHER SKIN INFECTIONS

PYODERMA (IMPETIGO).—Chafing, scratching, abrasion, insect bites, and altered host-response provide portals of entry for pathogenic bacteria present in the carrier state in a large portion of otherwise normal individuals. The usual agents are a *Staphylococcus* or β-hemolytic *Streptococcus* or both. This disease is characterized by thin-walled vesicles that rupture, leaving a reddened weeping spot that soon becomes crusted over and exudes pus from beneath. Clear vesicles and pustules are frequently clustered around the central lesion. Disease is readily spread to or from other parts of the body.

ECTHYMA.—Ecthyma resembles impetigo grossly, but invades the epidermis to involve the dermis. Because of the depth of penetration of the infection, subsequent scarring is common.

FOLLICULITIS.—Folliculitis occurs with infection of the hair follicles and nearby sebaceous glands and takes on the appearance of a papule, later becoming pustulated. The progression of this lesion to a boil that ultimately becomes fluctuant is not uncommon. Widespread involvement of tissue produces cellulitis and/or lymphangitis. The latter entities are accompanied by constitutional symptoms, including fever and chills.

ERYSIPELAS.—Erysipelas is a variant of streptococcal infection, being more superficial in nature than cellulitis but still accompanied by severe systemic symptoms, including headache, fever, and chills. One of the char-

acteristics of this lesion is a very sharp border that is mildly indurated.

Any of these entities requires culturing of free pus to obtain sensitivity studies. While awaiting culture reports, penicillin or erythromycin are good agents to start with. Cleaning of the affected areas with antibacterial soap and water is helpful and reduced activity will help to minimize spread. Instruction in scrupulous hygiene with washing of hands thoroughly after touching the area of infection is most important to minimize spread to other areas of the body. Any streptococcal infection may subsequently be associated with glomerulonephritis. Many types of infections are frequently superimposed on underlying dermatoses. Furthermore, aspects of this disease raise the possibility of syphilis and invasive carcinoma and failure of such lesions to respond to treatment rather rapidly must ultimately result in a biopsy. Serologic tests for syphilis must be done routinely.

ERYTHRASMA.—Erythrasma is an asymptomatic red lesion, usually symmetric in appearance, with distinct margins that are not elevated. The source of this lesion is a gram-positive intracellular bacteria, *Corynebacterium minutissimum*. The organism may be seen under the microscope using scrapings of the skin. It is extremely difficult to culture and requires special media. The lesion itself may fluoresce under Wood's lamp secondary to production of a porphyrin by the bacterium. Cure for this lesion is obtained using oral erythromycin or tetracycline over a ten-day period.

CYTOMEGALIC DISEASE.—The *Chlamydia* group, which is responsible for trachoma and infectious conjunctivitis as well as pelvic inflammatory disease, rarely will produce granulomatous lesions of the vulva. Antibody testing should be included in the differential diagnosis for any of these granulomatous or ulcerative diseases. Some indication of the presence of these organisms may be obtained by the cytopathologist, if intracellular inclusions and bizarre nuclei are present in cells obtained from scrapings of cervical lesions.

AMEBIC VULVOVAGINITIS.—*Entamoeba histolytica* produces multiple ulcerations of the labia and vagina resulting in a foul, bloody discharge and dyspareunia. There is almost always an antecedent history of uncontrolled diarrhea. Amebiasis may involve the urethra and be the underlying agent for fistulous tracts from rectum to the vagina and pelvic abscess formation. Intense local hygenic therapy coupled with antiamebic therapy will result in good outcome.

OTHER GRANULOMATOUS DISEASES OF THE VULVA.—Depending on the geographic area of origin of the patient, various less frequently encountered etiologic organisms should be considered, such as *Schistosoma haematobium* and *S. mansoni, Blastomyces dermatitidis, Coccidioides immitis,* and *Actinomyces israelii,* the latter being involved mainly with diseases of the uterus, fallopian tubes, and ovaries.

NECROTIZING FASCIITIS.—This potentially fatal disease is known for its ability to develop where there has been no apparent injury and also in areas of minor injury. A similar process known as *progressive bacterial synergistic gangrene* is most frequently associated with wound infection. Necrotizing fasciitis is frequently seen on a background of diabetes and preexisting vascular disease, and mortality rates as high as 70% have been reported in diabetics with the disease. Likely organisms in both entities belong to the coliform group and there is also a predominance of enterococci. Patients with progressive bacterial synergistic gangrene are much less ill, but are always potential candidates for the development of the more severe necrotizing fasciitis. Treatment must be very aggressive, with institution of antibiotic therapy and very wide surgical excision of all tissue back to margins that appear grossly normal and bleed easily. Frequently, more than one trip to the operating room for wide surgical excision is necessary, since initial attempts often fall short of what is ultimately required.

AUTOIMMUNE DISEASES

CROHN'S DISEASE.—This disease is primarily found in the colon and small bowel. Early symptoms are low abdominal and pelvic pain, which may mislead the gynecologist into believing that there is a gynecologic pelvic pathologic condition. On the other hand, this disease may present initially on the vulva as draining sinuses or abscesses or deep ulceration seemingly remote from rectum or anus. Constitutional symptoms are often present, including low-grade fever, diarrhea, fatigue, and weight loss. Differential diagnosis includes Behçets disease, tuberculosis, granuloma inguinale, and lymphogranuloma venereum. Radiographic evidence of bowel pathologic changes coupled with the appearance of communicating sinuses generally confirms the diagnosis. Surgical treatment alone is usually to no avail, and the disease may become progressively more destructive with creation of a cloaca. Treatment of the primary disease is mandatory and usually requires a daily dosage of steroids of up to 60 mg plus antibiotics of a systemic nature. Biopsy specimens of the vulvar lesions will reveal nonspecific granulomatous change. Ulcers should be debrided, and sinus tracts and ulcerated areas cleansed repeatedly with povidone-iodine. The addition of metronidazole to the regimen has been found to be helpful. Once healing is under way, wide excision of any sinus tracts usually results in good healing.

BEHÇET'S DISEASE (TRIPLE SYMPTOM COMPLEX).—Manifestation of this disease includes the ulceration of buccal mucous membrane, vulvar ulceration, and iritis or iridocyclitis. Biopsy of vulvar ulcers reveals a nonspecific picture of inflammation and vasculitis. Ulcers are more often small but very deep and tend to come and go almost on a spontaneous basis. Herpes and Stevens-Johnson syndrome should be ruled out. Herpes lesions come and go almost spontaneously in many individuals. The first line of defense is merely careful local cleansing measures and observation. The use of corticosteroids may be helpful and there have been reports that cyclic use of oral contraceptives, which are predominantly of an estrogenic nature, may be helpful. Surgery for this lesion is thought to be contraindicated unless the vulvar lesions are extremely destructive, with fenestration and scarring from loss of vulvar tissue.

DISEASE OF SWEAT GLANDS

HIDRADENITIS SUPPURATIVA.—Hidradenitis suppurativa is an infection resulting from mixtures of *Staphylococcus*, *Streptococcus*, and, occasionally, coliform organisms. This infection is unique in that it involves only the apocrine glands; therefore, the disease affects mainly labia majora, intercrural folds, occasionally the mons, and, extremely rarely, the clitoris or labia minora. A secretory and a suppurative phase may be exhibited simultaneously. Axillary sweat glands may be involved as well. Due to the cyclic nature of the disease, in early stages it may respond favorably to the use of intermittent oral estrogens or cyclic oral contraceptives. Once the disease progresses to the suppurative phase, multiple intercommunicating sinuses develop; it is typical at this stage that when one area is pressed pus will be seen extruding at a distance from another sinus. In early stages careful cleansing with Dial soap or Betadine solution may be helpful, and institution of intermittent courses of oral antibiotics may also help to diminish the progression of the disease. In spite of these measures, the chronic phase may develop, leading to multiple-abscess formation; these abscesses can be drained periodically but the end result is deep scarring beneath multiple recurrent sinuses. Ultimately, the treatment of choice for this condition is wide surgical excision with sparing of the labia minora, the clitoris, and the prepuce, and subsequent skin grafting. This approach will provide marked improvement and return a discouraged person to everyday activity within a relatively short time. This entity is frequently confused with folliculitis and also with lymphogranuloma venereum. However, lymphogranuloma results in massive edema and destruction of the labia minora as well as labia majora.

FOX-FORDYCE DISEASE.—This disease is also limited to the sweat glands, and is papular in appearance, secondary to plugging of these glands. It is believed that subsequent extravasation of the contents of the sweat glands into the epidermal tissue results in the intense pruritus that accompanies the lesion. The axilla may be simultaneously involved with the same process and there appears to be some relationship between the complaint of pruritus and a particular time in the menstrual cycle. Treatment may be successful using cyclic oral contraceptives; occasional relief with topical estrogen is noted.

CONTACT DERMATITIS

Contact dermatitis of the vulva may be caused by true primary irritants or by an underlying immunologic response to an external or, occasionally, internal agent. A detailed history must be taken to elucidate any of the many possible offending agents, including poison ivy, artificial fibers contained in clothing, toilet tissue (especially perfumed or colored), condoms, douches, contraceptives, nail polish, perfumes, deodorants, and sanitary napkins. Common causes of allergic contact sensitivity include para-aminobenzoic acid derivatives, azo dyes, chromates, cobalt, formaldehyde, lanolin, mercaptobenzothiazole, neomycin, nickel, oleoresins, phenothiazines, rubber compounds, and sulfa drugs. Common sources of primary irritant dermatitis are fatty acid and detergent molecules that are present in agents used to wash or bleach clothing. Some of these are not only irritants but may be allergens and/or photoallergens. The lesion takes the form of eczematous dermatitis with erythema, edema, vesicles, oozing, and crusting. In the chronic stage, it may be lichenified with hyperkeratotic scaling and, therefore, appear to be a white lesion. Excoriations and secondary infection are common. Treatment includes elimination of the offending agents, if one can be found, and during the acute phase, application of cool compresses of boric acid solution or saturated solution of aluminum acetate and aluminum subacetate 1%. Cornstarch and baking soda baths are helpful with the patient soaking one hour twice a day. Infection is irradicated with topical and/or systemic antibiotic. Corticosteroid cream and antihistamine or tranquilizers, or both, are very helpful in the acute phase. Additional lesions involved in the vulvar reaction may be purpura, vesicles, and, occasionally, ulceration.

ATROPHIC VULVITIS

Atrophic vulvitis is usually coexistent with a vaginitis of similar nature. Symptoms include vulvar burning, itching, and dyspareunia. Bleeding may occur from ulceration or telangiectasia. This physiologic, atrophic skin change usually starts at the climacteric or after artificial menopause, and the generally accepted cause is estrogen deficiency. The entire process is too complex, however, to be explained on this factor alone. Exogenous estrogen therapy will not reverse or prevent this ultimate change in most individuals. Other hormones and related factors presumably contribute to the general aging phenomenon. The mons pubis becomes less prominent and the labia majora shrink and flatten as the result of loss of subcutaneous fat. The adjacent skin becomes thin and shiny, the hair sparse, and tissue elasticity diminished. As a result, the vaginal orifice becomes narrowed or even stenotic, with resultant dyspareunia. A thin, watery discharge may be present. Diagnosis is evident by noting the degree of cornification of vaginal cells in a hanging-drop preparation or Papanicolaou smear. For the vaginal component of the disease, local applications of estrogenic creams or small oral doses of estrogens for short periods are quite effective. Combinations of estrogens with androgens will occasionally give superior results, especially when libido has been diminished. Emolient creams, starch baths, sedatives, and antipruritic lotions should afford relief in most cases.

SIMPLE KRAUROSIS.—Simple kraurosis of the vulva is a primary sclerosing atrophy limited to the labia minora, vestibule, urethra, and clitoris. It occurs most commonly in postmenopausal women. The labia majora, perineum, and perianal regions are not usually involved. In the early stages the skin may be red and glistening with isolated patches of dark red or dull purple (kraurosis rouge). In later stages the skin becomes pale yellow and has a smooth, glistening surface, obliterated labial folds, atrophic mons veneris, and scanty, broken-off pubic hairs (Fig 2–14). The vaginal orifice is narrowed and barely admits the index finger.

Histologically, there is hyperkeratosis (excess keratin above the epithelium) with flattening of the rete ridges, edema and homogenization of the cutis collagen, separation of the elastic fibers, and mild arteriosclerotic changes in the deeper blood vessels. Simple kraurosis bears no known relationship to carcinoma of the vulva.

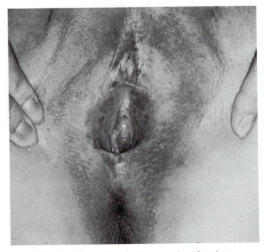

Fig 2–14.—Simple kraurosis of vulva.

WHITE LESIONS

White lesions of the vulva are the result of processes of depigmentation with loss or destruction of the melanocyte's ability to manufacture melanin, sclerosis of vessels that nourish skin, and/or the production of hyperkeratosis. Because of the occasional coexistence of white lesions of skin proximal with established cancer it has frequently been assumed that the white change is related to the onset of cancer. Bonney and Berkley have pointed out that malignant potential is more often related to the presence of hyperplastic lesions. Because of the general confusion, previous terminology such as kraurosis and leukoplakia have fallen into disrepute. Following the suggestion of Jeffcoat a decade earlier, the International Society for the Study of Vulvar Disease established a nomenclature in 1975 in an attempt to remedy the situation. This classification that is now in current use is as follows: (1) hyperplastic dystrophy *(a)* without atypia, *(b)* with atypia; (2) lichen sclerosus; (3) mixed dystrophy *(a)* without atypia, *(b)* with atypia. The atypia is graded as to whether it is mild, moderate, or marked. The exact relationship of atypia to the onset of carcinoma is still unclear, but certainly those with the most marked change are worthy of local surgical attention and follow-up. Associated intense pruritus with resulting self-inflicted trauma and attendant recurrent chronic healing processes may be related as much to development of atypias as to any other source. Treatment of the itch is to be conservative, with topical applications or appropriate agents once carcinoma has been ruled out by knife or punch biopsies. Vulvectomy is indicated for marked widespread atypism after failure of conservative therapy.

LICHEN SCLEROSUS.—This disease may be seen at any age, involving both the young and old. Neck, trunk, axilla, and extremities may be involved, or the lesion may present primarily on the vulva. The general skin background is pale and parchment-like, peppered

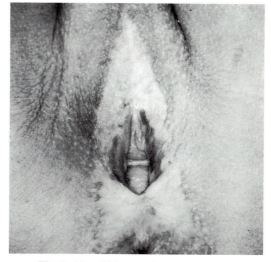

Fig 2–15.—Lichen sclerosus of vulva.

with whitish papular-appearing areas over the atrophic background (Fig 2–15). Mild edema and agglutination of the prepuce are not uncommon. Biopsy will reveal a thin epithelium, at times atrophic in appearance and at times with hyperkeratosis. Histologically there is loss of rete ridges, a collagenized subepithelial zone, and, beneath this, a layer of inflammatory cells (Fig 2–16). Treatment of lichen sclerosus is best accomplished using a 2% testosterone preparation in petrolatum or lanolin base. If itching and burning persist following this regimen, intermittent use of corticosteroid cream may be helpful. Application of testosterone should be done on a daily basis until the symptoms are brought under control; following this, intermittent use throughout the month will tend to keep symptoms under control. Vulvectomy with or without grafting cannot be expected to eradicate the process. It will always recur and be accompanied by the same symptoms.

HYPERPLASTIC DYSTROPHY.—This term embraces hyperkeratotic white lesions including lichen simplex chronicus and hypertrophic vulvitis, as well as neurodermatitis. The microscopic picture is nonspecific and characterized by elongation of rete pegs, hyperkeratosis, and the presence of dermal in-

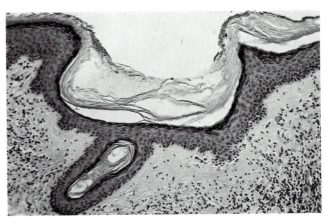

Fig 2–16.—Histologic appearance of lichen sclerosus.

flammation (Fig 2–17). One cannot assign significance to the lesion without biopsy, since it is what is going on at the depths of the lesion that is important (Fig 2–18), and not the appearance of the lesion. In any event, biopsy is mandatory to establish a diagnosis and assess the presence or absence of any atypia.

The treatment of choice for these lesions is the use of topical corticosteroids. Boric acid preparations are soothing and aid in alleviating the intense itch. With proper therapy the lesions should disappear. Failure of the original lesion to disappear or the reappearance of a new lesion warrants repeated biopsy.

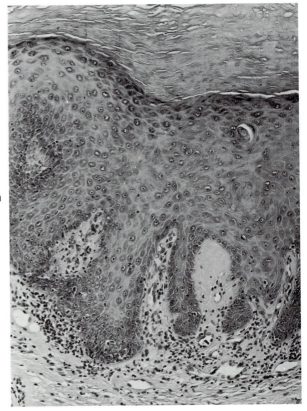

Fig 2–17.—Histologic changes in hyperplastic dystrophy.

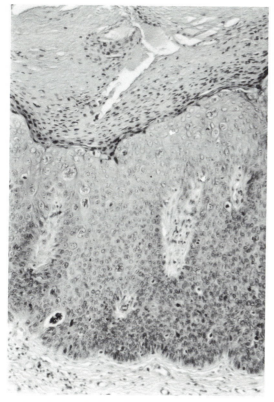

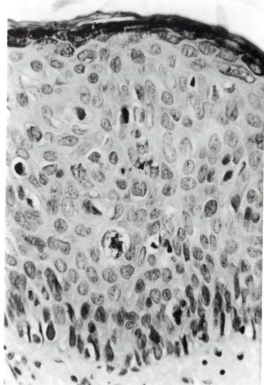

Fig 2–18 (left).—Carcinoma in situ of the vulva beneath a thick hyperkeratotic patch.
Fig 2–19 (right).—Carcinoma in situ of the vulva with well-keratinized surface epithelium. Note cellular disarray, abnormal mitoses, and dyskeratosis.

MIXED DYSTROPHY.—Mixed dystrophy is defined as the presence of both lichen sclerosus and hyperplastic dystrophy. Multiple biopsies are mandatory to rule out atypia and to determine the extent of atypia present. Aggressive topical therapy with alternating testosterone and corticosteroids usually results in regression of the disease.

OTHER WHITE DISORDERS

VITILGO.—This disease process may be present anywhere on the body and is characterized by a process in which melanocytes are destroyed. Commonly, dark hair may be seen growing from a white patch of skin. The disease is transmitted by dominant genes within families and its onset may be noted in early life.

ALBINISM.—Here, an enzyme deficiency prevents normal formation of the melanin pigment. A white forelock of hair is characteristic.

LEUKODERMA.—This entity is nonspecific and results from chronic trauma; it often follows inflammatory diseases of the vulva. Ultimately, the area will become repigmented.

INTERTRIGO.—This condition ensues from the presence of a constant moist environment, most often found in the depths of the skin folds, i.e., beneath a large panniculus or in the groin. Chronic low-grade dermatitis is most always present. Good hygiene, use of all-cotton underwear, and the application of drying powders are general aids in clearing the condition. If fungi or bacteria are present and do not respond to conservative measures, specific fungicidal or bactericidal topical agents may be necessary.

CARCINOMA IN SITU— INTRAEPITHELIAL NEOPLASIA

The criteria for the diagnosis of this disease as set forth by the International Society for the Study of Vulvar Disease include disorientation and loss of epithelial architecture that extends throughout the full thickness of the epithelium, not including keratinized or parakeratotic layers (Fig 2–19). Grossly, lesions may be white, red, or pigmented. They may be unifocal or multifocal, discrete or coalesced. It is important to note that approximately 20% of all vulvar carcinomas in situ will appear as dark spots. Other terms found in the literature that are basically synonymous include *Bowen's disease, erythroplasia of Queyrat,* and *Paget's disease.*

Recently, multifocal pigmented verrucous lesions have received added attention under the term *bowenoid papulosis.* This lesion is found usually in very young women who have either recently been pregnant or have had a prior history of herpes or condylomata acuminata. The true natural history of this lesion and its potential for invasion is as yet unknown.

In contrast to carcinoma in situ of the cervix, carcinoma in situ of the vulva has different histologic criteria. The relationship to invasive cancer is not strong. Only 20% of invasive cancers have adjacent carcinoma in situ. The interval between the peak ages for carcinoma in situ of the vulva and invasive carcinoma of the vulva is greater than that for cervical cancer. No series of untreated cases have been followed up and observed as to progress to invasive cancer of the vulva. Benedet and Murphy in a recent review of 81 patients with carcinoma in situ noted that there is an increasing incidence of this disease in young women with 42% being under the age of 25 years as contrasted to 14% in an earlier time period. The younger age group tended to manifest the disease with more multicentric and more frequent pigmented lesions as opposed to the older age groups, in which unifocal lesions dominated.

Caglar et al. reviewing a group of 50 patients note the occurrence of carcinoma in situ in 10% of patients who were in a state of immunosuppression. The same phenomenon has been pointed out by Sillman and others. In the series of Caglar et al., almost half the patients were asymptomatic; those with symptoms complained of itch. Sixty-five percent of the lesions were white in appearance.

Spontaneous regression of lesions has been noted in patients who were untreated including some lesions with aneuploidy. There has been an association between this lesion and the previous occurrence of sexually transmitted diseases including the granulomatous diseases and condylomata acuminata. This tends to suggest some sort of etiologic relationship that still remains to be proved. Studies of nuclear DNA obtained from biopsies of coalesced and unifocal lesions suggest the possible presence of different cell lines, with one possibly undergoing transformation from in situ to invasive cancer. This work needs confirmation by others. The association of other genital malignancies is reported as varying from 20% to 30%. In another series of 65 patients, Bernstein et al. reported that 84% of patients under the age of 40 years had multifocal disease and 65% of patients older than 40 years had unifocal disease. These authors also charted the site of recurrence of lesions and noted that the area most likely to be involved was the right lower labium majus, which was involved 50% of the time. Kaplan et al. have reported on ten patients with intraepithelial carcinoma extending to the anus. Lesions in this area may go unnoticed for some time.

Because of the rising incidence of intraepithelial neoplasia in young women, gynecologic surgeons have radically changed their approach to therapy in an effort to prevent disfigurement at an early age. Several options are available depending on the extent of disease and the patient's preference regarding surgery. Currently, wide local excision with or without skin grafting is preferred therapy. In the patient with multiple small lesions, several sittings using local anesthesia may be necessary to control the disease. Topical fluorouracil alone has not been satisfactory in the hands of many; however, Sillman has noted its usefulness as an adjuvant just prior to surgery, since it seems to help in demarcating the areas of epithelial involvement. The use of dinitrochlorobenzene appears to be an effective alternative for some who are unwilling to undergo surgery. It might be beneficial as well in patients with multiple lesions. Skin reaction to this treatment, however, is moderate to severe, and it is reported that patients are unwilling subsequently to undergo therapy. With very large lesions occupying most of the vulva a very careful histologic examination must be performed in order not to overlook a focus of invasive carcinoma. Such lesions are, of course, best dealt with using multiple knife biopsies prior to definitive surgery. However, it is still possible, even after many biopsies, to overlook a focus of invasion. Recurrence rates after conservative surgery are reported to 30%. Similar rates of recurrence are noted as well in patients treated by vulvectomy. Regardless of what form of therapy is instituted, extremely close follow-up examination is warranted over a long period.

BULLOUS DISEASES

Bullous diseases of the skin are usually present elsewhere on the body, including scalp and mucous membranes of the oral cavity as well as on the vulva. When bullae rupture, shallow oozing ulcerations are left.

Pemphigus vulgaris is the most common of the bullous diseases and, although rare, is usually fatal. Lesions are flaccid bullae and persistent ulcers appearing on normal skin and mucosal surfaces frequently appear first on the mouth or on the scalp, upper chest, and back. Vulvar involvement may occasionally be the primary site. As the disease progresses, anemia with leukocytosis and eosin-

ophilia are common. Without treatment, there is an 80% mortality rate. Cytologic examination of cells from cervical lesions as well as lesions elsewhere often reveal acantholytic cells with malignant characteristics. Circulating antibodies to intercellular antigens may be found in 80% of cases. Nearly 90% of skin biopsies will reveal deposits of IgG and/or complement. Treatment consists of the use of large doses of corticosteroids and/or cytotoxic agents, such as cyclophosphamide (Cytoxan).

The benign familial form of this disease is known as Hailey-Hailey disease. Immunofluorescent studies are negative and treatment consists of local injection of lesions with corticosteroids. Topical antibiotics and antifungal agents are also said to be helpful.

ERYTHEMA MULTIFORME.—This disease is believed to be an allergic and self-limited bullous involvement of skin and mucous membrane, confining itself to young people. The major form of the disease, Stevens-Johnson syndrome, usually has a prodrome consisting of fever, malaise, and pharyngitis, which precedes by a few days the appearance of cutaneous lesions that have a predilection for the palms, soles, the dorsum of the hands and feet, and extensor surface of the extremities. Precipitating causes include: drugs such as penicillin, barbiturates, and mecurials; bacteria; *Mycoplasma;* exposure to cold or sunlight; menstruation; and pregnancy. The typical lesion, when found, is a series of concentric rings of varying shades of red. Such a lesion is pathognomonic but rarely seen. Except for leukocytosis and elevation of the sedimentation rate there are no other abnormal laboratory findings. Pneumonitis occurs occasionally (Stevens-Johnson syndrome). Minor degrees of this disease are treated with topical corticosteroids. The major form of the disease requires systemic steroid therapy and other measures, such as antibiotic therapy, for the control of secondary pneumonia or pyodermal complications.

BULLOUS PEMPHIGOID.—Bullous pemphigoid exhibits lesions on the flexor surface of the extremities and intertriginous areas. The bullae are deeper and more tense and biopsy reveals subepithelial eosinophilic infiltrates.

HERPES GESTATIONIS.—Herpes gestationis is quite similar to bullous pemphigoid but occurs only in pregnant women. Circulating antibodies to basement membrane are usually lacking in the latter, as opposed to the former.

DERMATITIS HERPETIFORMIS.—Dermatitis herpetiformis may resemble both pemphigoid and erythema multiforme. These lesions, however, are located mainly on the knees, elbows, and buttocks, and IgA rather than IgG is found at the epidermal-dermal junction by immunofluorescence techniques. Dermatitis herpetiformis is an extremely pruritic papulovesicular eruption and most patients exhibit a spruelike enteropathy. A gluten-free diet will improve both the enteropathy and the lesions. However, treatment with sulfapyridine, 2 to 4 gm/day is usually also indicated.

DRY SCALY DERMATOSES

LICHEN PLANUS.—Lichen planus is an inflammatory dermatosis of unknown origin that is characterized by multiple, small, flat-topped, polygonal papules that have a peculiar violaceous color and are covered with an often umbilicated horny film, usually associated with lesions elsewhere on the body (wrists, ankles, inner thighs). It may be confused with dystrophy, kraurosis or neurodermatitis. Diagnosis is made by biopsy, which shows acanthosis, hyperkeratosis, absence of parakeratosis, saw-toothed rete ridges, and a bandlike infiltration of chronic inflammatory cells in the upper cutis (Fig 2–20). Treatment includes general measures such as sedatives, rest, avoidance of sweating and the use of tranquilizers. Locally, colloid baths, aluminum acetate solution, and an ointment such as:

Phenol	1.20
Salicylic acid	1.80
Liq/carbonis detergents	3.00
ung zinc oxide	60.00

may be tried. Corticosteroid creams are by themselves of little help, but their effect may be enhanced by an occlusive dressing of plastic material and cellophane tape. In hypertrophic lesions, injection of small amounts of triamcinolone acetate suspension may be efficacious.

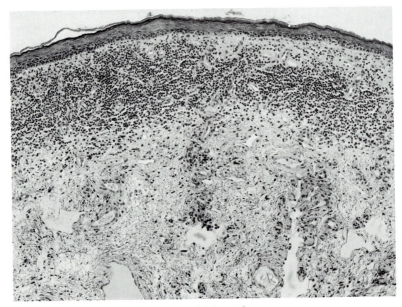

Fig 2–20.—Lichen planus.

PSORIASIS.—Psoriasis is an inflammatory dermatosis of unknown origin characterized by dry, scaling patches of various sizes covered by silvery-white or grayish-white scales. It may involve the vulva, although the sites of predilection are the scalp, nails, the extensor surfaces of the limbs, and the sacral area. If vulvar lesions are present, usually there are lesions on these other areas. The disease commonly has periods of exacerbation and remission, which may or may not be associated with subjective symptoms. The diagnosis may be obvious, but biopsy frequently is necessary. Microscopically there are a uniform parakeratosis, thin suprabasal epidermal plates, uniform rete ridge elongation with clubbing, and microabscesses in the stratum corneum. During periods of exacerbation, improvement may be noted with sunbaths, ultraviolet light, or the application of crude tar (2% to 5%) or salicylic acid (2% to 10%) ointments.

Topical use of fluorinated corticosteroids applied twice a day is helpful. Examples of such compounds include Valisone and Halog. Covering the area with a plastic film such as Saran Wrap may help to achieve a longer-lasting effect. In selected severe cases, the use of methotrexate has been helpful inasmuch as the disease is characterized by rapid cell turnover. Long-term use of topical corticosteroids must be avoided to minimize the likelihood of subepithelial fibrosis. Trauma and emotional stress are to be minimized.

SEBORRHEIC DERMATITIS.—Seborrheic dermatitis is a red rash appearing in areas of skin where there is a high concentration of sebaceous glands. It is not a disease of sebaceous glands per se. However, the skin does appear oily, and whitish-yellow plaques may occur. Common sites of involvement include the scalp (where the term *dandruff* is used), areas behind the ears, over the sternum, between the scapula, crural folds, perianal area, labia majora, mons, and intertriginous areas. With involvement of the vulva there is severe itching and the itch-scratch reflex may result in secondary excoriation and infection. The dis-

ease is not curable but may be ameliorated by use of tranquilizers, good hygiene, and topical steroids. The treatment of secondary infection is important. Avoidance of psychic stress and use of mild tranquilizers, especially at bedtime, is extremely helpful in moderating symptoms. Asymmetry of this lesion on the vulva is the exception and not the rule, and in such cases may be confused with chronic dystrophy or Paget's disease.

LICHEN SIMPLEX CHRONICUS AND NEURODERMATITIS.—Lichen simplex chronicus and neurodermatitis are grossly and microscopically similar. Clinical differentiation is often difficult, since these lesions seem to eventuate after many initiating factors, which bring into play the itch-scratch reflex and subsequent chronic trauma. Be that as it may, the important thing is to distinguish this from true dystrophies and biopsy is indicated more often than not. Cures for these entities do not exist, but amelioration of symptomatology and improvement in skin health can be effected by instituting scrupulously good hygiene, with use of all-cotton underwear; avoiding irritating substances; and periodically applying topical corticosteroid creams. The judicious use of tranquilizers, especially at bedtime, is very helpful and instruction in avoiding conscious scratching should be undertaken. The end result is a lesion with hyperkeratosis (a white lesion), which accounts for easy confusion with dystrophies; hence, the indication for early biopsy (Fig 2–21).

BENIGN NEOPLASMS

The most common benign neoplasms of the vulva are papillomas, lipomas, fibromas, and hidradenomas. Less common are neurofibromas, lymphangiomas, hemangiomas, and myxomas. Additionally, and rarer still, are glomus tumors, granular cell myoblastoma, angiolipoma, sebaceous adenoma, syringoma, and benign lymphoid hamartoma. Excision provides both diagnosis and adequate treatment.

Condylomata acuminata are benign and in-

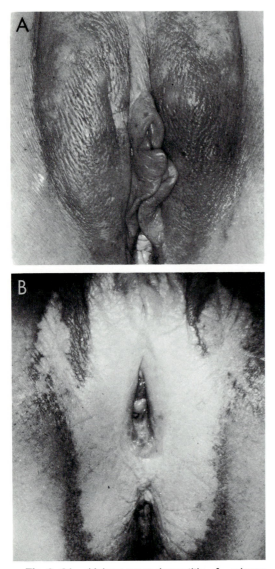

Fig 2–21.—Vulvar neurodermatitis. **A,** edema and lichenification of early stage. **B,** extensive hyperkeratosis in late stage.

Although the proper name for this lesion is nevus verrucosus, nevus cells are not present in the usual case. It is cured by simple excision.

LIPOMA.—A lipoma is a benign tumor that arises from the fatty tissue of the labia majora or mons veneris and usually grows slowly and causes no symptoms except when its size is excessive. When this occurs, the mass acquires a pedicle and hangs from the groin or vulva as a pendulum. If the pedicle is wide it may resemble a hernia (Fig 2–24). Some lipomas have attained gigantic size but the usual one is not larger than 10 to 12 cm. The histologic appearance is that of normal fat cells with a connective tissue framework and capsule. The incidence of liposarcoma is extremely rare. Nevertheless, the lesion should be excised, since difficulty in walking or in coitus will eventually occur.

FIBROMA.—A fibroma is a lesion that usually develops as a firm nodule on the labia majora, which then enlarges and develops a pedicle that may hang down for several inches (or feet), so that ulceration and necrosis of the distal portion may occur (Fig 2–25). The histologic picture is that of any dermatofibroma, with a well-circumscribed lesion made up of intertwined collagen bundles and fibroblasts. In rare cases the number of nuclei is excessive so that a suspicion of fibrosarcoma is raised. The circumscription of the lesion and absence of mitotic figures and giant cells is usually sufficient to indicate benignancy. These lesions should be surgically removed both for cosmetic effect and for their malignant potential, even though the latter is small.

fectious, and have been dealt with earlier in this chapter (Fig 2–22).

PAPILLOMA.—The dermal papilloma may occur on the vulva as a benign skin tumor of verrucous type, having a brown color. It may be single or multiple, and histologically it shows striking hyperkeratosis with acanthosis and elongation of the rete ridges (Fig 2–23).

HIDRADENOMA.—A hidradenoma is a benign, slow-growing, sweat gland tumor, whose histology simulates that of an adenocarcinoma. It is usually about 1 to 2 cm in diameter with a slightly raised, brown surface, which may be umbilicated. As seen in Figure 2–26, the lesion may become quite large and

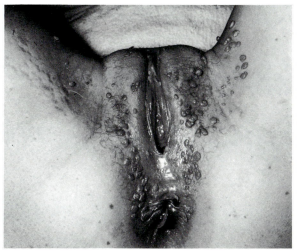

Fig 2–22.—Condylomata acuminata.

cystic change may occur. Histologically this is an adenoma of the vulvar apocrine glands. It is not connected with the epidermis and is usually well encapsulated. The basic pattern is that of a cystlike space in which numerous interlacing villous structures project (Fig 2–27). These structures, as well as the wall of the cyst, are lined by a single layer of high cylindrical cells with eosinophilic cytoplasm and a large, oval, pale-staining nucleus. The cells are regular and no anaplasia or atypism is evident. A characteristic finding is the layer of myoepithelial cells under the secretory cylindrical cells—a finding similar to that of apocrine tumors in the mammary gland. A rare variant is the clear cell hidradenoma. The lesion is almost always benign, but since a few hidradenocarcinomas have been reported, all should be excised and submitted to pathologic examination.

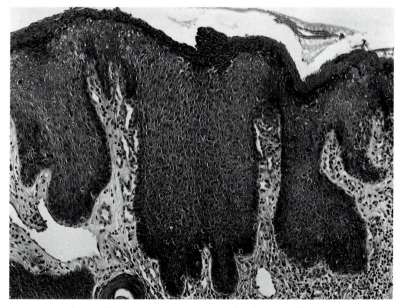

Fig 2–23.—Photomicrograph of vulvar papilloma.

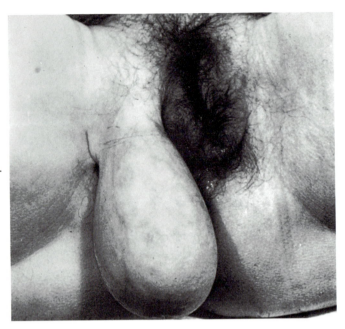

Fig 2–24.—Lipoma of vulva.

MALIGNANT NEOPLASMS

The broad terminology *malignant neoplasms* includes a variety of lesions of separate structure, the most common and most important of which are the squamous cell carcinomas of the labia majora, labia minora, and vestibule. Other lesions, fortunately rare, are carcinoma of the clitoris, adenocarcinoma of Bartholin's gland, adenocarcinoma of sweat glands, sarcomas, melanosarcomas, teratomas, and Paget's disease. The entire group is said to account for about 1% of all cancers in the female and for 5% to 10% of all cancers involving the female genitalia.

Carcinoma

Vulvar cancer usually occurs in postmenopausal women, about 70% of our patients being between 51 and 70 years, with an average age of 61.6 years. Youth does not afford complete protection, however, since Way has reported 18 patients between 21 and 40 years. Although postmenopausal bleeding will frequently bring the patient to the physician for examination, abnormalities of the vulva go unnoticed or, if discovered, are self-treated for long periods. A dangerous modesty seems to prevail that accounts for serious patient delay. Added to this is the unexplained hesitancy of many physicians to biopsy vulvar lesions when they are first seen and when

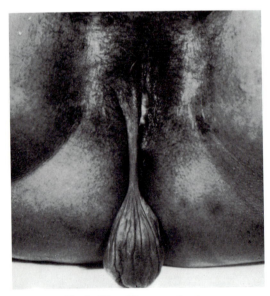

Fig 2–25.—Fibroma of vulva.

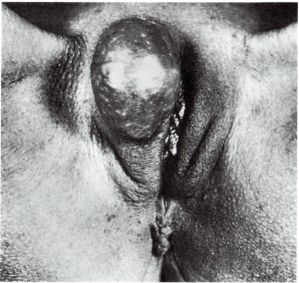

Fig 2–26.—Vulvar hidradenoma.

opportunity for cure is best. Many months are lost, during which time ointments, salves, lotions, and other medications are unsuccessfully tried.

It has become apparent that vulvar carcinoma is not only a disease of the aged but that, as age advances, the incidence of the disease rapidly increases. As the proportion of "old-age" individuals increases in our population, an ever-growing number of vulvar carcinomas will be seen. Thus, the importance of diminishing patient delay is obvious if increased survival is to be realized.

The symptoms complained of most commonly are a localized mass or lump, painful ulcer, discharge, vulvar irritation, dysuria, or bleeding. The duration of symptoms in some series has been as long as three or four years, but in the cases analyzed at the Brigham and Women's Hospital it was 13.8 months. Physical examination reveals the lesion to be extremely variable in appearance since in its early form it may merely be an elevated papule or small ulcer. The lesion may be a typical everting, ulcerating mass or it may be hypertrophic and resemble a papilloma. Another variety is the nonulcerating, superficial type, which produces severe edema and a peau

d'orange effect. About two thirds of the lesions are found on the labia majora and the remainder on the labia minora, clitoris, and posterior commissure. The majority of carcinomas are confined to the anterior half of the vulva, including the clitoris, and in most cases the external skin surfaces are far more commonly involved than are the medial surfaces of the labia.

Diagnosis is usually obvious except in very early and nonulcerated lesions. Condylomata acuminata, papillomas, ulcerated chancroid, gummata, and tuberculous ulcers may be confusing, but biopsy, gram-stain, and serologic tests will aid in the final diagnosis. The histology is usually that of a moderately well-differentiated, grade 1 or grade 2 squamous cell carcinoma. Way, however, found a rather large number of his cases to be of the anaplastic type and stated that these lesions are rapidly growing and rapidly metastasizing. In early lesions the microscopic pattern is that of irregular masses of epidermal cells invading the corium (Fig 2–28). These masses are composed of differentiated squamous and horn cells and dedifferentiated (atypical or dysplastic) squamous cells. Such dysplasia is expressed by variation in size and shape of the

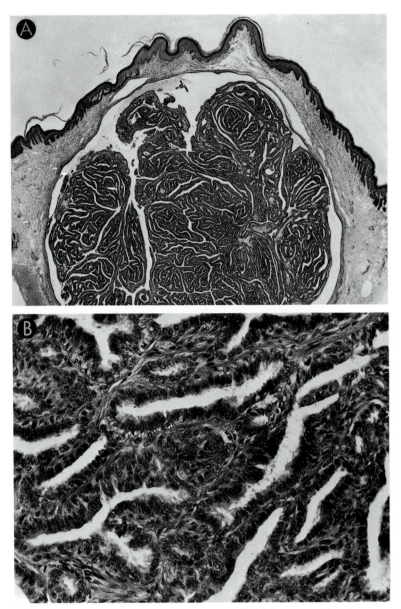

Fig 2–27.—Hidradenoma. **A,** low power; **B,** high power, showing myo-epithelial cells under the secretory cylindrical cells.

cells, hyperplasia and hyperchromasia of nuclei, loss of polarity, absence of prickles, keratinization of certain cells, presence of mitotic figures, and, particularly, atypical and bizarre mitoses. Differentiation is evident as an increased tendency toward keratinization with the formation of "pearls." These are composed of concentric layers of squamous cells with increased cornification toward the center. Extensive "pearl" formation is seen in Figure 2–29. In the Brigham and Women's Hospital series, 21% were classified as grade 1 tumors, 68% as grade 2, and 11% as grade 3.

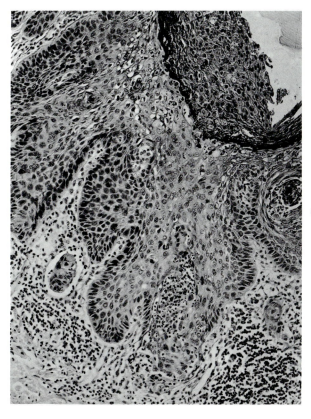

Fig 2–28.—Histologic appearance of early carcinoma of the vulva; low power.

Clinical staging of carcinoma of the vulva is important, since it refers to the degree of extension of the disease as determined by physical or x-ray examination. It is obvious that survival should be directly correlated with this staging, and this is true not only of carcinoma of the vulva but also of the cervix, breast, and endometrium.

Classification and Staging of Vulvar Carcinoma

The criteria for staging of epidermoid vulvar carcinoma were formulated by the International Federation of Gynecology and Obstetrics (FIGO) in 1967 and were subsequently approved in 1971. The rules for classification are similar to those at the other gynecologic sites. Tumors present in the vulva as secondary growths from either a genital or extragenital site should be excluded. Malignant melanoma should be separately reported. The femoral, inguinal, external iliac and hypogastric nodes are the sites of regional spread.

Clinical Stages of Carcinoma of the Vulva

FIGO Nomenclature—1971

Stage 0

Carcinoma in situ

Stage I

Tumor confined to vulva—2 cm or less in diameter. Nodes are not palpable or are palpable in either groin, not enlarged, mobile (not clinically suspicious of neoplasm).

Stage II

Tumor confined to the vulva—more than 2 cm in diameter. Nodes are not palpable or are palpable in either groin, not enlarged, mobile (not clinically suspicious of neoplasm).

Stage III

Tumor of any size with (1) adjacent spread to the

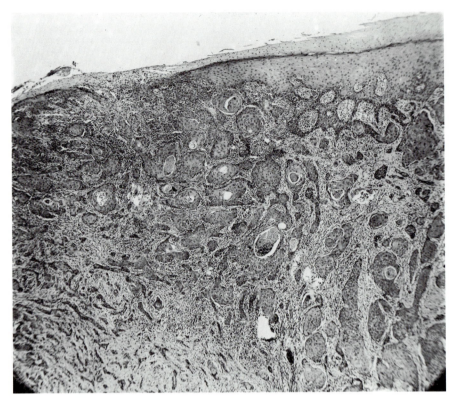

Fig 2–29.—High-power photomicrograph of carcinoma of the vulva. (Courtesy of Armed Forces Institute of Pathology; no. 70121.)

urethra and any or all of the vagina, the perineum, and the anus, and/or (2) nodes palpable in either or both groins (enlarged, firm, and mobile, not fixed but clinically suspicious of neoplasm).

Stage IV
Tumor of any size (1) infiltrating the bladder mucosa or the rectal mucosa or both, including the upper part of the urethral mucosa, and/or (2) fixed to the bone or other distant metastases. Fixed or ulcerated nodes in either or both groins.

Tumor-Node-Metastasis Nomenclature

Primary Tumor (T)
   TIS, T1, T2, T3, T4 See corresponding FIGO stages.

Nodal Involvement (N)
   NX Not possible to assess the regional nodes.

   N0 No involvement of regional nodes.

   N1 Evidence of regional node involvement.

   N3 Fixed or ulcerated nodes.

   N4 Juxtaregional node involvement.

Distant Metastasis (M)
   MX Not assessed.

   M0 No (known) distant metastasis.

   M1 Distant metastasis present.

Franklin evaluated this staging by retrospective application in a review of 164 patients treated at the M. D. Anderson Hospital from 1944 to 1968. His review of factors relating to tumor size, anatomic extent, and clinical evaluation of the possibility of metastatic inguinal lymphadenopathy proved them to be valid criteria for staging. Only minor exceptions to the adequacy of protocol for staging were noted. One was inability to confirm any adverse prognosis associated with perineal involvement by a lesion when it does not encroach on the anus or rectum. Another deficiency was the possibility that stage I and stage II did not adequately differentiate patient populations of favorable prognosis. Conclusions regarding the validity of these criteria must await further clinical trials.

Evaluation of accuracy of clinical staging has been addressed by other authors in recent years. Approximately 25% of the time, surgical staging does not agree with clinical staging. Reasons for this include the presence of palpable nodes with no disease, the presence of disease in nonpalpable nodes, and edema surrounding primary lesions, making assessment of lesion size inaccurate. In a recent review from the Mayo Clinic, Podratz et al. have concluded that clinical staging is of no value. In the same report, a decrease from a 90% five-year survival rate when lymph nodes are negative to about 45% when they are positive is noted. Furthermore, survival fell to 57% for single nodal involvement and to 37% when two or more nodes were involved. Survival for bilateral positive inguinal nodes was 29% at five years.

The natural history of vulvar cancer is, in general, that of a slowly growing lesion with spread to groin and pelvic nodes and localization in these areas for long periods. Remote metastases are not common until late in the disease when blood-borne spread may occur. If untreated, there is a subsequent fungating, ulcerative process that destroys the vulva, urethra, and anus, resulting in painful fistulas. Death may occur from ulceration of large blood vessels, from sepsis, or from widespread metastases.

Routes of Spread

Dissemination of vulvar carcinoma is usually by way of lymphatic metastases, probably by tumor emboli rather than by direct permeation. The commonest route of spread is via the superficial inguinal nodes to the node of Cloquet (the most superior deep femoral node that lies in the upper portion of the femoral canal under the inguinal ligament) and thence to the external iliac nodes. Lesions of the clitoris drain directly to Cloquet's node, and lesions that involve the posterior vulva and lower vagina may also bypass the superficial and deep inguinal nodes and drain directly to the external iliac nodes. It is important to realize that contralateral and bilateral spread may occur with a unilateral lesion.

Treatment

Since Taussig pioneered the radical surgical approach to the treatment of carcinoma of the vulva, there has been little doubt of its efficacy over the last 40 years. Gynecologic surgeons have come to realize that the standard treatment for the disease consists of radical vulvectomy with combined superficial inguinal and femoral lymph node dissection. The external iliac lymph node dissection (pelvic nodes) has become reserved for those patients in whom Cloquet's node was demonstrated to be positive for tumor. Omission of the deep pelvic node dissection has become acceptable for patients who are poor surgical risks and for those with minimal disease.

Curry has analyzed the chance of pelvic lymph nodes containing tumor according to the number and area of groin nodes involved. With fewer than four unilateral positive nodes, positive pelvic nodes were found in 8%. When four or more nodes were positive 50% of pelvic nodes were positive, and when bilateral inguinal or femoral nodes were positive 26% of pelvic nodes were positive. With clitoral involvement, 24 of 58 patients (41%) had positive nodes. However, there were no positive pelvic nodes without positive groin nodes.

Hacker believes that the low incidence of positive pelvic nodes in patients with fewer than three positive unilateral groin nodes does not justify pelvic lymphadenectomy. Whether or not contralateral groin dissection should be performed for lateral vulvar lesions remains controversial. Morris suggests that unilateral vulvar lesions may be best treated with groin dissection only on the same side as the lesion. The high incidence of inguinal and pelvic recurrences in patients with three or more positive nodes strongly suggests the need for adjuvant radiation therapy, and perhaps systemic adjuvant chemotherapy, since there is a high incidence of distant metastasis in such a group.

Macrometastases and Micrometastases

Iversen, reporting on a series of 258 patients, noted metastasis to superficial and/or deep inguinal lymph nodes in 38%. Only 64% of these were clinically suspicious. In 15% of the enlarged lymph nodes, no microscopic tumor was found. Five-year survival for patients with lymph node metastasis was 41%. Survival in the face of positive nodes depended on whether the metastatic disease was macrometastatic or micrometastatic. Those with micrometastasis had slightly fewer recurrences, 50% vs. 65%, and had a longer survival time and greater overall survival rates than those with macrometastasis, as might be expected. Donaldson et al. reported on a study of 66 patients noting that patients with regional lymph node metastasis had a 46% survival for three or more years as opposed to 76% survival for patients without nodal involvement. This study, however, highlights the fact that even the best prognostic groups that lacked lymph-space invasion or other unfavorable parameters had a 30% incidence of positive nodes.

Nodes and Stage

Frequency of positive nodes correlates directly with stage of disease. For stage I disease, recent reports vary from 10% to 15% having positive nodes; for stage II disease, 30% to 40%; for stage III disease, up to 80%; and for stage IV disease, 100%.

Tumor Grade

Histologic grade of tumor now appears to be an independent variable regarding survival. Mayo Clinic experience in this regard is 84% and 83% survival for grades 1 and 2, and 52% for grades 3 or 4.

Lesion Size

Krupp has noted that the critical size of the primary lesion is better placed at 3 cm as opposed to 2 cm, therefore confusing classical stage I and stage II definitions. The Mayo Clinic experience reports 90% five-year survival for lesions less than 1 cm, 89% for lesions 1 to 2 cm, 83% for lesions 2 to 3 cm, 63% for lesions 3 to 4 cm, and 44% for lesions greater than 4 cm.

Treatment of Late-Stage Disease

In the Mayo Clinic series, stage III disease did not appear to benefit when radical vulvectomy and inguinal-femoral lymphadenectomy was supplemented with deep pelvic node dissection. No case of pelvic node metastasis was noted without the presence of positive inguinal or femoral lymph nodes.

Patients with advanced disease continue to have poor survival in the face of radical surgery and lymphadenectomy. This suggests that the present approach to this disease is not adequate and therefore the application of adjuvant whole-pelvic radiation therapy, with or without central radiation, may be indicated. More clinicians are initially treating the primary lesion with vulvectomy and superficial and deep femoral and inguinal lymph node dissection, but are bringing the patient back at a later date for pelvic exploration and periaortic node biopsy; this will, hopefully, help the clinician to obtain more definitive information about the extent of the disease and to be able to make a combined attack on disease that has spread beyond the confines of the vulva and regional nodes. When the disease involves urethra, anus, or vagina, there is increasing likelihood of embolization being present in paravaginal and pararectal lymphatics. This may warrant more aggressive therapy, with selected cases being subjected to exenteration, both total exenteration and posterior exenteration with or without added radiation therapy.

Complications

Operative mortality is approximately 2% and is usually related to a cardiovascular complication, including pulmonary emboli. Necrosis of skin flaps, collection of lymph fluid, cellulitis, hematoma formation, urinary tract infection, phlebitis, leg edema, lymphangitis, urinary incontinence, fistula formation, and dyspareunia are occasionally encountered.

Recurrence

When local recurrences occur late following primary therapy, they respond well to local treatment. This suggests that skin of the neovulva subsequently undergoes malignant change, a theory embraced by Taussig.

VERRUCOUS CARCINOMA.—Verrucous carcinoma (Fig 2–30) is to be distinguished from condylomatous carcinoma, which has a more aggressive course. Grossly, it is often mistaken for condylomata acuminata and treated as such over a period of time. Subsequent biopsy may be misleading unless it is generous and deep. Invasive squamous cell carcinoma and intraepithelial neoplasia may coexist. Microscopically, the features that distinguish it from condyloma include swollen and velamentous rete pegs, absent fibrovascular stocks, and the presence of squamous "pearls" deep in the epithelium. Infiltrating margins are absent and individual malignant features of the cells throughout the tumor are also lacking, with good cytologic differentiation and uniformity of pattern. On the other hand, condylomatous carcinoma exhibits the hallmarks of invasive squamous carcinoma with infiltrating margins of cellular anaplasia and the presence of keratin "pearls." Treatment of this lesion is by wide local excision or vulvectomy. Radiation has been tried and found wanting. Inguinal lymph nodes are frequently enlarged, but in 27 cases reported in the literature lymph node metastasis has never been demonstrated. Local recurrences are common and should be treated surgically. The etiology of this variant is unknown.

Microinvasive Carcinoma of the Vulva— An Emerging Concept

In 1974, Wharton, Gallagher, and Rutledge reported on a group of 45 patients with invasive carcinoma of the vulva 2 cm or less in diameter. In this group, a subset of 25 patients was noted in which stromal invasion reached a depth of 5 mm or less. None of these patients had developed positive lymph nodes and, subsequently, no lesion recurred and no patient died from vulvar cancer. The authors concluded that their data suggested

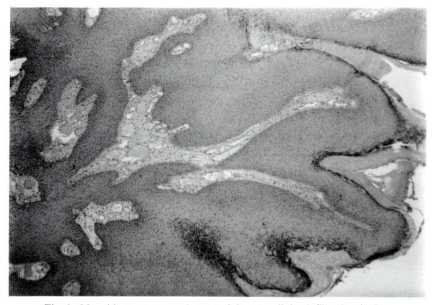

Fig 2–30.—Verrucous carcinoma. A hypercellular infiltrating lesion. Note the uniformly bland-appearing epithelium.

that patients with early invasion might be better treated with less than full radical surgical therapy.

In 1975, Parker et al. reviewed 60 patients with squamous cell cancers of the vulva of less than 2 cm in size. They noted that 58 of these patients had stromal invasion 5 mm or less in depth. Three of the 60 patients had pelvic lymph node metastasis. Two of the three had invasion of vascular channels, and the third patient exhibited cellular anaplasia. Subsequent interest in this subject has been intense, with at least 18 articles being published with data suggesting that criteria for lesser surgery were still inexact and that some patients with even 1 mm of invasion were known to have died of their disease.

Hoffman et al., in 1983, pointed out that there is still no widely accepted set of criteria to define the term *microinvasive* when pertaining to carcinoma of the vulva. In their experience with 90 patients with stage I squamous cell carcinoma of the vulva, they note that anaplasia and lymphovascular invasion are associated with nodal metastasis and that confluence with 3 mm or more of invasion may also be associated with spread to lymph nodes. These authors now recommend wide local excision and hemivulvectomy or total vulvectomy when the depth of invasion is 3 mm or less and nonconfluent. They believe that confluent tumor with less than 2 mm of invasion may also be treated more conservatively.

DiSaia has treated and prospectively followed up a group of 20 women meeting very rigid criteria including (1) a primary lesion less than 1 cm in diameter that is confined to the vulva or perineum, and (2) a lesion with invasion limited to 5 mm in depth measuring from the base of the overlying epithelium. Care was taken to evaluate other histologic criteria including confluency, invasion deeper than 1 mm, vascular-channel invasion, and high degrees of anaplasia. This surgical protocol consisted of careful study of the primary neoplasm after excisional biopsy. Definitive treatment was based on excision of superficial inguinal lymph nodes bilaterally with frozen section at the time. In the absence of metastasis, a wide local excision was carried out at the site of the primary lesion with either primary closure or skin grafting. If nodal disease was present at the time of inguinal dissection, formal superficial and deep inguinal and femoral node dissection was carried out along with standard radical vulvectomy. Subsequent follow-up has failed to reveal any recurrence.

To date, the literature is not in total agreement. Definitions and terminology employed vary widely. Therefore, great care must be taken in deciding which candidates are best for such a conservative treatment program. DiSaia now suggests that microinvasive carcinoma should be defined as a well-differentiated keratinizing squamous cell carcinoma, the diameter of the lesion being less than 1 cm, and stromal invasion not exceeding 3 mm in depth. There should be no evidence of confluence or lymphatic or vascular invasion. Although evidence is mounting that this is a reasonable approach, since it provides adequate therapy without mutilating anatomy, especially during the reproductive years, it is in no way universally accepted.

To summarize the literature, in 267 cases of microinvasive vulvar carcinoma, lymph nodes were positive in 8.2% of the cases. There were 28 recurrences and nine deaths (3.3%).

Other Vulvar Malignancies

CARCINOMA OF BARTHOLIN'S GLAND.—Carcinoma of Bartholin's gland is a rare finding, and its treatment is that suggested for other carcinomas. It may be mistaken for a benign tumor or a chronic bartholinitis because of its location. A high degree of malignancy exists because of the rich drainage of the gland lymphatics into the deep as well as the superficial lymphatics.

BASAL CELL CARCINOMA.—Basal cell carcinoma of the vulva is also rather rare, about 75 cases having been reported. It tends to recur locally rather than to spread by lymphatic and blood channels but, unlike basal cell carcinomas elsewhere on the skin, the prognosis is poor. Breen et al. recently reviewed the literature on basal cell carcinoma of the vulva and found a ratio of one basal cell for every 37 squamous cell carcinomas of the vulva. They added a series of 17 patients to the 96 already reported in the literature. The lesions were described grossly as ulcerations or masses located on the anterior labium majus. Etiologies were indeterminate, although two patients had previously received vulvar irradiation. Therapy consisted primarily of wide local excision and was effective in that follow-up studies in 16 patients revealed no deaths attributable to basal cell carcinoma. The data of these authors indicate that basal cell carcinoma is a locally invasive, nonmetastasizing tumor (Fig 2–31) best treated by wide local excision, provided the tumor edge does not extend to the margin of excision.

There is some evidence that these tumors do not arise from the basal cells of the epidermis but from hair sheaths or distorted primordia of dermal adnexae. Lever believes them to be nevoid tumors derived from arrested, embryonal, primary epithelial germ cells. No relationship between leukoplakia and basal cell carcinoma has been demonstrated. Treatment should include a wide and deep local excision.

SARCOMA.—This tumor may arise from the connective tissue of the vulva or from a fibroma. Several cases of reticulum cell sarcoma and lymphosarcoma have recently been added to the literature. The prognosis is poor, despite radical surgery.

MELANOMA.—Melanomas are, by definition, malignant; they account for between 5% and 10% of all vulvar malignancies. They are most often seen in women over the age of 50 years. The lesions may be brown or black in appearance. Larger lesions may have associated areas within them that are both red and white. Grossly, this disease cannot be distinguished from many benign lesions; therefore, a diagnosis must be made by biopsy of all pigmented lesions. Ideally, biopsy should be excisional, with an accompanying 1-cm margin of normal-appearing skin. When deeply invasive, melanomas metastasize by the lymphatic route and by hematogenous routes as well, the latter being attested to by recurrence at distal sites many years after primary surgery for the vulvar lesion. Depth of tumor invasion is the single best prognostic factor and in general should dictate the kind of surgical therapy to be undertaken. Tumor thickness is measured from the granular layer of the epidermis overlying the tumor to the deepest point of invasion. Tumors invading less than 0.7 cm have the best chance of cure by simple excision only. Tumors invading beyond 3 cm in general have a poor prognosis.

Until now, recommended treatment has always been radical vulvectomy, and deep and superficial inguinal and femoral lymphadenectomy combined with deep pelvic node dissection especially if the tumor involved the anterior vulva or clitoris. Such treatment is now

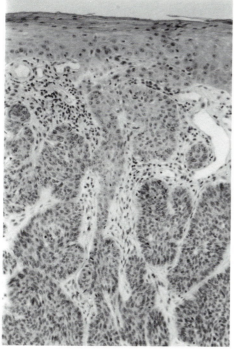

Fig 2–31.—Basal cell carcinoma: locally invasive, nonmetastasizing.

considered controversial. Retrospective studies of patients who underwent lymphadenectomy for melanoma at any site failed to show any value to the procedure. One study has demonstrated possible benefit from lymph node dissection when the lesion invades between 1.5 and 3.0 mm. Critics of these studies say they cannot be considered conclusive due to the retrospective nature of the study. No prospective randomized stratified studies exist. Still, others feel that the radical approach will provide local control of disease with better comfort. It is known that a vast majority of patients with tumor demonstrated in deep nodes will die of the disease. It is also known that most patients with minimal invasive disease will survive given only local therapy. Hence, critics of the radical surgical approach feel that such treatment is unnecessary in one group and constitutes overtreatment in the other group.

The classification of invasion according to level was first described by Mihm and Clarke in 1971 and modified by Chung et al. for adaptation to melanoma of the vulva in 1975. Depth of penetration may be correlated with the staging level system in that lesions up to 1.25 mm generally involve epidermis and papillary dermis and have the most favorable prognosis. Lesions extending from 1.25 to 2.25 mm involve the reticular dermis, and lesions extending below that usually involve fat and are designated as level 5 lesions.

PAGET'S DISEASE.—Paget's disease of the vulva is an intraepithelial carcinoma. As a disorder of the mammary gland, it is a well-known entity, having been described by James Paget in 1874. It is accepted that mammary Paget's disease is a primary duct cancer which has extended to the epidermis where it causes a cutaneous lesion. Woodruff, however, feels that Paget's disease of the vulva is an intraepithelial lesion and that Paget's cells arise de novo in the epithelium or in its appendages. It is entirely possible that this lesion may progress to invasive carcinoma in much the same fashion as Bowen's disease if

one accepts the histogenesis as being autochthonous, as suggested by Woodruff. Huber, in describing three new cases of vulvar Paget's disease, found a definite adenocarcinoma of the underlying apocrine sweat glands in one. Hart reported the first case of intraepithelial disease progressing to invasive carcinoma and lymph node metastasis.

In the vulva, the lesion occurs in women in the later decades of life whose presenting complaint is usually pruritus. Grossly, it is sharply demarcated, florid, red, and moist, with occasional crusting. It may appear eczematoid. Little islands of whitened skin appear between the reddened areas (Fig 2–32). The entire vulva may be involved, with spread to the perineum, mons, and thighs. The histologic appearance is characteristic (Fig 2–33). There is acanthosis with elongation and widening of the rete ridges. Paget's cells may be

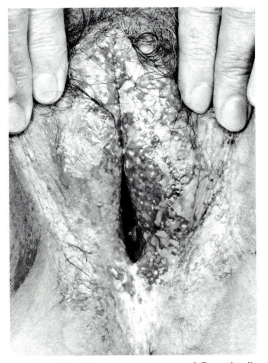

Fig 2–32.—Gross appearance of Paget's disease of the vulva. The dark areas are velvety red, and the white areas are as seen. (From Woodruff J.D., Williams T.F.: *Obstet. Gynecol.* 14:86, 1959.)

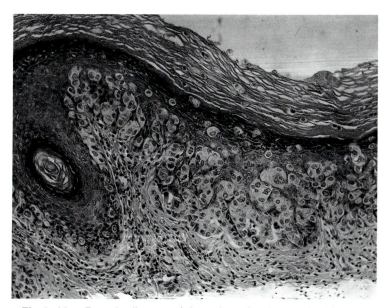

Fig 2–33.—Paget's disease of the vulva, showing marked hyperkeratosis and parakeratosis. Large, irregular cells are seen in the basal layer of the epidermis and infiltrating the upper layers as well. The Paget cells contain clear vacuolated cytoplasm and vesicular nuclei, which vary in size, shape, and staining quality.

scattered or grouped in clusters, usually in the basalis. They are large cells, lacking prickles, and are surrounded by clear spaces. The cytoplasm is very light and the nuclei are large, round, and pale. Pseudogland formation is common. Treatment should be that of wide and deep excision with careful follow-up, despite the long interval that usually elapses before definitive treatment is employed. For invasive disease, radical vulvectomy and bilateral lymph node dissection is mandatory.

Because local recurrences are common, repeated observations and biopsy of suspicious areas are suggested.

Vulvar Paget's disease is an intraepithelial adenocarcinoma that is locally recurrent and has an occasional propensity to invade and metastasize to lymph nodes.

Adenocarcinoma of the vulvar apocrine glands is the most commonly associated tumor. Another apocrine adenocarcinoma, carcinoma of the breast, either antecedent or concomitant, is the second most frequently associated tumor having been reported in 14 cases of vulvar Paget's disease. Therefore, preoperative breast screening procedures are indicated in all patients with vulvar Paget's disease.

Metastatic Vulvar Tumors

Metastatic and secondary tumors of the vulva constitute the third largest group of malignant tumors of the vulva. Epidermoid carcinoma of the cervix is the most frequent primary site, followed by the endometrium, kidney, and urethra. Most patients who subsequently develop vulvar metastases have signs of advanced primary tumor when initially diagnosed. Metastatic adenocarcinoma tends to invade the overlying squamous epithelium, whereas epidermoid carcinoma does not. The frequent occurrence of vascular involvement by metastatic tumor incriminates this as the mode of spread to the vulva. The prognosis is poor and death usually occurs within one year of the diagnosis. At the Brigham and Women's Hospital we have seen two patients with vulvar metastases from adenocarcinoma of the large bowel.

BIBLIOGRAPHY

Anatomy

Anson B.I.: *An Atlas of Human Anatomy.* Philadelphia, W.B. Saunders Co., 1950.

Lever W.F.: *Histopathology of Skin*, ed. 2. Philadelphia, J.B. Lippincott Co., 1954.

Nichols D.H., Milley P.S.: Clinical anatomy of the vulva, vagina, lower pelvis and perineum, in Sciarra J.J. (ed.): *Gynecology and Obstetrics.* Hagerstown, Md, Harper & Row, 1980.

Embryology

Koff A.K.: Embryology of the female generative tract, in Curtis A.H. (ed.): *Obstetrics and Gynecology.* Philadelphia, W.B. Saunders Co., 1933.

Patten B.M.: *Human Embryology*, ed. 2. New York, McGraw-Hill Book Co., 1953.

Robboy S.J., Welch W.R., Gang D.L., et al.: *Pathologic Basis of Intersex*, in press.

Welch W.R., Robboy S.J.: Abnormal sexual development: A classification with emphasis on pathology and neoplastic conditions, in Kogan S.J., Hafez E.S.E. (eds.): *Pediatric Andrology.* The Hague/Boston/London, Martinus Nijhoff Publishers, 1981.

Young H.H.: *Genital Abnormalities: Hermaphroditism and Related Adrenal Disease.* Baltimore, Williams & Wilkins Co., 1937.

Benign Diseases of the Vulva

Conway H., Stark R.B., Climo S., et al.: The surgical treatment of chronic hydradenitis suppurativa. *Surg. Gynecol. Obstet.* 95:455, 1952.

Friedrich E.G. Jr.: *Vulvar Disease*, ed. 2, vol. 9. Major Problems in Obstetrics and Gynecology Series. Philadelphia, W.B. Saunders, 1983.

Goodlin R.C., Frederick I.B.: Postpartum vulva edema associated with the birthing chair. *Am. J. Obstet. Gynecol.* 146:334, 1983.

Gordon S.W.: Hidradenitis suppurativa: A closer look. *J. Natl. Med. Assoc.* 70:239–343, 1978.

Kurman R.J., Sha K.H., Lancaster W.D., et al.: Immunoperoxidase localization of papilloma virus antigens in cervical dysplasia and vulvar condylomas. *Am. J. Obstet. Gynecol.* 140:931–935, 1981.

Leads from the *Morbidity and Mortality Weekly Report* (vol. 32/23, 24, 1983). *J.A.M.A.* 250:336, 1983.

Levine E.M., Barton J.J., Grier E.A.: Metastatic Crohn disease of the vulva. *Obstet. Gynecol.* 60:395–397, 1982.

Meltzer R.M.: Necrotizing fasciitis and progressive bacterial synergistic gangrene of the vulva. *Obstet. Gynecol.* 51:757–760, 1983.

Scott J.C. Jr., Smith M.L.: Benign neoplasms of the vulva, in Sciarra J.J. (ed.): *Gynecology and Obstetrics.* Hagerstown, Md, Harper & Row, 1980.

Tovell H.M.M., Young A.W. Jr.: Evaluation and management of diseases of the vulva. *Clin. Obstet. Gynecol.* 21:4, 1978.

Van Slyke K.K., Michel V.P., Rein M.F.: Treatment of vulvovaginal candidiasis with boric acid powder. *Am. J. Obstet. Gynecol.* 141:145–148, 1981.

Woodruff J.D.: Diagnosis and management of benign lesions of the vulva. *Curr. Probl. Obstet. Gynecol.*, vol. 1, no. 2, 1978.

Vulvar Intraepithelial Neoplasia

Benedet J.L., Murphy J.J.: Squamous carcinoma in site of the vulva. *Gynecol. Oncol.* 14:213–219, 1982.

Bernstein S.G., Kovacs B.R., Townsend D.E., et al.: Vulvar carcinoma in situ. *Obstet. Gynecol.* 60:304–307, 1983.

Caglar H., Tamer S., Hreshchyshyn M.M.: Vulvar intraepithelial neoplasia. *Obstet. Gynecol.* 60:346–349, 1982.

DiSaia P.J., Rich W.M.: Surgical approach to multifocal carcinoma in situ of the vulva. *Am. J. Obstet. Gynecol.* 140:136–145, 1981.

Foster D.C., Woodruff J.D.: The use of dinitrochlorobenzene in the treatment of vulvar carcinoma in situ. *Obstet. Gynecol. Surv.* 37:55–56, 1982.

Iversen T., Abler B., Kolstad T.: Squamous cell carcinoma in situ of the vulva: A clinical and histopathological study. *Gynecol. Oncol.* 11:224–229, 1981.

Kaplan A.L., Kaufman R.H., Birken R.A., et al.: Intraepithelial carcinoma of the vulva with extension to the anal canal. *Obstet. Gynecol.* 58:368–371, 1981.

Lifshitz S., Roberts J.A.: Treatment of carcinoma in situ of the vulva with topical 5-fluorouracil. *Obstet. Gynecol.* 56:242–244, 1980.

Sillman F.H., Boyce J.G., Macasaet M.A., et al.: 5-fluorouracil/chemosurgery for intraepithelial neoplasia of the lower genital tract. *Obstet. Gynecol.* 58:356–360, 1981.

Wilkinson E.J., Friedrich E.G. Jr., Fu Y.S.: Multicentric nature of vulvar carcinoma in situ. *Obstet. Gynecol.* 58:69–74, 1981.

Microinvasive Carcinoma of the Vulva

Barnes A.E., Crissman J.D., Schellhas H.F., et al.: Microinvasive carcinoma of the vulva: A clinical pathologic evaluation. *Obstet. Gynecol.* 52:234–238, 1980.

Buscema J., Stern J.L., Woodruff J.D.: Early invasive carcinoma of the vulva. *Am. J. Obstet. Gynecol.* 140:563–569, 1981.

Chu J., Tamimi H.D., Ek M., et al.: Stage I vulvar cancer: Criteria for microinvasion. *Obstet. Gynecol.* 59:716–719, 1982.

DiPaola G.R., Gomez-Rueda N., Arrighi L.: Relevance of microinvasion in carcinoma of the vulva. *Obstet. Gynecol.* 45:647–648, 1975.

DiSaia P.J., Creasman W.T., Rich W.M.: An alternate approach to early cancer of the vulva. *Am. J. Obstet. Gynecol.* 133:825–832, 1979.

DiSaia P.J.: A less radical approach to early vulvar cancer. *Contemp. Obstet. Gynecol.* 18:109–114, 1981.

Hacker M.S., Nieberg R.K., Berek J.S., et al.: Superficially invasive vulvar cancer with nodal metastasis. *Gynecol. Oncol.* 15:65–77, 1983.

Hoffman J.S., Kumar M.B., Molrey G.W.: Microinvasive squamous carcinoma of the vulva: Search for a definition. *Obstet. Gynecol.* 61:615–618, 1983.

Jafari K., Cartnick E.N.: Microinvasive squamous cell carcinoma of the vulva. *Am. J. Obstet. Gynecol.* 125:274, 1976.

Jafari K., Cartnick E.N.: Microinvasive squamous cell carcinoma of the vulva. *Gynecol. Oncol.* 4:158–166, 1976.

Kunschner A., Kanbour A.I., David B.: Early vulvar carcinoma. *Am. J. Obstet. Gynecol.* 132:599–606, 1978.

Magrina J.F., Webb J.J., Gaffey T.A., et al.: Stage I squamous cell cancer of the vulva. *Am. J. Obstet. Gynecol.* 134:453–459, 1979.

Nakao C.Y., Nolan J.F., DiSaia P.J., et al.: Microinvasive epidermoid carcinoma of the vulva with an unexpected natural history. *Am. J. Obstet. Gynecol.* 120:1122–1123, 1974.

Parker R.T., Duncan I., Rampone J., et al.: Operative management of early invasive epidermoid carcinoma of the vulva. *Am. J. Obstet. Gynecol.* 1:349–355, 1975.

Pickel T.H.: The early stages of vulvar carcinoma, diagnostic problems. *J. Reprod. Med.* 27:465–470, 1982.

Wharton J.T., Gallagher S., Rutledge F.N.: Microinvasive carcinoma of the vulva. *Am. J. Obstet. Gynecol.* 118:159–162, 1974.

Wilkinson E.J., Rice M.J., Pierson K.K.: Microinvasive carcinoma of the vulva. *Int. J. Gynecol. Pathol.* 1:29–39, 1982.

Yazigi R., Piver M.S., Tsukada Y.: Microinvasive carcinoma of the vulva. *Obstet. Gynecol.* 51:368–370, 1978.

Paget's Disease

Gunn R.A., Gallager H.S.: Vulvar Paget's disease: A topographic study. *Cancer* 46:590–594, 1980.

Hart W.R., Millman J.D.: Progression of intraepithelial Paget's disease of the vulva to invasive carcinoma. *Cancer* 40:2333–2337, 1977.

Jones R.E., Austin C., Ackerman A.B.: Extramammary Paget's disease: A critical re-examination. *Am. J. Derm. Pathol.* 1:101–132, 1979.

Lee R.A., Dahlin D.C.: Paget's disease of the vulva with extension into the urethra, vulva and ureters: A case report. *Am. J. Obstet. Gynecol.* 140:834–836, 1981.

Parmley T.H., Woodruff J.D., Julian C.G.: Invasive vulva Paget's disease. *Obstet. Gynecol.* 46:341–346, 1975.

Bowenoid Papulosis

Kao F.G., Graham J.H.: Bowenoid papulosis. *Int. J. Dermatol.* 21:445–446, 1982.

Wade T.R., Rorf A.W., Ackerman A.B.: Bowenoid papulosis of the genitalia. *Arch. Dermatol.* 115:306–308, 1979.

Melanoma

Day C.O. Jr., Mihm M.C. Jr., Sober A.J., et al.: Narrower margins for clinical stage I malignant melanoma. *N. Engl. J. Med.* 306:479, 1982.

Edington P.T., Monaghan J.M.: Malignant melanoma of the vulva and vagina. *Br. J. Obstet. Gynecol.* 87:422, 1980.

Nathanson L.: Update on melanoma. *Clin. Cancer Briefs* 4:3–13, 1983.

Silvers D.N.: What you need to know about tumors of melanocytes. *Contemp. Obstet. Gynecol.* 20:140–149, 1983.

Silvers D.N., Halperin A.J.: Cutaneous and vulvar melanoma: An update. *Clin. Obstet. Gynecol.* 21:1117–1133, 1978.

Sim S., Taylor W., Pritchard D., et al.: A prospective randomized study of the efficacy of routine elective lymphadenectomy in management of malignant melanoma, Abstracted. *Proc. Int. Cancer Cong.* 13:658, 1982.

Carcinoma of the Vulva

Breen J.L., Neubecker R.D., Greenwald E., et al.: Basal cell carcinoma of the vulva. *Obstet. Gynecol.* 46:122, 1975.

Buckingham J.C., McClure J.H.: Reticulum cell sarcoma of the vulva. *Obstet. Gynecol.* 6:121, 1955.

Chu J., Tamimi H.K., Figge D.C.: Femoral node metastasis with negative superficial inguinal nodes in early vulvar cancer. *Am. J. Obstet. Gynecol.* 140:337–338, 1981.

Curry S.L., Wharton J.T., Rutledge F.: Positive lymph nodes in vulvar squamous carcinoma. *Gynecol. Oncol.* 9:63–67, 1980.

Donaldson E.S., Powell D.E., Hanson M.B., et al.: Prognostic parameters in invasive vulvar cancers. *Gynecol. Oncol.* 12:184–190, 1981.

Hacker N.F., Leuchter R.S., Berek J.S., et al.: Radical vulvectomy and bilateral inguinal lymphadenectomy through separate groin incisions. *Obstet. Gynecol.* 58:574–578, 1981.

Hacker N.F., Berek J.S., Lagasse L.D., et al.: Management of regional lymph nodes and their prognostic influence in vulvar cancer. *Obstet. Gynecol.* 61:408–412, 1983.

Hertig A.T., Gore H.: *Tumors of the Female Sex Organs:* part 2. *Tumors of the Vulva, Vagina and Uterus.* Washington, D.C., Armed Forces Institute of Pathology, 1960.

Iversen T.: The value of groin palpation in epidermoid carcinoma of the vulva. *Gynecol. Oncol.* 12:291–295, 1981.

Morley G.W.: Infiltrative carcinoma of the vulva: Results of surgical treatment. *Am. J. Obstet. Gynecol.* 124:874–884, 1976.

Morris J.M.: A formula for selective lymphadenectomy: Its application to cancer of the vulva. *Obstet. Gynecol.* 50:152–158, 1977.

Plentl A.A., Friedman E.A.: *Lymphatic System of the Female Genitalia.* Philadelphia, W.B. Saunders Co., 1971.

Podratz K.C., Symmonds R.E., Taylor W.F., et al.: Carcinoma of the vulva: Analysis of treatment and survival. *Obstet. Gynecol.* 61:63–74, 1983.

Podratz K.C., Symmonds R.E., Taylor W.F.: Carcinoma of the vulva: Analysis of treatment failures. *Am. J. Obstet. Gynecol.* 143:340–351, 1982.

Rubin A.R.: Granular-cell myoblastoma of the vulva. *Am. J. Obstet. Gynecol.* 113:719, 1972.

Rutledge F.N.: Cancer of the vulva and vagina. *Clin. Obstet. Gynecol.* 8:1051, 1965.

Way S.: *Malignant Disease of the Vulva.* Edinburgh, Churchill-Livingston, 1982.

Zacur H., Genabry R., Woodruff J.D.: The patient at risk for development of vulvar cancer. *Gynecol. Oncol.* 9:199–208, 1980.

Verrucous Carcinoma of the Vulva

Japaze N., van Dinh T., Woodruff J.D.: Verrucous carcinoma of the vulva: A study of 24 cases. *Obstet. Gynecol.* 60:462–466, 1982.

Warty Carcinoma of the Vulva

Rastkar G., Okagaki T., Twiggs L.B., et al.: Early invasive and in situ warty carcinoma of the vulva: Clinical, histologic and electron microscopic study with particular reference to viral association. *Am. J. Obstet. Gynecol.* 143:814–820, 1982.

CHAPTER THREE

The Vagina

THE VAGINA (Latin, "sheath") is a tubular, fibromuscular structure, lined by stratified squamous epithelium, which extends from the vestibule to the uterus. Its function is to receive the penis during coitus and in so doing afford the seminal fluid protective entrance through the external os of the cervix. The reproductive function of the vagina is fulfilled during parturition, since it represents the lowermost part of the birth canal. A third function is that of an excretory duct for menstrual discharge. From the viewpoint of the clinician, a fourth function is the opportunity it provides for the examination of the internal genitalia.

EMBRYOLOGY

Embryologically the vagina may be looked on as having a double origin, i.e., from the urogenital sinus and from the müllerian ducts. As mentioned in Chapter 2, the terminal ends of the müllerian ducts impinge on the urogenital sinus at the termination of their caudad growth, thus forming the müllerian tubercle (Fig 3–1). Later, this tubercle disappears as two mesenchymal outgrowths appear on the dorsal surface of the posterior wall of the urogenital sinus. These are the sinovaginal bulbs from which the lower vagina develops. The epithelium of the caudal portion of the uterovaginal canal later proliferates and completely occludes the canal. Thus a solid cord of epithelium is formed, derived from the uterovaginal canal above and the sinovaginal bulbs below. When the embryo is about 150 mm in length, the central cells of this cord degenerate and a hollow tube is formed. Eventually penetration and invasion of this müllerian tube by urogenital sinus epithelium occurs and, when complete, the vagina is lined by stratified cuboidal epithelium derived from the urogenital sinus. The latter then differentiates into stratified squamous cells. A vaginal occlusion is thus the result of a failure of urogenital cells to invade the müllerian tube. Normally the replacement of müllerian with squamous epithelium ends at the external os of the cervix, but occasionally it ends distal to the os, leaving an area of columnar epithelium, the so-called congenital erosion or eversion. In other cases the squamous epithelium invades the endocervix for varying lengths and may remain there permanently. This process has been termed *epidermization*. By contrast, *squamous metaplasia* may occur in the endocervix and produce the same histologic effect, but here the columnar epithelium (müllerian) undergoes a change to a squamous type and is not actually replaced. To summarize the conclusions of Koff in relation to the development of the vagina, the following points are of importance:

1. The müllerian ducts appear in the 11-mm embryo as invaginations of the coelomic epithelium lateral to the cranial extremity of the mesonephros and lateral to the wolffian duct.

2. The solid tips of the müllerian ducts tunnel caudally through the mesenchyme, cross the wolffian ducts anteriorly at the level of the lower end of the mesonephros, approach each

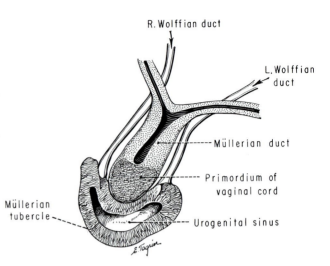

Fig 3–1.—Formation of the lower vagina. The müllerian tubercle is formed by impingement of the terminal ends of the müllerian ducts against the urogenital sinus. The vagina has a double origin, therefore, from the müllerian tubercle and from outgrowths of the urogenital sinus.

other in the midline, fuse, and reach the posterior wall of the urogenital sinus and push it forward to form the müllerian tubercle in the 30-mm embryo.

3. The fusion of the müllerian ducts is complete in the 56-mm embryo to form the uterovaginal canal.

4. In the 63-mm embryo the sinovaginal bulbs are formed by bilateral posterior evaginations of the urogenital sinus. Owing to the formation of these structures, the müllerian tubercle is obliterated. At the same period, there is a stratification of the cells lining this portion of the urogenital sinus, and the solid cells composing the tip of the uterovaginal canal show involutional changes due to compression by the paired sinovaginal bulbs.

5. The wolffian ducts show involutional changes throughout. When they do persist, their caudal ends migrate cranially with the growth of the sinovaginal bulbs.

6. The sinovaginal bulbs become solidified by proliferation of lining epithelium and fuse with the tip of the müllerian ducts, which later solidify by the same process and form the solid vaginal plate.

7. The solid primitive vaginal plate grows in all dimensions by the formation and fusion of trabeculae.

8. The central cells of the now solid vagina break down to form the cavity of the vagina.

9. The cranial end of the vagina is demarcated in the 151-mm embryo by the formation of the anterior and posterior fornices as solid epithelial projections (Fig 3–2). The caudal end expands, pushes in the posterior wall of the urogenital sinus, and extends along the posterior wall to form the caudal segment of the hymen; the anterior paired segment is formed where the evaginations of the urogenital sinus occur to form the sinovaginal bulbs.

ANATOMY AND HISTOLOGY

The anterior vaginal wall is in contact with the membranous urethra and bladder and is separated only by a thin layer of endopelvic fascia, the pubovesicovaginal fascia. The most cephalad portion of the anterior vaginal wall ends in a blind pouch, or fornix, and its epithelium is continuous with that of the anterior lip of the cervix, which projects forward into the upper vagina. The posterior vaginal wall is in contact with the structures of the perineal body and rectovaginal fascia but its upper extension, the posterior fornix, is more cephalad than its anterior counterpart and attaches to the cervix just below the uterorectal fold of peritoneum. The latter is known as the posterior cul-de-sac of Douglas and is of clinical importance since the peritoneal cavity may be easily entered through the posterior

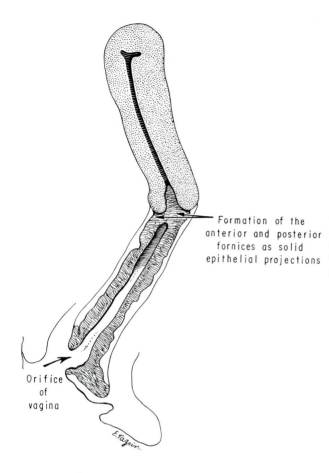

Fig 3–2.—Formation of the upper vagina in the 151-mm embryo. At this stage, the cranial end of the vagina contains two solid epithelial projections, which become the anterior and posterior fornices.

Formation of the anterior and posterior fornices as solid epithelial projections

Orifice of vagina

vagina without damage to adjacent organs or structures. The epithelium of the posterior fornix is also continuous with that of the posterior cervix. That portion of the cervix that juts forward into the vagina and is covered with stratified squamous epithelium is called the portio vaginalis (Fig 3–3).

The vagina is a potential cavity, but in the normal state the walls are in apposition. In multiparous women the potential space becomes an actual one due to the stretching and tearing of the vaginal supports. If the vagina is transected in its medial portion, it presents an H-shaped appearance, the lateral limits being moderately convex toward the midline. The vaginal length is variable but the posterior wall approximates 8 to 9 cm, and the anterior wall 6 to 8 cm. The bore follows the usual pattern of constriction at the outlet, dis-

tensibility in the midportion and narrowing at the fornices. This is exemplified at the time of delivery when the vaginal outlet must be incised to allow passage of the fetal head. The lateral aspects of the most cephalad portion of the vagina are known as the lateral fornices or vaults.

A longitudinal ridge is usually visible running along the anterior and posterior vaginal walls. These ridges are termed the vaginal columns and represent the line of fusion of the two müllerian ducts. Extending laterally from these columns are numerous elevations, the rugae, and between the rugae are intervening furrows. Seen in microscopic section these appear as simple elevations of the surface epithelium over the dermis. The rugae are formed by the ingrowth of numerous solid epithelial projections into the subjacent mes-

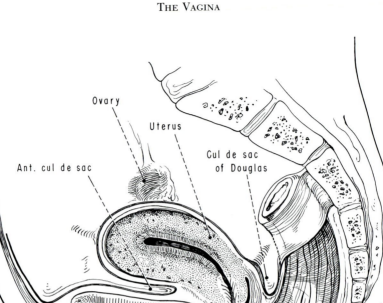

Fig 3–3.—Sagittal section of the human female pelvis showing the anatomic relations of the vagina.

enchyme when the vaginal lumen is not completely filled with epithelium. The rugated appearance of the vagina is prominent in young adolescents and adults but disappears with multiparity and senescence. Postmenopausally the vaginal mucosa is smooth and shiny.

The wall of the vagina is made up of three layers: (1) mucous membrane, (2) muscularis, and (3) adventitial connective tissue.

The mucous membrane consists of a lamina propria of dense connective tissue and a surface epithelium (Fig 3–4). The surface epithelium is made up of six to ten layers of strati-

fied squamous cells, which do not show cornification although keratohyalin granules may be present. The cells, even when desquamated, contain glycogen if adequate estrogen stimulation is present. In vaginal prolapse this is altered, and marked hyperkeratosis may be present. Under ordinary circumstances the glycogenated vaginal cells stain a deep brown with iodine (Schiller's) solution, whereas if hyperkeratosis has occurred this staining property is lost. Dermal papillae are rather prominent in the posterior wall together with irregular rete ridges, whereas in the anterior wall the epidermis is more regu-

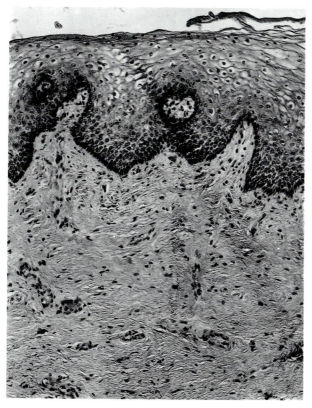

Fig 3–4.—Photomicrograph of the adult vaginal epithelium and stroma.

lar. Beneath the epithelium an interlacing network of elastic fibers is evident in the connective tissue. Interspersed are foci of lymphocytes and numerous blood vessels. There are no glands in the vagina under normal conditions, but occasionally misplaced endocervical glands, wolffian duct remnants, or epidermal inclusion cysts are found. The vagina is lubricated by secretions from the cervix and Bartholin's glands, although during sexual stimulation fluid has been described as originating from the vaginal epithelium.

The muscularis is made up of external longitudinal and internal circular layers. The latter are interspersed liberally into the fibroelastic tissue of the lamina propria.

The adventitial coat is an outer layer of dense connective tissue in which there are numerous blood vessels and nerves. It blends imperceptibly with the perivaginal (rectovaginal and vesicovaginal) fascia and is in itself supportive.

MALFORMATIONS

During the first three months of embryonic development there is a close association and correlation of development of the vagina, urinary system, urogenital sinus, cloaca, and rectum, so that abnormalities of one are commonly integrated with abnormalities in any or all of the others. It has been pointed out previously that the müllerian ducts normally fuse to form the uterus and vagina, but this process may be arrested at any point. Of particular importance is the process of differentiation of the müllerian tubercle. This structure opens into the urogenital sinus, as does the urinary tract. The process of separation of the two systems is brought about by the descent of this tubercle, creating a septum between the openings of the urethra and vagina in their normal position in the vestibule. The descent of the müllerian tubercle is believed to be a function of estrogenic stimulation so that if relative excesses of androgens are present (as in adrenal hyperplasia) the ultimate position of the vaginal orifice is altered. Thus the vagina may then connect with the urogenital sinus so that a common exit is present at birth. Another variant is due to incomplete fusion of the müllerian ducts, resulting in the formation of a double uterus (uterus didelphys), double cervix, and double vagina (Fig 3–5). In rare cases, canalization of the solid müllerian tube does not occur and total absence of the vagina results.

Congenital absence of the vagina seems to be a more common developmental defect in Finland than in other European countries. Turunen has seen more than 200 cases and has operated on 145 of them. Affected patients show normal constitutional development, though they are frequently of small stature. The secondary sex characteristics, breasts, and hair distribution are normal, as are the external genitalia in most cases. The uterus is usually of the rudimentary, bicornis separatus type but occasionally it is normal. In five patients Turunen was able to establish continuity between such a uterus and an artificial vagina with subsequent menstruation.

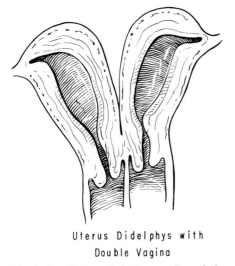

Uterus Didelphys with
Double Vagina

Fig 3–5.—Congenital abnormality of the vagina, showing a double uterus and double vagina.

Three of these patients became pregnant. This series also showed a large number of abnormalities of the thoracic spine, chiefly wedge vertebrae, fusions, and rudimentary and supernumerary vertebrae.

If the cells of the urogenital sinus do not penetrate the müllerian tube, there may be a total occlusion of the vagina. Occasionally both the vagina and rectum open into the urogenital sinus or into the urethra.

The first-mentioned abnormality, urovaginal connection, is seen frequently in patients with female hermaphroditism associated with adrenal hyperplasia. The findings include (1) a persistent urogenital sinus into which the vagina opens; (2) an enlarged clitoris; (3) hypoplastic or infantile uterus and ovaries; and (4) greatly enlarged adrenals with hyperplasia of the androgenic zone. Correction of these defects is possible by vaginal plastic surgery in combination with the administration of cortisone. Pregnancies subsequent to this therapy have been reported in such individuals. In those cases caused by adrenal neoplasm, surgery will be required, whereas in those due to hyperplasia or hyperfunction cortisone therapy alone may be effective. If the abnormality is that of a double vagina alone, this may be corrected by excision of the septum. If there is associated duplication of the uterus, serious difficulties may be encountered in the form of infertility, abortion, or dystocia. The construction of an artificial vagina in patients in whom it is completely lacking has become rather commonplace, and many recent reports indicate excellent results utilizing skin grafts and obturators of various types. Unfortunately, the uterus in most of these patients is not sufficiently well developed to allow menstrual function or conception. Although the uterus is frequently said to be absent, more often than not it may be found at laparotomy as a small rudimentary nubbin of tissue in the midline or along the lateral pelvic wall. For a complete description of these abnormalities and their treatment the reader is referred to the works of Wilkins et al.; Jones and Jones; and Young (see also Chapter 17, "Medical Genetics").

PHYSIOLOGIC ALTERATIONS

Before the various forms of vaginitis are considered, it is appropriate to review certain fundamentals of vaginal physiology that deal specifically with the subjects of acidity and bacterial flora. It has been known since 1877 that the vaginal discharge is acid and since 1892 that this acidity is due to the presence of gram-positive organisms, the Döderlein bacilli. The acidity is directly correlated with the amount of lactic acid present, although it has been suggested that perhaps other acids may be effective in certain cases. The exact origin of vaginal lactic acid is unknown but most evidence suggests that it represents a breakdown product of glycogen. Glycogen is deposited in the cells of the vaginal epithelium under the influence of estrogen although the administration of progesterone in castrates will accomplish the same effect. This is probably due to conversion of progesterone to estrogen. Diminution in the amount of estrogen results in the disappearance of cellular glycogen. Conversely, when estrogen levels are high, vaginal glycogen is abundant. Cellular glycogen may be converted directly to lactic acid by the action of Döderlein's bacilli or it may be fermented to simpler carbohydrates by vaginal enzymes and then reduced by bacteria to lactic acid. Other possibilities are that glycogen is converted to lactic acid by enzymes alone or that bacteria other than Döderlein's are capable of fermenting carbohydrates. Döderlein's bacillus is probably identical with *Lactobacillus acidophilus*, a facultative anaerobic, nonmotile, gram-positive rod.

The pH of the human vagina has been extensively studied with glass electrodes and various indicator dyes. The vagina of the newborn has a pH of about 5.7, the elevation presumably being due to the presence of alkaline amniotic fluid. Döderlein's bacilli appear about the fourth day and the pH falls to about 4.8. There is then a rise beginning on the eighth day to neutrality, and neutral values persist until the onset of puberty. Following onset of the menarche the pH varies between 4.0 and 5.0, depending on the stage of the menstrual cycle. Lowest values have been found at ovulation and premenstrually. This parallels the curves of estrogen excretion for the normal cycle. There is also a pH gradient, depending on the area of the vagina sampled. Thus, the lowest values are found near the anterior fornix, intermediate ones in the mid-vagina and highest ones near the vestibule. A pH of 4.0 or less is found during pregnancy, whereas in the postmenopausal woman neutral or alkaline values may be seen. The clinical importance of this maintained acidity is emphasized by the fact that most pathogenic bacteria disappear when the pH is kept between 4.1 and 4.9.

During pregnancy the vaginal epithelium reaches a maximum thickness, with concomitant increased glycogen content. Accordingly, the amount of lactic acid production is increased and the pH varies between 3.8 and 4.4. In the newborn infant the vagina is of adult histologic type as a result of maternal estrogen. After a few weeks, however, the epithelium diminishes in thickness and after a few months it is quite thin. This condition is maintained until puberty, with the result that the natural barriers to disease during this time are minimal and gonorrheal and nonspecific vaginitis are common. At puberty the epithelium thickens, glycogen is deposited, and the pH is lowered to about 4.0. A vaginal discharge may be noted at this time similar to that occasionally seen in the newborn infant. Microscopically, it is made up of precornified and cornified vaginal epithelial cells, leukocytes, and many Döderlein's bacilli. Menopause brings about changes in the vaginal epithelium similar to those found before puberty. The epithelial thickness is then greatly reduced and the surface appears smooth and shiny. The individual cells contain little glycogen and Döderlein's bacilli are scarce, so that a pH of 6.0 is common. Vaginal smears show mostly basal cells and leukocytes. The vagina during this stage is quite susceptible to infection and trauma. Interesting observations have been made on artificial vaginas constructed of homologous donor skin. In most cases the glycogen content, acidity, bacterial flora, and cytology closely resemble those of the normal vagina.

Cytology

The desquamated epithelial cells of the human vagina lend themselves to easy collection and have thus been extensively studied. This is a fortunate circumstance, since much may be learned by microscopic examination of either nonstained or stained material. From such observations one may determine the functional state of the ovaries in regard to the secretion of hormones, the presence of infection or carcinoma, the therapeutic responses to hormones, drugs, or radium, or even whether or not the membranes of a parturient are ruptured.

The cytologic examination of the vaginal desquamate is done by aspirating the so-called vaginal pool from the posterior fornix with a glass tube to which is attached a rubber bulb. The aspirate is immediately spread in a thin film on a glass slide and immersed in solution made up of equal parts of 95% alcohol and ether. Scrapings from the lateral vaginal wall may also be used. After fixation for 30 minutes the slide is allowed to dry and is stained by the method of Papanicolaou. The usual smear will show a preponderance of vaginal cells but also leukocytes, erythrocytes, fibrin, mucus, and a varied bacterial flora. Two major groups of cells are immediately recognizable: cornified cells (containing eleidin, a horny substance that gives the cells birefringence), which stain orange-red, and uncornified cells, which stain blue or various shades of blue-green. The cornified cells represent the maximum differentiation of the vaginal epithelium brought about by estrogen. The level of effective estrogen may be estimated by the proportionate number of cornified and precornified cells in stained smears, although vaginal infections will alter the cells and negate the importance of such determinations. Hormonal evaluation of cells is best obtained by scrapings from the lateral vaginal wall.

Typically, the cornified pyknotic cell is a large, thin, polygonal cell with smooth edges and a bright red-orange color. The cytoplasm is delicate, transparent, and homogeneous. The nucleus is small and pyknotic without definite clumping of the chromatin. These nuclei may have a vacuole beside them or may be surrounded by a clear perinuclear halo. Another characteristic of the cornified cells is the pyknotic nucleus, so that this group may be termed *cornified karyopyknotic* cells. The origin of these cells is the superficial and granular layer of the epithelium. Uncornified cells originate from three layers: superficial, intermediate, and deep. The karyopyknotic uncornified cells (sometimes called "pre-corns") are similar to the cornified cells except that their cytoplasm has an affinity for basic dyes, and stains clear blue or violet. The intermediate cells are polygonal in shape and rather large but have the nuclear pattern of the deep cells. They arise from the stratum spinosum where the presence of intracellular bridges is so marked as to give a spiny or prickle cell appearance. The deep cells are small in comparison with those just described but are larger than leukocytes. They are round or ovoid with well-defined edges. The nucleus is large and centrally placed and the cytoplasm forms a perinuclear zone, which lightly stains clear blue or violet.

Three types of smears are evident by examination of the cell types. They are (1) follicular, (2) progestational, and (3) atrophic. About the middle of the ovulatory cycle and corresponding with the peak of estrogen, the vaginal smear is characterized by a predominance of cornified cells. The cells are large, smooth, and polygonal with pyknotic nuclei, and the cytoplasm is free from folding or wrinkling. Mucus is scant and leukocytes are infrequent. After the corpus luteum is well formed and progesterone is being secreted in adequate amounts, the smear takes on a different appearance. Uncornified cells of the intermediate zone are predominant and they present themselves in groups with doubled-over edges and folded or vacuolated cytoplasm. There is an abundance of mucus, leukocytes, and bacteria. Certain unusual cells are evident during the progestational phase because of changes in morphology. The "oyster" or "navicular" cells are due to variations of the cell edges, with doubling over. They are especially common during pregnancy or when progesterone secretion is elevated. If neither estrogen nor progesterone is present in adequate amount, the smear has an atrophic appearance. The deep cells predominate here, and there may be complete absence of cornified cells. Considerable mucus, bacteria, and leukocytes are present. This smear is found during the prepubertal and menopausal periods and in patients with ovarian insufficiency. That these effects are due to lack of estrogen and progesterone has been shown in castrate females with atrophic smears. The sequential administration of estrogen and progesterone will produce both the follicular and the progestational smears followed by regression to the atrophic type after hormone withdrawal.

Exfoliative vaginal cytology has an important role in present-day obstetrics because it reflects the balance of the female hormones; it is simple to perform in the antenatal clinic; it does not inconvenience the patient: and it does not add an impossible burden to the work of the pathology department.

A reasonably constant feature in pregnancies threatening to abort is the persistence of a normal or nearly normal pregnancy smear. An increase of the pyknotic index from 15% (the normal level during pregnancy) to a figure around 25% carries a good prognosis. The persistency of cytolysis, the presence of navicular cells in clumps, the basophilic staining reaction, and a reasonably low pyknotic index (below 30%) all are favorable signs in a threatened abortion. These cytologic data indicate

that the amount of progesterone secreted by the corpus luteum or the placenta is sufficient to maintain the pregnancy. In contrast, the vaginal smear in cases of inevitable abortion shows a more or less uniform picture. The discrete arrangement of the cells, the low incidence of navicular cells, the clean background, the absence of cytolysis and high level of pyknosis are all distinctive features.

Morphologic changes in the vaginal cells have been used as a presumptive diagnostic criterion for ovulation. Since progesterone may be secreted from the theca interna cells of a luteinized follicle, however, this is not absolute. The use of vaginal and cervical cytology for the diagnosis and follow-up of cervical cancer is discussed in Chapter 4.

LEUKORRHEA

About one fourth of all patients who visit the average gynecologic clinic do so because of the vaginal discharge called *leukorrhea*. The majority of these discharges are due to infections of the vaginal epithelium, and the rest to malignancies of the cervix, uterus, or vagina, to cervical ectropions, and to senescent changes during menopause. With a decrease in vaginal acidity, bacterial invasion occurs and glycogen and Döderlein's bacilli are reduced. The pathogenic organisms that usually produce vaginitis prefer this elevated pH, so that the vaginal secretion with a pH of 5 to 6 favors continuation of the disease. These changes occur most frequently during menstruation, menopause, and following parturition.

The major causes of leukorrhea are: (1) *Trichomonas vaginalis* and (2) *Candida albicans* vaginitis, (3) nonspecific vaginitis, including *Hemophilus vaginalis* vaginitis, (4) senescent vaginitis, (5) chronic cervicitis, and (6) *Chlamydia trachomatis*.

Trichomoniasis

Trichomoniasis is an extremely common finding and frequently is asymptomatic. In a study of 1,197 pregnant women, examination of routine wet smears revealed trichomonads in 26.8%, and it has been demonstrated that one of every five adult women harbors the organism. In other women, however, it causes an acute vaginitis with a frothy, yellow-green or clear, sometimes watery discharge. Occasionally the discharge is mucopurulent. Usually it is profuse and produces an irritating vulvitis that results in marked pruritus, chafing, and dyspareunia. Even digital examination or the passage of a speculum may be painful, and there may be generalized complaints of headache, backache, or pelvic pressure. A characteristic fetid odor may be the only complaint noted by the patient. Examination reveals reddening of the labia minora, occasionally with intertrigo of the inner thighs, a typical discharge oozing from the introitus, and a vaginal membrane which may be fiery red. The portio vaginalis of the cervix is often involved and bleeds easily when wiped with a cotton swab. The vagina may be covered with multiple round, red papules giving a strawberry-like appearance to the epithelium. It has been definitely established that this vaginal inflammation is due to the protozoan flagellate, *Trichomonas vaginalis,* since bacteria-free cultures of the organism have produced the inflammation, whereas disappearance of the trichomonads from the vagina is associated with the cessation of symptoms and signs of the disease. The average pH of the vagina in affected patients varies from 5.1 to 5.4, and it has been found that cultures of trichomonads will not grow below pH 5.0 or above pH 7.5. The source of infection has not been definitely solved but various studies have suggested the gastrointestinal tract, the urinary tract, contamination from towels and water, and coitus as possible avenues. Although the male may have negligible symptoms or signs, there is little doubt that he may infect and reinfect his sexual partner. In a study of 246 men with nonspecific urethritis the incidence of *T. vaginalis* was 37%. In another report of 36 men whose wives had trichomoniasis, 58% of semen cultures showed trichomonads. The incidence of *Trichomonas* infestation in the male has been estimated at about 15%. Treatment should,

therefore, include the male as well as the female to be most effective. Other recurrences may be due to the presence of the organism in the endocervix, urethra, paraurethral glands, Bartholin's glands, or anus.

The diagnosis of trichomoniasis is made by placing a drop of the secretion on an ordinary or hanging-drop slide, adding a few drops of warm saline solution, and examining the preparation under high-dry magnification. The slide should be looked at immediately since the flagellate will no longer be motile if the preparation stands for any length of time. To aid in the visualization of the flagellate 1 drop of 1% brilliant cresyl blue solution in isotonic sodium chloride may be mixed with 1 drop of the discharge. This will separate the cells, and the vaginal cells will appear violet while only the trichomonads and a few living polymorphonuclear leukocytes will be white. Two precautions are necessary: the examination should not be made in an excessively cold place since cold suppresses trichomonal activity, and isotonic sodium chloride should be used rather than water since water causes the organism to become immobilized and swollen. Giemsa stains and cultures are useful in assessing cure and in detecting extravaginal sources of infection. *Trichomonas vaginalis* is morphologically similar to *T. hominis* with two exceptions: the marginal filament along the undulating membrane is not prolonged into a free flagellum and the parabasal body is well defined. The undulating membrane is about one third to two thirds the length of the body, and there are four anterior flagella and a thin projecting axostyle of the posterior end. The usual preparation will contain many desquamated vaginal cells and leukocytes (Fig 3–6). By comparison, *T. vaginalis* is larger than the leukocyte but about one half the size of a cornified epithelial cell. The average body length is about 15 to 20 μ and contains an oval nucleus in which are scattered chromatin granules.

TREATMENT.—Temporary relief from symptoms is usually accomplished easily, but per-

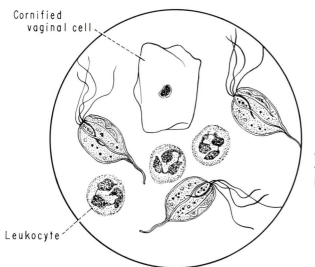

Cornified vaginal cell

Leukocyte

Fig 3–6.—Trichomonads as seen in the wet smear. They are about one half the size of a cornified vaginal cell, but larger than leukocytes.

manent cure is difficult and at times seems almost impossible. A combination of restoration of vaginal acidity and destruction of the parasite is desirable. This may be accomplished by mild acid douches (2 tablespoons of white vinegar or 2 teaspoons lactic acid per quart of warm water) and the concomitant use of a trichomonacide.

An oral preparation, metronidazole (Flagyl), has given excellent results when administered to both husband and wife for a ten-day period. It has been most effective in resistant cases. A single, 2-gm dose of Flagyl is used for primary trichomonal infections.

Clinical and experimental studies have shown metronidazole to be highly trichomonacidal in low concentration. It is readily absorbed from the intestinal tract. Metronidazole has been proved effective in the treatment of trichomonal vaginitis, cervicitis, urethritis, and prostatitis. Metronidazole is indicated in the treatment of trichomoniasis in both male and female patients when the presence of the trichomonad has been demonstrated by wet smear or culture, and for the sexual partners of those patients who have a recurrence of the infection, provided trichomonal infection is demonstrated in the urogenital tract of the sexual partner.

Although metronidazole has had no signifi-

cant effect on the blood or blood-forming elements in the patients studied to date, it should not be given to patients with evidence of, or a history of, blood dyscrasia because of its chemical structure. Also, it is recommended that metronidazole be withheld from patients with active disease of the central nervous system. At the present time, the use of metronidazole during pregnancy is contraindicated, since the preliminary studies have indicated that the drug passes the placental barrier and enters the fetal circulation rapidly.

Recent studies have shown that metronidazole is carcinogenic in rodents, mutagenic in bacteria, and should thus be regarded as potentially dangerous in humans. Although the risks associated with this drug are probably worth taking in some patients with amebiasis, it has been suggested that it should not be used for *Trichomonas* infections that can be made asymptomatic by other means. The difficulty with this admonition is that other methods of therapy presently available do not result in eradication of the organism with the same degree of effectiveness as does metronidazole.

For women, the recommended dosage is one tablet of 250 mg orally three times a day for ten days, or in stubborn cases two tablets orally and one vaginal insert of 500 mg daily for the same ten days. Vaginal inserts are not recommended as the sole treatment. In the male, metronidazole should be prescribed only when trichomonads are demonstrated in the urogenital tract. One 250-mg tablet two times daily for ten days is recommended as a course of treatment. When metronidazole is prescribed for the male in conjunction with the treatment of his female partner, the medication should be taken by both partners over the same ten-day period. When repeat courses of the drug are required it is recommended that an interval of four to six weeks elapse between courses and that leukocyte counts be made before, during, and after treatment.

It is equally important that instructions in personal hygiene be given. The patient is instructed (1) always to sweep toilet tissue in a posterior arc away from, rather than toward, the vagina, (2) to avoid use of enema tips for douching, (3) to use vaginal tampons rather than sanitary napkins during the menses, (4) to cleanse the vulva and perianal skin daily with Dial soap, then wash away all soap and dry. If the skin is excoriated, a bland ointment should be applied during therapy.

The treatment outlined seems to alleviate the vaginitis in about 90% of patients, and smears give negative results in the majority of individuals. In the other 10%, owing either to resistance of the parasite or to incompleteness of treatment, smears continue to show trichomonads and the patient is unimproved. About one fourth of all patients who are relieved of symptoms by initial therapy have recurrences. It is in these two groups that treatment must be varied and all possible efforts made to isolate the source of the infection. The following scheme has proved to be of value in the management of such cases. (1) The husband is referred to a urologist for a diagnostic survey and for treatment if he harbors the flagellate. (2) All possible foci (endocervix, periurethral glands, vulvovaginal glands, bladder, anus) are investigated and treated accordingly if trichomonads are found.

Particular attention should be paid to the possibility of an intravesical infection, and the urine should be carefully examined and cultures made to exclude infection in this organ. (3) Coitus is prohibited for several weeks and then is permitted only with the use of a condom. (4) Simultaneous treatment of the consort and patient is started with metronidazole, one tablet orally three times daily for ten days. (5) The possibility of a mixed infection must be entertained, proper diagnosis undertaken, and systematic treatment instituted. Streptococci, staphylococci, diphtheroids, or even *Candida albicans* may be involved. In postmenopausal or surgically castrated patients an atrophic vaginitis may be present. Preliminary treatment with an estrogenic vaginal cream should precede the active treatment of trichomoniasis. (6) There is recent evidence that recurrent vaginitis due to *T. vaginalis* may be correlated with emotional stress and is common in women who have symptoms of nervousness or fatigue, sleep disturbances, digestive upsets, headaches, menstrual irregularities, and painful breasts. An immature, dependent personality is often concealed by strong dominant drives and outward aggression. Treatment of such patients should include reassurance, explanation, and establishment of insight into the patient's problem. Sedation, diminished physical activity, daily rest periods, abstinence from coitus, and psychotherapeutic measures should be suggested. Hospitalization for intravenous administration of metronidazole is necessary to treat trichomoniasis that has not responded to increased oral dosage. Because metronidazole in high doses is neurotoxic, resistance should be confirmed by culture and sensitivity studies before empirically using large doses.

The status of the term "cure" in trichomoniasis has not been adequately defined. Most clinicians, however, are agreed that if examination for three consecutive months is negative for flagellates and the patient is asymptomatic, the patient may be said to be cured.

It has been recognized that the presence of *T. vaginalis* will produce morphologic changes in vaginal cells of sufficient degree to produce a class III or suspicious Papanicolaou smear. These abnormal cells disappear subsequent to adequate therapy. The clinician should not rush such a patient to the operating room for a conization of the cervix nor should he biopsy the cervix during the process of inflammation. After ten days of metronidazole therapy the smear should be repeated, the cervix stained with Schiller's solution, and then, if Schiller nonstaining areas are present, biopsies should be done.

A report by Szell et al. indicated a correlation of trichomonal vaginitis and the development of permanent atypical epithelium. In a study of 1,500 women, ages 15 to 82 years, carcinoma of the cervix was found in 3.3% of patients with chronic infection as against 0.6% of noninfected ones.

Candidiasis (Moniliasis)

Candidiasis (moniliasis) is the second most common cause of vaginal discharge. The vaginal mucosa is grayish or dull red, and there is a thick, caseous, yellow-white discharge that strongly resembles cream cheese. Candidiasis (moniliasis) is caused by a yeastlike organism, *Candida albicans*. Frequently the amount of discharge is small but the patient complains bitterly of vulvar and vaginal pruritus and burning. These complaints may be severe enough to interfere with ordinary activities and sleep. Intercourse causes severe pain. If the patient is obese or if the discharge runs down over the thighs a marked intertriginous rash may develop. Diabetes and pregnancy are predisposing factors. It has been estimated that in about 25% of all pregnant women fungi of some variety are present in the vagina, and this has been correlated with the increased vaginal glycogen during the pregnant state. The exact relationship between diabetes and candidiasis (moniliasis) has not been established. Thrush in the newborn may be etiologically related to vaginal candidiasis, the infant being infected at the time of delivery.

Another causative factor in the development of *Candida (Monilia)* vaginitis has been the extensive use of systemic antibiotics, particularly the tetracyclines. Their administration results in a reduction of the normal acid-forming vaginal bacilli, permitting fungi of the normal vagina to grow in abundance. A state similar to pregnancy may be produced by the use of oral contraceptives. It is important therefore in taking the history of a patient with pruritus vulvae to ascertain whether she (1) is pregnant, (2) is a diabetic, (3) has recently taken a wide-spectrum antibiotic, or (4) has been using oral contraceptives.

Examination reveals a hyperemic, edematous vulva, which may be covered with a gray-white frosting (see Fig 2–14) and which frequently bears evidence of marked scratching. When a speculum is introduced into the vagina, the typically cheesy or curdlike adherent discharge is evident. It may be difficult to "tease" the discharge from the underlying membrane, which may be red or violaceous. The vagina is usually edematous and tender. Its pH is acid and the vaginal smear characteristically shows mature, well-cornified epithelial cells without trichomonads.

The diagnosis is suggested by the history and examination but is corroborated by microscopic hanging-drop study of the caseous material. A small amount of the discharge is taken from the vagina and a drop of potassium hydroxide is added to thin out the preparation. It may be examined as a hanging drop or it may be stained with Gram's iodine. Characteristically *Candida albicans* is a thin-walled, yeastlike structure measuring 2 to 4 μ. Budding cells (conidia) are usually seen attached to fiberlike structures resembling bamboo shoots (mycelia). Frequently there is a tangled network of fine mycelia with clusters of conidia (Fig 3–7). The organism may be cultured on cornmeal agar or dextrose agar, mycelial development being best seen in colonies grown on the former. Individual culture tubes of Nickerson's medium are available for office use and do not need incubation. A small amount of discharge is placed

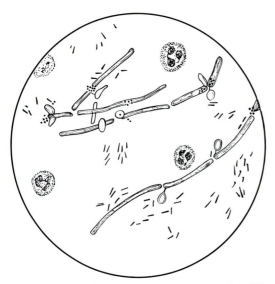

Fig 3–7.—Fiberlike mycelia of *Candida albicans* seen in a wet smear. Several leukocytes and Döderlein's bacilli are also shown.

on this medium, the cover replaced and in about 48 hours, if *Candida albicans* is present, multiple 1- to 2-mm black colonies will be evident. It should be remembered that nine varieties of *Candida (Monilia)* organisms have been described in cultures from man, but exacting cultural methods are necessary for this differentiation. Candidiasis (moniliasis) may also involve the nails, feet, webs of the fingers, oral mucosa, gastrointestinal tract, anus, and lungs. A generalized cutaneous form with meningeal involvement and death has been reported, although this is rare.

Women with *Candida albicans* infection appear to be more resistant to gonorrhea than are those without the yeast infestation. Recent studies suggest that the inhibition of gonococci by *C. albicans* occurs in vivo rather than on the transport medium, because all gonococci isolated from the patients with *C. albicans* were resistant to the strain of yeast with which they were found. Less gonorrhea is seen when *Candida* organisms are present because many of the sensitive gonococcal strains may be inhibited in vivo. Gonorrhea

may therefore be detected in these women only when they are infected with a strain resistant to their own *C. albicans.*

TREATMENT.—Treatment of *Candida (Monilia)* vaginitis is effective in producing a high percentage of cures except during pregnancy when mere palliation is achieved. If the patient is diabetic, excess glycosuria should be corrected and the general metabolic disorder controlled. If there has been excessive scratching with resultant vulvar edema, cool tap water or witch hazel compresses (or an ice cap) are applied locally and an antihistamine given orally. Occasionally codeine or codeine plus a barbiturate should be given for several nights so that the patient does not scratch the vulva during sleep. If tap water compresses alone do not bring about sufficient relief, the following prescription is applied to the vulva after the compresses:

Starch	6.0
Water	30.0
Polysorb	ad 60.0

Specific treatment of the vaginitis is best carried out with the use of nystatin (Mycostatin) vaginal suppositories, each containing 100,000 units of nystatin. The usual method is to insert one or two tablets high into the vagina every night before retiring, for 30 days. Clotrimazole (Gyne-Lotrimin) tablets may be utilized, but therapy is needed for only seven days. If the infection is severe, treatment should be repeated, utilizing seven days of therapy after each menstrual period for three consecutive months. Clotrimazole is also available in a 1% cream and solution for application to vulvar areas. If the infection is extensive or if there is reason to believe there is gastrointestinal involvement, the oral administration of Mycostatin tablets (500,000 units per tablet) three times daily is suggested. During pregnancy this treatment may have to be repeated several times, and there is no contraindication to the continuation of treatment until the onset of labor if the membranes have not ruptured. Other local therapy such as cleansing or douches is not necessary since relief is usually achieved within 48 hours. Occasionally a patient will not be helped by Mycostatin, and in this group the use of 2% aqueous gentian violet is effective. This solution is painted over the entire vaginal mucous membrane including the portio vaginalis of the cervix and over the vulva if this is affected. Since this treatment is rather messy, instructions are given to protect bed linen and lingerie from the medication. The patient is also given a prescription for gentian violet (Genapax) vaginal inserts and instructed to use one each night for six nights. Gentian Violet Supprettes are also available for home use. At the end of one week, examination is repeated in the office and the vagina is again painted with the solution. Home treatment is repeated for six additional nights, followed by an office visit for a final check. Usually by this time the vaginitis has cleared and smears give negative findings. Retreatment with gentian violet inserts or Supprettes is suggested for one week after the next three menstrual periods. The excessive use of gentian violet may prove to be locally irritating in some patients; simple withdrawal of the medication will suffice if this occurs.

In studies of patients with recurrent infections, the urine has been found to harbor *Candida (Monilia)* organisms in about 45% of cases, whereas the urine of the husbands gave positive cultures in about 30%. In such cases, the husband should be treated with oral Mycostatin and a careful search for a focus of infection in the urinary tract is initiated. The wife is treated simultaneously and coitus prohibited until improvement is noted. Alkaline medications are not recommended in the treatment of vaginal candidiasis (moniliasis), although *Candida* organisms grow easily in the highly acid vagina. The use of estrogens or estrogenic creams is not indicated since the vagina is already well glycogenated. It has been suggested that, during pregnancy, the relative deficiencies of vitamins B and C predispose to vaginitis, and thus these substances should be added to the diet.

A simple method of treatment for candidiasis (moniliasis) that has been used for years in rural areas in Kentucky has recently been revived. Capsules containing 600 mg of boric acid are placed high in the vagina two times daily for two weeks, and 5% boric acid ointment is applied to the irritated vulva three times daily. Several investigators have reported a cure rate with this regimen of 95% and this compares favorably with the rates obtained with all other agents. This treatment is readily accepted by most patients and the cost is less than with other agents.

In patients with chronic, recurrent fungal infection, further history about management of diabetes, personal hygiene, and occupational factors should be obtained. The patient should avoid tight trousers, panty hose, or synthetic fibers. The perineum should be kept clean and very dry. A hair dryer may be used for this purpose.

A few patients develop current *Candida (Monilia)* vaginitis while using oral contraceptives. In some patients it is necessary to have them repeat one of the anti-*Candida* agents each month, usually immediately after the withdrawal flow. Rarely, a patient will have to select another type of contraceptive because of the tendency to persistence or recurrence. All such individuals should have a two-hour postprandial blood sugar determination or a glucose tolerance test to exclude the possibility of diabetes. (See also the section concerning pruritus vulvae in Chapter 2, "The Vulva.")

Nonspecific Vaginitis

The discharge accompanying nonspecific vaginitis may be described as somewhere between those of *Trichomonas* and *Candida (Monilia)* infections. It is neither frothy and greenish like that of trichomoniasis nor cream-cheesy like that of candidiasis (moniliasis). The hanging drop reveals neither trichomonads nor mycelia and the Gram stain does not reveal gram-negative intracellular diplococci. The organisms usually found are staphylococci, streptococci, and *Escherichia coli.* There is evidence to support the fact that many of these "nonspecific" vaginal infections are due to *Gardnerella (Hemophilus) vaginalis.* This organism is a gram-negative, nonmotile, pleomorphic rod that may be isolated readily on proteose blood agar and has fulfilled Koch's postulates for pathogenicity. The organism has been cultured from the urethras of the majority of men whose wives harbor the infection. The commonest symptom associated with this entity is itching or burning of the vagina; also present is a moderate, gray-white frothy discharge.

In other patients, a specific streptococcal infection is evident. The inflammatory process may vary from a mild to a severe reaction and it may be acute or chronic. It is entirely possible for the pathogenic organisms to ascend through the uterus into the tubes and peritoneal cavity. Streptococcal infections produce generalized reddening of the vaginal walls with irregular patches of marked erythema and a thin discharge. The discharge associated with staphylococcal infections is usually sticky and purulent and the labia may be involved and matted together. *Escherichia coli* produces a greenish-yellow purulent exudate.

The diagnosis is usually not evident by hanging drop or Gram stain, and culture must be carried out. In many cases there is a mixed infection and anywhere from three to 12 organisms may be isolated in a given case. A good bacteriologic laboratory is necessary for adequate diagnosis in this group of vaginal infections, since sensitivity studies of various antibiotics will greatly aid rapid and complete treatment.

TREATMENT.—Specific therapy is determined by the type of offending organism and by its sensitivity to the available antibiotics and sulfonamides. Since alteration of the vaginal pH to alkalinity may predispose the mucosa to infection, this should be remedied by lactic acid douches or buffered vaginal creams. Occasionally this type of vaginitis follows use of a douching agent that has trau-

matized the vaginal mucosa. Removal of the offending agent plus cool tap-water douches produces rapid relief from symptoms. An impacted pessary or foreign body may be the inciting cause, and cure results promptly after removal.

In most streptococcal, diphtheroid, and colon bacilli infections treatment is best accomplished with vaginal jellies or creams containing sulfathiazole, sulfacetamide and sulfabenzamide (Sultrin); aminacrine, hydrochloride, allantoin, and sulfanilamide (AVC); or povidone-iodine (Betadine). The culture of the discharge should determine the most effective oral antibiotic to be given, on the basis of sensitivity tests. The antibiotic of choice for *Chlamydia* is doxycycline, a tetracycline. Staphylococcal infections have responded to the combined oral and local use of erythromycin. Systemic administration of ampicillin plus intravaginal Sultrin cream or metronidazole (Flagyl) have been reported as effective therapy in the treatment of *Hemophilus* infections.

Senescent Vaginitis

Senescent vaginitis is usually not a primary infection but consists of an inflammatory reaction together with ulceration and telangiectasia in a mucous membrane thinned by inadequate estrogenic stimulation. Occasionally, secondary infection by *T. vaginalis,* *Candida (Monilia)* or streptococci may supervene. Since the discharge is frequently blood tinged or mucoid, the possibility of cervical or endometrial cancer must be considered and diagnostic procedures accomplished. A thorough uterine curettage under anesthesia is mandatory in all patients who have postmenopausal bleeding or a bloody mucoid or watery pink discharge.

The usual symptoms are discharge, burning, itching, or perineal soreness. Frequently the only complaint is that of dyspareunia. Examination reveals the vagina to be smooth, shiny, and tender with the normal rugae lacking. The posterior commissure may be reddened or even ulcerated. The mucous membrane is pale with numerous red petechiae, ecchymoses, telangiectasia, or actual ulceration. Diagnosis is made by inspection and by a hanging drop of the secretion, which shows a typical "atrophic" smear with basal cells, leukocytes, and bacteria.

If cancer is not present, treatment should be twofold: the vaginal acidity should be restored with lactic acid douches or creams, and local estrogen should be given in the form of suppositories or creams. We have used dienestrol or conjugated estrogen (Premarin) vaginal cream successfully in such cases. The cream should be used every night for one week and then at regular intervals every six weeks. It should not be administered continuously for long periods since absorption of the estrogenic substance may lead to endometrial proliferation and irregular uterine bleeding. If the uterus is surgically absent, estrogens may be given orally (e.g., ethinyl estradiol, 0.05 mg daily), until a desired result is obtained.

Chronic Cervicitis

The discharge associated with a cervical erosion or ectropion is usually white or clear with an abundance of mucus. If infection is present, the discharge may be purulent. Although this entity is a common cause of leukorrhea, it will be discussed in detail in Chapter 4, "The Cervix."

Gonorrheal Vaginitis

Although the glandular epithelium of the periurethral glands and endocervix is the initial focus of growth in gonorrheal infection, the mucous membrane of the vagina may become secondarily involved, with resultant edema and inflammation. In immature females the commonest cause of vaginitis is the gonococcus. The thinness of the mucous membrane in this age group makes it particularly susceptible to this organism.

Although gonorrheal vaginitis is usually spread by sexual contact, in children it may be disseminated by direct contact with towels, toilet seats, fingers, etc. In institutions for young children it may become widespread before being detected and adequate therapy

instituted. The symptoms include a profuse, yellow or yellow-white discharge, vaginal itching, burning, and dysuria. In children the discharge may be slight and the symptoms minimal so that attention to the disorder is not immediate. In adults there is often involvement of Bartholin's glands, with an actual abscess occasionally found. Concomitant urethritis and skenitis may be present and should be looked for by gently exerting pressure under the terminal urethra and the openings of Skene's ducts. Pus, if present, can generally be expressed and smears and cultures obtained. The glands of the endocervix and the oviducts may be involved as part of either an acute or a chronic process. When the gonococcus reaches the internal genitalia, signs of pelvic peritonitis are frequently demonstrable.

The diagnosis of gonorrhea is made by placing a drop of secretion on a slide and examining it by Gram's method. A typical, coffee-bean, gram-negative, intracellular diplococcus is usually seen. Treatment should not be administered on the basis of the smear alone, since many other organisms may simulate the gonococcus. A culture should be taken at the time the smear is made and positive diagnosis should await this report. A complement-fixation test is available to settle the diagnosis in borderline cases. A fluorescent antibody technique has been introduced by L. H. Shapiro to aid in diagnosis. This involves the visualization of a specific antigen (e.g., *Neisseria gonorrhoeae*) under ultraviolet illumination. The specific antibody is "tagged" with a fluorescent dye. Thus, when antigen-antibody reaction occurs, the pathogen (*N. gonorrhoeae*) may be easily identified.

Most of the strains of gonococci now encountered are sensitive to adequate dosage of any of the following antibiotics: penicillin, streptomycin, chlortetracycline, oxytetracycline, chloramphenicol, and carbomycin. In the mature female (after positive findings on smear and culture) treatment now consists of an injection of 4.8 million units of penicillin G preceded by an injection of probenecid one hour previously to delay excretion. If the patient gives a history of penicillin sensitivity, tetracycline in a dose of 250 mg four times daily for four days is administered. All local therapy is avoided, and showers rather than tub baths are suggested during the first day or so of treatment. The patient is then asked to return at weekly intervals for follow-up smears and cultures. In the immature female, oral penicillin in a total daily dose of 400,000 units given for four days is usually adequate for cure. In most cases it has not been necessary to add estrogenic substances to this therapy, although the use of vaginal suppositories containing 100,000 units of estrogen for three to four weeks following antibiotic treatment is of value in certain patients. The oral or parenteral use of estrogen is not advised because of the possible side effects, namely, breast hypertrophy, uterine bleeding, and epiphyseal closure. (See also the discussion of gonorrhea in Chapter 18.)

VAGINAL RELAXATION

The most common abnormalities of the vagina are due to relaxations of the endopelvic and associated fascia, resulting in cystocele, urethrocele, rectocele, enterocele, or colpocele (Fig 3–8). Occasionally an obturator hernia or pelvic lipoma will protrude into the vaginal canal, but these are uncommon.

CYSTOCELE.—A cystocele results from a herniation of the bladder base into the vaginal canal and is best demonstrated by asking the patient to strain slightly. It is usually due to a laceration and retraction of the urogenital diaphragm and adjacent portions of the pubococcygeus muscle in association with relaxation of the musculofascial coverings of the bladder and anterior vaginal wall. The major etiologic factor is childbirth, but large cystoceles are occasionally seen even in nulliparous women. Complaints referable to a cystocele vary. Most women complain of a bulge, a lump, or a "dropping" in the region of the introitus. Some note only a sense of heaviness or pressure in the pelvis after being on their feet for

long periods, whereas others note symptoms of urinary frequency or dysuria. The latter symptoms are due to an increased amount of residual urine after voiding, with stasis and subsequent infection of the bladder trigone. Occasionally the symptoms are severe, yet only minimal displacement of the bladder is found at examination. It is important to examine these patients in the standing position, for only then will the cystocele be evident. The bladder should also be catheterized after voiding to determine if a large quantity (40 ml or more) of residual urine is present.

URETHROCELE.—A urethrocele is a protrusion of the inferior aspect of the urethra in an arc away from the pubis toward the vagina. It is frequently associated with a cystocele and is due to lacerations of the urogenital diaphragm with tearing of the pubococcygeal fibers and connective tissue that attach the urethra to the symphysis pubis. There is an associated flattening out and enlargement of the urethral bore as its musculofascial sheaths separate. The anatomic changes thus incurred bring about a change in the urethrovesical angle, so that urinary continence is impaired. Such incontinence is most marked when the patient strains, coughs, sneezes, or runs and is therefore known as *stress incontinence*. This should be differentiated from "urge" incontinence, which is characterized by preliminary loss of urine when the patient has a strong urge to void. The latter is associated with a chronic cystotrigonitis and may be due to a cystocele with a large amount of residual urine and long-standing bladder infection. In all urinary tract difficulties in the female, especially incontinence, the clinician must not be misled by obvious anatomic deformities, since the symptoms may be due to neurologic causes such as cord lesions, tabes dorsalis, or spina bifida. Therefore a thorough neurologic examination should be done in all patients with symptomatic cystourethrocele and cystometric studies done when indicated.

RECTOCELE.—A rectocele is a hernia of the lower rectum through its surrounding fas-

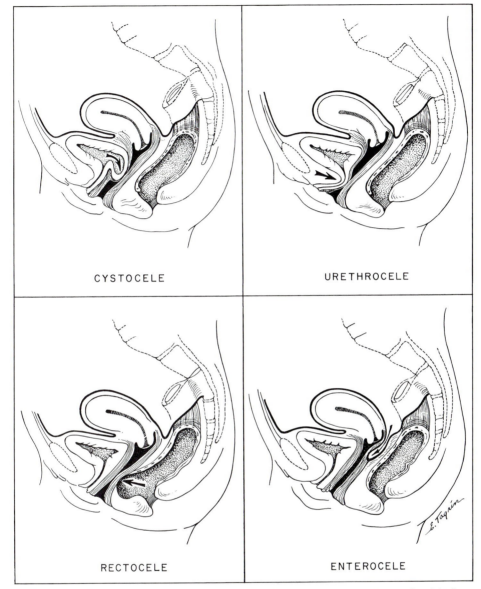

Fig 3–8.—Diagrammatic representation of the four most common types of pelvic floor relaxation: cystocele, urethrocele, rectocele, and enterocele. Arrows depict sites of maximum protrusion.

cial envelopes into the vagina. Injury sustained at the time of pelvic delivery is the predominant etiologic factor, although an innate developmental weakness combined with increased intra-abdominal pressure from hard physical work may bring about the same situation. The anatomic defect is due to stretching, tearing, and separation of the musculofascial sheaths of the rectum and vagina, the urogenital diaphragm, the levator ani, and, frequently, portions of the sphincter ani muscle. The perineal body may or may not show evidence of laceration. Frequently an episiotomy has been performed at delivery and the perineum and introitus appear normal, but if the patient is asked to strain or cough the posterior vaginal wall bulges out beyond the introitus. A high rectocele may not be evident unless the patient is examined in the erect position. A rectocele is frequently asymptomatic and, even when large, may cause no particular distress. In other cases there are symptoms of backache, protrusion, pelvic pressure or discomfort, heaviness, or perineal burning. These are aggravated by long hours in the standing position or by frequent constipation. Occasionally feces collect in the dilated lower rectum and become inspissated or impacted. It may sometimes be necessary for the patient to aid evacuation by digital pressure through the vagina. The diagnosis is obvious by inspection although a combined rectovaginal examination is often useful to delineate the extent of the rectocele. A high rectocele may be differentiated from an enterocele by placing a Sims speculum in the vagina with the blade held tightly in the posterior cul-de-sac, gently lifting the cervix. A finger in the rectum outlines the upper limits of the rectocele. If an enterocele is present, it will be seen to roll down from the apex of the vagina over the rectocele as the patient strains.

ENTEROCELE.—An enterocele is a herniation of the peritoneum lining the posterior cul-de-sac into the posterior vaginal fornix behind the cervix. Small bowel may be present in an enterocele but almost never becomes incarcerated therein. The condition is frequently associated with a congenitally deep or wide cul-de-sac with separation and attenuation of the uterosacral ligaments. In a primary enterocele the thin-walled peritoneal sac forms behind the cervix and lies between the posterior vaginal wall and the anterior rectal wall in the rectovaginal septum. A secondary enterocele is a herniation through the floor of the pelvis after total abdominal or vaginal hysterectomy. A small enterocele is usually asymptomatic, but after it gains sufficient size it may protrude beyond the introitus so that

the chief complaint is one of prolapse. This is especially disconcerting if it occurs after a vaginal hysterectomy and vaginal plastic repair since the patient cannot differentiate it from a cystocele or rectocele, the condition for which the original surgery was performed.

COLPOCELE.—A colpocele is a herniation of the vaginal wall beyond the introitus in association with a complete uterine prolapse. The symptoms are those of protrusion, although ulceration and infection of the vaginal mucosa may occur from long-standing eversion.

PERINEAL LACERATIONS.—Frequently, perineal lacerations are seen in association with a rectocele since the etiologic factor is usually difficult delivery. During the time the fetal vertex impinges against the pelvic floor, producing "bulging" and "crowning," there is a combined stretching and tearing of the fibromuscular support of the perineal body. If this stage of labor is prolonged or if episiotomy is not utilized to minimize the trauma, separation or avulsion of the superficial perineal muscles, both layers of the superficial fascia, and, usually, the deep perineal fascia occurs. When delivery is extremely difficult, there may actually be avulsion of the external anal sphincter, urogenital diaphragm, and levator ani muscle. These injuries should be repaired at the time of delivery, with particular attention to realignment of fascial layers without tension. Frequently, however, the obstetrician does not recognize the damage or feels incompetent to repair it. In other cases hematomas or infection supervene and a poor result follows. Simple, incomplete perineal lacerations, if unaccompanied by a rectocele, are usually asymptomatic. There is some gaping of the introitus, so that water enters the vagina rather freely during bathing and the patient may note dribbling for a short time after. In other cases a pinpoint fistulous tract occurs between the rectum and vagina so that gas (but not feces) enters the vagina and the patient complains of recurrent passage of gas per vagina. In complete perineal lacerations

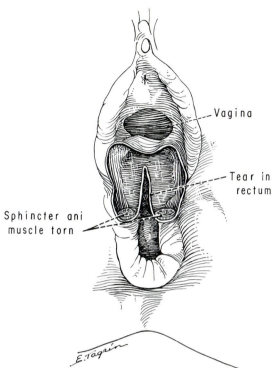

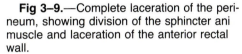

Vagina

Tear in rectum

Sphincter ani muscle torn

Fig 3–9.—Complete laceration of the perineum, showing division of the sphincter ani muscle and laceration of the anterior rectal wall.

(Fig 3–9) the sphincter ani muscle has been completely divided, a modified cloaca thus being formed. Although fecal incontinence may be noted during episodes of diarrhea, these patients are in general able to control bowel movements rather well. Vaginal contamination with feces is, however, unavoidable.

TREATMENT.—The management of vaginal relaxations, if asymptomatic, is surgical. The possible exception to this is a urethrocele with stress incontinence which, after a series of specific pubococcygeal exercises, will regain sufficient tone to be asymptomatic. In the surgical repair of vaginal relaxation, known as a vaginal "plastic" or colporrhaphy, basic surgical principles of hernia repair are employed. Thus, in a cystocele repair (anterior colporrhaphy) the bladder is freed from the vagina and mobilized from the cervix. The investing fascia that has spread laterally is mobilized and approximated in the midline with fine catgut sutures. Any excess vaginal mucosa is trimmed and the edges brought together. A urethrocele repair (urethroplasty) is somewhat more difficult, in that the urethra must be freed from scar tissue and its angle of entrance into the bladder base restored. This is usually accomplished by mobilizing musculofascial tissue and approximating it in a sling-like fashion under the proximal urethra. In recurrent cases this may be done by bringing a band of rectus fascia (obtained through an abdominal incision) retroperitoneally and directing it underneath the urethra, thus producing a supporting sling. Another method, entirely suprapubic, approaches the urethra through the space of Retzius. The urethra is suspended by suturing the periurethral fascia and vagina to the posterior aspect of the symphysis pubis and anterior rectus sheath.

A rectocele repair (posterior colporrhaphy) entails separation of the rectum from the vagina and interposition of the musculofascial layers, including the pubococcygeus and puborectalis, between the two structures. If a lacerated perineum is present, this is usually repaired simultaneously by excision of scar tissue and mobilization of the superficial perineal fascia (perineorrhaphy). In a complete perineal laceration the sphincter ani muscle must be dissected free and its ends approximated before the usual posterior colporrhaphy and perineorrhaphy are done.

An enterocele is corrected by incising the posterior vaginal wall to the level of the enterocele, isolating and mobilizing the peritoneal sac, which is excised, and repairing the defect by plication of the uterosacral ligaments and by mobilization and approximation of sufficient lateral fascia. If adequate structural support cannot be obtained vaginally, the abdomen may be opened and the posterior cul-de-sac partially obliterated by approximating the uterosacral ligaments. If a deep cul-de-sac is noted at the time of total abdominal hysterectomy and an incipient enterocele is anticipated, the posterior cul-de-sac should be obliterated by plication of the uterosacral ligaments. This produces a shelf behind the vagina with just sufficient space for the rectosigmoid to pass through. In a vaginal hysterectomy, steps should be taken to prevent the development of an enterocele by incising the posterior vaginal wall to an adequate level so that the important uterosacral ligaments may be brought together in the midline and thus form the apex of the posterior wall repair.

BENIGN NEOPLASMS

The two most common benign neoplasms of the vagina are cystic structures, one derived from remnants of the mesonephros and the other from surgically implanted fragments of perineal or vaginal epithelium. As shown in Figure 3–1, the wolffian ducts course along the superolateral aspect of the vagina, and occasionally some displaced fragments of tissue are stimulated to grow. In so doing, one or more small, cystlike structures are formed, and these are seen in the anterolateral portion of the vagina as clear-walled, soft, compressible masses *(Gartner's duct cyst)*. Rarely, one of these becomes extremely large and pedun-

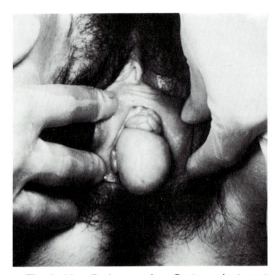

Fig 3–10.—Prolapse of a Gartner duct cyst through the introitus, simulating a large prolapsed enterocele.

culated and may appear to bulge through the introitus (Fig 3–10), resembling an enterocele.

Microscopically, these cysts have a variable lining, but usually the cells are tall, columnar to cuboidal, and are sometimes ciliated. Stratified squamous epithelium has occasionally been described as lining the cysts, but this may represent an inclusion of vaginal epithelium as the cyst forms. The cyst wall is made up of fibrous connective tissue, which sometimes is hyalinized, and the contents are usually a clear, colorless, or amber, serous or mucinous fluid. No malignancies have been reported to have developed in these cysts, but they should be differentiated from epidermal inclusion cysts, which usually occur in the distal, posterior vaginal wall and from endometriotic "implants." Treatment of Gartner's duct cysts consists of complete surgical excision.

Abnormal configurations of the bladder or urethra such as cystocele, diverticula, or urethrocele may usually be diagnosed by passing a catheter or metal probe into the urethra and noting its position. An enterocele may best be demonstrated by holding back the anterior and posterior vaginal walls with a Sims speculum and having the patient exert intra-abdominal pressure. Other conditions that rarely will present intravaginal masses are: hematocolpos, accessory ureteral cysts, and vaginitis emphysematosa.

Vaginitis emphysematosa is characterized by multiple gas-filled cysts in the vaginal and cervical mucosa. It is accompanied by a vaginal discharge, which may be the only symptom. It is more common in pregnancy, which may favor infection with *Trichomonas vaginalis* or *Hemophilus vaginalis* because of the altered physiology of the vagina. It is seldom diagnosed radiologically and needs to be distinguished from emphysematous cystitis, gangrene of the uterus, vaginal tampon, pelvic abscess, or pelvic bowel-gas shadows.

Vaginal *inclusion cysts* are quite common, but are of little significance unless large. They are formed by bits of stratified squamous epithelium that are buried under the vaginal mucosa at the time of an episiotomy repair or posterior colporrhaphy. The epithelium so displaced continues to desquamate cells and keratin, which undergo degeneration to form a yellow or yellow-white cheesy material. This becomes encased in a thin-walled structure, which is usually firm to palpation and is located in the lower third of the vagina on the posterior or posterolateral wall. The cysts are frequently discovered by the patient, but are otherwise asymptomatic unless they are so positioned as to cause dyspareunia. In general, no treatment is necessary but they are usually easily removed at the time of a subsequent episiotomy or vaginal repair.

Endometriotic cysts of the vagina may cause considerable pain and dyspareunia, especially if they contain functioning endometrial tissue. They are usually found behind the cervix in the posterior vaginal fornix and have a typical bluish color. During the premenstrual and menstrual phase of the cycle they may be acutely tender. Microscopically, the typical picture of endometriosis is found, although glands may be infrequent (Fig 3–11). The endometrial stroma shows varying amounts of hemosiderin-laden macrophages, lymphocytes, and old blood. In some areas

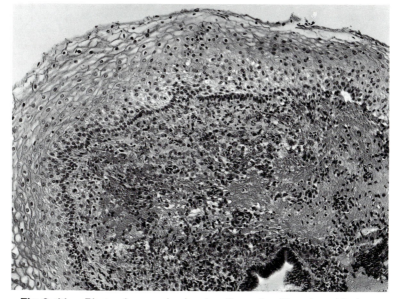

Fig 3–11.—Photomicrograph showing "menstrual" endometriosis under the vaginal epithelium. Biopsy was obtained from a typical "blueberry" nodule in the vaginal apex during the time of menstruation. (From Kistner R.W.: *Fertil. Steril.* 10:547, 1959.)

considerable fibrosis occurs. Such lesions may be treated hormonally or by surgical excision. Following menopause or oophorectomy, vaginal endometriosis regresses (see the section regarding treatment in Chapter 9, "Endometriosis").

CLEAR CELL ADENOMA

In 1971 a case-control epidemiologic investigation by Herbst, Ulfelder, and Poskanzer associated the occurrence of clear cell adenocarcinoma of the vagina in young women with intrauterine exposure to diethylstilbestrol (DES) administered to their mothers for the therapy of high-risk pregnancies. The results of this investigation were soon confirmed, and since then over 200 cases of vaginal and cervical clear cell adenocarcinoma have been collected with a definite history of maternal exposure to nonsteroidal estrogens in 65% of the investigated cases. Although these carcinomas have been encountered only rarely in females exposed to DES, a variety of other abnormalities of the lower genital tract have been reported to occur with great frequency. These include vaginal adenosis (the presence of glandular epithelium in the vagina), cervical erosion or ectropion (glandular epithelium on the portio of the cervix), and transverse fibrous ridges in the vagina and on the cervix ("cervical pseudopolyp," "cockscomb cervix," or "cervical hood"). Although most of these abnormalities were known to occur rarely in the pre-DES era, their prevalence in unexposed women examined as carefully as those who have been exposed has not been established.

In 1975 Herbst and associates published a prospective comparison of exposed female offspring with unexposed controls. The effects of prenatal exposure to DES were studied by a prospective cohort investigation of 110 exposed and 82 unexposed females. The general health characteristics of mothers and daughters in both groups were similar. Among the exposed, there were striking benign alterations of the genital tract, which included transverse ridges (22%), abnormal vaginal mucosa (56%), and biopsy-proved adenosis (35%). Among the unexposed, there were no ridges and one case of vaginal mucosal abnormality, including adenosis. Abnormal cervical epithelium occurred in almost all exposed subjects, but in only half of the unexposed. The incidence of vaginal adenosis was highest when diethylstilbestrol was begun in early pregnancy. It was not detected when treatment was initiated during the 18th week or later. Oral contraceptive use and prior pregnancy were associated with less adenosis and erosion, respectively. No cases of cancer were observed in this series. (See discussion in Chapter 4.)

Vaginal Adenosis

The lesion that is presently classified as adenosis has been recognized for many years, Von Preuschen being credited with the first description of this entity in 1877. Bonney and Glendining used the term *adenomatosis* to describe a similar change with extensive development of columnar epithelium in the vagina resulting in the copious secretion of mucus. Analogous changes have been referred to as "adenoma-like" lesions, vaginitis adenofibrosa, infiltrating diffuse adenoma with malignant change, and also as primary adenocarcinoma of the vagina. In a few reported cases, the changes were attributed either to adenomyosis of the vagina or to endocervicosis. The term *endocervicosis* was used to describe heterotopic rests of endocervical glands, which were originally considered to be a variation of endometriosis. In 1927, Plaut described a lesion known as *diffuse adenosis* and subsequently he and Dreyfuss, in 1940, described three new cases of this entity and presented a comprehensive review of the relevant literature pertaining to the lesion, which is presently designated *vaginal adenosis*.

Sandberg and associates, in 1965, described four cases of adenosis, one of which gave rise to an adenocarcinoma. At that time they accepted 76 cases of adenosis that had been reported in the literature and they were perhaps the first to suggest that this lesion was increasing in frequency, but they offered no explanation for this observation.

The information regarding the relative frequency of adenosis in women unexposed to DES in utero is sparse. Von Preuschen described the lesion in four of 36 women, whereas Ricci and associates were unable to find the lesion in any of the 14 vaginas studied. In 1968, Sandberg reported adenosis occurring in nine, or 25.7%, of the 35 vaginas examined. None of the vaginas from 13 prepubertal females showed the lesion, whereas nine, or 40.9%, of the vaginas from 22 postpubertal women had adenosis.

Adenosis is more common in females exposed to DES or dienestrol in utero, and Sherman et al. observed the change in over 90% of the women studied. Stafl et al. described adenosis in 91% of women with documented fetal exposure to DES. Burke and associates identified adenosis in 38, or 82.7%, of 46 women exposed to diethylstilbestrol in utero. These studies were based on colposcopic examination and biopsies or a comprehensive examination of the excised vaginas. Herbst et al., using inspection, Schiller's stain, and biopsy, detected vaginal adenosis in 13, or 38.2%, of 34 women studied.

While adenosis initially referred to the mucus-secreting columnar epithelium within or beneath the vaginal mucosa, the definition is now expanded to include the presence of mucus-secreting epithelium and its products. The epithelium exists on the surface of the vagina alone or may also occur within its submucosa. Sandberg has suggested a classification of the clinical forms of vaginal adenosis into occult, cystic, effluent, adenomatous, and adenocarcinomatous types. The epithelium involved in adenosis is believed to be of müllerian origin and may mimic the epithelium of the cervix, endometrium, or oviduct. Squamous metaplasia is frequently associated with adenosis and has been described in up to 95% of some cases reported. A variety of other changes may be observed in the presence of adenosis, such as cervical erosion, transverse cervical ridges, and a pericervical collar.

PREMALIGNANT NEOPLASMS

Carcinoma In Situ

Carcinoma in situ of the vagina is seldom diagnosed, except as a direct extension from carcinoma of the cervix. The epithelial changes adjacent to invasive carcinoma of the cervix are generally accepted, and involvement of the vagina is being reported with increasing frequency. The direct continuity of in situ lesions of the cervix involving the vagina is a more recent observation but at the Brigham and Women's Hospital diagnostic procedures to determine the presence of vaginal involvement has been routine prior to all hysterectomies for carcinoma in situ of the cervix. A Schiller test of the vagina is performed prior to surgery and all nonstaining areas are biopsied (see Chapter 4).

Intraepithelial carcinoma confined to the vagina without relation to cervical carcinoma is an apparent rarity. Fourteen patients who fulfilled this criterion have been observed at the Brigham and Women's Hospital. All but one case were detected by routine cytologic examination. The gross appearance of the lesions was not striking, having been described as "whitish" or "telangiectatic." The classic "blush" or "sugar coating" of cervical carcinoma in situ was not evident. The majority of patients were treated by local surgical excision some requiring simultaneous hysterectomy. Radium was utilized as adjuvant therapy in one, and was the primary treatment in two patients. Electrical and chemical coagulation was used in two others.

A patient with in situ vaginal carcinoma should be as curable as one with in situ cervical carcinoma. Partial vaginectomy is preferable to intravaginal radium in young patients. It is important to follow patients with cytologic tests every three months during the first year after a hysterectomy for cervical carcinoma in situ; cytologic examinations are then performed every six months during the next four years, and every 12 months thereafter.

MALIGNANT NEOPLASMS

Carcinoma

PRIMARY CARCINOMA.—Primary carcinoma of the vagina is almost always a squamous cell type, whereas adenocarcinoma is usually metastatic from another source. As a primary tumor, vaginal carcinoma makes up about 1% of all genital malignancies, and its relative incidence to that of cervical cancer is about 1:50. The average age is somewhere between 48 and 55 years, although this malignancy has been reported in patients in their late 20s.

There are no known predisposing factors that seem to affect the development of vaginal carcinoma. Thus the family history, parity, marital history, previous diseases, concomitant diseases, or exposure to irritants are of no etiologic significance. A vaginal cancer is found rarely in a patient who has been wearing a pessary for a long time, but this is believed to be coincidental.

The usual symptom is abnormal bleeding or a blood-tinged discharge. The bleeding is usually first noticed after intercourse or douching, but occasionally may begin as a severe hemorrhage. If the disease is extensive the discharge may be profuse, foul smelling, and cause a rather marked vulvitis with pruritus. A normocytic-hypochromic anemia may be found and generalized symptoms such as weakness, dizziness, and malaise may be secondary to it. If the tumor has invaded the bladder, symptoms of dysuria, frequency, and hematuria may be present, whereas with rectal involvement the patient may complain of tenesmus, diarrhea, melena, and pain.

The diagnosis of vaginal carcinoma is usually obvious by speculum examination but should be corroborated by tissue biopsy. Early lesions or carcinoma in situ may be diagnosed by cytologic methods before symptoms develop or before the lesion becomes obvious to the clinician. The value of routine vaginal cytologic examinations even in women who have had total hysterectomy has been demonstrated to us on several occasions by the finding of vaginal carcinoma in situ as a completely unexpected lesion. Biopsy of the vagina in cases in which the cytology is suspicious or positive may be aided by painting the entire vagina with Schiller's solution, since atypical epithelium, whether anaplastic, carcinoma in situ, or actual carcinoma, will not stain with this iodine solution. In differential diagnosis, consideration must be given to cervical cancer, sarcoma botryoides, endometriosis, and the granulomas. Biopsy is necessary for definitive diagnosis. Colposcopy-directed biopsies aid in detection.

The carcinoma may appear in several forms. It may be a large, fungating, cauliflower-like mass that fills the entire upper vagina or it may be flat, superficial, and locally infiltrative (Fig 3–12). A third type presents as a deep, ulcerating, locally destructive lesion. The tumor is most often found on the posterior wall in the upper third of the vagina. When the carcinoma involves the lower

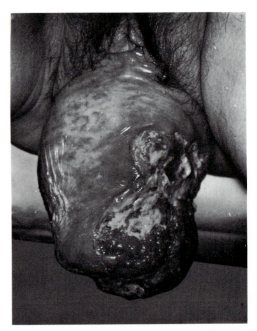

Fig 3–12.—Extensive primary carcinoma of the vagina in association with procidentia. (From Kistner R.W.: *Obstet. Gynecol.* 10:483, 1957.)

third, prognosis is poor. This is probably due to involvement of different lymphatics and quicker vascular dissemination. There is some evidence that the prognosis is better if the lesion is found on the anterior wall but this may be due to a higher incidence of less extensive tumor in that area.

The disease usually spreads upward toward the cervix and is confined for a fairly long time to the superficial portion of the vagina. If there is involvement of the cervix, it is difficult to determine whether the tumor is a primary cervical lesion with spread to the vagina or vice versa. If, however, the lesion is most extensive in the vagina and just involves the edges of the cervical portio, it may be properly termed a primary vaginal tumor. The growth pattern is usually one of rather localized spread, first up and then around the diameter of the vaginal tube before deep extension into the bladder or rectum occurs. In the ulcerative form, however, deep craters into the adjacent viscera may occur. Vesicovaginal and rectovaginal fistulas are usually late findings. The carcinoma spreads by contiguity and also by lymphatics. The upper vagina drains into the same lymphatic chain as the cervix (iliac, ureteral, hypogastric, and obturator nodes), whereas the lower vagina duplicates the drainage of the vulva (inguinal, femoral, Cloquet's nodes). Intermediate lesions may spread to the obturator or to either of the other pathways.

In 1971 the general assembly of the International Federation of Gynecology and Obstetrics approved the recommendations of the FIGO Cancer Committee for a classification and staging system of vaginal carcinoma. This classification is as follows:

Staging of Vaginal Carcinoma

Preinvasive carcinoma

Stage 0. Carcinoma in situ, intraepithelial carcinoma.

Invasive carcinoma

Stage I. The carcinoma is limited to the vaginal wall.

Stage II. The carcinoma has involved the subvaginal tissue but has not extended to the pelvic wall.

Stage III. The carcinoma has extended to the pelvic wall.

Stage IV. The carcinoma has extended beyond the true pelvis or has involved the mucosa of the bladder or rectum. A bullous edema as such does not permit allotment of a case to stage IV.

TREATMENT.—In the past it has been stated that vaginal carcinoma is the most difficult of female genital cancers to treat. Taussig is quoted as having said, "We acknowledge our total inability to do anything effective for primary carcinoma of the vagina." This statement does not coincide with the recent attitude of most gynecologists, who favor a radical surgical approach. Before 1945 only about 25% of patients were deemed suitable candidates for surgery, but in recent years an increasing number are being selected for this approach. In lesions that are apparently confined to the vagina, especially in the upper third, preliminary radium in the form of a plaque or surface mold may be applied to the carcinoma, followed in four to six weeks by a radical hysterectomy, extensive vaginectomy, and node dissection. If the lymph nodes are involved or there has been gross extension of the disease at the time of surgery, postoperative x-ray therapy is given. In tumors that involve the anterior vaginal wall extensively and that seem to involve the vesicovaginal septum or fascia, preliminary radium therapy is followed by anterior exenteration. This includes radical hysterectomy, cystectomy, vaginectomy, and node dissection. The ureters are best transplanted to an ileal conduit. When the posterior vaginal wall and adjacent fascia and/or rectum are involved, preliminary radium is given, followed by posterior exenteration (radical hysterectomy, node dissection, and abdominoperineal resection). In rare cases in which there is extension to bladder and rectum but not lateral fixation to the pelvic wall, a total exenteration is sometimes indicated. The ureters are transplanted to an ileal conduit whose stoma is brought out on the right side of the abdomen; a sigmoid colostomy is brought out on the left side. If the lower third of the vagina is involved, an extraperitoneal inguinal and femoral node dissection is also performed. It should be noted that these major surgical procedures are difficult and time-consuming, and usually the operative mortality is 15% to 25%. They should only be carried out in centers where blood replacement, electrolyte studies, and optimum postoperative care are possible. If these criteria cannot be met or if the patient is not a good risk for such operations, treatment should be accomplished with radium and x-ray.

Almost all studies have shown that the prognosis depends on the stage of the disease when it is first treated. Thus, prognosis is good for small lesions that are confined to the upper third of the vagina and that show negative nodes and clear lines of surgical excision. When the lymph nodes are positive or tumor has been transected, the results are poor. Radiation therapy alone has been disappointing, and a radical surgical approach is the treatment of choice in all operable lesions. An insufficient number of patients have been treated by radical surgery in our clinic to state an exact survival rate, but in other series a survival rate of between 30% and 40% has been reported although not all reports were five years after treatment. Merrill reviewed the treatment of 25 patients followed up for five years or longer and noted a survival rate of 28%. All but three of these patients were treated with radiation, but most did not have far-advanced disease when first seen. The five-year survival rate was 26.5%, and the ten-year survival rate was only 15.3% in the series of patients reported from the Radiumhemmet in Stockholm. Rutledge reported the highest survival rate in patients treated by radium and x-ray, with 44% of 70 patients living and well without evidence of disease after five years. As a result of his experience, Rutledge believes that radiation is the preferable initial therapy for vaginal cancer and, if the lesion fails to respond, surgery can be done later.

Radium therapy is ideally suited for the widespread, superficial polypoid lesion. The more common ulcerating or papillary growth usually has reached the rectovaginal or vesicovaginal septum by the time it is diagnosed. Thus, if radiation therapy is adequate, a fistula is practically assured.

When the tumor is located in the posterior vaginal wall, I prefer to do a posterior exenteration with total vaginectomy and pelvic lymphadenectomy. If the lesion involves the anterior wall, an anterior exenteration, total vaginectomy and pelvic lymphadenectomy is done. If the lesion involves the lower third of the vagina, a radical vulvectomy with inguinal and femoral node dissection is combined with the procedures already noted.

Death usually occurs from ureteral obstruction or wide dissemination of metastases, although, rarely, massive hemorrhage from erosion of a large blood vessel may be lethal.

Primary adenocarcinoma of the vagina is uncommon. As noted previously, most of the cancers arising in this site occurred during the fourth and fifth decades of life and are of the squamous cell type. Between the years of 1966 and 1969, eight patients aged 15 to 22 years were detected to have vaginal adenocarcinomas at the Massachusetts General Hospital in Boston. While similar neoplasms had been reported in older women, no such cancers were recognized in that institution prior to 1966. With one exception, the adenocarcinomas were characterized by tubules and glands lined by clear or "hobnail" cells containing glycogen. Vaginal adenosis was identified at the periphery of the neoplasms, whose structures suggested a müllerian origin. Since these neoplasms had not been previously identified in the second and third decades of life, an investigation was undertaken in an attempt to identify possible causative factors.

In the study group there was a history of maternal bleeding during pregnancy, and pregnancy loss was more often observed than in the control group. Seven of the eight mothers had been treated with DES during the first trimester of pregnancy. None of the women in the control group received comparable therapy. This led Herbst, Ulfelder, and Poskanzer to conclude that the administration of diethylstilbestrol during pregnancy increased the risk for the development of adenocarcinoma in females exposed to diethylstilbestrol in utero. Others reported similar adenocarcinomas in the offspring of women receiving DES during pregnancy, and a large series of cases were accumulated in a registry of clear cell adenocarcinoma of the genital tracts of young women.

Plaut and Dreyfuss concluded that primary adenocarcinoma of the vagina probably originates from adenosis in most instances. This conclusion was based on an evaluation of the accumulated cases in non–DES-exposed women. While this relationship may also exist between adenosis and clear cell adenocarcinoma of the vagina in the women exposed to DES in utero, the frequency of this outcome can only be postulated on the basis of present evidence, and to date no woman with adenosis has been observed to develop adenocarcinoma during the period of surveillance. The frequent coexistence of adenosis and clear cell adenocarcinoma would be consistent with the postulated cause-and-effect relationship.

Equally important are the other possible fates of vaginal adenosis. For example, involution was believed to occur in some lesions, although the frequency of this outcome has not been established. Cysts may evolve from the glandular epithelium in some instances, and the presence of associated squamous metaplasia suggests that the columnar epithelium may, in some cases, be replaced by squamous epithelium. Columnar epithelium occurring on the surface of the vagina may similarly be replaced by squamous metaplasia, giving rise to an epithelium so differentiated that it cannot be distinguished from the native squamous epithelium of the vagina. Both the metaplastic and the columnar epithelium relating to vaginal adenosis may be exposed to the same stimuli that induced precancerous changes in the uterine cervix. As a result, the lesions believed to be evolutionary changes of carcinogenesis may also occur in the vagina. Changes resembling dysplasia and carcinoma in situ have been described in association with adenosis, but the number of reported cases is small, and there is no conclusive evidence that they are more common in the DES-exposed woman than in unexposed controls. The available evidence suggests that there are several possible eventualities for the woman developing adenosis; the relative likelihood of an undesirable outcome, however, is still not established.

Many physicians used DES in the management of the high-risk pregnancy patient beginning in the late 1940s and early 1950s. In some institutions this practice has continued until a few years ago. In view of the recent studies establishing a relationship between DES exposure in utero and clear cell adenocarcinoma of the vagina and the increased likelihood for the development of adenosis, there is justification for examining all exposed women.

CLINICAL MANAGEMENT OF EXPOSED FEMALES.—Close follow-up and observation of the DES-exposed female population is indicated. Yearly follow-up should be required for those whose initial pelvic examination is normal. If adenosis or a significant cervical erosion is found, follow-up two or three times yearly appears reasonable. Preliminary evidence suggests that local progesterone therapy may accelerate the healing of vaginal adenosis, but this requires confirmation, and progesterone cannot be recommended as therapy at this time.

It has also been suggested that acidification of the vagina may promote the healing of adenosis but, again, no long-term confirmation of this observation has been published.

Excision of all areas of vaginal adenosis in DES-exposed females has been performed by some on the assumption that such a procedure is justified by the risk of the development of carcinoma in these areas. This procedure, however, does not seem appropriate at the present time. There is no evidence to suggest that this procedure protects the patient against the future development of cancer. Furthermore, the widespread adoption of such an approach would subject 90% to 95% of all DES-exposed females to extensive surgical therapy, much of which may be unnecessary. In cases in which nuclear atypicality or premalignant change in the epithelium of the vagina or cervix is apparent, locally destructive treatment by cautery, cryosurgery, or a cold-knife excision is indicated. Close follow-up of DES-exposed females who have no neoplastic genital changes, however, appears to be the most prudent approach.

SECONDARY CARCINOMA.—Secondary carcinoma is much commoner than primary cancer and is most often associated with metastases from the cervix, the endometrium, or the ovary. Cervical cancer may spread by direct contiguity, either along or underneath the epithelium, or possibly also by lymphatics. If it involves the upper vagina, the cervical cancer is then said to be stage IIa. The diagnosis must be made by visualization of the cervix, and exact details of the areas biopsied must be known, since the microscopic sections of the cervix and vagina may be identical. Frequently in cervical cancer there is spread along the uterosacral ligaments, which aids in making the differential diagnosis.

Endometrial cancer may also involve the vagina, although there is considerable speculation as to the exact mode of spread. These metastases are found most commonly in the vaginal vault and under the urethra and have been reported in about 10% of all patients with endometrial cancer. The tumor in the vault may be due to implantation at the time of hysterectomy or it may merely represent later growth of cancer cells that were under the vaginal mucosa in lymphatic or blood vessels at the time of surgery. The metastases under the urethra cannot be looked on as being due to implantation of cancer cells, but probably represent growth of tumor emboli that are trapped in the cross-circuit between the uterine and vaginal circulations. This is the area where the uterine blood supply ends and the pudendal begins. This same area is a common site for the metastatic vaginal lesions of hypernephromas, which must reach this area by vascular dissemination.

Ovarian carcinoma may occasionally invade the vagina by direct extension through the posterior cul-de-sac, and we have seen several large fungating masses that seemed to arise from the posterior vaginal wall but proved to be adenocarcinomas of a very anaplastic type. The finding of psammoma bodies in these microscopic sections suggested the ovarian origin of these lesions.

A variety of other metastatic carcinomas may be found in the vagina and will be diagnosed correctly only after biopsy, cystoscopy, proctoscopy, intravenous urograms, and x-rays of the colon. The commonest sites of the primary lesions are the rectum, bladder, urethra, breast, cecum, Skene's gland, Bartholin's glands, and left kidney. Blood-borne metastases from a hypernephroma of the left kidney may reach the vagina via the left ovarian vein, which drains into the left renal vein. The uterovaginal veins are secondarily involved from the ovarian vein. A choriocarcinoma may metastasize to the vagina; this lesion presents as a characteristic blue or dark red nodule or cystic mass, which may resemble a hemangioma. Biopsy of this mass may be the first indication of the exact nature of the disease process and may lead to diagnosis before pulmonary metastases are seen by x-ray. A malignant melanoma may occur in the vagina but is usually secondary to a melanoma of the skin, eye, or vulva. Although about a dozen apparently primary vaginal melanomas have been reported, it is imperative that a detailed search for another possible source be carried out. Teratomas also may involve the vagina but are usually secondary lesions.

Sarcoma

Sarcoma of the vagina is an extremely rare lesion, usually occurring as two major types: in childhood as sarcoma botryoides and in adult life as a dysontogenetic tumor of mixed-cell type. Sarcoma botryoides, a grapelike sarcoma, is usually found in infancy or early childhood although a few cases have been reported in later life. It is really a type of mixed mesodermal tumor with a rather loose-textured, but not too anaplastic, sarcomatous pattern mixed with embryonic striated muscle cells or masses of myxomatous tissue. It may arise from the cervix as well as from the vagina and it appears as a simple polypoid mass or a fungating, grape cluster protruding from the vagina. Despite the fairly differentiated cellular pattern the tumor is usually extremely malignant. Radical surgery has not

changed the poor prognosis. The incidence of polypoid masses of benign nature in the vaginas of children is so small that the mere presence should make one suspicious of sarcoma botryoides and biopsy should be done without hesitation.

The sarcoma occurring in adults is equally malignant although it may not be so easily discovered. It occurs as a mucosal type, which is raised, exophytic, and rapidly growing or as a deep or parietal type, which permeates the subvaginal mucosa rather extensively before ulcerating the surface. Histologically the tumor is of a mixed mesodermal variety and is thought to arise from displacements of embryonal anlage of the urogenital region. Thus it may contain striated muscle, smooth muscle, lipomatous material, cartilage, bone, and nerve tissue. In some cases the predominant cell type is of connective tissue variety, being either spindle cell, round cell, or a mixture. Hematogenous metastases usually occur to lungs, pleura, or brain and have fatal results in almost all instances.

BIBLIOGRAPHY

Anatomy

Anson B.J.: *An Atlas of Human Anatomy.* Philadelphia, W.B. Saunders Co., 1950, pp. 358–391.

Embryology

Jones H.W., Jones G.E.S.: The gynecological aspects of adrenal hyperplasia and allied disorders. *Am. J. Obstet. Gynecol.* 68:1330, 1954.

Koff A.K.: Development of the vagina in the human fetus, in *Contributions to Embryology.* Washington, D.C., Carnegie Institute, 1933, vol. 24.

Koff A.K.: Embryology of the female generative tract, in Curtis A.H. (ed.): *Obstetrics and Gynecology.* Philadelphia, W.B. Saunders Co., 1933.

Wilkins L., et al.: Further studies on treatment of congenital adrenal hyperplasia with cortisone. *J. Clin. Endocrinol. Metab.* 12:257, 1952.

Wilkins L.: Diagnosis of adrenogenital syndrome and its treatment with cortisone. *J. Pediatr.* 41:860, 1952.

Young H.H.: *Genital Abnormalities, Hermaphroditism and Related Adrenal Diseases.* Baltimore, Williams & Wilkins Co., 1937, pp. 23–45.

Physiology

DeAllende I.L.C., Orias O.: *Cytology of the Human Vagina.* New York, Paul B. Hoeber, Inc., 1950.

Lang W.H.: Vaginal acidity and pH: A review. *Obstet. Gynecol. Surv.* 10:546, 1955.

Infections

Gjonnaess H., Dalaker K., Anstead G., et al.: Pelvic inflammatory disease: Etiologic studies with emphasis on chlamydial infections. *Obstet. Gynecol.* 59:550, 1982.

Kistner R.W.: Vaginal infections, in Conn H.F. (ed.): *Current Therapy.* Philadelphia, W.B. Saunders Co., 1957.

Kundsin R.B.: Mycoplasma in genito-urinary tract infection and reproductive failure, in Sturgis S., Taymor M.L. (eds.): *Progress in Gynecology,* vol. 5. New York, Grune & Stratton, Inc., 1970.

McLennan M.T., Smith J.M., McLennan C.E.: Diagnosis of vaginal mycosis and trichomoniasis. *Obstet. Gynecol.* 40:231, 1972.

Pheifer T.A., Forsyth P.S., Durfee M.A., et al.: Nonspecific vaginitis—role of *Haemophilus vag-*

inalis and treatment with metronidazole. *N. Engl. J. Med.* 298:1429, 1978.

Zuspan F.: Management of patients with vaginal infections. *J. Reprod. Med.* 9:1, 1972.

Carcinoma

Bonney V., Glendining B.: Adenomatosis vaginae: A hitherto undescribed condition. *Proc. R. Soc. Med.* 4:18, 1911.

Burke L., Antonioli D., Knapp R.C., et al.: Vaginal adenosis: Correlation of colposcopic and pathologic findings. *Obstet. Gynecol.* 44:257, 1974.

Corcaden J.A.: *Gynecologic Cancer.* New York, Thomas Nelson & Sons, 1951.

Gilson M.D., Dibona D.D., Knab D.R.: Clear-cell adenocarcinoma in young females. *Obstet. Gynecol.* 41:494, 1973.

Greenwald P., Barlow J.J., Nasca P.C., et al.: Vaginal cancer after maternal treatment with synthetic estrogens. *N. Engl. J. Med.* 285:390, 1971.

Herbst A.L., Scully R.E.: Adenocarcinoma of the vagina in adolescents: A report of seven cases including six clear-cell carcinomas (so-called mesonephromas). *Cancer* 25:747, 1970.

Herbst A.L., Ulfelder H., Poskanzer D.C.: Adenocarcinoma of the vagina: Association of maternal stilbestrol therapy with tumor appearance in young women. *N. Engl. J. Med.* 284:878, 1971.

Herbst A.L., Kurman R.J., Scully R.E.: Vaginal and cervical abnormalities after exposure to stilbestrol in utero. *Obstet. Gynecol.* 40:287, 1973.

Herbst A.L., Robboy S.J., Scully R.E., et al.: Clear-cell adenocarcinoma of the vagina and cervix in girls: analysis of 170 registry cases. *Am. J. Obstet. Gynecol.* 119:713, 1974.

Kistner R.W.: Cervical carcinoma complicating procidentia. *Obstet. Gynecol.* 10:483, 1957.

Merrill J.A., Bender W.T.: Primary carcinoma of the vagina. *Obstet. Gynecol.* 11:3, 1958.

Plaut A.: Diffuse adenosis of vagina: A very rare disease, abstracted. *Am. J. Pathol.* 3:581, 1927.

Plaut A., Dreyfuss M.D.: Adenosis of vagina and its relation to primary adenocarcinoma of vagina. *Surg. Gynecol. Obstet.* 71:756, 1940.

Prangley A.G.: Premalignant lesions of the vagina. *Clin. Obstet. Gynecol.* 5:1119, 1962.

Ricci J.V., Lisa R.R., Thom C.H. Jr., et al.: The vagina in reconstructive surgery: A histologic study of its structural components. *Am. J. Surg.* 77:547, 1949.

Robboy S.J., Welch W.R., Young R.H., et al.: Topographic relation of cervical ectropion and vaginal adenosis to clear cell adenocarcinoma. *Obstet. Gynecol.* 60:546, 1982.

Rutledge F.: Cancer of the vagina. *Am. J. Obstet. Gynecol.* 97:635, 1967.

Sandberg E.C., Danielson R.W., Cauwet R.W., et al.: Adenosis vaginae. *Am. J. Obstet. Gynecol.* 93:209, 1965.

Sandberg E.C.: The incidence and distribution of occult vaginal adenosis. *Am. J. Obstet. Gynecol.* 101:322, 1968.

Sherman A.I., Goldrath M., Berlin A., et al.: Cervical-vaginal adenosis after in utero exposure to synthetic estrogens. *Obstet. Gynecol.* 44:531, 1974.

Smith F.R.: Primary carcinoma of the vagina. *Am. J. Obstet. Gynecol.* 69:525, 1955.

Stafl A., Mattingly R.F., Foley D.V., et al.: Clinical diagnosis of vaginal adenosis. *Obstet. Gynecol.* 43:118, 1974.

Tsukada Y., Hewett W.J., Barlow J.J., et al.: Clear-cell adenocarcinoma (mesonephroma) of the vagina: Three cases associated with maternal synthetic nonsteroid estrogen therapy. *Cancer* 29:1208, 1972.

Von Preuschen: Ueber Cystenbildung in der Vagina. *Archiv. J. Pathol. Anat. Physiol. Virchow* 70:111, 1877.

Way S.: *Malignant Disease of the Female Genital Tract.* Philadelphia, Blakiston Co., 1951.

Whelton J., Kottmeier H.L.: Primary carcinoma of the vagina. *Acta Obstet. Gynecol. Scand.* 41:22, 1962.

CHAPTER FOUR

The Cervix

HOWARD M. GOODMAN, M.D.
C. THOMAS GRIFFITHS, M.D.
ROBERT C. KNAPP, M.D.

EMBRYOLOGY

ALTHOUGH THE embryonic development of the cervix remains a poorly understood and controversial subject, newly acquired knowledge in this area provides some insight into the histologic and anatomic processes fundamental to its pathogenesis. The cervix as an embryologic entity does not begin to develop until the early fetal period at about 12 weeks' gestation, yet its origin is intimately associated with the earlier development of the entire müllerian system.

The müllerian (paramesonephric) duct system begins to develop in the fourth week as an invagination of the coelomic epithelium lateral to the wolffian (mesonephric) duct (see Chapter 3). Initially, these paired ducts run caudally, but they then turn medially to meet in the midline at six weeks' gestation, at which point they again run caudally to reach the urogenital sinus at approximately eight weeks' gestation (Fig 4–1). The point of contact between the now-fused müllerian ducts and the urogenital sinus enlarges to form the müllerian tubercle, with the wolffian ducts entering the sinus immediately lateral to the tubercle.

Evagination of the sinus between the wolffian ducts and the müllerian tubercle produces the sinovaginal bulbs, which proliferate to form the vaginal plate or vaginal cord. This solid plate advances in a caudal-cranial direction, obliterating the fused müllerian ducts (vaginal canal) as the müllerian epithelium degenerates. At 11 weeks' gestation, cavitation commences, again in a caudal-cranial direction, thereby creating the vaginal lumen. At the same time, a constriction appears between the developing corpus and cervix, with the cervix identifiable by a fusiform thickening of the surrounding mesenchyme (Fig 4–2). Cranial proliferation of the vaginal plate around the developing cervix forms the vaginal fornices, which are well delineated by the 21st week.

Just prior to the time of proliferation of the vaginal plate, the original müllerian epithelium of the vaginal canal is replaced by a pseudostratified epithelium, still of müllerian origin. Canalization of the vagina results in a stratified squamous epithelium, the origin of which remains in dispute. Koff suggested that the lower fifth of the vaginal epithelium is derived from the urogenital sinus and the remainder from transformed müllerian epithelium, whereas Bulmer proposed that sinus and müllerian epithelium are histologically distinct and that the vaginal epithelium is derived completely from sinus epithelium. Forsberg, using histochemical methods, postulated a wolffian origin for the vaginal lining. This investigator later showed in animals that inhibiting stratification of the original müllerian epithelium by estrogens caused heterotopic columnar epithelium to form in the

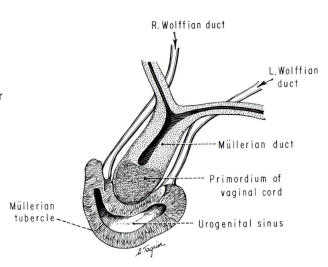

Fig 4–1.—Formation of the lower vagina. The müllerian tubercle is formed as the terminal ends of the müllerian ducts impinge on the urogenital sinus. Thus, the vagina has a double origin: from the müllerian tubercle and from outgrowths of the urogenital sinus.

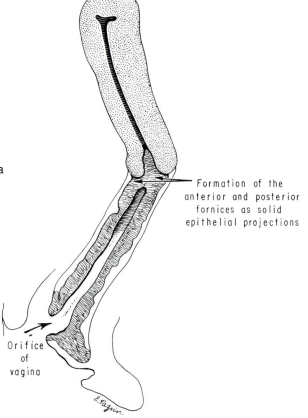

Fig 4–2.—Formation of upper vagina in the 151-mm embryo. At this stage the cranial end of the vagina contains two solid epithelial projections, which become the anterior and posterior fornices.

adult vagina—a response highly suggestive of the adenosis associated with diethylstilbestrol (DES) exposure. The origin of the adult vaginal epithelium would seem to play no part in this presumed mechanism of stilbestrol teratogenesis.

The origin of the endocervical mucosa is likewise controversial. Fluhmann postulated that the upward growth of vaginal squamous epithelium, which he believed was of sinus origin, extended into the endocervix, with subsequent columnar transformation. In contrast, Song felt that the endocervical columnar epithelium is a product of endocervical stromal cells that have been transformed from endometrial cells. Most authors, however, favor a müllerian origin for the endocervical mucosa.

Abnormalities in the development or fusion

of one or both müllerian ducts may result in malformations of the cervix. These include a double cervix with a septate or bicornuate uterus in conjunction with a normal or double vagina; a double cervix with uterus didelphys; or, rarely, complete atresia of the cervix (Fig 4–3).

In any discussion of the embryology of the cervix, mention should be made of the importance of *mesonephric remnants*. Characteristically, these structures are found as minute tubules or canaliculi in the lateral cervical wall. They are lined with nonciliated simple columnar or cuboidal cells having translucent cytoplasm and large, round nuclei. Huffman has confirmed the earlier work of Robert Meyer by examining serial sections of approximately 1,200 cervices and finding these remnants of the fetal mesonephros in about 1%;

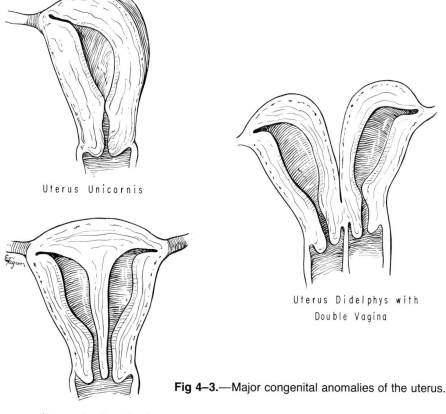

Uterus Unicornis

Uterus Septus Duplex

Uterus Didelphys with Double Vagina

Fig 4–3.—Major congenital anomalies of the uterus.

Meyer had previously reported an incidence of 20%. Bizarre tumors, both benign and malignant, may arise from these remnants and may prove to be histogenetically confusing if their origin is not appreciated.

ANATOMY

The cervix (Latin, "neck") is the narrowed, most caudad portion of the uterus (Fig 4–4). Somewhat conical in shape, it has a truncated apex that is directed downward and backward. It measures approximately 2.5 to 3.0 cm in length in the adult nulligravid and is contiguous above with the inferior aspect of the uterine corpus; the point of juncture is known as the isthmus. The vagina is attached obliquely around the center of the cervical periphery, thus dividing the cervix into two segments—an upper, supravaginal portion and a lower, vaginal portion. The cervix enters the vagina at an angle through the anterior vaginal wall and, in the normal situation, its vaginal portion is in contact with the posterior vaginal wall. The supravaginal segment of the cervix is separated anteriorly from the bladder by a layer of endopelvic fascia, the pubovesicocervical fascia. Laterally, at the same level, the cervix is in continuity with the paracervical ligaments or cardinal ligaments of Mackenrodt, which contain the uter-

ine blood vessels. Posteriorly, the supravaginal cervix is covered by peritoneum as it reflects off the uterosacral ligaments downward toward the vaginal apex.

The vaginal portion *(portio vaginalis, exocervix, ectocervix,* or *anatomic portio)* projects into the upper vagina between the anterior and posterior fornices as a convex prominence of elliptical shape. A small aperture, usually round or slitlike in the nullipara, is in the center of the projection and constitutes the anatomic external os. This orifice joins the uterine cavity with the vagina and is surrounded by the anterior and posterior lips.

The cervical canal extends from the anatomic os to the internal os, where it connects with the uterine cavity. It is somewhat fusiform, or spindle-shaped, measuring approximately 8 mm at its greatest width. Anterior and posterior longitudinal ridges may be evident on the walls of the canal, representing the lines of fusion of the müllerian ducts. Fanning out laterally from these ridges is a series of mucosal folds (plicae palmatae) that resemble the branches of a tree. When these are hypertrophied, insertion of a uterine sound or dilator may be hindered, since these longitudinal ridges may simulate a passage in the canal.

The isthmus is defined as that area of the uterus between the anatomic internal os

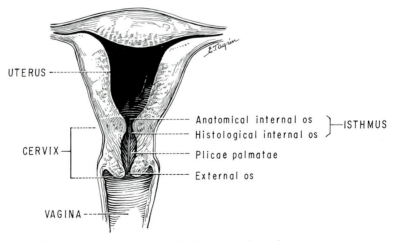

Fig 4–4.—Frontal section of uterine cervix and corpus.

above and the histologic internal os below. The latter is defined as the area of transition from endometrial to endocervical glands. The isthmic musculature is somewhat thinner than that of the corpus, thereby facilitating effacement and dilation during labor. This area is frequently referred to as the lower uterine segment during pregnancy and labor.

The uterine artery constitutes the major blood supply to the cervix, reaching its lateral walls within the cardinal ligaments (as noted previously). The venous drainage mirrors the arterial system. The cervical lymphatics, which are described in greater detail later, drain primarily laterally to the hypogastric, obturator, and external iliac nodes but also anteriorly to the posterior bladder wall nodes and posteriorly to the presacral nodes. Innervation of the cervix arises from the superior, middle, and inferior hypogastric plexuses and is primarily limited to the endocervix and the deeper areas of the exocervix. This accounts for the relative insensitivity to pain of the exocervix.

HISTOLOGY

An oversimplified consideration of the normal histology of the cervix would consist only of descriptions of its squamous and columnar epithelia and their subjacent stroma. However, of particular significance in the pathogenesis of cervical neoplasia is the area of transition between these two epithelial types. Thus, according to Johnson, it is most appropriate to discuss cervical histology and histopathology in terms of three histologic zones: the histologic portio, the transitional or transformation zone, and the histologic endocervix.

HISTOLOGIC PORTIO.—The histologic portio is defined as cervical stroma devoid of glands and covered by stratified squamous epithelium (Fig 4–5). This epithelium is 15 to 20 cells in thickness and demonstrates a progressive and orderly maturation from the lowermost basal layer through the prickle-cell layer to the superficial zone, where cornification occurs under estrogenic stimulation.

The basal layer (stratum germinativum), which is responsible for epithelial regeneration, consists of a single row of small cylindrical cells with large nuclei and scanty cytoplasm. Mitotic figures may occasionally be seen. Above the basal cells is a layer of larger polyhedral cells, four to ten cells in thickness, arranged in an irregular mosaic pattern and

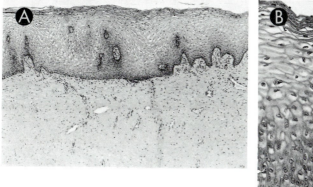
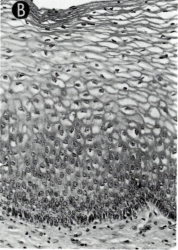

Fig 4–5.—A, normal exocervix (× 50). **B,** high-power magnification to show process of stratification and cornification (× 150).

interconnected by numerous tonofilament-desmosomal complexes. These characteristic intercellular bridges have led to the designation *prickle cells*, while their location has led to the designation *parabasal cells*. The cytoplasmic basophilia seen in these first two cell types is attributed to their ribonucleic acid (RNA) content. The beginning of cytoplasmic glycogenization is seen in the parabasal layer.

Above the prickle cells is a layer of larger oval or navicular cells with relatively small nuclei. These cells are involved in ascending maturation, during which nuclear size remains constant while cytoplasmic volume gradually increases. This layer has been called the intermediate, clear cell, or navicular zone. The most superficial layer, or stratum corneum, consists of flattened, elongated cells with small pyknotic nuclei. These are the cornified cells or squames seen in cytologic smears. The superficial and intermediate cells are rich in glycogen but appear clear in histologic sections, since the glycogen is washed out during fixation.

The basal layer is usually quite regular and does not show the rete peg formation seen in the vulva and vagina. The cervical squamous epithelium rests on a basement membrane, which is inconsistently seen under the light microscope and appears to consist of condensed stromal collagen. The underlying fibrous connective tissue stroma contains a lush capillary network at the epithelial junction, with scattered papillae extending upward into the epithelium.

TRANSFORMATION ZONE.—The transformation zone, found in the majority of uncauterized cervices during the childbearing years, lies between the histologic portio and the endocervical mucosa and consists of endocervical stroma and glands covered by squamous epithelium. The squamous epithelium comes to lie on the endocervical stroma as a result of several physiologic or pathologic processes to be described later. Although these processes cause upward displacement of the squamocolumnar junction, the junction between the

histologic portio and the transformation zone can be termed the original squamocolumnar junction. As can be seen in Figure 4–6, by the location of the numbered arrows, the transformation zone may lie above or below the anatomic external os.

HISTOLOGIC ENDOCERVIX.—The histologic endocervix is lined by a single layer of tall columnar epithelial cells characterized by dense, basal nuclei and pale pink-staining cytoplasm in standard hematoxylin-eosin preparations (Fig 4–7). Two cell types are present in this epithelium: the more prevalent mucus-secreting cells and scattered ciliated cells located in patches within the cervical canal and in gland orifices. The slight variation in height of these cells gives the appearance of a picket fence in histologic sections. These endocervical glands, as demonstrated by Fluhmann, are actually formed by complex, cleftlike infoldings of the epithelium, which appear as simple glandular units in histologic section. Although this concept renders the term "gland" a misnomer, reference to endocervical "glands" will most likely persist. The cleft arrangement increases the surface area of the endocervical mucosa, thereby permitting increased production of mucus, the secretion of which is dependent on estrogen. Maximal production and secretion occurs prior to ovulation, and in certain patients true mucorrhea exists.

For some years the location of cervical lesions, particularly those of a neoplastic nature, has been a matter of controversy between clinicians and pathologists. This is a consequence of the erroneous assumption that an anatomic area is synonymous with a histologic zone of the same designation. For example, the clinician defines a lesion of the portio as one existing on that area of the cervix that can be visualized with a speculum; the pathologist, on the other hand, defines a lesion of the portio as one arising in the squamous epithelium of the histologic portio. A lesion arising in the transformation zone (overlying endocervical glands) or in the columnar

HISTOLOGIC ZONES

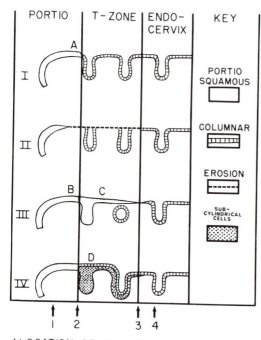

LOCATION OF ANATOMIC EXTERNAL OS

Fig 4–6.—Schematic relationship of the histologic zones to anatomic areas as determined by the location of the anatomic external os. The histologic zones are the portio, transformation zone, and endocervix. The anatomic areas are the portio (to the left of any given arrow) and the endocervix (to the right of any given arrow). The four types of squamocolumnar junction are: (I) normal; (II) pathologic erosion; (III) erosion healing by squamous epithelialization; and (IV) reserve (subcolumnar) cell metaplasia, which becomes squamous metaplasia after sloughing of the overlying columnar cells. Possible sites of origin of carcinoma in situ are: (A) basal cells of the portio epithelium; (B) basal cells of the portio epithelium at the margin of an old pathologic erosion; (C) basal cells of squamous epithelialization; (D) reserve cells within the transformation zone. (From Johnson L.D., et al.: *Cancer* 17:213, 1964.)

epithelium may thus be classified pathologically as endocervical even though it is located on the anatomic portio. Obviously the anatomic location of a lesion must be clearly distinguished from its histologic location.

This relationship between histologic zones and anatomic areas depends on the position of the external os with reference to the histologic zones (Fig 4–6). If the external os lies at arrow 2 in Figure 4–6, the anatomic portio and histologic portio are the same in all four variations of the squamocolumnar junction. If the external os lies at arrow 3, the anatomic portio will consist of histologic portio and either histologic endocervix (Fig 4–6,I) or transformation zone (Fig 4–6,III and IV). With the external os at arrow 4, all three histologic zones will be present on the anatomic portio.

It is important that clinicians be aware of the fact that the majority of early neoplastic cervical lesions in women of childbearing age occur on the anatomic portio, where they are readily available for biopsy. Again, it should be emphasized that histopathologic reports indicating that the majority of these lesions occur in the endocervix refer only to their histologic position.

From the anatomic and histologic characteristics described above, it is obvious that the cervix differs from the corpus in several important ways:

1. The cervix has only a small surface covered by peritoneum.

2. Approximately 85% of the cervix is made up of fibrous connective tissue.

3. There are no cervical venous sinuses.

4. Cervical mucosa does not undergo marked menstrual change as does the endometrium, although there are some cyclic changes dependent on estrogen and progesterone.

5. The vaginal cervix is covered by stratified squamous epithelium.

PHYSIOLOGY

The cervix functions passively as a segment of the birth canal and as a channel for the ex-

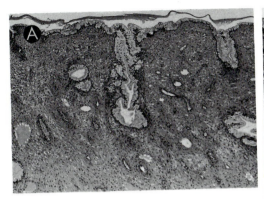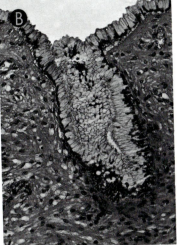

Fig 4–7.—A, normal endocervix (×50). **B,** high-power magnification to show typical high columnar epithelium (×150).

itus of menstrual discharge. Its primary physiologic function is the secretion of mucus, which facilitates the transport of spermatozoa and subsequently acts as a plug to seal off the gravid uterine cavity from the external environment.

This cervical mucus is subject to profound cyclic changes in relation to the levels of circulating ovarian hormones. In the immediate postmenstrual phase when the circulatory level of estrogen is low, and in the postovulatory period under the influence of progesterone, the cervical mucus is sparse, thick, and viscid. If allowed to dry on a slide, abundant vaginal and cervical cells, leukocytes, and mucus particles can be seen. From the eighth day of the cycle until ovulation, under the stimulation of rising levels of estrogen, the amount of mucus increases, its viscosity decreases, and it becomes highly permeable to spermatozoa. Just prior to ovulation, the mucus is glassy, transparent, and highly elastic. The term *spinnbarkeit* has been applied to this characteristic elasticity. If allowed to dry on a slide, the mucus assumes the form of fern or palm leaves with few notable cellular elements (Fig 4–8).

FERN TEST TECHNIQUE.—The specimen of mucus should be aspirated from the external

os after initial dry cleansing. The mucus is permitted to air dry for 10 to 20 minutes and is then examined under magnification of approximately ×100. False-positive fern test results are possible if (1) the aspirating tube is wet, (2) salt solution rather than distilled water has been used for cleaning or sterilizing the tube, or (3) excessive blood is mixed with the mucus.

Mucus secretions and most body fluids show the phenomenon of "ferning" or "arborization" in the dried state, which seems to represent a special form of crystallization of sodium chloride in the medium of drying cervical mucus. Although ferning per se is a nonspecific process, its occurrence in cervical mucus does depend on adequate estrogenic stimulation.

From a clinical point of view, examination of cervical mucus is a simple test of ovarian function. In the human castrate, small amounts of exogenous estrogen will cause arborization, whereas progesterone modifies this action of estrogen. In amenorrheic patients a persistently negative fern test result suggests insufficient estrogenic stimulation. In hypothalamic amenorrhea, this reaction may be reversed by the administration of estrogens, but in the amenorrhea of pregnancy exogenous estrogens will not produce ferning.

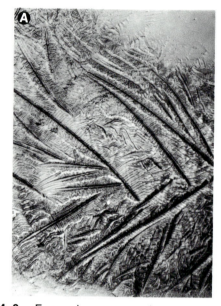

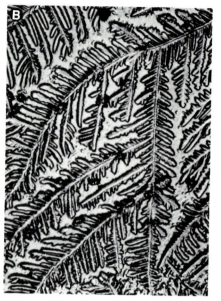

Fig 4–8.—Fern phenomenon in cervical mucus during the normal menstrual cycle between days 12 and 16. **A,** low power; **B,** high power. (Courtesy of Dr. Maxwell Roland.)

Although the logical conclusion as to the mechanism involved in pregnancy is that high progesterone levels negate the estrogen effect, investigation has shown that the cervical cells during pregnancy do not permit permeation of electrolytes. It may be that the effect of progesterone is to prevent imbibition of sodium chloride by the endocervical cells.

PHYSIOLOGIC ALTERATIONS

Changes in Endocervical Mucosa

Since the uterine cervix has become a focal point for the histologic and colposcopic study of oncogenesis considerable light has been shed on its response to several physiologic processes. Thus, many of the gross and microscopic variations previously considered to be pathologic are now regarded as normal physiologic alterations. Prominent among these are *prolapse of endocervical mucosa* onto the anatomic portio. It now appears that this cervical erosion is related to age, the first pregnancy, and estrogenic stimulation. The term *cervical erosion,* however, incorrectly implies

epithelial denudation and is more properly called *eversion* or *ectropion.*

One of the most significant contributions to our understanding of cervical eversions as well as to eliminating the confusion about anatomic areas vs. histologic zones was made by Schneppenheim and associates. They examined 853 unselected uteri and showed that the length of the gland-bearing endocervical mucosa is relatively constant throughout life; however, the location of endocervical mucosa in relation to the anatomic cervical canal varies with age. During the childbearing years, endocervical glands are found just below the internal os and extend to just below the external os, i.e., onto the anatomic portio, creating this so-called cervical erosion (Fig 4–6, arrows 3 and 4). After age 40 years, as a result of waning ovarian activity, the endocervical mucosa ascends the canal so that during the menopausal years the lowest glands, the original squamocolumnar junction, and the transformation zone are at or above the anatomic external os (Fig 4–6, arrows 1 and 2). Schneppenheim et al. attribute the downward shift

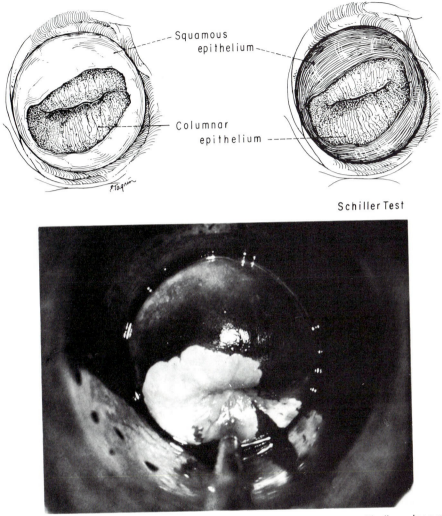

Schiller Test

Fig 4–9.—Application of Schiller's solution will stain the normal squamous epithelium dark brown. Endocervical epithelium does not stain.

and eversion of the endocervix to an increase in volume of the mucosa during the years when estrogen stimulation was maximal. This is certainly in agreement with Coppleson and Reid and with Song, and explains the increase in eversions noted after the first pregnancy (Fig 4–9).

During the latter part of intrauterine development, there is accelerated cervical growth activity, attributed to the high levels of cir-

culating estrogens; such growth is not shared by the corpus. At birth the cervix-to-corpus ratio may approach 3:1. After birth there is a rapid regression in cervical length, thereby returning to the more normal cervix-to-corpus ratio seen in the adult. During the third trimester the endocervical cells change from cuboidal to tall columnar with evidence of mucin secretion, and the mucosa deeply infolds into the stroma to form clefts or glands,

as previously described. This excessive *proliferation of endocervical mucosa* after the 28th week produces the congenital eversion seen in 50% of female neonates. In contrast, the endometrium is incompletely developed, usually inactive, and presents only a few tubular glands. Squamous cells of the endocervix in the newborn are likewise affected by maternal estrogens, since they are well stratified and contain abundant glycogen. At puberty, with the stimulation of estrogen from the developing ovarian follicles, these changes presumably occur again, although adequate morphologic studies in this age group are lacking.

Squamous Metaplasia and Epithelialization

In marked contrast is the cervix seen during childhood and during the menopause, two periods when circulating estrogen levels are low. The squamous epithelium is thin and atrophic, with loss of cellular maturation and an absence of glycogen. The squamocolumnar junction is out of view within the cervical canal (as described above).

Two mechanisms for replacement of the endocervical eversion by squamous epithelium have been proposed as the histogenesis of the transformation zone. Since virtually all cases of cervical squamous neoplasia originate in the transformation zone, its histogenesis provides insight into the oncogenesis of cervical neoplasia.

The first mechanism is termed *squamous metaplasia*, which is the result of a process known as subcolumnar "reserve cell" metaplasia. These reserve cells are undifferentiated spherical or polygonal cells with plump, centrally placed, dark-staining nuclei and scant cytoplasm. They come to lie beneath the columnar epithelium, and their origin is controversial. It has been proposed that they are derived from (1) embryonal rests of urogenital sinus epithelium, (2) direct or indirect metaplasia of columnar cells, (3) basal cells of the portio, or (4) stromal cells. Coppleson and Reid suggest that the metaplastic process is initiated by the exposure of the endocervical mucosa to the lower pH of the vagina and that estrogen plays a crucial role by promoting endocervical hyperplasia and prolapse and acidifying the vaginal environment. In support of this mechanism is work done by Hellman and associates who found a striking increase in reserve cell hyperplasia and metaplasia after the administration of large doses of estrogen to postmenopausal women.

The probable sequence of events in the metaplastic process may be outlined as follows:

1. Endocervical eversion.
2. Reserve cell hyperplasia (Fig 4–10,A).
3. Reserve cell metaplasia and stratification (Fig 4–10,B).
4. Sloughing of overlying columnar epithelium.
5. Differentiation into a multilayered immature squamous epithelium.
6. Differentiation into a mature stratified squamous epithelium.

The end point of the metaplastic process is differentiation into squamous epithelium that is indistinguishable from native squamous epithelium. The more commonly seen immature metaplastic epithelium is characterized by its lack of surface maturation and glycogen and is usually sharply demarcated from the adjacent portio. Particularly active squamous metaplasia filling multiple glands may be confused with carcinoma in situ, although hyperchromatism, nuclear atypia, and abnormal mitotic activity are not seen.

The second mechanism by which squamous epithelium comes to overlie endocervical stroma has been termed *squamous epidermization or epidermalization*. Since the analogy to skin is somewhat remote, Johnson's preference for the term *squamous epithelialization* is more appropriate. The initiating event may be a true pathologic erosion of the distal endocervix (see Fig 4–6,II) followed by an ingrowth or overglide of portio squamous cells.

In the early stages of this process, the squamous epithelium may be seen as a tenuous

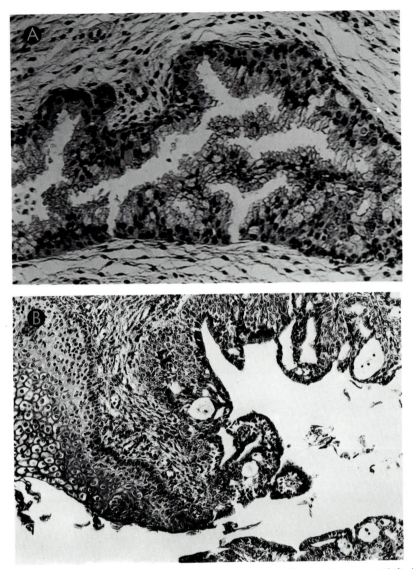

Fig 4–10.—A, hyperplasia of reserve cells in the endocervix. **B,** squamous metaplasia from reserve cells of the endocervix occurring at the histologic external os. Normal stratified squamous epithelium is seen at left. (Courtesy of Dr. Louis M. Hellman and Dr. Alexander Rosenthal.)

strand of immature squamous cells gradually decreasing in height as they are stretched over an otherwise denuded and inflamed stroma. Later observers have shown that the squamous epithelium of the portio may grow beneath the adjacent, intact endocervical epithelium, with loss of the overlying columnar cells on maturation and stratification of the squamous elements. As with many reparative and regenerative processes, mitotic activity with associated basal cell hyperplasia may be considerable, although the atypia of malignancy is absent. Extension of the new epithelium over the mouth of the endocervical gland may result in occlusion and formation of mucinous retention (nabothian) cysts. These are grossly visible on the portio as spherical elevations or small cysts 2 to 10 mm in diameter (Fig 4–11). Microscopically the cystic space is seen to be lined with low cuboidal or flattened endocervical cells.

PATHOLOGIC ALTERATIONS

Chronic Cervicitis

From the time of the earliest clinical and microscopic descriptions of cervical disease, inflammation or, more specifically, chronic cervicitis has been a ubiquitous finding. Either alone or coexisting with other diseases it has been implicated in the pathogenesis of cervical eversion, squamous metaplasia, basal cell hyperplasia, leukoplakia, polyps, and carcinoma. Although Song's criteria for the diagnosis of chronic cervicitis are the presence of epithelial necrosis and neutrophilic infiltration, leukocytic infiltration was found in 98% of 400 cervices examined by Howard. Chronic cervicitis is noted in nearly every specimen of cervical tissue examined at Brigham and Women's Hospital, and has been described in the cervices of newborns and young children. Extensive attempts to confirm bacteriologically that cervical infection is the etiology of chronic cervicitis have rarely revealed pathogenic organisms. Rather, a physiologic role for this infiltrate has been suggested—the removal of dead cells resulting from the metaplastic process.

Clinically the presenting symptoms of chronic cervicitis are a thick, tenacious yellowish-white vaginal discharge with postcoital or postdouche spotting or bleeding. Complaints of pelvic pressure, dyspareunia, or

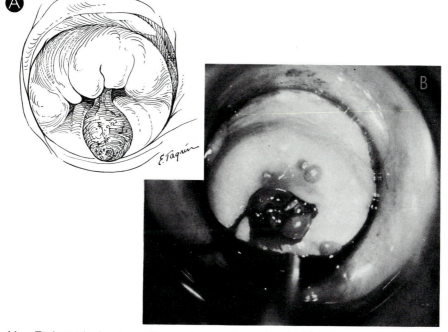

Fig 4–11.—Endocervical polyps. **A,** a solitary polyp protruding through the external os. **B,** several endocervical polyps occluding the exocervix. Several nabothian (mucous) cysts are seen on the portio epithelium.

dysmennorrhea suggest that the inflammatory process has extended to the paracervical tissues. Inspection reveals a beefy, friable cervix with a mucopurulent discharge. On culture this may reveal normal commensals or such organisms as *Staphylococcus, Streptococcus,* or *Escherichia coli,* the clinical significance of which remains in question.

A tentative diagnosis can be made on inspection; however, biopsy and tissue diagnosis are mandatory to rule out cervical neoplasia, which can present with a similar clinical picture. The inflammation and bleeding associated with chronic cervicitis render Papanicolaou smears unreliable in excluding carcinoma. Once carcinoma has been excluded, reassurance is usually all that is needed for the patient with the signs and symptoms of chronic cervicitis. If the symptoms are unacceptable or if this abnormal cervical mucus is felt to play a causative role in infertility, treatment is indicated. Radial hot cauterization, a previous method of treatment for this condition, has been replaced by cryocautery, which converts the boggy, friable cervix into one that closely resembles that of a nullipara (Fig 4–12).

Acute Cervicitis

Acute inflammation of the cervix may result from infection by specific microorganisms; as a response to trauma, malignant disease, or radiotherapy; or as one manifestation of a systemic inflammatory disease such as Behçet's syndrome or polyarteritis nodosa. The cervix appears hyperemic and swollen, and an accompanying purulent discharge is usually present. Histologically, stromal edema with a polymorphonuclear infiltrate and mucosal ulceration is seen. Treatment consists of avoiding instrumentation and interdicting coitus, limitation of activity, medicated douches or creams, or specific systemic antibiotic therapy depending on the type and sensitivity of the responsible organism.

The most common etiology of acute cervicitis is infection with *Neisseria gonorrhoeae.* Stratified squamous epithelium is relatively resistant to gonococcal infection, which is usually limited in uncomplicated cases to involvement of the endocervix, urethra, and rectum. Ascending infection may occur, with extension to the endometrium, fallopian tube, and ovarian and peritoneal surfaces producing pelvic inflammatory disease in approximately 15% of women with cervical infection. Gonococcal endocervicitis may be asymptomatic in as many as 50% of affected women. In the other 50%, the usual symptomatology includes vaginal discharge, dysuria, urinary frequency, labial tenderness, and dyspareunia.

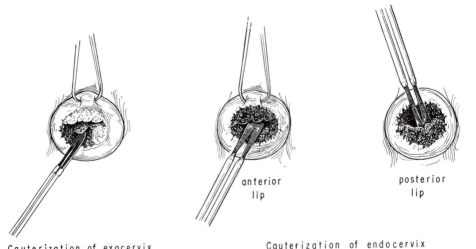

Cauterization of exocervix   Cauterization of endocervix

anterior lip   posterior lip

Fig 4–12.—Cauterization of the cervix using the hot cautery. This technique is of historical interest only, having been replaced by cryocautery and the carbon dioxide laser.

Speculum examination reveals an erythematous cervix with a thick, purulent discharge. Diagnosis requires culture techniques, since Gram stain has a sensitivity of only 50% in gonococcal cervicitis. Treatment consists of administration of the appropriate antibiotic.

During the past decade the role of *Chlamydia trachomatis* in the pathogenesis of genital tract disease has become well established. As many as 66% of women seen at venereal disease clinics may harbor *Chlamydia* in their cervices. Infection may be asymptomatic, may be limited to the cervix, or may ascend to cause pelvic inflammatory disease. Examination reveals a follicular cervicitis that can be seen histologically to be produced by subepithelial lymphoid follicles. Diagnosis requires culture techniques or the presence of the characteristic intracytoplasmic inclusion bodies seen on Giemsa stains of cervical smears. Of concern is the fourfold increase in cervical neoplasia reported by Paavonen in cervices harboring *Chlamydia*. Although no etiologic role for *Chlamydia* in cervical neoplasia has been suggested, this observation merits further study.

Trichomonas vaginalis is a flagellated protozoan that attacks the squamous epithelium of the vagina and cervix, destroying the epithelial cells on contact. In response there is an outpouring of polymorphonuclear leukocytes and marked proliferation of small blood vessels, yielding the characteristic colposcopic appearance of looped or hairpin capillaries. Although this infection may be asymptomatic, the classic presentation is a profuse greenish-gray frothy vaginal discharge with pruritus, dysuria, and, occasionally, vaginal bleeding. Diagnosis is easily made by the presence of the flagellate on microscopic examination of the discharge diluted in normal saline (Fig 4–13). Culture may be required, since wet mounts will miss approximately 30% of infected women. The pH of the vagina is frequently somewhat alkaline in the presence of *T. vaginalis*. The association of abnormal Papanicolaou smears with trichomonal infections

has been well described. Cytologic and colposcopic abnormalities revert to normal with appropriate treatment.

Tuberculous cervicitis is seen in approximately 3% to 5% of all cases of genital tuberculosis. The affected cervix may appear entirely normal, exhibit erythema with a mucopurulent discharge, or be invaded by a fungating mass suggestive of carcinoma. Histologically, caseating or noncaseating granulomas may be seen. Diagnosis requires the demonstration of acid-fast bacilli by suitable staining techniques or by culture. The differential diagnosis of granulomatous cervicitis includes syphilis, lymphogranuloma venereum, granuloma inguinale, chancroid, sarcoid, schistosomiasis, and pinworm.

Viral Cervicitis

Herpesvirus hominis types 1 and 2, the etiologic agents of genital herpes, belong to the large group herpesviruses, which have been found in almost every animal species studied. These are large DNA viruses, with five members associated with disease in man: herpes simplex virus types 1 and 2 (HSV-1 and HSV-2), varicella-zoster virus, cytomegalovirus, and Epstein-Barr virus. Infection requires direct contact, with an incubation period ranging from 2 to 20 days and averaging six days. Clinically, herpes genitalis may be conveniently divided into either primary or recurrent infection—the former reserved for infection resulting from the first exposure to either herpes simplex type 1 or 2 and the latter for any subsequent infection.

Primary infection is not infrequently heralded by a prodromal phase with symptoms of headache, myalgias, malaise, and fever. Multiple painful vesicles appear, usually 1 to 2 mm in size, on an erythematous background; these rapidly erode and coalesce to form large ulcers. Cervical involvement occurs in 80% of primary infections and presents as nonspecific inflammation, vesicles, ulcers, or occasionally as a fungating mass indistinguishable from invasive carcinoma. Symptoms include vulvar and pelvic pain, dysuria, and vaginal dis-

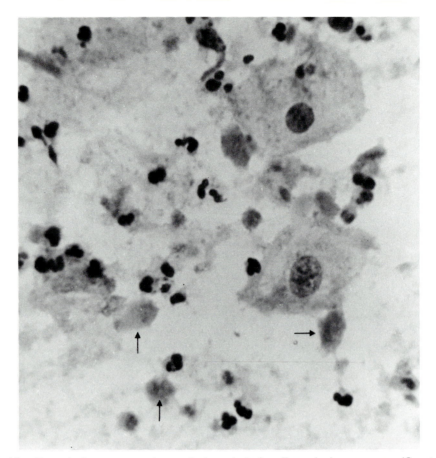

Fig 4–13.—Papanicolaou smear demonstrating *Trichomonas vaginalis* (×800). The characteristic pear-shaped protozoans with eccentrically placed, spindle-shaped nuclei are shown *(arrows).* The flagella are usually not well demonstrated on Papanicolaou smears. (Courtesy of Dr. Robert Ehrmann and the Division of Women's and Perinatal Pathology, Brigham and Women's Hospital, Boston.)

charge, the last seen especially with cervical involvement. Complete healing requires several weeks as symptoms and lesions slowly resolve.

Recurrent infection results from reactivation of latent virus thought to reside in sacral ganglia. Some 50% of patients experiencing an initial clinical episode of herpes genitalis will go on to suffer recurrences, with symptoms and signs usually less severe and of shorter duration than in the primary disease.

The clinical impression may be confirmed by culture technique, with characteristic cytopathic effects evident within one to two days; by serologic conversion following initial infection; or by cytologic methods demonstrating multinucleated giant cells or intranuclear viral inclusion bodies (Fig 4–14).

In addition to the neonatal risk associated with herpetic infection, Nahmias and others have implicated HSV in spontaneous abortion and premature labor. The association between HSV-2 and cervical neoplasia will be addressed later.

CONDYLOMAS.—The characteristic lesion

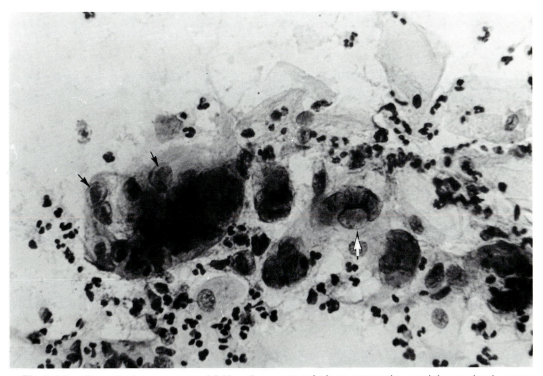

Fig 4–14.—Papanicolaou smear exhibiting the characteristic features of herpesvirus infection (×530). Intranuclear inclusions *(small arrows),* which may represent virus particles, and multinucleated giant cells are evident. Enlarged, ground-glass–appearing nuclei can also be seen *(large arrow).* (Courtesy of Dr. Robert Ehrmann and the Division of Women's and Perinatal Pathology, Brigham and Women's Hospital, Boston.)

of condyloma acuminatum, or venereal wart, is rarely found on the cervix (Fig 4–15). Only 254 cases were reported in the literature through 1974. It is caused by the human papillomavirus, a small DNA virus belonging to the Papovaviridae family, the only viruses proved to produce tumors in humans. Various subtypes have been associated with verruca vulgaris or the common wart, laryngeal papillomas, venereal warts, bladder papillomas, and epidermodysplasia verruciformis. The last is a rare disease in which large skin areas are covered with confluent flat warts that frequently undergo malignant degeneration. Microscopically the classic wart is characterized by papillomatosis, acanthosis, lengthening and thickening of the rete pegs, submucosal capillary proliferation, and the presence of koilocytes. Koilocytes were first described by Koss in 1956 and are now felt to be pathognomonic of human papillomavirus infection. They exhibit hyperchromasia, multinucleation, and perinuclear cytoplasmic vacuolization (Fig 4–16).

In 1977, Meisels et al. described two cervical lesions with koilocytotic atypia and other features suggestive of condylomas but without the typical gross papillary features. The "flat condyloma" is a flattened area of acanthosis with mild accentuation of the rete pegs and koilocytotic changes. They pointed out the striking contrast between the essentially normal-appearing deeper layers of the epithelium and the superficial areas that exhibit the koilocytosis. The second lesion he described is the endophytic or inverted condyloma,

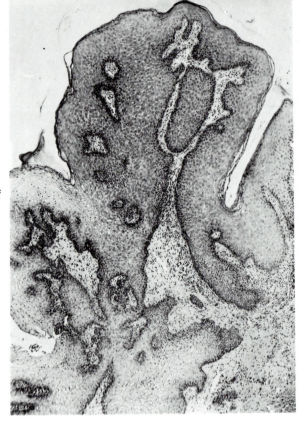

Fig 4–15.—Condyloma acuminatum of cervix. (From Kistner R.W., Hertig A.T.: *Obstet. Gynecol.* 6:147, 1955.)

which demonstrates gland involvement and may be mistaken for invasive carcinoma. These lesions are usually not visible without the aid of the colposcope, through which they can be seen to exhibit fine punctation on a white background.

Meisels reviewed 152 cervical smears diagnosed as mild dysplasia and found that 70% were suggestive of human papillomavirus infection, leading these authors to consider koilocytotic atypia to be an early phase in the natural history of cervical neoplasia. The relationship between condylomas and cervical carcinoma will be more fully discussed later. Condylomatous cervicitis is a very common disease, with 1% to 2% of all Papanicolaou smears exhibiting koilocytotic changes. Treatment consists of surgical excision or cauterization after invasive carcinoma has been adequately ruled out.

A special category of squamous papilloma is the giant condyloma of Buschke-Löwenstein. This rare tumor is grossly and microscopically similar to the classic venereal wart but clinically exhibits the features of a low-grade malignancy. Local therapeutic measures are usually inadequate; wide resection is the treatment of choice. It has been suggested that the giant condyloma represents an intermediate step in viral carcinogenesis between a benign condyloma and invasive carcinoma. The giant condyloma has not been reported to occur on the cervix.

Keratinization

Since keratinization is not a physiologic property of cervical squamous epithelium, any tendency in this direction must be considered abnormal, although some degree of

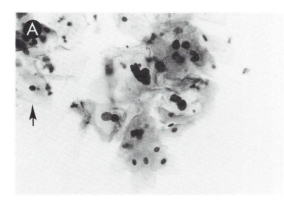

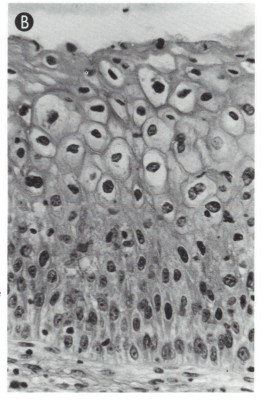

Fig 4–16.—A, koilocytes on a Papanicolaou smear (×320). The nuclei are hyperchromatic with characteristic perinuclear cytoplasmic vacuolization. Multinucleated forms are evident. A normal superficial cell is shown for comparison (arrow). **B,** flat condyloma (×530). Koilocytotic changes can be seen in the superficial layers. (Courtesy of Dr. Robert Ehrmann and the Division of Women's and Perinatal Pathology, Brigham and Women's Hospital, Boston.)

focal keratinization may occasionally be observed in the absence of other abnormalities. Hyperkeratosis and parakeratosis appear as white, raised plaques (leukoplakia), usually grossly visible on the portio. Hyperkeratosis microscopically exhibits a thickened layer of keratin, scant intraepithelial glycogen, and no cytologic atypia. It is not commonly seen except in cases of procidentia. Parakeratosis, the most common abnormality presenting as a white cervical lesion, exhibits similar features but with the retention of pyknotic nuclei in the keratin layer (Fig 4–17). There is no evidence to indicate that either hyperkeratosis or parakeratosis is premalignant; however, these histologic features may be associated with cervical neoplasia. Therefore, all white lesions of the cervix deserve biopsy for tissue diagnosis. Treatment of uncomplicated hyperkeratosis or parakeratosis is local excision or cauterization.

BENIGN NEOPLASMS

CERVICAL POLYPS.—Cervical polyps are usually derived from the endocervix as a result of a chronic papillary endocervicitis and present as soft, spherical, glistening red masses several millimeters to several centimeters in size (Fig 4–11). They are frequently quite friable and may be associated with profuse leukorrhea secondary to the underlying endocervicitis. Histologically, they are composed of endocervical epithelium with a fibrovascular stalk. The differential diagnosis includes (1) polypoid fragments of endocervical carcinoma or carcinosarcoma protruding through the os, (2) retained secundines, (3) the grapelike swellings of sarcoma botryoides that occasionally originate in the cervix, and (4) prolapsing submucous fibroids or endometrial polyps. Most cervical polyps can be grasped with a clamp and twisted free, with

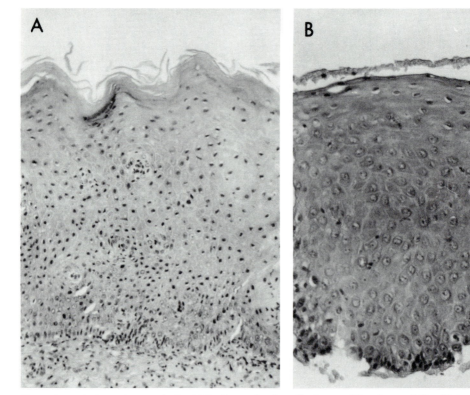

Fig 4–17.—A, hyperkeratosis (×120). Normal ascending cellular maturation with a thickened keratin layer can be seen. **B,** parakeratosis (×200). Pyknotic nuclei are evident within the keratin layer. (Courtesy of Dr. Robert Ehrmann and the Division of Women's and Perinatal Pathology, Brigham and Women's Hospital, Boston.)

the base cauterized for hemostasis. Certainly all cervical polyps should be submitted for pathologic evaluation, although malignant degeneration is extremely rare.

LEIOMYOMAS.—Leiomyomas or fibroids are the most common uterine tumors, with cervical involvement occurring in as many as 8% of cases. Cervical leiomyomas are grossly and histologically identical to those found in the corpus. Although they are frequently incidental findings on physical examination, they may cause bowel or bladder symptoms, dyspareunia, or dystocia in labor with excessive growth. Treatment for symptomatic fibroids is either myomectomy or hysterectomy.

ENDOMETRIOSIS.—Endometriosis of the cervix presents as red or reddish-blue vesicular lesions evident on the exocervix. They are usually asymptomatic but may cause dysmenorrhea or dyspareunia, which is most evident premenstrually. Biopsy specimens are best taken at this time for adequate pathologic interpretation. This pattern of endometriosis is frequently seen several months after cervical biopsy, cauterization, or trachelorrhaphy in menstruating women and thus suggests implantation as its etiology. However, areas of decidual reaction may occasionally be seen in the cervices of pregnant women who have not undergone any cervical procedures, suggesting that multipotential cells capable of responding to estrogen and progesterone are present in the cervical stroma. Infertility has been associated with extensive cervical endometriosis and is probably due to destruction of endocervical glands and decreased mucus production. After biopsy confirmation, treatment should consist of deep cauterization or excision.

Other less common benign tumors that may involve the cervix include hemangiomas, adenomyomas, fibroadenomas, fibromas, and lipomas.

CERVICAL NEOPLASIA

Five decades ago, carcinoma of the cervix was the leading cause of death from malignant disease in American women. Since 1940, however, the mortality rate from cervical carcinoma has declined by more than 50%, yet it still ranks sixth in cancer mortality, with estimates of 7,000 deaths each year in the United States. There are 16,000 new cases of invasive cervical carcinoma, with the peak in incidence between ages 45 to 55 years, and over 44,000 new cases of in situ cervical carcinoma discovered each year in the United States, accounting for over 60,000 women who require major and potentially morbid treatment annually. Despite the recognition of a significant preinvasive phase and availability of screening methods, cervical neoplasia remains a major health problem.

Epidemiology

Perhaps the earliest epidemiologic studies of cervical neoplasia were conducted in 1842 by Rigoni-Stern who showed that the incidence of cervical carcinoma was higher in married and widowed women and lower in never-married women and among nuns in certain religious orders. Since then, numerous epidemiologic studies looking at the association between cancer of the cervix and certain social factors have been reported (Table 4–1). In terms of greatest risk, the final common denominator seems to be related to *coitus* and more specifically to onset of regular sexual activity at an early age, and perhaps to

multiplicity of sexual partners. The higher incidence of cervical carcinoma in nonwhites compared with that in whites appears to be related to socioeconomic class, which may further be a function of early marriage and early childbearing. The interdependence of prostitution, sexually transmitted diseases, and coitus needs no clarification. Strongly supporting this concept is the rarity of cervical cancer in nuns, as noted by Rigoni-Stern and later by Gagnon.

The virtual absence of penile carcinoma among Jewish men suggested a relationship between *circumcision* and genital carcinoma, which was first studied in relation to cervical carcinoma by Handley in 1936. He demonstrated a lower incidence of this disease in one ethnic group of Fiji Islanders who practiced ritual circumcision compared with members of another ethnic group who did not. Support for this relationship came from work by Wahi in India, where, again, the incidence of this disease was significantly lower among ethnic groups practicing circumcision. The extremely low frequency of cervical carcinoma among Jewish women lends further support to the proposed protective effect of circumcision. It has been thought that the absence of smegma might account for this protective effect in that early studies indic-

TABLE 4–1.—ASSOCIATION
BETWEEN CERVICAL CANCER
AND SOCIAL FACTORS

Socioeconomic factors
  Poverty
  Race
Marital status
  Ever married vs. never married
  Marriage before age 20 years
  Multiple and broken marriages
Childbearing
  Multiparity
  First pregnancy before age 20 years
Sexual exposure
  First coitus before age 20 years
  Prostitution
  Sexually transmitted diseases
Smoking
Circumcision status

ated smegma to be carcinogenic in animals; however, later work has failed to confirm these findings. These epidemiologic observations have not as yet been adequately explained.

The role of the high-risk male was investigated by Kessler, who found a severalfold increase in risk for the development of cervical carcinoma among women whose husbands had previously been married to women with cervical carcinoma compared with a control population. Again, in reference to undefined social factors, wives of men of lower socioeconomic classes are several times more likely to be diagnosed as having cervical carcinoma than are women married to men in a higher socioeconomic class.

These epidemiologic studies clearly implicate a venereal transmission in cervical carcinoma. The recent interest in viral oncogenesis has suggested viruses as possible etiologic agents in cervical neoplasia.

The relationship between *HSV infections* and cervical cancer was first noted by Naib et al. in 1966 and has been examined intensively since then in an attempt to prove that HSV is an etiologic agent for cervical neoplasia. Numerous seroepidemiologic studies performed worldwide have revealed a significantly higher frequency and titer of HSV-2 antibodies in patients with cervical carcinoma compared with "controls." Criticisms of these earlier studies included the lack of suitable controls adequately matched for sexual history and the technical difficulty in differentiating exposure to HSV-1 from HSV-2, given the serologic techniques then available and the extent of antigenic cross-reactivity between these two viruses.

More recent studies using sensitive serologic methods and well-matched controls have confirmed this association. Nahmias and Sawanibani prospectively followed 870 women with a history of genital herpes and a control population of 562 women during a six-year period and found a twofold increase in cervical dysplasia and an eightfold increase in carcinoma in situ in the study population. Further serologic support came from the finding of antibodies to virus-associated antigens in those patients with cervical neoplasia compared with controls. Direct evidence for an association between cervical carcinoma and HSV-2 was the detection of viral DNA and RNA in carcinoma cells and, ultimately, the work of Aurelian, who demonstrated the release of infectious virus from carcinoma cells.

That herpesviruses may be oncogenic is no longer in question. Marek's disease, a lymphoproliferative disease of chickens, and Lücke's tumor, a renal adenocarcinoma in frogs, are now clearly related to herpes viruses. Although Wentz demonstrated malignant transformation in the mouse vagina by means of chronic exposure to HSV-2, absolute proof of the carcinogenicity of HSV-2 in humans has not been established.

Other investigators have looked at the role of *human papillomavirus* (HPV) in the pathogenesis of cervical neoplasia. This virus belongs to the Papovaviridae family, known to be oncogenic in numerous animal species as well as in humans. Malignant transformation of long-standing vulvar, vaginal, and rectal condylomatous lesions has been well described, as has that seen in epidermodysplasia verruciformis. These observations obviate mere postulation about a role for HPV in human carcinogenesis. The fact that condylomatous changes—koilocytotic atypia—are so frequently seen to coexist with cervical neoplasia as well as the histologic demonstration of transition between the two suggests a more than coincidental relationship between cervical neoplasia and HPV.

The epidemiology of cervical carcinogenesis suggests that the causative agent may be transmitted by or be associated with sexual intercourse and that the risk is inversely related to age and duration of exposure. According to the most popular theory, cervical carcinogenesis is thought to commence with an initiating event, such as exposure to an oncogenic virus, during the period of active squamous metaplasia. This is followed by promotion, which may represent continued exposure to the initiating factor or to a second carcinogen, yielding neoplasia. This theory would certainly explain why the vast majority of cervical neoplastic lesions are found in the transformation zone and correlates with the epidemiologic risk factors described.

Cervical Intraepithelial Neoplasia

Carcinoma in situ (CIS) may be defined as an intraepithelial lesion with cytologic atypia similar to that seen in invasive carcinoma but without evidence of invasion into the stroma (Fig 4–18). These atypical cells extend through the entire thickness of the epithelium and have enlarged, pleomorphic nuclei with dense, coarse chromatin and scant cytoplasm. The polarity of the cells as well as the polarity of the epithelium, i.e., the normal surface maturation and differentiation, is lost. Various degrees of parakeratosis may be seen.

Lesions composed of similar atypical cells but that retain some degree of surface maturation have been referred to as "dysplasias" by Reagan. Dysplastic epithelium spans a range of severity, from mild loss of polarity, a high degree of cellular differentiation, and few mitoses (mild dysplasia), to a lesion resembling carcinoma in situ in its marked cytologic and nuclear atypia and increased mitotic activity but retaining some degree of epithelial polarization (severe dysplasia) (Fig 4–19). In many cases, pathological differentiation of carcinoma in situ from severe dysplasia may be very difficult and may hinge on minimal cellular flattening in the most superficial cell layers of the epithelium.

The major significance of CIS lies in its role as a precursor to invasive cancer. Multiple series of untreated patients with CIS diagnosed on biopsy have been followed conservatively, with progression to invasive carcinoma, occurring in as many as 70% of cases. More controversial is the ultimate fate of cervical dysplasia and the question as to whether these lesions should be considered premalignant. Observed progression of dysplasia to carcinoma in situ has been reported in five to 60% of cases, and this variation in percentages appears to result from differences in the criteria used to define each lesion and varying periods of follow-up.

These reports also suggest that dysplastic lesions regress in as many as 50% of cases. It has been shown that biopsy may remove the dysplastic lesion entirely or that the inflammatory process accompanying repair at the biopsy site may destroy remaining areas of atypicality, thereby falsely giving the clinical impression of regression. More recent studies in which patients were diagnosed cytologically and then followed cytologically and colposcopically, thereby eliminating the "biopsy effect," confirm progression of dysplasia to carcinoma in situ in 40% to 60% of cases and spontaneous regression rates as high as 30% for mild or moderate dysplasia. The more severe the dysplasia, the higher the rate and speed of progression toward carcinoma in situ and the lower the rate of regression. The average age of patients with dysplasia is consistently five to ten years lower than that of patients with carcinoma in situ, which runs ten to 15 years behind the average age of patients with invasive squamous cell carcinoma.

The suggestion that these lesions represent a continuum of change that begins with mild dysplasia and advances through carcinoma in situ led Richart to introduce the concept of *cervical intraepithelial neoplasia*, with the following classifications: CIN I indicates mild dysplasia; CIN II, moderate dysplasia; and CIN III, severe dysplasia and carcinoma in situ. Evidence in support of Richart's classification of these lesions as a spectrum of one disease entity comes from the finding of aneuploid changes in the nuclei of dysplastic cells—the same chromosomal changes usually found associated with malignant tumors but not with benign tumors. Autoradiographic studies have demonstrated a steady increase in the mitotic activity of these lesions that

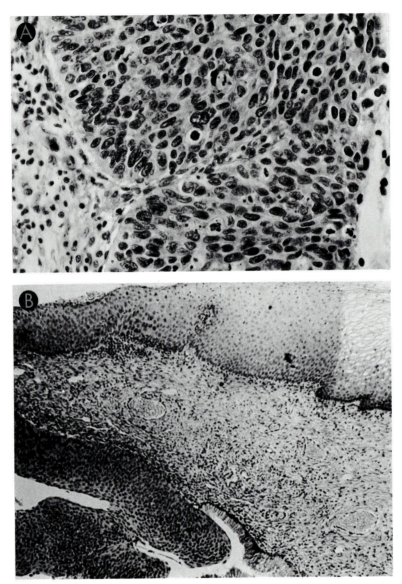

Fig 4–18.—A, carcinoma in situ of cervix. (From Hertig A.T., Gore H.M.: Tumors of the female sex organs, fasc. 33, *Atlas of Tumor Pathology.* (Washington, D.C., Armed Forces Institute of Pathology, 1960.) **B,** carcinoma in situ of cervix with gland involvement. An area of parakeratosis is seen at the upper right.

corresponds exactly to the degree of histologic dedifferentiation and maturation present; this observation is consistent with the postulate that cervical intraepithelial neoplasia represents stages in a continuum of disease.

Histologic and colposcopic observations have established the transformation zone as the site of origin of virtually all cervical intraepithelial neoplasia. These lesions are thought to arise from the basal cell of the transformation zone and, if progression occurs, to result in large-cell nonkeratinizing squamous cell

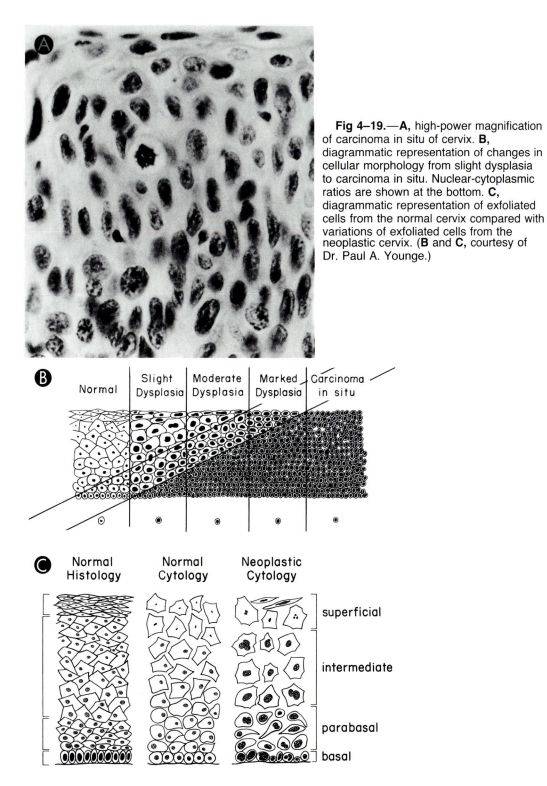

Fig 4–19.—**A,** high-power magnification of carcinoma in situ of cervix. **B,** diagrammatic representation of changes in cellular morphology from slight dysplasia to carcinoma in situ. Nuclear-cytoplasmic ratios are shown at the bottom. **C,** diagrammatic representation of exfoliated cells from the normal cervix compared with variations of exfoliated cells from the neoplastic cervix. (**B** and **C,** courtesy of Dr. Paul A. Younge.)

carcinoma. Small-cell carcinoma is thought to arise from the subcolumnar reserve cells of the endocervical canal, while large-cell keratinizing carcinoma is thought to arise from the basal cells of the native squamous epithelium. Large-cell nonkeratinizing squamous carcinoma is by far the most common histologic type seen, supporting the observation that the majority of cervical intraepithelial neoplasia originates in the transformation zone.

Although a small percentage of cases of cervical intraepithelial neoplasia will regress spontaneously or after biopsy, a finite percentage will progress to invasion. Until we can predict a priori instances in which cervical intraepithelial neoplasia will progress, regress, or remain stable, these lesions must be considered premalignant, and the patient must be evaluated, treated, and followed up appropriately. At the same time, each case must be individualized to take into account age, desire for fertility, and the presence or absence of other pelvic disease.

Diagnosis of Cervical Neoplasia

CYTOLOGY.—The outstanding contribution of recent decades to the field of cancer detection is that of the late George Papanicolaou. In studying cells exfoliated from the female genital tract, Papanicolaou, in the late 1920s, noted characteristic cellular changes associated with cervical carcinoma. These cellular abnormalities include anomalies of staining reaction, pleomorphism, nuclear irregularity, hyperchromasia, the presence of multiple nucleoli, and an increased nuclear-cytoplasmic ratio (Fig 4–20). As with so many important discoveries, fully 20 years elapsed before Papanicolaou's cytologic technique (the *Pap test*) was accepted as a cancer screening measure.

Papanicolaou's classification of the cytologic findings consisted of five grades:

I. Benign
II. Atypical benign
III. Suspect
IV. Probably positive
V. Positive

Although this classification applied to invasive cancer, it soon became apparent that it was possible to detect and identify specific abnormalities associated with carcinoma in situ and dysplasia by means of cytologic examination. It is the practice in many laboratories to equate dysplasia and carcinoma in situ with the class III and class IV designations, respectively.

An appreciation of both qualitative and quantitative variations in cell types found in abnormal smears has enabled cytopathologists to make reasonably accurate diagnostic interpretations. Okagaki performed differential cell counts on abnormal smears and found that, in cases of carcinoma in situ, 30% or more of the exfoliated abnormal cells were of the basal cell type. Although this approach is time-consuming, the rate of predictability was found to be 97.5% when results were correlated with the histologic diagnosis.

The earliest technique used for collecting cytologic material was aspiration from the posterior vaginal fornix via a glass pipette. Although various series reported failure rates of up to 60% in detecting documented cervical dysplasia and 45% in identifying carcinoma in situ using this technique, some practitioners continue to employ it. In 1947, Ayre devised a wooden spatula with which a "scrape biopsy" of the cervical epithelial cells could be carried out. He quoted 95% accuracy in screening for cervical neoplasms when this technique was used in conjunction with endocervical sampling.

Despite the overall success of exfoliative cytology, the significant incidence of *false-negative smears* has gradually become apparent. The practice of routinely performing a biopsy for every patient with an abnormal cervix was established at the Boston Hospital for Women by Younge in 1936, providing a controlled series from which the relative accuracy of cytology could be determined. If we consider the cases of carcinoma in situ diagnosed between 1962 and 1968, cytologic findings were negative in 16 of 113 cases, or 14.2%

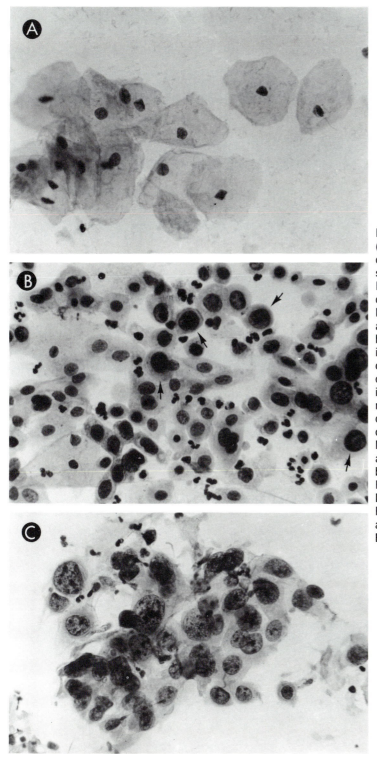

Fig 4–20.—A, class I Papanicolaou smear, benign (×320). Normal superficial cell, polygonal in shape, with small pyknotic nuclei **B,** class IV Papanicolaou smear, carcinoma in situ (× 320). Neoplastic cells are large and uniform in size, with hyperplastic nuclei and an increased nuclear-cytoplasmic ratio *(arrows).* **C,** class V Papanicolaou smear, invasive cancer (×320). The nuclei exhibit coarse, clumped chromatin and may contain multiple nucleoli. Marked pleomorphism and atypical mitotic figures may be seen. (Courtesy of Dr. Robert Ehrmann and the Division of Women's and Perinatal Pathology, Brigham and Women's Hospital, Boston.)

(Table 4–2). If we can presume that seven patients with carcinoma in situ diagnosed at a repeated examination one year later also had false-negative smears, the cumulative false-negative rate rises to 19.2%. The false-negative rate for dysplasia is shown to be 26%. Numerous subsequent reports in the literature confirm the false-negative rate for cervical cytologic diagnosis to be 15% to 20%.

TECHNIQUE OF OBTAINING VAGINAL AND CERVICAL SMEARS.—The following equipment is needed:

1. Clean glass (microscope) slides. Those with frosted ends permit easy labeling in pencil with the patient's name and also identify the "right side" or smeared side of the slide.

2. Glass pipettes measuring about 8 in. in length and having a slight curve, with a capillary opening for adequate suction of the cervical secretion.

3. Rubber suction bulb (1-oz or 2-oz size), with an opening that fits snugly over the pipette.

4. Spatula to be used for cervical scrapings and to prepare smear.

5. For fixative, any one of several dehydrating agents can be used:
   a. Half-and-half mixture of 95% ethyl alcohol and ether.
   b. Plain 95% alcohol or lesser dilutions to 75%.
   c. 75% to 95% methyl alcohol.
   d. 75% to 95% isopropyl alcohol or commercially available cytologic fixatives.

Smears are obtained prior to digital examination with the patient in the lithotomy position and without lubricants, which spoil the staining characteristics of the cells. Douches dilute and wet the cells so that a satisfactory smear cannot be obtained within 12 to 24 hours after douching. The glass pipette is used to aspirate the endocervical secretions, which are then blown out on the slide by compressing the aspiration bulb firmly, thereby creating a fine film. The slide is immediately fixed by immersion into a small stoppered bottle containing fixative or sprayed with commercially available fixative. The spatula is then used to scrape the portio circumferentially at the area of the transformation zone and a slide is rapidly smeared and fixed. Fixation is complete in 15 to 30 minutes, after which the slide may be dried and then secured in a cardboard or wooden holder for transport. Immediate fixation is possible with a cytologic fixative containing methyl alcohol, acetone, and polyethylene glycol.

The importance of endocervical sampling cannot be stressed too strongly. This was shown dramatically by Garite and Feldman, who randomized 710 patients into three groups to compare sampling techniques. The first group underwent sampling with a cervical smear only; the second group with an exocervical smear and endocervical sampling with a moistened cotton swab; and the third group with a method chosen based on the location of the squamocolumnar junction, as determined by the patient's physician. The addition of endocervical sampling doubled the

TABLE 4–2.—CORRELATIONS OF INITIAL CYTODIAGNOSIS WITH FINAL
DIAGNOSIS AT THE BOSTON HOSPITAL FOR WOMEN (1962 TO 1968)

SMEAR	PRECLINICAL CANCER	CARCINOMA IN SITU WITH EARLY STROMAL INVASION	CARCINOMA IN SITU*	DYSPLASIA*
Negative	2	0	16 (23)	60 (96)
Atypical	0	1	3	19
Dysplasia	0	1	40	133
Carcinoma in situ	3	5	45	12
Invasive	5	2	9	1
Total	10	9	113 (120)	225 (261)

*Figures in parentheses include cases detected at the first-year repeated examination.

detection rate of abnormal cytology. Rubio demonstrated that the cotton swab traps atypical cells, making the data of Garite and Feldman even more impressive.

The diagnosis rendered by the cytopathologist can be no better than an accurate interpretation of the cytologic abnormality present on the slide. Certainly the clinician can help to limit the number of false-negative smears by obtaining a proper smear from the area of the transformation zone as well as by obtaining an adequate endocervical sample—preferably with an aspiration technique, but at least with a swab—and assuring rapid fixation to give the examiner the best chance to provide an accurate diagnosis.

The effectiveness of *mass cervical screening programs* remains somewhat controversial with regard to their ability to decrease the incidence of and mortality from cervical cancer. Epidemiologists have described decreasing incidence and mortality rates of cervical carcinoma in countries where mass screening programs are not operating, suggesting that a change in the natural history of the disease might account for the benefits attributed to cervical cytologic screening. Excellent work done by Boyes et al. in British Columbia, Canada, where a screening program has been in operation since 1949, confirms the marked fall in the incidence and mortality rates of this disease (Table 4–3). They also show a rather dramatic increase in the incidence of cervical cancer among a group of unscreened women compared with women undergoing routine cytologic screening. Using data obtained from the other provinces, they directly related the decrease in mortality rate of cervical cancer to the level of screening activity. These observations seemingly establish a definite role for the Papanicolaou smear in contributing to the reduction in incidence and mortality rates for cervical cancer.

Recommendations are being made to re-

TABLE 4–3.—CERVICAL SCREENING IN BRITISH COLUMBIA*

YEAR	WOMEN SCREENED ANNUALLY	TOTAL CASES OF INVASIVE CERVICAL CANCER	INCIDENCE PER 100,000 WOMEN	MORTALITY RATE FROM CERVICAL CANCER PER 100,000 WOMEN
1952	4,140	. . .	. . .	. . .
1953	5,504	. . .	. . .	. . .
1954	8,848	. . .	. . .	. . .
1955	11,707	120	28.4	. . .
1956	15,106	119	27.2	. . .
1957	18,719	120	26.0	. . .
1958	29,869	112	23.7	. . .
1959	38,849	108	22.6	11.4
1960	54,844	96	19.7	10.6
1961	81,614	115	23.2	9.9
1962	106,176	78	15.5	10.3
1963	119,292	98	19.1	12.9
1964	138,700	86	16.3	11.0
1965	161,556	80	14.7	10.6
1966	182,375	77	13.6	7.7
1967	209,425	85	14.3	7.8
1968	236,234	80	13.0	6.4
1969	266,036	89	13.9	8.8
1970	297,407	82	12.3	7.1
1971	322,436	73	10.6	6.9
1972	336,351	66	9.2	8.0
1973	377,397	71	9.5	6.0
1974	385,303	67	8.6	5.6
1975	. . .	70	8.7	4.8
1976	. . .	69	8.4	5.2
1977	. . .	64	7.6	3.8

*Adapted from Boyes D.A., et al.: *Gynecol. Oncol.* 12S:143, 1981.

duce the frequency of cytologic screening in women identified to be at low risk for the development of cervical carcinoma. Until the efficacy of these conservative screening protocols has been established, we will continue to recommend annual screening for essentially all women. Women who have had hysterectomies for other than cervical neoplasia may probably undergo screening every other year or every third year, whereas those who have been treated for cervical neoplasia should undergo screening at least annually.

BIOPSY AND HISTOLOGIC DIAGNOSIS.—Clinicians have depended on the Papanicolaou smear as a screening method for detection of cervical neoplasia. Serial sampling over time provides a longitudinal look at the cervix, decreasing the impact of isolated false-negative smears. The Papanicolaou smear, however, must remain a *screening* technique. Biopsy and histologic diagnosis remain the cornerstones in the management of cervical neoplasia.

Every abnormal, visible cervical lesion must be biopsied. The literature is replete with cases in which a gross cervical abnormality was followed conservatively because multiple Papanicolaou smears were falsely negative or exhibited inflammatory changes only.

Random cervical biopsies were first used to obtain histologic material from cervices determined to be abnormal by Papanicolaou's smear in an attempt to obviate conization in all patients with abnormal smears. It has been shown that cervical intraepithelial neoplasms occur most frequently at the 6 o'clock and 12 o'clock positions in the transformation zone and less frequently toward the lateral angles on each side. Biopsy specimens taken at these two positions and then randomly from the remaining cervix may miss 15% of the invasive lesions present as determined by correlation with the subsequent cone or hysterectomy specimen.

A targeting technique developed by Schiller in 1938—now known as the *Schiller test*—may be used to "highlight" cervical abnormalities, making them visible for biopsy (Fig 4–9): A solution of sodium iodide and iodine is painted onto the cervix. The iodine reacts with glycogen to stain the normal squamous epithelium of the cervix and vagina dark brown. Nonstaining or Schiller-positive areas stand out from the dark background and represent surfaces lacking glycogen; these include columnar epithelium, true pathologic erosions, immature metaplastic epithelium, and neoplastic lesions.

The Schiller test is positive in at least 80% of cervices harboring carcinoma in situ, and with rare exception, positive biopsies are obtained from Schiller-positive areas. In conjunction with endocervical curettage, which is mandatory for evaluating any cytologically abnormal cervix, multiple Schiller-directed biopsies were shown by Griffiths and Younge to be positive in 95% of patients with carcinoma in situ and in virtually all patients with early invasion.

Colposcopy has superseded Schiller's technique in most centers as the initial step in evaluating abnormal Papanicolaou smears, although, as shown above, this simple test may be highly efficacious when employed properly. Hinselman developed the colposcope in 1925 in an attempt to localize small ulcerations that he theorized represented small cervical neoplasms. He found, however, that the low-power magnification of the colposcope ($\times 6$ to $\times 40$) revealed not the neoplastic cervical epithelium but alterations of the underlying stromal vasculature resulting from the neoplastic process, which could then be visualized through the thin epithelial layer. The degree of alteration in vascular pattern, in intercapillary distance, and in surface color and texture was found to correlate well with the severity of the neoplastic process. (For a detailed review of colposcopy, the reader is referred to a standard colposcopic atlas.)

Adequate colposcopic evaluation requires complete visualization of the transformation zone and the lesion in question as well as correlation between the cytologic and histologic diagnoses and the clinical impression of the.

colposcopist. Endocervical curettage should be performed as part of every colposcopic examination. An additional criterion of colposcopic adequacy is that the lesion must occupy less than 50% of the exocervix. This is based on the significant sampling error inherent in obtaining representative biopsies from such a large lesion. Almost 90% of women with abnormal cytologic findings may be adequately evaluated with colposcopy.

Cervical Biopsy

Cervical biopsy is perhaps the most frequent minor surgical procedure performed by the gynecologist. Simple and relatively painless, it may be performed as part of the routine office examination. Contraindications to cervical biopsy are limited to acute pelvic inflammatory disease and acute cervicitis. Certainly patients with coagulopathies should be managed in a hospital setting. Pregnancy is not a contraindication to biopsy.

TECHNIQUE.—The cervix is visualized with a speculum and adequately illuminated. Wiping the cervix with dry gauze frequently causes bleeding, so that the cervix should be cleansed with a cotton swab or ball soaked in an alkaline astringent solution (Alkalol) or aqueous benzalkonium chloride (Zephiran), or with 3% acetic acid, after which colposcopy may be performed. Schiller staining is mandatory for targeting the grossly normal cervix unless colposcopy is performed. A rectangular biopsy specimen is obtained using a Kevorkian or Younge biopsy punch and is then immediately fixed in Bouin's solution (Fig 4–21). Postbiopsy bleeding may be controlled by pressure, cauterization with silver nitrate or ferrous subsulfate (Monsel's solution), packing with Oxycel or Surgicel (oxidized regenerated cellulose), or suturing as required. The patient is instructed to avoid douching, use of tampons, and intercourse for two weeks after biopsy. Although the procedure is essentially

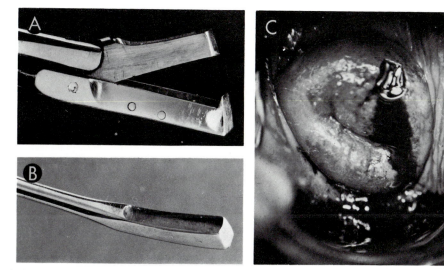

Fig 4–21.—A, Younge cervical biopsy forceps. Overall length is 10 in.; the narrow jaws facilitate insertion into the cervical canal. The front of the lower jaw is elevated and has fine teeth to anchor the bite on the precise area to be sampled. Serrations on the side of each jaw prevent slippage. A jaw opening of almost 90 degrees and sharp cutting edges insure adequate specimen size. **B,** Kevorkian biopsy curet, for detection of early endocervical lesions and for follow-up investigations. The narrow tip can be inserted without dilatation of the cervix, and the curet can be used without anesthesia. The rectangular cutting blade is slightly curved and obtains specimens that are easily oriented. Endometrial biopsies several centimeters in length may be obtained. **C,** typical biopsy site by Younge's method. (Courtesy of Dr. Paul A. Younge.)

painless, a paracervical block with lidocaine or chloroprocaine (Nesacaine) may be performed. Endocervical curettage may be added by vigorously curetting the canal with a narrow curet, obviating dilation.

Cervical Conization

Cervical conization remains the gold standard against which all outpatient evaluation techniques must be weighed. A properly performed conization removes the entire transformation zone and virtually the entire endocervical canal, providing the pathologist with the maximum amount of tissue to rule out invasive carcinoma absolutely. Drawbacks of this procedure include the need for anesthesia and a hospital stay, a complication rate approaching 10% in most series (primarily postoperative hemorrhage), and possible adverse effects on future fertility.

The vast majority of all patients may be completely and adequately evaluated for cervical intraepithelial neoplasia on an outpatient basis; however, the clinician must be assured that invasive cancer has been ruled out before consideration can be given to outpatient therapy. If the following conditions are not met, conization is required to rule out invasion:

1. Lesions seen colposcopically must be limited to the portio without extension into the endocervical canal.

2. The entire transformation zone must be visualized.

3. Results of endocervical curettage must be negative for neoplasia.

4. Biopsies and cytologic examination must reveal intraepithelial disease only.

5. Cytologic and histologic diagnoses must correlate.

TECHNIQUE.—Under adequate general anesthesia, the patient is placed in the dorsal lithotomy position, and the vagina and perineum are gently prepared with povidone-iodine (Betadine) to avoid traumatizing the delicate cervical mucosa. After the bladder has been catheterized, an examination is performed to rule out existing pelvic disease. A weighted retractor is placed in the posterior fornix, a Sims retractor is placed anteriorly,

and the cervix is visualized. Colposcopy or Schiller's test is performed to delineate the extent of disease on the portio. A tenaculum is placed on the portio anteriorly, above the planned limit of the cone biopsy. Lateral-angle sutures are placed into the stroma of the cervix at the 3 o'clock and 9 o'clock positions to ligate the descending branches of the uterine artery. These sutures are left long (for tying at the end of the procedure). The body of the cervix is infiltrated with a dilute solution of vasopressin in saline (20 units in 20 ml), or Marcaine hydrochloride (bupivacaine) epinephrine 1:200,000 which aids in hemostasis.

The mucosa is incised circumferentially, maintaining a margin of 2 to 3 mm beyond the lesions (as delineated via colposcopy or Schiller's staining). A cone-shaped specimen to a length of 1.5 to 1.8 cm is carefully excised encircling the endocervical canal. Care is taken to avoid prematurely entering the canal, since neoplastic tissue might then be left behind. A uterine sound may be placed within the canal to aid in the dissection. Manipulation of the mucosa of the specimen should be avoided. Traction may be attained by placing sutures within the stroma of the cone specimen or by grasping this area with forceps. A suture is placed at the 12 o'clock position in the stroma of the specimen to aid in pathologic orientation. The uterus is then sounded and dilated, and an endometrial sample is taken as desired.

Bleeding is usually minimal with this technique; however, persistent bleeding points may be electrocauterized or ligated with size 0 chromic sutures in a figure-of-eight pattern. The canal is then packed with Surgicel, which is gently tied into place with the long ends of the lateral sutures. The patient is usually observed overnight and then discharged home with instructions to avoid douching, use of tampons, and intercourse for two weeks.

Therapy for Cervical Intraepithelial Neoplasia

The approach to treatment of cervical intraepithelial neoplasia has undergone dramatic changes over the past several decades as the pathogenesis of cervical neoplasia has become better understood. In the past, extensive and potentially morbid procedures such as radical hysterectomy and pelvic irradiation were commonly employed to treat the high-grade dysplasias that are now treated on an outpatient basis at little cost and essentially without risk. Earlier lesions were occasionally ignored. The concept of cervical neoplasia as a continuum, as advanced by Richart, implies that these lesions may be treated in a similar manner, with the understanding that progression to invasive cancer is the natural history of a certain unpredictable percentage.

Treatment of CIN III (severe dysplasia and carcinoma in situ) perhaps remains most controversial. With the realization that radical surgery and irradiation were not necessary, simple hysterectomy has become the treatment of choice throughout the United States. Cone biopsy, as primary therapy, was limited to those patients desirous of retaining fertility. Several studies have been done comparing the results obtained from conization compared with hysterectomy. Boyes followed 3,688 women with carcinoma in situ. Of 808 treated with conization, 28 (3.4%) had a recurrence of in situ disease while three (0.3%) later manifested invasive carcinoma. A total of 2,819 patients were treated with hysterectomy with a recurrence of carcinoma in situ in almost 1.0% and invasion in 0.2%. In a later report by Kolstad of a series of 1,121 cases of carcinoma in situ, the lesion recurred in 2.3% and invasion later occurred in 0.9% after conization, while the corresponding rates after hysterectomy were 1.2% and 2.1%, respectively. He found that the in situ lesions recurred earlier and that a minimum follow-up of five years is essential when one is comparing therapeutic modalities in these diseases. Of further interest was a cure rate of almost 90% in those cases in which margins were positive for carcinoma in situ.

In a similar study, Ahlgren noted a cure rate of 98% when the margins of the surgical specimen were negative and 70% when the margins were positive. Certainly the risk of recurrence of cervical intraepithelial neoplasia after hysterectomy seems to be lower than that after conization, but the difference is not dramatic, indicating that conization may be considered a reasonable alternative to hysterectomy. Those favoring hysterectomy for CIN III point out the frequency with which hysterectomy specimens obtained immediately after conization contain residual disease—as many as 50% in some series. No mention is made as to whether or not the original cone margins had been adjudged negative, or whether the conization was performed to remove the entire transformation zone and endocervical canal for cure or merely to sample the canal with a narrow cone, obviously cutting through lesions on the exocervix with the intention of proceeding directly to hysterectomy after invasion had been ruled out.

Conization for any degree of cervical intraepithelial neoplasia—whether performed as part of the diagnostic evaluation or as primary therapy subsequent to outpatient evaluation—has a cure rate of 98% when surgical margins are negative, thus requiring no further therapy. Close follow-up is suggested, including Papanicolaou smears every three months for one year and every six months thereafter, a colposcopic examination yearly, and endocervical curettage in one year's time. Given the 70% to 80% cure rate reported after conization with positive margins, conservative management with serial endocervical sampling, colposcopy, and cytology is acceptable if patient compliance can be expected. Otherwise, reconization or hysterectomy is indicated. The latter may be relied on as primary management of cervical intraepithelial neoplasia when the pregnancy is undesired or when pelvic disease coexists. When the upper vagina is shown to be normal preoperatively on colposcopy or Schiller's staining, there is no need for a wide vaginal cuff. Certainly no procedure more extensive than simple hysterectomy is required for treatment of cervical intraepithelial neoplasia.

Perhaps 85% to 90% of all patients with cervical intraepithelial neoplasia may have lesions limited to the portio and at the same time fulfill all the criteria obviating coniza-tion. These patients are then candidates for outpatient therapeutic modalities, including electrocauterization, cryocauterization, and laser vaporization, which eradicate both the neoplastic lesion and the remainder of the transformation zone, allowing normal squa-mous epithelium to replace the epithelium that has been removed or destroyed.

ELECTROCAUTERIZATION.—This was at one time widely used, with cure rates approach-ing 90%. A complication rate of almost 10% (including bleeding, cervical stenosis, and pelvic inflammatory disease) as well as the de-gree of patient discomfort has detracted from its use, while other safer and virtually pain-less techniques have been developed.

CRYOCAUTERIZATION.—This technique ap-pears to be the simplest and safest outpatient modality developed. This technique employs a cryoprobe, cooled by carbon dioxide or freon, to necrose the surface epithelium that it contacts. Probes of various shapes are avail-able for different cervices. For large lesions, multiple applications may be required. After treatment, a watery discharge is common but resolves in several weeks. Reepithelialization begins immediately and is virtually complete in six weeks.

Creasman recently reviewed the efficacy of cryocautery in cervical intraepithelial neopla-sia and reported failure rates of 6% in CIN I, 7% in CIN II, and 14% in CIN III. Townsend found the failure rate in his study to be re-lated to lesion size rather than histologic grade, with a 96% cure rate in lesions 1 cm or less in diameter, but a 58% cure rate in lesions greater than 1 cm in diameter. This may be a function of the inability to necrose the entire lesion with overlapping applica-tions of the cryoprobe. Savage showed an 18% increase in the failure rate when the glands were involved, suggesting that the depth of cryonecrosis is limited. Anderson ex-amined 343 cone specimens and found glands to a maximum depth of 7.83 mm and involved glands to a maximum depth of 5.22 mm. Over 99% of the glands, however, were located within 4 mm of the epithelial surface. It has been well shown that when properly per-formed, cryocautery produces necrosis to a depth of 5 to 6 mm, which should theoreti-cally destroy well over 99% of the involved glands. The relative cryoresistance in the cases reported by Savage remains unclear, but suggests that gland involvement may be a relative contraindication to this technique.

Criticism of cryocauterization has resulted from reports of invasive carcinoma developing after the procedure, implying that residual neoplasia had been buried during the repara-tive process and had progressed to invasion while undetectable by cytologic or colpo-scopic techniques. Sevin reviewed eight such cases and found that seven of these patients had not undergone a pretreatment endocer-vical curettage, five had not undergone bi-opsy, one biopsy was misinterpreted and ac-tually represented invasive carcinoma, and only three patients underwent colposcopic ex-amination, implying that these failures were due to inadequate initial evaluation rather than a consequence of cryocauterization.

The most recent addition to the outpatient armamentarium against cervical intraepithe-lial neoplasia is the *carbon dioxide laser*. This device produces a coherent, or in-phase, par-allel beam of light of very high energy that is capable of instantaneously boiling water and, thus, vaporizing cells. Originally the laser was used to eradicate the lesion itself, thereby sparing the remaining cervix. However, fail-ure rates averaged 10% to 30%, and it be-came clear that the entire transformation zone could be vaporized safely to a depth of 5 to 7 mm to yield cure rates exceeding 90%. The major drawbacks of this technique are the cost of the laser apparatus and the greater skill required when compared with cryocau-terization. More experience with the carbon dioxide laser technique is required before it can be considered a replacement for cryocau-tery.

An acceptable clinical approach to evalua-tion of the abnormal Papanicolaou smear and subsequent management is shown in Figure 4–22.

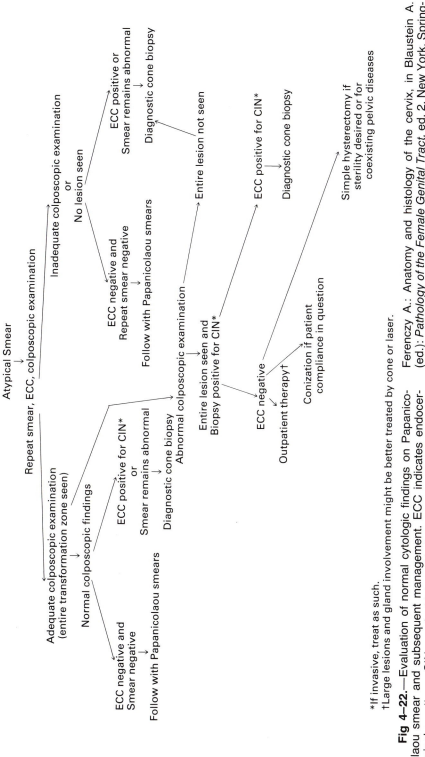

Evaluation and Management of the Abnormal Papanicolaou Smear

*If invasive, treat as such.
†Large lesions and gland involvement might be better treated by cone or laser.

Fig 4–22.—Evaluation of normal cytologic findings on Papanicolaou smear and subsequent management. ECC indicates endocervical curettage; CIN, cervical intraepithelial neoplasia. (Adapted from Ferenczy A.: Anatomy and histology of the cervix, in Blaustein A. (ed.): *Pathology of the Female Genital Tract*, ed. 2. New York, Springer-Verlag, 1982, p. 174.)

Invasive Cancer

Pathology

The gross clinical appearance of invasive cervical lesions is generally of two types: *exophytic* (proliferative) and *endophytic* (ulcerating). The exophytic lesion may involve the cervix totally and have a cauliflowerlike appearance, while the endophytic lesion has a predilection to invade upward into the endocervical canal, often expanding the lower uterine segment and giving rise to the so-called barrel-shaped cervix. Although an endophytic lesion may infiltrate the tissue adjacent to the cervix earlier than would an exophytic tumor, either type may extend into the parametrium and involve the uterosacral ligaments or may spread onto the vaginal mucosa and down the vaginal canal. This spread causes the tissues to feel firm and nodular. The rectum and bladder may likewise be infiltrated by tumor. Spread toward the bladder usually involves the vesicovaginal septum, with the formation of bullous edema of the bladder prior to actual involvement of the bladder mucosa. Posterior spread involves the rectovaginal septum, and only late in the course of the disease is there involvement of the rectal mucosa.

Microscopic Appearance

Squamous cell carcinoma accounts for 90% of invasive cervical cancer. Adenocarcinoma accounts for approximately 8%, while the remainder are sarcomas and primary or secondary lymphomas. Recently the incidence of adenocarcinoma has been reported to be as high as 25% in women younger than 35 years.

Wentz and Reagan have divided *squamous cell carcinoma* into three types: keratinizing, nonkeratinizing, and small-cell type. Keratinizing cells show foci of keratinization with cornified "pearls." Nonkeratinizing cells have well-demarcated tumor-stromal borders but no evidence of keratinization or cornified "pearls." The small-cell type consists of small, round, or spindle-shaped cells with poorly defined tumor-stromal borders.

The significant features differentiating invasive cancer from carcinoma in situ are the breakdown of the basement membrane and involvement of the stroma. Nests and clusters of epithelial cells can be seen scattered in an irregular pattern within a stroma infiltrated by inflammatory cells (Fig 4–23,A). Individual cells of invasive squamous cell carcinoma show the same characteristics described for in situ cancer, i.e., loss of stratification and polarity with numerous atypical mitotic figures, pleomorphism, nuclear hyperchromatism (Fig 4–23,B), and dyskaryosis. Tumor giant cells may be found along with areas of necrosis and cellular degeneration.

The typical appearance of cervical *adenocarcinoma* is shown in Figure 4–24. Adenocarcinoma arises from the columnar cells lining the endocervical canal and glands. The number of glandular elements is greatly increased, with marked variation in size and shape. Cellular pleomorphism, nuclear enlargement and hyperchromatism, and increased mitotic activity with areas of necrosis and degeneration are seen.

Adenosquamous carcinoma consists of intermingled malignant epithelial cell cores and malignant glandular structures. If the squamous component appears benign, the tumor is referred to as an adenocanthoma. The *glassy cell carcinoma* is a mixed carcinoma consisting of a poorly differentiated adenocarcinoma and squamous carcinoma. It is such a rare entity that Maier and Norris question whether it indeed represents a distinct clinical and pathologic entity. Although this tumor is believed to be poorly responsive to therapy, the number of reported cases is too small to allow any conclusions about survival to be drawn.

Histologic Grading of Cervical Cancer

The degree of differentiation of a cancer cell as viewed under high power determines its histologic grade. This should not be confused with stage, which defines the extent of disease as determined by physical and radiologic examinations. The grade classification

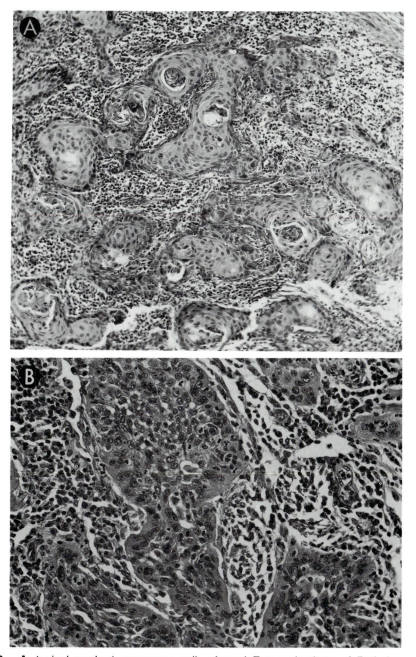

Fig 4–23.—A, typical grade 1 squamous cell carcinoma of the cervix. There is extensive keratinization with "pearl" formation and lymphocytic infiltration of the stroma. (From Hertig A.T., Gore H.M.: Tumors of the female sex organs, fasc. 33, *Atlas of Tumor Pathology.* Washington, D.C., Armed Forces Institute of Pathology, 1960.) **B,** grade 2 squamous cell carcinoma of the cervix. Several nests of malignant cells show pleomorphism, nuclear hyperchromatism, and atypical mitotic figures.

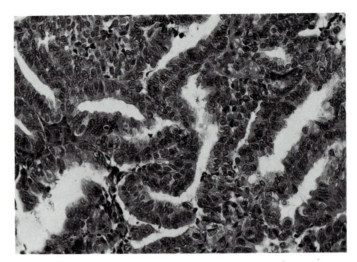

Fig 4–24.—Adenocarcinoma of the cervix. The malignant cells are arranged in a glandular pattern. The typical columnar appearance of the cell has been lost, and numerous cells show atypical mitoses.

most generally accepted is that of Broders, who in 1926 divided tumors into differentiated and undifferentiated groups and then assigned one of three grades depending on the relative amount of cellular differentiation present, with keratinization used as an index of differentiation. By this scheme, grade 1 would be the most differentiated and grade 3 the least differentiated, or most anaplastic. Since this original report, numerous publications have appeared concerning histologic grading and survival. Most of these reviews do not consider risk factors other than histologic grading that may influence prognosis. However, when Chung et al. evaluated histologic grade and prognosis, they noted that the more undifferentiated the primary tumor and the more bulky the primary lesion, the higher the incidence of pelvic node metastases. Poor prognosis may in fact relate more to the size and, ultimately, the stage of the lesion than to the degree of histologic differentiation.

Clinical Staging of Cervical Cancer

Clinical staging remains the most important prognostic criterion in determining the patient's response to therapy. In the early stages of cervical cancer, which are now being seen more often as a result of cytologic screening, it is important in any program in which clinical trials are carried out that information be obtained concerning size of lesion, depth of invasion, lymphatic or vascular permeation, and cellular characteristics to allow useful comparisons of treatment protocols to be made. Contiguous spread of cervical cancer into the vagina, adjacent parametrium, and pelvic organs is a rather characteristic course in the natural history of this disease and forms the basis for clinical staging.

Clinical staging of carcinoma of the cervix is described in Table 4–4. The gynecologist and radiation therapist should jointly evaluate and stage the tumor while the patient is under anesthesia by means of speculum and bimanual pelvic and rectal examinations. The cervix and vagina must be carefully visualized and biopsy specimens taken of any suspicious areas. Endometrial curettage should also be performed if the patient is to be treated with radiation therapy. Excretory urography is integral to the staging process, since ureteral obstruction almost always reflects extension of the tumor. Cystoscopy and proctosigmoidoscopy are recommended for advanced stages

TABLE 4–4.—STAGING OF CERVICAL
CARCINOMA*

Stage 0. Carcinoma in situ, intraepithelial carcinoma.
Stage I. Carcinoma is strictly confined to the cervix; (extension to the corpus should be disregarded)
    Stage Ia. Microinvasive carcinoma (early stromal invasion).
    Stage Ib. All other cases of stage I; occult cancer should be marked "occ"
Stage II. Carcinoma extends beyond the cervix but has not extended to the pelvic wall; involvement of the upper two-thirds of the vagina may be present
    Stage IIa. No obvious parametrial involvement
    Stage IIb. Obvious parametrial involvement
Stage III. Carcinoma extends to the pelvic wall; on rectal examination, there is no cancer-free space between the tumor and the pelvic wall; the tumor involves the lower third of the vagina; all patients with a hydronephrosis or nonfunctioning kidney are included
    Stage IIIa. No extension to the pelvic wall
    Stage IIIb. Extension to the pelvic wall and/or hydronephrosis or nonfunctioning kidney
Stage IV. Carcinoma has extended beyond the true pelvis or has clinically involved the mucosa of the bladder or rectum; bullous edema as such does not permit a case to be allotted to stage IV.
    Stage IVa. Spread to adjacent organs
    Stage IVb. Spread to distant organs

*Notes on staging: Stage Ia (microinvasive carcinoma) represents those cases of epithelial abnormalities in which histologic evidence of early stromal invasion is unambiguous. Diagnosis is based on microscopic examination of tissue removed by conization, portio amputation, or removal of the uterus. A punch biopsy specimen revealing microinvasion does not permit allocation to stage Ia as frank invasion in the remaining cervix cannot be ruled out. The remainder of stage I cases should be allotted to stage Ib. As a rule, these cases can be diagnosed by routine clinical examination. "Occult cancer" is a histologically invasive cancer that cannot be diagnosed by routine clinical examination. As a rule, it is diagnosed on a cone, on the amputated portio, or on the removed uterus. Such cancers should be included in stage Ib and marked "stage Ib, occ."

and if radiation therapy is planned; for stage I disease, however, the cost-effectiveness of these diagnostic procedures is questionable. These findings are recorded and the stage is determined. *Final staging cannot be changed once therapy has begun.*

Angiography has been used to determine aortic lymph node metastases but has recently been superseded by computerized axial tomography. This latter technique is particularly helpful in evaluating nodal enlargement. A percutaneous biopsy may then be performed to provide histologic evidence of metastatic spread. Results of thes[e] not be used to change the final scribed previously). Although rarely involves the colon, bariu... .... be helpful in ruling out benign disease, particularly if the patient is to receive radiation therapy.

Certain difficulties and misinterpretations are unavoidable in clinical staging. Frequently the examiner interprets pelvic inflammatory processes or scarring due to endometriosis as tumor and "overstages" the disease. Conversely, the lateral pelvis may be soft when palpated but at surgery positive lymph nodes may be found. Staging will thus vary somewhat with the experience and tactile prowess of the examiner. Discrepancy between the clinical staging and the surgical pathologic findings has been reported in as many as 25% to 40% of cases. It is for this reason that many investigators have elected to perform laparotomy prior to instituting therapy in order to determine the presence of metastases to the aortic nodes or other sites beyond the pelvis.

Mode of Spread of Cervical Cancer

Carcinoma of the cervix spreads principally by direct local invasion and via lymphatics. The number of tumors with a biologic propensity for hematogenous spread totals no more than 5%, but this may result in distant extrapelvic metastatic foci in spite of limited pelvic disease. Tumor growth commonly occurs by contiguous spread to the vagina, uterine cavity, and laterally through the cardinal and uterosacral ligaments. Lateral spread may occur within the substance of the ligaments or in the areolar tissue adjacent to them. Laterally extending carcinoma may encompass and obstruct the ureters as they traverse the paracervical region, causing hydroureter, hydronephrosis, and eventual loss of kidney function that may lead to uremia and, ultimately, death. The cancer may traverse the paravaginal fascia, with extension into the bladder or bowel resulting in vesicovaginal or rectovaginal fistulas.

Plentl and Friedman evaluated pelvic node metastases in cervical cancer by stage and found 15.4% positive nodes in stage I, 28.6% positive in stage II, and 47% positive in stage III. They further noted that the preferential metastatic spread is to the external iliac, hypogastric, and obturator lymph nodes. The next most commonly involved groups of nodes are common iliac, parametrial, and paracervical. Therefore, the lymphatic trunks leaving the cervix within the base of the broad ligament tend to be the preferred channels for lymphatic embolization. The posterior channels that drain to the sacral and then periaortic nodes are less frequently used pathways for tumor dissemination. It appears that the parametrial and paracervical nodes are frequently skipped in the transit of tumor emboli to the more preferred distal sites.

Widespread use of pretreatment laparotomy has afforded increased awareness of the spread of cervical carcinoma beyond the pelvis. The incidence of periaortic node metastases is about 5% in stage Ib, 10% in stage IIa, 18% in stage IIb, and 35% in stage IIIb. Buchsbaum reported 23 patients with positive aortic nodes who underwent left scalene node biopsies, of which eight (34.8%) were positive. The distribution sites of distant organ metastases in order of frequency are lung, liver, and bone. Recently we have observed patients with adenocarcinoma of the cervix that disseminated intra-abdominally in a manner similar to the spread of ovarian cancer. These were patients under 35 years of age whose tumors involved seedings throughout the peritoneal cavity. Diaphragmatic metastases and ascites were likewise noted.

Symptoms and Diagnosis

There are no specific symptoms that characterize cervical cancer, especially in its early stages. Frequently there are no symptoms whatever. Irregular vaginal and/or postcoital bleeding may be noted, or there may be only a pink discharge, occasionally odorous. Abnormal vaginal bleeding may first be noted as a prolonged menstrual period or as profuse flow at the time of a normal period. As the disease progresses and more blood vessels are eroded, an initially scant serosanguineous discharge may become grossly hemorrhagic. A common complaint is the daily appearance of a little blood, usually noted just after voiding and seen on the toilet tissue. In advanced cancer a characteristic bloody, malodorous discharge may be present together with pain from either fistula formation or nerve irritation. Pain is a late symptom and is typically of sciatic distribution, with radiation down the back of the buttock, thigh, and knee. Endophytic tumors may cause little or no bleeding or discharge; however, the cancer may spread rapidly to the sacral plexus and produce severe pain.

Obviously these symptoms, if due to cervical cancer, will become manifest when lesions are of moderate size. The patient should be advised to visit her physician regularly for proper diagnostic procedures at least once a year. Although age 35 years has been suggested as the minimum age for such examinations, this has been lowered to 20 years by many clinicians who have seen advanced cancer in women in their early 20s.

As noted earlier, carcinoma in situ presents no characteristic gross lesion and is detectable only by the judicious use of cervical cytologic studies and adequate biopsies. Similarly, in early invasive carcinoma, the cervix may appear normal or exhibit what seems to be an erosion. Any suspicious lesion on the cervix should always be biopsied. It should not be necessary to emphasize the importance of a digital and speculum examination in women in all age groups. No patient should be advised to take douches for abnormal discharges or bleeding without having a pelvic examination.

Differential Diagnosis

The lesions most commonly confused with cervical cancer are eversions, polyps, papillary endocervicitis, and papillomas. Tuberculosis, chancres, and granuloma inguinale rarely involve the cervix, although it may be impossible to differentiate these benign lesions from early invasive cancer by any method other than biopsy. In many cases repeat or multiple biopsies are necessary before a final diagnosis can be made. This has been particularly true in papillomas of the cervix, which are frequently difficult to distinguish from low-grade papillary carcinomas.

Secondary carcinoma of the cervix may occur by direct extension from the corpus or vagina. Metastatic ovarian, bladder, and breast carcinomas have also been reported, although the breast cancer may first spread to the ovary and secondarily involve the cervix. Lymphomas, particularly histiocytic lymphoma, may present as a cervical tumor.

Treatment

Radiation therapy is the basic treatment modality in the management of cervical cancer. However, surgery may be used to an advantage in early-stage malignancy and should be combined with radiation therapy in special situations.

Staging laparotomy, as noted above, has been used in several centers prior to radiation therapy to evaluate metastases outside the pelvis, particularly to periaortic lymph nodes. Although lymphangiography and particularly computerized axial tomography have been helpful for delineating periaortic nodes enlarged with metastatic cancer, these techniques have not been of value when microscopic metastases are present. This latter situation must be determined surgically and is the one in which radiation therapy offers the greatest potential for cure. It is hoped that extending the standard pelvic portals to include those nodal groups with documented metastases will improve survival. However, pretreatment laparotomy has not yet been shown to increase the survival of these patients. Also a high incidence of complications has been reported when periaortic node dissections have been carried out in patients subsequently treated with definitive radiation therapy.

RADIATION THERAPY.—Radiation therapy is administered in most clinics in two forms, radium and x-ray, with considerable variation as to types of applicators and sequence of administration. In the past the measurement of radium dosage was expressed in terms of milligram-hours, which was simply a computation of the amount of radium applied (in milligrams) times the number of hours it was in position. However, unless this figure is qualified by a statement of distance factors, filtration, arrangement of sources, and the volume of tissue irradiated, the term is quite meaningless for clinical therapy. A more logical method of expressing radium dosage is similar to that used in calculating x-ray dosage, i.e., in terms of the amount of ionization it produces. This may be expressed in terms of a roentgen (R), and for radium this is called the γ-roentgen. A roentgen may be defined as "that amount of x- or γ-radiation such that the associated corpuscular emission per 0.001293 gm (1 ml) of air produces, in air, ions carrying one electrostatic unit of quantity of electricity of either sign." A γ-roentgen has been accurately measured: 1 mg radium in equilibrium at a point source filtered with 0.5 mm platinum is accepted as giving 8.25 R/hr at 1 cm distance.

Numerous radium applicators have been devised, and practically every major clinic has made some change in their basic construction. The better known ones are the Stockholm, Fletcher, Paris, Manchester, Ernst, and Neary designs. In addition, cervical cancer may be treated by intravaginal cone (x-ray), interstitial needles, interstitial radon seeds, interstitial colloidal gold, or radioactive cobalt. All these methods strive to deliver a cancericidal dose throughout the tumor-bearing area without causing irreversible damage to normal tissues. This can be accomplished only if an understanding of pelvic anatomy and pathology is combined with a knowledge of the essentials of radiation physics and radiobiology.

Radiation therapy is not without a moderate incidence of *complications* due either to inherent sensitivity or to improper application. The commonest difficulties following radium treatment are cystitis and proctitis. Cystitis is usually delayed a year or more after treatment and is characterized by marked frequency, urgency with occasional incontinence, nocturia, dysuria, and, occasionally, hematuria. Urine specimens and cultures usually give negative results but the cystoscopic examination is diagnostic. The bladder mucosa is pale and smooth, blood vessels appear constricted, and there is a loss of normal elasticity, resulting in diminished bladder capacity. The entire process is due to the late effects of radium, namely, a gradual obliteration of capillaries and scarring of supportive tissues. Treatment is frequently unsatisfactory and protracted, but some relief may be obtained with antispasmodics and with bladder irrigations utilizing dilute silver nitrate or analgesic oily solutions.

Proctitis usually occurs shortly after radium administration but is transient in most cases. Symptoms include diarrhea, tenesmus, and painful defecation. Relief is obtained with a preparation of diphenoxylate hydrochloride and atropine sulfate (Lomotil) or with paregoric. Analgesic rectal suppositories are useful if tenesmus persists. In a few patients the radiation reaction may be delayed a year or more, and in these cases there may be constipation, diarrhea, and rectal bleeding. Extensive fibrosis may seriously diminish the caliber of the rectosigmoid region so that resection or colostomy is occasionally necessary. This condition, however, is due to a combined effect of radium and x-rays.

Vesicovaginal and rectovaginal fistulas are only rarely a result of radium therapy per se. Usually these are due to tumor or the destruction of tumor areas by irradiation. However, poor positioning of the radium applicator or overdosage may result in a fistula in the absence of cancer. This is not the fault of the methods but of the technique.

Pelvic inflammatory disease is a contraindication to the use of either radium or x-rays, since it may be markedly activated or aggravated and lead to tubo-ovarian abscesses, septicemia, and, occasionally, death. If pyometra is found at the time of uterine curettage, it should be drained and antibiotics given until evidence of infection has subsided. If inflammatory tubo-ovarian masses are present, a preliminary salpingo-oophorectomy should be carried out prior to radiation therapy. It has been our policy to administer a broad spectrum of antibiotics while the radium is in position and to remove the radium if the temperature exceeds 100° F.

Vaginal stenosis may develop after radium treatment. This may be prevented in younger women by frequent examinations and by breaking up the thin synechiae as they develop. Coitus will aid in keeping the vagina of normal size, and local application of an estrogen cream will prevent bleeding due to the changes that are inevitable with senescence. In older women the vagina usually closes off so that the cervix is no longer available for inspection or cytologic examination. Although this causes the patient no difficulty, it prevents adequate follow-up by means of vaginal smears.

The use of x-rays may cause nausea and vomiting (radiation sickness) and depression of the bone marrow, with subsequent mild leukopenia. It is our practice to have a complete blood count performed once weekly during the period of x-ray therapy. Similarly, if severe nausea or vomiting develops during treatment, hospitalization is recommended and phenothiazines and intravenous fluids are given. Skin hyperemia is an occasional result of x-ray therapy, and in some individuals with fair skin, blistering and ulceration may develop. Cessation of treatment for a few days and the use of a soothing ointment will usually permit adequate healing. The skin in these areas remains "tanned" for months, after which there is a gradual whitening with dilatation of capillaries, so that extensive telangiectasia may be evident. Use of the supervoltage technique has minimized this complication.

Other effects of x-ray and radium therapy include late small bowel obstruction and perforation, loss of libido, and menopausal symptoms. Bowel obstruction or perforation may occur as late as ten years after therapy. More often the patient may note vague lower abdominal crampy pain, irregular bowel habits, and blood in the stool. Roentgenograms may give entirely negative findings, but exploration will reveal multiple loops of small bowel adherent to each other and to adjacent structures. In the more severe forms, arteriolar occlusion may result in localized areas of necrosis with perforation. It is well to remember this possible complication of radiation therapy in the differential diagnosis of an acute abdomen.

Loss of libido is not common and may be prevented by a frank discussion of the problem with the patient during or at the conclusion of treatment. The use of estrogen creams to keep the vaginal mucosa soft and pliable has been mentioned. In addition, androgenic hormones in subvirilizing doses are frequently helpful. Hot flashes and sweats typical of the artificially induced menopause may be troublesome in some patients. Small doses of conjugated estrogens (Premarin, 0.625 mg) will relieve these symptoms and aid in the maintenance of a more normal extragenital endocrine balance. There is no evidence that such estrogenic therapy will bring about a recurrence of cervical cancer.

Appropriate Therapy Based on Clinical Staging

STAGE IA.—Considerable controversy continues to surround microinvasive squamous carcinoma of the cervix, not only regarding the implication of the term microinvasion, but also as to what constitutes appropriate treatment. Microinvasive carcinoma has been defined by some as invasion to 3 to 5 mm below the basement membrane (Fig 4–25), while others state that microinvasion applies to lesions no greater than 1 mm in depth and that all other lesions should be considered frank invasion. The Society of Gynecologic Oncologists has proposed the following definition: A microinvasive lesion should be defined as one in which neoplastic epithelium invades the stroma in one or more places to a depth of 3 mm or less below the base of the epithelium and in which lymphatic or vascular involvement is not demonstrated. Using this definition, Seski et al. evaluated the surgical tissues and clinical records of 54 surgically treated patients with microinvasive carcinoma of the cervix. In 37 of their patients in whom invasion was no greater than 3 mm and without lymphatic or vascular involvement, lymph nodes were not involved. Therefore, a total extrafascial abdominal hysterectomy without lymph node dissection may be considered adequate treatment for stage Ia disease.

Microinvasion can also be treated with intracavitary radioactive sources alone (7,000 to 9,000 mg-hr in one or two insertions). However, since many of these patients are young, surgical treatment is preferable to allow normal ovarian function to be maintained.

STAGES IB AND IIA.—In these stages either irradiation or radical surgery can be elected, since equally good results are obtained with either modality. Surgery has been preferred in young women because it allows ovarian conservation (the tumor rarely metastasizes to the ovaries) and causes less dyspareunia than does radiation therapy. Survival using either technique is about 85% to 90% for stage Ib and about 75% for stage IIa. The general medical status of the patient must be carefully evaluated before radical surgery is undertaken. Obesity is a major selection factor in that it renders dissection deep in the pelvis extremely difficult.

Bulky endocervical carcinoma (barrel-shaped cervix) has a high incidence of central recurrence, pelvic and periaortic metastases, and distant dissemination. Intracavitary radiation is unable to encompass all the cancer within a tumoricidal dose volume, and despite the use of external radiation in association with radium, central recurrence is not uncommon. Therefore, an extrafascial total abdominal hysterectomy should be combined with external radiation in this setting.

Invasive cervical carcinoma, stage Ib, that

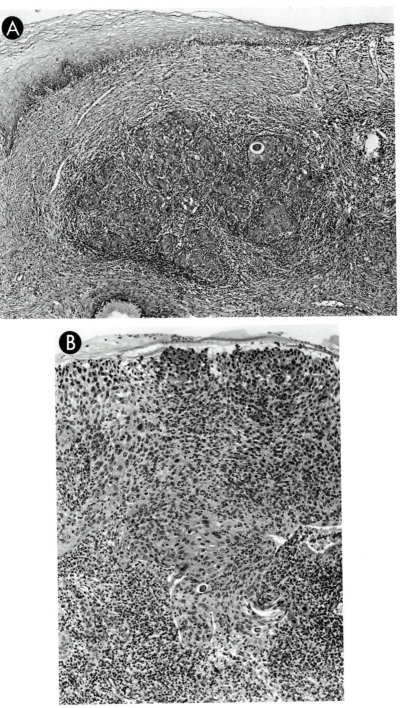

Fig 4–25.—**A,** microinvasive carcinoma under-lying normal portio epithelium. No other areas of invasion could be found in this cervix. Carcinoma in situ from which this miniature cancer must have arisen was found in the endocervix. **B,** late stromal invasion characterized by a confluence of invasive buds into an inflamed stroma. The sur-face epithelium is absent on the right but overly-ing carcinoma in situ is visible on the left.

has enlarged the diameter of the cervix to greater than 3 cm is associated with a high incidence of pelvic node involvement and poor prognosis. It is equally important to note the size of the cervical lesion within a given stage, since this has also been shown to be of prognostic value. Van Nagell found that for stage I lesions over 2 to 5 cm in diameter, the failure rate was 24% for surgery but only 11% for radiation. In one large series of women treated by radical hysterectomy, Piver and Chung reported a five-year survival of 85% for stage Ib lesions up to 3 cm in diameter but only a 66% survival for tumors 4 to 5 cm in diameter. These studies would suggest that stage I lesions larger than 3 cm in size are best treated with radiation therapy.

Radical hysterectomy for stage Ib and IIa is an extensive operation. It involves wide resection of the paracervical and vaginal tissues to the lateral pelvic side walls and to the floor of the pelvis. This requires dissection of the ureters to their insertion in the bladder, mobilization of the bladder neck as well as of the rectum to allow for extensive parametrial excision, and bilateral pelvic lymphadenectomy. Operative mortality is less than 1% in most series, but the morbidity rate approaches 35% to 45%. The most common complication is temporary paralysis of the urinary bladder, and it has become evident that the more radical the surgery, the more serious will be the impairment of bladder function. Although usually not permanent, the urinary stasis often results in chronic cystitis, ureteritis, and pyelonephritis. Some patients have permanent bladder paralysis but learn to control micturition by developing a semiautomatic bladder that will empty itself with the aid of voluntary abdominal pressure. Another serious complication is the development of urinary fistulas, usually of the ureterovaginal type. These occurred in 7% of the patients operated on by Meigs and in 19% in the series of Barber and Brunschwig. With better patient selection, improved surgical techniques, and the addition of suction drainage, the incidence of these complications has been reduced to less than 2% in most series.

The policy of treatment for invasive carcinoma of the cervix (stages I and IIa) at the Joint Center of Radiation Therapy at the Harvard Medical School combines radium and external radiation. Intracavitary radium giving 8,000 mg-hr divided in two applications is followed by 3,500 to 4,000 rads of external parametrial irradiation. A 15×15-cm portal is sufficient for stages Ib and IIa. A variety of applicators may be used for radium insertion, but we have found the Fletcher-Suit afterloading applicator particularly helpful (Fig 4–26).

STAGES IIB, III, AND IVA.—Patients with these stages of cervical carcinoma are best treated with radiation therapy techniques, since adequate dissection beyond the boundaries of tumor is not technically possible. An 18×15-cm portal for external radiation encompassing the common iliac nodes and the cephalad half of the vagina is employed. Stage IIb is treated with 3,500 to 4,000 rads of whole-pelvis irradiation along with 1,000 rads of additional parametrial irradiation followed in two weeks by one or two intracavitary radium insertions to 5,000 to 6,000 mg-hr. The five-year survival rate for stage IIb is 60% to 65%.

Stage III is treated with 4,000 to 5,000 rads of whole-pelvis irradiation plus 1,000 to 1,500 rads to one or both pelvic walls followed by intracavitary radium to 5,500 to 6,500 mg-hr. The five-year survival rate for stage III ranges from 25% to 40%.

Patients with stage IVa (bladder or rectal invasion) can be treated with either high-dose whole-pelvis external irradiation and intracavitary sources or with pelvic exenteration.

Recurrent Cervical Carcinoma

Cancer of the cervix, when it recurs, usually does so within two to three years of primary treatment. Symptoms may include vaginal bleeding, bloody discharge, hematuria, dysuria, constipation, melena, pelvic and leg pain, and fistulas. If sacral backache or pain of sciatic distribution occurs, it is invariably due to invasion of the sacral plexus by tumor. Costovertebral angle and flank pain may herald

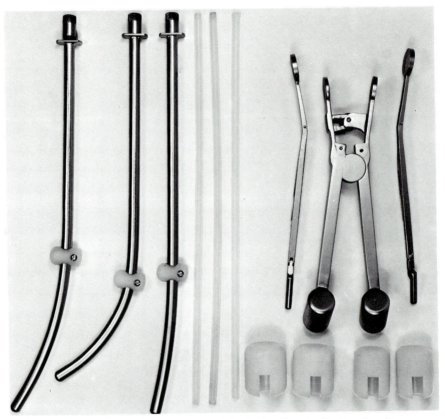

Fig 4–26.—Fletcher-Suit afterloading applicator showing vaginal colpostat and intrauterine tandems.

the development of ureteral obstruction and pyelonephritis. There is usually associated lassitude, anorexia, weight loss, and anemia.

Diagnosis may be simplified by routine cytologic studies on follow-up examination, since tumor cells may be detected before symptoms develop. This, of course, is applicable to recurrence in the vagina and cervix only, since tumor in the pelvic nodes or broad ligament will not exfoliate tumor cells. In most cases the diagnosis depends on an evaluation of symptoms and a careful pelvic examination. Progressive firm nodularity in the paracervical and uterosacral area, felt best on rectal examination, is usually pathognomonic of viable tumor. The anatomic sites of treatment failure in carcinoma of the cervix correlate closely with tumor stage. Cervical or vaginal vault (central) recurrences should always be confirmed by biopsy. Computerized axial tomography is useful for defining tumor in enlarged lymph nodes and distant metastases. Abnormalities on the excretory urogram, such as the development of hydroureter and hydronephrosis, suggest periureteral compression by tumor—although radiation fibrosis may on occasion produce the same condition—and may be amenable to surgical correction by means of ureteral implantation or urinary diversion.

Central recurrences are extremely rare in stages Ib and IIa. The usual cause of failure in patients with stage IIIb is parametrial infiltration that could not be controlled with external irradiation. In recent years, better local control has been achieved than in the past as a result of improved radiation technique. However, because of the high incidence of distant metastases in patients with stage III and IV cervical carcinoma, the development of adequate adjuvant therapy is needed to improve their prognosis. Local vault recurrence after radical surgery can be treated with radiation therapy with a salvage rate of about 50%. Usually recurrences after either surgery of radiation are too extensive to be treated with radiation alone. The usual type of recurrence includes spread to the vesicovaginal septum, bladder, rectum, and pelvic and central portion of the parametrium. Surgical therapy for this type of spread requires a multivisceral pelvic resection, commonly known as an exenteration. Prior to performing exenteration, one must explore carefully to determine the status of disease beyond the pelvis, including aortic and pelvic lymph nodes. If the tumor has spread to the lymph nodes or involves the parametrium with extension to the side walls, the cancer is considered inoperable. Morley reported on the use of pelvic exenteration for treating recurrent cervical cancer. Of more than 90 patients, 75% were treated with total pelvic exenteration; the remainder were treated with either resection of the bladder anteriorly or excision of the bowel posteriorly, depending on the location of the tumor. The five-year survival rate for recurrent carcinoma of the cervix in his series was 63%.

Ureteral compression either in the pelvis or near the kidney, with uremia and/or pyelonephritis, is a major cause of death and is found in about 50% of patients, whether treated or untreated. Other causes of death are infection (peritonitis, pelvic abscess, septicemia), uncontrolled hemorrhage, and extrapelvic metastases. Patients treated for cardiac failure will sometimes have severe pulmonary edema together with edema of the arms and neck. Usually, there is a plethora of the face and neck. This entity is due to superior vena caval obstruction from metastatic cervical cancer.

In 13% of deaths from cancer of the cervix

the cause was gastrointestinal tract involvement, usually manifesting itself as large bowel obstruction, particularly at the rectosigmoid level. Occasionally, perforation of the large or small bowel results in fatal peritonitis. Jaundice owing to extensive hepatic metastases may be noted terminally. In a few patients, diabetic acidosis due to extensive pancreatic metastases has been seen as a terminal event. If the blood count reveals thrombocytosis and nucleated red cells, splenic metastases should be strongly suspected.

CHEMOTHERAPY.—Based on the information obtained from pretreatment laparotomy, several attempts have been made to utilize adjuvant chemotherapy along with radical surgery or radiation therapy. To date, none of these regimens has been shown to be effective. In large bulky stage IIIb disease, combination chemotherapy consisting of methotrexate, bleomycin, and cisplatin has been used at our institution prior to radiation therapy. Although tumor response has been observed, this regimen has not significantly diminished recurrence rates or prolonged survival.

Chemotherapy used in patients with recurrent cervical carcinoma not amenable to radiation therapy or exenteration is usually more effective for distant metastases than for pelvic recurrence. A variety of single agents have been used, with cisplatin giving the highest objective response. Response rates with combination chemotherapy have exceeded those achieved with single agents. Regimens that include cisplatin appear to be more effective than those that do not. Since many of the patients have undergone radiation therapy, which compromises bone marrow function, or have impaired renal function, the ability to deliver adequate chemotherapy is often diminished.

Chemotherapy has also been used as a radiosensitizer to enhance the effect of radiation therapy. Piver reported significantly improved survival among patients with stage IIb and IIIb disease when hydroxyurea was used along with radiation therapy compared with a placebo and radiation therapy alone.

CLEAR CELL ADENOCARCINOMA OF THE CERVIX

Adenocarcinoma of both the cervix and the vagina in women with a median age of 19 years has been found to be associated with maternal ingestion of DES. As of June 1, 1980, 429 cases of both vaginal and cervical clear cell adenocarcinoma had been reported. Treatment for cervical adenocarcinoma is similar to that outlined for squamous cell carcinoma of the cervix. However, owing to the young age of these women the preferred therapy is radical hysterectomy and pelvic lymph node dissection in patients with stage I and IIa disease. Ovarian conservation is maintained, and if the vagina is involved, vaginectomy followed by reconstruction is performed and provides excellent functional results. Among 239 patients with stage I clear cell carcinoma, the overall survival rate was 90%. Most recurrences of clear cell carcinoma are within three years of the initial treatment. Pulmonary and supraclavicular nodal metastases are more frequent when compared with squamous cell carcinoma of either the cervix or the vagina. If there is local recurrence without side wall involvement, pelvic exenteration may be considered. If either aortic or pelvic nodes are involved, exenteration is contraindicated.

CARCINOMA OF THE CERVIX IN PREGNANCY

Carcinoma of the cervix complicates pregnancy in approximately 0.01% of patients. Therapeutic decisions are based on the stage of the cancer, the duration of the pregnancy, and the wishes of the mother. Although pregnancy does not appear to have a detrimental effect on the course of the disease, it is essential that the diagnosis be made promptly, since delay in treatment can alter prognosis.

Prior to the third trimester, treatment for the malignancy is carried out according to the stage of disease. For stage I and IIa lesions, radical hysterectomy with pelvic lymph node dissection is acceptable therapy. If radiation therapy is planned, the uterus may be evacuated at the time of the first radium application or whole-pelvis irradiation may be started. If abortion does not occur, surgical evacuation of the uterus follows the completion of external irradiation at the time of radium application.

For patients in the late second trimester, therapy may be delayed until fetal viability is assured. For stage I and IIa lesions, a classic cesarean section is performed, followed immediately by radical hysterectomy and pelvic lymph node dissection. In more advanced stages, external radiation is delivered after cesarean section. This usually requires a delay of a week to ten days until the abdominal incision has healed. After completion of the radiation therapy, intracavitary radiation is employed as outlined earlier for the appropriate stage.

BIBLIOGRAPHY

Embryology, Anatomy, and Histology
Bulmer D.: The development of the human vagina. *J. Anat.* 91:490, 1957.
Ferenczy A.: Anatomy and histology of the cervix, in Blaustein A. (ed.): *Pathology of the Female Genital Tract*, ed. 2. New York, Springer-Verlag, 1982.
Fluhmann C.F.: Developmental anatomy of the cervix uteri. *Obstet. Gynecol.* 15:62, 1960.
Fluhmann C.F.: *The Cervix Uteri and Its Diseases.* Philadelphia, W.B. Saunders Co., 1961.

Forsberg J.G.: Origin of vaginal epithelium. *Obstet. Gynecol.* 25:787, 1965.
Forsberg J.G.: Estrogen, vaginal cancer, and vaginal development. *Am. J. Obstet. Gynecol.* 113:83, 1972.
Forsberg J.G.: Cervicovaginal epithelium: Its origin and development. *Am. J. Obstet. Gynecol.* 115:1025, 1973.
Huffman J.: Mesonephric remnants in the cervix. *Am. J. Obstet. Gynecol.* 56:233, 1948.
Johnson L.D., et al.: The histogenesis of carcinoma

in situ of the uterine cervix: A preliminary report of the origin of carcinoma in situ in subcylindrical cell anaplasia. *Cancer* 17:213, 1964.

Koff A.K.: Development of the vagina in the human fetus. *Contributions to Embryology, Carnegie Inst.* 24:54, 1933.

Langman J.: *Medical Embryology.* Baltimore, Williams & Wilkins Co., 1981.

Meyer R.: In Stoeckel W. (ed.): *Handbuch der Gynäkologie.* Munich, J.F. Bergman, 1926, vol. 6, part 1, p. 651.

Prins R., et al.: Vaginal embryogenesis, estrogen, and adenosis. *Obstet. Gynecol.* 48:246, 1976.

Song J.: *The Human Uterus: Morphogenesis and Embryological Basis for Cancer.* Springfield, Ill., Charles C Thomas Publisher, 1964.

Physiology and Physiologic Alterations

Coppleson M., Reid B.L.: *Preclinical Carcinoma of the Cervix Uteri.* New York, Pergamon Press, 1967.

Ferenczy A.: Anatomy and histology of the cervix, in Blaustein A. (ed.): *Pathology of the Female Genital Tract,* ed. 2. New York, Springer-Verlag, 1982.

Hellman L.M., et al.: Some factors influencing the proliferation of the reserve cells in the human cervix. *Am. J. Obstet. Gynecol.* 67:899, 1954.

Johnson L.D.: Dysplasia and carcinoma in situ in pregnancy, in *The Uterus,* International Academy of Pathology monograph no. 14. Baltimore, Williams & Wilkins Co., 1973.

Langman J.: *Medical Embryology.* Baltimore, Williams & Wilkins Co., 1981.

Schneppenheim P., et al.: Die Beziehungen des Schleimepithels zum Plattenepithel an der Cervix Uteri in Lebenslauf der Frau. *Arch. Gynaekol.* 190:303, 1958.

Song J.: *The Human Uterus: Morphogenesis and Embryological Basis for Cancer.* Springfield, Ill., Charles C Thomas Publisher, 1964.

Speroff L., Glass R.H., Kase N.: *Clinical Gynecologic Endocrinology and Infertility.* Baltimore, Williams & Wilkins Co., 1983.

Pathologic Alterations

Borken M., Friedman E.A.: Duration of colposcopic changes associated with *Trichomonas vaginitis. Obstet. Gynecol.* 51:111, 1979.

Dawson M.E.: Cervicitis. *Clin. Obstet. Gynecol.* 8:201, 1981.

Ferenczy A.: Anatomy and histology of the cervix, in Blaustein A. (ed.): *Pathology of the Female Genital Tract,* ed. 2. New York, Springer-Verlag, 1982.

Howard L., et al.: A study of the incidence and histogenesis of endocervical metaplasia and intraepithelial carcinoma. *Cancer* 4:1210, 1951.

MacDonald-Burns D.C.: *Chlamydia* and other genital pathogens. *Clin. Obstet. Gynecol.* 8:215, 1981.

Oriel J.D., et al.: Infection of the uterine cervix with *Chlamydia trachomatis. J. Infect. Dis.* 37:443, 1978.

Paavonen J.: Colposcopic and histologic findings in cervical chlamydial infection. *Obstet. Gynecol.* 59:712, 1982.

Rein M.: Vulvovaginitis and cervicitis, in McCormack W.M. (ed.): *Diagnosis and Treatment of Sexually Transmitted Diseases.* Boston, John Wright PSG Inc., 1983, p. 67.

Rein M., Hart G.: Gonococcal infection, in Top F.H., Wehrle, P.F. (eds.): *Communicable and Infectious Diseases.* St. Louis, C.V. Mosby Co., 1976, p. 299.

Song J.: *The Human Uterus: Morphogenesis and Embryological Basis for Cancer.* Springfield, Ill., Charles C Thomas Publisher, 1964.

Viral Cervicitis

Kistner R.W., Hertig A.T.: Papillomas of the uterine cervix: Their malignant potentiality. *Obstet. Gynecol.* 6:147, 1955.

Koss L.G., Durfee G.R.: Unusual patterns of squamous epithelium of uterine cervix: Cytologic and pathologic study of koilocytotic atypia. *Ann. N.Y. Acad. Sci.* 63:1235, 1956.

Meisels A., et al.: Condylomatous lesions of the cervix: II. Cytologic, colposcopic, and histopathologic study. *Acta Cytol.* 21:379, 1977.

Nahmias A.J., et al.: Perinatal risk associated with maternal genital herpes simplex infection. *Am. J. Obstet. Gynecol.* 110:325, 1971.

Powell L.C.: Condyloma acuminatum: Recent advances in development, carcinogenesis, and treatment. *Clin. Obstet. Gynecol.* 21:1061, 1978.

Reid R.: Genital warts and cervical cancer: II. Is human papillomavirus infection the trigger to cervical carcinogenesis? *Gynecol. Oncol.* 15:239, 1983.

Syrajanen K.J.: Current views on the condylomatous lesions in uterine cervix and their possible relationship to cervical squamous cell carcinoma. *Obstet. Gynecol. Surv.* 35:685, 1980.

Cervical Neoplasia Epidemiology

Aurelian L., et al.: Herpes virus type II isolated from cervical tumor cells grown in tissue culture. *Science* 174:704, 1971.

Briggs R.M.: Dysplasia and early neoplasia of the uterine cervix. *Obstet. Gynecol. Surv.* 34:70, 1979.

Cancer Facts and Figures, 1983. New York, American Cancer Society, 1983.

Ferenczy A.: Cervical intraepithelial neoplasia, in

Blaustein A. (ed.): *Pathology of the Female Genital Tract*, ed. 2. New York, Springer-Verlag, 1982.

Ferenczy A., Fenoglio C.M.: Etiologic factors in cervical neoplasia. *Semin. Oncol.* 9:349, 1982.

Gagnon F.: Contribution to the study of the etiology and prevention of cancer of the cervix and of the uterus. *Am. J. Obstet. Gynecol.* 60:516, 1950.

Galloway D.A., McDougall J.K.: The oncogenic potential of herpes simplex viruses: Evidence for a "hit and run" mechanism. *Nature* 302:22, 1983.

Handley W.S.: The prevention of cancer. *Lancet* 1:987, 1936.

Kessler I.I.: Human cervical cancer as a venereal disease. *Cancer Res.* 36:783, 1976.

Kessler I.I.: Etiological concepts in cervical carcinogenesis. *Gynecol. Oncol.* 12:57, 1981.

Kessler I.I.: Epidemiologic aspects of uterine cancer, in Sciarra J.T. (ed.): *Gynecology and Obstetrics*. New York, Harper & Row, 1983, vol. 4, chap. 1.

Ludwig M.E., et al.: Cervical condylomatous atypia and its relationship to cervical neoplasia. *Am. J. Clin. Pathol.* 76:255, 1981.

Nahmias A.J., Sawanabani S.: The genital herpes-cervical cancer hypothesis—10 years later. *Prog. Exp. Tumor Res.* 21:117, 1978.

Naib F.M., et al.: Cytology and histopathology of cervical herpes simplex infection. *Cancer* 19:1026, 1966.

Reagan J.W., et al.: Concepts of genesis and development in early cervical neoplasia. *Obstet. Gynecol. Surv.* 24:860, 1969.

Reid R.: Genital warts and cervical cancer: II. Is human papillomavirus infection the trigger to cervical carcinogenesis? *Gynecol. Oncol.* 15:239, 1983.

Rigoni-Stern in The Walton Report. *Can. Med. Assoc. J.* 114:2, 1976.

Syrajanen K.J.: Current views on the condylomatous lesions in uterine cervix and their possible relationship to cervical squamous cell carcinoma. *Obstet. Gynecol. Surv.* 35:685, 1980.

Wahi P.N., et al.: Factors influencing cancer of the cervix in North India. *Cancer* 23:1221, 1969.

Wentz W.B., et al.: Induction of uterine cancer with inactivated herpes simplex virus types I and II. *Cancer* 48:1783, 1981.

Cervical Intraepithelial Neoplasia

Boyes D.A., et al.: Experience with cervical screening in British Columbia. *Gynecol. Oncol.* 12S:143, 1981.

Briggs R.M.: Dysplasia and early neoplasia of the uterine cervix. *Obstet. Gynecol. Surv.* 34:70, 1979.

Christopherson W.M., Gray L.A.: Dysplasia and preclinical carcinoma of the uterine cervix: Diagnosis and management. *Semin. Oncol.* 9:265, 1982.

Ferenczy A.: Anatomy and histology of the cervix, in Blaustein A. (ed.): *Pathology of the Female Genital Tract*, ed. 2. New York, Springer-Verlag, 1982.

Reagan J.W., et al.: Concepts of genesis and development in early cervical neoplasia. *Obstet. Gynecol. Surv.* 24:860, 1969.

Richart R.M.: A radioautographic analysis of cellular proliferation in dysplasia and carcinoma in situ of the uterine cervix. *Am. J. Obstet. Gynecol.* 86:925, 1963.

Richart R.M.: Influence of diagnostic and therapeutic procedures in the distribution of cervical intraepithelial neoplasia. *Cancer* 19:1635, 1966.

Spriggs A.I., Boddington M.M.: Progression and regression of cervical lesions: Review of smears from women followed without initial biopsy or treatment. *J. Clin. Pathol.* 33:517, 1980.

Rigoni-Stern in The Walton Report. *Can. Med. Assoc. J.* 114:2, 1976.

Diagnosis and Treatment

Ahlgren M., et al.: Conization as treatment of carcinoma in situ of the uterine cervix. *Obstet. Gynecol.* 46:135, 1975.

Anderson M.D., Hartley R.B.: Cervical crypt involvement by intra-epithelial neoplasia. *Obstet. Gynecol.* 55:546, 1980.

Ayre J.E.: Selective cytology smear for diagnosis of cancer. *Am. J. Obstet. Gynecol.* 53:604, 1947.

Boyes D.A., et al.: The results of treatment of 4,389 cases of preclinical cervical squamous carcinoma. *J. Obstet. Gynaecol. Br. Comm.* 77:769, 1978.

Briggs R.M.: Dysplasia and early neoplasia of the uterine cervix. *Obstet. Gynecol. Surv.* 34:70, 1979.

Creasman, W.T., et al.: Results of outpatient therapy of cervical intraepithelial neoplasia. *Obstet. Gynecol.* 12:5306, 1981.

Garite T.J., Feldman M.J.: An evaluation of cytologic sampling techniques: A comparative study. *Acta Cytol.* 22:13, 1978.

Griffiths C.T., Younge P.A.: The clinical diagnosis of early cervical cancer. *Obstet. Gynecol Surv.* 24:967, 1969.

Kolstad P., Klem V.: Long term followup of 1,121 cases of carcinoma in situ. *Obstet. Gynecol.* 48:125, 1976.

Okagaki T., et al.: Diagnosis of anaplasia and carcinoma in situ by differential cell counts. *Acta Cytol.* 6:343, 1962.

Rubio C.A.: A trap for atypical cells. *Am. J. Obstet. Gynecol.* 128:687, 1977.

Savage E.W., et al.: The effect of endocervical gland involvement on the cure rates of patients with cervical intraepithelial neoplasia undergoing cryosurgery. *Gynecol. Oncol.* 14:194, 1982.

Sevin B.U., et al.: Invasive cancer of the cervix after cryosurgery: Pitfalls of conservative management. *Obstet. Gynecol.* 53:465, 1979.

Townsend D.E.: Cryosurgery for cervical intraepithelial neoplasia. *Obstet. Gynecol. Surv.* 34:828, 1974.

Townsend D.E., Richart R.M.: Cryotherapy and carbon dioxide laser management of cervical intraepithelial neoplasia: A controlled comparison. *Obstet. Gynecol.* 61:75, 1983.

Wagner A.C., McElin T.W.: Colposcopy, in Sciarra J.T. (ed.): *Gynecology and Obstetrics.* New York, Harper & Row, 1983, vol. 1, chap. 84.

Invasive Cancer

Barber H.R.K., Brunschwig A.: Results of the surgical treatment of recurrent cancer of the endometrium, in Lewis G.C. Jr., Wentz W.B., Jaffe R.M. (eds.): *New Concepts in Gynecological Oncology.* Philadelphia, F.A. Davis Co., 1966.

Berkowitz R.S., et al.: Invasive cervical carcinoma in young women. *Gynecol. Oncol.* 8:311, 1979.

Broders A.C.: Carcinoma grading and practical application. *Arch. Pathol.* 2:376, 1926.

Buchsbaum H.J.: Extrapelvic lymph node metastases in cervical carcinoma. *Am. J. Obstet. Gynecol.* 133:814, 1979.

Chung C.K., et al.: Histologic grade and prognosis of carcinoma of the cervix. *Obstet. Gynecol.* 57:636, 1981.

Deutsch M., Parsons J.A.: Radiotherapy for carcinoma of the cervix recurrent after surgery. *Cancer* 34:205, 1974.

Jobson V.W., et al.: Chemotherapy of advanced carcinoma of the cervix with cyclophosphamide and cis-platinum. *Proc. Am. Soc. Clin. Oncol.* 22:475, 1981.

Knapp R.C.: Clear cell carcinoma of the vagina, in Heintz A.P.M., Griffiths C.T., Trimbos J.B. (eds.): *Surgery in Gynecological Oncology.* The Hague, Martinus Nijhoff Co., 1984, p. 30.

Lepanto P., et al.: Treatment of para-aortic nodes in carcinoma of the cervix. *Cancer* 35:1510, 1975.

Maier R.C., Norris H.J.: Glassy cell carcinoma of the cervix. *Obstet. Gynecol.* 60:219, 1982.

Meigs J.V.: Carcinoma of the cervix: The Wertheim operation. *Surg. Gynecol. Obstet.* 78:1, 1944.

Morley G.W.: Pelvic exenteration in the treatment of recurrent cervical cancer, in Heintz A.P.M., Griffiths C.T., Trimbos J.B. (eds.): *Surgery in Gynecological Oncology.* The Hague, Martinus Nijhoff Co., 1984, p. 174.

Piver M.S., Barlow J.J.: Para-aortic lymphadenectomy in staging patients with advanced local cervical cancer. *Obstet. Gynecol.* 43:544, 1974.

Piver M.S., Chung W.S.: Prognostic significance of cervical lesion size and pelvic node metastases in cervical carcinoma. *Obstet. Gynecol.* 46:507, 1975.

Piver M.S., et al.: Hydroxyurea and radiation therapy in advanced cervical cancer. *Am. J. Obstet. Gynecol.* 120:969, 1974.

Plentl A.A., Friedman E.A.: Clinical significance of cervical lymphatics, in *Lymphatic Systems of the Female Genitalia.* Philadelphia, W.B. Saunders Co., 1971, p. 98.

Seski J.C., et al.: Microinvasive squamous carcinoma of the cervix. *Obstet. Gynecol.* 50:410, 1977.

Van Nagell J.R., et al.: Therapeutic implications for patterns of recurrence in cancer of the uterine cervix. *Cancer* 44:2354, 1979.

Wentz W.B., Reagan J.W.: Survival in cervical cancer with respect to cell type. *Cancer* 12:384, 1959.

CHAPTER FIVE

The Uterine Corpus

GENERAL CONSIDERATIONS

THE NOUN *uterus* is of Latin derivation and is synonymous with the lay term *womb*. The Greek word *hystera*, however, has come to have wide acceptance, especially with regard to surgical terminology, and the word *hysterectomy* is well known to nonmedical as well as medical personnel. Hysteria was, at one time, believed to be of uterine origin since this organ was considered the anatomic site of the human mind. As far as is known at present, however, the uterus serves one function—childbearing. Menstruation occurs only when the process of ovulation is not followed by successful fertilization and should not be regarded as a primary function. Although suggestions have been made that the uterus secretes a hormone, there is no valid evidence to support this supposition.

The position and physiologic characteristics of the uterus lead to the development of numerous irregularities, mostly in the form of abnormal bleeding. Happily for the gynecologist, however, the uterine-cavity is readily available for thorough investigation by dilatation and curettage, and this has become the most common of all gynecologic operations. Because of this facility for early and complete diagnosis, together with the intrinsic physical characteristics of the uterus, malignant disease of this organ is attended by a five-year survival rate of at least 60%, a figure much superior to those for malignancy of the vulva, vagina, cervix, oviduct, and ovary.

The field of endocrinology is intimately correlated with the normal and pathologic physiology of the uterus. The mucosal lining of the uterus, the endometrium, is a sensitive end-organ that reflects both the effects of the ovarian hormones estrogen and progesterone and the stability of the hypothalamic-pituitary-thyroid-adrenal-ovarian axis. The secretions of these glands act in concert to produce a regulated, rhythmic pattern of endometrial change. Defects or deficiencies of any or all of these organs may result in abnormalities evidenced only as abnormal flow, amenorrhea, or irregular ovulation. Diagnosis and treatment depend on a clear understanding of basic physiologic principles.

The uterus consists of two portions, the corpus and the cervix. Attention will be given in this chapter to diseases and physiologic aberrations of the corpus.

ANATOMY

The uterus (Fig 5–1) is a muscular, hollow organ that lies in the true pelvis between the bladder and rectum. Its measurements are usually stated to be: length 7 to 7.5 cm; width 4.5 to 5 cm; thickness 2.5 to 3 cm. The cephalic portion of the corpus is known as the *fundus* and is characterized by lateral flarings known as horns or *cornua*. The oviducts enter the fundus in the region of these cornua and demarcate the fundus from the main body of the uterus. As the corpus approaches the cervix it becomes narrowed, giving a somewhat triangular appearance when viewed from both the front and the side. This constricted area

149

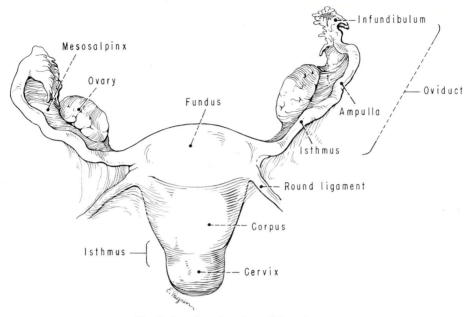

Fig 5–1.—Anterior view of the uterus.

separates the corpus from the cervix and is known as the *isthmus*. The cavity of the corpus is continuous with that of the endocervix and vagina and has an average depth of about 6 cm and a capacity of 3 to 8 ml. When the cavity is viewed in frontal section it appears triangular, with the base at the fundus and the two corners extending toward the orifices of the oviducts. In sagittal section the uterine cavity appears as a narrow cleft, whereas in transverse section it has the outline of a flattened ellipse.

The corpus possesses anterior and posterior surfaces, both of which are covered by visceral peritoneum. The anterior surface is slightly convex and, in the normally situated uterus, lies in contact with the most cephalad portion of the urinary bladder. As the uterine peritoneum approaches the region of the isthmus on the anterior uterine wall, it is reflected ventrally onto the bladder and thence continues as the parietal layer. The narrow space between these layers of reflected peritoneum is known as the anterior cul-de-sac. A sagittal section through the normal female pelvis (Fig 5–2) will show that the anterior

surface of the uterine isthmus is not covered by peritoneum. This anatomic fact is utilized in the performance of the *extraperitoneal* cesarean section in grossly infected patients since an adequate approach may be made by reflecting the bladder inferiorly and the peritoneum superiorly. The posterior surface of the corpus is slightly convex and is completely invested with a peritoneal covering. Caudally this peritoneal envelope is continued over the uterosacral ligaments, cervix, and upper portion of the posterior vaginal wall and is then reflected dorsally and cephalad over the rectum and lower sigmoid colon. The space between the reflected layers of peritoneum is known as the cul-de-sac of Douglas. It is of importance to the gynecologist for two reasons. (1) Blood or pus may be drained through the vagina by incising the posterior cul-de-sac, thus avoiding the major peritoneal cavity, and (2) various endoscopic instruments may be placed into this space through the vagina for a complete inspection of the oviducts, ovaries, and posterior uterine surface.

The anterior and posterior peritoneal cov-

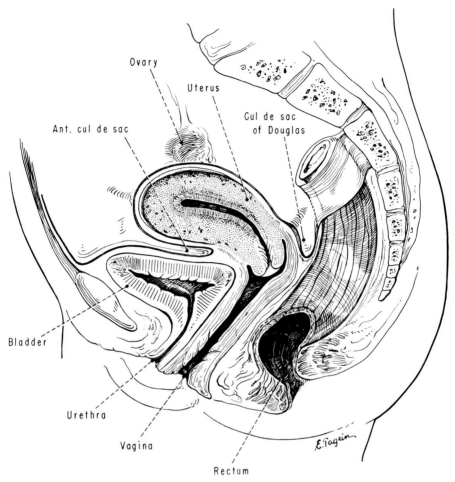

Ovary

Uterus

Ant. cul de sac

Cul de sac
of Douglas

Bladder

Urethra

Vagina

Rectum

Fig 5–2.—Sagittal section through normal female pelvis.

erings of the corpus join at the lateral uterine margin and form the leaves of the *broad* ligament (Fig 5–3). The peritoneal surfaces are in close proximity except where they diverge slightly to invest the *round* and *infundibulopelvic* ligaments. The broad ligament is, therefore, a double layer of peritoneum that extends from the lateral surface of the uterus outward to the pelvic wall. Its upper border consists of the peritoneal fold over the oviduct and the lateral extension from the ovary encircling the infundibulopelvic vessels. The midportion encompasses the round ligament, and the most inferior portion is thickened and contains a condensation of connective tissue

and muscle fibers called the *cardinal* ligament or lateral cervical ligament. The uterine vessels approach the lateral aspect of the cervix in the cardinal ligament, an anatomic point of importance in total hysterectomy.

The portion of the broad ligament between the ovary and the oviduct contains many small blood vessels and is termed the *mesosalpinx* or tubal mesentery. The vestigial remnants of the mesonephric tubules and duct are located within the leaves of the mesentery and are known as the epoophoron (lateral portion of the tubules) and the paraoophoron (medial portion of the tubules). All of these vestigial tubules are connected with the rem-

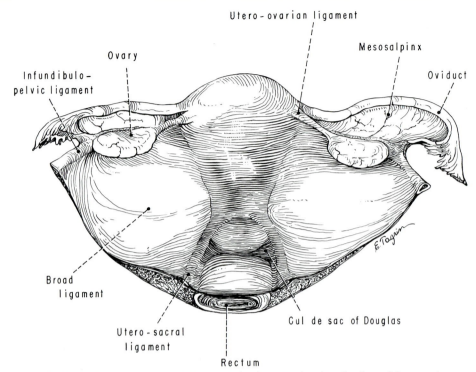

Utero-ovarian ligament

Ovary

Mesosalpinx

Infundibulo-
pelvic ligament

Oviduct

Broad
ligament

Utero-sacral
ligament

Cul de sac of Douglas

Rectum

Fig 5–3.—Posterior view of uterus and adnexae showing the broad ligament.

nant of the mesonephric duct (Gartner's duct). The blind upper extremity of the duct is occasionally dilated into one or more cystic structures known as hydatids of Morgagni. Cysts may develop from the main duct or from one of the smaller tubules and may be confused with ovarian cysts at the time of pelvic examination. These will be discussed further in Chapter 6.

The round ligaments consist principally of bands of muscle tissue that extend laterally from the anterolateral aspect of the fundus. They leave the peritoneal cavity through the internal inguinal ring, traverse the inguinal canal to the labia majora, and terminate by dissemination of fibers into the surrounding tissue. Although the round ligaments consist principally of muscle fibers prolonged from the uterus, there is also an admixture of fibrous and areolar tissue, blood vessels, lymphatics, and nerves. The round ligaments are about 10 to 12 cm long and 0.5 to 0.75 cm thick and are covered by the anterior and pos-

terior leaves of the broad ligament as far as the internal abdominal ring. In the fetus this duplication of peritoneum is prolonged as a short tubular process into the inguinal canal (canal of Nuck). It is generally obliterated in the adult, but occasionally it may persist and be the source of benign cystic structures that are frequently mistaken for hernias. Rarely, endometriosis occurs in this peritoneal projection.

The round ligaments were formerly believed to play a major part in uterine support, particularly the maintenance of the normal anterior position. Numerous operations have been devised that, in effect, shorten these ligaments with the hope that this will hold the fundus forward. The round ligaments may have some effect in returning the anterior uterus to its normal position after displacement by a full bladder or after pregnancy. They hypertrophy greatly during pregnancy and may be the source of localized lower-quadrant pain, which may simulate that of acute appendicitis. The lymphatics that traverse the ligaments are occasionally the route of metastases to the groin from endometrial carcinoma.

The uterosacral ligaments arise from the posterior wall of the uterus at the level of the internal cervical os. They are made up of connective tissue and involuntary muscle and contain blood vessels, lymphatics, and nerve filaments of the parasympathetic and sympathetic systems. Each ligament describes a posterior arc, passing dorsally around the rectosigmoid toward an insertion on the sacral wall at the level of the second and third sacral vertebrae. The peritoneum over the posterior uterine wall and cul-de-sac is reflected over the uterosacral ligaments throughout their course. The function of these ligaments is to exert tension on the cervix in a dorsal direction, in effect keeping the corpus anterior and the axis of the corpus and cervix at a right angle to the vagina. This prevents the uterus from assuming a position that would be in the axis of, and in direct line with, the vagina—a situation that is almost always associated with uterine prolapse.

The cardinal or transverse cervical ligaments (of Mackenrodt) have been mentioned as forming the inferior aspect or base of the broad ligament. They offer the chief support for the cervix and upper vagina and do so by integrating posteriorly with the uterosacral ligaments and anteriorly with the cervicovaginal portion of the endopelvic fascia. The cardinal ligaments are composed of muscle fibers and connective tissue that ensheath the uterine vessels, nerve fibers, and lymphatics. As they fan out laterally, the tissues of the ligaments insert into the fascia overlying the obturator muscles and the muscles of the pelvic diaphragm and, as pointed out by Anson, follow the course of the major vessels as a supporting framework. Careful dissection has shown that the effective dorsal fixation of the ligaments is provided by the perivascular fibrous tissue of the hypogastric and iliac vessels.

The utero-ovarian ligament (suspensory ligament of the ovary) extends from the lateral aspect of the uterus (between the round ligament and the oviduct) to the inferior pole of the ovary. It consists of connective tissue and smooth muscle in a rounded cord and is ensheathed between layers of the broad ligament. It is not known whether or not this ligament is capable of altering tubo-ovarian position at the time of ovulation, but some observations would indicate that this occurs.

UTERINE STRUCTURE.—The uterus is composed of three separate and distinct layers: (1) The perimetrium (serosa), an outer peritoneal covering; (2) the myometrium, an inner layer of smooth muscle; and (3) the endometrium, the mucous membrane lining the cavity (Fig 5–4). The perimetrium is continued laterally as the leaves of the broad ligament and is continued anteriorly and posteriorly as bladder and rectal reflections. The myometrium is composed of three rather indistinct layers of smooth muscle fibers. In each layer there is an interlacing and intermixture of the nonstriated muscle cells, which are held in juxtaposition by a connective tissue rich in elastic fibers. The outer muscular layer (stratum supravasculare) is chiefly longitudinal and is continuous with fibers entering the broad and round ligaments, whereas the middle layer is thicker and presents fibers in circular arrangement. The middle layer makes up the major portion of the myometrium and contains many blood vessels located between muscle bands (stratum vasculare). The inner layer represents an exaggerated muscularis mucosae and is composed of thin muscle strands arranged obliquely and longitudinally. The arrangement of the blood vessels between muscle bundles affords an ideal method for hemostasis following delivery. This is borne out clinically by patients whose uteri are atonic following parturition and in whom hemorrhage may at times prove fatal.

The endometrium is a soft inner layer of variable thickness made up of simple tubular glands, a stroma of resting cells in a fine connective tissue mesh, and a sensitive vascula-

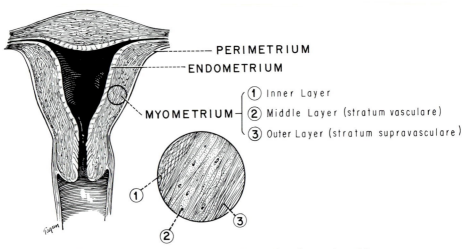

PERIMETRIUM
ENDOMETRIUM

MYOMETRIUM
1 Inner Layer
2 Middle Layer (stratum vasculare)
3 Outer Layer (stratum supravasculare)

Fig 5–4.—Structure of uterus, illustrating the endometrium, myometrium, and perimetrium.

ture. The histology and physiologic variations of this layer will be considered in the section "Menstruation."

BLOOD SUPPLY.—The uterus possesses a dual blood supply, receiving branches from both the uterine and ovarian arteries. The uterine artery is derived from the hypogastric trunk (Fig 5–5). It crosses over the ureter at the level of the internal os of the cervix and divides into ascending and descending limbs. The former runs tortuously upward between the leaves of the broad ligament, giving horizontal anterior and posterior branches to the cervix and corpus. As it reaches the cornu a branch is sent to the round ligament and then it is projected along the oviduct to anastomose with the ovarian vessels in the mesosalpinx. The descending branch of the uterine artery turns inferiorly and supplies the vagina from the lateral aspect. It anastomoses freely with the vaginal artery along its course.

The collecting veins from the corpus flow into two longitudinal trunks, which are usually distinct. The anterior surface is drained by the anterior uterine vein situated anterior to the ureter and lateral to the uterine artery. This vein empties into the hypogastric vein. The posterior uterine surfaces, however,

drain into a short and long trunk that pass posterior to the uterus and inferior to the uterine artery before joining either the hypogastric or obturator vein.

The processes of menstruation and pregnancy give singular importance to an understanding of the anatomic vascular pattern of the endometrium. As previously mentioned, a series of *radial* arteries are given off at right angles from the uterine artery as it courses along the corpus (Fig 5–6). These radial arteries branch in the inner third of the myometrium into *straight* and *spiral* (coiled) vessels. The straight arteries pass only as far as the basal layer of the endometrium and terminate in capillaries in that region. The spiral arteries, however, follow a coiled course throughout the thickness of the endometrium, give off a few branches in the endometrium, then fork and give rise to superficial capillaries just below the surface epithelium. These capillaries form plexuses in the stroma and a meshwork around the glands. In the superficial layer of the endometrium the capillaries form sinuslike dilatations known as "lakes." The blood is returned via small veins, which drain these vascular lakes and capillary plexuses. It should be remembered that the vascular pattern is a dynamic one, with constant prolifer-

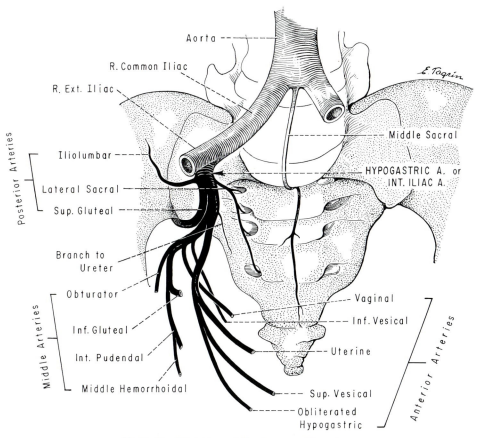

Fig 5–5.—Divisions of the hypogastric artery.

ation and regression. The specific morphologic details are considered in the section "Menstruation."

Although the prime function of the straight arteries is to supply the basal endometrium, they may also function to support regeneration of the lower portion of the functional layer. The coiled arteries alone supply blood to the superficial third of the endometrium and most of the blood to the middle third. Markee has shown in intraocular endometrial transplants, however, that some straight arteries may be converted into coiled ones and then later to the straight type. Thus it is possible that the blood supply of the endometrium could regenerate and develop specificity of function even after complete curettage.

The importance of the coiled arteries is not completely known. It should be pointed out, however, that they are absent or not fully developed in areas where extensive cyclic variations do not occur. Thus, in the lower uterine segment and lateral recesses of the endometrium the vascular supply is mostly through straight arteries.

NERVE SUPPLY.—The uterine extrinsic nerve supply is derived from three sources (Fig 5–7). (1) *Motor* fibers from the upper sympathetic thoracic ganglia course through the aortic plexus and the celiac ganglion to the *superior hypogastric plexus*. Fibers then diverge as they pass caudally to form the *inferior hypogastric plexus*, thence forward over the lateral surface of the rectal ampulla to join the *pelvic plexus* or *cervical ganglion*

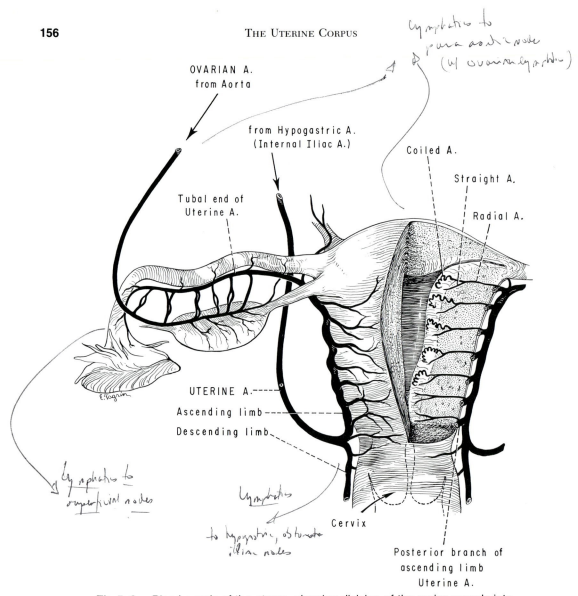

OVARIAN A.
from Aorta

from Hypogastric A.
(Internal Iliac A.)

Coiled A.

Straight A.

Radial A.

Tubal end of
Uterine A.

UTERINE A.

Ascending limb

Descending limb

Cervix

Posterior branch of
ascending limb
Uterine A.

Lymphatics to para aortic node (w/ ovarian lymphatics)

Lymphatics to superficial nodes

Lymphatics to hypogastric, obturator iliac nodes

Fig 5–6.—Blood supply of the uterus, showing division of the major vessels into radial, straight, and spiral (coiled) arteries and arterioles.

of Frankenhäuser. From this plexus, fibers pass along the uterosacral ligament to the smooth muscle of the uterus. Clinical evidence indicates that the motor fibers to the uterus leave the spinal cord at levels higher than the tenth thoracic nerve. (2) *Sensory* fibers are special visceral afferents that run through the hypogastric and aortic plexuses, through the 11th and 12th sympathetic ganglia without synapse, into the dorsal spinal root ganglia of these segments, thence up the dorsolateral fasciculus to the thalamus. The sensory supply to the cervix travels through the sacral parasympathetic chain communicating with the second, third, and fourth sacral nerves. (3) *Sensory and motor* fibers to the lower uterine segment and cervix are found in the sympathetic and parasympathetic plexuses, communicating with the second, third, and fourth sacral nerves. Visceral efferent fibers believed to be motor to the longitudinal muscle of the lower uterine segment and the

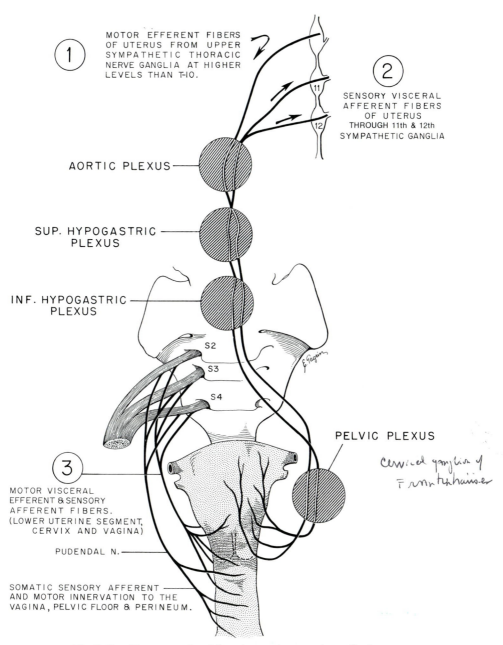

MOTOR EFFERENT FIBERS
OF UTERUS FROM UPPER
SYMPATHETIC THORACIC
NERVE GANGLIA AT HIGHER
LEVELS THAN T-10.

SENSORY VISCERAL
AFFERENT FIBERS
OF UTERUS
THROUGH 11th & 12th
SYMPATHETIC GANGLIA

AORTIC PLEXUS

SUP. HYPOGASTRIC
PLEXUS

INF. HYPOGASTRIC
PLEXUS

S2

S3

S4

PELVIC PLEXUS

Cervical ganglion of
Frankenhauser

MOTOR VISCERAL
EFFERENT & SENSORY
AFFERENT FIBERS.
(LOWER UTERINE SEGMENT,
CERVIX AND VAGINA)

PUDENDAL N.

SOMATIC SENSORY AFFERENT
AND MOTOR INNERVATION TO THE
VAGINA, PELVIC FLOOR & PERINEUM.

Fig 5–7.—Nerve supply of the uterus shown schematically.

circular fibers of the cervix and possibly inhibitory to the uterine fundus travel in the parasympathetic chain.

It should be remembered that although the sensory nerve fibers course through pelvic, hypogastric, and aortic plexuses before reaching the 11th and 12th thoracic nerves, they are functionally independent of the autonomic system. The sensory supply to the cervix, although traversing the sacral parasympathetics, is also functionally independent of the autonomic system.

LYMPHATIC SUPPLY.—The lymphatics of the uterine corpus proceed in four or five channels through the broad ligament just below the oviducts, thence upward along the ovarian vessels. In the course of their passage through the parametrium and ovarian ligament, they communicate with the ovarian lymphatics to terminate in the lumbar lymph nodes found in front of the aorta from its bifurcation to the diaphragm. The lymphatics from the lower uterine segment anastomose with adjacent lymph channels from the cervix and drain to the obturator, iliac, hypogastric, and sacral nodes. A third route of lymphatic drainage, especially from the fundal area, is via the round ligament to the superficial nodes.

EMBRYOLOGY

The normal uterus develops from the conjunction of two müllerian ducts of equal size, shape, and growth potential. The midline, unpaired structure is evolved as a result of three well-defined growth phases. These are (1) contact of the ducts, (2) fusion of the duct walls, and (3) involution of the created septum. If the ducts are not of equivalent size or have varying growth rates, a *uterus unicornis* may develop. If an abnormality of fusion occurs, a *uterus bicornis* or *didelphys* may develop. If the midline septum is not absorbed, the uterine cavity may be divided into two parts, forming a *uterus septus duplex*. The major developmental abnormalities are depicted in Figure 5–8. (For further detailed description of uterine abnormalities, see Chapter 10).

The lining of the prospective uterine cavity is columnar epithelium derived from the epithelium of the müllerian ducts. By a local downgrowth this epithelium forms the endometrial glands and these, in turn, provoke the development of an unusual stroma of a type found nowhere else in the body. Since organs (such as the uterus) derived from the müllerian duct epithelium and duct wall originate from the same germinal layer, the stroma and epithelium are more closely related in the internal genitalia than in most other organs. This is evident in the disease known as adenomyosis, in which islands of benign endometrial tissue "invade" the myometrium and seem to function just as normally as if they were lining the uterine cavity.

MENSTRUATION

Menstruation represents the effects of a fine interplay of gonadal and extragonadal hormones acting in concert on the endometrium in a sequential and cyclic fashion. It occurs usually about every 28 days, beginning at the menarche and continuing until menopause. It consists of the discharge from the uterus of fragments of endometrium, blood, and mucus with an admixture of vaginal epithelial cells. In this chapter the term *menstruation* will be considered to be the result of sloughing of secretory endometrium, i.e., an endometrium that has been acted on by progesterone subsequent to ovulation. Uterine bleeding from a nonsecretory endometrium is considered abnormal and will be discussed in the section "Dysfunctional Uterine Bleeding" in Chapter 14.

The age of onset of menstruation is variable, but in the Temperate Zone it is usually between 10 and 16 years. A number of cases have been reported of so-called idiopathic precocious puberty, in which children begin to ovulate and menstruate between the ages of 2 and 8 years, and some of these have become pregnant. No apparent endocrinologic disorder has been found in these children, but in others pituitary, midbrain, or ovarian tumors may bring about bleeding of an anovular nature. The onset of menstruation (*menarche*—"month beginning") may be delayed in some individuals until age 19 or 20 years. In such patients it should be remembered that many factors such as climate, heredity, health, and hygiene as well as social and economic background may delay the onset of the menses. It has been reported that warmer climates predispose to early menarche, whereas in extremely cold climates onset may be delayed. This, however, may

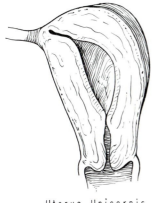

Uterus Unicornis

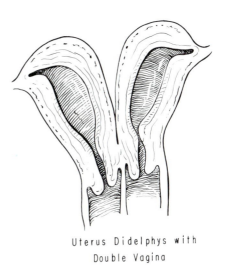

Uterus Didelphys with
Double Vagina

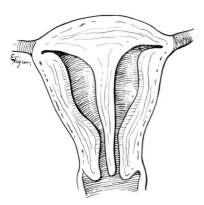

Uterus Septus Duplex

Fig 5–8.—Major congenital anomalies of the uterus.

merely be representative of variations in dietary and hereditary factors. Adolescents should not be subjected to vigorous hormonal treatment when the sole abnormality is the persistence of amenorrhea until age 18 or 19.

A plausible explanation of menstruation is now available from a study of current concepts of embryogenesis as well as a study of endometrial histology and biogenesis of steroids. The varying quality and quantity of the steroid hormones evoke growth and function of secretory tubules in endometrial tissue. These epithelial structures extend laterally, each joining its adjacent counterpart to form a complete lining of the uterine cavity. Under the influence of estrogen and progesterone an unbranched spiral artery of each endometrial segment expands into a terminal network of superficial capillaries. These arterioles and as-

sociated venules serve to make maternal blood accessible to the expectant trophoblast. The weak reticular matrix surrounding these vessels is converted into a buttressed tissue of contiguous stromal cells by their conversion into decidua, principally by the action of progesterone. Thus, the endometrium is primed and prepared for the arrival of the trophoblast.

The physiologic and morphologic changes responsible for the process of menstruation are (1) estrogen and progesterone withdrawal and slowed circulation, (2) vascular stasis and vasodilatation, (3) vasoconstriction, and (4) menstruation. These processes are under precise hormonal control, and specific conditions are essential for completion of endometrial sloughing. A reduction in the circulating levels of the endometrial-supporting steroids—

estrogen and progesterone—precipitate the morphologic events culminating in menses. There are four important conditions that are essential for this terminal event: (1) the hormonal stimulus must have been sufficiently intense; (2) the stimulus must have been present for an adequate duration of time; (3) the stimulus must be withdrawn relatively suddenly; and (4) the decrease must be sufficiently great. These conditions operate in all normal menstrual cycles and are the basis of the commonly used substitutional therapeutic schedules.

In the absence of trophoblastic implantation, and as a result of diminishing levels of estrogen and progesterone, the predecidua is deprived of nutriment. The decidual cells shrink, autolysis occurs, and the tissue becomes thinner. It has been suggested that a toxin derived from catabolism of stromal cells causes or potentiates tissue autolysis and arteriolar contraction. Superficial capillaries become devoid of stromal support and undergo autolysis. The caliber of spiral arterioles is diminished because of hormonal withdrawal, and intermittent contractions of these vessels eventuate in recurrent foci of ischemia. This slowed circulation is followed by a decrease in the thickness of the endometrium, mainly as a result of a fluid shift wherein a loss of extravascular fluid occurs.

As stromal shrinkage continues, the coiled arteries show further buckling with increased stasis. In intraocular transplants, the erythrocytes may not move for 60 to 90 seconds and a distinct bluing of the transplants is observable with the naked eye. A similar bluing of the human endometrium has been observed during the premenstrual period. Vasodilatation is sometimes seen during the period of stasis. It has been suggested that arteriovenous anastomoses play a role in the production of the stasis that leads to necrosis and menstrual bleeding. This theory assumes that acetylcholine-type compounds act on nerve fibers to control the opening and closing of the anastomoses. The presence of arteriovenous shunts has been confirmed, but that they play

a physiologic role in the menstrual process is not certain.

Some hours before menstrual bleeding begins, there is constriction of the basal part of the spiral arteries. This constriction is limited to that part of the artery that is located in the deepest part of the basalis or in the adjacent myometrium. The vasoconstriction affects individual coiled arteries in a random fashion. When vasoconstriction occurs it results in blanching of that part of the endometrium supplied by the constricted vessel. The constriction of the coiled arteries persists throughout the period of menstrual bleeding, being interrupted in individual vessels for only short periods.

Menstrual bleeding occurs when a previously constricted artery relaxes and blood again surges through it and its branches. It may be assumed that some weakening of the vessel's walls may have accompanied vasoconstriction. Several types of bleeding have been observed: (1) arterial or capillary bleeding with the formation of a hematoma; (2) direct hemorrhage from arterioles through the surface epithelium; (3) diapedesis through capillary walls; and (4) direct or retrograde blood flow from veins in the fields of previous hemorrhage and tissue destruction. Near the end of the first day of menstruation, fragments of endometrium slowly become detached and become part of the menstrual discharge.

The cessation of menstrual bleeding and endometrial desquamation usually occurs as the estrogen level begins to rise. Reepithelization occurs relatively rapidly and the vascular bed is restored.

Present evidence suggests that a hormonal substance, one of the prostaglandins known as $PGF_{2\alpha}$, is found in endometrial tissue in large amounts during the luteal phase of the cycle. This substance, one of nine prostaglandins derived from a carbon 20 compound known as prostanoic acid, is similar to the five known prostaglandins derived from human seminal plasma. When $PGF_{2\alpha}$ is infused intravenously or directly into the uterine lumen of the rat, a dramatic shift of the steroid pattern of ovaries occurs: progesterone levels are depressed, whereas the 20-hydroxyprogesterone levels are elevated. It has been suggested that $PGF_{2\alpha}$, a potent venoconstrictor, results in venospasms all along the venous pathway until the venoconstrictor is diluted in an ineffective concentration by venocaval blood. But the proximity of the ovary permits direct action on the production of steroids of the corpus luteum, thus causing a luteolytic effect. Thus a feedback mechanism between ovary and endometrium is established: $PGF_{2\alpha}$ is produced in the endometrium as a result of the effects of estrogen and progesterone; when the levels of $PGF_{2\alpha}$ reach a critical level during luteal phase, production of estrogen and progesterone are diminished by the potent venoconstrictor substance; diminution of estrogen and progesterone permits endometrial sloughing, reduction of $PGF_{2\alpha}$, and release of the hypothalamic blockade. This most attractive theory would explain the limitation of life of the corpus luteum, and support for this theory exists in cows, sheep, pigs, guinea pigs, and rats—animals that have shared venous drainage between the ipsilateral ovaries and the uterine cornua. These animals exhibit a unilateral effect on the ovary when a unilateral hysterectomy is performed. Proof of this mechanism in the human female has not been confirmed.

The average menstrual cycle is from 27 to 30 days and about 95% of ovulating women menstruate every 21 to 45 days. Therefore, if the cycle in a given individual is rhythmic (within a two- to three-day variation) and occurs within the interval mentioned, it should be considered normal. Bleeding at intervals of less than 21 or more than 42 days or with a total absence of rhythm should be considered abnormal and is frequently anovular. Menstrual flow usually lasts from three to six days, although many women bleed for only a day and a half and then have a day or so of staining. Others flow heavily for seven days but have always done so. Such variations should not be considered abnormal. About 30 to 100 ml of blood is lost during an average menstrual period, although many women may lose two to three times this amount and still have no physical or laboratory evidence of anemia.

Bleeding that is too profuse, too prolonged, or occurs at other than the usual regular intervals should be considered abnormal. Irregular or extremely long intervals are significant if they occur regularly. The degree of abnormality should be viewed in light of the patient's age. At the time of puberty or menopause the menstrual cycle is usually irregular—but only in respect to the length of intervals between periods. The duration and amount of bleeding should remain within the limits of two to seven days, with use of four to five pads a day. Prolonged or excessive bleeding is abnormal and should be investigated.

Menstrual discharge is characteristic in that it will not clot. This is probably due to a fibrinolysin and other factors prohibiting clotting rather than to the absence of some essential clotting factor, since if a small amount of menstrual discharge is added to fresh venous blood, clotting is speeded, then the clot dissolves. The average patient is aware of certain systemic changes for several days before the onset of flow. These include breast soreness or fullness, edema, backache, and leg ache, or just a sense of depression or lethargy. This group of symptoms has been termed *menstrual molimina* (Latin, "endeavor," "effort"). Exaggeration of these symptoms, plus a multiplicity of others, for ten to 14 days prior to menses has been described as *premenstrual syndrome,* or PMS.

Premenstrual syndrome has attracted extensive attention during the last two years, and it has been estimated that 10% of women in the United States are affected. The symptoms are breast swelling and tenderness, abdominal bloating, cravings for sweet and salty food, acne, asthma, constipation, nervousness, depression, and fatigue.

The cause of PMS is unknown but is probably multifactorial. About 40 "PMS centers" have been established in this country with emphasis on treatment with vaginal suppositories containing progesterone. Although several studies have failed to show diminished levels of progesterone during luteal phase, the administration of progesterone can, in some patients, relieve some symptoms and pelvic pain.

The various methods being used to help women cope with PMS suggests multiple causes, and every patient must be treated individually. It has been suggested that women could use PMS symptoms to excuse their own aberrant behavior. Others fear the condition could be used as a rationale to discriminate against women. Some medical professionals fear that PMS victims could be exploited by the unscrupulous physician.

Hormonal Aspects of Menstruation

A major part of the known relationships between the pituitary gland and the ovaries has been derived from animal investigation and therefore much of what follows is merely an application of this knowledge to the human female. Quantification of serum levels of the various hormones has led to a clearer understanding of the endocrinologic aspects of menstruation.

The first day of the *menstrual period* is considered as day 1 of the *menstrual cycle*. As the process of endometrial sloughing continues, a gonadotropic substance known as the *follicle-stimulating hormone* (FSH) is elaborated by certain basophilic cells of the adenohypophysis in progressively increasing amounts. In general, however, FSH may be regarded as a glycoprotein with a molecular weight of about 67,000, containing 1.5% hexosamine, 1.2% hexose, 15.1% nitrogen, and 1.5% sulfur. Follicle-stimulating hormone brings about a proliferation of the granulosa cells and formation of an antrum in an undetermined number of ovarian graafian follicles. In the male, FSH is a gametogenic agent, stimulating the seminiferous tubule system and spermatogenesis. The growth of the follicle prior to the antrum stage is controlled by extra-adenohypophyseal factors. The interstitial elements of the follicles are similarly stimulated to differentiate into the *theca interna*

and the *theca externa*. Available evidence suggests that the theca cells, not the granulosa, secrete an *estrogenic* (causing estrus) substance, probably estradiol-17β. Follicle-stimulating hormone alone is unable to bring about this secretion of estradiol by the follicle but will do so in the presence of a small amount of luteinizing hormone, a substance secreted by another distinctive basophilic adenohypophyseal cell.

Luteinizing hormone (LH) is responsible for luteinization of the theca interna and granulosa cells of the follicle. In recognition of this hormone's stimulating action on the interstitial cells of the testis, however, it is also appropriately called the interstitial cell–stimulating hormone, ICSH.

In a number of important respects LH (ICSH) acts as a physiologic complement to FSH. Luteinizing hormone, acting together with FSH, stimulates the follicle to full development and promotes the secretion of estrogen by the growing follicle. Luteinizing hormone at optimal levels is essential for ovulation and, in a sense, could rightly be considered the ovulating hormone. Following ovulation, LH induces the qualitative transformation of the cells of the theca interna and granulosa layers of the follicle to lutein cells and promotes the formation of the corpus luteum. The maintenance and activity of the corpus luteum may be dependent on a third gonadotropin, i.e., prolactin.

Prolactin, one of the first anterior pituitary hormones to be isolated in pure form, is a protein or proteinlike substance but, unlike FSH and LH, does not contain a carbohydrate moiety. The molecular weight is about 26,000 to 35,000.

Prolactin stimulates the alveolar cells of the mammary gland, resulting in the initiation and maintenance of milk secretion. This hormone also exerts an effect on corpus luteum maintenance and secretion of progesterone.

The effects of estrogens are twofold. (1) The endometrium begins to show *proliferative* changes characterized by glandular growth, regeneration of surface epithelium, and active mitoses in the stromal cells. These changes are considered in detail in the section "Dating the Endometrium." (2) A rise in the level of estrogen produces suppression of FSH, which is followed by a further rise in luteinizing hormone, perhaps stimulated by this particular level of estrogen. The normal range for estrogen production is usually between 60 and 200 μg per day for the follicular phase of the cycle, between 150 and 300 μg for the luteal phase of the cycle, and up to about 400 μg during the ovulatory rise. In summary, relatively pure FSH brings about only follicular development, whereas FSH plus LH effectively result in the secretion of estrogen from the follicle.

The ovary can be divided into four anatomic and functional subunits: the follicle, corpus luteum, stroma, and hilus. Each is a sort of endocrine gland of its own within the ovary, producing its own spectrum of hormones and having its own characteristic response to gonadotropin stimulation.

The developing follicle produces a wide variety of steroid hormones on the basis of assays of the follicular fluid and the incubation of the follicular apparatus with steroid precursors in vitro. The steroids isolated from ovarian tissue and follicular fluid are listed in Table 5–1. These include estrogens, androgens, and progestins, but the estrogens are quantitatively the most important constituents. Although not definitely established, it is assumed that well-developed and preovulatory follicles have the greatest steroid-producing potential. Isolation of these steroids from the ovary does not constitute proof of formation within the gland or follicle but is suggestive evidence due to the high concentration of hormones relative to other body fluids or tissues. It is evident that estrogens are the major hormones found, but progesterone, androstenedione, and even dehydroepiandrosterone are also formed.

Ryan has demonstrated that the granulosa cells can be separated from the theca cells of the follicle, and he has shown the capacity of each cell type in hormone synthesis. Both cell types have characteristic activity in steroid biosynthesis. The differences, thus far, seem more quantitative than qualitative but they may be of fundamental importance in the control of endocrine function. The granulosa has a clear superiority in progesterone accumulation. Ryan has also pointed out that in addition to their well-known histologic differences, the granulosa cell layer is an avascular tissue compared with the richly vascularized theca. Any hormone produced by the granulosa would no doubt have to traverse the theca before entering the bloodstream. These observations are the bases for the so-called two-cell theory of hormone formation.

In summary, it has been demonstrated that the follicular fluid contains a wide variety of steroids, that the follicular wall can synthesize hormones in vitro, and that stimulation with gonadotropins results in increased follicular size and hormone production. The follicular phase of the cycle can be correlated with increased levels of estrogen in urine, and the absence of follicles in the menopause can be correlated with a marked decline in estrogens. Although the follicle normally produces progesterone, androgens, and estrogens, its major secretory product appears to be estradiol.

Thus the stage is set for ovulation. An extremely delicate hormonal ovarian-pituitary

TABLE 5–1.—STEROIDS ISOLATED FROM THE HUMAN FOLLICULAR FLUID, OVARIAN TISSUE, AND CORPORA LUTEA*

ESTROGENS	ANDROGENS	PROGESTINS
Estradiol	Androstenedione	Progesterone
Estrone	Dehydroepiandrosterone†	20α-Hydroxypregn-4-en-3-one
Estriol†		17α-Hydroxyprogesterone

*From Ryan K.J.: Biosynthesis and metabolism of ovarian steroids, in Behrman S.J., Kistner R.W. (eds.): *Progress in Infertility*, ed. 2. Boston, Little Brown & Co., 1975, p. 277.
†Isolated predominantly from follicular tissue.

relationship has brought a graafian follicle to the surface of the ovary where it appears as a blisterlike elevation. Swelling of the entire structure occurs with expansion of the thinned granulosa and thecal elements. Simultaneously, the ovum is freed from its follicular attachment by the appearance of fluid in the cumulus cells. Within a short period thereafter the translucent edge of the follicle bulges from the ovarian surface as the *stigma* and, as a result of unknown factors, rupture occurs. This process is known as *ovulation* and usually occurs 14 ($\pm$ 2) days before the next expected menstrual period. The ovum is accompanied by the follicular liquor as it is released into the peritoneal cavity where it is enveloped by the fimbriated extensions of the oviduct.

The exact mechanism of ovulation is still unknown. Physical principles such as increasing intrafollicular tension, enzymatic destruction of the stigma, and variations in the adjacent muscle and fibrous connective tissue have been considered as ancillary factors. The regulation of ovulation by hormonal changes must be considered in light of present evidence to follow the following pattern: (1) FSH and LH mature the graafian follicle by specific action (FSH on granulosa cells, LH on theca cells); (2) a fully developed theca interna secretes estrogen; (3) low levels of estrogen stimulate FSH, thus increasing follicular growth; (4) higher levels of estrogen and/or its oxidation products are intimately involved in both the stimulation of the adenohypophysis and the release of LH (ICSH) from the pituitary gland; and (5) increased secretion of LH probably results in ovulation (definite lutein changes have been observed in the theca cells before ovulation, so the whole process is a gradual one). Since these preovulatory lutein changes may result in the secretion of small amounts of progesterone, the suggestion has been made that a proper balance of *estrogen* and *progesterone* effects adenohypophyseal secretion of LH through hypothalamic stimulation. This may be the final trigger mechanism necessary to rupture the stigma.

Ovulation, in the human, usually occurs from only one ovary, although more than one follicle may rupture at one time, resulting in dizygotic multiple pregnancy. There is no particular pattern of frequency as far as one ovary or the other is concerned, and studies in the monkey suggest a tendency for ovulation to occur in the proximity of the tubal end of the ovary and nearer the free edge than the hilum. Methods of detecting ovulation presently available are by direct observation at the time of laparoscopy and by certain presumptive laboratory methods. Included in the laboratory procedures are endometrial biopsy, basal body temperature, exfoliative cytologic findings, variations in hormone levels, and changes in the cervical mucus. The effects of progesterone on the endometrium may be reliably assayed by biopsy and results of the assay afford a fairly accurate estimate of the time of previous ovulation. Progesterone causes a rise in basal body temperature ranging between 0.4 and 1.0 F, which is usually maintained until menstruation. In general it is presumed that ovulation may be considered as occurring on or within two days before or after the day the temperature first rises. Exfoliative vaginal cytologic findings are not as applicable to clinical gynecology for the determination of the time of ovulation as biopsy or temperature charts, but they may serve as corroborative evidence. Progesterone produces a change in the cornification index of the squamous cells and, although the slides may be read rapidly, considerable training is necessary for correct evaluation. Studies on plasma progesterone indicate that free progesterone appears 24 to 48 hours before, or coincidental with, a prominent rise in waking temperature. Progesterone is excreted in the urine, in part, as pregnanediol, and current evidence indicates that the pregnanediol level rises significantly approximately 24 hours after ovulation (Fig 5–9).

The functional *corpus luteum* secretes both estrogens and *progesterone*. It usually lasts for about 14 days but begins to show degenerative changes from the ninth to 12th days. If pregnancy supervenes, the corpus luteum is maintained in an active state by gonadotro-

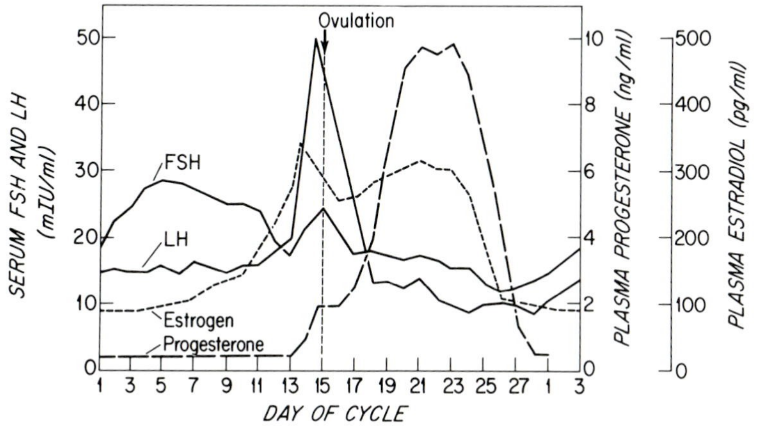

Fig 5–9.—Composite of normal menstrual cycle. The releasing factor stimulates gonadotropins, which in turn stimulate the secretion of estrogen. Rising estrogen levels stimulate the sharp rise in releasing factor and a rise in luteinizing hormone that triggers ovulation and the formation of the corpus luteum. High levels of progesterone and estrogen inhibit further output of gonadotropins, and the levels decline. The corpus luteum ceases to function, steroid levels drop, gonadotropin levels begin to rise, and the hormonal cycle starts over again. If pregnancy occurs, chorionic gonadotropin keeps the corpus luteum competent, estrogen and progesterone are secreted at high levels, and the cycle is broken. (From Taymor M.L.: *Reproductive Endocrinology,* New York, Medcom, 1974.)

pins derived from the cytotrophoblastic cells of the chorion. In the human female this state of preservation approximates 70 to 90 days.

The released ovum and its attached cells are about 150 μ in diameter, just visible to the unaided eye, and undergoes rapid degeneration in about 24 hours unless fertilized. The process of fertilization is said to occur in or near the fimbriated portion of the oviduct. Transfer of the fertilized human ovum along the oviduct usually takes about three days and implantation of the blastocyst occurs on the sixth or seventh day after fertilization.

The corpus luteum (yellow body) is formed from the remaining cells of the ovulated follicle. Following closure of the stigma, and as a result of increasing amounts of LH and luteotropic hormone (LTH), the granulosa cells enlarge, assume a polygonal shape with vesicular nuclei, and contain lipid vacuoles. They are now called *granulosa-lutein* cells. The theca-interna cells assume an epithelial appearance and migrate along newly formed vascular channels into the granulosa-lutein layer. The theca-lutein cells also contain lipid vacuoles and droplets and are believed to be the source of both estrogen and progesterone. Only small amounts of steroidal substances have been demonstrated in the granulosa-lutein cells during the active stage of the corpus luteum. Certain specialized and darker-staining cells derived from the theca interna have been demonstrated among the luteinized granulosa cells. They contain a high concentration of steroid substance, and it has been suggested that they are a major source of progesterone.

Numerous investigators have reported the levels of progesterone in plasma to vary from 0.1 to 1.6 μg/ml during the follicular phase of the cycle, and from 0.4 to 2.0 μg/ml during the luteal phase. The secretion rate of progesterone has been calculated as varying between 2.3 and 5.4 mg per day during the follicular phase of the cycle and from 22 to 43 mg per day during the luteal phase. A secretion rate of 1.3 mg/day was calculated for ovariectomized females, a secretion presumably of adrenal origin.

Direct assay of corpus luteum tissue has resulted in the identification of many of the same steroids isolated from follicular fluid.

The main distinguishing feature is the predominance of progesterone in the corpus luteum. The presence of the corpus luteum has been correlated with elevated levels of pregnanediol in urine and progesterone in blood. Such studies provide confirmatory evidence for an endocrine function of the corpus luteum during the second phase of the cycle.

The corpus luteum can readily be separated from the remainder of the ovary, and many studies have been performed by incubation of this tissue with steroid precursors in vitro. The corpus luteum can synthesize progesterone, androgens, and estrogens, but progesterone appears to be the major product. The estrogen produced during the luteal phase of the cycle is probably also produced by the corpus luteum but could in part be a product of developing follicles.

The ovarian stroma and hilus can be considered together, since they are essentially a continuum of ovarian tissue devoid of follicles and corpora lutea. The hilus is distinguished by greater vascularity and the presence of a Leydig-cell type, which sometimes forms the locus of an androgen-producing hilar cell tumor. The stroma and hilus can produce steroids in vitro with a spectrum of hormones qualitatively similar to those formed in the follicle and corpus luteum. In contrast to these other ovarian subunits, the stroma produces largely androgens. In the postmenopausal period, and when follicles are atretic, the stroma may be the site of significant hormone production. There is no evidence to suggest that these tissues are important during the normal cycle when either the follicle or the corpus luteum is active, but their role in this circumstance remains to be defined.

The effects of increased estrogen and progesterone secretion on the endometrium are discussed in detail in the next section ("Dating the Endometrium"). In general, there is an increased volume of blood carried to the glandular capillaries with the development of glycogen formation in the gland cells. This is followed by release of glycogen into the gland lumen—the "secretory" phase of the cycle. Stromal edema occurs at the midportion of the secretory phase and is followed by the collection of predecidual cells around the spiral arterioles.

Increased secretion of progesterone by the corpus luteum is probably responsible for the disintegration of that structure beginning about day 22 or 23 of the cycle. Progesterone has the ability to augment the conversion of estradiol to estrone and estrone to estriol and thus inhibits the formation of oxidation products of estrogen. It has been postulated that these oxidative products of estrogen (and not unchanged estrogen) are responsible for the release of LH and LTH. It becomes evident, then, that as the oxidative products diminish, LH and LTH are reduced and the corpus luteum begins to disintegrate with a resultant reduction in estrogen and progesterone secretion. Thus the support of the endometrium is withdrawn and within a few days bleeding—menstruation—occurs from the secretory endometrium.

The changes that take place in the endometrium have been studied by Markee in his classic experiments on transplanting monkey endometrium to the anterior chamber of the eye and observing the physiologic process with a dissecting microscope. He found that, following estrogen-progesterone withdrawal, the spiral arterioles undergo a process of constriction followed by dilatation. In addition, the number of capillaries supplying blood to the stroma decreases and the flow rate through these capillaries diminishes sharply. This is followed by a decrease in the total mass of endometrium with resultant increased stromal density. Shrinkage of the stroma withdraws lateral support from the coiled arterioles, causing them to buckle, and stasis results. This stasis is apparently caused by the increased resistance to flow resulting from the increased coiling of the arterioles. Stasis leads to diminished oxygenation of tissue with secondary necrosis. Tissue necrosis results in the production of *necrosin*, which brings about constriction of the undegenerated part of the coiled arterioles. Vasoconstriction begins slowly, then one coiled artery after another contracts during a one- to five-hour period, until all of those in a particular transplant show constriction. This period of a vasoconstriction precedes every menstrual period and always starts four to 24 hours before the onset of bleeding. When the amount of necrosin is reduced through diffusion, the coiled arteriole relaxes and hemorrhage occurs. Bleeding follows and continues as long as circulation through these arteries persists. These minute hemorrhages coalesce and grow and gradually effect a sloughing of the functional layer. The resultant endometrial slough, mucous secretion, and glands, together with the focal areas of hemorrhage, constitute the menstrual discharge.

Dating the Endometrium

Specific changes occurring in the stromal and glandular elements of the endometrium during the menstrual cycle have been of interest to both pathologist and clinician. By close scrutiny of these changes it has been possible to "date" the endometrium (within a range of about 48 hours), particularly in the postovulatory phase of the cycle. This correlation between the date of the cycle and the histologic appearance of the endometrium has particular importance in the study of the infertile patient. For purposes of simplicity a 28-day cycle, with ovulation occurring on the 14th day, will be described. The first day of the menstrual period will be considered the first day of the cycle, with the menstrual flow lasting four days. The *proliferative* phase of the cycle then begins at the termination of the *menstrual* phase. The postovulatory phase, or *secretory* phase, in this cycle extends from day 14 to day 28. Thus it is evident that the proliferative phase may persist for an indefinite period but the secretory phase is a constant 14 (± 2) days. It should be remembered that the changes to be described occur only in the functional layers of the endometrium and not in the basal layer or in the lower uterine segment. Biopsies of the endometrium therefore have significance only if an adequate amount of functional endometrium is obtained. It is recognized that all parts of the endometrium do not undergo simulta-

neous change since the tissue responsiveness may vary, depending on blood supply, adjacent leiomyomas, etc. In the normal cycle, however, an approximation of dating within 48 hours is frequently of considerable help.

Proliferative Phase

Under the stimulation of estrogen, the endometrium gradually rebuilds its substance. The *early* proliferative phase extends from the fourth through the seventh days, the *middle* proliferative phase extends from day 8 through day 10, and the *late* proliferative phase lasts from day 11 until the time of ovulation on day 14 (Fig 5–10). The characteristic histologic pattern of each phase (modified after Noyes, Hertig, and Rock) is as follows:

EARLY PROLIFERATIVE PHASE (FIG 5–11).— Glands: short, narrow, with mitotic activity (some glands remaining from menstrual phase may show secretory exhaustion). Surface epithelium: regenerating between openings of glands. Stroma: compact, few mitoses, cells stellate or spindle-shaped with scanty cytoplasm, nucleus large.

MIDDLE PROLIFERATIVE PHASE (FIG 5–12).—Glands: longer with slightly curved effect; beginning pseudostratification of nuclei (nuclei appear superimposed in layers, but actually all cells are attached at same level). Stroma: edema of variable degree; numerous mitotic figures; scanty cytoplasm and edema gives "naked nucleus" effect. Surface epithelium: covered with columnar epithelium.

LATE PROLIFERATIVE PHASE (FIG 5–13).— Glands: tortuous as a result of active growth; numerous mitoses; pseudostratification of nuclei. Stroma: dense with active growth pattern and numerous mitoses.

Secretory Phase

The changes after ovulation are due to the effects of estrogen and progesterone on an endometrium previously stimulated or "primed" with estrogen. As previously mentioned, this phase lasts about 14 days, the first seven of which are characterized by typical changes in

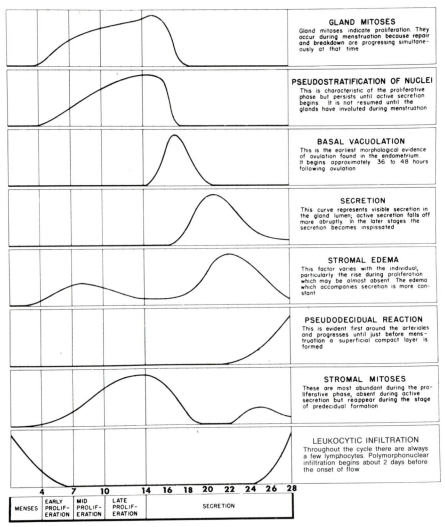

GLAND MITOSES
Gland mitoses indicate proliferation. They occur during menstruation because repair and breakdown are progressing simultaneously at that time

PSEUDOSTRATIFICATION OF NUCLEI
This is characteristic of the proliferative phase but persists until active secretion begins. It is not resumed until the glands have involuted during menstruation

BASAL VACUOLATION
This is the earliest morphological evidence of ovulation found in the endometrium. It begins approximately 36 to 48 hours following ovulation

SECRETION
This curve represents visible secretion in the gland lumen; active secretion falls off more abruptly. In the later stages the secretion becomes inspissated

STROMAL EDEMA
This factor varies with the individual, particularly the rise during proliferation which may be almost absent. The edema which accompanies secretion is more constant

PSEUDODECIDUAL REACTION
This is evident first around the arterioles and progresses until just before menstruation a superficial compact layer is formed

STROMAL MITOSES
These are most abundant during the proliferative phase, absent during active secretion but reappear during the stage of predecidual formation

LEUKOCYTIC INFILTRATION
Throughout the cycle there are always a few lymphocytes. Polymorphonuclear infiltration begins about 2 days before the onset of flow

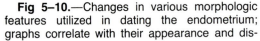

Fig 5–10.—Changes in various morphologic features utilized in dating the endometrium; graphs correlate with their appearance and disappearance during the menstrual cycle. (From Noyes R.W., et al.: *Fertil. Steril.* 1:3, 1950.)

the glandular epithelium. During the last seven days, specific stromal changes occur that may be utilized for dating purposes.

15TH DAY.—This is essentially a late proliferative pattern except for occasional vacuoles below the nuclei of the glands.

16TH DAY (FIG 5–14).—Basal vacuoles are seen in most glands; last day of pseudostratification; mitoses in glands and stroma.

17TH DAY (FIG 5–15).—Characteristic pattern of subnuclear glycogen vacuoles is evident, with homogeneous cytoplasm above nuclei of glands; position of nuclei rather regular; loss of pseudostratification of cells with increase in diameter and tortuosity; mitotic figures in glands and stroma rare.

18TH DAY (FIG 5–16).—Subnuclear vacuoles appear smaller as nuclei move back toward base of cell; beginning secretion of glycogen into lumen of gland; no mitoses.

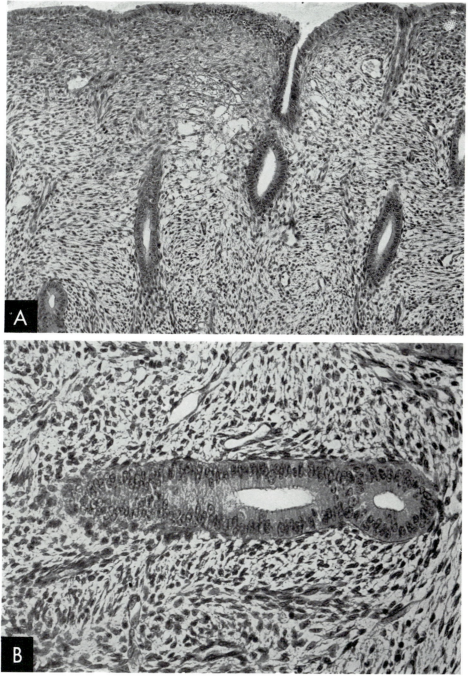

Fig 5–11.—Early proliferative endometrium. **A,** surface epithelium thin; glands sparse, narrow, and straight. **B,** few mitoses in glands and stroma; little pseudostratification of gland nuclei.

(Figures 5–11 to 5–21 from Noyes R.W., et al.: *Fertil. Steril.* 1:3, 1950. Low-power micrographs are magnified ×150; high-power, ×400.)

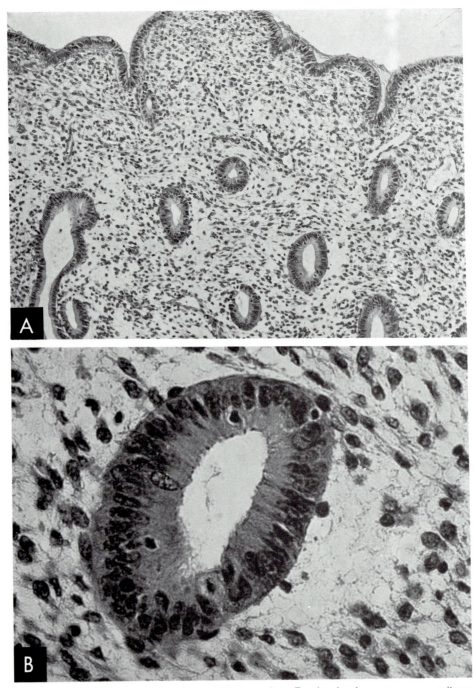

Fig 5–12.—Endometrium showing intermediate degree of proliferation. **A,** glands slightly tortuous; tall columnar surface epithelium. Extracellular fluid is not always as marked as in this section. **B,** glands show numerous mitoses with pseudostratification becoming marked. Note the "naked nucleus" type of stromal cell with fine anastomosing processes.

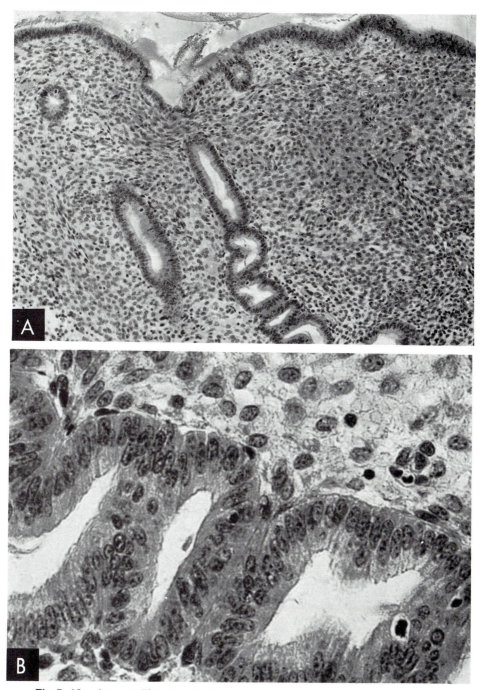

Fig 5–13.—Late proliferative endometrium. **A,** glands tortuous; stroma usually quite dense. **B,** epithelial nuclei are pseudostratified and oval in shape.

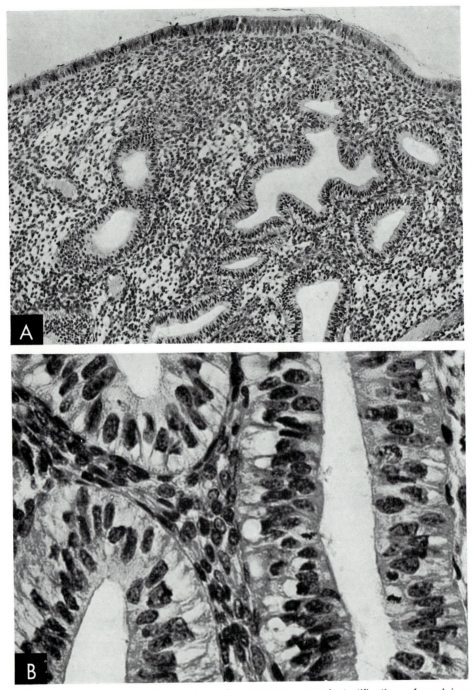

Fig 5–14.—Second postovulatory day. **A,** glands tortuous; stroma dense; cells consist of nearly naked nuclei. **B,** gland mitoses very numerous; pseudostratification of nuclei exaggerated by subnuclear vacuoles.

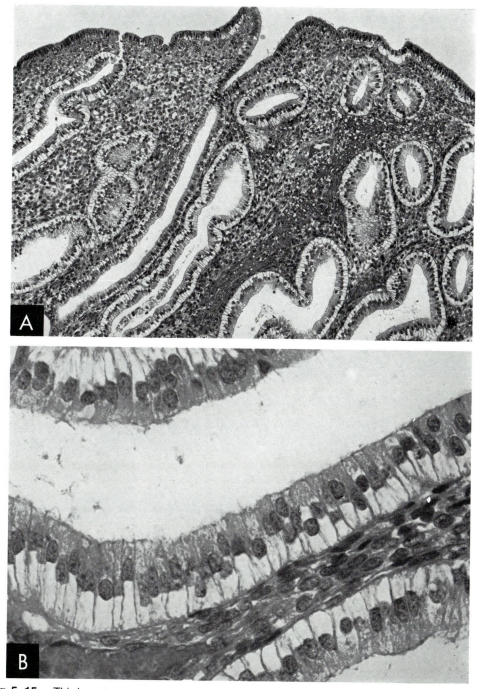

Fig 5–15.—Third postovulatory day. **A,** gland nuclei are pushed to the center of the epithelial cells with cytoplasm above and vacuoles below them. **B,** gland mitoses rare; pseudostratification decreasing.

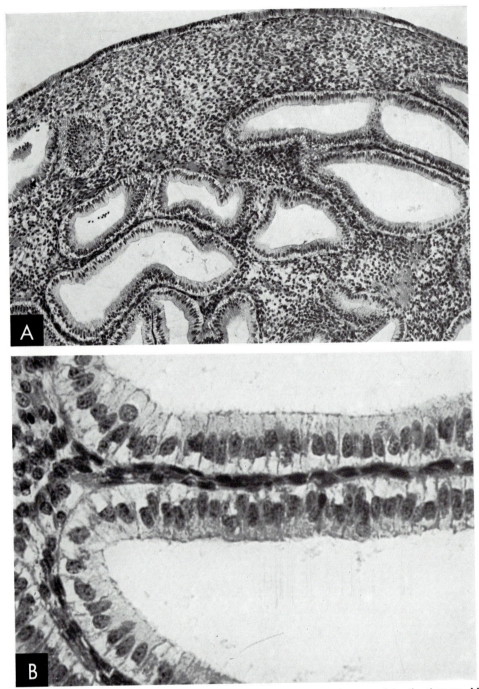

Fig 5–16.—Fourth postovulatory day. **A,** gland nuclei are returning to base of cells. Wisps of secretory material are present in lumina. **B,** some vacuoles are pushed past the nucleus on their way to empty glycogen into the lumen. Mitoses and pseudostratification of nuclei absent. This is the stage of arrival of ovum in the uterus.

19TH DAY.—Few subnuclear vacuoles are seen; resembles day 16 pattern except for secretion in lumen of gland and absence of pseudostratification and mitoses.

20TH DAY (FIG 5–17).—Occasional subnuclear vacuoles; acidophilic secretion is prominent in gland lumen.

21ST DAY.—Beginning stromal effects: cells of stroma have dark, dense nuclei with filamentous cytoplasm; beginning stromal edema.

22ND DAY (FIG 5–18).—Maximum point of stromal edema; thin-walled spiral arterioles may be seen. Secretion in gland lumen is active but subsiding and undergoing inspissation.

23RD DAY (FIG 5–19).—Edema of stroma persists but characteristic change is a condensation of the stroma around the spiral arterioles. This is due to an enlargement of stromal nuclei with an increase in cytoplasm and is called *predecidual* change.

24TH DAY (FIG 5–20).—Predecidual collections surrounding arterioles are marked; active stromal mitoses but lessening of stromal edema. The endometrium is now beginning to undergo involution unless maintained by pregnancy.

25TH DAY (FIG 5–21).—Predecidua is forming beneath the surface epithelium, and there is some edema around the arterioles; beginning lymphocytic infiltration of the stroma.

26TH DAY.—Gradual increase in predecidua is seen throughout stroma, with infiltration of polymorphonuclear leukocytes.

27TH DAY.—Predecidua is prominent around blood vessels and under surface epithelium; marked infiltration of polymorphonuclear leukocytes.

28TH DAY.—There is beginning focal necrosis of the predecidua with small areas of stromal hemorrhage. Stromal cells are clumped together; extensive polymorphonuclear leukocytic infiltration. Tortuous glands appear to have undergone secretory "exhaustion."

Certain specific changes in glands and stroma may be considered to indicate physiologic changes occurring in the endometrium. Thus, *gland mitoses* indicate active proliferation and growth and may be found from day 3 or 4 of the cycle until day 16 or 17. *Pseudostratification* of gland nuclei begins after the postmenstrual involution and usually disappears by day 17. It is an indication of proliferative glandular growth, and its appearance is due to crowding of nuclei when the gland is sectioned transversely. *Basal vacuolation* is the earliest morphologic evidence of ovulation discernible in the endometrium. Although occasionally one may be seen in the absence of progesterone, basal vacuoles are usually identified between day 15 and day 19, the glycogen being pushed into the gland lumen about day 19 or 20. The characteristic lining up of the nuclei above the vacuoles is best seen on day 17 and is an excellent indication of recent ovulation.

The secretory function of the glands is evident from day 18 until day 22 by the appearance of loose, feathery material in the lumina. If the blastocyst implants itself on the surface of the endometrium about six days after ovulation it would appear that morphology and function are well correlated, since days 20 to 22 would be critical ones from the standpoint of nutrient materials. The *edema* of the stroma, most striking between days 22 and 23, may represent an effort of the endometrium to simplify the implantation process by lessening tissue resistance. Periarterial *predecidual reaction* is evident beginning about days 23 and 24 and may represent a protective mechanism against premature vascular disruption. The predecidua is looked on as providing a supporting framework for newly developed blood vessels to aid in their increased load should pregnancy supervene. These changes in morphologic features are graphically summarized in Figure 5–10.

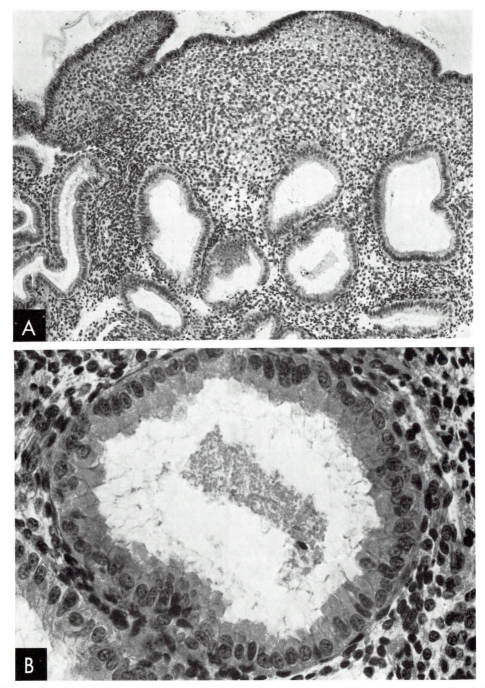

Fig 5–17.—Sixth postovulatory day, corresponding to beginning implantation in fertile cycle. **A,** secretion in gland lumen at peak; beginning of accumulation of extravascular fluid in stroma. **B,** subnuclear vacuoles rare; nuclei round and basally located.

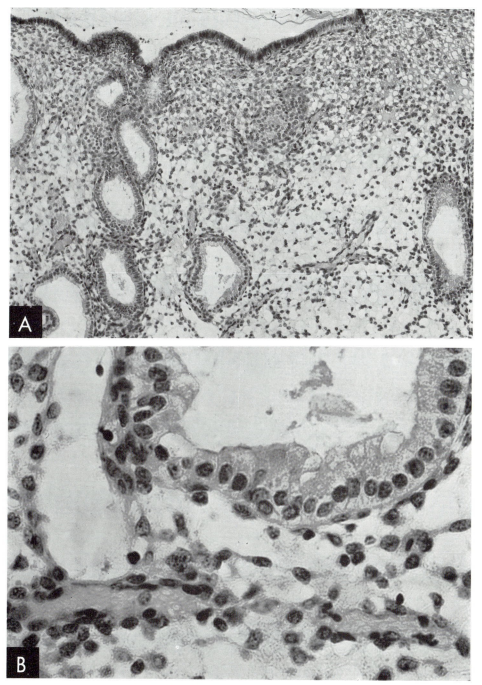

Fig 5–18.—Eighth postovulatory day. **A,** extracellular fluid maximal. Walls of spiral arterioles are not prominent. **B,** stromal cells still appear as small, dense "naked nuclei" widely separated by extracellular fluid. Glandular secretion still active but subsiding.

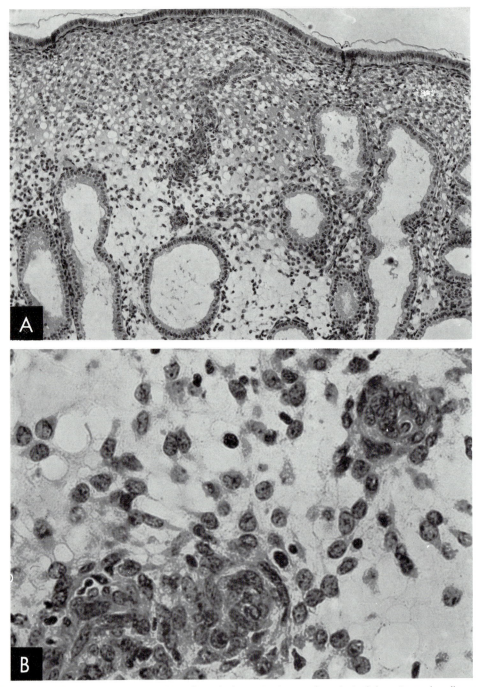

Fig 5–19.—Ninth postovulatory day. **A,** spiral arterioles become prominent because of condensation of surrounding stroma. **B,** both nuclei and cytoplasm of periarteriolar stromal cells are enlarging. This is the earliest predecidual reaction.

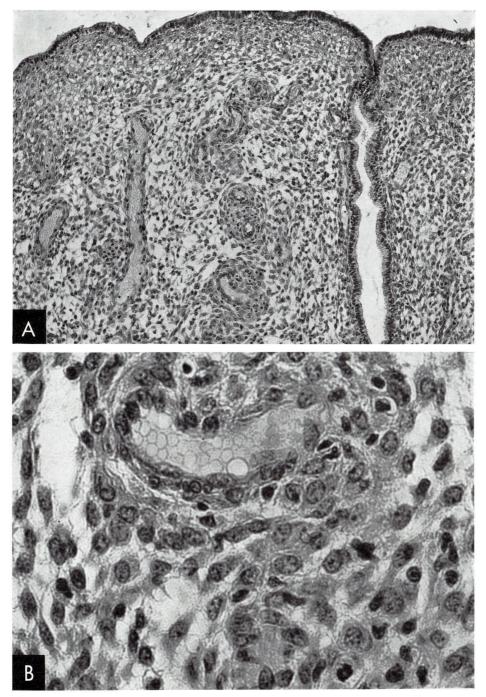

Fig 5–20.—Tenth postovulatory day. **A,** spiral arterioles and surrounding predecidua still more prominent; extracellular fluid subsiding. **B,** thick-ening of periarteriolar predecidual cuff; stromal mitosis evident.

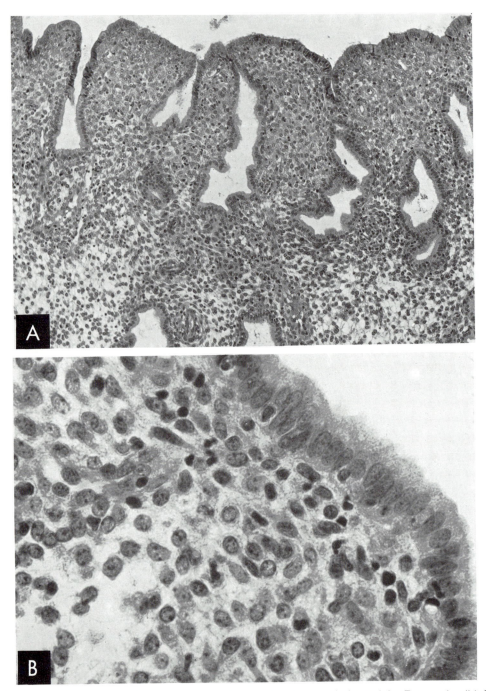

Fig 5–21.—Eleventh postovulatory day. **A,** pseudodecidua begins to differentiate under surface epithelium. Stroma of the stratum spongiosum still contains extracellular fluid except in areas near a spiral arteriole. **B,** round-cell infiltration accompanies predecidual differentiation. Stromal cells swell to become predecidual in type.

Systemic Changes Associated With the Menstrual Cycle

Certain phases of water and electrolyte balance occurring during the menstrual cycle have been studied using ^{131}I isotope-dilution techniques that measure total exchangeable body sodium. No evidence of a cyclic change in sodium balance or sodium retention was found in these experiments. This is at variance with previously accepted ideas of premenstrual sodium and water retention, which have been correlated with the syndrome of premenstrual tension. In other studies estrogenic substances have been shown to cause a *limited* storage of sodium and chloride together with an increase in the volume of extracellular fluid. A direct effect of estrogen on renal tubular reabsorption is believed to be the mechanism of this storage. Cyclic premenstrual edema in some individuals may represent a form of secondary aldosteronism. Antidiuretic hormone shows no variation during the menstrual cycle, and progesterone has been shown in castrate animals to increase urinary output.

The hematocrit declines and blood volume increases slightly at the end of menstruation. Plasma ester cholesterol diminishes at the time of ovulation and immediately before menstruation. The eosinophil count drops at the time of ovulation, with total counts being lower in the luteal than in the follicular phase.

Certain clinical correlations have been made by Rogers between diseases and menstruation. Thus, it has been noted that appendicitis rarely occurs during menses, whereas porphyria may show an exacerbation at the time of menstrual flow and may be brought on by exogenous progesterone. Epistaxis, nasal hyperemia, sinusitis, rhinorrhea, asthmatic bronchitis, and epilepsy have been noted as being brought on or worsened by menstruation. Several studies in penal institutions have shown that women in the childbearing age committed major crimes, including murder, most frequently during the premenstrual phase. Most females in this age group who attempt suicide do so during the postovulatory phase of the cycle.

The effects of impaired nutrition on the menstrual cycle, with the development of amenorrhea, have been observed and studied extensively. As a direct result of a diminished caloric intake, a lowering of FSH excretion is first observed, with subsequent hypothyroidism and hypoadrenocorticism. Although the release of gonadotropins into the circulation is restricted, the gonadotropic-hormone content of the adenohypophysis is normal or even increased. Obesity is similarly associated with abnormalities of menstruation, particularly amenorrhea, and weight reduction appears to effect resumption of normal menses in about half the patients. It has been suggested that both obesity and amenorrhea are symptoms of emotional disease that respond simultaneously to psychotherapy. It is also possible, however, that obesity is similar to inanition, both resulting in a diminished secretion of gonadotropin.

THE THYROID.—Disturbances of menstrual function may be associated with aberration of thyroid metabolism, although the precise pathophysiologic mechanisms are unknown. Thyrotoxic females may have perfectly normal menstrual cycles but, if untreated, may progress to states of oligomenorrhea and amenorrhea. Observations in the rabbit have indicated that thyroid hormone decreases FSH content and increases LH content of the pituitary, a possible explanation for the amenorrhea. In states of severe hypothyroidism, such as myxedema, variations of dysfunctional uterine bleeding may occur, with the development of subsequent endometrial hyperplasia. The administration of thyroid hormone to such patients will usually result in normal ovulatory cycles. The anovulation of myxedema may result from persistent FSH stimulation without the interplay of LH since, in thyroidectomized animals, estrogen is not effective in suppressing pituitary activity. When, however, thyroid is administered, FSH is diminished and LH is increased.

This effect of hypothyroidism, i.e., anovular ovarian function, is of great clinical significance since a number of important gynecologic problems may be associated with it. Amenorrhea, oligomenorrhea, hypermenorrhea, and polymenorrhea have all been associated with anovular ovarian activity. Obviously, ovulatory failure also leads to infertility.

The gynecologist's investigation of the cause of menstrual dysfunction should always include a thorough evaluation of thyroid function. In the true hypothyroid patient, replacement therapy produces very dramatic results. Such patients, however, are rarely seen in gynecology. More often the gynecologist is confronted with a patient complaining of menstrual dysfunction with only minimal symptoms of thyroid deficiency and laboratory findings that are somewhat equivocal. In such instances a so-called trial course of thyroid medication is often used. If the patient's gynecologic problem does not improve, the conclusion should not be drawn that she did not require thyroid medication. If the anovular pattern has not reached an irreversible stage, restoration of normal menstrual cycles may follow treatment. This appears to occur more often in the younger patient or where the dysfunction has existed for a relatively short time. On the other hand, if anovular ovarian function has existed for months or years, an irreversible stage of polycystic ovarian disease may develop. In such cases thyroid medication may improve the general health of the patient but have little or no effect on the menstrual dysfunction.

Other experiments have suggested that thyroid hormone may have a peripheral effect in decreasing the sensitivity of the ovary to the effects of adenohypophyseal hormones. The fine balance of such relationships has been reflected in the age-old custom of administering thyroid hormone to women who had noted irregularities of menstruation, in-

fertility, or both. Controlled investigations in euthyroid subjects have proved the fallacy of this reasoning, so that at present there is no valid reason for giving thyroid preparations to such patients.

THE ADRENAL.—It has been known for some time that the adrenal gland plays an integral part in the process of menstruation, and it was demonstrated in adrenalectomized rats that exogenously administered gonadotropins evoked no ovarian response. Gray and associates studied the aldosterone secretion rates, excretion of pregnanediol, and urinary sodium-potassium ratio during the menstrual cycle of 13 normal women. They found the mean value of aldosterone secretion to be 140 μg during the follicular phase and 233 μg/day during the luteal phase. This increase in the aldosterone secretion rate during the luteal phase was observed in subjects taking a diet unrestricted in sodium, as well as in subjects with a controlled high-sodium intake. When ovulation was suppressed with an estrogen-progestin combination, the rise in aldosterone secretion observed during the second half of the cycle was abolished.

Clinical evidence is seen in patients with Addison's disease who have persistent amenorrhea. Similarly, in the adrenogenital syndrome amenorrhea is a common symptom, and it has been postulated that the cause is an increased secretion of adrenal androgens and estrogens, which suppress the formation and secretion of adenohypophyseal gonadotropins. In such patients the administration of cortisone (or cortisonelike preparations) depresses ACTH production and results in a diminution of secretion of adrenal androgens and estrogens with increased secretion of FSH and LH. Ovulation and menstruation subsequently occur. The basic defect in this situation is thought to be an enzyme insufficiency in the adrenal zona reticularis, whereby there is a failure of hydroxylation of the 11 and 21 positions of a ^{21}C steroid. Thus, instead of formation of 17-hydroxycorticosterone there is produced an excess of 17-hydroxyprogesterone. Metabolites of 17-hydroxyprogesterone are not only androgenic (androsterone and etiocholanolone) but are unable to inhibit ACTH. There is thus set up a vicious circle, with further stimulation of the adrenal to produce more 17-hydroxyprogesterone. Cortisone inhibits the production of ACTH and removes the stimulus for the basic hyperplasia.

THE LIVER.—The liver is known to be an important site for the inactivation of estrogenic hormone. Thus, in animals estrus may be prevented by transplanting the ovaries into the mesentery or spleen. Estrogens are conjugated in the liver and apparently thereby inactivated. Progesterone is probably also similarly inactivated. Certain endocrine changes occurring in the premenopausal female with liver disease have therefore been attributed to delayed or incomplete estrogen deactivation. These are hypermenorrhea, polymenorrhea, endometrial hyperplasia, spider angiomas, and palmar erythema. Whether these are brought about by a specific vitamin B deficiency of the liver or by the effects of concomitant inanition has not been determined. In any event, administration of riboflavin, thiamine, protein, or a nutritious diet will frequently bring about clinical improvement in the symptoms of estrogen derangement.

DIABETES MELLITUS.—Although diabetes mellitus in the adult female may cause oligomenorrhea, amenorrhea, diminished libido, and infertility, the introduction and proper use of insulin has made these symptoms relatively uncommon. Menstruation has been noted to aggravate existing diabetes, and several reports have pointed out the relation of the menstrual period to an increased incidence of acidosis. This may be due to lowered levels of estrogen. Diabetes occurring before and during the menopause has been shown to improve following the administration of estrogen. The author has noted this clinically in postmenopausal diabetic patients who were given large amounts of diethylstilbestrol because of disseminated mammary carcinoma.

Animal experiments lend supporting evidence, in that diabetes induced in rats by subtotal pancreatectomy is made worse by oophorectomy. The mechanism by which estrogens improve diabetes is not known but two suggestions have been advanced. (1) Estrogen suppresses the growth hormone of the pituitary; (2) estrogen stimulates the islands of Langerhans to hypertrophy and hyperplasia. Progesterone or medroxyprogesterone acetate, however, when administered to patients with disseminated endometrial carcinoma has been noted to increase the severity of diabetes and increase the need for insulin. Clomiphene citrate, on the other hand, when administered to similar patients has been noted to diminish the need for insulin.

NERVOUS SYSTEM.—Epileptic seizures are more common at the time of the menses, and serial electroencephalograms have demonstrated increased cortical instability at this time. Studies of body water and sodium have negated a long-held idea that this increased convulsive tendency was due to salt and water retention. Seizures are uncommon during the luteal phase and the increased incidence just before, during, and after menstruation may be due to a lessened secretion of progesterone with its anticonvulsive effect. Migraine headaches may occur in association with the menses and are commonly relieved by periods of induced anovulation or by pregnancy. It has been suggested that the occurrence of migraine at the time of the menses is related to premenstrual retention of salt and water, but studies indicate no correlation between fluid retention and headache. The suppression of ovulation by estrogen-progestin combinations in the oral contraceptives does not protect against migraine, and some patients note aggravation of migraine subsequent to their use. The evidence suggests that the attack is related to *variations* in the levels of estrogen and progesterone rather than to excesses since the migraine headache seems to appear more frequently during the period when the oral contraceptive is *not* being taken. When these compounds are administered constantly, as in pseudopregnancy for endometriosis, migraine attacks are uncommon. Similarly, the use of a small amount of a synthetic progestin, administered constantly in a dose insufficient to suppress ovulation, is not attended by migraine attacks in women who experienced headache when the estrogen-progestin was used. This suggests an antiestrogenic effect of the progestin on the cerebral vessels, and there is evidence that a typical migraine attack may be initiated by the injection of estrogen in previously oophorectomized or postmenopausal females.

THE SKIN.—Acne vulgaris has been noted to become aggravated premenstrually, especially in adolescents. This is thought to be due to lowered estrogen and increased skin sebum. Improvement is frequently obtained by the administration of estrogenic substances. Chronic ulcerative vulvitis and stomatitis may relate to the menstrual cycle and mouth lesions such as necrotizing ulcerative gingivitis, aphthous stomatitis, and pyorrhea alveolaris have been reported to be exaggerated premenstrually. Increased pigmentation of the skin around the eyes, nipples, and perioral area may be noted during the week prior to menstruation, an effect of variations in the release of melanocyte-stimulating hormone from the pituitary.

THE BLOOD.—Thrombocytopenic purpura may be first evidenced by excessive uterine bleeding at the time of the menses. This is due to the rapid diminution in platelets and increased capillary fragility normally seen during the luteal phase of the cycle. Other blood dyscrasias that may result in hypermenorrhea are leukemia, erythrocytosis, and pseudohemophilia. A simple screening method in the evaluation of patients with abnormal bleeding at the time of the menses is the performance of a blood smear, a platelet count, and a determination of the bleeding time.

THE PSYCHE.—Depression, irritability, and, occasionally, aggression are commonly noted in the premenstrual phase of the cycle. Increased libidinous tendencies are frequently seen, and crimes of violence committed by women are much commoner during this phase. These symptoms and the entity known as *premenstrual tension* have been attributed to progesterone deficiency, abnormal estrogen-progesterone relationship, abnormal sodium and water retention, and abnormal psychodynamic processes. In the absence of a specific cause it is probably justified to consider these behavior patterns as abnormal manifestations of a normal physiologic process in susceptible or hyperreactive women.

Secondary amenorrhea is frequently psychogenic in origin and may be due to abnormalities of hypothalamic-adenohypophyseal function. Thus, LH may not be released or may not be sufficient to cause ovulation. Some patients with so-called hypothalamic amenorrhea may be resistant to exogenous estrogen and progesterone, suggesting a rapid neutralization or abnormal metabolism of these steroids. The gonadotropin excretion levels in psychotic patients have been found to be low, suggesting diminished pituitary function.

Hypermenorrhea may also occur in response to abnormal psychosomatic stimuli. Thus, it may follow periods of depression, shock, anger, fright, or similar stressful situations.

UTERINE RETRODISPLACEMENT

The enthusiasm for surgical correction of uterine retrodisplacement so prevalent for many years has now abated. Gynecologists generally regard the operation as of no value. Many have completed residencies without having performed a single suspension of the uterus. Similarly, the use of vaginal pessaries has received no more than token consideration.

We believe that there are certain patients with a particular symptom complex who may be helped by these simple gynecologic procedures. The selection of such a patient is difficult and necessitates taking a careful history and performing a meticulous examination, since studies in large gynecologic clinics have shown that approximately 20% of women examined for gynecologic complaints have uterine retrodisplacement. In many, the malposition is asymptomatic and merely of statistical interest. In others, however, striking improvement may be brought about by an appreciation of a few principles of pelvic anatomy and physiology.

The intrinsic muscular tone of the uterus itself, together with its configuration and vascular status, may be causally related. The flabby, boggy uterus associated with the syndrome of pelvic congestion is frequently displaced posteriorly. The situation may be congenital—purely a physical derangement—incorporating a short anterior vaginal wall and an upward tilting of the cervix. The lateral cervical attachments (cardinal ligaments) are the main long axis support of the cervix and uterus. Weakening of these ligaments is probably the principal cause of prolapse, although prolapse is almost always associated with some degree of retrodisplacement.

The round ligaments serve a definite function in retaining the normal anterior position of the uterus, although it is doubtful that they function alone. Even in severe retrodisplacement the round ligaments usually appear grossly normal. Given sufficient tension on the posterior aspect of the cervix by the uterorectosacral ligaments and normal intra-abdominal pressure on the posterior aspect of the fundus, the round ligaments aid in keeping the fundus anteflexed. Theoretically the round ligaments also function in the postpartum period of uterine involution to return the fundus to its anterior position. Similar function is presupposed after a full bladder has been emptied.

The uterorectosacral ligaments vary greatly in size, thickness, and consistency, but serve a most important function in keeping the cervix directed posteriorly. When the combination of ligamentous support is deranged, either by physiologic changes such as

pregnancy or by organic causes such as infection or endometriosis, retrodisplacement occurs.

Last, various tumors of the adnexa or bowel may displace the uterus from its normal position.

Uterine retrodisplacement may be considered under two general categories: (1) primary retrodisplacement, which is associated with congenitally deficient supporting structures and/or a short anterior vaginal wall; (2) secondary retrodisplacement brought about by childbirth, pelvic infection, endometriosis, or tumors.

PRIMARY RETRODISPLACEMENT.—The uterus is always retrocessed and occasionally retroverted in infancy and childhood. At puberty it usually assumes an anteverted, anteflexed attitude, but when there are other stigmata of infantilism, such as a short anterior vaginal wall and short uterorectosacral ligaments, the uterus remains retroverted. Cases have been described of incomplete ovarian descent with shortening of the infundibulopelvic ligament and posterior pull on the uterus. Many nulliparous patients who undergo routine pelvic examinations have asymptomatic, retroverted uteri unassociated with pelvic pathology. In these women this may be a manifestation of a generalized diminution in intrinsic tissue tone as evidenced by renal and intestinal ptoses, leg and vulval varicosities, hemorrhoids, hernias, and, occasionally, uterine prolapse.

SECONDARY RETRODISPLACEMENT (LIGAMENTOUS RELAXATION).—As previously noted, secondary uterine retroversion is commonly associated with laxity of the pelvic supporting tissue, whether due to repeated childbirth or to vascular aberrations resulting in pelvic congestion. The rigors of pelvic delivery and the puerperium probably are the leading causes of secondary retroversion. Sustained hard physical work during the pregnancy and long hours without rest or support in the erect position early in the puerperium undoubtedly are contributing factors. Repeated pregnancies may cause a change in the normal musculature with an increasing amount of vasculature, subsequent congestion, and, later, fibrosis. (Congenital factors must be considered as well, since many *grandes multiparas* have anteverted uteri.)

Postmenopausally this same uterine fibrosis occurs normally and results in atrophy and flaccidity. The uterus drops back and usually is found in the axis of the vagina—both anterior and posterior supports being, for the most part, inactive. The integrity of the cardinal ligaments and the pelvic diaphragm determines whether or not prolapse will occur at this stage.

Pathologic factors in retrodisplacement include endometriosis, pelvic infection, and tumors. In endometriosis the uterus is not infrequently found in deep, fixed retroversion. This process, involving as it does the peritoneum of the cul-de-sac and uterosacral ligaments, frequently produces areas of scarring across the posterior aspect of the fundus. The rectal serosa occasionally is involved and the adnexa may be implicated, producing a fixed, tender pelvic mass. In a recent study of a large group of patients with pelvic endometriosis, uterine retrodisplacement was noted in 28%.

The exudate of pelvic peritonitis may be etiologic in fixed retrodisplacement, since pelvic contour will cause such exudates to gravitate to the posterior cul-de-sac where organization and fibrosis occur. A large pyosalpinx is occasionally found anteriorly and adherent to the uterovesical space, with posterior displacement of the fundus. Post-abortive, postpartum, tuberculous, and gonorrheal infections are the major causes of such pelvic inflammation, although occasionally a ruptured appendix or diverticulum may produce the same situation.

Most adnexal tumors gravitate into the lateral pelvis or cul-de-sac and cause anterior rather than posterior displacement of the fundus. One exception to this is the dermoid cyst, which frequently is found anterior to the broad ligament with the corpus posterior (Küstner's sign). Pedunculated uterine leio-

myomas may reach sufficient size so that the fundus is displaced against the sacrum and may be independently palpated. Rarely, rectal carcinoma may force the cervix anteriorly, with subsequent posterior displacement of the fundus.

The idea that retroversion of the uterus may be caused by falls, injuries, or extensive athletic activity has generally been discarded by most gynecologists. Obviously, without a control examination before the accident or activity, conclusions would be hazardous.

PATHOLOGIC PHYSIOLOGY.—Following retrodisplacement of the uterine fundus, from whatever cause, vascular changes of great importance occur. The angles of entrance and exit of the uterine vessels are distorted, producing torsion and partial venous obstruction. The ovaries and tubes are drawn into a characteristic pelvic-wall prolapse attitude with increased pressure in the veins of the infundibulopelvic ligament. Laparotomy during the early puerperium strikingly reveals these changes, showing a large, congested, mottled, purple uterus, edematous tubes, and varicosities of the veins of the broad ligament. Microscopically, the veins of the myometrium are dilated and congested.

The endometrium associated with symptomatic retroversion has not been studied extensively, but Derichsweiler noted edema and overfilling of the vessels of the mucosa. Taylor, in his study of pelvic vascular congestion and hyperemia, examined the endometrium in 17 cases. The findings were not unusual except for three cases of chronic endometritis. The ovaries are frequently involved, cystic degeneration being noted in more than physiologic degree. Cortical fibrosis has been described. Taylor noted ovarian edema and vascular engorgement with a tough, unyielding capsule. It has been suggested that long periods of congestion result in connective tissue hyperplasia of the ovarian cortex with subsequent interference with normal ovulation. In his study of 105 cases of chronic pelvic hyperemia and vascular congestion, Taylor noted retroversion of appreciable degree in one third of the cases. Cotte, by iodized oil (Lipiodol) injection, demonstrated a reduction in uterine size following suspension of an enlarged, retroverted, congested uterus, so that there is adequate evidence for believing many of the changes are due to position alone.

SYMPTOMATOLOGY.—Probably the most common symptom noted by patients with acquired retrodisplacement is sacral backache, although it should be noted at the outset that retroversion frequently causes no symptoms whatsoever. Why this should be so is not clear. Variations in pain threshold, mental tension, and degrees of vascular abnormalities have been suggested as factors, but actually the physiopathology of this pain has not been adequately explained. In several series of cases of uterine retroversion the incidence of central, sacral backache has varied from 50% to 75%. Backache usually is aggravated by long hours in the erect position and commonly is worse in the late afternoon and evening. A backache that is noted in the morning and that seems to lessen as the patient goes about her housework probably is not caused by uterine malposition.

Many women complain of pelvic pressure or a bearing-down feeling and are unable to delineate their discomfort further. Occasionally lower quadrant pain is noted or the patient describes a "soreness in the ovaries." About half the patients with symptomatic retrodisplacement describe definite aggravation of their difficulties just before or at the time of the menstrual period. The premenstrual tension syndrome is common. Irregularities of menstrual flow, increased flow at time of periods with passage of clots, constipation, and leukorrhea may be associated with this syndrome. The leukorrhea is often due to an untreated cervical ectropion. Retroversion has been described as an etiologic factor in abortion, and King, in an analysis of a large series of cases of spontaneous abortion, found this statistically valid. Although retroversion is found in an appreciable number of cases of infertility, no conclusive evidence exists to support the idea that it is the position of the uterus that has prevented conception. The necessity for the cervix to "dip" into the seminal pool has received extensive considertion, but is apparently of minimum importance. Conception occurs whether the cervix is behind the symphysis, deep in the vault, or angulated forward or backward. As long as a film of seminal fluid with effective spermatozoa is placed across the os uteri, ascent into the uterine cavity will occur.

TREATMENT.—At the time of pelvic examination, the ease with which the retroverted uterus may be replaced is usually determined. Frequently replacement may be accomplished by simple bimanual examination, exerting sufficient force against the cervix to lift the fundus with the abdominal hand. If replacement is not easy, strenuous efforts should not be exerted. The presence of pelvic infection, tumors, or endometriosis, of course contraindicates further palliative measures and necessitates surgical correction. Frequently the uterus is soft and boggy and the vagina tender. These patients are instructed in a course of pelvic depletion. This consists of daily, hot, 15-minute douches, sitz baths, and knee-chest exercises for three or four weeks. At the end of this time replacement of the uterus usually is simplified, although occasionally it is necessary to use the tenaculum method of reposition. Should these methods prove unsuccessful, correct positioning may be accomplished by inserting a pessary and then having the patient assume the knee-chest position. In this way air opens the vagina, and intravaginal manipulation can be used to replace the uterus and obtain a good application of the pessary. We have routinely used the Smith-Hodge or Hodge hard rubber pessary to correct retrodisplacement (Fig 5–22).

It is in the group of patients with "married woman's complaint" that marked symptomatic improvement may be expected. Such a pa-

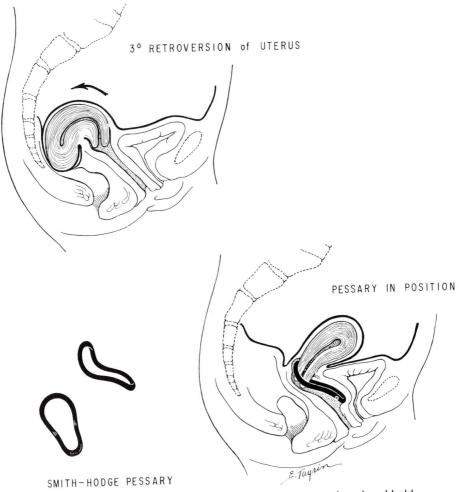

3° RETROVERSION of UTERUS

PESSARY IN POSITION

SMITH—HODGE PESSARY

E. Tagrin

Fig 5–22.—Third-degree retroversion of the uterus replaced and held anteriorly by a Smith-Hodge pessary.

tient is typically a hard-working housewife of moderate parity with one child or more under 4 years of age. Her complaints are those of backache, heaviness in the pelvis, aching thighs, vaginal discharge, chronic fatigue, and dyspareunia. Cervical cauterization may be necessary in certain cases after adequate cytologic and biopsy studies. The pessary is kept in place for five to six months with monthly examination, removal, and reinsertion. At the end of this time it may be removed and the patient observed for an additional two months. If symptoms recur and the fundus is again retroverted, repeated treat-

ment with a pessary may be tried. Uterine suspension occasionally may be considered, but is rarely indicated in this group of patients or as a primary surgical procedure. It is usually performed as part of a conservative laparotomy for infertility, endometriosis or the Stein-Leventhal syndrome. The use of estrogen-progestin combinations, particularly those containing a potent androgenic progestin with only 30 μg of estrogen, has simplified the management of "married woman's complaint." After two or three cycles of therapy, symptomatic improvement is usually noted. If the discomfort is exaggerated while taking these agents, adenomyosis or endometriosis should be suspected.

INFECTIONS

Infections of the uterine corpus are, for the most part, infections of the endometrium and are encompassed in the broad term *endometritis*. The most common etiologic factors are infected abortions, parturition, gonorrhea, tuberculosis, *Mycoplasma,* and *Chlamydia.* Certain office gynecologic procedures may occasionally be followed by endometrial infection. These include biopsy and cauterization of the cervix, endometrial biopsy, hysterosalpingography, and tubal insufflation. The use of a stem pessary for dysmenorrhea or insertion of gauze or radium into the uterine cavity may be followed by an acute or chronic endometrial inflammatory reaction. Cervical stenosis subsequent to conization, cauterization, or irradiation may diminish or prohibit uterine drainage and be a predisposing factor in the etiology of pyometra.

Postabortal Infection

The most serious, and occasionally fatal, type of endometrial infection is that associated with a septic abortion. The pathogenesis in this entity consists in the introduction of pathogenic bacteria into the uterine cavity by a catheter, bougie, sound, curet, or pack. The conceptus and its covering provide an ideal culture for growth of organisms, and the increased vascularity brought about by pregnancy permits rapid and widespread dissemination. The most common bacteria identified from cultures are the nonhemolytic, anaerobic streptococci, enterococci (*Escherichia coli, Pseudomonas aeruginosa, Bacterium aerogenes*) and *Clostridium perfringens.* An increasing number of pathogenic staphylococci have also been identified. These are presumably secondary invaders, which follow preliminary control of the original organism by antibiotics. The pathologic process usually begins as a necrotizing endometritis and deciduitis at the placental site with spread along the decidua and into the myometrium. Micro-

scopically, there is an acute inflammatory exudate, the decidua contains leukocytes and plasma cells, and there are extensive necrosis and thrombosis of small vessels. The inflammatory process may extend into the myometrium, forming multiple small abscesses, and dissemination into small veins and lymphatics may be extensive. The myometrium appears pale and flabby and microscopically shows cytolysis and edema.

The symptoms of an infected abortion are severe, rather constant (but occasionally crampy) pelvic pain, vaginal bleeding, chills, and prostration. A history of one or more missed menses may be obtained, but rarely, if ever, is the historian rewarded by being informed that an abortion has been performed. Examination reveals evidence of pelvic peritonitis with lower abdominal rigidity and rebound tenderness. The abdomen is usually distended because of ileus, and bowel sounds are hypoactive. Pelvic examination may disclose a foreign body (catheter or pack) in a cervical os that is soft and patulous. Occasionally necrotic decidua or membranes may be visualized coming through the cervix. The uterus is enlarged, soft, and acutely tender, and the broad ligaments feel thickened in the acute phase and ligneous in later phases of the process. The temperature is elevated, usually over 101 F, and there is tachycardia, leukocytosis, and a moderate anemia.

In certain severe cases, sudden hypotension occurs in the absence of blood loss and may rapidly result in death. The probable cause is the introduction of anaerobic, gramnegative organisms into the bloodstream following a decidual and placental bacteremia. These bacteria are capable, under such circumstances, of liberating a potent endotoxin, which possesses profound hemodynamic effects. The method of shock here has not been adequately explained but is probably correlated with a diminished peripheral resistance with visceral "pooling" and vascular sludging, together with a decreased cardiac output. Death may occur suddenly from shock or later from renal insufficiency.

TREATMENT.—Treatment of infected abortion cannot be didactically outlined—each case must be individually assayed. In general, however, the patient must be kept at complete bed rest and adequate hydration provided by intravenous fluids. Electrolyte balance should be maintained and anemia corrected by transfusions of whole blood. Culture specimens should be taken from the endocervix and from the blood, and antibiotics administered in adequate dosage depending on sensitivity. Anaerobic cultures should be made to rule out *C. perfringens* or anaerobic streptococci. It is our policy to give 2 gm of either tetracycline or chloramphenicol intravenously during the first 24 hours. This therapy is maintained until the drug can be taken orally, but is changed if the sensitivities indicate that another antibiotic is preferable. The patient is kept in a middle or high Fowler's position to promote the collection of pus in the posterior cul-de-sac. Repeated pelvic examinations are contraindicated; the patient's course may be followed by changes in temperature, pulse, sedimentation rate, and white blood cell count. Adequate analgesia and sedation should be provided, especially during the first 72 hours of illness. After five or six days, occasionally earlier, pelvic examination should be repeated to determine whether pus is localized in the posterior cul-de-sac. If so, it may be easily drained by posterior colpotomy. Postabortal infections usually spread laterally in the parametrial lymphatics, forming the typical "pelvic cellulitis," and in this way differ from gonorrheal infections. The latter frequently develop into tuboovarian abscesses, which fill the cul-de-sac and make vaginal drainage quite easy and thus expedite convalescence. Postabortal phlegmons may occasionally form between the leaves of the broad ligament and point above Poupart's ligament. These may be drained extraperitoneally, greatly aiding in resolution of the septic process. In longstanding cases of postabortal infection a thrombophlebitis of the pelvic veins may develop, with subsequent septic emboli. The diagnosis of this complication is difficult, but rapid and occasionally heroic treatment is necessary. Some authors suggest immediate ligation of the vena cava and infundibulopelvic veins, and cite a low mortality rate and minimal morbidity with this procedure. In patients with seemingly irreversible shock, hysterectomy offers the only hope of salvage. Less radical treatment consists of complete and rapid anticoagulation and the use of antibiotics. Should embolization occur while the patient is on anticoagulant drugs, caval ligation remains as a lifesaving procedure.

Anderson has noted a reduced mortality rate at the Los Angeles County General Hospital in patients with septic abortion since adoption of an aggressive therapeutic program. The regimen consists of massive doses of antibiotics, early curettage, and administration of cortisone. Steroid therapy has replaced the use of vasopressors in patients exhibiting hypotension, since observations in animals showed that the highest mortality rate in endotoxemic shock occurred in animals treated with blood-pressure–raising agents.

The criteria for beginning antibiotic treatment are (1) purulent material protruding through the cervix; (2) history of instrumentation; (3) signs of sepsis with no extrauterine source; and (4) shock out of proportion to blood loss. When the diagnosis is made, chloramphenicol, usually 500 mg, is given intravenously, followed by 1 gm in each liter of fluid given, so that 4 gm is given within a 24-hour period. Curettage is done immediately after the first injection. If shock is present or impending, 250 mg of hydrocortisone is given. During the next 24 hours, 500 mg of hydrocortisone is given in each liter of fluid, so that the patient receives a total of 1,750 mg the first day. Antibiotics are specific in their activity and the use of a particular agent should be based on an explicit assumption, even though provisional, of the nature and etiology of the disease process. A smear and Gram stain of infected cervical or vaginal exudates often provide an immediate guide to specific therapy and may save days while waiting for cultures. Furthermore, these observations may indicate a predominant organism or may help to resolve a dilemma of antibiotic selection. In addition, a simple Gram stain may suggest the need for special culture techniques when fastidious organisms fail to grow or cultures have been improperly processed.

Bacteremia of unknown type, particularly if accompanied by *endotoxin shock*, is a specific indication for antibiotic combinations. The dosage schedules (assuming normal renal function) for adults are: (1) 8 to 12 gm of cephalothin, daily, intravenously, plus 5 mg/kg of kanamycin every eight hours intramuscularly; (2) cephalothin, kanamycin plus 0.8 to 1.0 mg/kg of polymyxin B every eight hours intravenously; (3) cephalothin, plus polymyxin B; or (4) 1 gm of chloramphenicol every eight hours intravenously plus 4 million units of penicillin G every four hours intravenously (or 1 to 2 gm of ampicillin every four hours intravenously) plus polymyxin B. Clostridial infection is best treated with large doses of penicillin or tetracycline.

Vasopressors are used only if the blood pressure and urine output do not respond within six to eight hours. Antibiotics are continued until the patient has been afebrile for at least three days.

In severe cases or in patients not responding to these measures, hysterectomy is performed. Anderson has recommended that hysterectomy be performed under hypothermia (31 C) on the grounds that it lessens the insult by reducing metabolism and interfering with bacterial metabolism.

Tuberculosis

Tuberculosis of the female genital tract is not common in the United States and, when it does occur, is usually an incidental finding at laparotomy for pelvic inflammatory disease or infertility. Its incidence, therefore, is somewhat higher in hospitals or clinics where these entities are frequently seen. The diagnosis may be made, also unexpectedly, by endometrial biopsy in the routine workup of an infertility patient.

Genital tuberculosis is said to occur in from 3% to 8% of patients with pulmonary tuberculosis and is usually found during the child-bearing age, especially between 16 and 35 years. It is extremely rare in prepubertal and postmenopausal females. At the Brigham and Women's Hospital, tuberculosis has been diagnosed in only 1.8% of specimens removed surgically for salpingitis of various causes. This incidence is somewhat lower than the 5% cited by Novak and is less than the 2% to 10% cited in most pathologic reports. By comparison, in European countries tuberculosis may account for 20% to 50% of all salpingectomies.

Tuberculosis usually involves the female genital tract secondarily, the most common primary sites being the lung and the gastrointestinal tract. Dissemination may occur from caseous lymph nodes via blood or lymphatics or by contiguity from the peritoneal cavity. Primary tuberculosis of the vulva or cervix may be transmitted by coitus but this is extremely rare. The internal genitalia are then involved by direct ascending infection of the endometrium and oviduct. Proof of the primary site is lacking in well over one half the patients with proved genital tuberculosis.

Pelvic tuberculosis is discussed at length in Chapter 6.

BENIGN NEOPLASMS

Benign neoplasms of the uterine corpus will be considered under two general headings: (1) those involving the myometrium and (2) those involving the endometrium. The disease entities most often involving the myometrium are adenomyosis and leiomyoma. Both are of major importance to the gynecologist because they are the major indications for hysterectomy during the premenopausal years.

Adenomyosis

Adenomyosis is a serious, progressively disabling disorder of the premenopausal woman that has been described as "internal endometriosis" and is due to the presence of heterotopic endometrium in the myometrium. Such displaced endometrium must be at least two standard low-power fields beneath the endomyometrial junction and be associated with adjacent myometrial hyperplasia. It may occur focally or may be distributed throughout the uterus, producing generalized and symmetric enlargement. Since the diagnosis is made almost exclusively by examination of excised uteri, the true incidence of the disease is unknown. Adenomyosis is found in 8% to 20% of hysterectomy specimens in large gynecologic clinics, and its incidence at necropsy has been reported as high as 50%.

Adenomyosis is a disease of the childbearing period, the incidence being greatest between ages 41 and 50 years. In most reported series about 80% of the patients were multiparous and approximately 50% had associated leiomyomas. Salpingitis isthmica nodosa is found in 20% of these patients but simultaneously occurring endometriosis is uncommon. Benson, however, found endometriosis in 13% of patients who had hysterectomy for adenomyosis. A study by Marcus lends support to the idea that adenomyosis is encountered more often in the uterus with carcinomatous endometrium than in one with benign endometrium. Similarly it was found that adenomyosis uteri and endometrial hyperplasia occurred or coexisted more frequently with endometrial carcinoma than with benign endometrium. These interrelations suggest that a common denominator, possibly hormonal, may exist in these three lesions.

The pathogenesis of this disease is unknown. Numerous theories have been suggested, the most acceptable being that of direct invasion or extension of basal endometrium into the myometrium. An opposite, and less tenable, explanation postulates invasion of the myometrium from the serosal surface by endometriosis. Dedifferentiation of myometrium, mesothelial metaplasia, and misplaced müllerian or mesonephric duct tissue have also been suggested as possible etiologic factors. The stimulus for the benign invasion of glandular elements is unknown, although it

has been suggested that this process is the result of an excess of normally present growth factor or an exaggerated response to this factor. Estrogen, being the essential hormone for endometrial and myometrial growth, has been implicated in pathogenesis. A certain modicum of support is lent to this idea by the cyclic response to estrogen that the adenomyotic glands demonstrate and by the symptomatic improvement that usually occurs with the menopause. Growth and migration of the glands may actually lag behind the spread of endometrial stroma into the myometrium, and there is some evidence that glandular "invasion" can occur only after the way has been "paved" by the forerunning stroma.

Diagnosis

The clinical picture is difficult to evaluate, and correlation with the degree of adenomyosis is spurious because of associated leiomyomas or tubal disease. In most patients without these disease processes, however, the most common symptoms are hypermenorrhea, acquired dysmenorrhea, polymenorrhea, and premenstrual staining. Dyspareunia may be associated with a fixed third-degree uterine retroversion. The diagnosis should be suspected if one or more of these symptoms is described by a multiparous patient, aged 35 to 50 years, and pelvic examination discloses a moderately enlarged, globular, tender uterus that has a finely nodular surface. The tenderness seems to be increased if leiomyomas are present or if examination is done in the immediate premenstrual phase. In differential diagnosis, the entities to be considered are: (1) endometriosis, (2) multiple leiomyomas, (3) salpingitis isthmica nodosa with salpingitis, (4) idiopathic uterine hypertrophy of multiparity (fibrosis uteri), and (5) pelvic congestion syndrome. The diagnosis is not aided by uterine curettage, but hysterography will occasionally show pathognomonic changes (Fig 5–23). The symptoms of adenomyosis are exaggerated by estrogen-progestin combinations, particularly if these are given constantly in the form of pseudopregnancy.

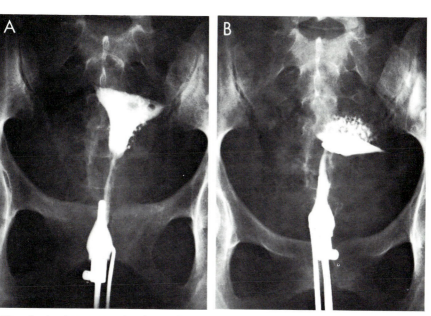

Fig 5–23.—A, hysterogram showing adenomyosis in a 20-year-old infertile woman. The diagnosis was later verified by biopsy at the time of hysterotomy. **B,** hysterogram of same patient with uterus anteverted showing extensive spread of radiopaque dye into areas of adenomyosis of the posterior uterine wall.

Pathology

The adenomyotic uterus is usually enlarged and heavier than usual, weighing about 125 gm (normal, 42 gm). Although symmetric enlargement (Fig 5–24) is the rule, focal adenomyomas may be found and these may occasionally protrude into the uterine cavity. When incised, the surface appears convex and bulging. The thickening of the uterine wall is seen to be made up of coarsely trabeculated areas, stippled or granular in appearance, with small yellow or darker cystic points, which may contain serous fluid or old blood. Close inspection of the cut surface will frequently reveal an irregularity of the endomyometrial junction with foci of down-dipping basalis. While the pathologist usually has no difficulty in making a diagnosis of adenomyosis by gross examination of the cut specimen, the surgeon cannot approach this degree of accuracy with the uterus "in situ." He may, however, suspect the disease if a focal area of adenomyosis is mistaken for a leiomyoma and a myomectomy attempted. Areas of

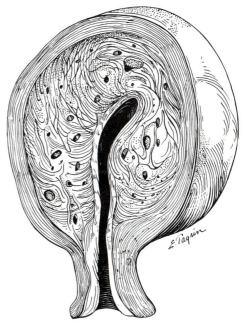

Fig 5–24.—Adenomyosis.

adenomyosis do not "shell" out or lend themselves to easy excision.

MICROSCOPIC APPEARANCE.—The pathognomonic feature of this disease is the occurrence of endometrial tissue, glands, and stroma within the myometrium (Fig 5–25), at least one low-power field (some authors demand two) from the endomyometrial junction. The misplaced endometrial tissue is similar to that of the basalis of the endometrial cavity and therefore does not always respond to hormonal stimulation. Occasionally, however, secretory change may be noted or there may be cystic or adenomatous hyperplasia. In several studies, a functional response in the aberrant endometrium was found in only about 50% of the cases in which the normally located endometrium was functional. Decidual changes in the stroma of adenomyotic areas have been noted during pregnancy and spontaneous ruptures of these areas have been reported. Symptoms of dysmenorrhea or constant pelvic pain might be anticipated if areas of adenomyosis demonstrated functional capacity, with edema and bleeding. The cause of symptoms in patients whose uteri do not show functioning areas of adenomyosis is unknown.

Malignant neoplasia may rarely occur in either the glands or stroma or both, about 30 malignant adenomyomas having been reported. These may be in the form of adenocarcinoma, sarcoma, or carcinosarcoma.

The myometrium is usually altered in uteri with extensive adenomyosis so that a surrounding zone of hypertrophy-hyperplasia is usually recognizable. Phagocytized hemosiderin may be seen deep in the myometrium, indicating previous extravasation of blood.

If the process of adenomyosis has extended into the cornua of the uterus and then laterally into the isthmic portion of the oviduct, a process may develop that is indistinguishable from salpingitis isthmica nodosa, except that inflammatory cells are usually present in the latter condition.

Correlation of Symptoms with Pathology

It has been axiomatic to consider adenomyosis as the most probable diagnosis when dysfunctional uterine bleeding and increasingly severe dysmenorrhea accompany an enlarging, firm, tender uterus in a woman of moderate parity in the 40- to 50-year age group. Yet this disease remains the most overdiagnosed when not present and the one most commonly missed when the process is moderately extensive. In the latter case the preoperative diagnosis is almost always "fibroids."

Ovarian dysfunction has been suggested as the major etiologic factor in the abnormal bleeding associated with adenomyosis. This has not been substantiated by pathologic studies, since there has been no evidence of ovarian failure, unusual cyst formation, stromal change, or "overactivity." Secretory endometrium is found in most cases and attests to the ability of the ovaries to ovulate normally even though many of these patients are in the late 40s or early 50s.

The vascular supply to the uterus has been shown to be appreciably increased in adenomyosis, and enormously so when the disease is extensive. Interference with myometrial contractility and subsequent inadequate vascular control of myometrial and endometrial vasculature have been advanced as a possible cause of the abnormal bleeding associated with adenomyosis. The hypermenorrhea may simply be due to the generalized enlargement of the uterus and the endometrial cavity with a larger area made available for bleeding. Overdistention of the uterine wall by this increased vascularity during the menses would also explain the dysmenorrhea. Both of these explanations would be more acceptable if a closer correlation with symptoms could be elucidated. Unfortunately, many patients with extensive anatomic findings are symptom-free, whereas others, with minimal or nonfunctional adenomyosis are incapacitated by pain.

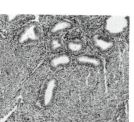

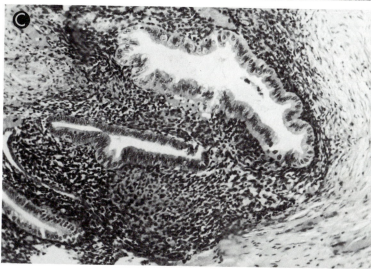

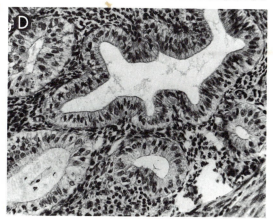

Fig 5–25.—A, typical adenomyosis in the wall of the uterus. Foci of basal type endometrium are located deep in the myometrium. The myometrium surrounding the areas of adenomyosis shows a whorled appearance similar to that seen in leiomyoma. (From Hertig A.T., Gore H.M.: Tumors of the female sex organs: part 2. Tumors of the vulva, vagina and uterus, sec. 9, fasc. 33, *Atlas of Tumor Pathology.* Washington, D.C., Armed Forces Institute of Pathology, 1960.) **B,** higher power of an area of adenomyosis showing cystic dilatation. The basal endometrium is at the top. **C,** adenomyosis in which the glandular element at the top right has undergone anaplasia. The glands are surrounded by typical endometrial stroma. **D,** adenomyosis showing secretory effect.

Treatment

The definitive treatment for adenomyosis should be total hysterectomy, with or without ovarian conservation. Various hormonal regimens have been tried but have been uniformly unsuccessful. The use of various progestational agents as a pseudopregnancy has resulted in an actual increase in pelvic pain. This was due, in all probability, to marked edema and distortion of the areas of adenomyosis with subsequent increased uterine motility. Androgens have not proved advantageous in adenomyosis. Since most patients are in the late 30s or early 40s and have completed their childbearing function, the loss of the uterus is not looked on with disfavor. If the patient has only minor complaints and a curettage has eliminated the possibility of endometrial abnormalities or a submucous leiomyoma, the use of analgesic agents together with explanation may be successful.

Leiomyoma

A leiomyoma is commonly but incorrectly termed a "fibroid." It is a well-circumscribed but nonencapsulated benign tumor composed mainly of muscle but with varying amounts of fibrous connective tissue. Synonymous descriptive terms are fibroma, fibromyoma, and myoma. Although the absolute incidence of leiomyoma is difficult to determine, varying reports suggest that they occur in from 4% to 11% of all women and comprise about 30% of the specimens seen in large gynecologic pathology laboratories. This lesion is most frequently found during the fourth and fifth decades of life and it has been estimated that approximately 40% of women aged 50 years or over harbor these tumors. They have not been reported before the menarche, and the incidence is three to nine times higher in blacks.

Numerous theories of histogenesis have been advanced but none has been adequately proved. It has been suggested that leiomyomas arise from totipotential primitive cells that normally give rise to muscle cells, connective tissue cells, and blood vessels. Other studies have indicated that the tumor may arise from adult muscle cells or from stromal connective tissue cells. Still other investigators have suggested that leiomyomas arise from the adventitial cells of the blood vessels or from the muscle cells of the arterioles and larger veins. A definite correlation with the presence of estrogen has been noted, since these tumors seldom, if ever, occur before the menarche and tend to disappear after the menopause. Furthermore, leiomyomas make their appearance during the years of maximum ovarian activity, enlarge during pregnancy, grow rapidly when exogenous estrogen is administered, and are often found in association with hyperplasia of the endometrium and with granulosa-thecal cell tumors of the ovary. Miller has suggested that these tumors occur in susceptible women who have a high incidence of anovular cycles with prolonged estrogen stimulation. He believes they arise from small, immature muscle cell nests in the myometrium.

There are three major types of leiomyomas—submucous, subserous, and intramural (Fig 5–26). The subserous variety may be attached by a broad or narrow base and is commonly pedunculated. Occasionally an intramural leiomyoma may extend laterally into the leaves of the broad ligament, in which case it is known as an intraligamentary tumor. The cervix may be involved, although this occurs in less than 5% of the total. A leiomyoma may become detached from its source and secure its blood supply from neighboring organs or omentum, in which case it is known as a "parasitic" myoma.

These tumors usually begin as minute seedings that may be seen scattered throughout the myometrium, each tumor measuring 3 to 4 mm in greatest diameter. They may grow to rather large proportions and some may weigh as much as 10 or 15 lb. The largest on record at the Brigham and Women's Hospital weighed 30 lb. The position of the leiomyoma is of clinical importance since a tumor that occludes the ostium of the oviduct may be an important factor in infertility, and one that

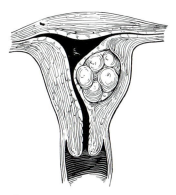

① SUBMUCOUS LEIOMYOMAS

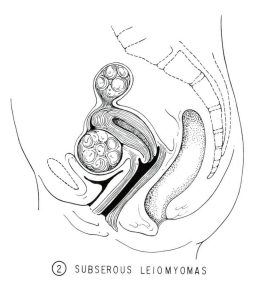

② SUBSEROUS LEIOMYOMAS

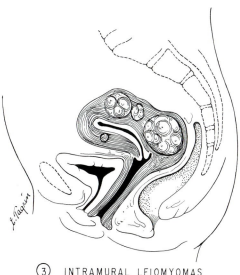

③ INTRAMURAL LEIOMYOMAS

Fig 5–26.—Leiomyomas classified according to location.

projects into the endometrial cavity may be a predisposing factor in habitual abortion. Similarly, the submucous variety is associated with abnormal bleeding, usually hypermenorrhea. Pressure symptoms may result from growth anteriorly or posteriorly, affecting the bladder or rectum.

Pathology

The gross appearance of a leiomyoma is somewhat variable, but in general the tumor is circumscribed and well demarcated from the surrounding muscle. A pseudocapsule is present that is merely flattened uterine muscle that has become compressed as the tumor increases in size. The consistency is usually firm or actually hard, except in cases in which degeneration or hemorrhage has occurred. The color is light gray or pinkish white, depending on the degree of vascularity. When the leiomyoma is cut across, the tissue will usually project above the level of the surrounding myometrium. When viewed in the fresh state, the smooth muscle bundles can usually be identified in a pattern of intertwining or whorl-like arrangement.

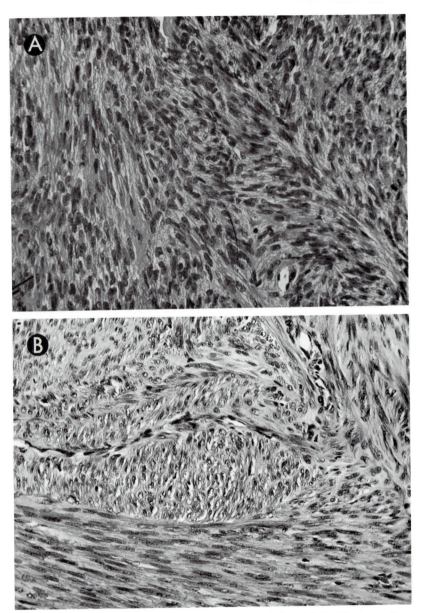

Fig 5–27.—A, high-power view of leiomyoma, showing typical structure. The tumor is composed of groups and bundles of smooth muscle cells arranged in twists and whorls in an interlacing pattern. It is relatively avascular. **B,** higher power shows cellular detail. The smooth muscle fibers in the central portion have been cut across their long axes. Note uniform appearance and lack of mitoses.

The microscopic appearance of a leiomyoma is usually rather characteristic, in that the nonstriated muscle fibers are arranged in bundles of varying sizes running in multiple directions (Fig 5–27), giving the pattern noted grossly. High-power examination reveals the spindle-shaped cells to have elongated nuclei, which are, for the most part, of uniform size and staining quality. Connective tissue elements of varying amounts may be noted between the muscle cells. In certain tumors the amount of the connective tissue element may be excessive, in which case the term *fibromyoma* may be more descriptive.

Degenerative changes may occur, the most common being hyalinization and cyst formation. These changes are due to diminished vascularity of the connective tissue element, so that the detail of connective tissue fibers is lost. The hyalin material presents no cellular detail, stains deeply with eosin, and may show remnants of muscle bundles interspersed between the homogeneous matrix. If the hyalinized connective tissue undergoes liquefaction necrosis, cystic degeneration then occurs. The cysts may then become filled with a gelatinous material that oozes forth when the tumor is cut across. This may be followed, especially in long-standing cases, by focal areas of calcification. In postmenopausal women these calcified leiomyomas may be evident on x-ray examination. Another type of degeneration is that known as acute red degeneration, occasionally seen as a complication of pregnancy. In this situation the cut surface simulates raw meat, this carneous change being due to hemorrhage into a par-tially hyalinized leiomyoma. This hemorrhagic complication is the result of accumulation of blood in the tumor because of venous obstruction and may occur during the rapid growth associated with pregnancy or immediately post partum, when the venous drainage is occluded. Acute red degeneration of leiomyomas has also been reported in association with the use of massive medroxyprogesterone acetate (Depo-Provera) therapy in the treatment of endometriosis.

Sarcomatous change may occur in a leiomyoma (Fig 5–28) but is extremely rare, the incidence being somewhere between 0.1% and 0.6%. This malignant change should be suspected if a myoma undergoes rapid enlargement, especially after the menopause, or if postmenopausal bleeding occurs in the presence of known leiomyomas. During pregnancy a certain degree of pleomorphism, which simulates the morphology of leiomyosarcoma, is seen in 10% to 15% of excised tumors. Although the tumor may appear very fleshy and microscopically appears quite cellular, the cells are all of equal size, mitotic figures are absent, and giant cells are not prominent.

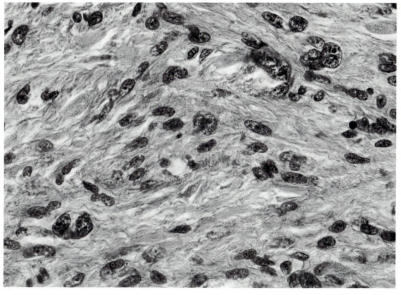

Fig 5–28.—Leiomyosarcoma, showing resemblance to cells in Figure 5–27, A and B, but with pleomorphism and variation in size and staining density.

Symptomatology

The most important symptom associated with uterine leiomyomas is abnormal bleeding. This is usually in the form of hypermenorrhea and may be associated with the passage of large clots. Secondary anemia may therefore be present. The myoma per se does not cause bleeding. This is usually due to an abnormal endometrial pattern—frequently hyperplasia—overlying a submucous tumor. Bleeding may occur from the thinned endometrium overlying an intracavitary, pedunculated myoma. The presence of the tumor in the endomyometrium may so affect the normal hemostatic mechanism that extensive flow occurs. It is important to remember, however, that bleeding from other sources, such as carcinoma of the endometrium or cervix, may coexist and definitive therapy should not be carried out until malignancy has been excluded. If the bleeding is intermenstrual or postcoital, carcinoma should be strongly suspected even though extensive myomas are present.

If a myoma reaches a size such that it practically fills the pelvic cavity it may, by encroachment on other organs, cause certain pressure symptoms. Pressure on the bladder may be evidenced by suprapubic discomfort, frequency, urinary retention, or overflow incontinence. If the rectosigmoid is encroached on by the growing tumor, constipation may result. A generalized feeling of discomfort, edema of the legs, or increased varicosities may result from an enlarging tumor. In many patients no symptoms are noticed until the mass becomes sufficiently large to become an abdominal structure. The patient may then notice a firm, nodular mass or may simply complain of an increase in abdominal girth. Myomas usually do not produce pain unless they become twisted or undergo degeneration with subsequent hemorrhage and infection. When pain does occur in the presence of a myoma, it is likely to be caused by other pathologic disorders, e.g., tubal inflammation, endometriosis, diverticulitis, or even ovarian cancer.

Diagnosis

A presumptive diagnosis of a leiomyoma of the uterus may be made by abdominal palpation if the uterus is displaced out of the pelvis or if the tumors are large. They may be palpated as firm, irregular nodules or masses arising from the pelvis and extending into the lower abdomen. Usually these masses are movable without causing pain. Occasionally a firm, nodular mass may be felt almost to the level of the umbilicus without any symptoms having been noted by the patient. Bimanual pelvic examination is more helpful in making the diagnosis since the uterus can usually be outlined easily and the distortion of its normal contour is readily appreciated. The myomas may be small irregularities on the surface of the uterus, no larger than 1 cm, or they may incorporate and distort the fundus to such an extent that separation of tumor from uterus is impossible.

The differential diagnosis is not always easy. During the childbearing period an intrauterine gestation should always be suspected, particularly if some degree of diminished flowing has occurred. A leiomyoma may occasionally be soft and the associated pelvic congestion may produce softening of the cervix. Conversely, an early intrauterine pregnancy may exist without softening of the cervix and when a leiomyoma occurs in a pregnant uterus it may undergo softening and enlargement. When in doubt a pregnancy test should always be obtained.

Another aspect of pregnancy may interfere with accurate diagnosis. During the early weeks of pregnancy the uterus may enlarge asymmetrically and if there is a tendency toward a bicornuate development, there will be a pronounced enlargement of one uterine horn. This may be mistaken for an ovarian mass or a myoma. Moderate degrees of this asymmetric enlargement are normal in all pregnancies, presumably because of lateral placental implantation. Such a growth pattern is known as Piskacek's sign. Similarly, pregnancy occurring in the interstitial portion of the oviduct may give rise to an asymmetric enlargement of the uterus that may be confused with a myoma or ovarian lesion.

A subserous, pedunculated myoma is frequently mistaken for an ovarian tumor, either a fibroma or dermoid cyst, particularly if the pedicle has become elongated. Such leiomyomas are generally freely mobile, but careful examination will usually reveal an attachment to the uterus. In such patients it is important that the ovary be palpated and differentiated from the myoma, since surgical exploration is indicated for an enlarged, solid ovarian mass, whereas observation is suggested as optimum therapy if the mass is a simple, uncomplicated myoma. Frequently, a parasitic or intraligamentous myoma cannot be delineated adequately, since such lesions are usually fixed and may coalesce with the adnexal structures.

Other pelvic masses that may be mistaken for myomas are: (1) a redundant or distended cecum filled with feces, (2) a redundant sigmoid, (3) appendiceal abscess, (4) diverticulitis, and (5) carcinoma of the sigmoid. Cleansing enemas and radiographic studies of the bowel will assist in diagnostic precision. Occasionally a pelvic kidney may rest close to the uterus but urography will detect this congenital abnormality. X-ray films of the urinary tract are also indicated if a myoma is intraligamentous, to ascertain ureteral deviation prior to surgery. A full bladder or urachal cyst may rarely be mistaken for a myoma, but routine voiding prior to pelvic examination will eliminate this obvious error. Cystograms are indicated if bladder involvement is suspected. As a matter of fact, the radiologist is frequently suspicious of a myoma by the indentation it and the uterus make on the dome of the bladder as seen on the intravenous urogram. Calcification in a myoma may also be detected on the same films. Ultrasonography is a valuable diagnostic aid in the detection of all pelvic tumors, and this technique is advantageous in the diagnosis of leiomyomas as well.

A pedunculated submucous myoma may be evident as a mass that protrudes through the cervix as a gray-pink smooth mass. The usual submucous myoma may be detected at the time of curettage or by hysterogram.

Treatment

The treatment of uterine leiomyomas cannot be standardized. Each patient presents individual variations that must be assayed before suggesting extirpation. If the tumor is discovered at routine pelvic examination, is asymptomatic, and is not of excessive size, no specific treatment is indicated. This is especially true if the patient is premenopausal, since the tumor will diminish in size after the menses cease. Close observation is suggested with pelvic examinations at about six-month intervals. Surgery is sometimes advisable on the basis of size alone, but exact measurements cannot be given. In general, if the leiomyoma fills the true pelvis, i.e., if it equals or exceeds the size of a 12-week gestation, surgery is usually indicated.

Conservative measures may also be followed if symptoms are minimal. Thus if the patient has noted only slight hypermenorrhea or pressure symptoms and is nearing the menopause, treatment may include oral or intramuscular administration of iron, vitamins and a high-protein diet. The use of androgenic substances has been suggested but should not exceed 300 mg per month. If there is associated anovular bleeding with endometrial hyperplasia, treatment with an androgenic progestin, such as norethindrone 10 mg daily for 20 consecutive days, may reduce the amount of flowing and this may be continued indefinitely if successful. This has proved to be effective temporizing therapy in preparing patients for hysterectomy in whom blood loss has been excessive. Medroxyprogesterone acetate (Depo-Provera) has been used similarly in a dose of 100 mg intramuscularly every three to five days while the patient is being prepared for surgery. In a few patients in whom hysterectomy was contraindicated because of serious medical disease, I have used Depo-Provera in a continuing dose of 200 mg per month for as long as three years until the patient entered menopause and spontaneous regression of the myomas occurred. Oxytocic substances have little, if any, effect on the bleeding associated with leiomyomas.

Surgery is indicated in the following situations: (1) excessive size or excess rate of growth except during pregnancy; (2) submucous location if associated with hypermenorrhea; (3) if the tumor is pedunculated; (4) if the bladder or rectum is encroached on to a degree that produces pressure symptoms; (5) if the tumor is intraligamentous or if differentiation from an ovarian mass is not possible; (6) if there is associated pelvic pathology such as endometriosis or pelvic inflammatory disease; or (7) if infertility or habitual abortion seems due to the anatomic location of the tumor.

Conservative surgery for leiomyomas may be performed in younger women if there is no other indication for removal of the uterus. The mere presence of a myoma that does not compromise tubal function or the integrity of the endometrial cavity, however, should not be an indication for myomectomy. Uterotubograms may be utilized to demonstrate distortion of the endometrial cavity or obstruction of the intrauterine ostia of the oviducts. Preliminary curettage may reveal endometrial hyperplasia or polyps. Hysteroscopy has recently been utilized in the diagnosis of intrauterine synechia and tumors. It is of particular value in the diagnosis of partial or complete obstruction of the intrauterine ostia of the oviducts in patients with infertility. Large cervical myomas may produce distortion and tortuosity of the cervical canal with obstruction to spermatozoa. In addition, before a planned laparotomy for a myomectomy, the cervix and endometrial cavity should be adequately studied by cytology and biopsy to rule out malignant or premalignant disease. If a myomectomy is planned because of infertility, the husband should have been studied thoroughly, the patency of the oviducts determined, and the endometrium biopsied to make certain of ovulation and to exclude endometrial disease.

Myomectomy may be single or multiple.

Pregnancies have followed the removal of large, solitary tumors that completely distorted the endometrial cavity as well as the removal of multiple small tumors. The incidence of pregnancy following myomectomy approximates 40%. The patient should be informed, however, to attempt pregnancy soon after surgery, since the recurrence rate of leiomyoma is considerable, in some series being as high as 10%.

The morbidity and mortality after myomectomy are minimal if the usual care is given to secure hemostasis and prevent infection. Delivery following myomectomy need not be by cesarean section unless the endometrial cavity was entered at the time of original surgery or the postoperative course was febrile and the myometrial scar possibly weakened.

TECHNIQUE OF MYOMECTOMY.—The uterine fundus is grasped with double hooks or traction sutures and drawn toward the abdominal wound in such a position as to expose the myoma to be removed. An incision (Fig 5–29, A) is made through the wall of the uterus parallel with the axis of the uterus over the most prominent part of the tumor. Hemostasis may be aided by placing a tourniquet such as a small Penrose drain around the uterus at the level of the uterine vessels. This can be done simply by merely piercing the broad ligament bilaterally and clamping the tourniquet posteriorly. The local injection of oxytocin (Pitocin) or phenylephrine hydrochloride (Neo-Synephrine) has also been advocated for securing hemostasis. We have not utilized these methods if the myomas are small but have found them advantageous in the treatment of large and multiple leiomyomas. The incision is then carried down to the surface of the myoma (Fig 5–29, B), which can be readily recognized by the difference in the direction of its fibers.

When the surface of the myoma is exposed the tumor is grasped either with a double hook or by a traction suture placed through its substance. With firm traction the tumor can be readily "shelled" out by means of

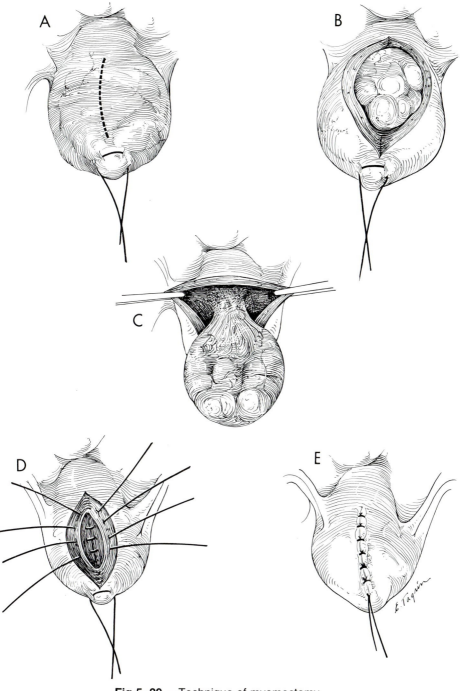

Fig 5–29.—Technique of myomectomy.

blunt dissection, exposure being provided by placing Allis' clamps on the lateral aspects of the myometrium (Fig 5–29,C). The individual blood vessels are then clamped and ligated as necessary. The enucleation should be done carefully to prevent excessive laceration of the uterine wall and to avoid opening the uterine cavity if possible. If the tumor is an adenomyoma, it will not "shell" out with this facility and sharp dissection will be necessary.

Careful control of the bleeding is then important, and all bleeding points should be isolated and ligatured as completely as possible. The tourniquet may be released intermittently in order to identify such vessels. The dead space brought about by the removal of the tumor is obliterated by approximating the myometrium with interrupted (Fig 5–29,D) or figure-of-eight sutures of chromic catgut. The peritoneum is then closed with sutures of fine catgut (Fig 5–29,E) or by a subserosal continuous suture. When it is found necessary to remove a large number of myomas, it is important to make the incision in the uterine wall in such a way that multiple tumors may be removed through the same incision. Following the myomectomy, a suspension operation should always be performed to prevent the possibility of an adherent retroversion. If the myomectomy incision has involved the posterior wall of the uterus, adhesions to ileum or sigmoid colon are quite common. This complication may be prevented by meticulous closure of the uterine serosa or by attaching an omental graft to the uterine wall.

Hysterectomy

Simple total hysterectomy is, in the hands of the well-trained specialist, a safe operation. Numerous reviews cite morbidity rates varying from 10% to 48%. The extreme variation depends on whether or not the author has adhered to the strict interpretation of minor febrile reactions or has reported only what he considers to be morbid states. Mortality rates reported in these same reviews approximate 0.3%, with variation from 0.1% to 0.9%.

Most of the serious complications were caused by inadequate hemostasis, ureteral, bladder, and rectal trauma and pulmonary disease. Methods of preventing the first two categories are outlined herein.

Two basic surgical principles are of major importance in the performance of the abdominal hysterectomy. They are (1) good visualization and (2) adequate hemostasis. The former is provided by a combination of proper positioning of the patient, well-chosen incisions, and relaxing anesthesia. The latter is a result of careful dissection in proper cleavage planes, meticulous ligature of major vessels, and elimination of needless steps. The actual procedure of removal of the uterus should never be started until the operative field has been freed of adhesions and the specimen mobilized.

TECHNIQUE OF HYSTERECTOMY.—*Position.*—Most gynecologists prefer a modified Trendelenburg position of about 25 to 35 degrees for pelvic surgery. When spinal anesthesia is utilized, lesser degrees are usually provided but because of excellent muscular and intestinal relaxation this seems adequate. Our own preference is for so-called accentuated Trendelenburg positioning of about 45 to 55 degrees with the table being broken at knee level. This has been used continuously for over 60 years at the Free Hospital for Women, and surveys of morbidity have not indicated a greater incidence of pulmonary complications following its use. This position greatly facilitates visualization of the pelvic viscera.

Incision.—The advantages of the transverse incision over the midline or paramedian approach have been well documented. The choice depends on the training of the operator, and if he performs the transverse incision with ease and rapidity this is then superior for him. The amount of visualization and facile approach to the pelvic viscera with the transverse incision certainly equals and frequently exceeds that obtained with a vertical one, especially if the recti muscles are divided. The cosmetic result is better, wound healing is improved, physiologic stress patterns are diminished and postoperative hernias are extremely rare. The sole disadvantage seems to be that its opening and closure takes somewhat more time, although this should not be a serious deterring factor. A retrocecal appendix may also be more difficult to mobilize but in most cases appendectomy is not hindered.

Hemostasis.—The principles of securing hemostasis have been previously noted, but reiteration of one point is essential: the uterus and adnexa are completely mobilized before actual removal of the specimen is begun. Occasionally this entails more ingenuity and surgical skill than the hysterectomy itself but is rewarding by prevention of ureteral, bladder, and rectal injury. In extensive pelvic inflammatory disease the adnexa must be dissected from their attachment to the posterior peritoneum and serosa of the rectosigmoid. Frequently this may be carried out by blunt finger dissection, but if a good cleavage plane is not available sharp dissection with good visualization of the posterior pelvis is mandatory. This will prevent penetration of the rectosigmoid by the exploring finger. It has been found valuable to divide the uterosacral ligaments in such cases (after the rectum has been displaced) before actually starting the hysterectomy, since the entire uterus then "rides up" into the superior strait of the pelvis and makes approach to the lateral ligaments easier.

In endometriosis of severe degree, extensive uterine fixation frequently exists. Division of the posterior peritoneum and uterosacral ligaments will secure a line of cleavage inside the endopelvic fascia, which will enable the operator to perform a total hysterectomy in almost every case.

The ligaments.—The ligaments opposite the operator are usually ligated and divided first, and these may be put on stretch by removing the retractor on the surgeon's side and exerting strong traction on the uterine fundus by means of a toothed hook. This may be done by the second assistant on the operator's side while the opposite retractor is held directly over the ligaments to be divided. Many authors have suggested starting the operation by clamping and dividing the round ligaments, then perforating the posterior leaf of the broad ligament with the finger and mobilizing the infundibulopelvic ligament in this fashion. They place two clamps across this ligament and replace each with a ligature of no. 0 or 00 chromic catgut. An alternative, and perhaps simpler, method is to place a suture around the infundibulopelvic ligament first (if the ovaries are to be removed), without clamping, and tie it. (A half-length Kelly clamp has previously been placed adjacent to the corpus and lateral to the ovary to prevent backflow. This clamp also includes the round ligament at its uterine margin.) Using the same suture, the needle is placed directly through the round ligament and the suture tied in such a fashion as to include the infundibulopelvic ligament, thus securing it for the second time. The needle is then placed through the broad ligament about 0.5 cm below the round ligament. As the round ligament is divided the anterior peritoneum is easily picked up and a transverse incision carried halfway toward the midline (Fig 5–30, A–C).

Following bilateral ligation of the round and infundibulopelvic ligaments, attention is usually turned to the uterine vessels, and there is general agreement that they should be dissected cleanly of all adjacent areolar tissue and peritoneum. If this is carefully done the vessels may be secured by one or two ligatures without clamping. One important point that has not received adequate attention is the division of the posterior peritoneum and the uterosacral ligaments prior to uterine vessel ligation. This is usually carried out by cutting transversely with the scalpel beginning at the peritoneal edge developed by division of the round ligaments and exposure of the uterine vessels and continuing across the uterosacral ligaments superior to their insertion into the uterovaginal fascia. These ligaments usu-

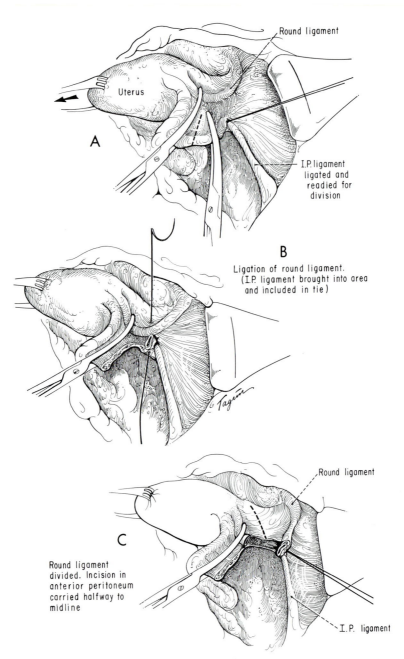

Round ligament

Uterus

A

I.P. ligament
ligated and
readied for
division

B

Ligation of round ligament.
(I.P. ligament brought into area
and included in tie)

C

Round ligament
divided. Incision in
anterior peritoneum
carried halfway to
midline

Round ligament

I.P. ligament

Fig 5–30.—A, a Kelly clamp is placed over the round and infundibulopelvic ligaments to control backflow bleeding; a suture is placed around the infundibulopelvic ligament and a second Kelly clamp is applied medial to the suture; the infundibulopelvic ligament is then divided between the clamps. **B,** after division of the infundibulopelvic ligament, a suture is placed through the round ligament and tied so that the infundibulopelvic liga- ment is brought into proximity; the same suture is then placed through the broad ligament caudad to the round ligament as shown; when this suture is tied it encompasses the infundibulopelvic liga- ment, thus doubly securing it. **C,** the round liga- ment is divided and the incision is continued through the anterior leaf of the broad ligament curving toward the midline. *(Continued)*

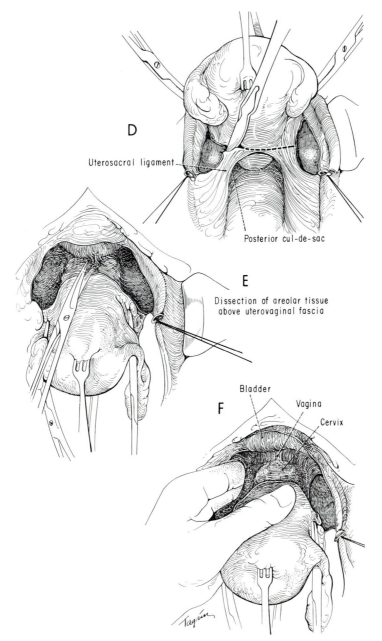

D

Uterosacral ligament

Posterior cul-de-sac

E

Dissection of areolar tissue
above uterovaginal fascia

F

Bladder

Vagina

Cervix

Fig 5–30 (cont.).—D, after the posterior leaf of the broad ligament has been divided and the uterine vessels exposed and skeletonized, the posterior peritoneum and uterosacral ligaments are divided with a knife. **E,** the anterior peritoneum of the vesicouterine fold has been completely divided and the vesicocervical ligaments are divided; note that the scissors are turned away from the bladder; dissection should be in the plane of the areolar tissue between the fascial layers. **F,** traction cephalad is placed on the uterus and two fingers are placed below the cervix; a gentle rolling motion with the thumb displaces the bladder below the cervicovaginal junction. *(Continued)*

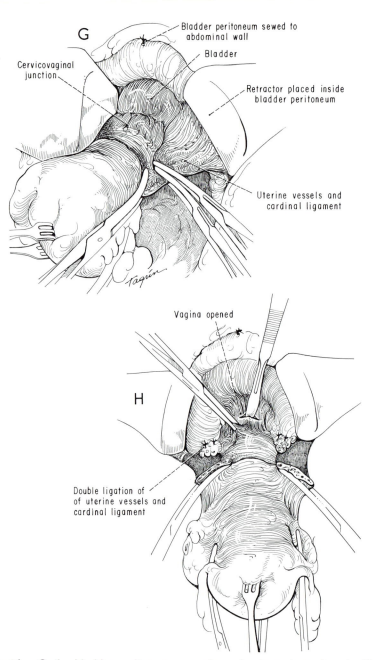

Fig 5–30 (cont.).—G, the bladder peritoneum is sutured to the abdominal wall and retractors are placed inside the reflected bladder; the lower clamp incorporates the lateral aspect of the endopelvic fascia as it is placed over the uterine vessels; a second clamp is placed over the vessels and they are divided with care to include some of the endopelvic fascia in the medial as-pect; each clamp is replaced with a suture. **H,** unless the cervix is elongated a separate division and ligation of the cardinal ligament is not necessary; a Kocher clamp is placed across the vagina at the cervicovaginal junction and the vagina is entered with a knife; a second clamp then picks up the lower vaginal edge. *(Continued)*

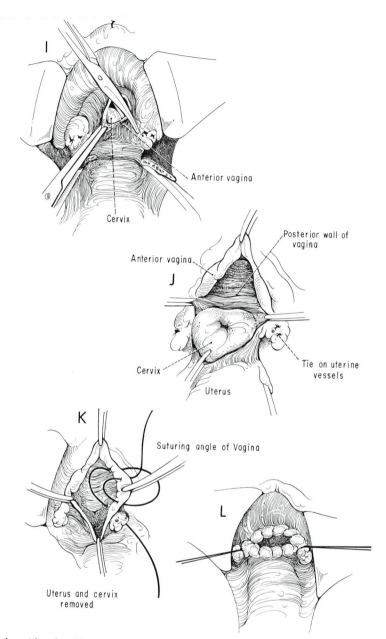

Fig 5–30 (cont.).—I, with medial traction on the vaginal edges, the vagina is incised with a scissors directed toward the lateral angle. **J,** Kocher clamps are placed at each vaginal angle and the cervix is drawn cephalad; the posterior vaginal wall is divided under direct vision. **K,** the vaginal angle suture is placed through the utero-sacral ligament, posterior vaginal wall, anterior vaginal wall and then is looped around the lateral clamp; the suture is then brought through the posterior and anterior vaginal walls lateral to the first loop; when the suture is tied the loop lateral to the vagina encircles the uterine vessels thus placing a third tie around them. **L,** the angle sutures are held with clamps and provide traction, a running, unlocked suture is begun in the midline of the posterior vaginal wall and is carried around the circumference of the vagina for hemostasis; the vagina is left open for drainage.

ally do not need clamping and ligation. The posterior leaf of fascia, together with the uterosacral ligaments, is dissected or pushed off the posterior aspects of the cervix, thus opening the posterior fascial envelope around the cervix. This also serves the important function of displacing the ureter posteriorly so that ligation of the uterine vessels is accomplished without danger (Fig 5–30,D).

Bladder peritoneum.—After the round ligaments have been divided bilaterally and the medial extension of the anterior peritoneum brought to the midline, the anterior peritoneal dissection is complete. Scissor dissection in the areolar tissue above the uterovaginal fascia serves to displace the bladder from the vagina for a distance of 2 to 3 cm. It is then technically easy with the thumb above the cervix and two fingers under it to displace the bladder digitally below the level of the cervicovaginal junction. If the bladder peritoneum is then sewed to the abdominal wall and retractors are placed *inside* the bladder peritoneum, ready access to the vessels and cervix is easily obtained. Whether the dissection of the anterior peritoneum is done before that of the posterior peritoneum or after is not important. The importance lies in preparing the uterine vessels for complete ligation (Fig 5–30,E and F).

Uterine vessels.—As previously noted, the uterine vessels may be either doubly clamped, divided, and ligated, or simply ligated without preliminary clamping. Various techniques of management of the anterior leaf of the uterovaginal fascia (pubovesicocervical fascia) have been published previously. It has been suggested that this fascia be divided transversely, split through three quarters of its circumference, or incised in the form of an inverted "T." The advantages cited are: (1) by any of these techniques the cardinal ligaments may be clamped and divided *inside* the endopelvic fascia, thus protecting the ureter, and (2) the resulting fascial envelopes may be utilized for vaginal closure and support. These fascial techniques, while anatomically sound, have

been found by others to be unnecessary and time-consuming.

A simplified method of management has been described, which merely includes the endopelvic fascia (cardinal ligament) in the clamp on the uterine vessels. Thus, if the ureter is well displaced by the development of the posterior peritoneum and subjacent fascia and the bladder is adequately advanced beyond the cervix, the first clamp on the uterine vessels can be placed much lower than usual. This clamp is placed at the level of the uterosacral attachment posteriorly, then swings anteriorly, biting into and including a good portion of the anterior and lateral expanse of the fascia (Fig 5–30,G). A second clamp is placed above the first, and the usual backflow clamp is applied. The vessels and fascia are then divided and the suture ligatures placed so that the needle enters the medial portion of the fascia (Fig 5–30,H). Double ligation is recommended.

This step secures the cardinal ligament in apposition to the vessels, eliminates the fascial incisions (which sometimes bleed), and makes separate bites of paracervical tissue for the most part unnecessary. It seems to aid in hemostasis since the uterine vessels are anchored securely.

Entering the vagina.—Anterior, lateral, and posterior entrance have all been suggested and each author cites reasons why his particular method seems easier for him. For most gynecologists, however, it seems reasonably simple to identify the anterior longitudinal striations of the vagina, elevate them with a Kocher clamp in the midline, and make a transverse thrust into the vaginal space with a knife just above the clamp. If another Kocher clamp is placed on the anterior lip of the cervix, the incision may be everted so that by simply laying the curved scissors against the cervix it may be easily "circumcised." Kocher clamps may be placed at each angle and in the midline posteriorly as the specimen is removed. Care should be taken to include the vaginal mucosa in the angle clamps since, if it

pulls away, postoperative hemorrhage from the cuff may occur (Fig 5–30, H–K).

Treatment of the vagina.—Most gynecologists favor closure of the vaginal cuff with catgut sutures, with considerable importance being given to everting the vaginal mucosa into the vaginal space. The bothersome vascularity at the angle is usually managed by a figure-of-eight suture, which frequently serves the double purpose of securing the cardinal ligament to the vaginal cuff as a major means of support. If the fascial envelopes have been developed, they are frequently brought together over the closed cuff and closed with a running transverse suture. This, it is felt, adds further support to the vaginal apex.

Another group favors leaving the vagina open and simply running a hemostatic suture around the periphery of the cuff, making certain to include a good bit of the mucosa with every bite (Fig 5–30, L). Before placement of this stitch, an important figure-of-eight suture is utilized to close the angle. This suture begins posteriorly, picking up the divided uterosacral ligament, goes obliquely through the posterior vaginal wall, and also through the anterior vaginal wall (and its fascia) somewhat more medially. It is then looped around the angle clamp and is directed laterally through the posterior and anterior vaginal walls. As it is tied, the loop incorporates the uterine vessels and the cardinal ligament. This places a third tie around these important vessels and secures the cardinal ligament to the vagina for support. The proponents of the open vagina feel that it results in a longer, more functional structure than if closed, that less granulation tissue develops, and that early bleeding is easily diagnosed and treated. Pelvic retroperitoneal hematomas are said to be less common. Advocates of the closed vagina state that by this method hemostasis is superior, support is better, and, if care is taken with the mucosal edges, granulation tissue is minimal.

The ovaries.—The problem of ovarian salvage at the time of hysterectomy for benign conditions has not been satisfactorily solved.

It is generally agreed that when extensive endometriosis or pelvic inflammatory disease exists and the uterus is removed the ovaries should be extirpated. If the patient is over the age of 45 years, many gynecologists prefer to remove what are apparently "normal" but nonfunctioning ovaries. It is now known that even after bilateral oophorectomy at this age measurable amounts of estrogenic substances continue to be excreted in the urine. This is presumably of adrenal origin since bilateral adrenalectomy will result in a marked diminution or total absence of such material as measured by present methods. Under the age of 45 years, or as long as the patient is having apparently normal ovulatory cycles, most authorities favor leaving one or both ovaries. A report from a large Boston clinic, however, favors bilateral oophorectomy with every hysterectomy (regardless of age) with immediate postoperative replacement therapy. This management was based on a study in which 6% of patients who had apparently "normal" ovaries left in at the time of hysterectomy had subsequent symptoms referable to the remaining ovary, and 3% had later oophorectomy because of recurrent pain. An additional group had severe mastodynia with retained ovaries, and of major interest was the fact that the patients whose ovaries were left in had a greater incidence of vasomotor symptoms (flushes and sweats) than those who had bilateral oophorectomy and who received adequate replacement therapy.

If the ovaries are left in, it seems wiser not to fix the round and utero-ovarian ligaments to the lateral aspect of the vaginal vault, since this may drop the ovary into the posterior cul-de-sac and result in dyspareunia. It is also possible that by stretching the infundibulopelvic ligament the ovarian blood supply may be compromised. If the ovaries are removed and the untied infundibulopelvic and round ligaments are loose and long they may be tied into the vaginal angle suture. This simplifies peritonization but does not increase support of the vaginal vault to any degree. If the ligaments are short they are best left in position

and peritonization begun by carefully picking up the lateral peritoneal edges with a running suture of no. 00 or 000 chromic catgut. Most ureteral injuries and angulations have occurred at this point and during this step the ureter should be visualized on the medial leaf of peritoneum with the placement of every suture.

Endolymphatic Stromal Myosis

The disease process known as endolymphatic stromal myosis should be differentiated from adenomyosis since there is evidence that it may have malignant potential. It has been called variously stromatous endometriosis, perithelioma, hemangiopericytoma, and stromatoid new growth of the uterine wall. It consists pathologically of strands and masses of noncollagenous connective tissue that is usually regarded as being of endometrial origin. The disease is found most often during the fourth and fifth decades of life and is associated with symptoms of menorrhagia, metrorrhagia, or postmenopausal bleeding. Other symptoms include dysmenorrhea and weight loss. The one constant physical finding is a diffuse uterine enlargement.

The pathogenesis of endolymphatic stromal myosis is unknown but three theories of development have been advanced. The generally accepted concept suggests direct extension or invasion of stroma from the basal endometrium. Other theories indicate that the tissue develops from undifferentiated cells between myometrial fibers or from lymphatics and/or blood vessels of the endometrial stroma. Several authors have suggested that the tumor arises from *vasoformative cells* such as pericytes, and therefore the term *hemangiopericytoma* has gained prominence. The fact that late recurrence of endolymphatic stromal myosis has a pattern similar to the original tumor strongly supports this concept.

Gross examination of the uterus reveals diffuse enlargement, usually symmetric with white or yellow rubbery masses extending throughout the myometrium. Small yellow nodules may occasionally project above the cut surface or section of the freshly cut specimen. Occasionally the tumor masses may extend into the endometrial cavity as polypoid excrescences.

Microscopically, the tissue is made up of round or oval cells of uniform and moderate size (Fig 5–31). The cells resemble endometrial stromal cells of the mid-to-late proliferative phase. The cytoplasm is scanty and irregular. Mitotic figures are rare and vascularity is variable. In some cases the tumor cells blend into the myometrium and its limits may be determined only by special stains.

Novak interpreted endolymphatic stromal myosis as a stage in the development of uterine malignancy. The simple infiltration of the myometrium by glands and stroma is represented by adenomyosis. A more advanced phase embraces endolymphatic and extravascular ex-

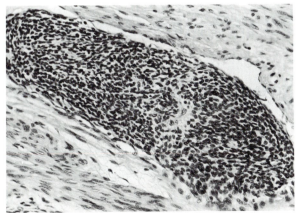

Fig 5–31.—Endolymphatic stromal myosis, showing a lymphatic space in the uterine wall filled with benign endometrial stroma.

tension (endolymphatic stromal myosis), and a third group, more advanced, resembles endometrial stromal sarcoma.

The treatment of this unusual process usually consists of total hysterectomy and bilateral salpingo-oophorectomy. In most cases, this treatment has already been completed by the time diagnosis is made. There is no evidence at present that postoperative x-ray therapy increases the survival rate.

The prognosis is good if the treatment just mentioned is carried out and dissemination has not already occurred. The five-year survival rate in most series has approximated 85%. Metastases have occurred to the lungs, peritoneum, and ovary. Pleomorphism and mitotic activity indicate an increased liability to recurrence but an inactive histologic appearance is no guarantee against recurrence.

Endometrial Polyps

Endometrial polyps are hyperplastic overgrowths of the glands and stroma of rather localized extent that form a projection above the surface. Such polyps may be sessile or pedunculated and rarely show foci of neoplastic growth. These tumors are relatively common and usually occur between ages 29 and 59 years, with the greatest incidence after age 50 years. Symptoms are variable and, since polyps may exist with other abnormalities, are difficult to ascribe to the polyp per se. In general, the patient may note intermenstrual spotting or, more commonly, postmenstrual staining of four to five days' duration. Usually this discharge is dark brown and somewhat mucoid. In postmenopausal patients irregular staining and bleeding may ocur. Occasionally a history of oral ingestion of estrogenic substances for months or years may be elicited. It should be remembered that many unsuspected and asymptomatic polyps are discovered by the pathologist when hysterectomies are performed for other indications, such as leiomyomas or adenomyosis. This is particularly true in the postmenopausal patient who undergoes a vaginal hysterectomy for uterine prolapse. Similarly, approximately 10% of uteri of postmenopausal women examined at autopsy harbor asymptomatic, benign polyps.

The diagnosis should be strongly suspected if a premenopausal patient notes recurrent postmenstrual staining without other symptoms of dysfunctional bleeding. Hysterograms will frequently demonstrate large polyps but smaller ones will not be visualized. Hysteroscopy is of particular value in the diagnosis of small intracavitary polyps, particulrly those in the fundus of the uterus or near the intrauterine ostia of the oviducts. Endometrial biopsy is inadequate for complete diagnosis, since the polyp moves about so easily it may be brushed aside by the curet. A thorough uterine curettage is necessary for diagnosis and the operator should assiduously curet all portions of the endometrial cavity and then explore further with a polyp extractor, a modified placental forceps that grasps the polyp securely. Most gynecologists have had the experience of performing a "thorough" curettage prior to hysterectomy only to be surprised when the opened specimen is shown by the pathologist. Large, fleshy polyps are easily missed if not sought for repeatedly. If bleeding persists following a curettage for dysfunctional uterine bleeding, the physician should assume that a polyp remains in the endometrial cavity.

Gross examinations of the excised polyp reveals a smooth, usually red or orange, velvety mass varying from 0.3 to 12.0 cm in diameter, although most have a diameter of 2 to 4 cm. Although usually solitary, polyps may be multiple, especially if exogenous estrogen has been administered for long periods. Most polyps arise in the fundal region and extend downward (Fig 5–32), occasionally prolapsing through the cervix. Since the base of the polyp is located high in the corpus and is broad and vascular, removal should not be attempted in the office or clinic. In this respect endometrial polyps differ from those arising in the endocervix.

Microscopically, most endometrial polyps show a histologic pattern of basal endometrium of an immature type usually not reac-

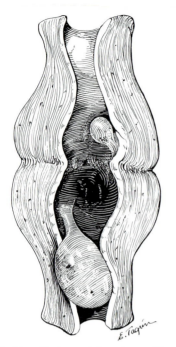

Fig 5–32.—Endometrial polyps. The uterus has been bivalved to show the interior of cavity.

tive to hormonal stimuli. The great majority are composed of cystically dilated glands, lined by a single layer of flattened cells, surrounded by relatively inactive stroma. The typical polyp found in the senescent uterus is of this type (Fig 5–33). The thin-walled, cystically dilated glands may represent foci of previous hyperplasia, the "retrogressive hyperplasia" of Novak and Richardson. In some polyps, the stroma shows extensive fibrosis and hyalinization, representing a diminution in vascular supply following the onset of the menopause. Other polyps demonstrate much more epithelial activity, with rather extensive cystic hyperplasia and foci of adenomatous hyperplasia as well. The stroma here is loose and edematous, and mitotic figures are common. These are frequently seen and associated with extensive cystic and adenomatous endometrial hyperplasia. A third type, which poses problems for both clinician and pathologist, demonstrates a mixture of hyperplasia, carcinoma in situ, and questionable areas of invasive carcinoma. The accompanying endometrium may be perfectly normal so that, in most cases, cure is brought about by removal

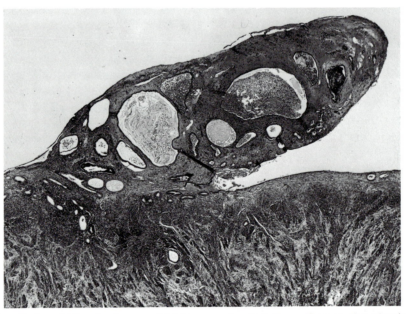

Fig 5–33.—Endometrial polyp in a postmenopausal uterus. The glands within the polyp show cystic dilatation, whereas the glands of the endometrium are senescent and inactive.

of the polyp alone. One should remember, however, that up to 15% of women with endometrial cancer will also have polyps in the endometrial cavity at the time of hysterectomy. This finding makes thorough curettage mandatory in the postmenopausal age group.

Polyps are generally believed to develop as the result of prolonged anovulation together with persistent estrogen stimulation. Yet polyps are frequently found at autopsy in the uterine cavity of many women who have not taken estrogenic substances and whose ovaries are atrophic. The epithelium may, in patients who ovulate irregularly, exhibit secretory change on the surface. The finding of unequivocal invasive carcinoma in a polyp is extremely rare, especially when the remainder of the endometrial cavity is free from malignancy. Peterson and Novak found acceptable evidence of carcinoma in only 0.36%. Hertig and Sommers noted that in 31% of patients with invasive endometrial cancer, polyps had been discovered at prior curettage. This does not necessarily implicate polyps as being premalignant, since these findings were based on a selective group of patients in a retrospective study. In general, polyps do not recur and most patients proceed through menopause without further difficulty. As previously noted, about 10% of all uteri examined at autopsy show asymptomatic benign polyps.

Management

The majority of patients with endometrial polyps are cured by thorough curettage. This is particularly true in the postmenopausal group. Therapy must be guided by the histologic pattern of the polyp itself as well as by that of the endometrium. If the polyp contains areas of dysplasia or carcinoma in situ and the endometrial curettings show a similar hyperplastic pattern, hysterectomy may be performed if the patient is beyond the childbearing age. An equally acceptable, although more conservative approach, would be to await another episode of abnormal uterine bleeding or to perform a second curettage within six months.

Since the changes in the polyp and the endometrium may represent only a temporary derangement of pituitary-ovarian function at menopause, with prolongation of estrogen stimulation and absence of progesterone differentiation, a single curettage may prove curative. Continued secretion of estrogenic substances by ovarian tumors of the granulosa-thecoma group would result in recurrence of the hyperplastic process and abnormal bleeding. In the postmenopausal patient, recurrence of uterine bleeding following removal of a benign polyp is an indication for hysterectomy. Uteri removed for this reason frequently show other polyps, missed at the first curettage, as well as foci of endometrial hyperplasia, and, rarely, a minute area of carcinoma in a relatively inaccessible position. Such areas are in the fundus near the junction of the oviduct or behind a submucous leiomyoma. One should make certain, however, that the bleeding has its origin in the endometrial cavity and is not due to senescent or inflammatory vaginitis. Furthermore, it is imperative that the patient be questioned about the use of estrogenic substances in the form of tablets, injections, vaginal creams, or suppositories and the use of the popular "hormonal" face creams.

Treatment in younger patients may be both expectant and hormonal. If the basic problem is one of anovulation or oligo-ovulation, adequate investigation of the causes of these problems should be performed. Therapy will depend on the specific endocrine derangement. (See Chapter 13, "Endocrine Disorders.") In certain patients, no cause for ovulatory failure can be found, but episodes of hypermenorrhea, irregular flow, and endometrial hyperplasia may be avoided by continued cyclic use of estrogen-progestin combinations. This therapeutic regimen, although administered solely for the relief of symptoms, is occasionally followed by a return to normal ovulatory cycles. Furthermore, it prevents the prolonged growth stimulation of the endometrium by estrogens, adds the differentiating effect of progesterone, and allows for regular shedding of the glands and stroma.

Endometrial Hyperplasia

Endometrial hyperplasia includes a varied group of histologic patterns characterized by overgrowth of glandular and stromal elements together with increased vascularity and lymphocytic infiltration. The process may be generalized throughout the uterine cavity or localized to one or more areas. It may occur in any age group and is occasionally seen in teenage patients who have persistent estrogen stimulation without intermittent progesterone. Similarly, it is commonly observed during the menopause when the process of ovulation is waning. It is obvious, then, that hyperplasia is seen frequently at the two extremes of the reproductive period and is associated with the clinical entity called dysfunctional uterine bleeding.

Endometrial hyperplasia may be produced in animals (monkey, hamster, rabbit) and in human subjects by the administration of estrogenic substances for prolonged periods. We produced varying degrees of hyperplasia (including dysplasia) in normally ovulating females by administering a synthetic estrogen for periods up to 90 days. This process was temporary, however, since the endometrium returned to normal as soon as the estrogen was discontinued and ovulation permitted to occur. Prophylactically, therefore, it is important to preserve the function of ovulation and the differentiating effect of progesterone.

Pathology

Grossly, the appearance of the endometrial cavity containing hyperplastic tissue is quite variable. In some cases it is markedly thickened or polypoid (Fig 5–34) and large quantities of tissue may be removed at the time of uterine curettage. This gross appearance is occasionally confused with that of the very thick and succulent endometrium removed on day 27 or 28 of the normal secretory cycle. In some patients, particularly menopausal ones, the curettings may be scanty and only a small focus will be found to contain areas of hyperplasia, and very often if a hysterectomy is performed within a few days or weeks after the

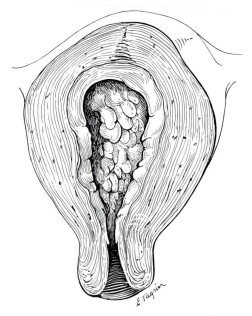

Fig 5–34.—Endometrial hyperplasia.

curettage, the uterus will be found to harbor only atrophic endometrium. Thus, it is possible, at least temporarily, to remove all hyperplastic endometrium by curettage. In this older age group, however, one should strongly suspect that invasive carcinoma may be present in an area ajacent to the hyperplasia.

HISTOLOGIC PATTERNS.—Three major types of endometrial hyperplasia are recognized histologically. These are the cystic, the adenomatous, and the dysplastic. Mixtures of all three frequently coexist in the same endometrial cavity and may coexist in the curettings. The typical hyperplastic pattern that follows estrogen therapy in the human female is of the cystic variety. This usually takes four to six weeks to develop and will do so only if moderately large doses of estrogens are administered. Cystic hyperplasia is characterized by a glandular pattern that resembles Swiss cheese, i.e., irregular enlargement and dilatation of some glands and preservation of normal architecture in others (Fig 5–35). The epithelium lining the dilated glands is usually cuboidal or cylindrical, with darkly stained nu-

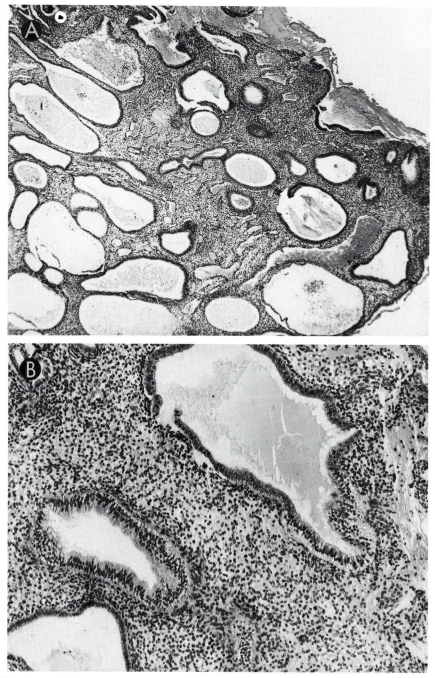

Fig 5–35.—A, cystic hyperplasia of the endometrium, showing cystic dilatation of glands and an increase in the number and size of the blood vessels. (From Kistner R.W., Smith O.W.: *Fertil. Steril.* 12:121, 1961.) **B,** cystic endometrial hyperplasia showing secretory effect ten days after administration of a single dose (100 mg) of medroxyprogesterone acetate. The dilated gland at top right is lined by tall cells of high cuboidal and columnar type, but the lowermost fragment shows subnuclear vacuoles, the effect of the progestin. The gland at lower left shows pseudostratification with extensive subnuclear vacuoles. In this postmenopausal patient, endometrial hyperplasia resulted from the administration of estrogens.

clei and scant cytoplasm. The smaller glands are usually of proliferative type with numerous mitoses and pseudostratification of nuclei. The stroma is quite cellular and dense and the stromal cells show extensive mitotic activity. Aggregates of lymphocytes are frequently found in the stroma, together with dilated and engorged vascular spaces. It is not difficult in the usual case to distinguish cystic hyperplasia from a cystic gland that occasionally results from obstruction of the gland lumen or from one that is lined by atrophic flat cells found in the endometrium of the postmenopausal patient.

Adenomatous hyperplasia is characterized by an increased number of glands (Fig 5–36), many of which have small outpouchings or budlike glandular projections into the stroma. A typical finger-in-glove appearance frequently results, and eventually these outpouchings become pinched off and lie in groups with a back-to-back pattern and very little or no intervening stroma. The nuclei are usually darkly stained and the cytoplasm is scant.

Dysplasia, or lessened differentiation, has a typical histologic appearance. The lining cells of the glands exhibit a pronounced variation in size, shape, cytoplasmic staining, and polarity. Similarly, the nuclei are usually irregularly shaped and show marked variation in size and staining qualities. There is a generalized pallor of the cells, but this may not be uniform.

Symptomatology

The usual symptom associated with the process of endometrial hyperplasia is that of irregular, occasionally profuse, uterine bleeding. There may be lower abdominal, cramplike pain, which is due to the accumulation of blood in the endometrial cavity. This pain is usually relieved by the expulsion of several large blood clots. Endometrial hyperplasia may exist in the teenage patient because of constant estrogen stimulation. This process disappears as soon as cyclic ovulation and menstruation begin. In the middle-aged patient hyperplasia is

associated with an interruption of ovulation either because of intrinsic disease (granulosa cell tumors, thecomas, Stein-Leventhal syndrome, adrenocortical hyperplasia) or because of constant administration of estrogenic substances. The history in these patients reveals an interruption in cyclic menses, usually with skips and delays of flow or with prolonged periods of amenorrhea. The usual premenstrual moliminal symptoms are absent. In postmenopausal patients endometrial hyperplasia is characterized by postmenopausal bleeding. If ingestion of exogenous estrogenic substances has been excluded, hyperplasia is due, in most patients, to ovarian lesions, which are presumed to secrete steroidal substances of varying estrogenic potency. These lesions are cortical stromal hyperplasia, thecomatosis (thecosis), granulosa-theca tumors, and gynandroblastoma.

Management

The management of endometrial hyperplasia is similar to that outlined for endometrial polyps. Of prime importance are the age of the patient and the histologic pattern of the hyperplastic process. It is obvious that treatment of the teenage girl with cystic hyperplasia will always be conservative, whereas in the postmenopausal patient adenomatous or dysplastic hyperplasia is usually treated by hysterectomy and bilateral salpingo-oophorectomy. Between these two extremes there exist multiple variations of therapeutic regimens. They depend, in large measure, on the relationship of hyperplasia to carcinoma of the endometrium—unfortunately an unsettled and frequently disputed correlation.

It has been suggested that if ovulation could be brought about in certain patients who have a syndrome of obesity, hypertension, diabetes, and endometrial abnormalities, the eventual development of carcinoma in such patients might be avoided. Hertig has stated that optimum treatment for these patients is ovulation, menstruation, and pregnancy; most patients in this particular group never accomplish this goal.

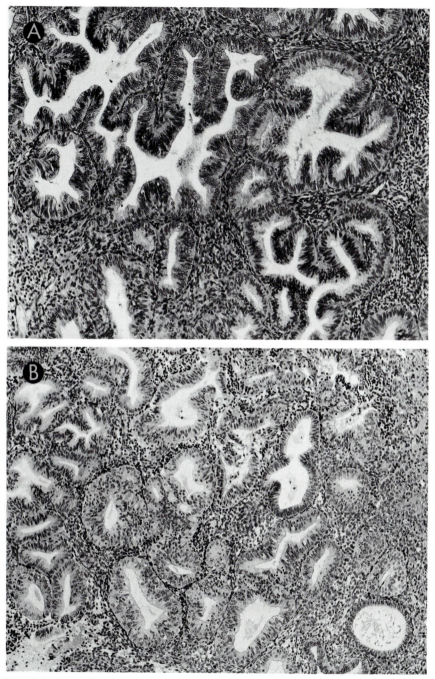

Fig 5–36.—Adenomatous hyperplasia of the endometrium. **A,** note outpouching of glands into a dense stroma. The epithelium lining the glands is of active proliferative type and tends to form budlike projections, which may be pinched off to form small nests of closely packed glands. These do not vary in staining qualities from the surrounding proliferative endometrium. Specimen was obtained by curettage from a woman, 42 years old, who had received exogenous estrogens for several years. (From Kistner R.W., Smith O.W.: *Fertil. Steril.* 12:121, 1961.) **B,** focal carcinoma in situ in central area of adenomatous hyperplasia. (From Kistner R.W.: *Cancer* 12:1106, 1959.)

The association of hyperplasia and carcinoma of the endometrium was first noted by Backer in 1904, but prior to the report of Taylor in 1932 the simultaneous occurrence of these two lesions was believed to be one of chance alone. The review by Taylor and that by Novak and Yui in 1936 suggested that a definite correlation between these entities did exist and, furthermore, that estrogenic substances might, under favorable circumstances, be carcinogenic. In 1954, Larson reviewed the literature on the relationship of estrogens in endometrial hyperplasia to carcinoma and was able to formulate five distinctly different points of view held by various groups of investigators. Briefly, these are as follows.

1. Endometrial hyperplasia does *not* have any tendency toward malignant change in the *reproductive* years but when it occurs as a result of postmenopausal estrogenic stimulation of the endometrium, it *may* predispose toward malignant disease (Novak).

2. Endometrial hyperplasia (and hence excess estrogen) predisposes to carcinoma at any age (Dockerty et al., Morrin and Max).

3. Endometrial hyperplasia and cancer are not associated but "the unopposed action of estrin, with its resultant effect on the endometrium, is the basic principle at work in the development of malignancy of the endometrium of those individuals who possess the genetic factor necessary for the development of cancer" (Herrell).

4. Endometrial hyperplasia may be followed by anaplasia, carcinoma in situ, and adenocarcinoma of the uterus, but "no convincing studies are available to show that estrogen stimulation alone will produce this picture, and many excellent estrogen studies failed to mention such histological changes" (Hertig and Sommers).

5. Neither hyperplasia nor prolonged estrogen stimulation is associated with corpus cancer other than on a chance basis (Fahlund and Broders; Jones and Brewer).

The available data from human material would suggest that: (1) there is little, if any, evidence that estrogenic substances are carcinogenic in the premenopausal woman; (2) only meager evidence is available to indicate that cystic (Swiss-cheese) hyperplasia is causally related to endometrial carcinoma; (3) in *predisposed* individuals, the unopposed action of estrogenic substances for considerable periods of time will result in endometrial adenomatous hyperplasia, dysplasia, carcinoma in situ, and, eventually, carcinoma. We produced varying degrees of hyperplasia and dysplasia in young, normally menstruating women by the administration of an estrogen for 45 to 100 days. After the exogenous estrogen was stopped, all patients subsequently had normal menstrual periods and normal endometrium as determined by biopsy. Gusberg classified "atypical" hyperplasia as being histologically identical with adenomatous hyperplasia, carcinoma in situ, and stage 0 cancer. He followed up 64 patients with this entity for five years and subsequently found invasive cancer in only 3, or 4.6%. In a later study Gusberg noted that carcinoma developed in 12% of patients with atypical hyperplasia treated only by curettage and followed for at least five years. He concluded that adenomatous hyperplasia might be present in the same endometrium with adenocarcinoma or might be a precursor to cancer.

The specific morphologic changes preceding the development of carcinoma of the endometrium are not completely known. Some evidence has already been advanced by the work of Hertig and Sommers, based on retrospective study of prior curettings, that adenomatous (atypical) hyperplasia precedes carcinoma. There is also evidence to support the fact that adenomatous hyperplasia does not *always* proceed relentlessly toward unequivocal carcinoma, and the prediction of which hyperplasia will and which will not become malignant is presently impossible. It is probably true, however, that many endometria in which there is carcinoma have passed through the various phases shown in Figure 5–37. On the other hand, carcinoma of the endometrium has been found in a few women who have had bilateral oophorectomy many years

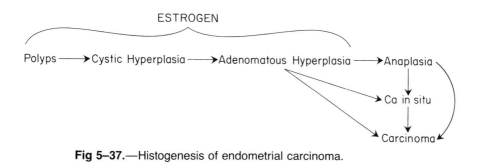

Fig 5–37.—Histogenesis of endometrial carcinoma.

prior to diagnosis and in whom estrogenic substances had not been administered. In some instances endometrial carcinoma seems to arise in an atrophic endometrium, in a patient whose ovaries are also atrophic. Yet how can one be certain that the area of carcinoma was not an area of carcinoma in situ or atypical hyperplasia five years previously? Areas of carcinoma are occasionally found in basically secretory or proliferative endometrium, but I know of only one report of endometrial carcinoma that coexisted with an intrauterine pregnancy.

Several reports indicate that cystic and adenomatous hyperplastic glands may undergo regression, and actively growing stroma may be converted to decidua by the action of synthetic progestational agents. These changes are noted even in the usually stable basal layer of the endometrium and are more pronounced after prolonged, constant therapy. In the younger patient, optimum treatment would seem to be the cyclic administration of these newer progestins in the regimens outlined for dysfunctional uterine bleeding. Similarly, in older patients who are not good candidates for surgery, constant administration of large doses of either 17α-hydroxyprogesterone caproate (Delalutin) or medroxyprogesterone acetate (Depo-Provera) for periods of up to six months will bring about adequate hemostasis and endometrial atrophy. A succinct summary by Speert emphasizes the importance of an evaluation of prospective as well as retrospective studies: "Glandular hyperplasia of the endometrium was a common precursor of carcinoma, but carcinoma occurs in only a small proportion of women with en-

dometrial hyperplasia." Therefore, because of the reversibility of glandular changes that heretofore were thought to be premalignant, the often-quoted dictum of Halban, *"Nicht Karzinom, aber besser heraus!"* ("Not carcinoma, but better out!") is not wholly acceptable.

PREMALIGNANT NEOPLASMS

Carcinoma In Situ

The earliest stage of endometrial carcinoma that is not invasive has been termed *carcinoma in situ.* Although this term is not acceptable in many clinics throughout the country, it has been so designated for a specific lesion, first described by Hertig, in the Pathology Laboratory at the Free Hospital for Women since about 1940. The diagnosis is based on the presence of glands composed of large eosinophilic cells with abundant cytoplasm (Fig 5–38). The nuclei tend to be pale with small chromatin granules and slightly irregular, folded, or scalloped nuclear membranes. Cytologic dysplasia is present, but there is no stromal invasion. The region of carcinoma in situ is usually focal, sharply in contrast in morphologic and staining characteristics with adjacent unaffected glands. In other clinics this same histologic picture has been designated as *atypical hyperplasia* or *carcinoma stage 0.*

There is no characteristic symptom associated with carcinoma in situ of the endometrium other than that of irregular bleeding in the premenopausal woman or postmenstrual staining in the older patient. It is occasionally described as an incidental finding in endo-

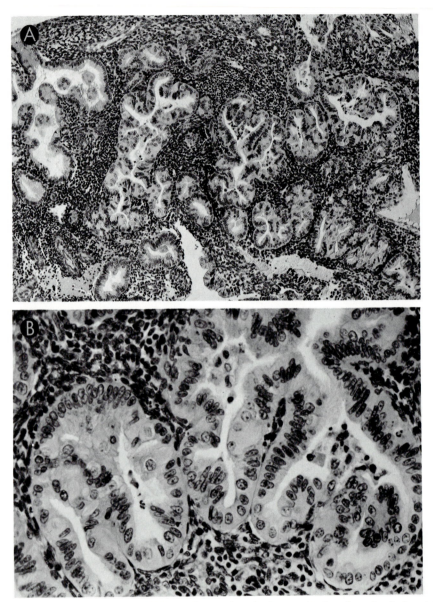

Fig 5–38.—**A,** carcinoma in situ of the endo-metrium. The glands are composed of large cells with abundant, clear, eosinophilic cytoplasm. The nuclei are pale, with fine granular chromatin and slightly wrinkled or irregular nuclear membranes arranged in irregular palisades. **B,** higher power shows cellular disorientation and dyspolarity with intraluminal tufting. Carcinoma in situ is often sharply demarcated and easily distinguished from adjoining normal, senescent, or hyperplastic glands. There is moderate crowding of affected glands but not necessarily a back-to-back pattern or invasion or displacement of the endometrial stroma. (From Kistner R.W.: *Cancer* 12:1106, 1959.)

metrial hyperplasia or invasive carcinoma. Until 1960 it was believed that endometrium with this particular histologic picture did not revert to normal, hyperplastic, or senescent endometrium and that, unless completely removed or destroyed, it would be followed in time by invasive endometrial carcinoma. The highest incidence of carcinoma in situ was noted in the three to five years before invasive cancer. The impact of the retrospective study of patients with invasive carcinoma has prevented adequate observation of the life history of this lesion in our clinic. Thus, Steiner and Craig have reviewed the material for 222 patients in whom a diagnosis of carcinoma in situ of the endometrium was made. Two hundred were treated by hysterectomy and only 15 were followed up. Seven were lost to follow-up. Only two of the patients who were followed up without further therapy developed invasive carcinoma and in one other patient the hysterectomy specimen showed a "questionable invasive" lesion. Invasive carcinoma was not found in any of the 200 hysterectomies done for carcinoma in situ of the endometrium.

Active therapeutic measures should be instituted without delay in the treatment of the adolescent female whose endometrium shows evidence of hyperplasia, dysplasia, or carcinoma in situ (Fig 5–39). An effort should be made to secure ovulation and cyclic secretory differentiation followed by shedding. It is important to ascertain the precise etiology of the anovular process by a complete diagnostic survey. Subsequent therapy with cortisone, progestins, clomiphene, or ovarian wedge resection should be selected, depending on the diagnosis. Ovarian wedge resection should be the last, not the first, therapeutic measure employed in patients having Stein-Leventhal syndrome since the ovary in this disorder seems unusually responsive to clomiphene. If ovulation cannot be regularly established, substitutional therapy may be administered in the form of cyclic or constant progestins. The clinician should realize that the situation is not acute and that immediate hysterectomy is

neither necessary nor indicated. This is of particular importance in the young, infertile woman. It is imperative, however, that a thorough curettage be performed in all patients prior to therapy in order to exclude the presence of simultaneously occurring endometrial carcinoma. Although the progestins are capable of bringing about striking changes in the morphologic features of the endometrial glands, they should not be regarded as a panacea and should not be used as a substitute for usual and accepted diagnostic procedures and appropriate therapy.

Since it is impossible for the pathologist, at present, to predict the malignant potential of atypical endometrium, it is necessary that the clinician select the optimum method of therapy on the basis of other factors. The presence of other pathologic processes involving the internal genitalia or the inability to follow the patient adequately are valid reasons for hysterectomy. In the young, the infertile, or the very old patient with serious medical disease, a more conservative approach is now possible. Although the patient most likely to benefit from a conservative regimen is the young woman with irregular or absent ovulation, it should also be remembered that the endometrial hyperplastic process may occur in women approaching the menopause, as a result of constant estrogen stimulation.

The following recommendations for therapy can be made. In the premenopausal or menopausal patient with adenomatous hyperplasia, in whom carcinoma has been excluded by uterine curettage, cyclic progestins may be given for six to 12 months. An androgenic-type progestin should be selected that will result in scanty flow and eventual endometrial atrophy. In patients having carcinoma in situ, constant intramuscular progestins may be given for six to 12 months. Hysterectomy may subsequently be performed, depending on the age of the patient, her medical status, and the response of the endometrium noted at the time of curettage. I have not seen persistence of the carcinoma in situ process when therapy has been given for at least six months. The

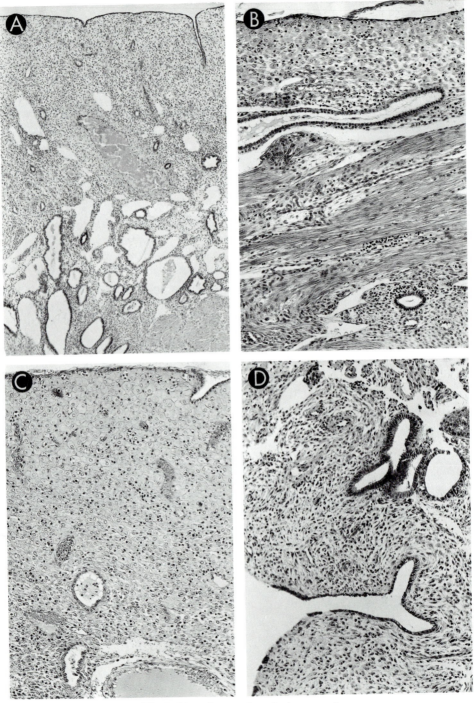

Fig 5–39.—*(Legend on facing page)*

medications used for constant therapy are as follows: medroxyprogesterone acetate (100 mg/week for four weeks, followed by 400 mg/month for the next five months) or 17α-hydroxyprogesterone caproate (500 mg/day for two weeks, followed by 2 gm/week for six months).

MALIGNANT NEOPLASMS

Adenocarcinoma

Adenocarcinoma of the body of the uterus is a common disease. In the past it was said to occur only about one eighth to one tenth as frequently as cervical carcinoma. There has been a marked increase in the incidence of carcinoma of the corpus and a marked decrease in the incidence of cervical cancer during the past two decades. Adenocarcinoma is a malignant neoplasm arising from the epithelial elements of the endometrium. Although it is usually glandular, squamous metaplastic elements occasionally are noted and, rarely, the lesion may be of a pure squamous cell type. In an analysis of the incidence of various cancers in the female in the state of New York, Corscaden reported an incidence of 11.9 cases per 100,000 female population for corpus cancer and a comparable figure of 34.3 for carcinoma of the cervix. During the interval 1957 to 1967 the number of patients admitted to the Free Hospital for Women with endometrial cancer was 404 and the number with cancer of the cervix was 400, a 1:1 ratio.

This is in marked contrast to the ratio of 6:1 noted in this hospital during the interval 1930 to 1940. During the interval 1968 to 1975 there were 432 new cases of endometrial carcinoma and 219 new cases of cervical cancer. The cause for the increasing incidence of endometrial carcinoma is unknown but may be due to improved diagnostic methods, more precise histologic criteria, or simply an aging population. Increased use of estrogenic hormones during the last 20 years has been suggested as a possible etiologic factor.

The studies of MacDonald and Siiteri have recently provided the first strong scientific evidence for a causal relationship between *endogenous* estrogen production and endometrial carcinoma.

The role of *exogenous* estrogen as an etiologic agent is less clear. Conclusive studies regarding cause and effect are unavailable. Part of this controversy involves the incidence of endometrial carcinoma in recent years. Results comparing the data of the Second and the Third National Cancer Survey showed essentially no change in the incidence of endometrial cancer between the years 1947 and 1970. Recent data collected by the California Tumor Registry, however, reveal an apparent increase in endometrial cancer incidence of 50% for invasive lesions and 100% for in situ lesions from 1953 to 1974.

A recent study by Smith et al. compared 317 hospital cases of endometrial carcinoma with an equal number of other gynecologic

Fig 5–39.—Effect of progestational agents on endometrial hyperplasia and carcinoma in situ. **A,** hysterectomy specimen from patient with carcinoma in situ after 44 days' therapy with mestranol and norethynodrel (Enovid). In the superficial endometrium the glands are small, circular, and lined by a single layer of cuboidal epithelium. Glands are inactive in a layer of dense decidual stroma. Cystically dilated glands in an edematous stroma are seen in the basalis, but even here the epithelium is inactive. A portion of the myometrium is seen at lower right. **B,** hysterectomy specimen obtained after 80 days of continuous therapy with Enovid in a patient with carcinoma in situ (seen in Fig 5–38). There is an extremely thin layer of endometrium with decidual effect. A single, thinned-out basal gland is seen with intraluminal secretion. **C,** another section of endometrium from same specimen as **B.** The compact and superficial layers show well-preserved decidua. Two inactive glands of the basalis are seen below and to the left of a dilated blood vessel. (**A-C** from Kistner R.W.: *Cancer* 12:1106, 1959). **D,** curettage specimen from a patient with extensive carcinoma in situ of the endometrium obtained after 55 gm of hydroxyprogesterone caproate (Delalutin) was given over nine months. Only scanty curettings were obtained and the glands were inactive. Focal decidual reaction is seen in the stroma. (From Kistner R.W.: *Clin. Obstet. Gynecol.* 5:1178, 1962.)

malignancies in matched controls. Estrogen was much more frequently used among the endometrial cancer patients than among the controls, leading to an estimated relative risk of endometrial cancer of 4.5 among women exposed to estrogen therapy. This study, however, did not address itself to dosage of estrogens, specific estrogens, or treatment schedules. Certainly if these patients received high doses of estrogens continuously, for prolonged periods of time, one would expect all to have developed adenomatous hyperplasia of varying degree and 10% to 12% of these with atypical hyperplasia might subsequently develop carcinoma. Thus, the average risk factor in the order of 5, as calculated from their data, must be viewed with the consideration that dosage schedules, length of administration, and compounds of varying estrogenicity may affect the ultimate risk.

Another retrospective study by Ziel and Finkle revealed that 82% of patients with endometrial cancer used estrogenic substances, compared with 22% of matched controls. The increased risk of endometrial cancer for all patients taking conjugated estrogen was 7.4. This risk ratio increased with duration of estrogen exposure to 8.0 in patients with three or more years' exposure. In this report, conjugated estrogens appeared to be the prime culprit; since the principal steroid component of these preparations is sodium estrone sulfate, estrone was considered to be a possible carcinogen. The authors concluded that high levels of estrone, either endogenously derived from androstenedione, or exogenously administered in conjugaged estrogen, create an environment that may trigger endometrial cancer in the genetically susceptible patient. Speert reviewed the nine major series of endometrial carcinoma reports in 1948 and noted that the mean age varied from 54.0 to 58.6 years, with an average of 55.5 years. At the Free Hospital for Women, Hertig found the mean age to be 57.2 years in a study of 500 patients. The range was 25 to 88 years, with a peak incidence of 40.6% in the sixth decade.

Cancer of the corpus is the predominant genital malignancy in white women over age 50 years, though it remains second to cancer of the cervix in blacks. The highest rates for corpus cancer among whites were found in western regions of the United States, and lowest rates were found in the South. Cancer of the corpus is now the predominant site of invasive gynecologic cancers among whites, although it is not believed that this increased incidence is due to an actual increased number of cases but rather to the decreased incidence of cervical cancer in whites.

PATHOLOGY.—Adenocarcinoma may arise from any part of the uterus and has been separated into two major anatomic types, the diffuse and the localized. In addition, invasive carcinoma has been described in the tip of an endometrial polyp.

The discrete or circumscribed variety of endometrial carcinoma may arise anywhere in the cavity but is generally believed to be found more commonly on the posterior wall. This form may merely represent an earlier variety of the disease than the extensive, diffuse form. The lesion may be papillary, polypoid, or only slightly raised from the surrounding endometrium. Frequently it can be diagnosed only by microscopic examination and may then be called a *microcarcinoma*. Although the discrete variety may be localized to the endometrium, more often it has invaded the myometrium to a rather considerable degree. Despite this fact, as pointed out by Javert, tumor tends to remain localized in the myometrium in slightly over one half the cases, and this particular feature accounts in large measure for the relatively good prognosis. In many patients the disease process is so localized that it is entirely removed at the time of curettage, the subsequent hysterectomy specimen being completely devoid of tumor. Needless to say, the prognosis in such a patient is excellent. Minute focal carcinomas are occasionally found in the region of the cornua and these are notoriously difficult to diagnose by routine curettage. Approximately one fifth arise in the isthmus or lower uterine segment and frequently spread to the endocervix. It is for this reason that a "fractional" curettage is done routinely at the Brigham and Women's Hospital in an effort to localize the tumor, since endocervical involvement makes it mandatory to treat the patient as if she had primary cervical cancer.

The diffuse form of endometrial carcinoma may be quite superficial and may be difficult to distinguish from polypoid hyperplasia. Grossly, however, the carcinoma is paler, firmer, more friable, and less likely to have a glistening mucosal surface. Since this tumor is notoriously slow to invade the myometrium and since it invades the stroma before spread to the myometrium, prognosis is proportionately better than for other genital cancers. In patients with tumor localized in the endometrium, only one of 51 had metastases within a five-year follow-up. Javert reported that usually the tumor grows out into the uterine cavity as a cauliflowerlike mass faster than it invades the myometrium. In some cases ulceration may be extensive and it is then difficult to make a definite diagnosis from the curettage, since only necrotic tissue is recovered. In advanced cases the endometrium is markedly thickened with large exophytic masses protruding into the cavity of the uterus, and invasion of the muscular wall and the serosa is frequently obvious. The cervical canal may be blocked by the extension of tumor, with resulting pyometra. Since many endometrial carcinomas produce excessive mucus it is not unusual to find a bloodstained mucoid vaginal discharge as a distinctive sign. The finding of pyometra with endometrial carcinoma alters the prognosis significantly, not only because of the intrinsic septic nature of the pyometra but also because of the more extensive lymphatic permeation of the cancer. In fact, pyometra as the primary cause of death was noted by Henriksen in 28.8% of 208 patients with pyometra complicating uterine cancer.

The microscopic picture varies considerably according to the degree of malignancy and the gross extent of the tumor. All grades of undifferentiation are seen, from a simple increase in the number of glands to extensive arborization of solid tumor. Usually the diagnosis can be made on low-power examination simply by the obvious glandular pattern. Examination of the specific epithelial cells shows various changes, and in the low-grade type the cells grow regularly in a single layer, are larger, and stain more deeply than normal cells, and there is an increase in the number of mitotic figures. All degrees of undifferentiation beyond this simple picture are seen, with extensive piling up of cells in layers even filling the lumina of glands and invading the stroma. It should be remembered that although the disease fundamentally is an adenocarcinoma, in approximately 20% of the cases there is an accompanying squamous element, such tumors being called *adenoacanthomas* (Fig 5–40). In adenoacanthomas, the glandular carcinoma is usually fairly well differentiated but seems to be less malignant. The squamous element is usually well differentiated also and is not necessarily microscopically malignant. It is an integral part of the tumor, however, as is indicated by the fact that metastases show both glandular and squamous elements. Recent emphasis has been given to the clinical and morphologic features of adenosquamous (mixed) cancer of the endometrium. Compared with routine endometrial adenocarcinoma, adenosquamous cancers are more readily detected by cellular methods, occur at an older age, have a shorter symptomatic period, are associated with less-differentiated glandular components, are more advanced at detection, and have a poor five-year survival (less than 20%).

Classification and Staging of Endometrial Carcinoma

Carcinoma of the endometrium does not lend itself well to strict microscopic grading because of the extreme variability of the tumor in different areas of the endometrial cavity. In general, however, it may be said that the prognosis is much better in well-differen-

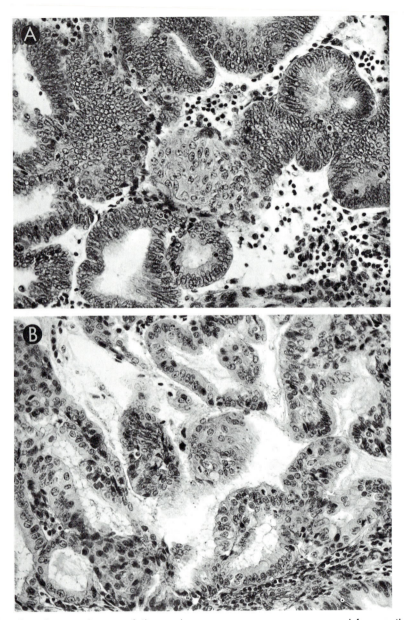

Fig 5–40.—A, adenocarcinoma of the endometrium with squamous metaplasia, also called adenoacanthoma. **B,** adenocarcinoma showing a secretory pattern. Note the pale vacuolated cells and intraluminal secretion. Secretory adenocarcinomas are uncommon and frequently appear innocuous morphologically. Nevertheless, they are capable of extension and metastasis. Occasionally a corpus luteum may be found in the ovary in such cases.

tiated tumors. Several series have indicated a survival rate of approximately 75% in grade 1 tumors, with a gradual decline to approximately 25% in grade 4 tumors. The five-year survival is also correlated with the clinical staging of the disease, and it is obvious that undifferentiated tumors are found more commonly in patients with stage III and stage IV disease.

The following classification has been recommended by the International Federation of Gynecology and Obstetrics (1971).

Clinical Stages of Carcinoma of the Corpus

Stage 0. Carcinoma in situ. Histologic findings suspicious of malignancy. Cases of stage 0 should not be included in any therapeutic statistics.

Stage I. The carcinoma is confined to the corpus.

Stage Ia. The length of the uterine cavity is 8 cm or less.

Stage Ib. The length of the uterine cavity is more than 8 cm.

The stage I cases should be subgrouped with regard to the histologic type of the adenocarcinoma as follows:

G1. Highly differentiated adenomatous carcinomas.

G2. Differentiated adenomatous carcinomas with partly solid areas.

G3. Predominantly solid or entirely undifferentiated carcinomas.

Stage II. The carcinoma has involved the corpus and the cervix.

Stage III. The carcinoma has extended outside the uterus but not outside the true pelvis.

Stage IIIa. Cases with microscopic adnexal pelvic metastases.

Stage IIIb. Cases with pelvic extension by invasion.

Stage IV. The carcinoma has extended outside the true pelvis or has obviously involved the mucosa of the bladder or rectum. Bullous edema as such does not permit allotment of a case to stage IV.

Stage IVa. Involvement of adjacent organs.

Stage IVb. Involvement of distal organs.

NOTE: On occasion, it may be difficult to decide whether the cancer actually is of the endocervix, or a carcinoma of the corpus and endocervix. If a clear differentiation is not possible from the findings at fractional curettage, then those that are adenocarcinoma should be classified as carcinoma of the corpus, and any epidermoid carcinoma as carcinoma of the cervix.

A case should be classified as carcinoma of the endometrium (corpus) when the primary site of the growth is in the corpus. Cases of mixed mesenchymal tumors and so-called carcinosarcoma should be excluded.

STAGE 0.—Carcinoma in situ. Histologic findings suspicious of malignancy.

Cases of stage 0 should not be included in any therapeutic statistics.

STAGE I.—The carcinoma is confined to the corpus. The great majority of cases of carcinoma of the corpus will be allotted to stage I. The factors that decide the prognosis in carcinoma of the corpus stage I are: (1) the age and general condition of the patient, (2) the size of the uterine cavity, and (3) the histologic pattern.

Several years ago, the Annual Report of the Results of Treatment in Carcinoma of the Uterus recommended a subdivision of the stage I cases with regard to operability. Patients of advanced years and patients suffering from extragenital disease were considered poor operative risks. Experience has obviously shown that no absolute criteria can be given for "poor operative risk." Such a judgment depends on the ability and skill of the surgeon. The Cancer Committee of FIGO considers a subdivision with regard to operability of limited value. We will not deny, however, that—especially in presentations of therapeutic results in carcinoma of the corpus—it is of value to know the number of patients suffering from serious extragenital disease (e.g., nephrocardiovascular disabilities) and the number of patients of 70 or 80 years of age, respectively.

Studies of large series of endometrial carcinoma limited to the corpus have shown that the prognosis, to some extent, is related to the size of the uterus. Enlargement of the uterus, however, may be caused by fibroids, adenomyosis, or other factors. Therefore, the size of the uterus cannot serve as a basis for subgrouping stage I cases. The length of the uterine cavity, however, measured with a sound from the external os, may give information of value for therapy. The Cancer Committee recommends a subdivision of the stage I cases with regard to the length of the sound. Cases with a sound depth of 8 cm or less should be allotted to stage Ia, and cases with a depth of more than 8 cm to stage Ib.

The histopathology as such should not serve as a basis for clinical stage grouping. Experience, however, has demonstrated that highly differentiated adenocarcinoma, frequently with papillary structures, as well as differentiated carcinomas with partly solid areas, have a tendency to grow exophytically in the uterine cavity, while predominantly solid and entirely undifferentiated dysplastic tumors frequently tend to deeply invade the myometrium at an early stage of development. Thus, these last-mentioned tumors are more malignant, and experience has shown that they have a worse prognosis than the differentiated ones. A subdivision of the stage I cases with regard to the histologic structures will facilitate the interpretation of a series of carcinoma of the corpus stage I. Therefore, the Cancer Committee recommends a subdivision of the stage I cases into:

G1. Highly differentiated adenomatous carcinomas.
G2. Differentiated adenomatous carcinomas with partly solid areas.
G3. Predominantly solid or entirely undifferentiated carcinomas.

STAGE II.—The carcinoma has involved the corpus and the cervix.

As far as prognosis and therapy are concerned, it is important to know whether the cancer has extended to the cervix. The extension of the carcinoma to the endocervix is confirmed by fractional curettage or hysteroscopy. The scraping of the cervix should be examined separately. Occasionally, it may be difficult to decide whether the endocervix is involved by the cancer. In such cases, simultaneous presence of normal cervical glands and cancer in the same piece will give the

final diagnosis. In questionable cases, the histologic examination of the curettage should decide whether the origin of the cancer is in the corpus or in the cervix. If a clear decision cannot be made, an adenocarcinoma should be allotted to carcinoma of the corpus and an epidermal carcinoma to carcinoma of the cervix.

STAGE III AND STAGE IV.—Extension of the carcinoma outside the uterus should refer a case to stage III or stage IV.

The presence of metastases in the vagina permits, as such, the allotment of a case to stage III.

Every gynecologist and pathologist knows that there are cases in which it is clinically as well as histologically impossible to decide whether the cancer is primarily a cancer of the corpus uteri or a cancer of the ovary. Previously, such cases were diagnosed as carcinoma uteri et ovarii, but this is not adequate. As a rule, it is possible, from the history of the patient and from the clinical examination, to decide which tumor is likely to be the primary one. In rare cases this may, however, be impossible. Such rare cases should be included in the statistics on carcinoma of the corpus as well as in the statistics on ovarian cancer. They should be reported separately.

Three major lymphatic channels have been described by Henriksen as draining the corpus uteri. One of these effects drainage from the lower uterine segment and midportion of the corpus into the same lymphatic channels as those from the cervix; the second channel, mostly from the fundus of the uterus, drains through the broad ligament and the infundibulopelvic ligament to hypogastric, external iliac, common iliac, and aortic nodes. The third channel drains along the course of the round ligament and into the superficial and deep inguinal nodes. It is primarily because of this lymphatic drainage that surgical treatment of carcinoma of the endometrium by radical hysterectomy and lymph node dissection is not looked on with favor. Distant metastases occur in approximately 40% of patients, and the organs most commonly involved are the lungs, liver, peritoneum, ovary, bowel, pleura, adrenal, and bones. The peritoneal implantations are the result of direct extension of the tumor cells to the peritoneal cavity by way of the oviduct, whereas ovarian metastases, occurring in approximately 4% of cases, are usually due to lymphatic spread.

Certain histochemical features have been described in carcinoma of the endometrium and may bear some relation to methods of treatment, particularly in regard to progestational agents. Studies have been reported by Atkinson, Hall, and McKay. Alkaline phosphatase reaches a peak in the cytoplasm during the proliferative phase of the cycle and has been described in endometrial hyperplasia and well-differentiated carcinoma. It seems to be correlated with growth patterns and differentiation. Glycogen is scanty during the proliferative phase but increases markedly in the progestational phase of a normal cycle. Glycogen has been found to be scanty and variable in distribution in both hyperplasia and carcinoma in situ, whereas in actual adenocarcinoma all variations of glycogen content have been described. Ribonucleic acid (RNA) has been found in large amounts in both hyperplasia and carcinoma. During the progestational phase of the normal cycle, RNA progressively declines. Acid phosphatase is minimal in the proliferative phase of the normal cycle but increases during the progestational phase. It is present in rather marked degree in carcinoma in situ, but its amount in invasive carcinoma is variable.

Studies have indicated a variation in content of deoxyribonucleic acid (DNA) in presumed precursors of endometrial carcinoma. Wagner and associates carried out microspectrophotometric measurements of Feulgen-stained gland-cell nuclei in 16 patients with presumed precursors (six cystic hyperplasia, ten adenomatous hyperplasia) and six adenocarcinomas of the endometrium. In all patients with cystic hyperplasia a diploid-to-tetraploid DNA distribution was found that was indistinguishable from that of a normal proliferating endometrium. The same diploid-to-tetraploid DNA distribution was found in eight of the ten adenomatous hyperplasias. Only two cases of adenomatous hyperplasia had an aneuploid DNA distribution pattern, and this was similar to that of invasive carcinoma. The six patients with adenocarcinoma had aneuploid DNA distribution. Since every group of precursor lesions in other organs studied in a similar way have been reported to have aneuploid DNA-distribution patterns, the results of this study suggest that most of the lesions now diagnosed as precursors of endometrial carcinoma either deviate from the pattern of other epithelia or that the morphologic criteria that traditionally are used in the diagnosis of these lesions are insufficiently precise.

Vaginal metastases from adenocarcinoma of the endometrium have been described in from 10% to 15% of patients. These metastatic areas are frequently found on the anterior vaginal wall, usually in the suburethral area. Although it has been felt that vaginal metastases were due to implantation of tumor cells at the time of surgery, in all probability they represent lymphatic permeation.

PATHOGENESIS.—Although the precise etiology of endometrial cancer is unknown, considerable evidence from clinical, endocrinologic, and pathologic studies has accumulated that indicates that the lesion develops as a result of long-continued estrogen stimulation without the interposition of progesterone. This general concept is true in the young patient under age 35 years with a history of dysfunctional bleeding, in the premenopausal patient with a similar history, and even in the postmenopausal patient with a granulosa cell tumor of the ovary or thecomatosis.

Other stigmata of endocrine dysfunction in these patients are the increased incidence of obesity, diabetes, thyroid malfunction, breast cancer, and infertility. As described in the section "Endometrial Hyperplasia," there may be a gradual progression through the various processes of cystic hyperplasia, adenomatous hyperplasia, dysplasia, carcinoma in situ, and, finally, invasive carcinoma. Any one of these entities may regress at any time if the constant stimulation of estrogen is removed or if the differentiating effects of progesterone or pregnancy supervene. It is true that a carcinoma may arise in the endometrium in a young patient who is cyclically ovulating and who may have menstrual endometrium adjacent to the cancerous area. It is probable that such carcinomas originate in a focus of hyperplasia or a polyp that does not respond to the secretory stimulation of progesterone.

A gradual morphologic transition from benign hyperplasia to neoplasia has been observed in sequential biopsies and also in multiple curettings obtained at the same time from the same endometrium. As long ago as 1923, Meyer emphasized that the morphologic differences between hyperplasia and cancer were those of degree only and described the concomitant finding of hyperplasia and cancer in the same tissue sections.

The studies of Wagner and associates suggest, therefore, that the endometrial lesions conventionally regarded as being precursors of endometrial adenocarcinoma may be divided into two types—a unimorphous type and a polymorphous type. Unimorphous hyperplasia is seen commonly in patients to whom estrogenic drugs have been administered for relatively long periods and in anovular patients. The association between this type of alteration with estrogenic states and the epidemiologic studies suggesting the possible association of estrogenic hormones with endometrial carcinoma provides a tentative hypothesis for the development of endometrial carcinoma in which estrogen may be regarded as an essential cocarcinogen that produces true hyperplasia that is diploid in character. This hyperplasia may progress to a true neoplasm by the continual action of another carcinogen or, in the absence of such additional stimuli, may remain unaltered. Our reports of the successful treatment of patients with adenomatous hyperplasia or carcinoma in situ by the administration of progestins suggests that some of these lesions may be reversible. It seems entirely possible that the reversible cases might fall into the unimorphous or diploid class.

Since an aneuploid DNA distribution, found in all other recognized groups of in situ neoplasms in other epithelia, was found in only two of ten patients reported by Wagner, one must conclude that adenomatous hyperplasia deviates from this general pattern or that the usual morphologic criteria for diagnosis are insufficiently precise. This failure of differentiation would place both benign abnormalities and preinvasive neoplasms in the same diagnostic category. Such a mixture of hyperplastic and neoplastic lesions in the same group might account for the relatively low incidence of invasive carcinoma eventually found in those patients followed without therapy. It remains to be determined, however, either by prospective or retrospective studies of patients with adenomatous hyperplasia, whether the prognosis is truly different in the subdivisions of this group as defined by DNA content. Even if such a difference can be demonstrated, the clinical application may be difficult because of the coexistence of both types of adenomatous hyperplasia in the same patient and the notoriously inadequate sample of the endometrium obtained by biopsy or curettage.

We have been able to produce invasive carcinoma of the endometrium in the rabbit by the insertion of a cotton string impregnated with a known carcinogen, 3-methylcholanthrene. But it is necessary to leave the string in place for at least a year to produce cancer. A control of the experiment was made possible by the use of a string coated in beeswax and placed in the opposite uterine horn. The tendency to carcinogenesis was absent in the control uterine horn. The necessity of estrogen in the experiment was emphasized by repeating the same plan in oophorectomized rabbits. No cancer developed in these animals. Based on the work of Wagner, it might be concluded that the addition of 3-methylcholanthrene to the estrogen-stimulated endometrium was sufficient to convert DNA distribution from a diploid or tetraploid pattern to the aneuploid pattern. Furthermore, when endogenous estrogen was removed by oophorectomy the DNA distribution of the atrophic endometrium was not affected by the carcinogen. Finally, the administration of synthetic progestins to rabbits with intact ovaries significantly inhibited the carcinogenesis in the methylcholanthrene uterus and caused regression of established carcinomas. We have theorized that the progestin, acting locally as an antiestrogen and producing glandular atrophy, acts in the same fashion as oophorectomy.

SYMPTOMATOLOGY AND DIAGNOSIS.—The commonest symptom is that of intermenstrual or postmenopausal bleeding. Occasionally this may be profuse, although at the outset symptoms may be those of excessive flow at the time of the normally expected period and some bloody discharge, frequently mucoid, between the flows. After the menopause, irregular bleeding or just spotting may be the primary symptom; as the tumor becomes more extensive and necrotic, there is a constant bloody discharge.

Certain patients are at high risk for the development of endometrial carcinoma. Identifiable risk factors include:

Postmenopausal bleeding, endometrial hyperplasia and/or polyps.

Heavy or irregular bleeding after age 40 years.

Large somatic size (fat or tall).

Prior breast or ovarian carcinoma.

Presence of a state of prolonged unopposed estrogen exposure, endogenous or exogenous.

Management of patients at high risk should embody two basic principles: (1) frequent visits and (2) adequate endometrial sampling. Return office visits two, three, or four times per year should be planned for these patients. Uterine curettage or adequate office endometrial biopsy are recommended. Postsound-

ing aspirations, cytologic examination, and suction curettage are sometimes helpful adjuncts. Exogenous hormone therapy should be discouraged. For patients with severe vasomotor symptoms, continuous unopposed estrogen therapy should be avoided. Acceptable alternatives include cyclic low-dose estrogen, cyclic estrogen-progestin, cyclic estrogen-androgen, or injectable progestin.

Until recently a reliable diagnosis of adenomatous hyperplasia was possible only by dilatation and curettage or endometrial biopsy. The cytologic sample, obtained by placing a uterine sound into the cavity and spreading the adherent material over a glass slide, is frequently unreliable in the diagnosis of hyperplasia. Improved diagnosis may be facilitated by use of the Vabra* aspirator—a sterile, disposable, vacuum curette that permits rapid, routine office histologic screening for endometrial carcinoma and its precursors. The technique is reliable and accurate; investigators report diagnostic correlation ranging from 90% to 100% between aspiration and conventional dilatation and curettage. Obviously, if the aspiration is negative and irregular bleeding continues, it is imperative that undiagnosed endometrial cancer, submucous leiomyomas, endometrial polyps, or other intrauterine pathologic findings be excluded by thorough curettage.

Fractional uterine curettage and microscopic examination of the curettings is the only acceptable method of diagnostic survey in endometrial carcinoma. Although the disease may be suspected by positive results of cytologic examination and even diagnosed by endometrial biopsy, a thorough curettage is mandatory for proper management. It has been customary at the Brigham and Women's Hospital to perform a so-called fractional curettage in these patients. The endocervix is first thoroughly curetted and this tissue placed in a separate fixative. The cervix is then carefully dilated and the uterine cavity is

*Vabra aspirator, Cooper Laboratories, Inc., Wayne, NJ, 07470.

sounded to determine its extent and direction. Following this, the entire endometrial cavity is systematically and thoroughly investigated, and special attention is paid to the uterine cornual areas, since corpus carcinoma may be hidden in these areas. If pyometra is discovered at the time of cervical dilatation, drainage is instituted and the purulent material is cultured. Fractional curettage may be done later, following treatment with an appropriate antibiotic. Accidental perforation of the uterus in elderly women should lead to a suspicion of endometrial carcinoma. Occasionally leiomyomas are so situated that the curet cannot reach the malignant area, but fortunately such cases are rare. At the conclusion of the curettage, polyp forceps or a Kelly clamp should be used since the sharp curet may miss a polyp harboring carcinoma.

It should be emphasized that the size of the uterus is no absolute criterion for the presence or absence of carcinoma. In the average case the uterus is larger when tumor is present, but a well-developed cancer may be found in a small or even atrophic uterus. Tissue removed from the uterus may be screened through a gauze sponge that has been soaked in saline solution, since frequently the fragments of tumor are small and mixed with blood. With such a maneuver the tissue fragments will remain on the sponge and the liquid blood will drain through. If no readily discernible tissue is identified, we routinely fix the entire sponge in Bouin's solution. The fixed tissue is then removed by the pathologist. Although we do not routinely perform frozen section for diagnosis at the time of curettage, this method will obviate a second anesthesia if intracavitary radium therapy is planned. In general, there is an error of about 5% with frozen-section diagnosis, but this error may be reduced practically to zero by the use of rapid semipermanent or permanent sections utilizing polychrome methylene blue stain. If this technique is perfected, diagnosis may be made at the time of the original curettage and immediate therapy carried out. As previously mentioned, the use of endometrial or suction biopsy is advantageous provided carcinoma is found, but it is of no value as negative evidence, since a good-sized area of tumor may be missed. It has been my experience that when nothing but necrotic tissue is obtained, carcinoma of the endometrium is usually present and the patient should be treated accordingly. If hyperplastic endometrium is removed, the operator must decide whether hyperplasia is present alone or is accompanied by carcinoma or whether the hyperplasia is related, especially in the postmenopausal patient, to a tumor of the ovary. If endometrial tissue of any extent is removed in the postmenopausal patient, exclusive of a solitary polyp, the presence of a thecoma or granulosa-thecoma is strongly suspected and immediate hysterectomy may be carried out at this time. It seems unwise to advocate routine hysterectomy in all patients who have postmenopausal bleeding simply on the supposition that since cancer is frequently a cause it is better to operate rather than run the risk of causing metastases by doing a curettage.

The differential diagnosis includes dysfunctional (endocrine) uterine bleeding, submucous leiomyomas of the uterus, carcinoma of the cervix, polyps of the cervix and endometrium, and ovarian tumors. Cancer of the endometrium is exceedingly rare before age 40 years, only 5% of cases occurring prior to that age. Sixteen per cent of endometrial cancers occur before age 50 years. It is imperative, therefore, that curettage be done in all patients between age 35 and 50 years who are suspected of having ovarian dysfunction as the cause of abnormal bleeding. Hormonal therapy administered prior to precise diagnosis may seriously delay early cancer detection.

When excess bleeding or bloody mucoid discharge occurs after the menopause, it indicates that cancer is present somewhere in the genital tract in about 50% of cases.

The postmenopausal patient in whom careful examination and curettage fail to reveal a cause for the bleeding should be followed and, if bleeding recurs, should undergo hysterectomy. A neoplasm of the endometrium, oviduct, or ovary may be present that cannot be demonstrated by other methods. One should never be satisfied, particularly in the postmenopausal patient, to assume that the bleeding is due to a senescent vaginitis or a cervical polyp even if these have been demonstrated. Many postmenopausal patients may have bleeding as a result of overenthusiastic use of various estrogenic preparations given for menopausal symptoms. Hysterectomy is not indicated in such patients, in the absence of carcinoma, since the iatrogenically induced hyperplasia will disappear after the exogenous use of estrogens is discontinued.

A thorough curettage should always precede a pelvic operation, whether it be performed via the vaginal or abdominal route, in order to exclude cancer of the endometrium before proceeding with the definitive procedure. However, if one swipe of the curet produces obvious endometrial carcinoma, further curettage is not necessary and may disseminate tumor cells. Clusters of metastatic tumor cells are frequently seen on the ovarian surface when surgery is deferred for three weeks after curettage and radium treatment. If a diagnosis of carcinoma has been made by prior endometrial biopsy a subsequent curettage is unnecessary, but the endocervix should be adequately sampled. Tissue that is suspicious should be given to the pathologist and an immediate frozen section performed. This is particularly true when vaginal plastic operations or combined procedures such as the Manchester-Fothergill operation are to be performed.

Vaginal cytologic examination may prove to be a valuable aid in diagnosis of early carcinoma of the endometrium, but owing to the rather high incidence of false-negative results vaginal smears should never be relied on as final diagnostic tests. The diagnostic accuracy of cytologic examination may be greatly improved by the use of endometrial suction or endometrial lavage.

The commonest errors in diagnosis of endometrial carcinoma have been summarized as follows by Finn: (1) failure to investigate irregular bleeding in a woman who is still menstruating, (2) correction of only the obvious causes of postmenopausal bleeding, (3) failure to curet when a cervical stenosis is dilated and hematometra is drained, (4) disregard of the significance of perforation in an older woman, (5) reliance on cytologic smears alone to detect endometrial carcinoma, (6) complete reliance on endometrial biopsy to detect endometrial carcinoma, and (7) inadequate curettage.

TREATMENT.—The basic and fundamental treatment of carcinoma of the endometrium is surgical, but various combinations of x-ray therapy and radium have been used as adjunctive measures by most gynecologists throughout the country. Several clinics, however, have continued to utilize surgery alone, whenever this is possible, and report five-year cure rates from 47% to 66%. It is obvious that the cure rate will depend on the clinical stage of the disease, and therefore if a particular clinic is fortunate enough to have most of their patients in stage I or stage II, the cure rate by surgery alone should approach 60% to 70%. With newer techniques of radium and x-ray administration followed by hysterectomy and bilateral salpingo-oophorectomy, five-year salvage rates from 75% to 94% have been reported. In these later series an average of 84% salvage was secured. It is important to realize that, because of the complicating factors of obesity, hypertension, diabetes, and heart disease, death due to causes unrelated to the malignancy will occur in about 15% to 20% of patients. During the years 1955 through 1960 at the Free Hospital for Women nine different treatment methods were utilized in the management of patients with endometrial carcinoma. It is difficult to standardize treatment in a disease of this type, yet is is not adequate to state simply that treatment should be individualized in each patient.

If the diagnosis is made at the time of curettage, the generally accepted plan has been to insert intracavitary radium and to do a total hysterectomy and bilateral salpingo-oophorectomy in approximately three weeks. Beginning in 1945 a so-called modified radical hysterectomy was introduced. This consists of removal of the external iliac, hypogastric, obturator, and periureteral lymph nodes together with the adjacent areolar tissue. The ureters are not usually dissected although if the patient is in good general condition and is not too obese, the ureters may be displaced and a wide parametrial and cervical cuff removed, together with the upper third of the vagina. If the excised lymph nodes contain tumor or if there is extension of tumor to the oviduct, ovaries, outer portion of the myometrium, or uterine serosa, postoperative x-ray therapy is administered.

It has been suggested that if the uterus is small and the contained tumor minute, intracavitary radium need not be administered. It is impossible, however, to know how extensive the tumor is; also, if the uterine cavity is capacious, all parts of it may not receive the same intensity of radiation. This argument may be overcome, to a certain extent, by the use of multiple, small radium tubes together with adequate packing. The presence of submucous myomas will distort the contour of the uterine cavity and will also prevent the full application of radium to the tumor area. Despite these difficulties it is believed that irradiation appreciably decreases the size of the tumor and the uterus, reduces congestion, and probably devitalizes a certain number of cells so that there is less chance of spreading viable tumor cells during operation. Previous studies have indicated that residual carcinoma is found in approximately 50% of uteri at hysterectomy after at least 3,600 mg/hour of radium. With the use of Heyman capsules the incidence of tumor in removed uteri has been reduced to approximately 25%.

A further reduction in the incidence of residual tumor may be obtained by the adjunctive use of progestational steroids with radium. For the last ten years it has been my policy to give medroxyprogesterone acetate

for three weeks prior to surgery, beginning at the time radium is inserted. The following regimen is used: 400 mg intramuscularly daily for seven days (2,800 mg); then 400 mg three times weekly for two weeks (2,400 mg). If the excised specimen shows viable tumor beyond the inner third of the myometrium, medroxyprogesterone acetate is given along with cobalt therapy in the following regimen: 400 mg daily for seven days; then 400 mg three times weekly as long as x-ray therapy is given. Figure 5–41 illustrates the morphologic changes effected by the progestational agent.

Frick and associates at the Presbyterian Hospital in New York published a review of 348 cases of primary adenocarcinoma or adenoacanthoma of the uterine corpus in 1973. Whereas hypertension and cardiovascular disease were present in 25% of patients, diabetes was found in only 8%. It is of interest that a false-negative Papanicolaou smear was obtained in 67% of 193 cases. The five-year survival for stage I adenoacanthomas was 88% compared with 86.1% for stage I, grade 1 adenocarcinomas. Survival rates range from 81.5% in stage Ia to 3.2% in stage IV. Of 48 patients without disease in the specimen, 91.6% survived five years.

Austin and MacMahon reviewed all cases of invasive carcinoma of the uterine corpus admitted to the Free Hospital for Women between 1920 and 1959. Cases of in situ cancer were not included. During this interval 941 patients were classified as having invasive cancer but 180 were excluded because of prior treatment, lack of histological confirmation, mixed tumors, and lack of follow-up. A total of 761 patients were then available for analysis. For the series as a whole, the crude five-year survival rate was 67.3%, and the relative survival ratio was 76.5%. Among patients in stage I, the assignment of nuclear grade appeared to have considerable prognostic value since the survival was 93.3% in well-differentiated nuclear grade 1 tumors, but only 39.8% in grade 4. This differential was maintained in patients not classified in stage I. Clinical and postoperative staging were

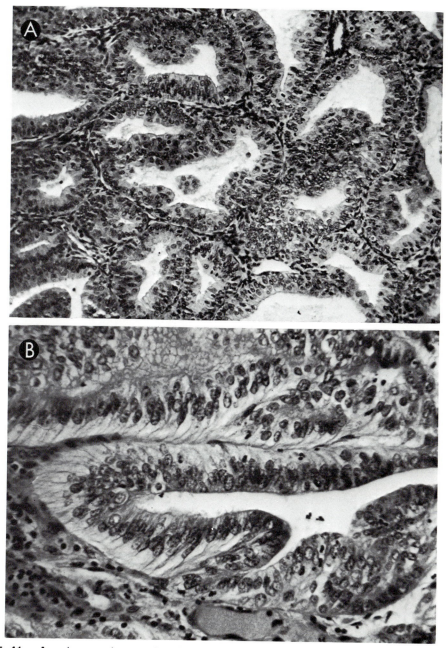

Fig 5–41.—A, adenocarcinoma classified as grade 3 in a 61-year-old patient. **B,** hysterectomy specimen in patient noted in **A** after four days of intrauterine medroxyprogesterone acetate. The glycogen secretion in the glands of the basal endometrium simulates 17-day secretory pattern. (From Kistner R.W., et al.: *Cancer* 18:1563, 1965.)

highly correlated with the probability of survival. Of the 761 patients clinically staged, 86% were in stage I, and 70% remained in stage I after examination of the excised uterus. The five-year survival in this group was 89.9%. Austin and MacMahon noted no significant difference in survival based on uterine size if the enlargement was due to tumor. The five-year survival rate was 94.1% in patients without uterine enlargement due to tumor and 87.4% in patients with enlarged uteri. Involvement of the myometrium was significant only if the tumor invaded deeply, since 91.2% survived five years if only the endometrium was involved and 81.2% survived if deep myometrial involvement was noted. Patients having an adenoacanthoma had slightly better survival rates than those with adenocarcinoma, with 79.8% of 191 patients with adenoacanthoma surviving five years as compared with 75.2% of 570 patients with adenocarcinoma. The crude cumulative survival rate for the 761 patients diminished from 68.8% at five years to 36.5% at 20 years, but the *relative* cumulative survival rate dropped only from 76.5% at five years to 70.8% at 20 years.

It has been shown that patients who do not have residual carcinoma in the cavity of the uterus at the time of hysterectomy have a better prognosis. In certain clinics preoperative external irradiation has been utilized in all patients with operable endometrial carcinoma. This has been found to be a valuable adjunct to surgical treatment in these series, the reported five-year survival rate being 89.6%. Surgery is usually performed approximately six weeks after the conclusion of external x-ray therapy and this combined method has not increased the incidence of postoperative fistulas. Not only has the overall five-year survival rate been increased, but the incidence of recurrences seen in the vagina has been reduced from an average of 15% to less than 1%.

There has been some effort to treat endometrial carcinoma by a radical surgical approach in exactly the same manner in which cervical cancer is treated. The results, however, have not warranted a continuation of this program. Unfortunately, this disease occurs in the later decades when obesity and cardiorenal disease are common. These factors and the number of inoperable cases reduce the total number that can be treated by surgery. Furthermore, several studies have indicated that the operative mortality rate and postoperative morbidity rate preclude the usual radical hysterectomy for this disease.

RECOMMENDATIONS FOR PRIMARY THERAPY.—The primary therapy for operable adenocarcinoma of the endometrium at the Brigham and Women's Hospital is surgery. Radiation therapy may be combined with surgery as an adjunctive modality, depending on the histologic findings and extent of disease. Primary radiotherapy should be reserved for medically inoperable patients, stage IIIb following inadvertent hysterectomy, and for palliation.

Treatment program

1. Medically operable
   a. Apparent stage Ia or Ib with histologic findings uncertain and incomplete information concerning cervix: Examination under anesthesia, fractional dilation and curettage (D&C), insertion of "afterloading" Fletcher-Suit tandem and ovoids with "rush" preparation of final histologic slides. When information concerning histology is available within 24 hours, patient treated as follows, depending on stage and grade of lesion.
   b. Stage Ia G1: Simple hysterectomy followed by postoperative vaginal radium if surgical specimen shows deep invasion (more than one half the depth of the myometrium).
   c. Stage Ia G2–3, Ib G1, 2, or 3: Preoperative intrauterine and intravaginal radium application followed by simple hysterectomy with limited vaginectomy. If deep invasion is demonstrated in specimen or G3 tumor is present, add postoperative whole-

pelvis irradiation. *Alternative management* for large or anaplastic tumors is whole pelvis irradiation plus presurgical radium exposure to uterus and vagina in either order followed by simple hysterectomy with limited vaginectomy.

d. Stage II: Intrauterine and intravaginal radium followed by radical hysterectomy, *or* whole-pelvis irradiation and preoperative intrauterine and intravaginal radium in either order, followed by extended simple hysterectomy with limited vaginectomy.

e. Stage IIIa: Add external irradiation to whole pelvis or postoperative radium exposure, whichever is necessary to complete the full adjunctive radiation program.

f. Stage IIIb: Whole pelvis irradiation with possible parametrial and/or para-aortic boost combined with intrauterine and intravaginal radium, *or* laparotomy with appropriate surgery followed by combined external pelvic irradiation and suitable radium application, *or* presurgical radium exposure followed by laparotomy plus such subsequent pelvic irradiation as indicated by surgical findings.

2. Medically inoperable

a. Stages Ia-b G1–2 intrauterine canal up to 10 cm in depth: Multiple radium applications with tandem and/or Heyman capsules plus ovoids.

b. Stage Ib with intrauterine canal greater than 10 cm and any G; also Ia G3: Combined external pelvic irradiation and intrauterine and intravaginal radium applications to radical dose levels.

c. Stage II: Combined whole-pelvis irradiation and intrauterine and intravaginal radium applications to radical dose levels.

d. Stage III: Combined whole-pelvis ir-

radiation and intrauterine and intravaginal radium applications to radical dose levels.

3. Inadvertent hysterectomy

a. Ia G1: No additional radiation.

b. Ia G2 and Ib G1 and 2 with superficial invasion: Vaginal radium cylinder.

c. G3 and/or deep myometrial invasion in Stage Ia-b: Combined whole-pelvis irradiation and vaginal radium application.

d. Surgical stages II, IIIa, IIIb: Combined whole-pelvis irradiation with appropriate "booster" dose and vaginal radium application.

e. In certain cases, further surgical exploration may be indicated.

4. Perforation of uterus prior to or during treatment

Whole-pelvis irradiation followed by radium application and appropriate surgical procedures. *Immediate* surgery may be imperative, depending on clinical factors such as evidence of intraperitoneal bleeding, "surgical" abdomen, or other factors.

At the Brigham and Women's Hospital radical hysterectomy and pelvic lymphadenectomy is not utilized in the treatment of endometrial cancer unless the cervix is involved. In a series of 78 patients previously treated by this method between 1945 and 1959, ten patients were found to have positive lymph nodes and only two of these survived five years. During the same period of time, however, two operative deaths occurred as a direct result of the radical procedure.

At the Brigham and Women's Hospital the following recommendations for preoperative workup have been made:

1. Fractional curettage. The cervix should be curetted separately before uterine sounding or dilatation. This should be done with a small curette (Duncan or Kevorkian). All diagnostic curettages should be done in this fashion. The endocervical specimen is to be submitted in toto with blood and mucus labeled " endocervical curettings." The patient

is examined under anesthesia by the radio-therapist and gynecologist.

2. Chest roentgenogram.

3. SMA 20 blood analysis.

4. Cystoscopy and proctosigmoidoscopy if the endocervix is involved.

5. Urography and blood chemistries are recommended for clinical indications (e.g., evidence of pelvic or advanced disease).

6. Hysterogram for anatomic details if the patient is to be treated by primary radiotherapy.

When surgery is strictly contraindicated, the patient is usually given two applications of intracavitary radium followed by full x-ray therapy, the external irradiation being administered to four pelvic ports, with the beams angled so that the body of the uterus is in the center of the cross fire. If radium and x-ray are used without surgery it is essential to do a thorough curettage about six months following first treatment to determine the presence of persistent disease. If disease is present, the patient may have become operable either by reduction in size of the pelvic organs or by an improvement of her general condition.

Kottmeier has reported on 1,123 patients treated by primary radiotherapy. The five-year cure rate in 864 patients in stage I was 71%; in 103 patients in stage II it was 44%; in 135 patients in stage III the survival was 19% and in 21 patients in stage IV the five-year salvage was also 19%. The overall five-year cure rate was 61%.

Since 1960 I have treated patients in the inoperable group by adding medroxyprogesterone acetate to the radiation plan. There is evidence, not as yet conclusive, that the progestin may increase the sensitivity of the tumor cell to radiation. This progestin is given in the following regimen: 400 mg intramuscularly daily for seven days beginning at the time of the first radium insertion; then 400 mg is given three times weekly during the next two weeks, giving a total "loading dose" of 5,200 mg during the first three weeks. During the period of x-ray therapy the same progestin is continued in a dose of 400 mg

weekly. If a repeat curettage fails to reveal viable tumor, progestin therapy is discontinued. If tumor remains or if there is evidence of distant metastases, however, the progestin is continued indefinitely in a dose of 400 mg monthly.

Recurrent endometrial carcinoma is found in approximately 15% of all patients treated, the rate of recurrence being directly proportional to the histologic grade of the carcinoma. In patients with undifferentiated cancers the recurrence rate is about five times as high as in those with well-differentiated cancers. The most common sites of recurrence are the remaining pelvic organs, the vagina, the bladder, the ureters, the pelvic lymph nodes, and the pelvic peritoneum. The incidence of recurrence is high during the first three years following initial treatment, but thereafter approximates 1% annually. The curative effect of x-ray or radium irradiation on recurrences has not been encouraging. In specific cases extensive pelvic surgery for solitary, localized recurrences has shown encouraging results, even though the number of patients treated has been small.

Approximately 25% of all carcinomas of the endometrium in metastatic sites will respond to the use of 17α-hydroxyprogesterone caproate (Delalutin) or medroxyprogesterone acetate (Depo-Provera). Dramatic results have occurred in some patients, with complete disappearance of lesions in the vagina, mediastinum, pelvis, and lung parenchyma (Fig 5–42). Biopsy material, when available, has shown increased differentiation of tumor cells together with secretory activity as a result of the progestational agent in those patients with objective remissions. Subjective remissions have occurred in approximately 75% of patients. The exact mode of action of progestational agents in endometrial carcinoma is not known but it is surmised that, because endometrium is a tissue normally under strong progestational control, endometrial carcinoma (and its metastases) may also have such sensitivity. It is important that such patients be treated with rather massive doses of 17α-

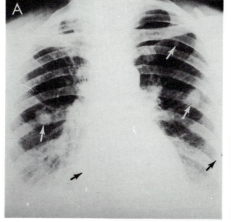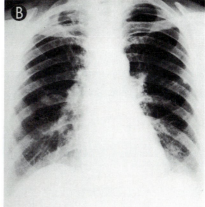

Fig 5–42.—A, roentgenogram of chest in an 82-year-old patient with metastatic foci of endometrial carcinoma in both lung fields. The larger lesions in the midthoracic area are noted by arrows. **B,** roentgenogram showing almost complete resolution of pulmonary metastases. The patient had received between 400 and 700 mg of medroxyprogesterone acetate (Depo-Provera) weekly for three months and during this interval had marked subjective and objective improvement.

hydroxyprogesterone caproate, i.e., from 3 to 7 gm weekly. The steroid substance is without toxic effects, and in some instances remissions have lasted for over six years. Well-differentiated lesions in patients in whom there has been a long hiatus between original treatment and the discovery of the metastases will respond with lower doses, whereas maximum amounts should be given to other patients. The optimum dosage of medroxyprogesterone acetate for endometrial carcinoma seems to be in the range of 400 to 1,000 mg monthly as a maintenance dose. Our results, however, indicate that an original loading dose of 3 to 5 gm given during the first three weeks of therapy is advisable. This may be accomplished by giving 400 mg of medroxyprogesterone acetate daily for seven days, then 400 mg three times weekly for the next two weeks. Therapy should be given for at least six weeks before a decision is reached regarding the presence of an objective response. If a remission is obtained, it should be continued indefinitely and not diminished in amount. We have advised a maintenance dose of 400 mg monthly although several authors have suggested doses in the range of 2 gm per month. In a

few patients receiving progestins, recurring carcinoma has responded to the use of estrogen or an alkylating agent given along with the progestin.

The mechanism of action of progestational agents in effecting remissions has not been precisely defined. There is evidence to favor a local effect as a result of the marked changes brought about by the direct instillation of progestins into a vaginal metastasis or endometrial cavity (see Fig 5–41). It has been suggested that the progestins alter the receptor site in the endometrial cell for estrogen, thus diminishing its potential for growth.

Sarcoma

Sarcoma may occur in the corpus of the uterus and may arise in the muscle tissue, in the connective tissue between the muscle, or in the connective tissue of the endometrium. Further, it may originate per se in leiomyomas. Sarcoma occurs five times as often in the corpus as in the cervix. In general, it constitutes about 3% of all malignant diseases of the uterus. The highest incidence is in the sixth decade, and therefore it may be said to be a disease of the postmenopausal female.

There is always much speculation as to whether the sarcoma has actually arisen in a leiomyoma or in the normal tissues of the uterus, especially when the disease is extensive. Although different authors have a variance of opinion in regard to the percentage of leiomyomas that become sarcomatous, the average has been somewhere between 0.4% and 0.8%. In a series of 5,000 leiomyomas at the Free Hospital for Women the incidence of sarcomatous change was quoted as 0.81%. The variation in incidence is due to a disagreement among pathologists as to the exact criteria for sarcoma. If a leiomyoma is rapidly growing and if the nuclei are rather closely packed together, a mistaken diagnosis of sarcoma may be forthcoming. Various changes of a degenerative nature occur in leiomyomas, and sarcomatous change occurs most often at the center of the tumor. It has been described as having a raw-pork appearance in the early stages when the whorl-like arrangement of the fibers is lost. Eventually the tumor becomes necrotic and softened, with cavities formed by liquefaction of tissue.

A leiomyosarcoma may arise either in a preexisting leiomyoma or in the uterine wall or from muscle or connective tissue in either site. It has recently been suggested that some tumors of this type may actually arise in the muscle and connective tissue of the uterine blood vessels. The gross appearance of a leiomyosarcoma is extremely variable and may be that of a simple, solitary nodule, which cannot be distinguished from an ordinary leiomyoma. Occasionally the tumor may extend through the serosa and be adherent to the omentum and intestines. In other types, growth has occurred beneath the mucosa with actual projection into the endometrial cavity. Grossly, the cut surface of the leiomyosarcoma may be difficult to distinguish from that of an ordinary leiomyoma. Usually, however, when the surface is cut the tumor area bulges above the surrounding tissue, loses its whorl pattern and appears homogeneous in color, with some mixture of pink and gray. Vascularity is prominent and there is no sharp line of demarcation between the tumor and the myometrium.

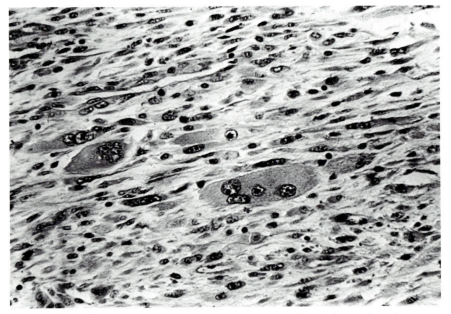

Fig 5–43.—Leiomyosarcoma showing pleomorphism of muscle cells and multinucleated giant cells.

Microscopically, a leiomyosarcoma presents the characteristic spindle, round, or giant cell types (Fig 5–43). In some areas the cells blend with mature muscle cells, and frequently more than one type of tumor cell is present. Prognosis depends on the "mitotic activity," and evidence has shown that when counts exceeded 2,000 mitoses per cubic millimeter of tissue the patients died, whereas they survived when counts were less than 800 per cubic millimeter. Novak pointed out that when mitotic counts were over 30 per high-power field the patient died, and, in general, that low mitotic counts were usually found in sarcomas arising in a leiomyoma.

ENDOMETRIAL STROMAL SARCOMA.—Endometrial stromal sarcoma is a sarcoma which apparently arises from the stromal cell of the endometrium. Grossly, these tumors are polypoid, fleshy masses that arise from the uterine fundus. Invasion of the myometrium often occurs despite the endometrial origin. Microscopically, endometrial stromal sarcomas are made up of spindle-shaped cells with varying amounts of cytoplasm, so that the cells frequently resemble the stromal cells of the proliferative phase of the menstrual cycle (Fig 5–44). In other cases the cytoplasm is abundant and a resemblance to decidual cells is striking. Tumor giant cells are commonly seen since the tumor cells themselves exhibit marked pleomorphism. They may be confused with placental-site giant cells or even foreign-body giant cells. The degree of malignancy of the tumor depends on the number of mitoses identified.

There are no characteristic symptoms, most patients having episodes of irregular bleeding and abdominal or pelvic pain. A mass is frequently palpable and surgery is carried out for this reason.

The only known treatment for endometrial stromal sarcomas is complete hysterectomy and bilateral salpingo-oophorectomy. X-ray therapy has not been of value except for palliation. The prognosis is poor, five-year survival rates being in the range of 14% to 16%.

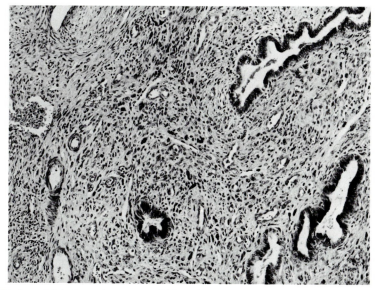

Fig 5–44.—Endometrial stromal sarcoma. This is a well-differentiated tumor showing neoplastic endometrial stroma with whorled pattern, pleomorphism, and giant cells scattered about normal proliferative glands. (From Hertig A.T., Gore H.M.: Tumors of the female sex organs: part 2. Tumors of the vulva, vagina, and uterus, sec. 9, fasc. 33, *Atlas of Tumor Pathology.* Washington, D.C., Armed Forces Institute of Pathology, 1960.)

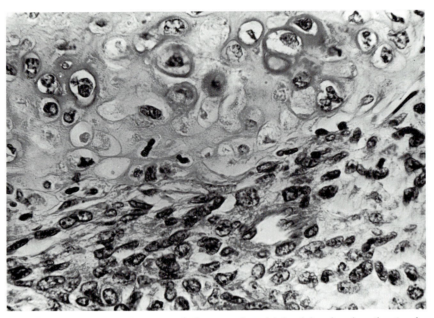

Fig 5–45.—Mixed mesodermal tumor of the endometrium. This is predominantly a sarcoma of endometrial origin showing the tendency of the tumor to form cartilage in this area.

By comparison, five-year survival rates for sarcomas arising in leiomyomas have ranged from 15% to 75%.

MIXED MESODERMAL TUMOR.—The mixed mesodermal tumor is an uncommon tumor of endometrial stromal origin containing both sarcomatous elements of mesenchymal origin and carcinomatous elements of müllerian potential. Some doubt has been cast on the validity of these tumors as a biologic entity and they have been explained as originating: (1) as a "collision" tumor from two independent lesions invading one another; (2) as a "combination" tumor resulting from two blastomatous elements derived from one stem cell, or (3) as a "composition" tumor resulting from blastomatous conversion of stroma and parenchyma. Synonyms for this tumor are carcinosarcoma, combined mesenchymal, sarcoma-carcinoma of the uterus, and the preferred description, *malignant mixed mesodermal tumor.*

Eleven patients with this lesion have been treated at the Free Hospital for Women. All were postmenopausal and five gave a history of artificial induction of menopause by radiation. The uterus is usually enlarged and filled with multiple polypoid masses, which are attached by broad masses to the endometrium. Such masses have been described as having a phalluslike appearance contained in the endometrial cavity. Microscopically, these polypoid masses are made up of intermingled carcinomatous and sarcomatous elements with varying degrees of differentiation. The carcinoma is usually an adenocarcinoma, but occasionally squamous elements may be found. There is frequently a tendency to form thin-walled blood vessels with associated areas of hemorrhage and necrosis. In some tumors, striated muscle fibers, osteoid elements, or cartilage may be identified (Fig 5–45).

The treatment of this lesion is total hysterectomy and bilateral salpingo-oophorectomy followed by x-ray therapy. The value of adjunctive x-ray therapy is unknown, since most patients do not survive two years. Chemotherapeutic agents have not increased the length of survival of patients with this lesion.

BIBLIOGRAPHY

Anatomy and Physiology

Allan F.D.: The embryology of the reproductive system, in Velardo J.T.: *Endocrinology of Reproduction.* New York, Oxford University Press, 1958.

Anson B.J., Curtis A.H.: Anatomy of the female pelvis and perineum, in Curtis A.H. (ed.): *Textbook of Gynecology.* Philadelphia, W.B. Saunders Co., 1946.

Gillman J.: The development of the gonads in man, with a consideration of the role of fetal endocrines and the histogenesis of ovarian tumors, in *Contributions to Embryology*, vol. 32. Washington, D.C., Carnegie Institute, 1948.

Gruenwald P.: The relation of the growing müllerian to the wolffian duct and its importance for the genesis of malformations. *Anat. Rec.* 81:1, 1941.

Gruenwald P.: The development of the sex cords in the gonads of man and mammals. *Am. J. Anat.* 70:359, 1942.

Koff A.K.: Development of the vagina in the human fetus, in *Contributions to Embryology*, vol. 24. Washington, D.C., Carnegie Institute, 1933.

O'Rahilly R.: The embryology and anatomy of the uterus, in Norris H.J., Hertig A.T., Abell M.R. (eds.): *The Uterus*, Int. Acad. Pathol. Monogr. no. 14. Baltimore, Williams & Wilkins Co., 1973.

Menstruation

Amoss M., Guillemin R.: Hypothalamus and anterior pituitary, in Behrman S.J., Kistner R.W. (eds.): *Progress in Infertility*, ed. 2. Boston, Little Brown & Co., 1975.

Barlow J.J., Logan C.M.: Estrogen secretion, biosynthesis and metabolism: Their relationship to the menstrual cycle. *Steroids* 7:309, 1966.

Bartelmez G.W.: Menstruation. *Physiol. Rev.* 17:28, 1937.

Bartelmez G.W.: Factors in the variability of the menstrual cycle. *Anat. Rec.* 115:101, 1953.

Bartelmez G.W.: Premenstrual and menstrual ischemia and the myth of endometrial arteriovenous anastomosis. *Am. J. Anat.* 98:69, 1956.

Bartelmez G.W.: The phases of the menstrual cycle and their interpretation in terms of the pregnancy cycle. *Am. J. Obstet. Gynecol.* 74:931, 1957.

Dignam W.J.: Progestins, in Behrman S.J., Kistner R.W. (eds.): *Progress in Infertility*, ed. 2. Boston, Little Brown & Co., 1975.

Goebelsman U.: Estrogen assay, in Behrman S.J., Kistner R.W. (eds.): *Progress in Infertility*, ed. 2. Boston, Little Brown & Co., 1975.

Gray M.J., Strausfield K.S., Watanabe M., et al.: Aldosterone secretion rates in the normal menstrual cycle. *J. Clin. Endocrinol. Metab.* 28:1269, 1968.

Hamolsky M.: Thyroid factors, in Behrman S.J., Kistner R.W. (eds.): *Progress in Infertility*, ed. 2. Boston, Little Brown & Co., 1975.

Kistner R.W.: The use of progestational agents in obstetrics and gynecology. *Clin. Obstet. Gynecol.* 3:1047, 1960.

Lipsett M.B.: Evaluation of androgen metabolism, in Behrman S.J., Kistner R.W. (eds.): *Progress in Infertility*, ed. 2. Boston, Little Brown & Co., 1975.

Markee J.E.: Menstruation in intra-ocular endometrial transplants in rhesus monkeys, in *Contributions to Embryology*, vol. 28. Washington, D.C., Carnegie Institute, 1939.

Noyes R.W., Hertig A.T., Rock J.: Dating the endometrial biopsy. *Fertil. Steril.* 1:3, 1950.

Ryan K.J.: Biosynthesis and metabolism of ovarian steroids, in Behrman S.J., Kistner R.W. (eds): *Progress in Infertility*, ed. 2. Boston, Little Brown & Co., 1975.

Schneeberg N.C.: Adrenal cortical factors, in Behrman S.J., Kistner R.W. (eds.): *Progress in Infertility*, ed. 2. Boston, Little Brown & Co., 1975.

Selenkow H.A.: Clinical laboratory appraisal of thyroid function, in Behrman S.J., Kistner R.W. (eds.): *Progress in Infertility*, ed. 2. Boston, Little Brown & Co., 1975.

Taymor M.L.: Methods of gonadotropin assay, in Behrman S.J., Kistner R.W. (eds.): *Progress in Infertility*, ed. 2. Boston, Little Brown & Co., 1975.

Ovulation

Gemzell C.A.: The induction of ovulation in the human by human pituitary gonadotropin, in Villee C.A. (ed.): *Control of Ovulation.* New York, Pergamon Press, 1961.

Gemzell C.A., Diczfalusy E., Tillinger K.G.: Clinical effect of human pituitary follicle-stimulating hormone. *J. Clin. Endocrinol. Metab.* 18:1333, 1958.

Gemzell C.A., Roos P., Loeffler F.E.: Follicle stimulating hormone extracted from human pituitary, in Behrman S.J., Kistner R.W. (eds.): *Progress in Infertility*, ed. 2. Boston, Little Brown & Co., 1975.

Greenblatt R.B.: Experimental studies using clomiphene citrate, in Behrman S.J., Kistner R.W. (eds.): *Progress in Infertility*, ed. 2. Boston, Little Brown & Co., 1975.

Greenblatt R.B., et al.: Induction of ovulation with MRL-41. *J.A.M.A.* 178:101, 1961.

Kistner R.W.: Further observations on the effects of clomiphene citrate (Clomid) in anovulatory females. *Am. J. Obstet. Gynecol.* 92:380, 1965.

Kistner R.W.: Induction of ovulation with clomiphene citrate (Clomid). *Obstet. Gynecol. Surv.* 20:873, 1965.

Kistner R.W.: Use of clomiphene citrate, human chorionic gonadotropin, and human menopausal gonadotropin for induction of ovulation in the human female. *Fertil. Steril.* 17:569, 1966.

Kistner R.W.: Induction of ovulation—clinical aspects, in Balin H., Glasser S. (eds.): *Human Reproductive Biology.* Amsterdam, Acta Obstetricia et Gynaecologicia, 1971.

Kistner R.W., Smith O.W.: Observations on the use of a non-steroidal estrogen antagonist: MER-25. *Surg. Forum* 10:725, 1959.

Rock J., et al.: The use of estrogens and gestogens to induce human ovulation. *Fertil. Steril.* 11:303, 1960.

Rogers J.: *Endocrine and Metabolic Aspects of Gynecology.* Philadelphia, W.B. Saunders Co., 1963.

Rogers J., Mitchell G.W. Jr.: The relation of obesity to menstrual disturbances. *N. Engl. J. Med.* 247:53, 1952.

Smith O.W.: Chemical induction of ovulation: Letter to the Journal. *J.A.M.A.* 179:99, 1962.

Smith O.W., Smith G.V., Kistner R.W.: Action of MER-25 and of clomiphene on the human ovary. *J.A.M.A.* 184:878, 1963.

Zarate A., Canales E.S., Jacobs L.S., et al.: Restoration of ovarian function in patients with amenorrhea-galactorrhea syndrome after long-term therapy with L-dopa. *Fertil. Steril.* 24:340, 1973.

Infections

Douglas R.G., Birnbaum S.J.: Intrapartum and puerperal infection. *Clin. Obstet. Gynecol.* 2:693, 1959.

Goodno J.A., Cushner I.M., Molumphy P.E.: Management of infected abortion: An analysis of 342 cases. *Am. J. Obstet. Gynecol.* 85:16, 1963.

Mead P.B., Louria D.B.: Antibiotics in pelvic infections. *Clin. Obstet. Gynecol.* 12:219, 1969.

Mickal A., Sellman A.H.: Management of tubo-ovarian abscess. *Clin. Obstet. Gynecol.* 12:252, 1969.

Neuwirth R.S., Friedman E.A.: Septic abortion: Changing concept of management. *Am. J. Obstet. Gynecol.* 85:24, 1963.

Snaith L.: Chronic pelvic inflammation and infertility. *Clin. Obstet. Gynecol.* 2:862, 1959.

Benign Neoplasms

Benson R.C., Sneeden V.D.: Adenomyosis: A reappraisal of symptomatology. *Am. J. Obstet. Gynecol.* 76:1044, 1958.

Brown A.B., Chamberlain R., Te Linde R.W.: Myomectomy. *Am. J. Obstet. Gynecol.* 71:759, 1956.

Colman H.I., Rosenthal A.H.: Carcinoma developing in areas of adenomyosis. *Obstet. Gynecol.* 14:342, 1959.

Cullen T.S.: *Adenomyoma of the Uterus.* Philadelphia, W.B. Saunders Co., 1908.

Davids A.M.: Management of fibromyomas in infertility and abortion. *Clin. Obstet. Gynecol.* 2:837, 1959.

Emge L.A.: Adenomyosis. *West. J. Surg.* 64:291, 1956.

Finn W.F., Muller P.F.: Abdominal myomectomy: Special reference to subsequent pregnancy and to the re-appearance of fibromyomas of the uterus. *Am. J. Obstet. Gynecol.* 60:109, 1950.

Hertig A.T., Gore H.: Tumors of the female sex organs: part 2. Tumors of the vulva, vagina and uterus, sec. 9, fasc. 33, *Atlas of Tumor Pathology.* Washington, D.C., Armed Forces Institute of Pathology, 1960.

Marcus C.C.: Relationship of adenomyosis uteri to endometrial hyperplasia and endometrial carcinoma. *Am. J. Obstet. Gynecol.* 82:408, 1961.

Novak E.R.: Benign and malignant changes in uterine myomas. *Clin. Obstet. Gynecol.* 1:421, 1958.

Pedowitz P., Felmus L.B., Grayzel D.G.: Hemangiopericytoma of the uterus. *Am. J. Obstet. Gynecol.* 67:549, 1954.

Sehgal N., Haskins A.L.: The mechanism of uterine bleeding in the presence of fibromyomas. *Am. Surg.* 26:21, 1960.

Hyperplasia and Carcinoma

Anderson D.G.: Management of advanced endometrial adenocarcinoma with medroxyprogesterone acetate. *Am. J. Obstet. Gynecol.* 92:87, 1965.

Andrews W.C.: Estrogens in endometrial carcinoma. *Obstet. Gynecol. Surv.* 16:747, 1961.

Andrews W.L., Andrews M.C.: Stein-Leventhal syndrome with associated adenocarcinoma of the endometrium: Report of a case in a 22-year-old woman. *Am. J. Obstet. Gynecol.* 80:632, 1960.

Atkinson W.B., Gall E.A., Gusberg S.B.: Histochemical studies on abormal growth of human endometrium: III. Deposition of glycogen in hyperplasia and adenocarcinoma. *Cancer* 5:138, 1952.

Austin J.H., MacMahon B.: Indicators of prognosis

in carcinoma of the corpus uteri. *Surg. Gynecol. Obstet.* 128:1247, 1969.

Barber K.W. Jr., Dockerty M.B., Pratt J.H.: A clinicopathologic study of surgically treated carcinoma of the endometrium with nodal metastases. *Surg. Gynecol. Obstet.* 115:568, 1962.

Bateman J.C., Carlton H.N., Thibeault J.P.: Chemotherapy for carcinoma of the uterus. *Obstet. Gynecol.* 15:35, 1960.

Blaikley J.B., et al.: Classification and clinical study of carcinoma of the uterus. *Am. J. Obstet. Gynecol.* 75:1286, 1958.

Corscaden J.A., Fertig J.W., Gusberg S.D.: Carcinoma subsequent to the radiotherapeutic menopause. *Am. J. Obstet. Gynecol.* 51:1, 1946.

Cox L.W., Kirkland J.A.: *Effect of Ethynodiol Diacetate on Endometrial Cancer*, Symposium on Recent Advances in Ovarian and Synthetic Steroids. Sydney, Australia, 1964.

Cramer D.W., Cutler S.J.: Incidence and histopathology of malignancies of the female genital organs in the United States. *Am. J. Obstet. Gynecol.* 118:443, 1974.

Cramer D.W., Cutler S.J., Christine B.: Trends in the incidence of endometrial cancer in the United States. *Gynecol. Oncol.* 2:130, 1974.

Dockerty M.B., Lovelady S.B., Foust G.T. Jr.: Carcinoma of corpus uteri in young women. *Am. J. Obstet. Gynecol.* 61:966, 1951.

Dockerty M.B., Mussey E.: Malignant lesions of the uterus associated with estrogen-producing ovarian tumors. *Am. J. Obstet. Gynecol.* 61:147, 1951.

Ehrmann R.L., McKelvey H.A., Hertig A.T.: Secretory behavior of endometrium in tissue culture. *Obstet. Gynecol.* 17:416, 1961.

Finn W.F.: A clinicopathological classification of endometrial carcinoma based upon physical findings, anatomical extent, and histological grade. *Am. J. Obstet. Gynecol.* 62:1, 1951.

Griffiths C.T., et al.: Effect of progestins, estrogens and castration on induced endometrial carcinoma in the rabbit. *Surg. Forum* 14:399, 1963.

Griffiths C.T., Craig J.M., Kistner R.W., et al.: Effect of castration, estrogen, and timed progestins on induced endometrial carcinoma in the rabbit. *Gynecol. Oncol.* 3:259, 1976.

Gusberg S.B.: Precursors of corpus carcinoma: Estrogens and adenomatous hyperplasia. *Am. J. Obstet. Gynecol.* 54:905, 1947.

Gusberg S.B.: Developmental stages of uterine cancer and their diagnostic appraisal. *Clin. Obstet. Gynecol.* 1:559, 1958.

Gusberg S.B.: Standard practices at Sloane Hospital. The management of carcinoma of the corpus. *Bull. Sloane Hosp. Women* 5:53, 1959.

Gusberg S.B., Moore D.D., Martin F.: Precursors of corpus cancer: II. Clinical and pathological study of adenomatous hyperplasia. *Am. J. Obstet. Gynecol.* 68:1472, 1954.

Gusberg S.B., Hall R.E.: Precursors of corpus cancer: III. The appearance of cancer of the endometrium in estrogenically conditioned patients. *Obstet. Gynecol.* 17:397, 1961.

Gusberg S.B., Jones H.C. Jr., Tovell H.M.M.: Selection of treatment for corpus cancer. *Am. J. Obstet. Gynecol.* 80:374, 1960.

Gusberg S.B., Kaplan A.L.: Precursors of corpus cancer: IV. Adenomatous hyperplasia as stage 0 carcinoma of the endometrium. *Am. J. Obstet. Gynecol.* 87:662, 1963.

Hertig A.T., Sommers S.C.: Genesis of endometrial carcinoma: I. Study of prior biopsies. *Cancer* 2:946, 1949.

Hertig A.T., Sommers S.C., Bengloff H.: Genesis of endometrial carcinoma: III. Carcinoma in situ. *Cancer* 2:964, 1949.

Hulka B.S., Fowler W.C. Jr., Kaufman D.G.: Estrogen and endometrial cancer. *Am. J. Obstet. Gynecol.* 137:92, 1980.

Kaufman R.H., Abbott W.P., Wall J.A.: The endometrium before and after wedge resection of the ovaries in the Stein-Leventhal syndrome. *Am. J. Obstet. Gynecol.* 77:1271, 1959.

Kelley R.M., Baker W.H.: Effects of 17-alpha-hydroxy progesterone caproate on metastatic endometrial cancer, in *Conference on Experimental Clinical Cancer Chemotherapy*, monograph no. 9. Bethesda, Md., National Cancer Institute, 1960.

Kennedy B.J.: Progestogen for treatment of advanced endometrial cancer. *J.A.M.A.* 184:758, 1963.

Kistner R.W.: Histological effects of progestins on hyperplasia and carcinoma in situ of the endometrium. *Cancer* 12:1106, 1959.

Kistner R.W.: Treatment of carcinoma in situ of the endometrium. *Clin. Obstet. Gynecol.* 5:1166, 1962.

Kistner R.W.: Carcinoma of the endometrium—a preventable disease? *Am. J. Obstet. Gynecol.* 95:1011, 1966.

Kistner R.W.: *The Effects of Clomiphene Citrate on Endometrial Hyperplasia in the Premenopausal Female*, Proceedings of the Fifth World Congress on Fertility and Sterility, Stockholm, 1966. Amsterdam, Excerpta Medica, no. 81, 1967.

Kistner R.W.: Further observations on the effects of progestational agents on hyperplasia and carcinoma in situ of the endometrium: Symposium on Oral Gestogens and Their Uses in General Medicine and Public Health. *Clin. Trials J.* 5:57, 1968.

Kistner R.W.: Endometrial and cervical cancer, in Stoll B.A. (ed.): *Endocrine Therapy in Malignant Disease.* Philadelphia, W.B. Saunders Co., 1972.

Kistner R.W.: Estrogens and endometrial cancer. *Obstet. Gynecol.* 48:479, 1976.

Kistner R.W., Griffiths C.T.: Use of progestational agents in the management of metastatic carcinoma of the endometrium. *Clin. Obstet. Gynecol.* 11:439, 1968.

Kistner R.W., Griffiths C.T., Craig J.M.: The use of progestational agents in the management of endometrial cancer. *Cancer* 19:1563, 1965.

Kistner R.W.: Treatment of hyperplasia and carcinoma in situ of the endometrium. *Clin. Obstet. Gynecol.* 25:63, 1982.

Kottmeier H.L.: Individualization of therapy in carcinoma of the corpus, in The University of Texas M.D. Anderson Hospital and Tumor Institute: *Cancer of the Uterus and Ovary.* Chicago, Year Book Medical Publishers, Inc., 1969.

Kottmeier H.L.: Carcinoma of the corpus uteri: Diagnosis and therapy. *Am. J. Obstet. Gynecol.* 78:1127, 1959.

Larson J.A.: Estrogens and endometrial carcinoma. *Obstet. Gynecol.* 3:551, 1954.

MacDonald P.C., Siiteri P.K.: The relationship between the extraglandular production of estrone and the occurrence of endometrial neoplasia. *Gynecol. Oncol.* 2:259, 1974.

McKay D.G.: Ovarian cortical stromal hyperplasia, in Meigs J.V., Sturgis S.H. (eds.): *Progress in Gynecology,* vol. 3. New York, Grune & Stratton, Inc., 1957.

McKelvey J.L., Prem K.A.: Adenocarcinoma of the endometrium, in Meigs J.V., Sturgis S.H. (eds.): *Progress in Gynecology,* vol. 3. New York, Grune & Stratton, Inc., 1957.

MacMahon B., Austin J.H.: Association of carcinomas of the breast and corpus uteri. *Cancer* 23:275, 1969.

Meissner W.A., Sommers S.C., Sherman G.: Endometrial hyperplasia, endometrial carcinoma and endometriosis produced experimentally by estrogens. *Cancer* 10:500, 1957.

Miller N.F.: Carcinoma of the endometrium: Some facts, figures and fancies. *Obstet. Gynecol.* 15:579, 1960.

Nolan J.F., Harrison L.A. Jr.: Carcinoma of the endometrium and an evaluation of preoperative radiation therapy. *Obstet. Gynecol.* 17:601, 1961.

Nordqvist R.S.B.: Hormone effects on carcinoma of the human uterine body studied in organ culture: A preliminary report. *Acta Obstet. Gynecol. Scand.* 43:296, 1964.

Novak E.R.: Cancer of uterus. *J.A.M.A.* 135:199, 1947.

Novak E.R.: Relationship of endometrial hyperplasia and adenocarcinoma of the uterine fundus. *J.A.M.A.* 154:217, 1954.

Novak E.R., Yui E.: Relation of endometrial hyperplasia to adenocarcinoma of uterus. *Am. J. Obstet. Gynecol.* 32:674, 1936.

Roxier J.C., Underwood P.B.: Use of progestational agents in endometrial adenocarcinoma. *Obstet. Gynecol.* 44:60, 1974.

Siiteri P.K., Schwarz B.E., MacDonald P.C.: Estrogen receptors and the hypophysis in relation to endometrial and breast cancer. *Gynecol. Oncol.* 2:228, 1974.

Smith D.C., Prentice R., Thompson D.J., et al.: Estrogen and endometrial carcinoma. *N. Engl. J. Med.* 293:1164, 1975.

Sommers S.C., Hertig A.T., Bengloff H.: Genesis of endometrial carcinoma: II. Cases 19–35 years old. *Cancer* 2:957, 1949.

Steiner G.J., Kistner R.W., Craig J.M.: Histological effects of progestins on hyperplasia and carcinoma in situ of the endometrium—further observations. *Metabolism* 14:356, 1965.

Wagner D., Richart R.M., Terner J.Y.: Deoxyribonucleic acid content of presumed precursors of endometrial carcinoma. *Cancer* 20:2067, 1967.

Wentz W.B.: Effect of a progestational agent on endometrial hyperplasia and endometrial cancer. *Obstet. Gynecol.* 24:370, 1964.

Yahia C., Benirschke K., Sturgis S.H.: Carcinoma of the endometrium, in Meigs J.W., Sturgis S.H. (eds.): *Progress in Gynecology,* vol. 4. New York, Grune & Stratton, Inc., 1963.

Ziel H.K., Finkle W.D.: Association of estrone and other estrogens with the development of endometrial carcinoma. *Am. J. Obstet. Gynecol.* 124:735, 1976.

Ziel H.K., Finkle W.D.: Increased risk of endometrial carcinoma among users of conjugated estrogens. *N. Engl. J. Med.* 293:1167, 1975.

Sarcoma

Aaro L.A., Dockerty M.B.: Leiomyosarcoma of the uterus. *Am. J. Obstet. Gynecol.* 77:1187, 1959.

Bell H.G., Edgehill H.: Sarcomas developing in uterine fibroids: Review of literature and presentation of three cases. *Am. J. Surg.* 100:416, 1960.

Radman H.M., Korman W.: Sarcoma of uterus. *Am. J. Obstet. Gynecol.* 78:604, 1959.

Schwartz A.E., Brunschwig A.: Radical panhysterectomy and pelvic node excision for carcinoma of the corpus uteri. *Surg. Gynecol. Obstet.* 105:675, 1957.

Sternberg W.H., Clark W.H., Smith R.C.: Malignant mixed müllerian tumor (mixed mesodermal tumor of the uterus): A study of 21 cases. *Cancer* 7:704, 1954.

CHAPTER SIX

The Oviduct

ANATOMY AND HISTOLOGY

THE OVIDUCTS (fallopian tubes) are paired muscular canals that extend from the uterus to the ovaries, each measuring about 12 cm. Since these structures transport the ova into the uterine cavity they may be considered as ovarian excretory ducts, but, unlike other efferent ducts, the oviduct is not in continuity with the ovary—it is only in apposition with it. Both tubes are covered with peritoneum and lined with mucous membrane and, except for a short intrauterine portion, are enveloped in the free margin of the broad ligament known as the mesosalpinx.

The oviduct emerges from the uterine wall at the junction of the corpus and fundus. The proximal segment arches laterally and posteriorly, adjacent to the lower pole of the ovary, then assumes a tortuous course along the mesovarial border of the ovary to the fimbriated end. At this point the tube is in direct relation to the medial ovarian surface. Normal variations from this description are common, especially if there is a marked uterine retroversion. In disease states such as gonococcal salpingitis, both tubes may be displaced behind the uterus into the posterior cul-de-sac, whereas with adhesions due to a ruptured appendix the oviduct may be displaced laterally and fixed to the lateral pelvic wall or cecum. In endometriosis the fimbriae are usually patent but the rest of the oviduct may be densely adherent to the ovary or to the posterior peritoneum.

Four subdivisions of the oviduct are described (Fig 6–1). (1) The *interstitial* portion is short and begins at the superior angle of the uterine cavity, communicating with the latter by a minute ostium. It extends through the thickness of the myometrium, angulating through the fundus to exit at the uterine cornu just superior to the attachments of the round and utero-ovarian ligaments. (2) The *isthmic* portion is a relatively straight, narrow but thick-walled segment. It gradually increases in luminal diameter and shows a diminution in thickness of the wall as it progresses laterally. (3) The *ampullar* portion is the longest segment of the oviduct. In its normal state it is slightly convoluted and has a relatively thin, dilatable muscular wall. (4) The *infundibular* portion is the terminal portion of the oviduct. It is somewhat trumpet-shaped at its ovarian end and is divided into numerous delicate folds or fimbriae, which give a fringed appearance. One of these folds is prolonged and is attached to the mesosalpinx. Frequently it lies in apposition to the tubal pole of the ovary.

The wall of the oviduct consists of three layers, an external or serous, an intermediate muscular, and an internal mucous layer. The serous covering is an extension of the broad ligament peritoneum and invests the tube completely except for the attachment of the mesosalpinx and the intrauterine portion. Beneath the mesothelial cells of the serosa is a connective tissue layer containing mostly blood vessels and nerves, which intermingle with the subjacent muscular layer. The outer layer of the muscularis is arranged longitudi-

249

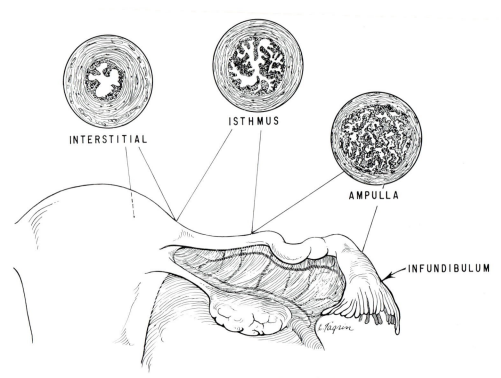

Fig 6–1.—Anatomic divisions of the oviduct.

nally, whereas the inner layer is arranged circularly. The mucous membrane lining presents a characteristic folded, somewhat arborescent pattern, which is most pronounced toward the fimbriated portion (plicae tubariae). These longitudinal folds begin as four duplications of the mucosa in the interstitial portion of the tube enclosing a small lumen. The lumen of the oviduct becomes larger as it approaches the fimbriated portion and thus affords added space for increased mucosal folding. As the ampullary portion of the tube is reached, the plicae are extremely complicated and present numerous reduplications and outpouchings (Fig 6–2). The mucosa is lined with a columnar epithelium containing ciliated and nonciliated or "secretory" cells. Intercalary or "peg" cells are most easily identified in the premenstrual and menstrual period. The endosalpinx, like the endometrium, exhibits a cyclic morphologic variation depending on hormonal stimulation. During the proliferative phase of estrogen stimulation, the epithe-

lium is uniformly tall with prominent ciliated cells and narrow nonciliated cells. During the late secretory phase the ciliated cells are much lower, and the secretory cells are quite prominent, giving a rather uneven surface to the mucosa. During the menstrual phase the epithelium is rather low, since the secretory cells have now been depleted of their cytoplasm. Intercalary cells (Fig 6–3,A) are numerous during the menstrual phase and their appearance at this time suggests that they may merely be remnants of emptied secretory cells. The immediate postmenstrual phase presents a low epithelial surface in the oviduct, but regeneration is rapid during the proliferative phase.

During the postmenopausal period the epithelium is low and flat, the tubal folds become rounded and fibrous and their cilia disappear (Fig 6–3,B and C). The tubal epithelium in patients with endometrial hyperplasia is usually high, with uniform, narrow cells, most of which are ciliated. This

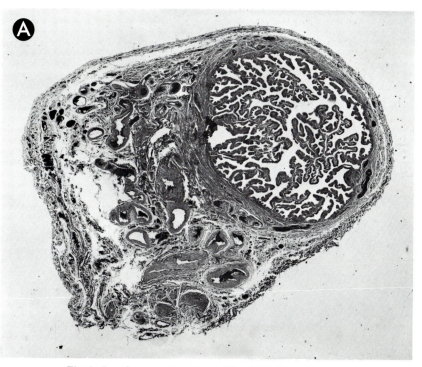

Fig 6–2.—A, normal oviduct. *(Continued)*

represents the effects of persistent estrogen stimulation without the normal cyclic intervention of progesterone. The hormonal effect is even more evident during pregnancy when a decidual reaction in the stromal cells may be extensive.

EMBRYOLOGY

The oviducts are formed by differentiation of the unfused paramesonephric ducts. (The fused portions form the uterus and a significant portion of the vagina.) The paramesonephric (müllerian) ducts arise early in the seventh week, lateral and parallel to the mesonephric duct, by a process of invagination of the coelomic epithelium opposite the cranial end of the mesonephros. The solid portions of the ducts extend caudally through primitive mesenchyme and cross the mesonephric duct anteriorly at the level of the caudal end of the mesonephros.

The most common type of congenital anom-aly of the oviduct is the absence of the ampullary portion (or a rudimentary one), which probably occurs because of torsion and subsequent ischemic atrophy. Supernumerary oviducts are rare, but duplication of the ampullary region and accessory tubal ostia are relatively common. Accessory tubes that arise along the course of the oviduct never communicate with the lumen but the accessory ostia located near the main ostium always do. Unilateral absence of the oviduct is uncommon but when it does occur it is associated with ureteral and renal abnormalities on the involved side. Bilateral tubal absence is rare and is usually associated with uterine and vaginal agenesis. In such cases, there may be normal ovaries that are attached laterally to the free edge of the empty broad ligament. Segmental atresia and persistence of the coiled fetal pattern are rare anomalies but may be seen occasionally when large numbers of laparotomies are done for so-called idiopathic infertility.

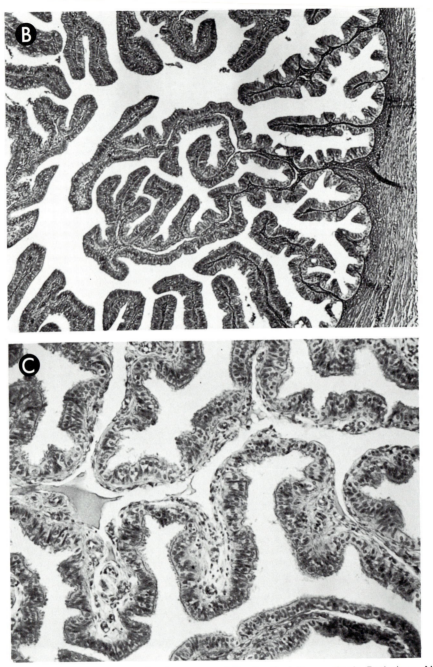

Fig 6–2 (cont.).—B, higher power to show epithelium in proliferative phase. **C,** higher power to show epithelium in secretory phase. (From Hall J.E.: *Applied Gynecologic Pathology.* New York, Appleton-Century-Crofts, Inc., 1963, p. 197.)

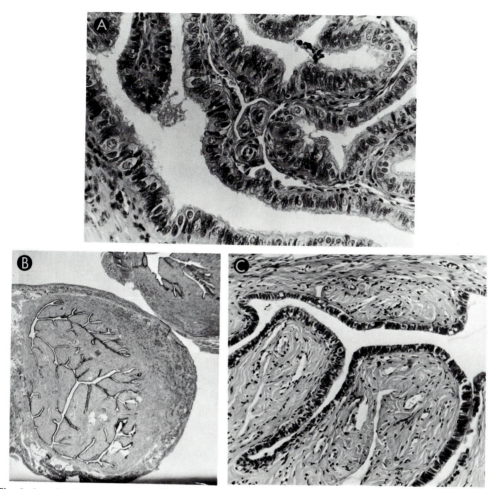

Fig 6–3.—A, high-power magnification of epithelium covering the plicae of the oviduct. The darkly stained "peg" or intercalary cells are easily identified. **B,** cross-section through ampullar portion of a senescent oviduct. The epithelial element is sparse and there is extensive replacement by fibrous connective tissue. **C,** high power of senescent oviduct. The epithelium is flat and cuboidal, the tubal folds are rounded and ciliated cells are not present.

CORRELATION OF STRUCTURE AND FUNCTION

Although it had generally been accepted that the human fallopian tube consisted of two layers of musculature between the serosa and the mucosa, work by Horstmann in 1952 revealed three distinct muscular layers. He described a subperitoneal layer running along the long axis of the tube; a middle or vasomotor layer with fibers paralleling the blood vessels that encircle the tube; and an inner, spirally arranged layer, which takes origin from multicentric areas in the tube. Stange described in detail the muscular arrangement of the fimbriated extremity. He noted that the subperitoneal fibers continue along to the fimbria and extend for greater lengths at the upper and lower tubal edge than on the sides. Thus a mechanism for grasping is accomplished. These fibers are anchored to the subperitoneal blood vessels at the neck of the infundibulum, which in general is extremely well vascularized. The inner muscle layer also ends at the infundibulum with an intertwining of its fibers with the circular fibers of the vascular layer. In effect there is formed a functional sphincter at the fimbriated portion of the tube. Stange further suggested that the muscular component of the paraovarium actually lifts the ovary while the projected tubal frond (muscle attrahens tubae) brings the fimbriated end of the oviduct onto the ovary.

Westman has described the mechanism of ovum pickup in the rabbit and in the monkey. In these animals the fimbriated portion of the oviduct actually embraces the ovary. Decker observed this same phenomenon with the culdoscope and, in addition, described a shortening of the utero-ovarian ligament at this time. Doyle reported similar observations at culdotomy, noting a trumpet-shaped cone of contraction at the fimbriated opening. Both noted that the ovary and fimbriae were brought in close apposition to the uterus in a fossa on the posterior aspect of the broad ligament. Ovum pickup is probably assisted by tubal suction, since a current of fluid within the tube has been demonstrated by von Ott, who recovered a dye from the cervix after placing it into the cul-de-sac, and by Decker, who made a similar observation using starch.

Ovum transport within the oviduct has been extensively studied in animals, but only a few thorough investigations have been accomplished in women. It has been noted in animals that there is a rather striking increase in ciliary activity at the time of ovulation. Such action has also been described in the human oviduct, demonstrating that spermatozoa are dispersed over the luminal surface by to-and-fro action of the cilia. Larger particles (such as the ovum) are permanently in contact with the mucosal cells, a steady movement toward the uterus being effected. An increase in muscular activity has been noted at the ovulatory phase of the menstrual cycle as well as slower, more uniform contractions during the premenstrual phase. These muscular contractions begin at the ampulla and proceed to the isthmus. Further, the frequency of the ampullary contractions is higher than those found in the isthmus. In all probability the action of the cilia provides the primary mechanism for ovum transport within the tube, aided and abetted by the muscular contractions.

It is known from studies of early implantation sites in the human subject that the fertilized ovum resides within the oviduct for approximately three days. The reason for this delay in transit is presently unknown. Although fertilized ova are retained in the ampullary portion of the tube in the rabbit, this is accomplished by a physiologic closure of the isthmus. There is no evidence of a similar mechanism in the human female. Furthermore, administration of estrogen to experimental animals will cause a diminution in the rate of descent of ova so that ovum retention may actually be produced in the absence of an anatomic occlusion of the isthmus. The delay in the oviduct is probably related to maturation of the ovum. Chang demonstrated a definite relation between the age of the ovum and the ability to implant. Thus, if rabbit ova were transferred from the oviduct to the uterus within 24 hours of fertilization, implantation did not occur. After 48 hours a small number of implantations occur, but the majority implanted when transfer was effected after three days.

After ovulation the ovum is surrounded by a mass of cells termed the *cumulus oophorus*. These cells may be made to disintegrate rapidly simply by exposing the freshly ovulated ova to spermatozoa in vitro. The *corona radiata*, however, is not removed by the exposure. There is evidence that complete dispersion of the corona radiata is brought about by some influence within the oviduct. Mansani and Mazzella found that either high hyaluronidase levels or semen merely loosened the cells of the cumulus oophorus, but that either of these combined with extracts of tubal mucosa caused complete denudation. This strongly suggests that a tubal enzyme is necessary for fertilization.

The morphologic variations that occur during the menstrual cycle has been described.

Recent histochemical studies confirmed the earlier work and further demonstrated that periodic acid-Schiff (PAS) reactive material (presumably glycogen) was present in the supranuclear and infranuclear areas of the ciliated cells. The supranuclear material disappears in the early luteal phase, coinciding with increased ciliary activity. Fredricsson has shown large amounts of PAS-reactive material in the tubal lumen in the midluteal phase. He postulated that this may provide the uterus with amylase to digest endometrial glycogen and nourish the newly implanted ovum.

There is evidence that early development of the ovum is greatly influenced by tubal environment. It has been known for years that in rabbits castrated shortly after ovulation the ova were fertilized but displayed degenerative changes after three days. Since the ova were lying free in the tubal lumen during this time, it was reasoned that the degeneration resulted from changed secretions of the tubal mucosa. Similar degeneration may be produced in rabbits by administering 5 μg of estradiol daily, beginning an hour after mating. Such degeneration was coincident with a reduced deposition of mucin in the oviduct. Whereas progesterone increases the thickness of this mucin layer, the effect of estrogen is to reduce it. There is evidence also that the developing ovum is capable of incorporating specific substances elaborated by tubal mucosal cells. It has been demonstrated that a tubal fluid is secreted in the rabbit oviduct and that this fluid contains glucose, phospholipid, and lactic acid. Castration reduces the rate of secretion but administration of estrogen causes a reversion to the precastration level. Progesterone brings about a diminished rate of secretion and during the first three days of pregnancy the secretion rate is diminished by one half.

Present evidence strongly suggests that the oviduct functions in more than just a passive nature and serves as more than a simple conduit for ova and sperm. The changes in tubal morphology and fluid accumulation are ob-

viously under hormonal regulation. The formation and elaboration of specific substances needed for growth and development of the ovum are similarly controlled by estrogen and progesterone.

INFLAMMATION

Surface Extension—Gonorrhea

Gonorrhea affects the oviducts as an infection ascending from the lower genital tract and is usually secondary to an acute infection of Bartholin's gland, the endocervix, or the urethra. This organism has an affinity for glandular epithelium and therefore in its ascent through the female genital tract usually does not involve the squamous epithelium of the vagina or exocervix. Transient endometritis may occur but, because of the recurrent sloughing of the endometrium, the disease process usually extends into the oviduct where its most extensive manifestations occur. The physical force or trauma of intercourse may be sufficient to introduce the organism into the female genital tract and within a rather short period an acute inflammatory process may arise in the tubal epithelium. The initial infection may then extend to the ovary, resulting in an acute perioophoritis followed by a perisalpingitis.

In these earlier stages of the disease process the musculature of the oviduct is usually uninvolved. Grossly, the tube is slightly reddened or glistening with rather marked edema and fine, nonadherent adhesions of the tubal serosa to the ovary. The fimbriated portion of the oviduct may be similarly involved by edema and acute inflammation but the ostium is usually patent. With recurrent infection the tubal plicae adhere and form typical adenomatous spaces, which may, on occasion, be confused with an early malignancy. The microscopic picture, however, is rather typical and has been termed *follicular salpingitis*. Eventually the entire tubal wall becomes involved, with subsequent occlusion of the fimbriated end as repeated exacerbations occur. Secondary bacterial invaders complicate the original gonococcal infection and lead to partial or complete sealing of the isthmus with subsequent retention of pus within the tubal lumen followed by varying degrees of distention.

At this stage the ovary is frequently involved in the total disease so that bilateral pyosalpinges very commonly embrace the ovary in a collective mass, the so-called tubo-ovarian abscess. It is probable that leakage of pus from the partially occluded ostium infects the contiguous ovary, the port of entry being provided by the periodic rupture of follicles. An enlarging ovarian abscess may eventually destroy all the normal ovarian parenchyma. Eventually, in the most advanced cases, the ovary is converted into a mass many times its original size. Further increase in the size of the abscess causes progressive thinning of the fibrous wall, which explains the ease with which these tubo-ovarian abscesses rupture. Similarly, the tube may become enormously distended, with extensive inflammatory involvement of the wall and subsequent ischemia (Fig 6–4). This compromise of the vascular supply results in focal areas of necrosis and ultimate perforation. In long-standing infections the tubo-ovarian abscess may become densely adherent to the bladder, rectosigmoid, or vaginal vault, and perforation of the abscess with evacuation of the contents into these organs may occur. As might be expected, this frequently results in a dramatic relief of symptoms and eventual recovery.

These adnexal abscesses may rupture spontaneously or after trauma. In several cases, rupture has been reported following the use of purgatives, too vigorous bimanual examination, coitus, uterine curettage, and barium enemas. Although the etiologic agent in most cases of pelvic inflammatory diseases is believed to be the gonococcus, this organism is usually not found in cultures taken at the time of surgery for advanced inflammatory disease. As a matter of fact, positive culture results are found in less than 15% of patients with ruptured tubo-ovarian abscesses and generalized peritonitis. While the positive organism of the primary infection is probably the gonococcus, in most cases secondary bacterial invaders are responsible for continued growth of the abscesses as well as the occasionally fatal peritonitis. Nonhemolytic streptococci and *Escherichia coli* have been the organisms most often recovered from the peritoneal fluid and the abscess cavities.

A significant number of cases of acute pelvic inflammation have been noted following the insertion of an intrauterine device. Symptoms usually occur within one week of insertion, and ten deaths have been reported.

Microscopically, the acute phase of the salpingitis is characterized by edema of the plicae, the presence of polymorphonuclear leu-

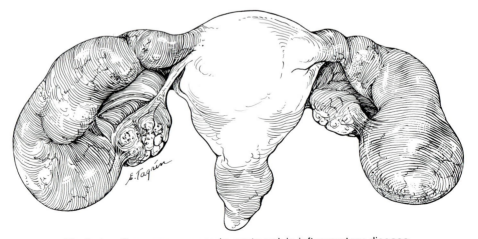

Fig 6–4.—Gross appearance in acute pelvic inflammatory disease.

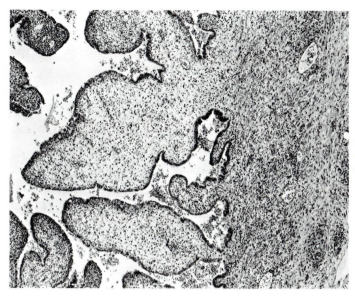

Fig 6–5.—Acute salpingitis. Note edema of tubal plicae and inflammatory exudate. (Courtesy of Dr. J.D. Woodruff.)

kocytes in the stroma of the plicae, leukostasis (stasis of leukocytes within the capillaries), and polymorphonuclear leukocytes in the tubal lumen (Fig 6–5). When the inflammatory process is somewhat more intense there are leukocytic infiltration of the inner muscularis and necrosis of tubal epithelium. Depending on the length of time the tube has been involved in the inflammatory process, extension to the outer muscularis and serosa may be evident. During the acute phase, special stains will reveal bacteria in the tubal lumen, the plical connective tissue, and muscularis.

SYMPTOMATOLOGY.—The commonest symptom of acute salpingitis is that of pelvic pain. Although occasionally this is acute in onset and of a lancinating type, usually it is of a dull, aching variety more commonly described by the patient as discomfort. The pelvic pain may begin on one side with involvement of the opposite side within 24 or 48 hours. Frequently the onset is associated with a sensation of lassitude, occasionally with chills and low-grade fever. The pain frequently occurs in the immediate postmenstrual phase. It is usually exaggerated by intercourse and physical exertion.

Abnormal vaginal bleeding may occur in the form of intermittent staining of dark blood or spotting. Profuse vaginal bleeding is not common, although subsequent menstrual periods may be more profuse than normal if the disease process is protracted.

Involvement of the urethra and Bartholin's glands may result in urinary frequency and dysuria together with an increased vaginal discharge. The latter may also be associated with involvement of the endocervical glands by the offending organism.

The most constant clinical sign is abdominal and pelvic tenderness. Examination of the abdomen reveals tenderness in both lower quadrants on deep palpation. There is usually no rectus muscle rigidity or spasm even in the presence of a rather well-marked pelvic peritonitis. Although the disease process is usually bilateral, abdominal findings may be confined to the side more extensively involved. Pelvic examination may reveal a copious, yellow discharge, and pressure on the urethra will frequently bring forth purulent material from the urethral meatus and the periurethral glands. Speculum examination reveals an acutely inflamed cervix with a profuse exudate from the glandular epithelium. Material should be obtained from the cervix and the periurethral glands and submitted for routine staining and culture in order to identify gram-negative intracellular diplococci. Occasionally there will be an acute bartholinitis, and purulent material expressed from this gland should also be submitted for study.

The most common sign on pelvic examination is that of tenderness elicited on motion of the cervix. The uterus is usually of normal size and consistency but is also tender when manipulation is attempted. Adnexal tenderness is a characteristic finding but it varies in degree, depending on the duration and extent of the inflammatory process and on the pain threshold of the patient. In the early stages of the disease the tenderness may be elicited only on one side and the tube may be felt as a rubbery, cordlike structure with little, if any, fixation. As the disease process becomes more extensive and there is bilateral involvement with edema, the pelvic findings become more characteristic. At this stage, pelvic examination will reveal bilateral, tender, enlarged tubes, which are found fixed in the posterior cul-de-sac.

During the acute phase of the disease and immediately following, there may be a slight elevation in temperature, usually not exceeding 101 F. There may be a moderate leukocytosis and a moderate increase in the erythrocyte sedimentation rate. It has been our custom to rely more on increases in the sedimentation rate since we have seen numerous patients with pelvic inflammatory disease, proved at surgery, who had normal white blood cell and differential cell counts. Similarly, after treatment has been initiated, the course of the disease may be followed by sequential sedimentation rates.

When the disease is more extensive, but still acute or subacute, the pelvic findings may be characteristic. Thus, large tubo-ovarian masses may be palpated either posterior or anterior to the uterus. An intermittent fever of 101 to 102 F may be present, together with rather marked leukocytosis and elevations of the sedimentation rate.

When an adnexal abscess leaks into the peritoneal cavity, a pelvic peritonitis or occasionally a generalized peritonitis results. If the perforation is small, adhesions may form around it and seal off the opening. This episode may be indistinguishable from an acute exacerbation of pelvic inflammatory disease. The patient usually has noted lower abdominal pain, weakness, rectal tenesmus, and diarrhea. Examination reveals pelvic peritonitis with direct and rebound abdominal tenderness, and mild degrees of shock may even be present. On bimanual examination pus may be palpable in the posterior cul-de-sac or masses may be felt anterior or posterior to the uterus. Since these masses may be quite firm they are frequently mistaken for leiomyomas and the abdomen may be opened because of a mistaken diagnosis of "degenerating fibroids." Even in such cases the temperature may be normal but there is usually a moderate tachycardia. The examiner should reconsider carefully the diagnosis of uterine myomas if the history of intermittent pelvic pain and the palpation of tender masses are combined findings.

Massive perforation of an adnexal abscess gives a characteristic clinical picture. The onset is abrupt, with severe lower abdominal pain usually referred to the side of rupture. Within a short time the entire abdomen is involved because of the development of a generalized peritonitis and, especially if the amount of purulent material discharged is excessive, a rapid state of shock ensues. This may be initiated with symptoms of nausea and vomiting and the findings of extreme tachycardia, cold, clammy skin, and hypotension. Abdominal distention secondary to paralytic ileus occurs rather rapidly and the patient appears severely ill or even moribund. Immediately following rupture of the mass the temperature may be normal or even subnormal. Within a matter of hours, however, it rises abruptly and may reach levels of 107° to 108° F. The resulting shock is due to a combination of peritoneal insult and endotoxemia. The hypotension therefore does not respond in full measure to the administration of blood or blood replacements or to corticosteroids. Pelvic examination may be important in that a previously described adnexal mass will no longer be palpable. As a matter of fact, such catastrophes may actually occur within two to three hours of repeated examination. Laboratory aids are of no help diagnostically since the white cell count may be markedly elevated to 30,000/cu mm or more or even depressed to 6,000/cu mm or less. At this stage of the disease the erythrocyte sedimentation rate is of no value in diagnosis.

DIFFERENTIAL DIAGNOSIS.—Pelvic inflammatory disease must be differentiated from ectopic pregnancy, septic abortion associated with an inflammatory process, torsion or rupture of an ovarian cyst, endometriosis, acute appendicitis and other acute inflammatory processes of the small and large intestine such as regional ileitis and diverticulitis.

TREATMENT.—Treatment of acute pelvic inflammatory disease is basically medical, with surgical procedures being reserved for the treatment of complications and sequelae. During the acute phase of the illness, especially if the gonococcus has been isolated, treatment should be supportive and should include bed rest, analgesics, and antipyretics, together with specific antibiotics such as penicillin or the tetracyclines. For uncomplicated gonococcal infection the optimum therapeutic regimen is aqueous procaine penicillin G, 4.8 million units intramuscularly, divided into at least two doses and injected at different sites during one visit. One gram of probenecid is given, by mouth, just before the injection. For patients allergic to penicillin, tetracycline or spectinomycin should be used. For additional details of antigonococcal therapy, see the section entitled "Treatment" in Chapter 2. Coitus should be interdicted, and cultures should be repeated following completion of therapy.

When the disease process has become more extensive and may be termed subacute, the same treatment is indicated, but, in addition, the use of pelvic heat in the way of hot douches and hot sitz baths is advantageous. Since the gonococcus is usually not the offending organism at this time, the use of a broad-spectrum antibiotic such as chlortetracycline is usually more effective, although in certain instances the specific gram-negative organism may be more susceptible to penicillin and streptomycin. It has been our routine to give 10 million units of penicillin daily together with 0.5 gm streptomycin two times daily for five days. The streptomycin is then discontinued to reduce the risk of eighth nerve complications, but the penicillin is continued until the sedimentation rate becomes normal. The antibiotic of choice in *Bacteroides* infections is chloramphenicol, although erythromycin, tetracycline, and lincomycin are also effective. For *Pseudomonas* infections, colistin, polymyxin, or gentamicin may be used. If renal disease complicates the pelvic infection, carbenicillin should be used for *Pseudomonas* and *Proteus* infections.

Large adnexal masses have been noted to decrease considerably during a therapeutic regimen of this type, although the functional integrity of the endosalpinx may never return to its normal state. During this so-called subacute phase of the disease the patient should be kept hospitalized and only minor activities permitted. Pelvic and rectovaginal examination should be done gently every three or four days to determine whether a cul-de-sac abscess has developed. Should one develop, drainage of the abscess by cul-de-sac incision will greatly expedite the recovery rate. When a posterior colpotomy is performed, a split Penrose drain should be placed in the posterior cul-de-sac to prevent premature closure of the incision.

Numerous strains of gonococci have become resistant to penicillin, and therapy has assumed geographic limitations. For example, in California 60% of gonococci are penicillin resistant, whereas in Maine almost all strains are penicillin sensitive. Therefore, the tetracyclines are first choice in many areas of the United States and Asia. Doxycycline (Vibramycin) has been shown to be particularly effective in a regimen of 200 mg to start, followed by 100 mg two times daily for five days. Acute gonococcal urethritis in males is usually cured by a single dose of 300 mg of Vibramycin.

The treatment of ruptured adnexal abscesses is primarily surgical and the urgency and extent of the procedure will depend on the size of the perforation. Similarly, if a lack of response to conservative treatment is evidenced by persistent pelvic pain, fever, tachycardia, leukocytosis, and particularly by elevation of the sedimentation rate, a small perforation with persistent leakage of an adnexal abscess should be suspected. Many of these patients may be managed by drainage of the abscess through a posterior colpotomy together with transfusions of whole blood, intestinal suction, supportive intravenous fluids, and antibiotics. Following recovery from the acute phase, and with improvement of the patient's general condition, hysterectomy and bilateral salpingo-oophorectomy may be performed without unnecessary risk. Failure to operate at this time may be hazardous since subsequent rupture of the abscess will probably occur if the patient is exposed to repeated infections.

Treatment of large ruptures of adnexal abscesses demands immediate and major surgery. It has been shown that the interval between rupture of the abscess and operative treatment is an important factor in prognosis. The lowest mortality rate will obviously be associated when surgery is performed during the first six to 12 hours, and the sooner the better. If the offending organism is not known, penicillin, cephalothin, and colistimethate sodium (Coly-Mycin) should be given; or cephalothin may be combined with gentamicin. If the organism is gram-negative, ampicillin plus kanamycin or gentamicin should be administered. Pedowitz and Felmus reported treatment of 19 patients without a single fatality and attribute their success to the combination of radical surgery, blood transfusions, excellent anesthesia, and antibiotics. They pointed out that these patients do not respond to the usual remedial measures for shock, and recovery may be expected only when the source of contamination has been removed. They advise hysterectomy and bilateral salpingo-oophorectomy provided the technical difficulties are not too great. If it is necessary to do a supracervical hysterectomy, the cervix should be split or coned since drainage through the vagina will result in fewer postoperative complications. In some patients it may be technically easier to open the posterior vaginal wall behind the cervix and lead a rubber drain into the vagina. Surgical procedures for ruptured tubo-ovarian abscesses are difficult technically because of extreme edema, pus, and distortion of structures. In order to prevent damage to the ureter, I usually open the retroperitoneal space bilaterally after dividing and ligating the infundibulopelvic ligaments. Both ureters are dissected free to the level of the uterine vessels. These vessels should be clamped, divided, and ligated with the ureter in direct vision. In order to prevent postoperative hemorrhage due to tissue necrosis, I have taken advantage of the retroperitoneal approach to ligate both hypogastric arteries before beginning the hysterectomy. The mortality rate has been lower when both tubes and ovaries are removed than when residual infected material is allowed to remain. Oophorectomy also eliminates the need for subsequent surgery since, if recovery occurs, the ovary does not function normally and frequently becomes cystic.

The treatment of tubal disease caused by pelvic inflammation is discussed in Chapter 10. There is evidence that mycoplasma infections do indeed greatly influence the possibility of conception, implantation and demise of human embryos. Nonclinical *Mycoplasma* infection may be the causative factor in recurrent vaginitis and cervicitis, chronic cystitis, nonspecific pelvic inflammatory disease, and chronic endosalpingitis leading to tubal pregnancies and pelvic peritonitis.

Mycoplasma organisms, especially the T-strain, are difficult to culture and the transfer from the patient to the culture medium must be prompt. Although most tetracyclines seem to be at least partially effective in treating *Mycoplasma* infections, Horne advises demeclocycline (Declomycin), 300 to 1,200 mg daily, depending on weight, for husband and wife for ten days. Reculture should be done in four to six weeks or at the onset of pregnancy.

In the United States, at all socioeconomic levels, *Chlamydia trachomatis* plays an important role in pelvic inflammatory disease. Recently, the Centers for Disease Control in Atlanta issued new recommendations for treatment based on the increasing incidence of *Chlamydia* infection (Table 6–1).

Puerperal or Postabortal Salpingitis

The usual organisms causing the type of infection known as puerperal or postabortal salpingitis are the anaerobic streptococcus and

TABLE 6–1.—COMBINATION REGIMENS
FOR PELVIC INFLAMMATORY DISEASE*

Hospitalized patients
  Give doxycycline, 100 mg intravenously (IV) twice a day, plus cefoxitin, 2 gm four times a day; continue drugs for at least four days and at least 48 hours after patient's temperature drops; continue doxycycline, 100 mg by mouth twice a day after discharge from the hospital to complete ten to 14 days of therapy
    or
  Give clindamycin, 600 mg IV four times a day, plus gentamicin or tobramycin, 2 mg/kg IV, followed by 1.5 mg/kg IV three times a day for patients with normal renal function; continue drugs IV for at least four days and at least 48 hours after patient defervesces; continue clindamycin, 450 mg by mouth four times a day, after discharge from the hospital to complete ten to 14 days of therapy
    or
  Give doxycycline, 100 mg IV twice a day, plus metronidazole, 1 gm IV twice a day; continue drugs IV for at least four days and at least 48 hours after patient defervesces; then continue both drugs at same dosage orally to complete ten to 14 days of therapy
Ambulatory patients
  Give cefoxitin, 2 gm intramuscularly; amoxicillin, 3 gm by mouth; or aqueous procaine penicillin G, 4.8 million units at two sites—each along with probenecid, 1 gm by mouth—followed by doxycycline, 100 mg by mouth twice a day for ten to 14 days.
  Tetracycline hydrochloride, 500 mg by mouth four times a day is less active against certain anaerobes and requires more frequent dosing—two drawbacks

*From *M.M.W.R.* 31:435, 1982.

the staphylococcus. Occasionally the offending organism may be *E. coli, Clostridium perfringens, Proteus, Bacteroides,* or certain mycoses. These organisms are disseminated through lymphatics or thrombosed venous sinuses as well as by the interstitial tissues of the pelvic supporting structures. Occasionally β-hemolytic streptococcal puerperal infection may spread via the mucosa of the tubes to the peritoneum. Before 1940 the commonest cause of this disease was an infection occurring during the early puerperium, and thus the term *childbed fever* was a common one. During the past two decades this type of salpingitis has occurred most frequently following septic abortion. In the fully developed state, the gross appearance of the uterus and adnexal structures is characteristic. The uterus is softened and subinvoluted and may be focally necrotic and pultaceous. The tubal serosa is similarly involved because of the marked perisalpingitis, so that the peritoneal coverings of the uterus and tubes appear dull and are flecked with areas of thrombosis and subserosal abscesses. The cut surface of the uterus is boggy and gray, resembling certain sarcomas. There may also be multiple small abscess cavities. The vessels and lymphatics of the broad ligament are similarly involved. Microscopically, the endometrium shows a mixture of an acute and chronic process with remnants of placental tissue and decidua. The superficial areas are completely necrotic and colonies of bacteria may be identified in the stroma and in perivascular spaces.

SYMPTOMATOLOGY.—During the acute phase of postabortal salpingitis, symptoms of the acute process will be evident. The patient usually complains of constant or intermittent pelvic pain and irregular vaginal bleeding, which may be dark brown and odorous. Backache, generalized lassitude, and a chilly sensation or frank shaking chills frequently occur. There may be associated dysuria and a history of dyspareunia. The temperature is usually above 101 F and may be as high as 106 or 107 F. If the offending organism is of the gram-negative variety, endotoxemic shock may occur. In this case the pulse will be rapid and thready, the blood pressure hypotensive, and the urinary output minimal. If the abortion has been induced with a paste abortifacient, jaundice of severe degree may be noted. This results from the extravasation of certain soap contents into the generalized circulation with massive intravascular hemolysis. *Clostridium perfringens* may occasionally be introduced into the uterine cavity during the performance of an abortion. Owing to the biochemical characteristics of this organism, gas may form in and around the vagina and cervix, with large submucosal bullae resulting. Cases have actually been reported of massive collections of air and pus (pyophysometra), especially if drainage through the cervix is inadequate. The full syndrome of clostridial sepsis, rare but fatal in 50% to 75% of patients, results from the systemic effects of endotoxins with intravascular hemolysis and renal failure. Early recognition and the presence of gram-positive, club-shaped rods on the clinical specimen are important for cure. Treatment consists of surgical debridement with hysterectomy and bilateral salpingo-oophorectomy. *Clostridium* is susceptible in vitro to penicillin, cephalothin, chloramphenicol, erythromycin, lincomycin, clindamycin, and tetracycline.

Pelvic examination reveals the cervix to be soft and frequently slightly patulous. Blood, seropurulent material, or actual fragments of placental tissue or membranes may be seen protruding through the external cervical os. The uterus is usually subinvoluted and tender and both adnexal areas are acutely tender, with a doughy consistency. The characteristics of the pelvic examination will depend on the extent of the disease, the organism involved, and the temporal relationship to the onset of infection and the type of treatment utilized. Thus, early in the disease process the tube feels edematous and is distinct from the ovary. After a week or ten days, however, the entire lateral aspect of the broad ligament and paracervical areas takes on the characteristics of a soft tissue phlegmon. At this stage of the disease the tissues are firm and characteristically stony hard. It is difficult to distinguish the ovary from the tube.

The differential diagnosis is essentially the same as that noted under gonococcal salpingitis, but the precise diagnosis is usually simplified by the presence of placental tissue or membranes protruding through the cervix. Occasionally the patient will even volunteer the information that an abortion has been done or telltale marks of the tenacula may be seen on the anterior lip of the cervix.

TREATMENT.—Treatment consists in combating the infection with the appropriate antibiotic, supporting normal metabolic processes, correcting shock, and evacuating the uterus at the opportune time. If the patient is not bleeding excessively and her general condition is good, initial therapy consists of either penicillin, streptomycin, chlortetracycline, cephalothin, kanamycin, polymyxin B, or combinations thereof, intravenous fluids and oxytocic drugs. Anemia is corrected by transfusion and when the temperature has returned to normal and evidence of lateral infection has abated, a gentle uterine curettage is performed with extreme care taken not to perforate the wall of the subinvoluted uterus. Antibiotics should not be discontinued too quickly following curettage since residual infection frequently remains in the endometrium and in the perisalpingeal tissue.

Conservative management cannot be continued in the presence of hemorrhage, a lack of response to treatment or massive gram-negative endotoxemia. If bleeding is profuse and does not respond to oxytocic drugs, immediate curettage should be performed despite the presence of parametrial extension of the disease. This curettage must be gentle but thorough and uterine contractility may be improved by the use of a continuous intravenous drip of oxytocin (Pitocin) or methylergonovine maleate (Methergine). At the same time, ampicillin plus kanamycin or gentamicin is given. The latter is effective against all bacteria found in postabortal sepsis except group B streptococci. The uterine cavity should not be packed and, rarely, a hysterectomy may be necessary to control bleeding. Two other approaches have been suggested in an effort to save the uterus and to control uterine bleeding. These are (1) bilateral ligation of the uterine arteries by the vaginal approach and (2) bilateral ligation of the hypogastric arteries via an abdominal transperitoneal route or an extraperitoneal approach through an inguinal incision.

Hysterectomy may be the only procedure that will save a patient with overwhelming gram-negative endotoxemic shock from a persistent uterine focus. It has been suggested that, in such patients, the uterus is merely a "bag of pus" and the only certain method of cure is rapid hysterectomy. The patient must be supported before, during, and after surgery with transfusions of whole blood since there is frequently intravascular hemolysis. Massive doses of antibiotics and potent vasopressor agents should be given to support the blood pressure and maintain cardiac output. In severely ill patients (assuming that renal function is normal) we have utilized combinations of antibiotics as follows: (1) 8 to 12 gm of cephalothin daily, intravenously, plus 5 mg/kg of kanamycin every eight hours intramuscularly; (2) cephalothin plus kanamycin as in (1), plus polymyxin B in a dose of 0.8 to 1.0 mg/kg every eight hours intravenously; (3) penicillin G, 4 million units every four hours, intravenously, plus chloramphenicol, 1 gm every eight hours, intravenously, plus polymyxin B as in (2); (4) ampicillin, 1 to 2 gm every four hours, intravenously.

Tuberculosis

The incidence of pelvic tuberculosis varies considerably with the geographic location being studied and with the type of patient under consideration. Thus, in some areas of Scotland pelvic tuberculosis is discovered in 0.5% to 1.0% of all female hospital admissions. When the incidence of pulmonary tuberculosis in a particular area is above nor-mal, one may expect a high incidence of pelvic tuberculosis, since it is found in approximately 10% of patients with pulmonary disease. The incidence will also be higher in clinics where patients are studied extensively because of infertility. For this reason the Brigham and Women's Hospital, because of the association of the fertility and endocrine clinic, has a greater than normal incidence of pelvic tuberculosis. This increased incidence may be attributed in part to the large number of endometrial biopsies performed on infertile patients. Most patients with pelvic tuberculosis are in the childbearing age group, and the diagnosis in our clinic has often been made as a result of an unexpected finding in endometrium removed by biopsy or at the time of laparotomy for pelvic inflammatory disease.

The pathogenesis of the tuberculous process in the oviduct is usually believed to be via hematogenous spread, although occasional cases have been reported in which the infection is presumed to have been transmitted by the male. In the latter cases no extragenital site was discovered in the female and the male partner was known to have genital tuberculosis. It is believed that the oviduct is the primary site of genital tuberculosis and that subsequent spread is by direct continuity or via lymphatics. The endometrium is usually secondarily involved but is more resistant to extensive development of disease because of cyclic sloughing. The ovary is involved only when there is extensive salpingitis.

We have utilized progestational drugs to create a pseudopregnancy for two to three months in patients with suspected pelvic tuberculosis. This prevents the cyclic shedding of the superficial and intermediate layers of the endometrium, and subsequent endometrial biopsies have shown abundant tubercles when the previous material, obtained during the normal luteal or menstrual phase, gave negative findings. The resultant histologic picture is a most unusual one, since the progestational agent exerts its usual effect on the stroma and an extensive decidual reaction is formed. In addition, the glandular elements proceed through secretion and then begin to regress after approximately six to eight weeks of constant therapy. In some of the biopsies or curettages performed after such a pseudo-pregnancy abundant glandular atypia has been found. This is probably due to the inflammatory reaction set up by the tuberculous process. The routine use of such a procedure could conceivably increase the number of early diagnoses in infertile patients.

Pathology.—The gross findings are extremely variable, depending on the duration and extent of the disease. In early cases the oviducts may appear normal to gross inspection or only a few small, elevated tubercles may be identified on the serosal surface. When the disease is more advanced, the tube is markedly thickened and firm and there are numerous adhesions to adjacent bowel and ovary. At this stage a hysterectomy and bilateral salpingo-oophorectomy may be done under the mistaken diagnosis of postgonococcal inflammatory disease. In later stages the diagnosis is obvious, since the oviduct and ovary are usually involved in a conglomerate mass that is soft, pultaceous, and tortuous with numerous gray nodulations on the surface (Fig 6–6). The lumen of the tube contains caseous material and the peritoneum of the pelvis is usually involved with small white tubercles varying in size from 0.1 to 0.2 cm. The fimbriated portions of the oviduct are usually patent even in the extensive tuberculous process, but the peculiar eversion of the fimbria has an appearance that has been likened to a tobacco pouch.

Microscopically, the tubal mucosa presents a rather typical follicular salpingitis in which the tubercles characteristic of tuberculosis are seen. In addition, when the disease is extensive, areas of caseous necrosis are common. The epithelium may on occasion exert an exuberant growth pattern, resembling the glandular arrangement seen in adenocarcinoma. The tubercles, however, will usually distinguish the process as being nonmalignant.

There are certain conditions that may mimic the microscopic picture seen in tuberculous salpingitis, and it is therefore mandatory that the organism be identified by specific staining techniques and by culture. Culture may be done in tissue removed from the endometrium at the time of curettage, but the number of positive results will be greatly increased if the curettage is done just at or prior to the onset of the menstrual period. Although tuberculous peritonitis is a common complication of tuberculous salpingitis, rupture of the tube is uncommon. Tubal pregnancy in an oviduct showing tuberculous involvement is rare, fewer than 100 cases having been reported. Our study of 197 cases of tuberculous salpingitis at the Boston Hospital for Women during 54 years revealed ectopic pregnancy coexisting in only one patient. During this same period 313 patients were operated on for tubal pregnancy.

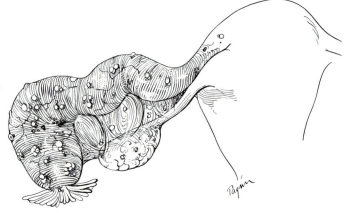

Fig 6–6.—Tuberculosis of oviduct. There is thickening of the serosa with tubercles scattered over the surface.

DIAGNOSIS.—The pelvic examination in women having early tubal tuberculosis is usually completely normal. When the disease process has been present for some time, palpation of the abdomen may reveal a characteristic doughiness, a result of the matting together of the intestines and peritoneum from the tuberculous process. Ascites in young women is highly suggestive of tuberculous peritonitis. Bimanual examination may reveal the tube to be completely normal or slightly thickened. Occasionally large tubo-ovarian masses are present. If the introitus is virginal and bilateral tubo-ovarian masses are discovered, pelvic tuberculosis should be suspected.

To confirm the diagnosis of genital tuberculosis certain bacteriologic, roentgenographic, and histologic examinations are necessary.

The tuberculin test should be performed routinely, except in the presence of fever, pregnancy, influenza, or measles since these conditions produce a temporary false-negative reaction. A positive tuberculin reaction (an area of edema and redness measuring 5 mm or more 48 hours after the injection) signifies only that the patient has been sensitized to the foreign protein of the tubercle bacillus. Therefore if the results are negative, except as just noted, one may be quite certain that the patient does not have pelvic tuberculosis.

An x-ray of the chest should be taken routinely although *active* pulmonary tuberculosis is not frequently associated with pelvic tuberculosis. Endometrial curettage is preferable to endometrial biopsy and should be performed in the immediate premenstrual phase of the cycle. Tissue obtained from the cornual regions is most likely to show tubercles. Endometrial biopsy may be performed, as noted previously, after creating a pseudopregnancy with progestational agents. Tissue removed at curettage should be inoculated into several culture mediums, into a guinea pig, and the rest examined by a direct smear using the Ziehl-Neelsen method. Since it is necessary to wait six or eight weeks before a definite result is obtained from cultures and guinea-pig inoculation, it is important to prepare and examine numerous fragments of tissue by the Ziehl-Neelsen method.

Menstrual discharge has been collected in a plastic cup and submitted to routine culture. Halbrecht reported positive results in almost 90% of patients when menstrual blood was cultured, compared with 63% when an endometrial biopsy specimen was cultured.

Whenever the tubogram reveals evidence of blockage in the course of a sterility workup and the oviducts appear irregular or shaggy with multiple filling defects in the lumen, tuberculosis is suspect. In addition, especially in the disease process that has been present for some time, the oviducts are straight, rigid, and have the appearance of a pipestem. Calcified areas in the tubal lumen, pelvic lymph nodes, or in one or both ovaries may also be visible, and vascularization of the radiopaque material may occur in the uterine and ovarian vessels (Fig 6–7). Endoscopy is not particularly advantageous as a diagnostic adjuvant measure.

TREATMENT.—Schaefer has suggested the following summary of treatment. The optimum treatment for genital tuberculosis combines surgery with preoperative and postoperative use of the antituberculosis drugs. When the patient is over age 40 years, complete removal of the uterus and adnexa serves the best interest of the patient. In selected cases in the younger woman, more conservative surgery may be indicated. Schaefer feels that once a tuberculous lesion has progressed to the stage of caseation, antibiotic therapy will not bring about a cure and such tissue should be completely removed. The radical extirpation of diseased tissue should be preceded by a course of streptomycin and para-aminosalicyclic acid. The dose of streptomycin is 1 gm daily, administered intramuscularly for two weeks, and then 1 gm two times a week for six to eight weeks preoperatively. Para-aminosalicyclic acid is given orally in doses of 12 gm daily in four divided doses. Postoperatively this medication is continued for three to four weeks or even longer, depending on

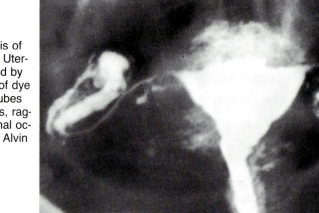

Fig 6–7.—Tuberculosis of endometrium and tubes. Uterine shadow is surrounded by lymphatic extravasation of dye in a fine network. Both tubes have multiple sinus tracts, ragged contours, and terminal occlusion. (Courtesy of Dr. Alvin M. Siegler.)

the presence of active extrapelvic tuberculous lesions. Isoniazid in a dose of 100 mg three times a day may be added to the streptomycin and para-aminosalicyclic acid regimen.

The question of whether to do conservative or radical surgery is, to a certain degree, still unanswered. It has been shown that the effectiveness of streptomycin is in direct proportion to the blood supply of the lesion. Streptomycin produces temporarily excellent results in the earlier type of tuberculosis and in those lesions to which the blood supply is relatively good. Poor results have been obtained in the chronic fibrocaseous type of lesions, which are less vascular. Experiments with radioactive isoniazid, however, indicate that isoniazid and its metabolites diffuse into dense caseous lesions and are actually present there in high concentrations three to five hours after administration. It has also been noted that adnexal masses present before the start of chemotherapy may show no significant alteration at the termination of treatment. In certain cases, however, when unsuspected genital tuberculosis is found to be associated with infertility and no palpable adnexal lesions are present, chemotherapy should be instituted and the patient checked at intervals of three months for persistent activity of disease.

The indications for surgery are: (1) abdominal pain persisting during or recurring after treatment, (2) persistence or development of adnexal masses following treatment, and (3) recurrence of endometrial infection or excessive bleeding following treatment. Sutherland suggests admitting the patient to the hospital for one or two weeks prior to operation at which time a course of streptomycin, para-aminosalicyclic acid, and isoniazid is started. Surgery is timed for the middle of the ovarian cycle and a complete hysterectomy and bilateral salpingo-oophorectomy is performed whenever possible. Sutherland also suggests continuation of therapy for six months after surgery and for one year if the extirpated tissue shows active disease.

The chances of pregnancy and its normal progression to term are better in patients treated for tubal tuberculosis than in patients treated for endometrial tuberculosis. Prior to antibiotic therapy, ectopic pregnancies were frequently reported (from geographic areas where tuberculosis is common) in patients with active or even spontaneously healed tubal tuberculosis. Since the advent of antibiotics there has been an increase in both ectopic and intrauterine pregnancies, but the latter seldom reach term delivery. Before the use of antibiotics intrauterine pregnancies did not occur in patients with endometrial tuberculosis. Use of the newer drugs has brought about a small but appreciable increase in intrauterine pregnancies, although early abortion is still common. Halbrecht and Blinick reported a full-term pregnancy after antibiotic treatment of proved endometrial tuberculosis and noted that four other instances had been reported in the literature up to 1960. In the series of 446 patients treated from 1950 through 1966 at the David Elder Infirmary in Glasgow, Scotland, Sutherland reported 34 pregnancies as having occurred in 23 patients. There were 15 ectopic pregnancies and nine abortions. Ten live babies were delivered, including two to one patient. At the Brigham and Women's Hospital only one full-term delivery has occurred subsequent to treatment, but the incidence of tuberculosis of pelvic organs is only a fraction of that seen in Scotland.

Although there is still considerable disagreement as to whether all three drugs should be used simultaneously or whether a combination of any two is adequate, it is certain that short-term chemotherapy for pelvic tuberculosis is worthless. Schaefer showed evidence of tuberculosis in from 75% to 100% of oviducts removed from patients who had received antimicrobial drugs for two to six months. Therefore, a period of therapy of at least one and probably two years is optimal. Schaefer suggests that all three drugs be used in treating advanced active disease and that the patient be examined every few weeks to note any change in the size of the adnexal masses. Some decrease in size will occur in six to eight weeks. Antimicrobial therapy should be continued for three to four months. Then, if further improvement has not occurred, surgery should be performed. If the patient is over age 40 years, a complete hysterectomy and bilateral salpingo-oophrectomy should be done. In younger women in whom it is desirable to retain childbearing function, or even menstrual function, the extent of the surgery must be governed by the extent of the pathologic findings.

In long-term treatment of minimal tuberculosis Schaefer has indicated a preference for isoniazid combined with streptomycin or para-aminosalicyclic acid, or both. Since some patients will refuse to take streptomycin two times weekly for prolonged periods, they may be continued on the other two preparations. Other patients cannot tolerate para-aminosalicyclic acid and therefore may be carried on a regimen of streptomycin and isoniazid. Although Halbrecht noted healing and cicatrization after antibiotic treatment in 80% of the patients, the end results may show complete obliteration of the oviduct or other changes in the endosalpinx that favor the development of a tubal pregnancy. Ryden has stated that tuberculosis salpingitis produces lasting infertility in the vast majority of patients, particularly when the oviducts have been closed at the beginning of treatment. At the end of one year of therapy a repeat tubogram may be obtained to study the effect of the conservative program. Sutherland has reported the results of 80 patients utilizing the following triple therapy regimen: streptomycin, 1 gm; para-aminosalicyclic acid, 15 gm; and isoniazid, 300 mg, daily for 120 days. Para-aminosalicyclic acid, 12 gm, and isoniazid, 300 mg, daily are then continued for 18 months. Of 69 patients having endometrial infection prior to treatment, 34 (49%) had a persistently negative endometrium following therapy—with an average duration of follow-up of 11 months.

If the diagnosis of genital tuberculosis is made at the time of surgery, and the disease is extensive, a bilateral salpingo-oophorectomy and hysterectomy should be performed and postoperative chemotherapy administered for 12 months or longer. If the uterus and adnexa cannot be removed because of technical difficulties, the abdomen should be closed and a course of chemotherapy be given for three to four months. The disease process may then abate so that complete surgery may be performed.

Physiologic Salpingitis

In the course of routine examination of fallopian tubes removed at the time of hysterectomy at the Brigham and Women's Hospital, numerous cases of salpingitis associated with menstrual endometrium have been encountered. While the inflammatory reaction was of the acute variety and was associated with an infiltration of polymorphonuclear leukocytes, it did not have the precise pathologic appearance of acute salpingitis due to bacterial infection. Nassberg et al. described this inflammatory process in 43 of 69 patients who had hysterectomy and salpingectomy at the time of menstruation. The inflammatory reaction was characterized by polymorphonuclear leukocytes *within* the lumen of the tube (Fig 6–8), in the stroma of the tubal plicae, but only rarely in the muscularis. The plicae showed edema, stasis of leukocytes within their capillaries and dilatation of the lymphatics. The inflammatory process was confined to the mucosal part of the oviduct, and the muscle walls were seldom involved. There was no associated evidence of healed follicular salpingitis as characterized by infiltration of lymphocytes, plasma cells, or fusion of the tips of the plicae. No bacteria were demonstrated and the patients showed no evidence of infection clinically. Since the inflammation was superficial and submucosal and since endometrial debris as well as leukocytes and red blood cell debris were found in the lumina it was suggested that the cause of this reaction was related to the regurgitation of menstrual blood into the oviducts during the menstrual period. Although this inflammatory reaction appears to be quite severe, there is no evidence that residual damage to the tube occurs. Even during the acute phase neither necrosis nor destruction of any portion of the tubal structure is noted.

This same process had been produced by G. V. Smith by the injection of human menstrual discharge into one horn of a rabbit uterus. The histologic picture in this experiment and that seen in the human oviducts at the time of menstruation are practically identical.

Hellman described an acute salpingitis that appeared to be histologically identical with the morphology described by Nassberg. The oviducts studied by Hellman, however, were obtained at the time of sterilization on various days of the puerperium. He found a nonbacterial, inflammatory reaction in approximately 30% of the oviducts removed on the sixth to eighth puerperal day. It was rarely discovered during the first four days postpartum.

Since it has been previously demonstrated that the oviducts are the most sensitive of all the pelvic organs to pain stimuli, it is interesting to note that in Nassberg's series 25% of the patients complained of dysmenorrhea at the time of operation and several of these had had dysmenorrhea during previous menses. These observations suggest the possibility that the pain in certain cases of dysmenorrhea may be initiated by a transient acute physiologic salpingitis.

Nontuberculous Granulomatous Salpingitis

Nontuberculous granulomatous salpingitis is a rather common type of salpingitis, which seems to be increasing in incidence because of the large number of salpingograms performed with iodine-oil preparations. The granulomatous lesion produced by the deposition of this oil in the tubal mucosa may stimulate tuberculosis. The tubercle, however, is atypical, organisms are not identified by proper staining and cultures are negative. Furthermore, caseation necrosis is not seen.

Deposition of talc granules into the peritoneal cavity at the time of surgery may lead to a similar granulomatous salpingitis (Fig 6–9). Apparently the talc granules are ingested by the fimbriated portion of the oviduct and become embedded in the endosalpinx. These are most commonly seen in the fimbriated and ampullary portion of the tube. Certain generalized diseases (such as sarcoid) or fungal infections (such as actinomycosis) may occasionally give rise to a granulomatous salpingitis, which may be confused with that of tuberculosis.

TUBAL ECTOPIC PREGNANCY

Ectopic pregnancy continues to be a major diagnostic problem and is responsible for approximately 2% to 3% of all obstetrically

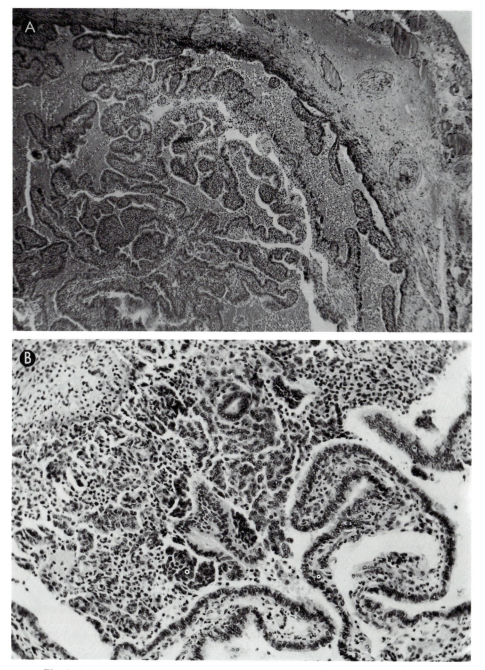

Fig 6–8.—Physiologic salpingitis. **A,** low-power view. **B,** high power to show leukocytes and cellular debris in tubal lumen.

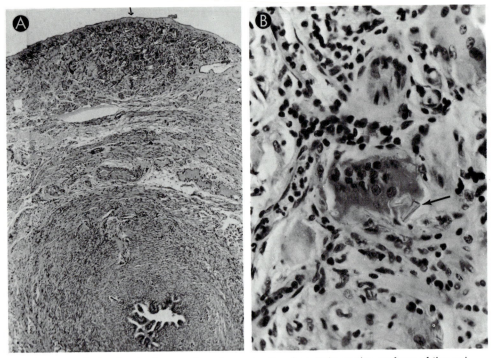

Fig 6–9.—A, foreign-body granulomatous reaction from talc on the surface of the oviduct. **B,** higher power showing a crystal (talc) adjacent to the foreign-body giant cell.

caused maternal deaths in the United States each year. The incidence of ectopic pregnancy is variable, depending on the type of hospital reporting the data. Thus, the incidence has been noted to be 0.6% of all pregnancies at the Charity Hospital of New Orleans, whereas at the Mayo Clinic it is 2.5%. The use of antibiotics and conservative treatment of pelvic inflammation has undoubtedly increased the incidence of tubal gestation. The ages of patients with tubal ectopic pregnancy vary from 15 to 45 years but in most reported series the average age is 30 years.

Diagnosis

PRESENTING SIGNS AND SYMPTOMS.—*Pain.*—Pain is the most common and consistent symptom associated with ectopic pregnancy, but the type is variable depending on the duration of the gestation and the extent of hemorrhage. Most of the patients with ectopic pregnancy complain of cramplike pelvic or lower abdominal pain on the affected side

early in the gestation. This pain may be due to uterine contractions and distention of the tubal serosa.

Lancinating pelvic pain associated with fainting is frequently seen in patients with acute rupture of an ectopic pregnancy, whereas dull, aching pain occurs in those having an organized hematoma around an unruptured ectopic pregnancy. About 10% of the patients have shoulder pain in addition to pelvic pain, an almost certain indication of intraperitoneal spill of blood and diaphragmatic irritation.

Abnormal vaginal bleeding.—A careful, accurate history of the recently menstrual periods is of extreme importance in diagnosis. The exact dates of the previous three bleeding episodes together with the character and duration of flow should be ascertained. Frequently, it will be discovered that the most recent bleeding did not occur at the expected time in the cycle and that it was slightly diminished in amount. In approximately 50% of patients the menstrual history will be normal. Most of these patients, however, will have noted spotting or intermittent slight vaginal bleeding since the last normal menstrual period, and in about 10% of patients the bleeding begins simultaneously with the onset of pain. Profuse bleeding with passage of large clots is not a common symptom unless the patient has associated leiomyomas. Continued diminished bleeding and the absence of large clots is helpful in distinguishing ectopic pregnancy from threatened or incomplete abortion.

Amenorrhea of two or three months' duration may be associated with an ectopic pregnancy occurring in the interstitial portion of the oviduct or in a rudimentary uterine horn, since rupture in these areas is delayed.

Pregnancy signs and symptoms.—Nausea, vomiting, and breast engorgement are not usually seen because of the early termination of the gestation. They may be present in pregnancies occurring in the uterine cornua or interstitial portion of the oviduct.

PHYSICAL EXAMINATION.—*General.*—The condition of the patient may vary from normal to one of extreme shock with pallor, clammy skin, sweating, tachycardia, and hypotension. The majority of patients, however, do not present this typical "textbook" picture, which is associated with acute loss of blood into the peritoneal cavity. An exception to this is seen in rupture of a rudimentary horn or interstitial pregnancy. The intraperitoneal hemorrhage in these patients is massive because of the vascularity of the area and its double blood supply.

Temperature.—A ruptured ectopic pregnancy, even with a large pelvic hematoma, will cause only a slight elevation in temperature. In patients having acute rupture the temperature is frequently found to be subnormal, and it is uncommon to find it exceeding 101 F (38.3 C). This characteristic of the temperature to remain subnormal or only slightly

elevated is a valuable sign in differentiating pelvic inflammatory disease and septic abortion.

Pulse rate.—The pulse rate is characteristically rapid when the ectopic pregnancy has ruptured but otherwise is normal.

Blood pressure.—The blood pressure reflects both the acuteness of the process and the degree of blood loss. In patients with unruptured ectopic pregnancies as well as those with slowly leaking ruptures with hematoma formation, the blood pressure is normal. Systolic pressures below 80 mm Hg are seen in only about 10% of patients.

Abdomen.—Examination of the abdomen usually yields negative findings in patients with an unruptured or locally confined process. There may be lower quadrant tenderness if a large peritubal hematoma has formed. In the presence of massive intraperitoneal bleeding the abdomen is diffusely tender and presents typical muscular rigidity. If the intraperitoneal bleeding is of several days' duration, abdominal distention due to small bowel ileus may be noted. Occasionally a periumbilical blue discoloration is noted in patients with massive intraperitoneal bleeding (Cullen's sign).

Pelvic examination.—Findings are extremely variable, depending on the duration of pregnancy and the amount of intraperitoneal bleeding. The cervix and uterus are usually of normal size and consistency, but manipulation of the cervix causes pelvic pain in most patients if there is leakage of blood or rupture of the tube. In early unruptued tubal pregnancy, the tubal enlargement may be too slight to be detected by bimanual examination and is frequently missed. If the adnexa on the opposite side are normal to palpation, the chances of tubal pregnancy are greater. Since chronic salpingitis is a predisposing factor to the development of ectopic pregnancy, the finding of contralateral disease does not eliminate the possibility.

After tubal abortion or rupture the adnexal

area is exquisitely tender. If the tube has ruptured, it is apt to be less markedly enlarged than when tubal abortion has taken place. Liquid blood in the cul-de-sac produces a doughy or "full" feeling although frequently both adnexal areas will be thought to be normal even when bathed in liquid blood. After the blood has clotted it is easily felt as a soft, somewhat indefinite, tender mass in the cul-de-sac or adnexal region.

The importance of limiting bimanual examinations and observing extreme gentleness in doing this procedure must be emphasized. Examination under anesthesia is frequently desirable since the pain associated with manipulation of the internal genitalia limits the examiner considerably. Shock following a pelvic examination under anesthesia is suggestive of a ruptured ectopic pregnancy but may also occur subsequent to rupture of a tubo-ovarian abscess.

DIAGNOSTIC PROCEDURES.—*Laboratory. Blood examination.*—Determination of the leukocyte count is not of particular assistance. Approximately half of the patients with ectopic pregnancy have a white blood cell count below 10,000/cu mm and in three quarters it is below 15,000/cu mm. A leukocytosis exceeding 20,000/cu mm has been noted in only about 10% of patients, and a persistent leukocytosis of this degree favors a diagnosis of pelvic inflammatory disease. There is an initial leukocytosis immediately following tubal rupture, but this usually returns to normal within 24 hours unless there is recurrent bleeding.

The erythrocyte count and hematocrit reflect the extent of bleeding, but the initial determination is modified by preexisting anemia and the state of hydration. In hospitals having a large indigent population, about 50% of the patients have an erythrocyte count below 3 million per cubic millimeter prior to bleeding from ruptured ectopic pregnancy. Of more importance than the initial count are *sequential* determinations of the hematocrit and erythrocytes. A gradual decrease is frequently associated with persistent leakage of blood into a peritubal hematoma.

In patients with a chronically leaking ectopic pregnancy and gradual absorption of blood, the serum bilirubin and icteric index may be elevated.

Biologic tests for pregnancy.—Biologic tests are negative in approximately half of the patients with ectopic pregnancy. When they are positive (as in tubal rupture or combined intrauterine and extrauterine gestation), they are indicative only of living trophoblastic tissue. The test is of no value in differentiating an intrauterine from an extrauterine pregnancy. These determinations are likely to be negative in patients with tubal abortion, particularly when the symptoms suggest recurring tubal bleeding with hemorrhagic disruption of the villi. A β-subunit test for human chorionic gonadotropin should be obtained if tubal pregnancy is suspected.

Surgical. Examination under anesthesia.—When surgical examination under anesthesia is performed the operating room should be ready for immediate laparotomy. Under anesthesia it is frequently possible to differentiate an early intrauterine pregnancy from an ectopic one by more detailed examination of the cervix, uterus, and adnexa. The well-circumscribed outlines of the corpus luteum or follicular cyst are usually readily distinguished from the indefinite mass formed by the distended tube and adjacent hematoma. In many patients the localized enlargement of the oviduct may be delineated from the ovary even before rupture. In early tubal pregnancy, however, more precise diagnostic methods such as culdocentesis, posterior colpotomy, culdoscopy, or laparoscopy are necessary.

Culdocentesis.—Culdocentesis is of particular value if the cul-de-sac is bulging. It may be done without general anesthesia, using a long 15- to 18-gauge needle on a 10- or 20-ml syringe. A dry tap is unusual and should warrant another attempt. The fluid obtained may suggest: (1) if clear, serous, and straw-colored—a normal, negative pelvis; (2) if turbid but serous—pelvic inflammatory disease; (3) if blood-tinged and serous—ruptured ovarian cysts, ovulation bleeding or, occasionally, pelvic inflammatory disease; (4) if bright red and grossly bloody—recently bleeding corpus luteum, recently ruptured ectopic pregnancy with fresh bleeding, or a traumatic cul-de-sac aspiration; (5) if *old blood, brownish-colored*—ectopic pregnancy with intraperitoneal bleeding over a few days or weeks. *Blood does not clot*, or at times tiny clots may be aspirated.

Posterior colpotomy.—Colpotomy is safer than culdocentesis in patients without definite bulging of the cul-de-sac. If tubal abortion or rupture with intraperitoneal bleeding has occurred, usually sufficient blood is in the cul-de-sac to make it apparent as soon as the peritoneum is opened. When the vagina is roomy and the uterus is retroverted, visualization of the adnexa is easily accomplished. In other patients, with chronic salpingitis or previous pelvic surgery, adequate visualization is difficult or impossible. Endoscopy is preferable in such cases.

Endoscopy.—Culdoscopy requires considerable experience and technical skill on the part of the operator but it is of extreme value in differentiating a corpus luteum or follicular cyst from an unruptured tubal pregnancy. If an organized blood clot is present in the cul-de-sac, culdocentesis may be negative, whereas the culdoscope will usually traverse the clot and the diagnosis can be made. If visualization by culdoscopy is not adequate, the incision may be extended and posterior colpotomy performed. If there is a large pelvic mass or obliteration of the cul-de-sac from endometriosis or inflammatory disease, culdoscopy is neither indicated nor advantageous. Moreover, injudicious attempts to introduce the trocar in such patients may result in damage to the rectosigmoid or small bowel. Laparoscopy is the optimum diagnostic procedure in patients with a suspected unruptured ectopic pregnancy. Ultrasonography is frequently of value in differentiating an intrauterine pregnancy from an unruptured tubal gestation.

Uterine curettage.—If chorionic tissue is found either grossly or microscopically, the presence of an intrauterine pregnancy is obvious. The rare combination of intrauterine and extrauterine pregnancy, however, is still a possibility. If the curettings show only decidua, a diagnosis of ectopic pregnancy must be considered. It is possible, however, to curet a pregnant uterus and miss the ovum so that only decidual tissue is obtained. Similarly, a decidual reaction in the endometrial stroma may be brought about by a corpus luteum cyst, a luteinized follicular cyst, or granulosa cell tumor, or by the administration of potent synthetic progestational agents.

In general, it may be concluded that when decidua without chorionic tissue is found by curettage, there is a good possibility of an ectopic pregnancy, but the absence of decidua does not exclude tubal pregnancy, especially if the bleeding is of several weeks' duration. The endometrium in such patients may be secretory, proliferative, or menstrual.

Specific morphologic changes in the epithelium of the endometrium have been described in association with either intrauterine or extrauterine pregnancy. This *Arias-Stella* reaction has been called an anaplasia of pregnancy and, if found, should alert the clinician to the possibility of an ectopic pregnancy. This morphologic pattern has not been described in the endometrium of patients receiving synthetic progestational agents for pseudopregnancy.

Since the findings from curettage are equivocal in so many patients and since a normal intrauterine pregnancy may be interrupted, this procedure is not advised as a routine diagnostic procedure.

TREATMENT.—The optimum treatment for ectopic pregnancy is surgical removal. This should be performed as rapidly as possible after diagnosis has been made, and supportive therapy, if necessary, should be administered in the operating room. Expectant treatment of ectopic pregnancy is extremely hazardous since the gestational sac and adjacent oviduct may rupture without warning and the patient may die from massive hemorrhage. Despite inconvenience, it has been advised that "the sun never set on a possible ectopic pregnancy." Transfusions of whole blood should be given to patients who are in shock, the patient transferred to the operating room as soon as possible and transfusion continued throughout the procedure.

The management of ectopic pregnancy demands that hemorrhage be prevented or arrested. Therefore, treatment usually consists of excision of the involved tube. If the patient has been in shock or if there is massive intraperitoneal hemorrhage, operation should be limited to removal of the ectopic pregnancy and control of hemorrhage. In many patients who are operated on for ectopic pregnancy and whose condition is good, a hysterectomy may be indicated. This is true if one oviduct has been previously removed and the present ectopic pregnancy is in a part of the tube that cannot be salvaged. Since the development of in vitro fertilization, hysterectomy is usually not performed. An ovarian malignancy or an extensive inflammatory process involving the opposite tube is an adequate indication for hysterectomy at the time of surgery.

When the ectopic gestation involves the fimbriated portion of the tube or even the ampulla (Fig 6–10), and particularly if a patient has been infertile, conservative procedures may help preserve the childbearing potential. Both lateral incisions of the tubes and salpingostomy have been suggested as methods of tubal preservation (Figs 6–11 and 6–12). After such a procedure the patient must be observed closely since the risk of repeat ectopic pregnancy is increased, both in the repaired and in the opposite tube, especially if follicular salpingitis is present.

Other ancillary surgical procedures may be performed without increasing morbidity if the patient's general condition is good and if massive intraperitoneal hemorrhage has not occurred. Appendectomy has been performed in many patients in this group and abdominal myomectomy has been carried out in a few nulliparous patients desirous of having children. Several studies have indicated that a patient who has an ectopic pregnancy has an increased potential for a second ectopic pregnancy, the incidence ranging from 5% to 11%. It is important in performing a salpingectomy that the interstitial portion of the tube be removed to prevent implantation of a subsequent gestation in this particular area.

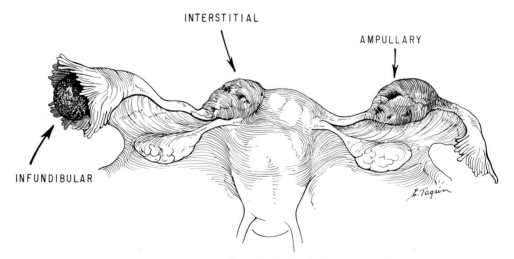

INTERSTITIAL

AMPULLARY

INFUNDIBULAR

Fig 6–10.—Anatomic sites of tubal ectopic pregnancies.

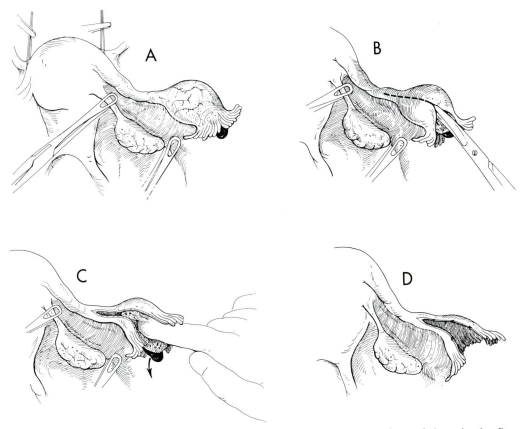

Fig 6–11.—Operative approach to distal tubal pregnancy. **A,** distal tubal pregnancy showing dilatation and protrusion of blood clot from the fimbriae. **B,** the tube is incised with a fine scissors along the antimesenteric border to a point well above the distended portion. **C,** the blood clot, sac, and placental elements are gently "teased" from the mucosal surface of the tube by finger dissection or by a pledget of gauze placed over the finger. **D,** the linear salpingostomy is left open. Closure may result in a localized hematoma or subsequent phimosis. (From Patton G.W., Kistner R.W.: *Atlas of Infertility Surgery,* ed. 2. Boston, Little Brown & Co., 1984.)

Fertility After Ectopic Pregnancy

There is no doubt that the occurrence of an ectopic pregnancy is a major accident for a patient who wishes subsequently to become pregnant. It has been estimated that only about one third of such patients will ever succeed in delivering a living child. More than one third will become pregnant but many will lose the gestation either by miscarriage or by recurrent ectopic pregnancy. It has been estimated that such patients are seven to eight times more likely to have a subsequent misplaced pregnancy than are women who have not had ectopic gestations. It is imperative

therefore that every patient who undergoes surgery for an ectopic gestation be left with a normally patent residual tube. When infertility follows an operation for ectopic pregnancy, the possibility arises that the infertility is due to damage of the residual tube as a result of the surgical procedure itself. Grant suggests that the remaining tube is iatrogenically damaged by residual blood or subsequent infection in the peritoneal cavity in almost 50% of cases.

To avoid this difficulty, Grant suggested the following principles: (1) early operation, (2) removal of the blood clot and the free

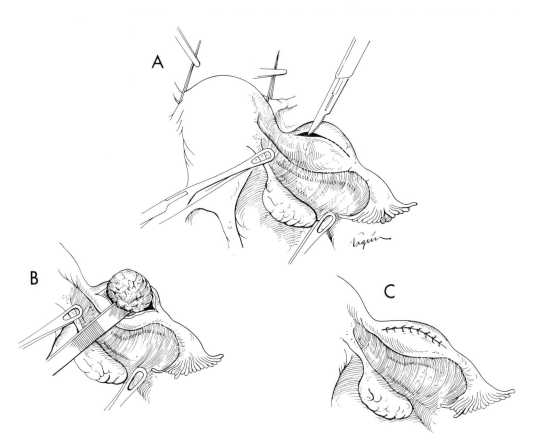

Fig 6–12.—Operative approach to midsegment tubal pregnancy. **A,** unruptured pregnancy is shown in midsegment. A linear incision is made along the antimesenteric border and is carried slightly beyond the area of dilatation. **B,** the knife handle is used to free and displace the ovisac and placenta from their attachments to the tubal mucosa. **C,** after hemostasis is secured, the incision is closed with interrupted sutures of 6–0 polyglycolic acid (Dexon). (From Patton G.W., Kistner R.W.: *Atlas of Infertility Surgery,* ed. 2. Boston, Little Brown & Co., 1984.)

blood from the peritoneal cavity, (3) conservation of the residual tube, and (4) a patency test of the residual tube within a few weeks of operation. Grant emphasized the importance of removing the numerous blood clots and free blood from the peritoneal cavity since he feels that this may reduce the incidence of later adhesions. Furthermore, it is suggested that a broad-spectrum antibiotic be administered routinely after surgery for a ruptured ectopic pregnancy. Grant also emphasized the importance of testing the residual tube for patency within one month of the operation. If it is found to be blocked, some nonsurgical therapy for tubal blockage may be instituted.

Thus, repeated insufflations with carbon dioxide even at pressures exceeding 200 mm Hg may be desirable. Hydrotubation with a solution of cortisone and antibiotics has been utilized successfully in a large number of patients. Timonen and Nieminen reported subsequent pregnancy in about 50% of patients undergoing radical or conservative surgery for tubal pregnancy. Term pregnancies occurred in over half of the patients in both groups, and recurrent ectopic pregnancy was noted in 11.5% after radical surgery, compared with 15.7% following conservative surgery. These results are similar to the collected data of Grant who recorded a 43%

postoperative pregnancy rate, with 22% term and 9% recurrent ectopic pregnancies.

Tubal plastic surgery for a tubal pregnancy is justified only when the opposite tube is absent or blocked. With our presently available techniques it is probable that tubal plastic surgery at the time of an ectopic pregnancy in a single residual tube is of greater psychologic than reproductive benefit to the patient. The pregnancy salvage is approximately 25%, with a high recurrence rate of ectopic pregnancy. If the pregnancy is in the proximal half of the oviduct it seems advisable to excise the affected area and to reimplant the normal portion of the tube at a later date. Immediate tubal implantation into the uterus at the time of operation for ectopic pregnancy is time-consuming and not advised. Conservative operations in selected cases of tubal pregnancy seem feasible and safe and do not further impair tubal function.

It has been suggested that removal of the ovary on the side of the ruptured ectopic pregnancy at the time of salpingectomy results in a 12% increase in the subsequent pregnancy rate. Although the placement of the remaining patent tube immediately adjacent to the only source of ova seems logical, it may occasionally result in a protest from the patient. It has not been our routine to remove the ovary on the side of the ectopic pregnancy unless that ovary is abnormal. In certain patients it may be a desirable procedure. Bender published a series in which postoperative pregnancy occurred in 58% of patients undergoing salpingo-oophorectomy, compared with 42% following salpingectomy alone. Douglas also noted an increased pregnancy rate, 53.5%, following salpingo-oophorectomy, compared with 42.3% after salpingectomy. The term pregnancy rate, however, was not statistically different. A series by Franklin revealed equal fertility following these two procedures, but increased recurrent ectopic pregnancy in the salpingo-oophorectomy group. This is probably due to the greater incidence of pelvic infection in patients having salpingo-oophorectomy.

Combined Intrauterine and Extrauterine Pregnancies

The diagnosis of combined pregnancy should be considered if the patient gives a history of ectopic pregnancy or has unilateral lower abdominal tenderness with concomitant evidence of an intrauterine pregnancy. If the uterus is enlarged, the cervix closed, and there is minimal vaginal bleeding the physician should always be suspicious of this combination. The persistence of lower abdominal pain following spontaneous abortion of an early uterine pregnancy should suggest that an ectopic pregnancy may coexist. Sonographic examination will usually show both intrauterine and extrauterine pregnancies. The treatment for combined pregnancy should be a laparotomy with removal of the extrauterine pregnancy. Postoperative attention should be directed toward the preservation of the intrauterine gestation. Routine curettage in extrauterine pregnancy is not advised because of the possibility of interruption of an intrauterine pregnancy.

SALPINGITIS ISTHMICA NODOSA

Salpingitis isthmica nodosa is a disease process of unknown etiology, characterized by nodular thickenings in the intramural and isthmic portions of the oviduct. Microscopically, the nodules are noted to be in the muscular wall of the tube and to contain nests of glandlike tissue. Frequently the lumina of these glands are connected to the central tubal lumen. This disease process is also known variously as diverticulosis adenomyosis of the tube, adenosalpingitis, and endosalpingiosis. The incidence is variable and depends on the detailed examination of the pathologist and on the number of microscopic sections taken through this portion of the oviduct. The disease occurs most commonly between the ages of 25 and 50 years, with an average age of 35 years. It is more common among blacks than among the white population.

The pathogenesis of this disease is controversial but several theories have been advanced as to its origin. The most commonly accepted suggests that this disease is the sequel of inflammation either of gonorrheal or of tuberculous type. The support for the inflammatory origin is provided chiefly by the fact that associated inflammation is found in 75% to 80% of cases. Bilateral lesions are also quite common. Finally, certain patients who had grossly normal oviducts at the time of laparotomy later were found, following an attack of gonorrhea, to have typical salpingitis isthmica nodosa. It has been suggested that the islands of glandular tissue are formed as a result of an extension of the mucosa during the acute inflammatory process. Thus, minute intraluminal abscesses may rupture or dissect into the softened muscularis. This process is abetted by the absence of a typical muscularis mucosa in the oviduct. Some time later these fragments of displaced epithelium form glandlike spaces, which subsequently undergo proliferation and set up an irritative process. Hypertrophy and hyperplasia of the muscle fibers result.

In several reports of patients with salpingitis isthmica nodosa, fewer than 50% had an associated inflammatory process. In such patients the lesion was thought to be of noninflammatory origin, and it was suggested that the process arose from a proliferation or hyperplasia of the epithelial lining cells of the isthmus or possibly by a contiguous spread of uterine adenomyosis.

The congenital origin of salpingitis isthmica nodosa was championed by numerous authors at the turn of the century but many discrepancies in this theory of histogenesis have been noted. In the first place, the condition has been found only in the adult female and not in the fetus. Second, the connections between the glandlike spaces and the tubal lumen have definitely been demonstrated, proving that they are diverticula. Third, the condition has been shown to be present only where there is evidence of a chronic inflammatory process. The German pathologist Robert Meyer also denied the congenital origin of this disease after he had examined 100 uteri from all ages of fetal development. He found adenomatous structures of this variety to be rare in the fetus, whereas in adults glandular proliferation in the oviducts occurred rather frequently.

The gross appearance of salpingitis isthmica nodosa (Fig 6–13) is usually characteristic. The lesions are bilateral in about 35% of patients. Usually the nodules are multiple and irregularly distributed, presenting a somewhat beaded appearance. The nodules vary in size from a few millimeters to 2.5 cm in diameter and frequently are sharply circumscribed, firm, irregular but with a smooth surface. The mucosa and the serosa are generally smooth and essentially normal. On cut surface the nodules are seen to be white or brownish yellow, generally solid but occasionally with a central lumen.

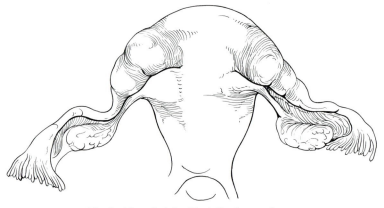

Fig 6–13.—Salpingitis isthmica nodosa.

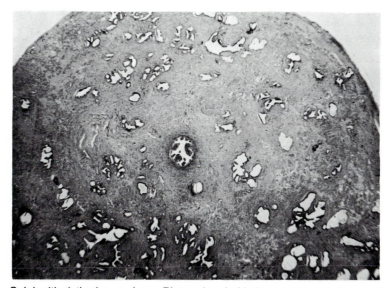

Fig 6–14.—Salpingitis isthmica nodosa. Photomicrograph shows multiple islands of epithelium in tubal isthmus. The tubal lumen is evident in the center of the section.

The microscopic appearance of salpingitis isthmica nodosa (Fig 6–14) is variable, depending on the duration of the lesion. In its earliest form there is a simple outpocketing of the tubal mucosa into the musculature. In its fully developed state, glandlike spaces are scattered throughout the myosalpinx and are associated with hyperplasia and hypertrophy of the muscle fibers. The spaces are extremely variable in size and shape and some appear cystically dilated. The epithelial connection with the tubal lumen may or may not be apparent. The epithelium is usually cuboidal or columnar, of one cell-layer thickness, with cells typical of those ordinarily seen in the normal oviduct. In cystically dilated glands there is flattening of the epithelium, whereas in the smaller glandular spaces the epithelium is a mixture of that seen in the tube and endometrium. The epithelium usually does not show the cyclic changes seen in the endometrium, but on occasion certain glands may simulate the secretory phase of the endometrial epithelium. There is a surrounding stroma of collagenous fibrous connective tissue, which is usually infiltrated with plasma cells, leukocytes, or eosinophils. In certain cases the stroma may closely resemble the stroma of the endometrium. In adjacent areas there may be evidence of a chronic salpingitis.

DIAGNOSIS.—The diagnosis of salpingitis isthmica nodosa is usually made at the time of laparotomy for infertility or pelvic inflammatory disease. With the use of the laparoscope, however, this diagnosis has been made in a large number of patients in our clinic prior to definitive surgery. In 1951, Bunster demonstrated that this lesion, which he called tubal diverticulosis, could be diagnosed by means of salpingography and he published hystero-salpingograms revealing such diverticula. Siegler, in 1955, was able to diagnose tubal diverticulosis in 1.6% of 1,160 hysterosalpin-gograms performed on patients whose primary complaint was infertility. He suggested that the diagnosis should be suspected in a woman in the fourth decade of life who has had a history of unexplained involuntary sterility for five years or more and in whom no previous pelvic inflammatory disease had occurred. The temperature, leukocyte count, and sedimentation rate are usually normal, and on pelvic examination adnexal masses are usually not palpable. Siegler further cautioned that the x-ray picture of tubal diverticulosis must be differentiated from that of tubal tuberculosis. In the latter condition, the oviducts are usually rigid, devoid of peristalsis, and are often occluded at the proximal end of the ampulla. Fistulous tracts seen in tuberculosis, however, may be confused with diverticulosis. Calcification of pelvic lymph nodes or calcified areas in the tubal lumen or in one or both ovaries are diagnostic of genital tuberculosis. The endometrial biopsy may reveal typical tuberculous endometritis.

TREATMENT.—The lesions per se are innocuous and require no specific treatment. The prognosis is good and might be compared with the prognosis in a nonspecific salpingitis. The lesion is not considered to be premalignant. If tubal diverticulosis is discovered as an incidental finding at laparotomy and the tubes are grossly normal, nothing need be done. A patient with a long-standing history of infertility, however, who has bilateral isthmic occlusion due to diverticulosis could be considered a candidate for reconstructive surgery. In this case, bilateral reimplantation of the oviducts would be the procedure of choice.

BENIGN NEOPLASMS

Benign tumors of the oviduct are rare entities, yet a large variety of neoplasms have been reported as having originated in the fallopian tube. Tumors may be located in the wall or within the lumen or occasionally may be pedunculated and project from the fimbriated portion of the tube. In a consideration of benign tumors of the oviduct, lesions such as salpingitis isthmica nodosa, endometriosis, and adenomyosis should be excluded. Similarly, the hydatids of Morgagni are so commonplace that they should not be considered as a tumor mass. The following benign tumors have been reported in the literature: cystic and solid teratomas, papilloma, fibroadenoma, fibroma, leiomyoma, lipoma, hemangioma, lymphangioma, mesothelioma, and mesonephroma.

Somewhat more common is the adenomatoid tumor (Fig 6–15), sometimes called an angiomyoma or a reticuloendothelioma. This is a small circumscribed tumor of the tube usually confined to the muscle wall and found incidentally at the time of laparotomy. It has a characteristic microscopic appearance, being composed of small glandlike spaces lined by cells of mesothelial, endothelial, or even epithelial appearance. Grossly, the tumors appear as gray, gray-white, or yellow discrete nodules occupying the muscularis and rarely exceeding 3 cm in diameter. Because of the glandular arrangement of the cells, the microscopic picture has occasionally

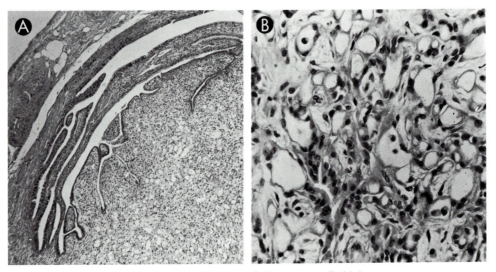

Fig 6–15.—Adenomatoid tumor. **A,** low power. **B,** higher power.

been confused with a low-grade adenocarcinoma. The histogenesis of these tumors is not clearly defined. Hertig and Gore consider this tumor to be of peritoneal origin and therefore support its origin from mesothelial cells. It is not believed that these adenomatoid tumors possess malignant potential.

Leiomyomas of the tube are usually asymptomatic lesions that are discovered at laparotomy performed for another indication. Approximately 50 cases have been reported in the literature, but since these tumors are usually solitary and small it is entirely probable that many have been unreported. Occasionally they have enlarged and produced acute torsion of the oviduct, and degenerative changes similar to those occurring in uterine leiomyomas have been reported.

Approximately 35 cystic teratomas of the oviduct have been reported, most having been discovered accidentally. These cystic teratomas may become infected and give rise to a clinical situation simulating pelvic inflammatory disease. Intraperitoneal rupture may occur, producing the same clinical and pathologic picture as a ruptured dermoid cyst of the ovary. A few solid teratomas of the oviduct have been reported. In one, reported by Henriksen, the entire tumor consisted of adult thyroid tissue, a so-called struma salpingii. Hertig and Gore have suggested that these dermoid tumors of the oviduct arise from primordial germ cells that have been arrested in their migration from the mesentery of the gut to the ovary.

MALIGNANT NEOPLASMS

Primary Carcinoma

The rarest carcinoma of the female genital tract is primary carcinoma of the oviduct. Since the report of the first patient in 1888, approximately 500 cases of this entity have been documented. In relation to the overall incidence of genital cancer, the incidence of tubal carcinoma varies from 0.1% to 0.5%. This is in marked contrast to carcinoma of the cervix, which accounts for approximately 45%, and carcinoma of the corpus, which accounts for approximately 30% of the total. At the Boston Hospital for Women, Hu et al. found that tubal carcinoma constituted 0.31% of all genital cancers. This was based on a report of 12 patients operated on between 1909 and 1948. An additional 26 patients with primary tubal carcinoma have been seen since 1948, a total of 38 cases in 52 years. At the state cancer hospital in Pondville, Mass., 18 cases have been seen (0.1% incidence), and at the Massachusetts General Hospital 16 tubal carcinomas have been treated (incidence 0.4%).

The age incidence has varied from 18 to 80 years, but most patients have been between 40 and 65 years, with an average of approximately 52 years. Infertility has been a common finding in patients with tubal carcinoma and, in a review by Wechsler, 32% of the patients had never given birth to a full-term child. At the Boston Hospital for Women the incidence of sterility was 44%.

Two factors have been suggested in the histogenesis of this tumor. Chronic salpingitis has long been held as a predisposing cause, and tuberculosis has also been suggested as being a possible forerunner of the disease. At the Brigham and Women's Hospital during the past five years, three patients were found to have, as incidental findings, carcinoma in situ in the tubal mucosa. Neither tuberculosis nor chronic salpingitis was found in these patients. Crosson states that the "preceding chronic tubal infection is the most important single etiologic factor" in the development of this disease, whereas Ayre doubts the validity of this statement, since salpingitis is so common and malignancy so rare. Hu et al. found that salpingitis was present in all but three of their 12 cases. Finn and Javert reported six cases and stated that the opposite tube was free from salpingitis in all five instances, one patient having bilateral carcinoma. In all probability the tumor itself produces a chronic inflammatory reaction, which eventually seals off the fimbriated portion of the tube and actually may simulate a hydrosalpinx.

DIAGNOSIS.—While there are no distinctive symptoms that might be called pathognomonic, the most consistent sign is a watery and frequently blood-tinged vaginal discharge. Intermittent or colicky, low abdominal pain associated with abnormal bleeding may also be present. The latter may be manifested as irregular bleeding or spotting during the postmenopausal era and as menstrual irregularities during the childbearing period. Occasionally the discharge may be profuse, although the occurrence of *hydrops tubae profluens* as a characteristic symptom is quite rare. The latter may occur with the release of a watery or blood-tinged fluid from a hydrosalpinx through the uterus and vagina, regardless of whether or not tubal carcinoma is associated.

The physical findings include abdominal enlargement, if ascites is present, and a palpable abdominal mass or more commonly a palpable, firm mass found during pelvic examination. The finding of a tubal carcinoma is so rare that it is only occasionally listed as the primary preoperative diagnosis. According to Martzloff, in only 6% of the cases reported in the literature had the correct diagnosis been made preoperatively, and in the series at the Boston Hospital for Women only one patient had a preoperative diagnosis of tubal carcinoma. In postmenopausal patients the usual diagnosis is ovarian tumor, and in premenopausal patients the most common diagnoses are leiomyomas and pelvic inflammatory disease. If, however, there is recurrent bleeding—or particularly a bloody, watery discharge—in a postmenopausal patient in whom biopsies of the cervix and endometrial curettage have given negative findings, the suspicion of tubal cancer should be strongly entertained. Vaginal smears may disclose neoplastic cells characteristic of tubal cancer, particularly when there is a loss of fluid from the uterus. Culdocentesis may also reveal suspicious or definite malignant elements. Occasionally hysterosalpingography has suggested a cancer of the tube, and endoscopy or culdotomy may verify the diagnosis. A dilatation and curettage may reveal tubal cancer metastatic to the endometrial cavity. In one of our patients the presenting complaint was that of an inguinal mass, which, on biopsy, revealed an undifferentiated adenocarcinoma. Laparotomy subsequently revealed the primary carcinoma to be in the fallopian tube, and the endometrial cavity was not involved.

PATHOLOGY.—The lesion is usually unilateral, only about 30% of the patients having had bilateral tumors. If the fimbriated portion of the tube is closed, the gross appearance (Fig 6–16) of the mass may simulate that of a hydrosalpinx or pyosalpinx. The serosal surface is frequently roughened and adherent to the large and small intestines. Lesions have been described as large as 17 cm in diameter

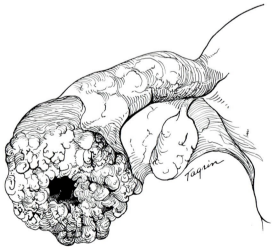

Fig 6–16.—Typical gross appearance of carcinoma of the oviduct.

although the association of a hydrosalpinx or pyosalpinx may make the gross appearance much larger. Cross-section of the tumor reveals granular tissue that is gray or yellow-tan, with a marked tendency to friability. The lesion is usually situated in the distal third of the tube, from where it may extend through the fimbriated portion. The tubal lumen is usually distended with fluid, and a papillary mass of friable or hemorrhagic tumor lines the mucosal surface.

The pathologic diagnosis of primary carcinoma of the oviduct is based on proof that the tumor arises from the endosalpinx. The criteria suggested by Hu et al. for differentiating between primary and metastatic tumors are as follows: (1) Grossly, the main tumor is in the tube. (2) Microscopically, the mucosa should be chiefly involved and should show a papillary pattern. (3) If the tubal wall is involved to a great extent, the transition between benign and malignant tubal epithelium should be demonstrated.

The following microscopic classification of tubal carcinomas is used at the Brigham and Women's Hospital.

Microscopic Classification of Tubal Carcinomas

PAPILLARY (Grade 1): The pure papillary growth is confined to the tubal lumen and transition between normal and malignant epithelium is clearly seen. The cells are fairly well differentiated and columnar in shape, and there are scanty mitotic figures (Fig 6–17,A).

PAPILLARY-ALVEOLAR (Grade 2): This group shows beginning glandular formation and invasion of the tubal muscularis. The cells are undifferentiated, with a moderate number of mitoses (Fig 6–17,B).

ALVEOLAR MEDULLARY (Grade 3): The growth pattern is more solid, in contrast to the papillary type. The cells are arranged in medullary or glandular pattern and there is definite invasion of the tubal lymphatics. The cells are poorly differentiated, with vacuolation and abundant and atypical mitoses.

The usual method of spread of tubal carcinoma is via the lymphatics, but tumor growth may occur via the tubal lumen along the mu-

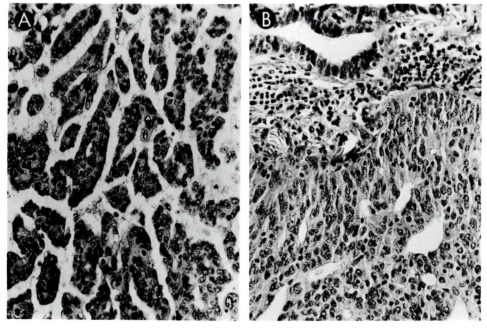

Fig 6–17.—A, typical papillary carcinoma of oviduct. **B,** alveolar carcinoma of oviduct.

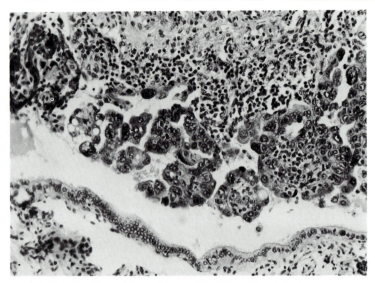

Fig 6–18.—Carcinoma of the oviduct involving tubal mucosa.

cosal surface (Fig 6–18). Generalized peritoneal implants are uncommon, due in all probability to closure of the fimbriated portion of the tube. The iliac, lumbar, and preaortic nodes may be involved by lymphatic permeation (Fig 6–19), and occasionally dissemination via the round ligament to the inguinal nodes may occur. Hematogenous spread accounts for metastases to the liver, lungs, stomach, and supraclavicular lymph nodes. The ovary, uterine corpus, and vagina may be involved by direct extension.

The clinical staging of carcinoma of the tube is as follows:

Clinical Staging for Fallopian Tube Carcinoma*

Stage I.	Growth limited to the tube.
Stage Ia.	Growth limited to one tube, no ascites.
Stage Ib.	Growth limited to two tubes, no ascites.
Stage Ic.	Growth limited to one or both tubes, ascites present with malignant cells in fluid.

*Adapted from Turunen A.: *Int. J. Obstet.* 7:24, 1969.

Stage II.	Growth involving one or both tubes with pelvic extension.
Stage IIa.	Extension and/or metastases to the uterus or ovary.
Stage IIb.	Extension to other pelvic tissues.
Stage III.	Growth involving one or both tubes with widespread intraperitoneal metastases to abdomen.
Stage IV.	Growth involving one or both tubes with distant metastases extraperitoneally.

TREATMENT.—The optimum method of treatment is total hysterectomy with bilateral salpingo-oophorectomy followed by x-ray therapy. If there is extension to the endocervix or upper vagina a radical hysterectomy and pelvic lymphadenectomy is advisable. If a primary cancer of the tube is discovered early and removed promptly, the prognosis is good. The prognosis in general is considered to be poor although the five-year survival rate is directly related to the extent of the disease. The prognosis is also worse in poorly differentiated lesions, but it is in this particular group that metastases are found at the time of

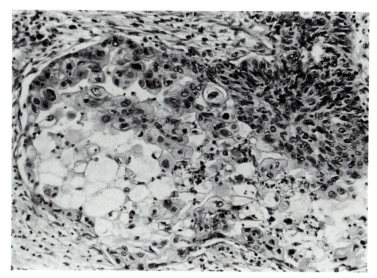

Fig 6–19.—Carcinoma of the oviduct metastatic to peritubal lymphatic.

surgery. Prior to 1926 only three five-year survivals were reported in the first 200 cases in the literature. The five-year salvage rate has varied from 5% to 48%, the latter figure being noted in the 38 cases from the Boston Hospital for Women in which a five-year follow-up was possible. The average five-year survival rate for primary fallopian tube cancer the world over is between 10% and 15%. Alertness to the possibility of tubal cancer, prompt intervention, and adequate treatment will improve this discouragingly low "cure rate." The precise value of postoperative x-ray therapy is difficult to determine since the number of cases in each series is small and, in addition, x-ray has not been given to all patients who had a very localized lesion.

Phelps and Chapman treated 15 patients referred for postoperative radiotherapy. Nine patients had stage I or stage II disease, and six patients had stage III. Eighty-nine percent of patients with disease confined to the pelvis survived; all patients with stage III disease have died. These authors recommend postoperative irradiation for all patients with primary tubal carcinoma, including intraperitoneal instillation of radiocolloid when large masses of tumor are not present. Patients presenting with advanced disease may achieve significant palliation with radiotherapy followed by chemotherapy.

Boutselis and Thompson reported the clinical data of 14 primary carcinomas of the tube. Only one was diagnosed correctly before surgery, and vaginal cytologic findings was negative in 12 instances. A diagnostic triad of pain, vaginal discharge, and palpable adnexal mass was present in eight of 14 patients. Minimal therapy should include total hysterectomy and bilateral salpingo-oophorectomy, but Boutselis noted significant beneficial effect in seven of eight patients after postoperative external radiation. More extensive pelvic operation is indicated on a selective basis, and chemotherapy deserves further consideration as adjuvant treatment. Five of 14 patients are living without disease, two to ten years after adequate therapy.

Sarcoma

Sarcomas are extremely rare tumors, less than 30 cases having been reported in the literature. The ratio of sarcoma to carcinoma of the oviduct is of the order of 1 to 25. The age incidence and clinical picture are similar to those in carcinoma of the tube. If the disease is extensive, the most common symptoms are pelvic pain, abdominal enlargement, and malaise. Physical examination may reveal abdominal distention, a pelvic mass, and emaciation. The tubal tumor varies in size from 2 to 20 cm and the cross-section reveals a soft, papillary or pultaceous intraluminal mass. Microscopically, the sarcoma is most commonly of the spindle-cell type but other variations such as round cell, myosarcoma, myxosarcoma, perithelioma, and endothelioma have been described.

This most malignant tumor may spread via the bloodstream, lymphatics, or by direct extension to adjacent pelvic organs. The optimum method of treatment is total hysterectomy with bilateral salpingo-oophorectomy followed by x-ray therapy. The prognosis is poor and it is doubtful whether therapy of any type retards the eventual outcome in advanced cases.

Carcinoma Metastatic to the Oviduct

As might be expected, the two organs responsible for most metastatic lesions in the oviduct are the ovary and the endometrium. The method of spread may be either by direct extension or via the lymphatics. Carcinoma of the stomach and pancreas may also metastasize to the tube. The lesions may be unilateral or bilateral, and there is no characteristic gross appearance. Histologically, the tumors are identical with the primary tumor (Fig 6–20) and, in contrast to primary carcinoma

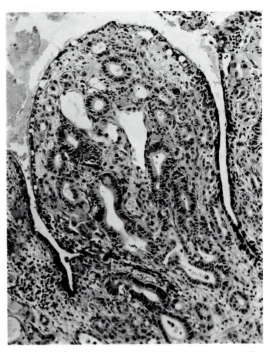

Fig 6–20.—Carcinoma of the pancreas metastatic to the oviduct.

of the tube, the serosa of the oviducts as well as the lymphatics of the muscularis and of the mesosalpinx are usually involved. The treatment is that of the primary disease, usually complete hysterectomy and bilateral salpingo-oophorectomy. Postoperative x-ray therapy is advisable, but the prognosis for five-year survival is poor.

BIBLIOGRAPHY

Structure and Function

Borell U., Nilsson O., Westman A.: Ciliary activity in the rabbit fallopian tube during estrus and after copulation. *Acta Obstet. Gynecol. Scand.* 36:22, 1957.

Chang M.C.: Development and fate of transferred rabbit ova or blastocysts in relation to the ovulation time of recipients. *J. Exp. Zool.* 114:197, 1950.

Clewe T.H., Mastroianni L.: Mechanisms of ovum pickup: I. Functional capacity of rabbit oviducts ligated near the fimbria. *Fertil. Steril.* 9:13, 1958.

Decker A.: Culdoscopic observations on the tubo-ovarian mechanisms of ovum reception. *Fertil. Steril.* 2:253, 1951.

Inflammation

Centers for Disease Control: Sexually transmitted diseases treatment guidelines, 1982. *M.M.W.R.* 31:435, 1982.

Hellman L.M.: The morphology of the human fallopian tube in the early puerperium. *Am. J. Obstet. Gynecol.* 57:154, 1949.

Horne H.W., Kundsin R.B., Kosasa T.S.: The role of mycoplasma infection in human reproductive failure. *Fertil. Steril.* 25:380, 1974.

Ledger W.J., Hackett K.A.: Significance of clostridia in female reproductive tract. *Obstet. Gynecol.* 41:525, 1973.

McGruder C.J.: Surgical management of chronic pelvic inflammatory disease. *Obstet. Gynecol.* 13:591, 1959.

Mead P.B., Louria D.B.: Antibiotics in pelvic infections. *Clin. Obstet. Gynecol.* 12:219, 1969.

Mickal A., Sellman A.H.: Management of tubo-ovarian abscess. *Clin. Obstet. Gynecol.* 12:252, 1969.

Mishell D.R., Moyer D.L.: Association of pelvic inflammatory disease with the intrauterine device. *Clin. Obstet. Gynecol.* 12:179, 1969.

Nassberg S., McKay D.G., Hertig A.T.: Physiological salpingitis. *Am. J. Obstet. Gynecol.* 67:130, 1954.

Pedowitz P., Felmus L.: Rupture of tubo-ovarian abscesses. *Am. J. Surg.* 83:507, 1952.

Schaefer G.: Female genital tuberculosis: A review of the literature. *Obstet. Gynecol. Surv.* 8:461, 1953.

Sutherland A.M.: The treatment of genital tuberculosis in women. *Geneesk. gids* 45:362; 386, 1967.

Tubal Ectopic Pregnancy

Beacham W.D., Webster H.D., Beacham D.W.: Ectopic pregnancy at New Orleans Charity Hospital. *Am. J. Obstet. Gynecol.* 72:830, 1956.

Bender S.: Fertility after tubal pregnancy. *Br. J. Obstet. Gynaecol.* 63:400, 1956.

De Cherney A.H., Maheux R.: Modern management of tubal pregnancy. *Curr. Probl. Obstet. Gynecol.* 6:4–38, 1983.

Douglas E.S., Shingleton H.M., Crist T.: Surgical management of tubal pregnancy: Effects on subsequent fertility. *South. Med. J.* 62:954, 1969.

Franklin E.W., Zeiderman A.R., Laemmle P.: Tubal ectopic pregnancy: Etiologic and obstetric and gynecologic sequelae. *Am. J. Obstet. Gynecol.* 117:220, 1973.

Grant A.: The effect of ectopic pregnancy on fertility. *Clin. Obstet. Gynecol.* 5:861, 1962.

Kistner R.W.: Ectopic pregnancy in Conn H.F. (ed.): *Current Diagnosis.* Philadelphia, W.B. Saunders Co., 1966, p. 668.

Kistner R.W., Hertig A.T., Rock J.: Tubal pregnancy complicating tuberculous salpingitis. *Am. J. Obstet. Gynecol.* 62:1157, 1951.

Kistner R.W., Patton G.W.: *Atlas of Infertility Surgery.* Boston, Little Brown & Co., 1975, pp. 152–159.

Langer R., et al.: Conservative surgery for tubal pregnancy. *Fertil. Steril.* 38:427, 1982.

Schenker J.G., Evron S.: New concepts in the surgical management of tubal pregnancy and the consequent postoperative results. *Fertil. Steril.* 40:709, 1983.

Timonen S., Nieminen U.: Tubal pregnancy: Choice of operative method of treatment. *Acta Obstet. Gynaecol. Scand.* 46:327, 1967.

Inflammation

Ledger W.: New concepts in the management of pelvic inflammatory disease. *J. Reprod. Med.* 28:10, 1983.

Neoplasms

Boutselis J.G., Thompson J.N.: Clinical aspects of primary carcinoma of the fallopian tube. *Am. J. Obstet. Gynecol.* 111:98, 1971.

Golden A., Ash J.E.: Adenomatoid tumors of the genital tract. *Am. J. Pathol.* 21:63, 1945.

Green T.H., Scully R.E.: Tumors of the fallopian tube. *Clin. Obstet. Gynecol.* 5:886, 1962.

Grimes H.G., Kornmesser J.G.: Benign cystic teratoma of the oviduct. *Obstet. Gynecol.* 16:85, 1960.

Herbut P.: *Gynecological and Obstetrical Pathology.* Philadelphia, Lea & Febiger, 1953.

Hertig A.T., Gore H.: Tumors of the female sex organs: part 3: Tumors of the ovary and fallopian tube, sec. 9, fasc. 33, *Atlas of Tumor Pathology.* Washington, D.C., Armed Forces Institute of Pathology, 1961.

Hu C.Y., Taymor M.L., Hertig A.T.: Primary carcinoma of the fallopian tube. *Am. J. Obstet. Gynecol.* 59:58, 1950.

Phelps H.M., Chapman K.E.: Role of radiation therapy in treatment of primary carcinoma of the uterine tube. *Obstet. Gynecol.* 43:669, 1974.

Turunen A.: Carcinoma of fallopian tube. *Int. J. Gynecol. Obstet.* 7:294, 1969.

CHAPTER SEVEN

The Ovary

C. THOMAS GRIFFITHS, M.D.
ROSS BERKOWITZ, M.D.

THE HUMAN OVARY is an organ of complex embryologic derivation that provides ova for reproduction and functions as an intricate endocrine gland during half a lifetime. Throughout a woman's life, however, the organ is susceptible to a variety of neoplastic transformations and acute surgical conditions. As a result, the ovary has been an organ of extreme interest to geneticists, gynecologists, surgeons, endocrinologists, and pathologists. As the target organ for pituitary and placental hormones it may exhibit marked variations in appearance that closely simulate neoplastic processes. For this reason it is imperative that the physician recognize normal physiologic variations as well as pathologic states so that inappropriate surgical intervention will not be substituted for conservative or expectant therapy. In the past, ill-advised and overenthusiastic pelvic surgical procedures in the child or young adult have been a major cause of sterility. On the other hand, failure to recognize an acute surgical process or an ovarian malignancy is likely to result in loss of life.

ANATOMY

The human ovary undergoes variations in size, shape, and position during its lifetime in addition to extensive histologic changes brought about by hormonal stimuli and repetitive ovulation.

The ovary of the newborn is an elongated structure approximately 1.5 cm long, 0.5 cm wide, and 2.5 cm in thickness. The ovarian surface is pinkish white, smooth, and glistening. Occasionally, small cystic structures, the primordial follicles, may be seen through the surface epithelium. The ovaries in the term fetus lie in the posterior segment of the false pelvis, directly adjacent to the posterior uterine surface.

Between birth and pubescence the ovaries move into the true pelvis and enlarge to about $3.0 \times 1.8 \times 1.2$ cm, assuming an almond shape. The number of cystic structures seen beneath the surface increases although they are only 2 to 3 mm in diameter. The smooth gray appearance of the pubescent ovary resembles that of the Stein-Leventhal ovary of later life.

The onset of puberty brings about many changes in the histologic anatomy of the ovary, which in turn alter the gross appearance. The organ now measures 2.5 to 5.0 cm in length, 1.5 to 3.0 cm in width, and 0.6 to 1.5 cm in thickness and lies close to the lateral pelvic wall. The anterior margin of the ovary is thin and attached to the posterior surface of the broad ligament by a fold of tissue, the mesovarium. Blood vessels and nerves enter the hilus through the mesovarium.

In addition to the mesovarium, the ovary is supported by two other structures. The inferior or uterine pole is attached to the uterus

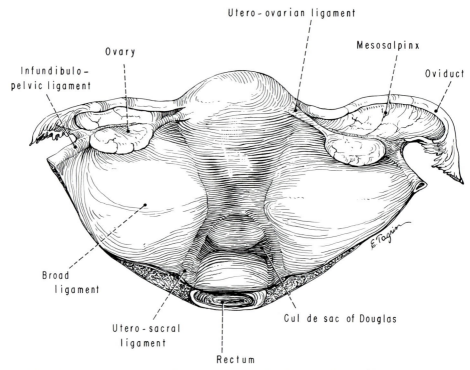

Utero-ovarian ligament

Ovary

Mesosalpinx

Infundibulo-
pelvic ligament

Oviduct

Broad
ligament

Utero-sacral
ligament

Cul de sac of Douglas

Rectum

Fig 7–1.—Posterior view of the internal genitalia showing the position
and ligamentous support of the ovaries.

by a fibromuscular cord, the utero-ovarian ligament. The upper or tubal pole is embraced
by the fimbria of the oviduct and is supported
by the infundibulopelvic or suspensory ligament. The latter represents the upper margin
of the broad ligament lateral to the tubal ostium and contains the ovarian vessels (Fig
7–1).

Various functional activities impart an uneven, occasionally nodular appearance to the
ovarian surface. The persistence of fetal mark-
ings, scars of previous ovulation, and atretic
follicles produce anatomic variations. An
ovary that has not been scarred by ovulation
usually presents a smooth and glistening surface. Single or multiple reddish elevations
represent recently ruptured follicles of recently formed corpora lutea, whereas older
corpora lutea are yellow. These structures
vary from a few millimeters to several centimeters in diameter and occasionally a large

yellow corpus luteum occupies one third of
the ovary.

The normal ovarian cortex is usually tense
and elastic. When cut, fluid escapes from cystic follicles, exposing a pink, moist surface.
Follicular cysts are smooth, thin-walled cavities and vary from 3 to 5 cm in diameter.
Theca-lutein cysts have a crenated border
with a yellow wall. Corpora albicantia are
white or slightly yellow, crenated, fibrous
structures that may be scattered throughout
the stroma. They represent the final involution of corpora lutea and atretic follicles.

The arterial supply of the ovary is derived
from both the ovarian artery and a branch of
the uterine artery, which anastomose with the
latter vessel within the mesosalpinx. The
ovarian arteries arise from the aorta opposite
the lower second or upper third lumbar vertebrae and diagonally cross the psoas muscle
in their descent to the pelvic brim. After

passing through the infundibulopelvic ligament they divide, giving off a branch to the
oviducts. The main ovarian trunk runs in the
folds of the broad ligament and mesovarium,
freely anastomosing with the ascending division of the uterine artery. As it passes
through the ovarium hilus, paired medullary
branches are given off that traverse the entire
ovary. Each medullary artery runs in a
straight-line fashion to the opposite pole of
the ovary, giving off *cortical* branches during
its course.

The venous drainage is similar to the arterial arrangement, the veins emerging at the
hilus as two major vessels. These represent
both the uterine and ovarian venous systems,
and in pregnancy or extreme venous congestion a pampiniform plexus of enormously distended veins may form. Although the ovarian
veins accompany the arteries in their downward course from the midabdomen, the right
ovarian vein terminates in the inferior vena
cava, whereas the left empties into the left
renal vein.

The nerve supply arises from a sympathetic
plexus intimately enmeshed with the ovarian
vessels in the infundibulopelvic ligament. Its
fibers are derived from branches of the renal
and aortic plexuses as well as from the celiac
and mesenteric ganglia.

During pregnancy, the ovaries are lifted
out of the true pelvis by the enlarging uterus
and thus become abdominal rather than pelvic organs. During the early weeks of gestation the corpus luteum is large and usually exceeds in size the remainder of the ovary.
Regrettably, the unusual appearance of the
corpus luteum of pregnancy, which may produce unilateral pelvic pain, has too frequently
led to the removal of the entire ovary under
the mistaken impression that a neoplasm exists. At the time of cesarean section the ovaries are usually of normal size but covered
with a pink, irregular frosting. This tissue
represents a pseudodecidual reaction in totipotential germinal epithelium due to the prolonged and continuous stimulation of cho-

rionic estrogen and progesterone. During the
puerperium the ovary diminishes in size and
the pseudodecidual reaction disappears. The
cystic follicles have undergone atresia, and
some time may elapse before gonadotropic
function brings about follicular maturation
and ovulation.

Postmenopausally the ovary undergoes
rapid regressive changes. As it becomes
smaller, the surface becomes wrinkled, frequently resembling the gyri and sulci of the
cerebrum. Perhaps the most striking change
is in the size of the organ, since it may be
only $2.0 \times 1.5 \times 0.5$ cm or less. The postmenopausal ovary is so rarely palpable on pelvic examination that Barber has justifiably
proposed that palpability connotes enlargement and the probability of a neoplasm.

EMBRYOLOGY

Although the sex of an embryo is determined genetically at the time of fertilization,
the genital systems of both sexes are indistinguishable until six weeks' gestation. Consequently this early period of genital development has been termed the *indifferent stage*.
The gonads are derived from three distinct
embryonic tissues, the coelomic epithelium of
the urogenital ridge, the mesenchyme underlying the coelomic epithelium, and the primordial germ cells. Although the specific contributions of these embryonic tissues to the
cellular components of the mature ovary has
been a subject of heated controversy, the following sequence of events appears to be currently accepted by most embryologists.

The initial event in gonadogenesis is apparent at four weeks' gestation and consists of a
thickening of coelomic epithelium overlying
the urogenital ridge anterior to the preexisting mesonephros. Rapid proliferation of this
coelomic or germinal epithelium and its underlying mesenchyme results in a distinct
protuberance, the genital ridge. By five
weeks, fingerlike projections from the germinal epithelium have extended into the mes-

enchyme to form the primary sex cords. At the same time, the paramesonephric duct (müllerian duct) is formed by the invagination of a strip of coelomic epithelium along the lateral opposing aspect of the urogenital ridge.

The primordial germ cells are first visible at 22 days' gestation intermixed with the endodermal cells of the caudal yolk sac wall, which ultimately form the hindgut. After infolding of the embryo, the primordial germ cells migrate along the dorsal mesentery of the hindgut, and by eight weeks' gestation all have entered the mesenchyme of the genital ridges. Rapid proliferation of the germ cells, now termed *oogonia*, occurs by mitotic division between eight and 20 weeks and then tapers off and ceases by birth. By six weeks' gestation a number of oogonia have been incorporated into the primary sex cords, and the indifferent stage of gonadal development

ends at this time. The primary sex cords under the influence of the Y chromosome separate from the germinal epithelium and occupy the medullary portion of the gonad where they differentiate, ultimately to form the seminiferous tubules. The male oogonia accompany the primary sex cords, and the cortex of the indifferent gonad condenses to form a dense fibrous layer, the *tunica albuginea*.

The ovary, in the absence of a differentiating chromosome, develops more slowly. By 12 weeks' gestation secondary or cortical sex cords have extended from the germinal epithelium to expand the cortex, and the primary sex cords have been displaced into the regressing medulla or hilus, where they become the *rete ovarii* (Fig 7–2). Also occupying the hilus until shortly after birth are a number of oval or polygonal cells with central round nuclei known as hilus cells. Presum-

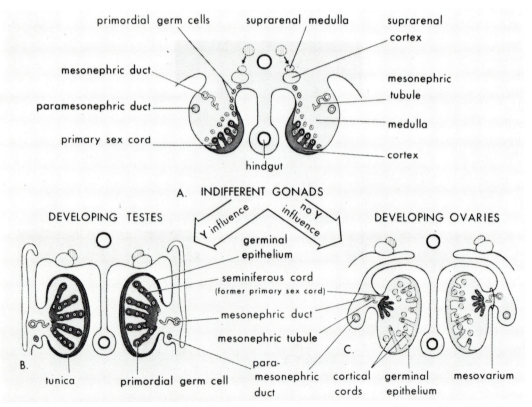

Fig 7–2.—Diagrammatic representation of early testicular and ovarian development from the indifferent gonad. (From Moore K.L.: *The Developing Human,* ed. 2. Philadelphia, W.B. Saunders Co., 1977.)

ably derived from the medullary mesenchyme, they are the analogue of the testicular Leydig cells and reappear in the ovarian hilus at puberty. They are present in at least 80% of adult women and may give rise to the virilizing hilus cell tumor.

The oogonia in the cortex are gradually incorporated into the cortical cords, which separate from the germinal epithelium and form isolated cell clusters at about 16 weeks' gestation. On completion of mitotic activity, an oogonium differentiates into a *primary oocyte,* which progresses into prophase of the first meiotic division. Shortly thereafter the oocyte is surrounded by flattened follicular cells, which are derived from cortical cord cells and are destined to become granulosa cells. The resultant structures are termed *primordial follicles.* Within the primary oocyte each of the 46 chromosomes has replicated and exists as two sister chromatids united by a common centromere. Pairing of homologous chromosomes has occurred as well as crossing over, with the resultant exchange of certain genetic loci between homologous chromatids (Fig 7–3). At this point maturation is arrested for well over a decade, and the first meiotic division is not completed until just prior to ovulation. Consequently, primary oocytes are diploid, and reduction to a haploid number of chromosomes by the second meiotic division occurs only in those primary oocytes destined to become *secondary oocytes* and then *ova.* The process of follicular atresia begins as soon as primordial follicles are formed. At birth there are about 2 million primordial follicles of which 50% are atretic. By seven years of age they number less than 300,000.

Several aspects of ovarian development bearing specific relevance to pathologic states deserve special comment.

1. Although the ovarian coelomic epithelium is no longer thought to be the source of primordial germ cells, embryologists continue to use the term *germinal epithelium.* In the mature ovary, however, this tissue is modified peritoneum and is in fact mesothelium. Until there is an official change in terminol-

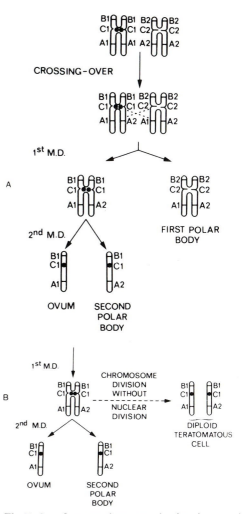

Fig 7–3.—A, normal oogenesis showing a pair of homologous chromosomes that are heterozygous at loci *A* and *B* and have heteromorphic centromeric markers. Crossing over has occurred in the region between the centromere and *A* locus but not between the centromere and *B* locus. **B,** Linder's proposed abnormality of the second meiotic division, resulting in a parthenogenic teratomatous cell. The homologous chromosome is homomorphic at the centromere and homozygous at locus *B,* but is heterozygous at locus *A.* (From Gerald P.S.: *N. Engl. J. Med.* 292:103, 1975. Reprinted by permission.)

ogy we will continue to refer to the *germinal epithelium.*

2. Both the germinal epithelium of the ovary and the internal genitalia are derived from the coelomic epithelium of the urogenital ridge. As will be described further, these derivatives retain the potential for a recapitulation of embryogenesis.

3. A homologous relationship between granulosa cells and Sertoli's cells and between theca cells and Leydig's cells, has been accepted. A major controversy in gonadogenesis, however, concerns the proposed origin of Sertoli's and granulosa cells from the coelomic epithelium by the downgrowth of the sex cords. There is general agreement that the follicular theca cells are derived from the ovarian mesenchyme, and the usual coexistence of both granulosa cells and theca cells in the same tumor suggests a common origin of both cell types. Scully (1970) has proposed that granulosa and theca cell tumors be categorized as "sex cord—mesenchyme tumors" rather than simply as gonadal stromal tumors.

4. There is no evidence that adrenal or mesonephric cells occupy the developing gonads and thus persist as embryonic rests.

5. The primary oocyte may persist to middle life in the human female. It contains a diploid number of chromosomes but each has replicated into two chromatids. This concept is relevant to the genesis of ovarian teratomas.

HISTOLOGY

In the newborn, the germinal epithelium of the ovary is made up of a single layer of low, cuboidal or cylindrical cells, each having a large nucleus. The primordial follicle measures about 50 to 60 μ in diameter and is composed of a primary oocyte surrounded by a single layer of follicular cells. A portion of the parenchyma around the follicle is differentiated into spindle-shaped cells and fibrils.

In proximity to the medulla is a zone of growing follicles, and in the newborn well-developed graafian follicles have matured under the stimulus of chorionic gonadotropin. During infancy, growth of follicles and stroma is rapid, but then tapers off until pubescence when rapid development again occurs. The number of primordial follicles diminishes from birth, and there is no evidence that formation of new follicles subsequently occurs. The number of ova in the newborn ovary has been estimated at about 2 million. In the average female not more than 300 to 400 will proceed through ovulation and be released, with the potential of fertilization.

During pubescence the follicles of the hilus develop first. Initially there is an increase in size and number of the follicular cells as they become cuboidal with an increase in cytoplasm. Eventually the follicular cells become multilayered and a fluid—the *liquor folliculi*—accumulates eccentrically. The precise origin of this fluid is unknown in the human, but it is presumably a combination of cell secretion, cell degeneration, and vascular transudate.

In follicles under 0.3 mm the ovum (oocyte) is centrally placed, but larger follicles are vesicular and the ovum is placed eccentrically (Fig 7–4). The follicle cells, now known as granulosa cells, are arranged about the ovum in a covering eight to 12 rows in thickness. The mound of granulosa cells containing the ovum, which projects into the cavity of the follicle, is known as the *cumulus oophorus.* As the growth of granulosa cells continues, the cumulus moves to a more peripheral position and the cells around the ovum increase in number. The layer of granulosa cells immediately adjacent to the ovum is known as the *corona radiata.* There is a gradual increase in cytoplasm of the ovum, so that a 2 mm follicle will contain an ovum of 90 to 100 μ. During this stage of development the *zona pellucida,* a hyaline band around the ovum, begins to appear.

Whereas the primordial follicle is devoid of a connective tissue covering, the fully developed follicle has two coverings. The inner layer, the *theca interna,* is made up of fine, fibrillar, connective-tissue cells with abundant

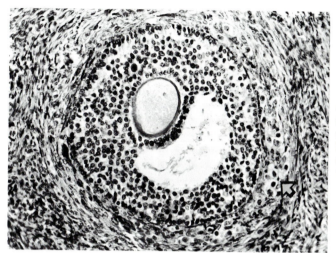

Fig 7–4.—Maturing graafian follicle. A developing layer of theca cells *(arrow)* is seen external to the granulosa cells. (From Morris J.M., and Scully R.E.: *Endocrine Pathology of the Ovary.* St. Louis, C.V. Mosby Co., 1958.)

blood vessels (see Fig 7–4). There is evidence that these cells contain steroid substances, which probably are precursors in the production of estrogen and progesterone. An outermost layer, the *theca externa*, contains many coarse fibers that intertwine around the follicle and form a thick capsule.

The medulla of the ovary contains numerous blood vessels with cellular tissue. Follicles are usually absent. The remnant of the *rete ovarii* is found in the medulla and is identified as a group of irregular tubules lined with cuboidal, cylindrical, or ciliated epithelium. As noted in the previous section, a cluster of hilus cells is often seen in the medulla.

The mature ovary does not differ appreciably from the description of the ovary at pubescence except for the changes associated with ovulation. The germinal epithelium retains only a tenuous single layer of flattened cuboidal cells, but there are furrows and folds in areas of previous ovulation. Occasionally the germinal epithelium dips into the cortical area and may become pinched off to form inclusion cysts or "cortical glands" (Figs 7–5 and 7–6). The thin tunica albuginea lies subjacent to the surface epithelium and is composed of interlacing, coarse fibers with minimal cellularity. Scattered throughout the parenchymatous zone are maturing follicles of all ages, together with atretic follicles and recent and old corpora lutea. Several ripe follicles may be seen at the surface just prior to rupture. They actually protrude a bit beyond the surface and may measure up to 20 mm in diameter.

Follicular Atresia

Since not all primordial follicles reach maturity, the vast majority undergo a degenerative process known as atresia. This process begins in the fifth month of fetal life and continues past the menopause, when the last remaining follicle either ovulates or becomes atretic. The zona pellucida first becomes hyalinized and crenated. After degeneration of the ovum the follicular epithelium undergoes specific necrobiotic changes. In a well-developed follicle, atresia begins with resorption of the *liquor folliculi* and infolding of the peripheral layers. Both the granulosa and the theca layers are replaced by fibrous connective tissue, which is later hyalinized. The scar may persist for long periods and is known as a *corpus fibrosum* or *corpus atreticum*. Large follicles may not undergo complete regression and, if the liquor is not completely absorbed, a cystic structure persists.

The Postmenopausal Ovary

After cessation of ovulation the ovary becomes quiescent and shrinks greatly in size. The remaining follicles undergo atresia and it

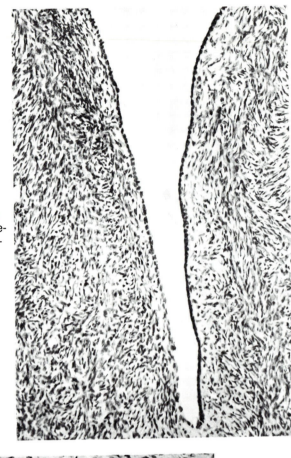

Fig 7–5.—Histogenesis of ovarian tumors. Surface of ovary showing a groove lined by coelomic epithelium, which has the potential to develop into serous, mucinous, or endometrial epithelium. (From McKay D.G.: *Clin. Obstet. Gynecol.* 5:1188, 1962.)

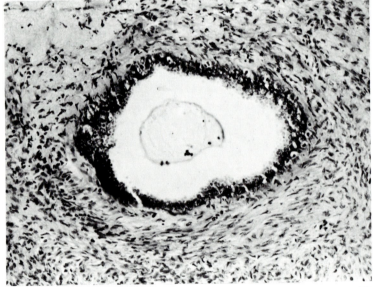

Fig 7–6.—Histogenesis of ovarian tumors. Coelomic epithelial inclusion cyst formed by "pinching off" of epithelium noted in Figure 7–5. (From McKay D.G.: *Clin. Obstet. Gynecol.* 5:1118, 1962.)

is unusual to find residual follicles after four or five years of menstrual inactivity in this age group. Occasionally, however, an episode of bleeding may occur in a postmenopausal patient and, if hysterectomy with bilateral salpingo-oophorectomy is performed for this reason alone, the operator may be surprised to find a recent corpus luteum in the ovary and secretory endometrium in the uterus.

The surface epithelium persists in the senile ovary as a single layer of flattened cells, and the tunica albuginea is composed of dense connective tissue cells and a few inactive spindle cells. Below the tunica are numerous corpora fibrosa and corpora albicantia, together with areas of hyalinization and calcium. The stromal cells are relatively inactive, although groups of theca cells may persist near the hilus.

Vestigial Remnants

The tubular system of the primitive mesonephros may persist in the adult as a series of convoluted tubules that run radially from the hilus within the mesovarium. This structure is known as the *epoophoron* and may occasionally give rise to cystic or papillary growths known as Kobelt's cysts. The caudal glomeruli of the mesonephros may persist as tubules between branches of the ovarian artery in the broad ligament and is known as the *paraoophoron*. The mesonephric excretory canal is represented by Gartner's duct, which extends from the caudal pole of the ovary to the lateral vaginal wall. Cystic dilatation of this duct may occur and usually presents as an intravaginal cyst in the upper third of the vagina (see Fig 3–10).

Ovulation and Corpus Luteum Formation

The precise physical and chemical factors initiating ovulation in the human are unknown, but evidence in the rat indicates that ovulation is not due to, or associated with, increased intrafollicular pressure (Blandau).

Follicular rupture is associated with an escape of the liquor and extrusion of the ovum into the fimbria of the oviduct or into the peritoneal cavity. Following rupture, there is

hemorrhage into the theca interna and the stigma is sealed by a blood clot from the thecal vessels as well as by a central coagulum in the cavity. Examination at this stage reveals active mitoses in both the granulosa and theca cell layers, and the structure is rapidly converted into the *corpus luteum*. It is possible, however, for ovulation to occur without release of the ovum. Ovarian pregnancies and certain cases of idiopathic infertility may be explained on this basis.

Four stages in the life cycle of the corpus luteum are recognized: proliferation, vascularization, complete development, and regression. During the *proliferative* stage, both granulosa cells and theca cells show active mitotic activity, and growth is rapid. The theca cells enlarge even more than the granulosa cells, and deposits of lipid are seen in the cytoplasm. This stage lasts about four days and results in the formation of an epithelial gland with secretory activity.

The stage of *vascularization* is characterized grossly by the appearance of a raspberrylike protuberance on the ovarian surface. The endothelial capillaries now extend through the entire granulosa layer to the central coagulum. Eventually fibrin is deposited in the core, and connective tissue cells begin to invade the coagulum. The stigma is healed by a similar process.

The stage of *full development* is evidenced by a moderate increase in size of the total structure, firmness of the central core, and a scalloped border, which assumes a brown or yellow color. Liquefaction of the central coagulum may give rise to cyst formation. At this stage the granulosa cells have a characteristic pale, clear cytoplasm and the theca cells are diminished in number and are arranged in groups between the granulosa cell columns and around the periphery of the granulosa layer (Fig 7–7).

The stage of *regression*, beginning about day 26 of a normal cycle, proceeds rapidly. The core becomes fibrotic, the granulosa layer diminishes in size, and the cells become granular and vacuolated and lose their colum-

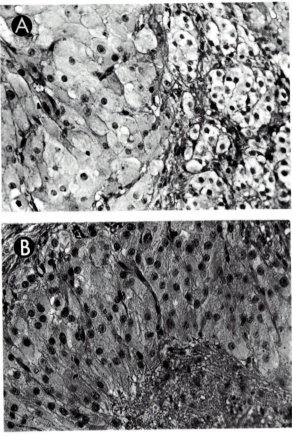

Fig 7–7.—A, high-power magnification of mature corpus luteum. The larger, rounded cells at left are granulosa-lutein cells; the smaller, clearer cells are theca-lutein cells. (From Morris J.M., Scully R.E.: *Endocrine Pathology of the Ovary.* St. Louis, C.V. Mosby Co., 1958.) **B,** wall of corpus luteum cyst, showing luteinized granulosa cells.

nar arrangement. The theca cells are loosely arranged in groups, with dark nuclei and pale cytoplasm. There is progressive fibrosis and hyalinization of the core and atrophy of the lutein layers. The resultant scar, known as a *corpus albicans*, requires about 70 days to develop.

OVARIAN NEOPLASMS

Of all gynecologic cancers, malignant disease of the ovary ranks first as a cause of death in the United States. Nearly 11,000 American women die from ovarian cancer annually and more than eight to ten times that number undergo operative procedures for both benign and malignant ovarian neoplasms each year. Even though the uterus and ovaries are the only abdominal organs normally accessible to palpation, early diagnosis of ovarian cancer is the exception. In the United States, fully 72% of ovarian carcinomas have metastasized by the time of diagnosis. For this reason the early recognition and management of abnormal ovarian enlargement are imperative. Proper concern for malignancy, however, must be tempered by an attitude of conservatism toward reproductive function in the younger patient. In this regard, a planned period of observation or noninvasive diagnostic procedures may constitute optimal management.

A consideration of ovarian neoplasms must encompass not only the wide range of benign and malignant tumors but also those tumor-like conditions of the ovary that are actually non-neoplastic. Familiarity with physiologic and pathologic conditions of other pelvic and lower abdominal organs that may simulate ovarian enlargement obviously is essential to the logical formulation of a differential diagnosis.

Classification

A formidable number of histologic tumor types derived from the various cellular components of the ovary have both fascinated pathologists and confounded clinicians responsible for optimal management and an estimate of prognosis. Numerous classifications of ovarian tumors have been proposed, each having certain advantages and disadvantages. Classifications based on presumed histologic origin allow broad grouping into similar clinical and histologic types from which more specific subgroups may be derived.

The usefulness of histogenetic classifications in predicting survival has been limited by a substantial group of unclassifiable tumors, by the frequent heterogeneity of cell types, and by variability in the malignant behavior within these histologic types. Since these drawbacks apply primarily to the common epithelial tumors (germinal epithelial origin), which also constitute 90% of ovarian malignancies, the International Federation of Gynecology and Obstetrics (FIGO) has adopted (1971) a detailed classification for the epithelial group.

Histological Classification of the Common Primary Epithelial Tumors of the Ovary

I. Serous cystomas
  a. Serous benign cystadenoma
  b. Serous cystadenomas with proliferating activity of the epithelial cells and nuclear abnormalities, but no infiltrative destructive growth (low-potential malignancy)
  c. Serous cystadenocarcinomas

II. Mucinous cystomas
  a. Mucinous benign cystadenomas
  b. Mucinous cystadenomas with proliferating activity of the epithelial cells and nuclear abnormalities, but no infiltrative destructive growth (low-potential malignancy)

  c. Mucinous cystadenocarcinomas

III. Endometrioid tumors (similar to adenocarcinomas in the endometrium)
  a. Endometrioid benign cysts
  b. Endometrioid tumors with proliferating activity of the epithelial cells and nuclear abnormalities, but no infiltrative destructive growth (low-potential malignancy)
  c. Endometrioid carcinomas

IV. Mesonephric tumors
  a. Benign mesonephric tumors
  b. Mesonephric tumors with proliferating activity of the epithelial cells and nuclear abnormalities, but no infiltrative destructive growth (low-potential malignancy)
  c. Mesonephric cystadenocarcinomas

V. Concomitant carcinoma, unclassified carcinoma (tumors that cannot be allotted to one of the groups I, II, III, or IV)

For many years pathologists and gynecologists have been aware of a specific group of papillary ovarian tumors with atypical proliferative activity but without the other histologic hallmarks of malignancy. The clinical course is compatible with the histologic appearance of a tumor of low-grade malignancy despite the occasional occurrence of superficial peritoneal metastases. This group with low-potential malignancy has also been termed *borderline* and *grade 0*. Although the FIGO histologic classification includes a low-potential malignancy category for each of the epithelial tumors, the designation is applicable primarily to the serous and mucinous cell types. Aure et al. found that whereas 21% of serous and 39% of mucinous carcinomas were considered to be of low-malignant potential, only 3% of endometrioid and none of the clear cell carcinomas were noninvasive.

The World Health Organization (WHO) Committee on Ovarian Neoplasms under the leadership of Serov and Scully have proposed an extremely detailed histogenetic classification that allows both for variability within cell types by adding additional subtypes and for the frequent admixture of cell types. It is hoped that this classification will be universally adopted and replace the multiplicity of classifications that have been shrouded in controversy and confusion.

WHO Histological Classification of Ovarian Tumors*

  I. Common "epithelial" tumors
     A. Serous tumors
        1. Benign
           a. Cystadenoma and papillary cystadenoma
           b. Surface papilloma
           c. Adenofibroma and cystadenofibroma
        2. Of borderline malignancy (carcinoma of low-malignant potential)
           a. Cystadenoma and papillary cystadenoma
           b. Surface papilloma
           c. Adenofibroma and cystadenofibroma
        3. Malignant
           a. Adenocarcinoma, papillary adenocarcinoma, and papillary cystadenocarcinoma
           b. Surface papillary carcinoma
           c. Malignant adenofibroma and cystadenofibroma
     B. Mucinous tumors
        1. Benign
           a. Cystadenoma
           b. Adenofibroma and cystadenofibroma
        2. Of borderline malignancy (carcinoma of low-malignant potential)
           a. Cystadenoma
           b. Adenofibroma and cystadenofibroma
        3. Malignant
           a. Adenocarcinoma and cystadenocarcinoma
           b. Malignant adenofibroma and cystadenofibroma
     C. Endometrioid tumors
        1. Benign
           a. Adenoma and cystadenoma
           b. Adenofibroma and cystadenofibroma
        2. Of borderline malignancy (carcinoma of low-malignant potential)
           a. Adenoma and cystadenoma
           b. Adenofibroma and cystadenofibroma
        3. Malignant
           a. Carcinoma
              i. Adenocarcinoma
              ii. Adenoacanthoma
              iii. Malignant adenofibroma
           b. Endometrioid stromal sarcomas
           c. Mesodermal (müllerian) mixed tumors, homologous, and heterologous
     D. Clear cell (mesonephroid) tumors
        1. Benign: adenofibroma
        2. Of borderline malignancy (carcinomas of low-malignant potential)
        3. Malignant: carcinoma and adenocarcinoma
     E. Brenner tumors
        1. Benign
        2. Of borderline malignancy (proliferating)
        3. Malignant
     F. Mixed epithelial tumors
        1. Benign
        2. Of borderline malignancy
        3. Malignant
     G. Undifferentiated carcinoma
     H. Unclassified epithelial tumors

---

*From Serov S.F., Scully R.E.: *Histological Typing of Ovarian Tumors*, International Histological Typing of Tumors no. 9. Geneva, World Health Organization, 1973.

II. Sex cord stromal tumors
  A. Granulosa-stromal tumors
    1. Granulosa cell tumor
    2. Tumors in the thecoma-fibroma group
      a. Thecoma
      b. Fibroma
      c. Unclassified
  B. Androblastomas: Sertoli-Leydig cell tumors
    1. Well differentiated
      a. Tubular androblastoma; Sertoli cell tumor (tubular adenoma of Pick)
      b. Tubular androblastoma with lipid storage; Sertoli cell tumor with lipid storage (folliculome lipidique of Lecene)
      c. Sertoli-Leydig cell tumor (tubular adenoma with Leydig cells)
      d. Leydig cell tumor; hilus cell tumor
    2. Of intermediate differentiation
    3. Poorly differentiated (sarcomatoid)
    4. With heterologous elements
  C. Gynadroblastoma
  D. Unclassified
III. Lipid (lipoid) cell tumors
IV. Germ cell tumors
  A. Dysgerminoma
  B. Endodermal sinus tumor
  C. Embryonal carcinoma
  D. Polyembryoma
  E. Choriocarcinoma
  F. Teratomas
    1. Immature
    2. Mature
      a. Solid
      b. Cystic
        i. Dermoid cyst (mature cystic teratoma)
        ii. Dermoid cyst with malignant transformation

    3. Monod[...] speciali[...]
      a. Stru[...]
      b. Car[...]
      c. Stru[...] carci[...]
      d. Others
  G. Mixed forms
V. Gonadoblastoma
  A. Pure
  B. Mixed with dysgerminoma or other form of germ cell tumor
VI. Soft tissue tumors not specific to ovary
VII. Unclassified tumors
VIII. Secondary (metastatic) tumors
IX. Tumor-like conditions
  A. Pregnancy luteoma
  B. Hyperplasia of ovarian stroma and hyperthecosis
  C. Massive edema
  D. Solitary follicle cyst and corpus luteum cyst
  E. Multiple follicle cysts (polycystic ovaries)
  F. Multiple luteinized follicle cysts and/or corpora lutea
  G. Endometriosis
  H. Surface-epithelial inclusion cysts (germinal inclusion cysts)
  I. Simple cysts
  J. Inflammatory lesions
  K. Parovarian cysts

Incidence

Since the occurrence of benign ovarian tumors within a definable population has not been a matter of record, the true incidence of these tumors has been unknown. The only information available is that provided by Bennington et al. who determined the incidence of selected benign and malignant ovarian neoplasms occurring among members of the Kaiser Foundation Health Plan between the years 1958 and 1963. Since two thirds of the women in the study population were under the age of 45 years the overall incidence cannot be compared with that in the general population. The incidence of serous cystadeno-

which constituted 53% of the benign tumors, began to rise rapidly in adolescence and reached a maximum of about 38 per 100,000 per year by age 30 years. Thereafter, the incidence remained stable until it declined sharply at about age 70 years. Mucinous cystadenomas, which constituted 12% of the group, slowly increased in incidence during adolescence and reached a peak of 13 per 100,000 per year at age 50 years. The incidence of benign cystic teratomas, which constituted 30% of the group, reached a maximum of 30 per 100,000 per year at about age 30 years and then steadily declined to 0 by age 70 years. The international incidence rates for selected ovarian cancers as modified from Berg and Baylor are listed in Table 7–1.

As pointed out by Berg and Baylor, the number of countries represented is small, as are the number of cases reported from many individual areas. Unfortunately a number of the individual reports failed to differentiate between the various epithelial tumors and they are thus reported under the single category "adenocarcinoma."

Based on a number of published series, several general comments may be made regarding the relationship of benign to malignant ovarian neoplasms. Approximately 20% of all ovarian tumors are malignant, but the ratio of benign to malignant tumors declines after age 40 years. In the series reported by Bennington et al. only 6% of ovarian tumors were malignant below the age of 45 years,

TABLE 7–1.—INTERNATIONAL INCIDENCE RATES FOR SELECTED OVARIAN CANCERS*

| REGISTRY | INCIDENCE OF ALL OVARIAN CANCERS† | INCIDENCE OF SPECIFIC TYPES† | | | | NO. OF CASES IN HISTOLOGY SERIES |
		ADENOCARCINOMAS‡	GRANULOSA CELL CANCER	DYSGERMINOMA	MALIGNANT TERATOMA	
Sweden	14.4	11.8	1.2	0.14	0.17	3,060
Alameda County, California (white)	12.6	10.6	0.3	. . .	0.22	286
Southwest region, England	12.2	7.0	0.6	0.20	0.07	846
Connecticut	11.3	13.2	0.7	0.30	0.21	915
Birmingham, England	10.8	7.9	0.3	0.05	0.16	1,235
Alameda County, California (black)	10.4	9.9	0.5	. . .	0.69	27
El Paso, Texas (non-Latin)	9.8	6.7	0.8	. . .	0.11	48
Cali, Colombia	9.2	6.5	1.1	0.19	0.10	88
Vas, Hungary	9.0	2.3	0.1	0.92	0.10	57
El Paso, Texas (Latin)	8.8	5.2	0.2	0.19	0.20	30
Scotland	8.8	4.4	0.3	0.06	0.04	1,206
Slovenia	8.6	5.5	0.2	0.10	0.02	335
Jamaica	8.3	4.9	0.3	0.13	0.32	47
Rural Poland	7.8	3.1	0.5	0.04	. . .	19
Natal, South Africa (African)	6.4	3.1	0.6	. . .	0.20	23
Cracow, Poland	6.3	3.4	0.2	0.14	0.25	118
Bombay, India	6.1	1.7	0.1	0.06	. . .	103
Natal, South Africa (Indian)	3.3	1.2	. . .	. . .	0.45	6

*Modified from Berg J.W., Baylor S.M.: Hum. Pathol. 4:537, 1973.
†Rate per 100,000—age-standardized to world population.
‡Includes all cystadenocarcinomas—mucinous, serous, and unspecified.

whereas 33% were malignant between the ages of 45 and 74 years. The relative frequency of the more common malignant tumors based on recently reported series is given in Table 7–2.

About 4% of ovarian neoplasms are discovered in children under 10 years, and approximately 50% of these are malignant. These are usually solid teratomas or carcinomas, but occasionally a dysgerminoma or granulosa cell tumor may be found. The benign varieties are usually dermoid or epithelial cysts.

Diagnosis

Symptoms

Ovarian neoplasms are frequently asymptomatic. Unfortunately, subjective complaints are likely to occur only after complications arise or the tumor has reached considerable size or, in the case of malignancy, after dissemination has taken place. A recent nationwide survey (Cutler et al., 1976) indicated that 72% of ovarian cancers have disseminated by the time of diagnosis.

Specific symptoms depend on the size, location and type of the tumor, as well as on the presence of complicating factors such as torsion, hemorrhage, infection, or rupture. The usual presenting complaints include lower abdominal pain or pressure or concern for a mass or abdominal enlargement (Table 7–3). Unfortunately, these symptoms are related either to the accumulation of ascites, the size and weight of the tumor, or adherence to surrounding structures with resultant traction

TABLE 7–2.—OVARIAN CANCER—COMMON CELL TYPES AND RELATIVE FREQUENCY

Serous cystadenocarcinoma	40%
Mucinous cystadenocarcinoma	12%
Endometrioid carcinoma	15%
Undifferentiated adenocarcinoma	15%
Clear cell carcinoma (mesonephroma)	6%
Granulosa-theca cell tumor	3%
Dysgerminoma	1%
Malignant teratoma	1%
Metastatic carcinoma*	5%
Others	2%

*Undetected primary cancers mostly of the Krukenberg type.

TABLE 7–3.—SYMPTOMS IN OVARIAN NEOPLASMS

	CASES	
SYMPTOM	NO.	%
Pain or discomfort	198	56.7
Distension or mass	177	50.7
Abnormal uterine bleeding	120	34.4
Urinary	59	16.9
Gastrointestinal	57	16.3

or pressure. In other words, the usual symptoms are those of advanced growth. In some instances, particularly with benign tumors, the diagnosis is made during a routine pelvic examination. When pain is present it is usually not severe and may be described as a mild discomfort in the lower quadrants of the abdomen. The observation that vague digestive disturbances such as flatulence, eructations, and abdominal discomfort may precede other symptoms by many months has led the well-known English gynecologist Stanley Way to query, "How many early carcinomas of the ovary have been nurtured in a sea of bicarbonate of soda. . . ?" The combination of moderate anorexia or indigestion and slight abdominal enlargement should alert the physician to the possibility of ovarian cancer even if a pelvic mass is not readily apparent.

Abnormal uterine bleeding was noted in 34% of patients with ovarian tumors reported from the Boston Hospital for Women (Kent and McKay), and a similar incidence has been reported in other series (see Table 7–3). In a few instances, endometrial metastases and coexistent lesions such as leiomyomas, polyps, and even primary endometrial carcinomas are responsible, but the cause of bleeding is often obscure. Uterine bleeding associated with gonadal stromal tumors known to be hormonally active is easily explained on the basis of endometrial stimulation. It now appears that a number of benign and malignant tumors considered hormonally inactive may also be associated with increased sex steroid production. The origin of these sex steroids has been attributed to the stimulation of normal thecal tissue to produce androstenedione (MacDonald et al.) by adjacent tumor. In a study of 38 postmenopausal patients with ovarian tumors, Rome et al. assessed uterine bleeding and ovarian histology in relation to urinary excretion of estrogens and pregnanediol. Evidence of ovarian hormone production was present in 50% of patients with epithelial and metastatic tumors, and 50% of these experienced postmenopausal bleeding. Stromal proliferation with and without luteinization was noted in 60% of those with elevated hormone levels but in only 13% of those without evidence of hormone production. About 50% of hormonally inactive tumors may increase ovarian steroid production by stimulation of benign stroma. Postmenopausal bleeding associated with a proliferative, hyperplastic, or even an inactive endometrium may be the result of an undetected ovarian tumor.

Other specific complaints may relate to the location, size, and weight of the primary tumor or its metastases. Tumors expanding in the anterior pelvis can exert pressure sufficient to compromise bladder capacity or provide some degree of outflow obstruction. Pressure at the pelvic brim may produce ureteral obstruction and secondary pyelonephritis. In addition to vague digestive complaints, compression of the rectosigmoid by an expanding posterior pelvic mass can cause significant constipation or even partial large bowel obstruction. Similarly, adhesion formation between the tumor and sigmoid colon or terminal ileum may result in torsion and intermittent obstructive symptoms.

Severe pain of sudden onset is indicative of an acute complication. The most common of these is torsion of the ovarian pedicle. Tumors with a narrow or elongated pedicle are most prone to this complication. Benign cystic teratomas (dermoid cysts) are particularly susceptible since they are freely mobile with a slender pedicle and are disproportionately heavy. Twisted ovarian cysts cause severe, localized pain often accompanied by nausea and vomiting. A precedent history of unusual physical activity may be obtained. If the torsion is incomplete, partial occlusion of the blood supply results in venous stasis with extravasation of serum and blood into the cyst cavity. The mass rapidly enlarges, becomes exquisitely tender and is susceptible to rupture or hemorrhage (Fig 7–8). On physical examination there may be abdominal rigidity with local and rebound tenderness. Pelvic examination discloses a firm, tender mass, but the findings may be variable, depending on the size and location of the cyst. If torsion is sufficient to produce obstruction of the arterial supply, infarction and necrosis of the cyst wall may result in perforation and peritonitis. Inadvertent rupture may follow vigorous pelvic examination or handling of the mass at laparotomy. It is generally recommended that ovarian cysts with a twisted pedicle not be unwound prior to removal because of the possibility of venous embolization by thrombi or necrotic debris. Thin-walled cysts of the follicular or corpus luteum type may rupture into the peritoneal cavity and, if accompanied by significant bleeding, symptoms of intraperitoneal hemorrhage and shock may ensue. Ovarian cysts with thicker walls do not often rupture, but perforation of endometriomas may follow a fall or mild abdominal trauma. The release of old blood and debris promptly causes a severe local peritonitis. The rupture of a benign cystic teratoma (dermoid cyst) is catastrophic. An immediate, severe chemical peritonitis produces a clinical picture even more dramatic than that associated with perforation of a hollow viscus.

Hemorrhage into an ovarian cyst is a common complication and may occur spontaneously or as the result of physical trauma. Bleeding can be profuse, filling and enlarging the cystic cavity in the manner of a hemorrhagic corpus luteum. Intermittent hemorrhage with slow growth and thickening of the capsule is common with an endometrioma. Soft, pultaceous tumors such as granulosa cell tumors are particularly prone to vessel rupture and hemorrhage within their substance.

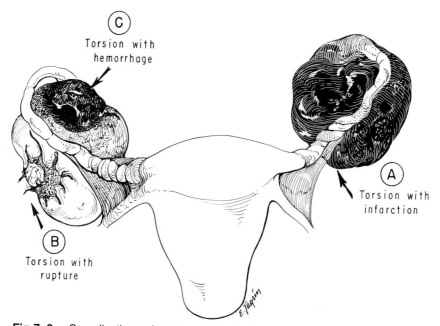

Fig 7–8.—Complications of ovarian cysts: torsion with **A,** infarction; **B,** rupture; and **C,** hemorrhage.

Physical Signs

The diagnosis of an ovarian neoplasm is usually made on bimanual pelvic examination. In order to clearly outline adnexal masses the bladder and lower bowel should be empty and the abdominal musculature relaxed. Rectovaginal examination is essential and allows palpation of the suface of a mass in the posterior cul-de-sac. By displacing the cervix anteriorly, nodularity of the uterosacral ligaments may be detected, suggesting endometriosis or local metastases. A precise preoperative diagnosis of an ovarian neoplasm may be difficult. In our patients with ovarian carcinoma a pelvic mass was noted in 86%, and an abdominal mass in 76%. Huge cysts that fill the abdomen are usually mucinous or serous cystadenomas, but these may be confused with mesenteric cysts or cysts of the kidney or retroperitoneal space. Thin-walled physiologic cysts of the corpus luteum or follicle range from 3 to 6 cm in diameter and because of their mobility may be difficult to palpate. It is generally agreed that these cysts rarely exceed 6 cm in diameter, whereas neo-plastic tumors are rarely smaller than this. This "6-cm rule" is far from infallible. Epithelial carcinomas and granulosa cell tumors, particularly in the older age groups, may be found in ovaries of near-normal size.

A number of palpable characteristics are helpful in differentiating benign from malignant ovarian masses. A smooth, regular surface suggests a benign cyst, whereas an irregular or nodular surface is indicative of malignancy or at the least a multiloculated, serous cystadenoma. Adhesions to the omentum or adherent loops of small bowel mask the size and consistency of an ovarian mass and also suggest malignancy. If there is fixation, the examiner should suspect malignancy, endometriosis, interligamentous growth, simultaneous inflammatory process, or adhesions secondary to necrosis. Otherwise, benign tumors tend not to form adhesions and unless they reach gigantic proportions are quite mobile on manipulation. Consistency can be of diagnostic importance. A soft or somewhat flaccid cystic mass is likely to be a physiologic cyst in the premenopause

or a simple cyst in the postmenopause. A uniformly firm or tensely fluctuant cyst suggests a benign neoplasm. Malignant epithelial tumors often contain cystic areas interspersed with hard nodules or they have a solid consistency. The presence of firm nodules in the cul-de-sac or nodularity along the uterosacral ligaments in association with an ovarian mass strongly suggest either endometriosis or carcinoma with cul-de-sac metastases.

Most ovarian neoplasms are in a position lateral or posterior to the uterus. The benign cystic teratoma (dermoid cyst) is a notable exception and is usually found anterior to the broad ligament. A tumor situated in the posterior pelvis may displace the uterus anteriorly so that the cervical portio lies behind the symphysis pubis. With expanding tumor growth the cervix may actually produce bladder neck obstruction.

Bilateral involvement is indicative of malignancy. In the series reported by Bennington et al., 9% of benign tumors and 42% of malignant tumors were bilateral. In considering benign and malignant tumors as a whole, 16% were bilateral, and of these 53% were malignant.

Clinically evident ascites is present in 25% of patients with malignant ovarian tumors. The aspiration of ascitic fluid for cytologic examination may provide useful information prior to laparotomy. Rarely, benign ovarian tumors, particularly fibromas and serous cystadenomas, are associated with nonmalignant ascites and right pleural effusions. This clinical picture is known as Meigs' syndrome, and the mechanism by which the serous effusions form is unknown. A pleural effusion does not necessarily connote inoperability and should always be tapped for cytologic examination. Occasionally, malignant ovarian tumors are associated with nonmalignant serous effusions ("pseudo-Meigs' syndrome").

Differential Diagnosis

Before proceeding to the various lesions that may be confused with ovarian neoplasms, it should be emphasized that common midline "tumors" that on occasion may simulate an ovarian cyst are a distended urinary bladder and enlargement of the uterus due to an intrauterine pregnancy. The urinary bladder that is tensely distended simulates a large cyst since it displaces the uterus backward, giving the impression of a mass anterior to the broad ligament. It is imperative, therefore, that all patients void before pelvic examination. During the first eight to 12 weeks of pregnancy the uterine corpus is smooth, soft, cystic, and freely mobile. Since the lower uterine segment is particularly soft, the corpus may be palpated as a separate mass unless particular care is taken during examination.

Several conditions involving the colon frequently simulate ovarian neoplasms. These include a low-lying, distended cecum, a redundant sigmoid colon, an appendiceal abscess, impacted feces in the rectosigmoid, carcinoma of the sigmoid, and diverticulitis. A cecum distended with gas, particularly if associated with pain, may simulate a right ovarian cyst (Fig 7–9,A). Careful examination, however, usually reveals marked flaccidity and obvious fluid and gas on compression of the mass. A redundant sigmoid colon may present a similar picture and when filled with fecal material the diagnosis of a firm ovarian neoplasm may be entertained (Fig 7–9,B). A thorough catharsis or enema will resolve the problem.

A localized appendiceal abscess (Fig 7–9, C) may be confused with an ovarian neoplasm undergoing hemorrhage, rupture, or torsion. A previous history of upper abdominal or periumbilical pain associated with nausea, vomiting, and subsequent localization of the pain in the right lower quadrant together with local peritoneal signs will aid in diagnosis. Occasionally, however, the initial symptoms of acute appendicitis are obscure and the abscess develops gradually with the formation of a thick, adherent capsule.

A firm, fixed mass in the left pelvis of women over age 50 years strongly suggests carcinoma of the ovary or rectosigmoid (Fig 7–9,D). A history of altered bowel habits, col-

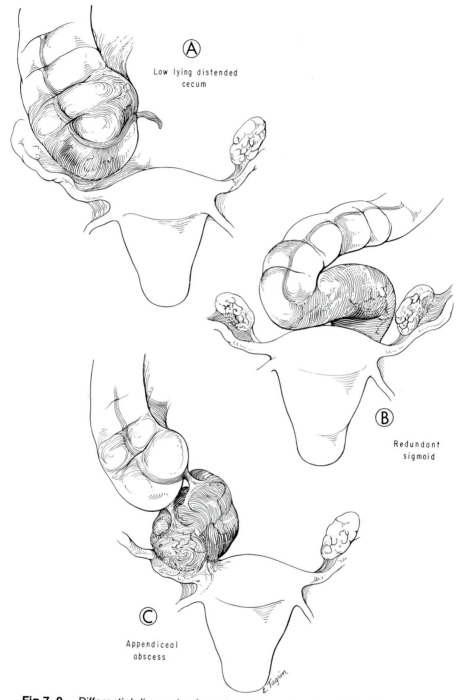

Fig 7–9.—Differential diagnosis of ovarian lesions. **A,** redundant or distended cecum; **B,** redundant sigmoid colon; **C,** appendiceal abscess. *(Continued)*

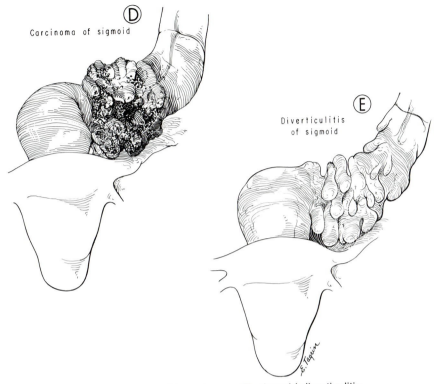

Fig 7–9 (cont.).—D, sigmoid carcinoma; **E,** sigmoid diverticulitis.

icky pain, blood or melena, or diminution in the caliber of the stool suggests sigmoid cancer. The diagnosis is confirmed by barium enema or sigmoidoscopy and biopsy of the tumor mass. In some cases, however, the sigmoid colon and left ovary are so intimately adherent in a carcinomatous process that even the pathologist finds it impossible to determine the primary site.

Diverticulitis of the sigmoid colon (Fig 7–9,E) is a frequent cause of erroneous gynecologic diagnoses. Although many women over age 40 years have asymptomatic diverticulosis, a mass in the left side of the pelvis following rupture of a diverticulum may be difficult to distinguish from ovarian cancer. A typical attack of diverticulitis is manifested by intermittent cramplike abdominal pain, usually in the left lower quadrant, associated with diarrhea, and small amounts of blood and mucus in the stool. Evidence of peritoneal irritation together with leukocytosis and fever aid in the differential diagnosis. Pelvic examination will elicit localized tenderness but otherwise is not of great value since perforation results in a firm mass that lodges in the left side of the pelvis or iliac fossa. Diagnosis will depend on a barium enema, which should be done during a quiescent period of the disease and should reveal diverticula, an irritable colon, and areas of stenosis.

The oviduct or mesosalpinx may also give rise to cystic structures, which must be differentiated from those arising in the ovary. A parovarian cyst may arise from the rudimentary structures in the mesosalpinx and develop between the leaves of the broad ligament. These cysts are usually unilateral, somewhat fixed, ovoid, and thin walled. A tubal ectopic pregnancy may closely simulate an acute accident arising in an ovarian tumor, such as torsion or hemorrhage. Symptoms

suggesting pregnancy and a chorionic gonadotropin level by β-subunit assay will aid in the correct diagnosis. The signs associated with a ruptured ectopic pregnancy may be exactly the same as those associated with a ruptured ovarian cyst; in this case the diagnosis can be made by operative means. Perhaps the lesion most commonly mistaken for an ovarian tumor is a pedunculated uterine leiomyoma, particularly if the tumor is solitary and somewhat soft. Such leiomyomas ("fibroids") are usually freely mobile, but careful examination will reveal an area of attachment to the uterus. It is impossible to delineate adequately a parasitic or intraligamentous fibroid (Fig 7–10,A) since these lesions are relatively fixed and may be situated in areas directly adjacent to the ovary. If the pedicle of a pedunculated fibroid undergoes torsion and infarction, the presenting signs and symptoms will be indistinguishable from those of a twisted ovarian cyst.

Other lesions that, although rare, may simulate ovarian tumors are a hematoma of the rectus muscle, a desmoid tumor, urachal cyst, and a retroperitoneal neoplasm or abscess. A hematoma of the rectus muscle (Fig 7–10,B) usually follows trauma or unusual strain, but there may be no antecedent history of the latter, particularly in patients receiving anticoagulants who appear to be predisposed. The superficial location of the mass usually can be demonstrated by tensing the abdominal muscles. A desmoid tumor may arise in the suprapubic portion of the anterior abdominal wall and in this location may closely simulate a fixed, firm ovarian mass lying anterior to the broad ligament. A urachal cyst (Fig 7–10,C) in the same area may present a similar clinical picture. An ectopic kidney situated in the pelvis deserves special comment (Fig 7–10,D). The use of intravenous urograms before laparotomy for a suspected ovarian cyst is of great importance in delineating the position of the kidneys and ureters. Retroperitoneal pelvic tumors such as fibromas, sarcomas, dermoids, and malignant teratomas may extend into the lower pelvis. Their presence may be suspected by intravenous urography but exact diagnosis can only be made after surgical exploration. Similarly, certain abscesses originating in the spine or perivesical areas may be confused with firm ovarian masses.

The accumulation of ascitic fluid within the peritoneal cavity may give the impression of a large, thin-walled ovarian cyst. In the presence of ascites, however, the small intestine is located centrally, resulting in a tympanitic percussion note in midabdomen and shifting dullness in the flanks. In addition, a definite fluid wave should be present. By comparison, a large ovarian cyst will displace the small intestine laterally so that percussion reveals tympany laterally.

Roentgenography should always be employed in the preoperative evaluation of patients with pelvic masses. Foci of calcification representing teeth are pathognomonic of a benign cystic teratoma. Diffuse, hazy calcification over the tumor area strongly suggests multiple psammoma bodies within a serous tumor. Intravenous urography often reveals a pressure effect of the tumor on bladder or ureter and, on occasion, obviates further diagnostic or therapeutic procedures by the disclosure of a pelvic kidney that has simulated an adnexal mass. A contrast study of the colon also should be performed for the reasons just noted.

In some instances laparoscopy may differentiate between a pedunculated leiomyoma and an ovarian mass or between a physiologic cyst and an ovarian neoplasm. The external appearance of an ovarian mass may be deceiving, however, and when any doubt exists endoscopic procedures must not replace exploratory laparotomy.

As with most disease processes, routine laboratory determinations are of importance. Anemia may be secondary to abnormal uterine bleeding or hemorrhage into a cystic mass or the peritoneal cavity. On the other hand, severe anemia may be associated with ovarian carcinoma and represent inhibitory effects of the tumor on bone marrow that cannot keep pace with normal or accelerated red cell de-

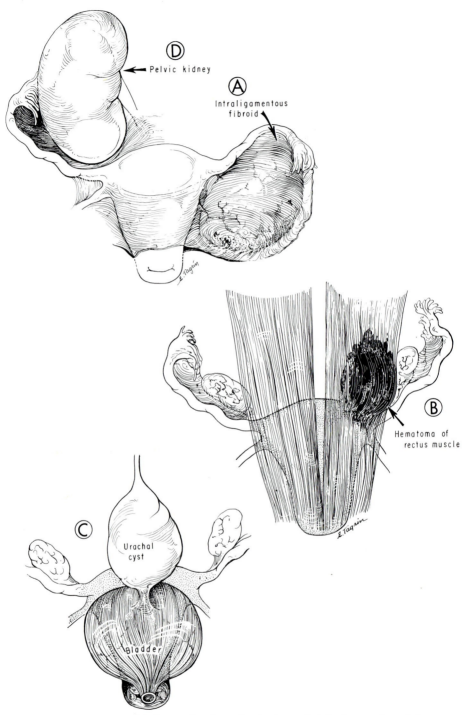

Fig 7–10.—Differential diagnosis of ovarian lesions. **A,** intraligamentous leiomyoma; **B,** hematoma of the rectus muscle; **C,** urachal cyst; **D,** ectopic kidney.

struction. Although neoplasia may be associated with mild elevations of the leukocyte count and sedimentation rate, marked elevations of these above-normal values suggest a pelvic inflammatory process. The elevation of certain nonspecific oncofetal tumor markers and products of tumor catabolism have been noted with ovarian malignancies, and their determinations may assist in preoperative evaluation as well as postoperative follow-up. For example, among patients with advanced ovarian carcinoma, carcinoembryonic antigen is elevated in 21%, alkaline phosphatase (Regan isoenzyme) in 46%, chorionic gonadotropin in 34%, lactic dehydrogenase in 100%, and fibrin split products in 72%.

Non-neoplastic Cysts of Graafian Follicle Origin

In any consideration of ovarian neoplasms the student and clinician must be familiar with the physiologic variations of the ovulatory cycle that occasionally result in a non-neoplastic cyst. By definition, physiologic cysts are incapable of autonomous growth, but on the basis of clinical signs and symptoms as well as gross appearance they may be indistinguishable from true ovarian neoplasms. The normal ovary from a fertile patient usually has as many as eight to ten follicles visible on midsagittal section, which vary from 3 to 5 mm in diameter and show varying degrees of congestion, hemorrhage, and luteinization. In patients who ovulate infrequently the ovary may contain multiple cystic

follicles, each about 1 to 2 cm in diameter, which are thin-walled and project above the ovarian surface. Since all follicles are cystic to some degree, we have arbitrarily adopted a diameter of 2.5 cm as the dividing line between a cystic follicle and an actual follicle cyst.

Follicle cysts may occur at any age before the menopause and on occasion reach a diameter of 7 to 8 cm. An ovary containing a single large follicle cyst is usually asymptomatic, but may give rise to a sense of pelvic discomfort or heaviness on the affected side. Because of associated hormonal activity, the patient may have noted irregularity of the menstrual cycle such as delayed flow followed by irregular and intermittent spotting. The latter symptoms are likely to induce the patient to seek medical consultation, at which time the cyst is discovered. Occasionally, spontaneous rupture and subsequent bleeding, which is usually self-limited, produces acute pelvic pain.

Grossly, follicle cysts are thin-walled and translucent, although occasionally intracystic bleeding may impart a dark-brown appearance. Granulosa and theca-interna cells show varying degrees of luteinization. The granulosa cells may be slightly pleomorphic and have relatively large nuclei (Fig 7–11). In larger cysts only a few granulosa cells may be identified, and the cells of the theca interna and externa show areas of luteinization and hyalinization, respectively, depending on the age of the cyst (Fig 7–12).

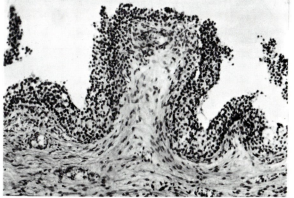

Fig 7–11.—Wall of follicle cyst, showing pleomorphism of the inner granulosa cells and a moderately well-preserved theca layer. (From Hertig A.T., Gore H.: Tumors of the female sex organs: part 3. Tumors of the ovary and fallopian tube, sec. IX, fasc. 33 of *Atlas of Tumor Pathology.* Washington, D.C., Armed Forces Institute of Pathology, 1961.)

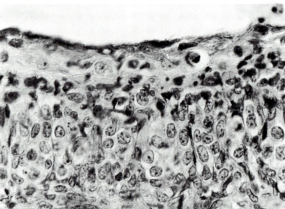

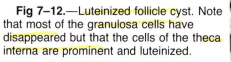

Fig 7–12.—Luteinized follicle cyst. Note that most of the granulosa cells have disappeared but that the cells of the theca interna are prominent and luteinized.

On pelvic examination follicle cysts are mobile and somewhat soft on compression. Occasionally they are inadvertently ruptured during examination. Treatment of a follicle cyst should be conservative unless rupture and hemorrhage warrant surgical intervention. If the cyst is less than 6 cm in diameter the patient should have a pelvic examination every three or four weeks. If examination is performed after the next menstrual period, the cyst will often have disappeared. For cysts 6 cm or larger or those that persist through two or more menstrual cycles, laparoscopy may clarify the diagnosis. When doubt exists, laparotomy is indicated. Since follicle cysts are dependent on pituitary gonadotropic stimulation, we have used oral contraceptives to hasten their disappearance. With this program, all non-neoplastic cysts of this type have regressed within 20 days.

Cystic Structures Derived From the Normally Ruptured Follicle

Corpus Luteum Cyst

The mature corpus luteum has a central core filled with blood. After resorption, the cavity normally may be distended with hemorrhagic or clear fluid, making the corpus luteum itself a cystic structure. A corpus luteum cyst results from an abnormal persistence or exaggeration of this physiologic process. If the normal organization of the coagulum by fibroblasts is prevented or if there

is extensive bleeding into the cavity, an abnormally functioning cyst will result. Such a *corpus luteum hematoma* may cause local pain, amenorrhea, and signs closely resembling a tubal ectopic pregnancy. Although most hematomas of the corpus luteum do not exceed 7 or 8 cm, several as large as 11 cm in diameter have been described. Following the resorption of the blood, a typical corpus luteum cyst may evolve.

The diagnosis of a corpus luteum cyst cannot be made with exact precision but should be suspected in a patient who has noted delayed menses followed by irregular staining and a constant discomfort or sense of heaviness in one side of the pelvis. A positive diagnosis of a corpus luteum cyst or hematoma can usually be made by laparoscopy.

A ruptured hemorrhagic corpus luteum may result in all the signs and symptoms of intraperitoneal bleeding. Rupture may occur following pelvic examination, strenuous exercise, or even coitus. The clinical picture includes lower abdominal pain, nausea and vomiting, rectus muscle spasm, and rebound tenderness. Pelvic examination will reveal an enlarged, tender ovary or, if bleeding has been extensive, a doughy or fluctuant cul-de-sac. The temperature may be elevated to 100.4 F, and moderate leukocytosis is usually present. The blood loss occasionally is severe, exceeding 1,000 ml.

Gross examination of a corpus luteum cyst

or hematoma reveals the yellowish color in the thin wall of the cyst. Microscopically, the typical cyst will show all the elements of the normal corpus luteum (see Fig 7–7). Both granulosa and theca-lutein cells will be found in the wall, together with organizing fibrous connective tissue and erythrocytes. If a corpus luteum hematoma is small, spontaneous regression will occur, giving rise to a corpus albicans cyst. The corpus luteum of early pregnancy is a cystic structure that occasionally gives rise to unilateral pain and is sometimes confused with an unruptured ectopic pregnancy. During pregnancy the corpus luteum functions for a variable time, usually six to nine weeks, occasionally somewhat longer.

Physiologic ovarian cysts of large size may be associated with hydatidiform mole, chorioadenoma destruens, or choriocarcinoma. They result from the stimulus of excessive chorionic gonadotropic hormone secreted by these trophoblastic tumors. Bilateral lutein cysts occur in about one third of these patients. Surgical extirpation of the ovaries is not necessary, however, since lutein cysts gradually regress and the ovaries return to normal size and function after removal of the trophoblastic tissue. These cysts may reach rather large proportions, filling the pelvic cavity on both sides. Each large cyst is made up of multiple locules varying from 1 to 2 cm in diameter. Each locule contains a clear yellow fluid, and each cystic cavity is lined by luteinized theca-interna cells, which resemble the lutein cells of the corpus luteum.

Luteoma of Pregnancy

The pseudotumors known as luteoma of pregnancy were first described by Sternberg in 1963. They consist of hyperplastic nodules of luteinized theca cells, which are multiple in 50% of reported cases, and involve both ovaries in 30% of cases. In contrast to the theca-lutein cyst, which is a physiologic response to elevated levels of chorionic gonadotropin, the luteoma represents an exaggerated response to normal levels of chorionic gonadotropin. Although the pregnancy lu-

teoma may obtain a diameter of 16 cm, most have been discovered at cesarean section. Spontaneous regression of the nodules has been noted consistently during the postpartum period. In 1975 Garcia-Bunuel et al. contributed 20 cases of pregnancy luteoma to the literature, bringing the total number of reported cases to 74. The most dramatic feature of the pregnancy luteoma has been the frequent association with maternal and fetal virilization. In 22 of the 74 reported cases maternal virilization was evident; among these, seven of 11 female neonates were also virilized. In all instances, virilizing signs regressed post partum.

The Simple Cyst

The simple cyst rarely arouses the interest of pathologists but is of considerable importance to clinicians in light of its frequent occurrence during the menopausal years. These cysts are translucent, thin-walled structures that contain a thin serous fluid and are somewhat soft to palpation. They rarely exceed 10 cm in diameter. Their internal surface is impeccably smooth and free of papillary projections. Although simple cysts are almost always unilateral, the opposite ovary usually contains a number of germinal inclusion cysts.

Microscopically, the internal surface is lined by flattened mesothelial cells resembling peritoneum, but areas of cuboidal cells consistent with coelomic metaplasia are often present. Simple cysts are most likely derived from germinal inclusion cysts in which the reversionary coelomic epithelium has undergone complete or partial regression after cystic enlargement. In the event of differentiation rather than regression, cysts of identical gross appearance are lined by tubal-type epithelium. These serous cystomas are usually categorized with the serous cystadenomas despite their lack of proliferative activity.

Simple cysts are surprisingly persistent and since they occur in postmenopausal women early laparotomy is required to exclude a malignant process. Both ovaries should be removed because of the possibility that a second simple cyst or cystadenoma will arise in the contralateral ovary.

Cystomas of Germinal Epithelial Origin (Common Epithelial Tumors)

Most clinically important ovarian neoplasms fall into the category of cystomas of germinal epithelial origin (see Table 7–2). These tumors include the serous and mucinous cystadenomas and cystadenocarcinomas, benign and malignant endometrioid tumors, the clear cell carcinomas, and the rarely malignant Brenner tumor. Hertig's all-inclusive term, *cystoma*, is appropriate since, to a varying degree, cyst formation is a histogenetic characteristic. With progressive epithelial proliferation, however, all of the cystomas, particularly endometrioid and clear cell carcinomas, tend to become solid in nature. Those epithelial tumors in which the stroma predominates, such as cystadenofibromas and Brenner tumors, have a solid morphology from the outset.

The histogenesis of the ovarian cystomas represents one of the more curious phenomena in human biology. McKay (1962) and Lauchlan (1972) have described graphically the process whereby germinal epithelium recapitulates the embryogenesis of the müllerian duct with which it shares a common derivation from the coelomic epithelium of the urogenital ridge. The germinal epithelium of the adult ovary consists of a flattened layer of mesothelial cells indistinguishable from other visceral peritoneum. Although the mechanism is unclear, the surface of the aging ovary becomes progressively convoluted, forming irregular gyri and sulci. Cystoma histogenesis begins with metaplasia of mesothelium within the sulci to form cuboidal epithelium that resembles primitive coelomic epithelium (see Fig 7–5). This process has been called "reversionary metaplasia" by McKay, and the invaginated "coelomic epithelium" is a simulation of the initial step in müllerian-duct formation. In most instances the surface continuity of deep mesothelial invaginations is closed off by intervening stroma, thereby forming germinal inclusion cysts or "cortical glands," a common finding in the postmenopausal ovary (see Fig 7–6).

In the event of neoplastic transformation, the new coelomic epithelium undergoes proliferation, and concurrent cellular differentiation to specific cell types completes the embryologic recapitulation of the müllerian duct lumen. Consequently, the tumor epithelium may resemble endosalpinx (serous cystoma), endocervix (mucinous cystoma), or endometrium (endometrioid cystoma) (Fig 7–13). Scully (1970) has suggested that the clear cell carcinoma is an endometrial variant, although benign and malignant aggregates of the component cells may be found at other locations in the female genital tract. Despite a probable derivation from germinal epithelium, the Brenner tumor is not a convincing example of müllerian differentiation since its characteristic cell resembles urinary bladder epithelium. Nevertheless, the epithelial elements of Brenner tumors and mucinous tumors are frequently mixed. It is apparent that müllerian differentiation from reversionary coelomic epithelium may proceed in several directions simultaneously since a number of tumors containing various mixtures of serous, mucinous, endometrioid, and clear cell components within a single cyst have been described.

The stages of cystoma histogenesis may be summarized as (1) invagination, (2) coelomic metaplasia, (3) occlusion and cyst formation, (4) proliferation, and (5) differentiation. These steps may not always follow the sequence, and they may not all take place. Without deep invagination or isolation from the surface, cyst formation fails and the result is a papillary epithelial tumor on the surface of the ovary. Should proliferation not take place, a unilocular cyst lined by a single cell layer is formed—the simple serous cyst. The end result of proliferation without differentiation is the highly anaplastic undifferentiated carcinoma.

Both misunderstanding and controversy have resulted from frequent reference to the "müllerian origin" of the common epithelial

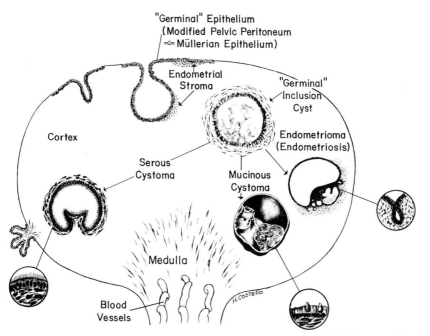

Fig 7–13.—Schematic diagram of origin of ovarian cystomas from surface or "germinal" epithelium. On the surface are a papillary outgrowth of germinal epithelium, an early infolding, a later stage of infolding, and a small focus of endometrial-type stroma lying beneath the germinal epithelium. A germinal inclusion cyst is lying within the cortex and is surrounded mainly by ovarian cortical stroma and partly by endometrial stroma. The three main derivatives are shown. (From Hertig A.T., Gore H.: *Rocky Mt. Med. J.* 55:47–50, 1958.)

tumors. This concept is clearly incorrect since these tumors do not arise from the müllerian duct but rather represent metaplastic müllerian epithelium at ectopic sites. Woodruff and Telinde have pointed out that the ovarian cystomas arise from mesothelium and that histologically identical tumors occasionally arise from extragonadal pelvic peritoneum. As pointed out by Hertig and Gore, the peritoneal mesothelium of the pelvis has the potential for coelomic metaplasia and müllerian differentiation. In an excellent review of the subject, Lauchlan has suggested that the term *secondary müllerian epithelium* be used to denote any epithelium derived from peritoneum that closely resembles one of the cell types lining the müllerian duct. These cell types include the endosalpinx, endometrium, and endocervix, but not the squamous epithelium of the exocervix. The propensity of peritoneum for *secondary müllerian* differentia-

tion is greatest overlying the ovary and is decremental as the distance from the ovary increases. Consequently, small serous inclusion cysts are most frequently found on the ovary, tube, uterine serosa, anterior and posterior cul-de-sacs, and lateral pelvic peritoneum, in that order. As a rule, these cysts are barely visible and this condition, known as endosalpingiosis, is usually an independent finding of the pathologist. In summary, the ovarian cystomas and their peritoneal counterparts consist of secondary müllerian epithelium derived by metaplasia from certain areas of mesothelium that have retained a specific embryonic potential.

Serous Cystadenomas and Cystadenocarcinoma

The serous cystomas are the most common of all benign and malignant ovarian neoplasms. They are characterized by an epithelium that closely resembles that of the oviduct, although the degree of resemblance is dependent on differentiation of the tumor epithelium. Variations within this cell type, however, depend on the architectural pattern of tumor growth as well as the degree of epithelial differentiation.

Serous cystadenomas constitute about 25% of benign ovarian tumors. They may be unilocular or multilocular and are bilateral in 15% of cases. They usually do not exceed 10 cm in diameter; rarely, they may become enormous, filling the entire abdomen. The surface is smooth and tends to be grayish white with multiple, fine blood vessels visible beneath the serosal surface. Intracystic bleeding may impart a purplish hue. In its most simple form, the inner surface is lined by epithelium indistinguishable from that of the fallopian tube (Figs 7–14 and 7–15). Multiple, small papillary structures that barely project above the cyst wall give the internal surface a roughened or velvety appearance. The cyst fluid is usually thin and serous but it may be slightly mucoid, indicating that some mucinous epithelium is present. Although tumor

enlargement occurs by fluid accumulation and expansion into newly formed locules, intracystic proliferation may proceed with the formation of larger and more complex papillary structures. It is at this point that the potentially malignant nature of a serous cystadenoma may for the first time become apparent. In those tumors destined to remain benign, the papillary structure is simple and consists of a broad, dense fibrous stroma covered by a single layer of columnar cells (Fig 7–16). The presence of ciliated, secretory, and peg cells maintains the resemblance to tubal epithelium. At the time of operation a serous cystadenoma rarely arouses suspicion of malignancy. The operative procedure performed depends on the age of the patient and her preference regarding ovarian conservation. In women over 40 years of age a complete hysterectomy and bilateral salpingo-oophorectomy are indicated. In younger patients the cyst should be enucleated and opened by the pathologist in the operating room. Gross inspection should reveal the papillary nature of the cyst, although on occasion a rapid histologic section is required. Rapid histologic sec-

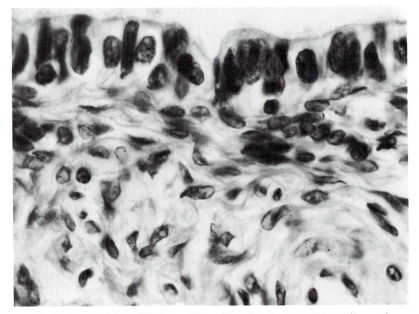

Fig 7–14.—Tubal epithelium. Note ciliated cells, secretory cells, and peg cells. The epithelium of serous cysts simulates this epithelium.

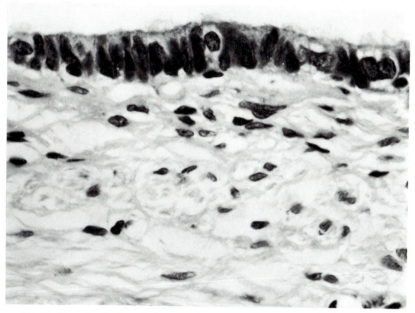

Fig 7–15.—Epithelium lining a serous cyst. Compare with Figure 7–14. (From McKay D.G.: *Clin. Obstet. Gynecol.* 5:1189, 1962.)

tions, however, are unreliable in assessing the degree of proliferation and the possibility of malignancy. After the diagnosis of a papillary tumor has been established, the remainder of the ovary should be removed. The opposite ovary has a 15% chance of containing a similar, though inapparent, cyst and therefore should be bisected and carefully inspected. Other than complete abdominal exploration, any further treatment should await examina-

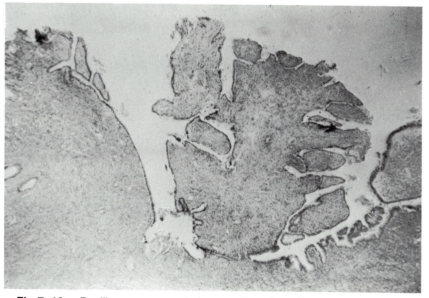

Fig 7–16.—Papillary serous cystadenoma. Broad papillae are covered by a single layer of columnar epithelium.

tion of the permanent histologic sections and discussion with the patient. The prognosis is excellent following surgical extirpation of these lesions and even the threat of a retained contralateral ovary appears minimal.

The malignant potential of a serous cystadenoma is first manifested by a proliferation of the epithelium of the small papillae. The epithelium lining the cyst wall usually retains its original appearance, whereas the papillary epithelium becomes pseudostratified or stratified with a loss of differentiation (Fig 7–17, A). With progressive growth, cellular pleomorphism and increased numbers of mitotic figures become prominent. As the epithelial growth exceeds that of the stroma, tufts of malignant-appearing cells become detached from the papillae and float freely in the cyst

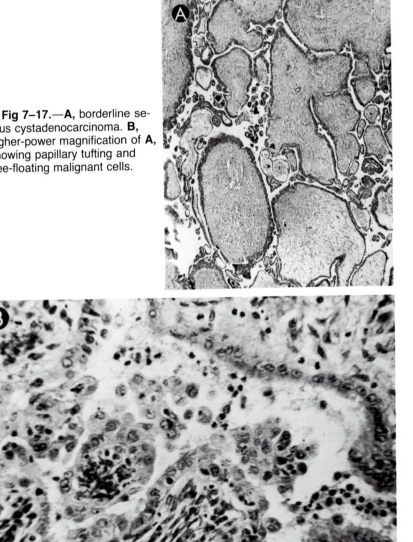

Fig 7–17.—A, borderline serous cystadenocarcinoma. **B,** higher-power magnification of **A,** showing papillary tufting and free-floating malignant cells.

fluid (Fig 7–17,B). Rapid proliferation of serous epithelium is often accompanied by the formation of microscopic calcospherites known as psammoma bodies. These tiny spherical laminated structures are usually found in areas of cellular degeneration. Aure et al. have described an improved prognosis if serous cystadenocarcinomas contain psammoma bodies. Most serous cystadenomas of low-potential malignancy (borderline serous cystadenocarcinomas) fit this description. Most important, there is no evidence of infiltrative growth into the tumor stroma. The justification for this intermediate category is based on clinical outcome. In the series reported by Santesson, the ten-year survival rate in cases of borderline serous cystadenoma was 76%, whereas the corresponding figure for serous cystadenocarcinomas was only 13%. Aure et al. found that 21% of the proliferating serous tumors were of the borderline category and that more than half of these women were under age 45 years. The relative frequency of borderline serous tumors among women during the childbearing years has been noted by others who have demonstrated that removal of the involved ovary has provided adequate therapy if the tumor was confined to that ovary. Approximately one third of borderline serous cystadenomas are bilateral; thus, wedge biopsy of the contralateral ovary is an essential part of a conservative therapeutic regimen.

In the case of serous cystadenocarcinomas, the papillary growth pattern, though similar to that just described, is more extensive. Invasion of the papillary stroma or the tumor capsule may occur even when the cystic tumor is small (Fig 7–18,A). The stroma itself is diminished by rapid epithelial proliferation, and long, thin branching papillae tend to coalesce and form friable, cauliflower-like masses. About one fourth of the serous cystadenocarcinomas are primarily cystic; two thirds are semisolid; and one twelfth are entirely solid. Papillary growth on the external surface of the cyst usually follows perforation of the capsule by invasive tumor. Microscopically, the epithelium shows varying degrees of differentiation. In the well-differentiated tumors the epithelium continues to resemble that of the oviduct, and ciliated cells may occasionally be found. In addition, the architecture consists of well-formed, frondlike papillary structures. The coalescence of the papillae and formation of solid areas is accompanied by a loss of epithelial differentiation (Fig 7–18,B). The cellular layer increases in thickness with increasing mitotic activity and the resemblance to tubal epithelium diminishes. In the poorly differentiated tumors, the papillary architecture may be barely evident within large solid areas, and the diagnosis of a serous tumor can be made only by a thorough search for better differentiated epithelium. Approximately 25% of serous cystadenocarcinomas are well differentiated (grade 1), 35% are moderately well differentiated (grade 2), and 40% are poorly differentiated (grade 3). The prognosis of patients with this tumor is related to the degree of differentiation. This relationship and treatment of serous cystadenocarcinomas are discussed in the section, "Carcinoma of the Ovary."

SEROUS CYSTADENOFIBROMA.—A cystadenofibroma is usually defined as a cystadenoma in which at least one fourth of the tumor mass consists of fibrous stroma. Although the cystadenofibroma has been considered a distinct cell type in the past, we agree with Scully and Lauchlan that it is an architectural variant of the serous cystadenoma. The epithelial component is almost always tubal in character, and the connective tissue originates from the cortical stroma, the tunica albuginea, or both. These tumors vary considerably in size but may reach 20 cm in diameter. They are bilateral in 15% of cases. The proportion of stroma to epithelium is extremely variable. Thus, the microscopic appearance may be that of a cystic tumor with broad polypoid papillae or that of a solid fibrous tumor interspersed with spherical glandlike structures (Fig 7–19). Occasionally, large luteinized theca cells have been found in the stroma and

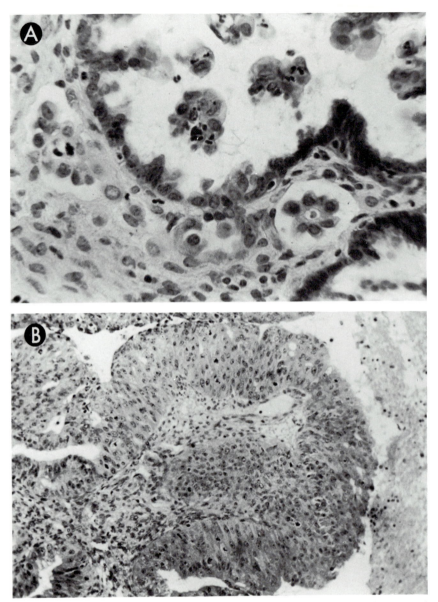

Fig 7–18.—A, early stromal invasion in a well-differentiated serous cystadenocarcinoma. **B,** massive stromal invasion in a poorly differentiated serous cystadenocarcinoma.

may be responsible for the estrogen secretion frequently attributed to cystadenofibromas. Papadiki and Beilby demonstrated a number of stromal cells with the ultrastructural characteristics of steroid-producing theca cells. These tumors are rarely malignant. In comparing 34 cystadenofibromas with 39 cystadenomas, Czernobilsky et al. found no epithelial proliferation or atypia among the former tumors, whereas 6% of the cystadenomas demonstrated epithelial tufting, mitotic activity, and nuclear atypia.

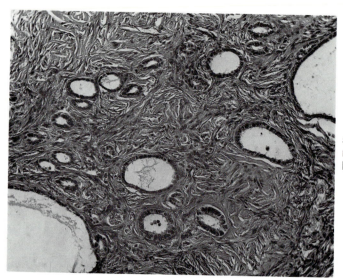

Fig 7–19.—Cystadenofibroma, showing a dense connective tissue matrix containing cysts lined by cuboidal or columnar epithelium.

Mucinous Cystadenoma and Cystadenocarcinoma

Mucinous cell types constitute 12% of the common epithelial tumors, and 12% of these are malignant. Although a germinal epithelial origin with endocervical differentiation has been generally accepted, considerable doubt has been cast on the concept of a uniform histogenetic pathway. Nevertheless, the frequent admixture of mucinous epithelium with serous, endometrioid, and clear-cell elements within individual cystomas supports a germinal epithelial origin (Fig 7–20). On the basis of both light and electron microscopy, Fenoglio et al. classified benign mucinous cystadenomas into two types: a pure endocervical type and a mixed intestinal endocervical type. Ten of 14 tumors studied were of the former type, and four tumors were of the mixed variety. Since most mucinous tumors contained pure endocervical epithelium, whereas none contained pure intestinal epithelium, the authors concluded that a germ cell origin was unlikely. They admit, however, that the presence of mature intestinal epithelium in the mixed type requires accep-

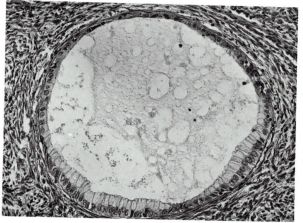

Fig 7–20.—Early mucinous cystoma arising in a germinal inclusion cyst. Note tall columnar epithelium gradually merging into the indifferent cuboidal germinal epithelium of the cyst. (From Hertig A.T., Mansell H., in Anderson W.A.D. [ed.]: *Pathology*, ed. 3. St. Louis, C.V. Mosby Co., 1957.)

tance of a difficult concept: that metaplasia in a structure of mesodermal origin can result in an endodermal derivative. The authors support this concept by drawing a parallel with a metaplastic process commonly seen in chronically irritated urothelium. The conditions known as cystitis cystica, ureteritis cystica, and pyelitis cystica represent areas of mesodermally derived urothelium that have undergone metaplasia to mature intestinal epithelium.

Although mucinous cystadenomas occur most often during the third to fifth decade, rare instances have been reported in infants and children, and about 10% are found in postmenopausal patients. The malignant variety is most common during the fourth to sixth decades.

Grossly, the outer surface is generally smooth, lobulated, and gray-white in color. Seventy percent of the benign and malignant mucinous cystadenomas are multilocular. Although mucinous tumors range from microscopic size to 50 cm in diameter, most are between 15 and 30 cm and weigh between 2,000 and 4,000 gm. The largest tumor on record is said to have weighed 328 lb. The serosal surface of the malignant form may show extracystic papillary growth, which becomes densely adherent to adjacent structures, particularly

the bowel and bladder. When invasion of the capsule is extensive, rupture of the tumor may occur. Benign tumors are usually not fixed to adjacent structures and are therefore susceptible to torsion. This complication has been reported in as high as 20% of cases.

On section, the number and size of the cystic cavities vary with the amount of stroma. The internal surface of the mucinous cystadenoma is smooth or velvety and does not contain solid or nodular areas. Almost 25% of benign tumors and the greater proportion of malignant tumors will contain intracystic papillary projections, which arouse the suspicion of malignancy. Solid areas and firm nodules are found in about 50% of borderline mucinous tumors and in about 75% of obviously malignant tumors.

Microscopically, the mucinous cystadenomas contain cysts lined by a single layer of well-differentiated mucinous epithelium, which closely resembles that of the endocervix except for the absence of ciliated cells (Fig 7–21). Goblet cells and argentaffin cells are present in approximately 30% of tumors. The presence of papillary processes does not connote malignancy, provided there is neither nuclear atypism nor stratification of the epithelium (Fig 7–22).

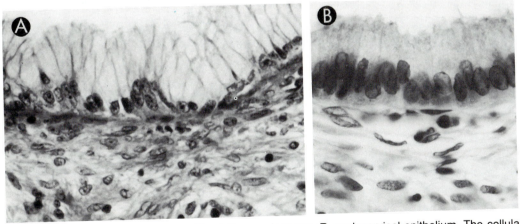

Fig 7–21.—**A,** mucinous cystoma. The tall columnar "picket" cells resemble the secretory cells of the endocervix. The intracytoplasmic mucin and basal location of the nuclei are characteristic features. **B,** endocervical epithelium. The cellular arrangement is slightly more orderly than in **A,** and occasional cells are ciliated. (From McKay D.G.: *Clin. Obstet. Gynecol.* 5:1186, 1962.)

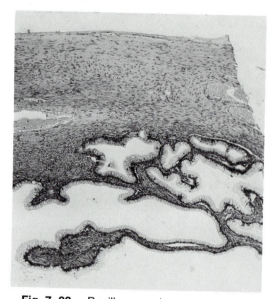

Fig 7–22.—Papillary mucinous cystadenoma with a single layer of well-differentiated mucin-secreting cells. (Compare with Fig 7–21, B). The secondary cysts in connective tissue wall do not represent invasion. (From Hertig A.T., Gore H.: Tumors of the female sex organs: part 3. Tumors of the ovary and fallopian tube, sec. 9, fasc. 33, *Atlas of Tumor Pathology*. Washington, D.C., Armed Forces Institute of Pathology, 1961.)

In considering the borderline and malignant mucinous tumors as a whole, the borderline group constituted 39% in the series reported by Aure et al. and 71% of the stage I cystadenocarcinomas in Hart's and Norris' se-

ries. Microscopically, the borderline tumors contain secondary cysts and short papillary infoldings. The papillary projections tend to be fine and branching and are supported by a delicate connective tissue stroma (Fig 7–23). The cysts are lined by atypical cells, which are stratified into two or three layers and contain variable amounts of intracytoplasmic mucin. The nuclei are irregular and hyperchromatic, and mitotic figures may be abundant. Papillary formation is somewhat greater in the mucinous cystadenocarcinomas and the marked proliferation of epithelial cells results in a thick, stratified epithelium composed of atypical cells (Fig 7–24). Because a glandular pattern within the stroma is common, invasion has been difficult to determine without reservation. Hart and Norris have suggested that even though invasion is not demonstrable, stratification of atypical epithelium exceeding three cells in thickness should indicate that the lesion is in fact malignant. In their series of 27 patients with stage I cystadenocarcinomas, stromal invasion was identified in only 56%, but the five-year survival rate was 65%. In contrast, the five- and ten-year survival rates for patients with borderline tumors were 98% and 96%, respectively.

As a group, the mucinous cystadenocarcinomas are less malignant than their serous counterparts. In the series reported by

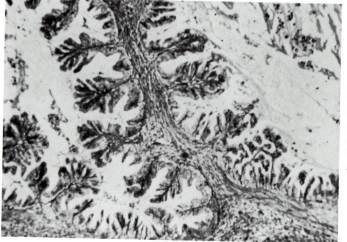

Fig 7–23.—Borderline mucinous cystadenocarcinoma. The papillary projections are fine and branching. In many areas the epithelial layer is two or three cells in thickness. (From McKay D.G.: *Clin. Obstet. Gynecol.* 5:1190, 1962.)

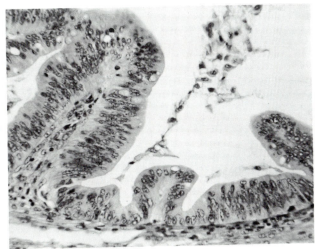

Fig 7–24.—Mucinous cystadenocarcinoma. The epithelial layer is greater than three cells in thickness. Although a suggestion of the mucinous character is present, the cells are anaplastic, with increased mitotic activity.

Decker and associates from the Mayo Clinic, only 25% of mucinous cystadenocarcinomas had spread beyond the ovary at the time of diagnosis and only 6% were poorly differentiated histologically. In contrast, 73% of serous cystadenocarcinomas had disseminated and 52% were poorly differentiated.

The treatment of mucinous tumors is identical to that of serous tumors. Since mucinous tumors are bilateral in only 8% of cases, conservation of childbearing capacity in younger women is possible with greater frequency.

PSEUDOMYXOMA PERITONEI.—Pseudomyxoma peritonei refers to the process of mucinous ascites secondary to mucinous tumors of intra-abdominal organs. Although this condition has been associated with primary mucinous carcinomas of the urachus, bowel, and common bile duct, the ovary and the appendix have been the sites of origin in nearly all reported cases, with the ovary predominating. Although pseudomyxoma may arise, rarely, from apparently benign mucinous tumors of the ovary and appendix, there is general agreement that the process is indeed malignant. Confusion has resulted from the fact that the primary tumors are highly differentiated and the mucinous ascites itself contains strips of actively secreting, but benign-appearing, epithelium. In the recent report of

ten cases by Limber and associates, all six of the ovarian tumors contained areas of stromal invasion. The ascites form of the tumor, however, is rarely invasive, and a protracted clinical course is characterized by progressive mechanical interference with gastrointestinal function frequently resulting in partial bowel obstruction.

The treatment of ovarian pseudomyxoma peritonei consists of surgical excision of the primary tumor (both ovaries are usually involved) and evacuation of as much of the mucinous material as possible. Recurrence within 18 months is frequent, but an aggressive initial operation as well as repeated surgical evacuation has resulted in an overall five-year survival rate of 45%. The highly differentiated epithelium portends not only slow growth but also relative resistance to adjuvant radiotherapy and chemotherapy. Nevertheless, thorough evacuation of mucin followed by the intraperitoneal infusion of ^{32}P chromic phosphate during the early postoperative period may significantly delay or prevent recurrence, provided a uniform distribution of the isotope is obtained.

Endometrioid Carcinoma

Sampson first described endometrioid carcinoma in 1925 and at the same time proposed rigid diagnostic criteria that required

direct origin from endometriosis. In August, 1961, a conference of the Cancer Committee of FIGO was held in Stockholm for the purpose of standardizing a histologic classification of the common epithelial ovarian tumors. Surprisingly, Santesson of Sweden proposed that a new group termed *endometrioid* tumors be added because of their prevalence. Santesson presented 616 histologically reviewed primary ovarian cancers of which endometrioid tumors constituted 24.4%. For inclusion in this category, Santesson did not require evidence of origin from endometriosis but only that the tumors resemble endometrial adenocarcinoma or adenoacanthoma. Since that time, endometrioid carcinomas have been reported to constitute 15% to 20% of all ovarian cancers. A major problem in diagnosis has resulted from the fact that 25% of endometrioid carcinomas are associated with a histologically similar carcinoma of the endometrium. In this instance, Scully has suggested that if the endometrial carcinoma is less than 2 cm in diameter, is well differentiated, and only minimally invades the myometrium, the assumption of synchronous primary tumors in the ovary and endometrium can safely be made.

Grossly, endometrioid carcinomas may be cystic with a velvety inner surface and resemble the benign "chocolate" cyst with an intrinsic tumor mass. More commonly they are semicystic, but they may be entirely solid. Although intrinsic tumor may penetrate the cyst wall, the external papillary excrescences of serous cystadenocarcinomas are absent. Endometrioid carcinomas vary in size from 10 to 25 cm in diameter. About 30% are bilateral, a figure exceeded only by serous cystomas.

Microscopically, endometrioid carcinomas have a glandular pattern that closely resembles that of endometrial carcinoma (Fig 7–25). Areas of squamous metaplasia are common. A mixed papillary pattern is observed frequently, but the papillae are blunt and short in contrast to the fine-branching papillarity of serous cystadenocarcinomas. In the series reported from the Boston Hospital for Women by Kurman and Craig, 13 of the 37 endometrioid carcinomas contained other sec-

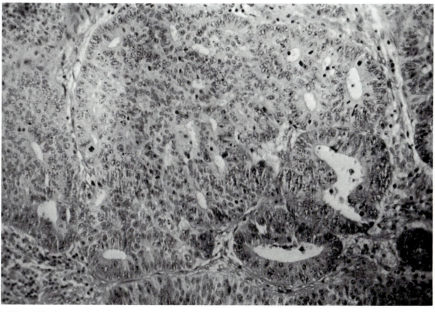

Fig 7–25.—Endometrioid carcinoma of the ovary indistinguishable from a primary carcinoma of the endometrium. The tumor was unilateral and the uterine cavity was uninvolved.

ondary müllerian elements, and in 11% endometriosis was demonstrated in the same ovary.

The prognosis associated with endometrioid carcinoma is better than that of serous cystadenocarcinomas because of an increased percentage of localized and well-differentiated tumors in the former group. In the Boston Hospital for Women series, 47% of patients had stage I tumors; 28%, stage II; and 26%, stage III and stage IV. The overall five- and ten-year survival rates were 46% and 37%, respectively. For stage I tumors the five- and ten-year survival rates were 69% and 63%, and the corresponding figures for stage II disease were 50% and 30%. There were no survivors in the stage III and stage IV categories. Kurman and Craig found that the influence of histologic grade was significant. Patients with stage I, grade 1 tumors had a 100% five- and ten-year survival rate, which diminished steadily with increasing grade. Among patients with stage II disease, 80% of those with grade 2 tumors survived five years and 60% ten years, whereas only 20% with less differentiated tumors survived five years and none survived ten years.

The treatment of endometrioid carcinoma of the ovary is the same as for the other malignant cystomas. Preservation of childbearing capacity is less feasible in light of the 30% bilaterality, but these tumors tend to be more common in older women. The mean age in the Boston Hospital for Women series was 57 years, with a range of 36 to 86 years.

Clear Cell Carcinoma

The checkered history of the *clear cell carcinoma* regarding its birthright is still evident in the FIGO classification where it is termed a *mesonephroid tumor*. In 1939 Schiller described a tumor that contained structures resembling mesonephric glomeruli. Schiller called this tumor *mesonephroma ovarii* and postulated an origin from mesonephric rests within the ovary. Unfortunately Schiller included in the same report a second tumor type, which consisted of cystic or tubular

structures lined by large clear cells that also formed solid masses (Fig 7–26,A). Teilum clarified Schiller's original article by pointing out that two distinct, unrelated tumors had been described. Teilum also demonstrated a resemblance between Schiller's mesonephroma and the endodermal sinuses of the rat placenta and suggested an extraembryonic germ cell origin of this tumor type. A mesonephric origin for Schiller's second type (the clear cell tumor) was challenged in 1967 by Scully and Barlow who described an association with endometriosis in 53% of 17 cases. Also citing the occurrence of clear cell carcinomas within the müllerian system at some distance from mesonephric remnants, these authors proposed that these tumors were derived from primary or secondary müllerian epithelium. Kurman and Craig at the Boston Hospital for Women have added credence to Scully's thesis by demonstrating endometrioid, serous and mucinous elements in five of their 12 cases of clear cell carcinoma. As a corollary, these authors found clear cell elements within seven endometrioid carcinomas, eight serous carcinomas, and one undifferentiated carcinoma.

On gross examination, clear cell carcinomas vary from a predominantly cystic to a predominantly solid architecture. The cystic spaces usually are filled with chocolatelike fluid and contain pale-brown polypoid masses. Clear cell carcinomas are bilateral in less than 10% of cases. Microscopically, they are made up of masses of large polyhedral epithelial cells, which contain a small nucleus and abundant clear cytoplasm (see Fig 7–26,A). Cystic spaces or tubules are lined by clear cells and by "hobnail" cells (Fig 7–26,B). Scully suggests that the hobnail cells may, in fact, be clear cells that have discharged their cytoplasmic content.

Clear cell carcinomas constitute approximately 5% of the malignant ovarian tumors. Although a number of clinical reports have been published, the largest representative series consists of 95 cases reported from the Emil Novak Ovarian Tumor Registry by Rogers et al. The ages ranged from 10 to 79 years,

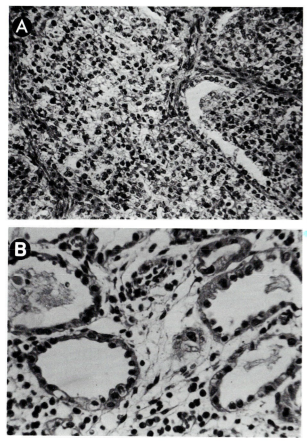

Fig 7–26.—A, clear cell carcinoma. Solid masses of large clear cells are interspersed with tubular structures. **B,** hobnail cells, a characteristic of clear cell tumors throughout the female genital tract.

but 78% of patients were between the ages of 40 and 70 years. In 63% the tumor was confined to one ovary, and 68.2% of patients fell into the stage I category. In 19% of cases the tumor had spread to the pelvic peritoneum (stage II), and in 11.6% the upper abdomen was involved (stage III). The tumor had disseminated beyond the abdominal cavity in only one instance (stage IV). While a five-year survival rate of 63% was obtained with stage I tumors, only 17% of patients with stage II and none of the patients with stage III and stage IV disease survived. These figures are consistent with smaller reported series and indicate that (1) a greater number of clear cell carcinomas are confined to the ovaries at the time of diagnosis than with the other malignant cystomas: (2) the five-year survival rate for stage I clear cell carcinomas is similar to that of other malignant cystomas; and (3) once

the tumor has disseminated beyond the ovary the survival rates are much lower than with the other malignant cystomas. These observations are inconsistent with the parallel often drawn between endometrioid and clear cell carcinomas. Although a high percentage of both tumor types appear to remain localized for protracted periods, the malignant behavior of the clear cell carcinoma is much greater than that of an endometrioid carcinoma. The initial surgical procedure should be the same for clear cell carcinomas as for the other epithelial tumors, but aggressive postoperative adjuvant therapy must be instituted in any case of extraovarian spread.

Brenner Tumor

The Brenner tumor consists of multiple nests of benign transitional-type epithelium (urothelium) distributed throughout a dense

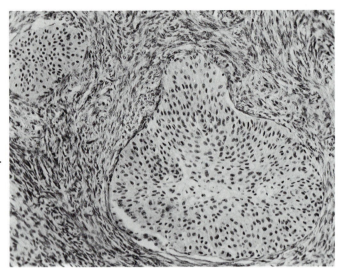

Fig 7–27.—Brenner tumor. Nests of epithelial cells resembling urothelium surrounded by a fibromatous connective tissue matrix.

fibrous stroma (Fig 7–27). Brenner tumors are relatively uncommon, accounting for no more than 0.5% of ovarian tumors. Although several histogenetic theories have been advanced, an origin from germinal epithelium has now been generally accepted. Arey demonstrated by three-dimensional reconstructions that the epithelial component consists of intricately branching cords, which radiate from a common stalk, which in turn arises from an epithelial plaque at the ovarian surface. The similarity between the epithelial cells of the Brenner tumor and those of the Walthard rest have led to the widely held view that Brenner tumors arise from Walthard's rests. Since Walthard's rests are most commonly found on ovarian and tubal surfaces in continuity with peritoneum, they would qualify as secondary müllerian epithelium except for their transitional cell differentiation. Even a müllerian connection is retained since 20% of Brenner tumors coexist with mucinous cystadenomas. Moreover, in about 30% of Brenner tumors the epithelial islands cavitate and a mucin-containing cystic structure lined by endocervical-type epithelium develops. It is apparent that mucinous cystadenomas may, in some instances, develop from preexisting Brenner tumors.

The finding of a Brenner tumor is usually incidental to hysterectomy for other indications in premenopausal women in their late 30s and 40s. As a consequence of their slow growth rate, larger and symptomatic Brenner tumors tend to be discovered after the menopause. Symptoms are related to the size of the tumor and are those characteristic of any benign ovarian neoplasm. Several cases of Meigs' syndrome have been reported. As with other tumors in which stromal proliferation is prominent, luteinized thecal activity may result in estrogen secretion. Coexistence of endometrial hyperplasia has been reported in 5% to 20% of patients.

Although usually small (3 to 8 cm in diameter), Brenner tumors may reach large proportions. They are bilateral in only 8% of cases. On gross examination these tumors are smooth, slightly lobulated, and quite firm, though cystic areas may be palpated.

More than 35 malignant Brenner tumors have been reported, and a potentially malignant or proliferating group has been identified. In contrast to the usual benign form, the proliferating tumors tend to be cystic. Because of more rapid growth, they are larger and more frequently symptomatic. In the series reported by Miles and Norris the average size was 16 cm in diameter. The microscopic picture is one of multiple cystic spaces lined by well-differentiated but proliferating urothelium, which forms papillary projections into the cyst cavities. Squamous metaplasia is common, and moderate focal cellular atypia has been described. Stromal invasion is absent and metastases have not been observed. Miles and Norris compare the proliferating Brenner tumor with a low-grade papillary transitional cell carcinoma of the bladder.

Malignant Brenner tumors are characterized by foci of papillary transitional cell carcinoma intermixed with benign and proliferating urothelium. Marked cellular pleomorphism and stromal invasion are obvious. Squamous metaplasia is common and squamous cells may also be histologically malignant. Metastatic disease and death have been reported.

As pointed out by Miles and Norris, malignant Brenner tumors exhibit a clear-cut progression from benign to proliferating to malignant urothelium. In addition, the mean age of patients in this study's malignant group was 68 years, whereas the mean age of patients with proliferative tumors was 50 years. This difference in age provides further evidence that malignancy in Brenner tumors develops by a slow transition from the benign form.

In light of the rarity of malignant change, particularly in younger women, and the infrequency of bilaterality, unilateral oophorectomy is adequate treatment in the younger age group. Perimenopausal and postmenopausal women, however, should undergo hysterectomy and bilateral salpingo-oophorectomy. The relative frequency of mucinous cystadenomas in the opposite ovary as well as the possibility of a metachronous Brenner tumor militates against ovarian conservation without good cause.

Carcinosarcoma and Mixed Mesodermal Sarcoma

Carcinosarcoma and mixed mesodermal sarcoma are highly malignant tumors that are histologically identical to their endometrial counterparts. Although considered quite rare, they are being reported with increasing frequency. At the time Dehner et al. published their report in 1971 only 17 cases had been reported; by 1975 when Hernandez et al. submitted their review the total had risen to 93 cases.

Carcinosarcomas and mixed mesodermal sarcomas occur with nearly equal frequency and predominantly affect postmenopausal women. The median age for the 93 reported patients was 58 years, with a range from 18 to 86 years. The incidence of nulliparity exceeds that of the general population.

The gross appearance is similar for both tumor types. The size varies from 3 to 30 cm in diameter, with an average of 15 cm. The tumors consists of large multilocular cysts interspersed by solid tissue. Capsular penetration by tumor is common. Microscopically, the carcinosarcomas consist of malignant stromal cells and aggregates of malignant glandular structures. Papillary excrescences made up of both epithelial and mesenchymal elements commonly project into the cystic cavities. The mixed mesodermal sarcoma differs only by the presence of heterologous mesodermal elements within the sarcomatous stroma. Dehner and associates found cartilage in 57%, striated muscle in 50%, and osteoid elements in 21% of tumors.

The mode of dissemination is consistent with that of the other cystomas, predominantly by diffuse implantation on peritoneal surfaces. In reviewing the 93 reported cases, Hernandez et al. found that 29% were localized to the ovary at diagnosis whereas 51% had spread beyond the pelvis. The prognosis is bleak. Seventy-seven percent of all patients were dead within one year of diagnosis, and only 29% of patients with stage I disease survived more than two years.

Optimal treatment consists of hysterectomy, bilateral salpingo-oophorectomy, and the excision of as much metastatic tumor as is feasible. Radiation therapy has been ineffective. Chemotherapy, incorporating doxorubicin (Adriamycin) should follow operation in all cases. Unfortunately, only 4 of 35 patients with mixed mesodermal sarcoma of the ovary responded to various chemotherapeutic regimens in a series reported by Lele et al. (1980).

Dehner et al. found the median survival time of their 13 patients with carcinosarcoma to be 15 months, whereas that for their 14 patients with mixed mesodermal sarcoma was only six months. These authors postulate that the homologous form of the tumor is somewhat less malignant than the heterologous variety.

Gonadal Stromal Tumors

The designation *gonadal stromal tumor* is applied to all tumors that arise from the ovarian stroma without regard to the embryonic origin of specific precursor cells. Although the term *mesenchymal tumors* has been proposed, the WHO designation *sex cord-stromal tumors* maintains the connotation of embryonic precursors while avoiding the controversial assumption that the sex cords are derived from the mesenchyme.

Most gonadal stromal tumors contain recognizable ovarian cell types and are termed *granulosa-theca cell tumors*. A smaller proportion consists of testicular cell types and these are called *Sertoli-Leydig cell tumors*. There is general agreement that granulosa cells and Sertoli cells are homologous, as are theca cells and Leydig cells. It must be emphasized that testicular-type cells in the ovary are sex chromatin-positive. A very small percentage of tumors, classified as lipid cell tumors, consists of several clinically and histologically similar subtypes. Ten percent of gonadal stromal tumors cannot be classified because of intermixtures of poorly differentiated cellular elements.

For the most part, granulosa-theca cell tumors secrete estrogens, whereas Sertoli-Leydig cell and lipid cell tumors produce androgens. At least 15% of gonadal stromal tumors are said to be hormonally inert, but this estimate is based on clinical interpretations rather than on laboratory evidence. The type of hormonal production is also variable. A small percentage of granulosa-theca cell tumors cause virilization, whereas a few Sertoli-Leydig cell tumors secrete estrogen. In some instances both estrogen and androgen are produced by the same tumor. These variations probably relate not only to the functional tissue type but also to the extraglandular conversion of an estrogen and androgen precursor, namely, androstenedione. Within the follicular apparatus, granulosa cells appear necessary for the aromatization of androstenedione to estrone and thence to estradiol (Savard et al.). It is therefore not surprising that estradiol is the primary hormone product of granulosa-theca cell tumors. As demonstrated by Savard and associates, androstenedione, although a by-product of follicular steroidogenesis, is the primary secretory product of pure ovarian stroma. Without the capability of aromatization, testosterone production, which is unique to the stroma, exceeds that of estrogen. For this reason, stromal tumors tend to be androgenic in the absence of granulosa cells, although estrone may be derived from the peripheral conversion of androstenedione (MacDonald et al.). Virilism with granulosa-theca cell tumors is probably related to testosterone production by isolated stromal components.

Granulosa-Theca Cell Tumors

Granulosa-theca cell tumors are composed of the cellular constituents of the graafian follicle wall in varying proportion. Approximately 20% are predominantly granulosa cell tumors, 20% are mixed granulosa-theca cell tumors and 60% are relatively pure thecomas. Granulosa-theca cell tumors constitute 4% to 9% of all ovarian tumors, and about 3% of ovarian cancers are malignant granulosa cell tumors.

The histogenesis of granulosa-theca cell tumors remains unclear and, as previously noted, controversial. Whereas Teilum is insistent that all gonadal stromal tumors (excepting the hilus cell tumor) arise from undifferentiated ovarian mesenchyme, others have proposed that the granulosa cells are derived from germinal epithelium (secondary sex cords) and the theca cells from cortical stroma. Furth and Butterworth (1936), and McKay and associates (1953), have advanced the theory that these neoplasms originate from persisting remnants of follicular epithelium in atretic follicles. Animal experimentation lends support to the idea that, following the death of the ovum, tumors may arise from residual follicular elements in the presence of constant gonadotropin stimulation. In the classic experiment of Biskind and Biskind (1949), autologous ovarian transplantation into the spleens of castrated rats resulted not only in the death of ova but in the shunting of ovarian estrogen directly to the liver where it was inactivated. With removal of the negative feedback mechanism, persistently elevated levels of gonadotropin uniformly resulted in granulosa cell tumor formation in the ovarian grafts.

These tumors have been observed at all ages from birth to 90 years. Fifty percent are found in postmenopausal women, whereas fewer than 5% are discovered before puberty. In most series the median age is early in the sixth decade. The initial symptoms are usually related to the endocrine activity of the tumor and vary with the amount of hormonal secretion as well as with the age of the patient. Perhaps the most dramatic effect is the development of precocious pseudopuberty in the prepubertal child. During the reproductive years the clinical picture is less striking, but irregular menses and even amenorrhea are common. In the postmenopausal era the characteristic symptoms are a resumption of uterine bleeding and occasional enlargement of the breasts. Virilization has been described in 1% to 3% of patients with granulosa cell tumors. As the tumor becomes progressively larger, symptoms of pelvic pressure and pain supervene. An unusual characteristic is the propensity of soft pultaceous granulosa cell tumors to rupture spontaneously and result in intraperitoneal hemorrhage. As many as 15% of women with this tumor during their reproductive years present with the picture of an acute abdominal catastrophe, which may mimic that of a ruptured ectopic pregnancy.

Granulosa-theca cell tumors are nearly always unilateral, and most series report bilaterality in only 2% to 6%. The tumors may vary in size from 0.4 to 40.0 cm in diameter and weigh as much as 35 lb. Grossly, they are mobile, oval, and encapsulated with a smooth, lobulated surface and a soft, solid, or semicystic consistency. On section, 90% have cystic cavities and more than half of these contain old blood. This characteristic appearance makes a tentative diagnosis possible by gross inspection alone.

Microscopic examination may reveal a variable architectural structure, but the granulosa cells have a characteristic and monotonously uniform appearance. They are rounded or polygonal with a slightly granular eosinophilic cytoplasm and poorly defined cytoplasmic borders. Nuclei are small and round and are often folded, resulting in the longitudinal groove characteristic of ovarian stromal cells. Nuclear atypia and mitotic figures are rare. Interspersed theca cells are spindle shaped with ovoid nuclei and contain cytoplasmic lipid droplets or are occasionally luteinized (Fig 7–28,A). Theca cells are surrounded by supporting reticulum fibers, which are easily demonstrable by a reticulum stain. Multiple architectural patterns of granulosa cell tumors have been described and have been termed folliculoid, adenomatoid, cylindroid, sarcomatoid, and trabeculoid (Fig 7–29). These patterns have borne no relationship to malignant behavior and ultimate prognosis, and, as pointed out by Norris and Taylor, have led to imprecision in the definition of a distinct clinicopathologic entity. The most common pattern, which has been called folliculoid or microfolliculoid, is characterized by the arrangement of granulosa cells in a rosette fashion with the nuclei at right angles to a central area of pink inspissated material. These structures are termed *Call-Exner bodies* and are pathognomonic of granulosa cell tumors (see Fig 7–29).

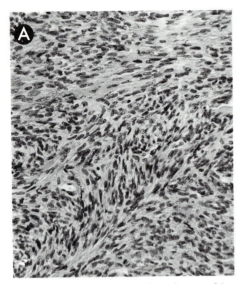 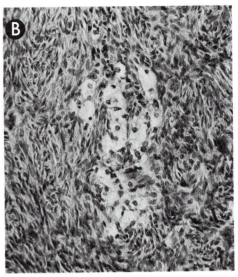

Fig 7–28.—A, thecoma showing cluster of luteinized granulosa cells. **B,** thecoma showing fibrillar appearance of cellular cytoplasm and interlacing bundles of fibrous connective tissue.

Since histologic appearance has not been predictive of malignant behavior, estimates of malignant potential have been based on the observed incidence of metastases or mortality from the disease. These observations have varied markedly as exemplified by the survival rates from five recent series listed in Table 7–4. In the Ovarian Tumor Registry (OTR) series reported by Novak et al., 25% of tumors were malignant by virtue of primary metastases or recurrence. The corresponding figure reported by Fox et al. (Manchester, England) was 30%, whereas only 10% of patients with granulosa-theca cell tumors reported by Norris and Taylor from the Armed Forces Institute of Pathology (AFIP) were demonstrably malignant. Norris and Taylor propose that the marked variability in reported rates of malignancy and mortality stems from (1) the inadvertent inclusion of malignant tumors not meeting the criteria for granulosa cell tumors (Fig 7–29,D); (2) the inclusion in some series of the rarely malignant thecomas; (3) the use of crude mortality rates in a population of aging women prone to die of other causes; and (4) failure in some series to report long-term follow-up of a disease in which

TABLE 7–4.—GRANULOSA-THECA CELL TUMOR SURVIVAL RATES*

| | | SURVIVAL RATES, % | |
SERIES	NO. OF PATIENTS	5-YR	10-YR
Norris and Taylor (1968)†	68	97	93
Novak et al. (1971)	86	64	. . .
Fox et al. (1975)†	74	68	59
Stenwig et al. (1979)	118	95	88
Björkholm and Silfverswärd (1981)	197	96	89

*Excluding unrelated deaths.
†Actuarial survival rates.

most tumor-related deaths occur after five years. In an attempt to explain the relatively low five-year survival rate among the OTR patients, Novak et al. suggest that either more anaplastic or bizarre cases were registered with the OTR, or undifferentiated carcinomas and sarcomas were inadvertently included. Many tumors included in the Manchester series were highly malignant since more than half the deaths accrued during the first two

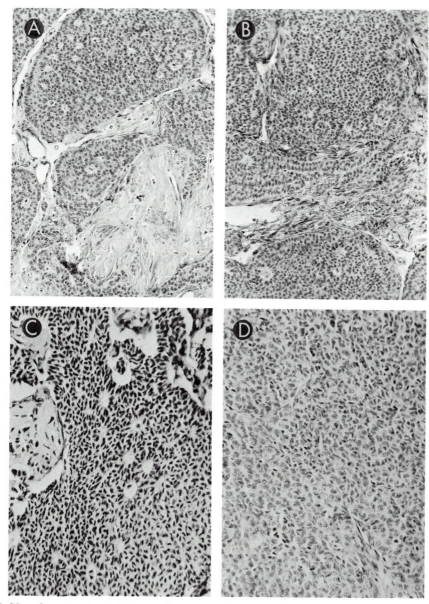

Fig 7–29.—A, granulosa-theca cell tumor showing folliculoid pattern of granulosa cells and collagenous hyalinization of the thecal stroma. **B,** granulosa-theca cell tumor showing a diffuse pattern *(above),* cylindroid pattern *(center)* and folliculoid pattern *(below).* (**A** and **B** from Hertig A.T., Gore H.: Tumors of the female sex organs: part 3. Tumors of the ovary and fallopian tube, sec. 9, fasc. 33, *Atlas of Tumor Pathology.* Washington, D.C., Armed Forces Institute of Pathology, 1961.) **C,** granulosa-theca cell tumor showing typical Call-Exner bodies in a folliculoid pattern. **D,** poorly differentiated granulosa-theca cell tumor showing pleomorphism and numerous mitoses in upper right. This tumor was malignant and death occurred two years after surgical excision.

years. As previously noted, the usual growth of malignant granulosa cell tumors is leisurely and is manifested by late recurrences and death after five years.

Norris and Taylor, and Fox et al. have delineated several clinical and pathologic factors that relate to prognosis. Both groups noted fewer overt malignancies in women under age 40 years, and a worsened prognosis for women whose tumor exceeded 10 to 15 cm in diameter. Fox et al. found that survival was diminished among patients with abdominal symptoms and bilateral tumors. Both groups agree that the histologic growth pattern bears no influence on outcome and deplore the misleading "sarcomatoid" designation often applied to the diffuse growth pattern. Neither group could correlate atypia with malignant behavior, but Fox et al. found that abundant mitotic figures were an ominous sign. Contrariwise, Norris and Taylor were unable to demonstrate a relationship between mitotic activity and outcome.

The diagnosis of granulosa-theca cell tumors is often made at laparotomy indicated by reason of a palpable mass or an acute complication. When signs and symptoms of inappropriate estrogen secretion are unaccompanied by a palpable adnexal mass, the diagnosis may be obscure. In the prepubertal child, urinary and plasma estrogen levels are considerably higher than normal adult values and fail to show cyclic variation or response to pituitary suppression. In the postmenopause, endometrial hyperplasia is an associated finding in 25% to 50% of patients, and endometrial carcinoma has been described in from 3% to 21%. Endometrial hyperplasia in the presence of other estrogen effects such as breast tenderness and vaginal cornification in a postmenopausal woman strongly suggests a granulosa-theca tumor, provided an exogenous source of estrogen has been excluded.

The treatment of granulosa-theca cell tumors usually consists of a hysterectomy and bilateral salpingo-oophorectomy. In light of the relative benignity of these tumors—particularly below the age of 40 years—and the infrequency of bilaterality, excision of the tumor and involved ovary is sufficient treatment for young women. In the event of disseminated or recurrent disease, metastases should be excised when possible. Since granulosa-theca cell tumors have been relatively radioresponsive, pelvic or abdominal irradiation may have a beneficial effect. Complete clinical remission has been recently reported in two patients with metastatic granulosa cell tumors treated with cisplatin and doxorubicin (Jacobs et al., 1982). This combination regimen shows promise and deserves further evaluation.

THECOMA.—Although included in the granulosa-theca cell group, these tumors are set apart by possible differences in histogenesis and their almost invariable benignity. The prevalence of thecomas varies widely, depending on histologic criteria. A granulosa-theca cell tumor predominantly composed of theca cells may be considered a thecoma by some, whereas others reserve that diagnosis for tumors composed purely of theca cells. Even in the latter instance a granulosa cell component is usually found if sufficient histologic sections are examined. At the other end of the spectrum, thecomas may be indistinguishable from fibromas, and many pathologists include thecomas and fibromas in a single category.

There is reason to believe that the histogenesis of thecomas may differ from that of granulosa cell tumors. Woll et al. noted a change in the aging ovary, which they termed *cortical stromal hyperplasia* (Fig 7–30). In some ovaries the process occurs locally and the resultant nodular masses are histologically identical to thecomas. Transitional stages between cortical stromal hyperplasia and thecomas have also been observed, and patients with thecomas of one ovary almost invariably have cortical stromal hyperplasia of the contralateral ovary.

Thecomas have been reported in females from 1 to 90 years of age, but most are found in postmenopausal women. The presenting

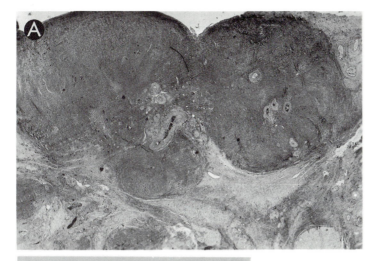

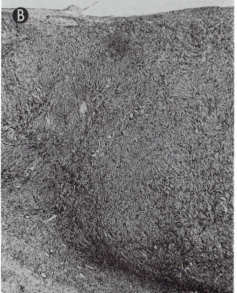

Fig 7–30.—Cortical stromal hyperplasia. **A,** section of ovary of postmenopausal patient. The surface of the ovary is nodular, because of the proliferation of stromal cells into the periphery of the cortex. Occasionally the areas of stromal hyperplasia extend into the medulla and occupy almost the entire sectioned surface of the ovary. **B,** low-power view of ovarian surface, showing marked thickening of the cortex. Note the absence of ova and follicles and the fascicular arrangement of stromal cells. In left center are several foci of lutein cells. **C,** high-power view, showing characteristic large stromal cells with plump, blunted nuclei. In the central area is a focus of lutein cells arranged in clumps. These lutein cells are indistinguishable from those seen in some polycystic ovaries of patients with the Stein-Leventhal syndrome. (Courtesy of Drs. Arthur T. Hertig and Hazel Gore.)

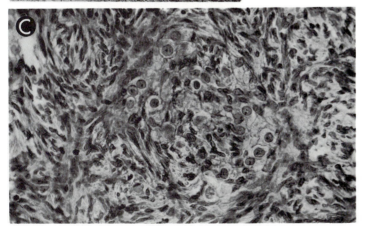

symptoms, hormonal activity, and the association with endometrial carcinoma are similar to those of the granulosa-theca cell group as a whole. Thecomas have been as frequently associated with the Meigs' syndrome as have fibromas.

Thecomas vary from microscopic size to 15 cm in diameter, although most range from 6 to 10 cm in diameter. In contrast to the granulosa-theca cell tumors they are more likely to be solid than cystic, and internal hemorrhage is infrequent. The cut surface is firm and white, but yellow areas representing luteinization are visible. Microscopically, the tumor is composed of plump, oval, or spindle-shaped cells arranged in a whorled or trabecular pattern (see Fig 7–28,B). Although thecomas resemble fibromas, they may be distinguished by areas of luteinized granulosa or theca cells (see Fig 7–28,A), cytoplasmic vacuoles identifiable as fat globules, and intercellular reticulum.

Malignant behavior has been reported in 1% to 15%; again this variability depends on the histologic definition of a thecoma. Probably most "malignant thecomas" have actually been undifferentiated gonadal stromal tumors or fibrous sarcomas. One of the 99 clearly defined thecomas reported by Norris and Taylor was malignant.

Sertoli-Leydig Cell Tumors

The Sertoli-Leydig cell tumor is the most common virilizing tumor of the ovary although its prevalence is only one tenth that of the granulosa-theca cell tumor. Sertoli-Leydig cell tumors are also known as arrhenoblastomas and androblastomas. The former term proposed by Robert Meyer and used in previous editions of this text, *arrhenoblastoma,* has been discarded because tumors of this type are not uniformly virilizing, and a pure derivation from ovarian "blastema" remains conjectural.

Sertoli-Leydig cell tumors are most frequently found during the childbearing era; 75% have occurred between the ages of 15 and 45 years, with a median age of 32 years.

More than 95% of Sertoli-Leydig tumors are unilateral, and they vary in size from 0.5 to 10.0 cm in diameter. Both the external and cut surfaces resemble those of the granulosa cell tumors, but cystic and hemorrhagic areas are somewhat less common. The histologic picture is variable but suggests a recapitulation of early testicular gonadogenesis. The Sertoli cells are represented by cuboidal or columnar cells arranged in cordlike or tubular structures reminiscent of the sex cords or seminiferous tubules of the fetal testis. The most differentiated form of the tumor consists entirely of tubules lined by a single layer of Sertoli cells with clear cytoplasm (tubular adenoma of Pick) and tends to be either hormonally inactive or productive of estrogens. In its most common form, the tumor consists of less–well-defined tubules within a stroma containing both undifferentiated stromal cells and large polygonal cells with round central nuclei and abundant eosinophilic cytoplasm (Figs 7–31) and 7–32,D). These polygonal cells strongly resemble testicular Leydig cells and may contain crystals of Reinke. These intracytoplasmic bodies are characteristic of Leydig cells and are visible as eosinophilic rodlike structures whose blunt ends may project beyond the cell membrane. In the least-differentiated form of the tumor only a suggestion of a cordlike or tubular pattern remains (Fig 7–33).

Although the histologic appearance of 10% to 15% of Sertoli-Leydig cell tumors suggests malignancy, recent reports indicate that less than 5% manifest malignant behavior by metastases or recurrence (Norris and Chorlton; Ireland and Woodruff). Undoubtedly the inclusion of poorly differentiated but virilizing gonadal stromal tumors in previously reported series has resulted in the oft-quoted malignancy rate of 25%. The diagnosis of a Sertoli-Leydig cell tumor must be made with caution in patients with bilateral tumors or primary metastases unless the histologic diagnosis is unequivocal.

Approximately 75% of Sertoli-Leydig cell tumors are associated with androgen produc-

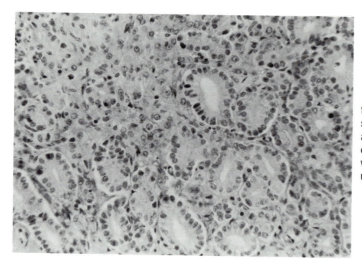

Fig 7–31.—Sertoli-Leydig cell tumor with simple tubular structures lined by columnar cells at the right, and a stroma containing large polygonal cells with round central nuclei in the upper left.

tion. The endocrinologic effect usually begins as a gradual process of defeminization, and anovulation followed by complete amenorrhea may be the initial event. Some women, however, continue to have ovulatory cycles despite marked virilism. Gradually the feminine sex characteristics regress and excessive androgen production is manifested by a male habitus, marked hirsutism, acne, temporal balding, voice deepening, and clitoromegaly (Fig 7–34). In the absence of a palpable adnexal mass (40%), the diagnosis depends on differentiation between the adrenal gland and ovary as a source of androgen production. Androgenicity secondary to adrenal hypersecretion is typically associated with marked elevation of the urinary 17-ketosteroids. Sertoli-Leydig cell tumors are accompanied by normal or only slightly elevated levels of 17-ketosteroids, since the primary hormone secreted is testosterone. When initially elevated, levels of plasma testosterone consistently return to normal following treatment of patients with Sertoli-Leydig cell tumors. In addition, testosterone levels obtained from the venous drainage of the involved ovary have been 30 times that of peripheral venous blood.

Since less than 5% of Sertoli-Leydig cell tumors are bilateral, unilateral oophorectomy appears to be adequate treatment for this tumor, which predominantly afflicts younger women. On the other hand, nearly 10% of tumors are either bilateral or malignant, and hysterectomy and bilateral salpingo-oophorectomy is optimal therapy for women in their 30s no longer desiring pregnancy. Insufficient experience has accumulated to comment on the efficacy of radiotherapy or chemotherapy in advanced or recurrent cases.

Gynandroblastomas

Gynandroblastomas are rare tumors that demonstrate a biphasic differentiation toward both ovarian and testicular structures and thus contain histologic elements of both the granulosa cell and the Sertoli-Leydig cell tumor. Although many authors have recommended that gynandroblastomas be included in the category of nonspecific gonadal stromal tumors (Scully; Norris and Chorlton; Ireland and Woodruff), we have reserved the latter category for poorly differentiated cell types irrespective of a tendency to form ovarian or testicular elements alone or in combination. The histologic criteria for diagnosis of a gynandroblastoma must include aggregates of granulosa cells forming Call-Exner bodies and either well-defined tubules or Leydig cells identifiable by Reinke crystals. A case re-

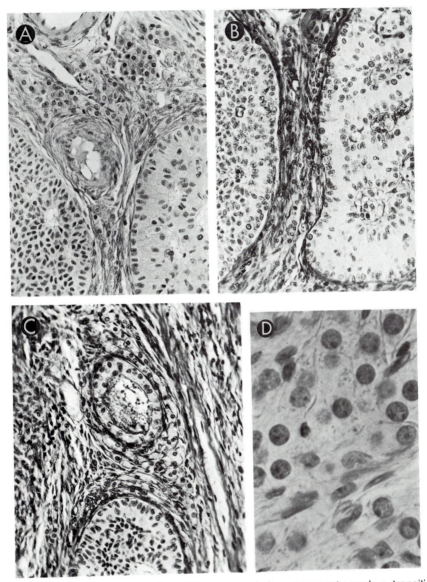

Fig 7–32.—Gynandroblastoma. **A,** Sertoli-like epithelium is seen at lower right and granulosa cells at lower left. Multiple interstitial (Leydig) cells are scattered throughout the stroma but are clearly seen in the upper part of the photograph. **B,** high-power view shows an area of typical granulosa cells *(left)* and early tubule formation *(right)* in which the cells are of the Sertoli type. **C,** high-power view shows gradual transition between granulosa cells and Sertoli's cells. The area below represents such a transitional area. The tubule above is surrounded by epithelial cells with stroma. The latter cells may be the prototype from which either theca interna or Leydig's cells are derived. (**A** to **C** from Emig O.R., Hertig A.T., Rowe F.J.: *Obstet. Gynecol.* 13:135, 1959; Armed Forces Institute of Pathology photomicrographs). **D,** higher-power view shows interstitial cells of Leydig. Pigment granules are seen in the clear cytoplasm.

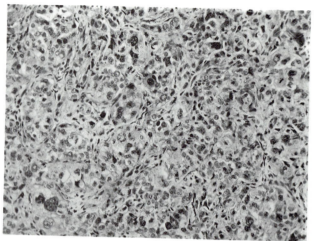

Fig 7–33.—Poorly differentiated Sertoli-Leydig cell tumor with a suggestion of a cordlike pattern and an interspersion of large cells with round dark nuclei reminiscent of Leydig cells.

ported from the Boston Hospital for Women that met these criteria is depicted in Figure 7–32. In this case, the homologous relationship between granulosa cells and Sertoli cells is demonstrated by the apparent transition from Call-Exner bodies to tubules lined by Sertoli cells.

These rare tumors are usually found during the childbearing years, and a disruption of the normal menstrual pattern may precede the diagnosis by several years. Despite the presence of ovarian elements and the occasional finding of endometrial hyperplasia, virilism is the dominant effect of these tumors. In general the gross appearance, biologic behavior, and optimal therapeutic approach are identical to those of the Sertoli-Leydig cell tumors.

Lipid Cell Tumors

Lipid cell tumors include cell types previously designated as hilar, or hilus, cell tumors, Leydig cell tumors, stromal luteomas, and adrenal rest tumors. Despite the histogenetic implications of these cell types, none

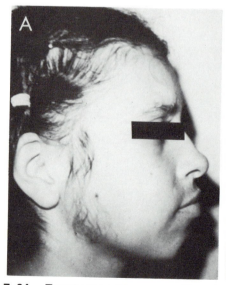

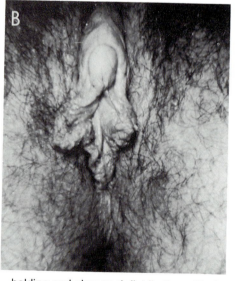

Fig 7–34.—Twenty-year-old woman with a virilizing Sertoli-Leydig cell tumor. **A,** note temporal balding and abnormal distribution of facial hair. **B,** marked clitoromegaly in the same patient.

has been clearly defined as an independent entity. The presence in the ovarian hilus of Leydig-type cells indistinguishable from those of the testis (except for sex chromatin) has been accepted as a normal condition. Most tumors designated as hilar cell tumors not only are located in the medulla rather than in the hilus but less than half contain Reinke crystals, the specific hallmark of Leydig cells. Characteristically, tumors of the hilar type are composed of closely packed polygonal cells of uniform size that contain a round, centrally placed nucleus within a finely granular eosinophilic cytoplasm (Fig 7–35). In the absence of Reinke crystals, these cells also resemble luteinized stromal cells.

Lipid tumors of the adrenal type consist of sheets of large, round, or polyhedral cells with clear, vacuolated cytoplasm containing a small, pyknotic, eccentrically placed nucleus. Adjacent aggregates of Leydig or hilar-type cells are usually visible (Fig 7–36). When the cells are arranged in strands or fascicles with intervening capillaries, the resemblance to the zona fasciculata of the adrenal gland is striking. Nevertheless, the previously held view that tumors of this cell type arise from adrenal rests has been largely discarded. Moreover, the concept that most hilar- and adrenal-type cells have a common origin has

been amply supported (Hughesdon; Taylor and Norris) and remains unrefuted (Teilum).

The most compelling reason for including both cell types within a single category is their usual intermixture within the same tumor. In fact, Taylor and Norris found both hilar- and adrenal-type cells in all 30 of their lipid cell tumors. Hilar-type cells predominated in 14, adrenal-type cells predominated in seven, and the two types were equally admixed in nine. Reinke crystals were seen in both types but were most frequently present in the predominantly hilar-type tumors. Only three of the latter were located in the ovarian hilus.

Only 1% to 2% of lipid cell tumors are bilateral. They range from 0.4 to 20.0 cm in diameter, with a median size of about 5 cm. Grossly, they are smooth, soft, lobulated tumors that project above the ovarian surface. The cut surface is solid and yellow orange in color.

Although most lipid cell tumors occur after age 45 years, the ages range from 3 to 80 years. Seventy-five percent of tumors induce virilizing signs or symptoms, but oligomenorrhea or amenorrhea may precede the diagnosis by many years. Estrogenic activity has been noted in 20% of tumors, and postmenopausal bleeding may be an early symptom. In

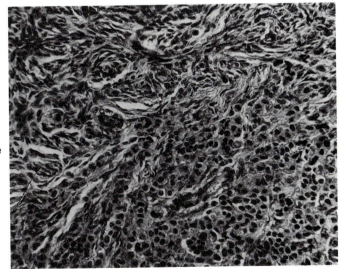

Fig 7–35.—Lipid cell tumor of hilar cell type. The cells, closely resembling the Leydig cells of the testis, are ovoid or polygonal with round central nuclei. There are fine connective tissue strands between the cells.

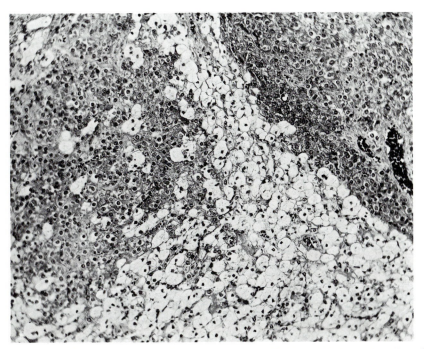

Fig 7–36.—Lipid cell tumor of adrenal type. The large cells with clear cytoplasm and a small nucleus resemble those of the adrenal zone fasciculata. Clusters of hilar or Leydig cells can be seen in the upper portion of the illustration.

10% of patients, Cushing's syndrome is suggested by virilism, hypertension, and abnormal glucose tolerance curves. In contrast to patients with Sertoli-Leydig cell tumors, 17-ketosteroid excretion (including the 11-oxygenated fraction) may be significantly elevated, suggesting adrenal hyperfunction.

An extremely low prevalence of malignant behavior has been noted. In the series reported by Ireland and Woodruff, only one of 22 "adrenal rest" tumors recurred with subsequent death of the patient, and none of the 20 "hilar cell" tumors was malignant. In contrast, Taylor and Norris observed six tumor-related deaths among their 30 patients. In three instances, extraovarian spread was evident at initial laparotomy, and two tumors considered malignant on histologic grounds (cellular pleomorphism and mitotic activity) subsequently proved to be so. The predominant cell type was unrelated to prognosis but no tumor containing Reinke crystals was malignant—an observation confirmed in other series.

These tumors may be treated in the same manner as other gonadal stromal tumors. Appropriate treatment for metastatic lesions has not been defined. Since nearly all malignant lipid cell tumors are virilizing, hormonal assays may provide tumor "markers" to assist in therapeutic evaluation and the early detection of recurrence.

Nonspecific Gonadal Stromal Tumors

Norris and Chorlton estimate that 10% of all gonadal stromal tumors fall into the category of nonspecific gonadal stromal tumors, whereas Ireland and Woodruff have assigned fully 50% of their virilizing stromal tumors to a group simply termed *gonadal stromal*. It is clear that the proportion of nonspecific gonadal stromal tumors in any series will vary inversely with the proportion of tumors that meet the pathologist's criteria for assignment to specific cell types. Most of these tumors consist of a predominantly undifferentiated stroma, although partial differentiation toward structures characteristic of specific cell types may be identified. As suggested by Norris, these tumors are best referred to descriptively as gonadal stromal tumors with differentiation toward whatever cell type is suggested. The tumors illustrated in Figures 7–29,D and 7–33 properly belong in this category although they show slight differentiation toward a granulosa cell or Sertoli-Leydig cell pattern, respectively.

Presumably, these tumors tend to display a more malignant behavior than their well-differentiated counterparts. Nevertheless only five of the 67 patients reported by Ireland and Woodruff died of this disease.

Gonadoblastomas

The gonadoblastoma is a rare neoplasm that contains both gonadal stromal and germ cell elements. The tumor develops almost exclusively in the abnormal gonads of individuals with pure or mixed gonadal dysgenesis or male pseudohermaphroditism.

The tumor is composed of discrete aggregates of primordial germ cells intermixed with, or surrounded by, immature Sertoli cells and granulosa cells. In 85% of postpubertal tumors, elements resembling Leydig or luteinized stromal cells are also present. The germ cells exhibit mitotic activity in 85% of tumors and have begun to overgrow the stromal elements in about 50%. In most instances the germinomatous component is indistinguishable from the usual dysgerminoma. In nearly 20% of the cases reported by Scully, however, more malignant germ cell types, including the endodermal sinus tumor, were not only present but often resulted in the patient's death. Other microscopic characteristics are the formation of hyaline bodies within the granulosa cell nests and calcifications in the form of expanding psammoma bodies (Fig 7–37). Calcification is present in 80% of tumors and is frequently visible on pelvic roentgenograms.

In Scully's series of 74 cases, 22% of gonadoblastomas originated in a gonadal streak, 18% in a cryptorchid dysgenetic testis, and the remainder in gonads of indeterminate type. They were bilateral in one third of the cases. Eighty percent of patients were phenotypic female, and more than half of these were virilized. Eighty-nine percent of patients were sex chromatin-negative. Chromosomal analysis carried out in 30 patients revealed 46 XY karyotypes in 57%, 45 XX/46 XY mosaicism in 30%, and a 45 X karyotype in one patient.

At the very least, gonadoblastomas repre-

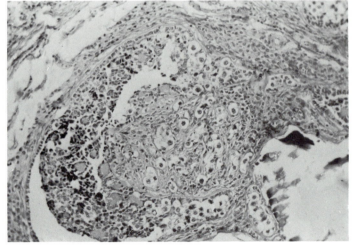

Fig 7–37.—Gonadoblastoma showing a central aggregate of germ cells with abundant clear cytoplasm and round, centrally placed nuclei. Granulosa cells are seen in the crescent-shaped area to the left. The Call-Exner bodies tend to contain more than the usual amount of central secretion, and the dark-staining psammoma bodies are intermixed.

sent a germ cell malignancy in situ. Since they are frequently bilateral, and dysgenetic gonads are valueless, treatment should include removal of all gonadal tissue. The uterus, though "hypoplastic" or even rudimentary, contains endometrium susceptible to the prolonged estrogen therapy that will be necessary. It therefore seems prudent to perform a hysterectomy as well.

Germ Cell Tumors

Dysgerminomas

Dysgerminomas make up less than 2% of primary ovarian cancers, but they are the most common ovarian malignancy found in postpubertal girls and young women. Although the ages range from 2 to 78 years, 85% of these tumors occur before age 30 years.

The dysgerminoma is morphologically identical to its homologue, the testicular seminoma, and both are believed to arise from the primordial germ cells of the indifferent stage of gonadogenesis.

Dysgerminomas have varied in size from a diameter of 3 cm to extremely large tumors that entirely fill the abdomen. Approximately 11% are bilateral. They are spherical or lob-

ular and predominantly solid, with areas of necrosis or hemorrhage in 50%. The histologic appearance is characteristic. The tumor cells that are uniformly large and polygonal with distinct margins and abundant clear cytoplasm are morphologically identical to primordial germ cells. The nucleus tends to be centrally placed and contains clumped chromatin and one or two prominent nucleoli. Mitotic activity and nuclear atypia are variable. The architectural pattern varies somewhat but usually consists of aggregates of tumor cells arranged in an alveolar pattern separated by strands of connective tissue that are infiltrated by lymphocytes (Fig 7–38). A linear arrangement of tumor cells to form cords is also common. In fewer than 15% of dysgerminomas a noncaseating granulomatous reaction with giant cells of the Langhans type is present and resembles the lesions of sarcoidosis. Isolated syncytiotrophoblastic giant cells are occasionally seen and account for the excretion of chorionic gonadotropin in the absence of choriocarcinomatous elements.

Several gross and microscopic findings of prognostic significance have been described. As expected, extraovarian tumor spread diminishes the chance for survival, but with

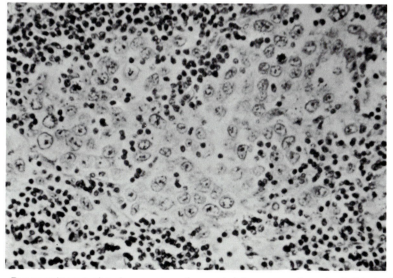

Fig 7–38.—Dysgerminoma showing groups of large, round cells with clear cytoplasm and nuclei containing several nucleoli. Marked lymphocytic infiltration is present.

carefully planned radiation therapy more than 50% of these patients can be salvaged. Bilaterality due to a synchronous tumor does not affect survival. Gross penetration of the tumor capsule and the presence of ascites, particularly if hemorrhagic, adversely affect prognosis. Microscopically, marked lymphocytic infiltration or a granulomatous response are associated with a favorable outcome. Asadourian and Taylor observed 6.7% mortality in a group of patients with marked lymphocytic infiltration, whereas 20% of patients whose tumors had minimal lymphocytic reaction died. These authors also found that mitotic figures in excess of eight per 5 high-power fields were associated with a 23% mortality rate as opposed to a 10% mortality from tumors with fewer mitotic figures. The tumor recurred in four of the seven patients in this series in whom vascular invasion was recognized.

The most important microscopic determinant of survival is the presence of other germ cell elements. In Asadourian and Taylor's study, the five-year survival rate of 98 patients with pure dysgerminomas was 90%, whereas all 12 patients with admixtures of other cell types were dead within two years. Nine of the 30 mixed germ cell tumors recently analyzed by Kurman and Norris were predominantly dysgerminomas. The authors concluded from their entire series that if more than one third of a stage I neoplasm was composed of endodermal sinus tumor, choriocarcinoma, or grade 3 immature teratoma, the prognosis was poor. On the other hand, if the tumor contained less than one third of these elements or was composed of dysgerminoma combined with embryonal carcinoma or grade 1 or 2 teratoma, the prognosis was excellent.

By the time of diagnosis the tumor has extended beyond the ovaries in 15% to 30% of cases. Metastases may occur by local tumor implantation consistent with epithelial tumors, but dysgerminomas also have a propensity for lymphatic dissemination. Pelvic and aortic nodes have been the only sites of metastatic disease in nearly 50% of patients with extraovarian spread. Metastases to liver, spleen, kidney, pancreas, lung, heart, and thyroid gland have been observed late in the course of the disease.

Although dysgerminomas are considered uniformly malignant, wide variations in reported survival rates have led to disagreement regarding the optimal management of tumors confined to one ovary. The implications of conservative therapy in the age group usually affected are obvious. The contralateral ovary poses a definite risk for recurrence; occult involvement by a synchronous dysgerminoma has been noted in only 6% to 15%, but undetected metastases may occur more frequently. In the 1955 series of Pedowitz et al. the remaining ovary was the primary site of recurrence in 36% of patients following conservative operation. The outlook has been far more optimistic during the past two decades by virtue of a greater proportion of localized cases and the clear-cut demonstration that radiation therapy can effect cure in more than 50% of recurrent cases. Consequently, attention has again been focused on the preservation of childbearing capacity and the corresponding risk of conservative treatment. Malkasian and Symmonds in 1964 reported an 80% five-year survival rate among 21 patients with unilateral encapsulated dysgerminomas treated by unilateral salpingo-oophorectomy alone. The tumor recurred in 11 patients (52%), but seven of these were salvaged by radiation therapy. The disease recurred in only one of six patients treated by irradiation or more extensive operations and this recurrence was successfully irradiated. The results reported by Asadourian and Taylor in 1969 are even more encouraging. Unilateral oophorectomy was the primary treatment in 46 of 71 patients with dysgerminomas confined to one ovary. The tumor recurred in ten of these (22%) but was successfully controlled in six, resulting in a five-year survival rate of 91%. Three recurrences were observed among 25 patients who underwent bilateral oophorectomy with and without irradiation (12%), but since these three patients died the survival rate was 88% for this group. Gordon et al. (1981) have also reported five-year survival in 67 of 72 patients (94%) with dysgerminoma confined to one ovary and treated by unilateral adnexectomy. The marked radiosensitivity of dysgerminomas was demonstrated by Afridi et al. who successfully treated metastatic tumor even at distant sites in six of seven patients. Radiation doses of only 2,000 to 3,000 rads were required. Krepart et al. (1978) have also reported three-year survival in ten of 13 patients (77%) with dysgerminoma and aortic nodal metastases treated with radiation therapy.

The optimal therapeutic approach to this disease must be based on the operative findings and a thorough histologic examination of all tumor tissue. For patients in whom childbearing is not an issue, hysterectomy and bilateral salpingo-oophorectomy should be accompanied by omental and aortic-node biopsy and the excision of gross tumor when dissemination has taken place. Adjuvant radiation therapy to the abdomen, pelvis, and para-aortic nodes should be used, and when tumor involvement of aortic nodes has been demonstrated the mediastinum and supraclavicular areas must also be irradiated.

Unilateral salpingo-oophorectomy is adequate therapy for most unilateral dysgerminomas, but a number of recurrences must be anticipated. In the young nullipara, this procedure should be performed in conjunction with intraperitoneal saline irrigation for cytologic study, wedge biopsy of the contralateral ovary, distal omental biopsy, and aortic node sampling at the level of the duodenum. Any palpable aortic or pelvic lymph nodes should be removed. The final decision to elect conservative therapy must await thorough histologic examination of the tissue and discussions with the patient and her family. Although the risk of recurrence and the need for intensive follow-up during the initial two years must be explained, the surgeon sincerely offering conservative management must maintain an optimistic and empathic attitude. Since the patient's life depends on the early detection of recurrence, an intensive program of surveillance must be designed to cover the first two years during which most dysgerminomas recur. A postoperative lymphangiogram will provide an outline of the aortic-node chain for 12 months. Plain films of the abdomen at specific intervals should reveal changes in configuration resulting from intranodal tumor growth. In all cases, β-subunit HCG and α-fetoprotein determinations should be carried out immediately after operation, if not before. Not only may the presence of endodermal sinus tumor or choriocarcinomatous elements be revealed, but a useful serum marker may be provided for assessment of therapeutic effect and detection of early recurrence.

Immature (Malignant) Teratomas

The immature teratoma is composed of both embryonal and adult tissues derived from all three germ layers. Although a specific precursor cell has not been identified, there is reason to believe that both immature and mature teratomas are similarly derived. Consequently, the initial event—inappropriate division of a secondary oocyte— is followed by repetitive mitotic division and incomplete differentiation into ectodermal, mesodermal, and endodermal elements. Kurman et al. described admixtures of extraembryonic elements (endodermal sinus tumor, choriocarcinoma, embryonal carcinoma) in seven of ten predominantly teratomatous mixed tumors, the remaining three containing a dysgerminomatous component. Since the presence of extraembryonic elements adversely affects survival, these mixed germ cell tumors must be excluded from the group containing only teratomatous tissue.

The largest series of "pure" immature teratomas has been reported from the Armed Forces Institute of Pathology (AFIP) by Norris and associates, and most of the information presented herein is derived from the 58 patients included in that study. The ages ranged from 14 months to 40 years, with a median of 19 years. The symptoms were consistent with those of other malignant ovarian neoplasms.

Eighty percent of patients had a palpable abdominal or pelvic mass, and fever and leukocytosis were noted in 25%.

The tumors were all unilateral except one that had metastasized to the opposite ovary. Sixty percent were confined to one ovary (stage I), 15.5% involved other pelvic structures (stage II), and 15.5% involved extrapelvic abdominal structures (stage III). The mode of spread is by implantation on serosal surfaces and aortic nodal involvement at the level of the renal vessels has been noted. Hematogenous metastases are rare.

Immature teratomas are firm with an irregular contour, and range from 5 to 35 cm in diameter. Although usually considered solid tumors, all contain multiple cystic spaces, which vary from 0.5 to 10.0 cm in diameter. The cut surface reveals small cystic spaces interspersed throughout solid tissue that is soft and rubbery and may contain areas of necrosis and hemorrhage. Neural tissue may be visible grossly. Norris et al. found cartilage in all specimens, bone or calcification in 64%, and hair in 41%.

The histologic picture is variable. Mesodermal elements often predominate, depending on the maturity of the tumor (Fig 7–39). Endoderm may be represented by tubules lined with columnar epithelium, and the ectoder-

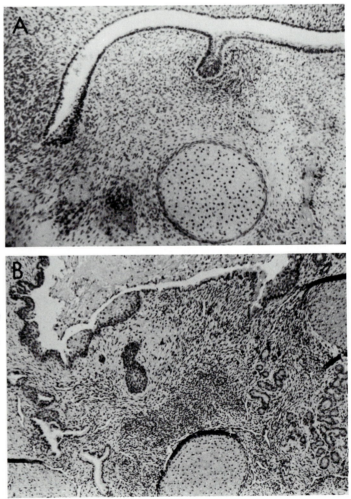

Fig 7–39.—A, sagittal section through a 25-mm embryo showing a branchial cleft and a section of immature tracheal cartilage within an undifferentiated mesenchyme. **B,** section of an immature teratoma showing a cleft lined by mature respiratory epithelium undergoing squamous metaplasia. In addition to immature cartilage and undifferentiated mesenchyme, mature mucinous glands are seen on the left and immature glandular structures on the right. (Courtesy of R.L. Ehrmann, M.D.)

mal component usually consists of hair, rudimentary teeth, and neural tissue. These structures are contained within a loose stroma of primitive mesenchyme. The degree of malignancy is closely correlated with the proportion of immature tissue. Robboy and Scully and the AFIP workers (Norris et al.) have adopted similar grading systems that are predictive of malignant behavior and eventual outcome. Grade 0 tumors are constituted of mature tissue only, whereas grade 1 through 3 are characterized by an increasing proportion of poorly differentiated embryonal tissue intermixed with the mature components. Mature tissue elements are infrequent in grade 3 tumors in which a primitive neuroepithelial component is prominent within a highly cellular sarcomatous stroma. Mitotic activity increases with the tumor grade.

Both the stage of the disease and the tumor grade are important and independent determinants of prognosis. The influence of these factors on survival in the AFIP series is demonstrated in Table 7–5.

The histologic grade of metastases may differ from that of the primary tumor; it also bears a relationship to prognosis. In the AFIP study, five of six patients with grade 0 metastases survived, whereas two of five with grade 1, three of six with grade 2, and none of seven patients with grade 3 metastases survived. Robboy and Scully have reported 12 patients with solid teratomas (two with grade 0; ten with grades 1 through 3) and peritoneal implants composed entirely or predominantly of mature glial tissue. None of these patients died, although persistent tumor was presumed or palpated in seven asymptomatic patients followed for five to 38 years after primary operation. In considering these two series as one, metastases consisted only of mature glial tissue in 14 of the 18 stage II and III survivors. Two explanations for the paradoxical occurrence of mature and benign metastases originating from a basically immature and malignant primary tumor have been offered. Robboy and Scully proposed that defects in the tumor capsule at areas occupied by glial elements are responsible for the selective dissemination and implantation of these cells. Other investigators, however, have presented presumptive evidence that immature elements are capable of differentiation to mature teratomas after dissemination (Favara and Franciosi; Nogales and Oliva). Recently Piver et al. described the transition of immature teratomatous metastases to solid mature teratomas in two patients during chemotherapy (cyclophosphamide and vincristine). These authors suggest that the drugs either selectively destroyed the immature elements, induced maturation, or were unrelated to the maturation phenomenon. In these two cases, the sequence of events favors chemotherapeutic destruction and the first hypothesis seems most logical.

For stage I immature teratomas, surgical treatment consists only of unilateral salpingo-oophorectomy. Combination chemotherapy consisting of vincristine, dactinomycin (actinomycin D), and cyclophosphamide (VAC) has been effective in some cases and should be administered over a 12-month period for stage I, grade 3 lesions. Rupture of the tumor capsule before or during operation has carried an 80% risk of tumor recurrence, and adju-

TABLE 7–5.—INFLUENCE OF STAGE AND GRADE ON ACTUARIAL SURVIVAL*

| GRADE | STAGE I | | STAGE II | | STAGE III | | TOTAL % SURVIVAL |
	NO. OF PATIENTS	% SURVIVAL	NO. OF PATIENTS	% SURVIVAL	NO. OF PATIENTS	% SURVIVAL	
1	14	100	4	50	4	50	82
2	20	70	2	50	2	0	62
3	6	33	2	0	2	50	30
Total	40	74	8	38	8	38	64

*From Norris H.J., Zirkin H.J., Benson W.L.: *Cancer* 37:2359, 1976.

vant chemotherapy is advisable under this circumstance. Patients with stage I, grade 1 or 2 tumors require close observation during the first 12 to 18 months, and periodic intraperitoneal surveillance by laparoscopy will provide early recognition of recurrence. Patients with stage II or III disease or recurrence are best managed by excision of tumor masses when feasible, followed by combination chemotherapy. Two-year disease-free survival was achieved in six of 11 patients (55%) with stage III immature teratoma treated with combination chemotherapy (Curry et al., 1978). In the absence of tumor involvement, extirpation of the uterus and contralateral adnexa is needless and should be avoided. Normal full-term pregnancy has been reported following successful combination chemotherapy for ovarian immature teratoma (Jahaveri et al., 1983). Radiation therapy has been ineffective in the management of this disease.

Mature (Benign) Teratomas

Benign or adult cystic teratomas constitute the vast majority of tumors in the category of mature teratomas. Solid mature teratomas referred to in the previous section as grade 0 are exceedingly rare and although their solid nature carries a malignant connotation they are invariably benign.

The benign cystic teratoma, which is often called a dermoid cyst because of a preponderance of epidermal elements, is the second or third most common ovarian neoplasm, depending on the age of the population base. Although cystic teratomas have been found in neonates and octogenarians, they occur predominantly during the reproductive years. Bennington et al. noted a steeply rising incidence from childhood that peaked at about 29 per 100,000 per year in the 20 to 44-year age group and then rapidly declined to zero by age 75 years. The benign cystic teratoma is the most commonly encountered ovarian neoplasm during adolescence and during pregnancy.

Although these tumors have been recognized from antiquity, the term *teratoma*, meaning "monstrous growth," was introduced by Virchow in 1863. The name *dermoid cyst*, which antedated Virchow's description by 30 years, has persisted and common usage has made it an acceptable, though unofficial, synonym. Despite the ectodermal implication of this term, many pathologists believe that all three germ layers can be identified by a diligent search of multiple histologic sections.

The theory of a parthenogenic origin has been in and out of favor for more than a century, but the recent contribution of Linder and associates appears to have settled the question once and for all. Utilizing chromosome banding techniques and electrophoretic enzyme analysis, these workers compared the cytogenetic markers of cells from five benign cystic teratomas with those of the normal host cells (see Fig 7–3). All teratomatous tissue had a 46 XX karyotype. The only possible explanation for the findings of Linder et al. is that cystic teratomas arise by parthenogenesis from secondary oocytes.

Benign cystic teratomas have varied widely in size from 4 mm in diameter to huge masses weighing 40 lb, but the vast majority are less than 15 cm in greatest diameter. Only 12% are bilateral, although multiple dermoid cysts rarely are found in both ovaries. The cyst wall tends to be thick and pearly gray, but the color varies, depending on the thickness of the capsule and the hue of the contents. The consistency is doughy, but hard areas representing cartilage or bone may be palpated. The cystic cavity is usually unilocular and contains a thick, greasy fluid made up of sebum and desquamated cells. The fluid of a cyst containing intestinal epithelium may be mucinous or, if brain tissue is a prominent component, clear and watery. Occasionally the cavity contains laminated pellets made up of lipids such as palmitin, stearic acid, and other fatty acids (Fig 7–40,B). Tangled masses of hair are often present and teeth have been reported in from 10% to 30% of tumors. When the contents of a cyst have been emptied, a discrete nodule that projects into the cavity can be found attached to the cyst wall.

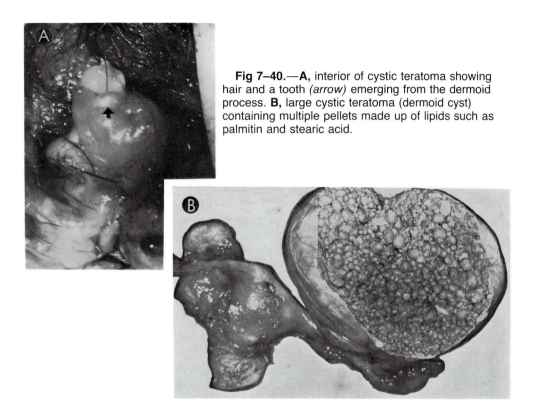

Fig 7–40.—A, interior of cystic teratoma showing hair and a tooth *(arrow)* emerging from the dermoid process. **B,** large cystic teratoma (dermoid cyst) containing multiple pellets made up of lipids such as palmitin and stearic acid.

This structure is known either as *Rokitansky's protuberance* or as the *dermoid process* (Fig 7–40,A). The cyst wall is smooth, but islands of epidermis or other differentiated tissue may be evident. Complex dermatoid cysts have been described that contain rudimentary fetal structures such as cranium and brain, ear anlage, mandible with teeth, arm and forearm, ribs, pelvic bones, vertebrae, and phalanges of a finger or foot.

Microscopically, a wide variety of tissues has been found. The cyst wall is lined by stratified squamous epithelium with irregular clusters of underlying dermal elements (Fig 7–41). The skin over the dermoid process is composed of stratified squamous epithelium without dermal papillae. Sebaceous glands, sweat glands, and hair follicles are present within a typical dermis. Although dermal structures are the most common component of Rokitansky's protuberance, all three germ layers are often represented. In their histo-logic examination of 295 benign cystic teratomas, Caruso et al. found fat in 67%, nervous tissue (well-differentiated glia, ganglion cells, and brain tissue) in 32%, cartilage in 39%, and bone in 19%. Respiratory tract epithelium was present in 18% of tumors, and gastrointestinal epithelium in 7% (Fig 7–42). Organs of special senses are occasionally discovered, particularly anlage of the eye.

Benign cystic teratomas tend to be asymptomatic, but Peterson and co-workers in reviewing 1,007 reported cases noted complaints of pain in 47% of patients and an abdominal mass in 15.4%. In addition, 15% of patients complained of abnormal uterine bleeding. Complications of dermoid cysts include torsion, rupture, and malignant transformation. Torsion is the most frequent of these and has been discussed previously (see the section "Diagnosis"). If twisting of the pedicle results in venous obstruction only, congestion and hemorrhage of the cyst wall

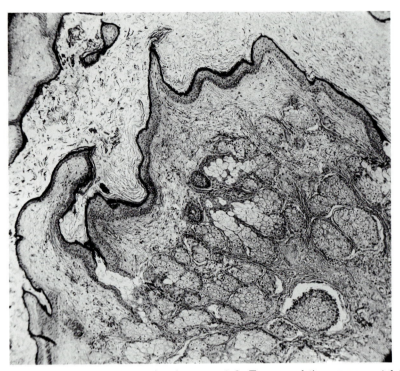

Fig 7–41.—Lining of cystic teratoma, showing desquamation of keratin, normal skin, and sebaceous glands. (Figs 7–41 to 7–43 from Hertig A.T., Gore H.: Tumors of the female sex organs: part 3. Tumors of the ovary and fallopian tube, sec. 9, fasc. 33, *Atlas of Tumor Pathology.* Washington, D.C., Armed Forces Institute of Pathology, 1961.)

induces an inflammatory reaction and adherence to surrounding structures. In this manner a new blood supply may be acquired by the tumor and if eventual dissolution of the pedicle occurs a so-called parasitic dermoid is the result. The omentum is the usual source of neovascularization.

Rupture of benign cystic teratomas is a rare but interesting phenomenon. According to the well-documented historical review by Pantoja and associates, the manifestations of rupture into hollow organs have been recognized for centuries. These include the expulsion of teeth, bones, and hair from the rectum and bladder. Intraperitoneal rupture is probably a more common occurrence. When released into the peritoneal cavity the cystic contents produce a chemical peritonitis; although sudden widespread peritoneal contamination is a catastrophic event, the clinical picture varies with the degree and rate of spillage. Consequently, slow leakage through a small defect in the cyst wall often causes chronic abdominal pain, which may be intermittent and diagnostically obscure. A granulomatous peritoneal reaction follows the deposition of neutral fat, fatty acid, and cholesterol crystals and the detritus of exfoliated cells. Microscopically, the granulomata are composed of lipid-laden macrophages, lymphocytes, plasma cells, and foreign body giant cells.

The percentage of benign cystic teratomas containing a malignant tissue component has been generally accepted as 1.9%, based on Peterson's extensive review in 1957. As might be expected, squamous cell carcinomas constitute the majority of these, and transitions from dysplasia and carcinoma in situ have been described. In reviewing the 272 re-

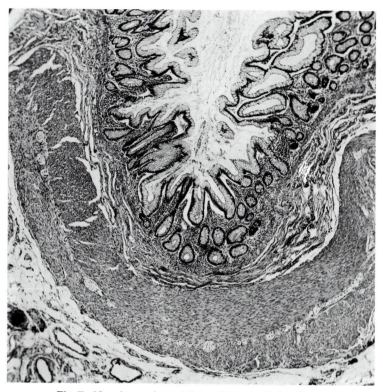

Fig 7–42.—Large-bowel tissue in a cystic teratoma.
A mucinous cystoma or adenocarcinoma could arise from this epithelium.

ported cases through 1967, Climie and Heath found that 75% were squamous cell carcinomas, 6% adenocarcinomas, 6% carcinoid tumors, 1.5% malignant melanomas, and 7% sarcomas. Squamous cell carcinomas usually arise from the skin covering Rokitansky's protuberance. Both the squamous cell carcinomas and adenocarcinomas metastasize by implantation on serosal surfaces, and a poor prognosis has been associated with the preoperative or intraoperative rupture of dermoid cysts containing these elements. Like their somatic counterparts, melanomas and sarcomas within dermoid cysts are likely to metastasize by way of the bloodstream. The prognosis is relatively good for all of these if the cyst wall is intact and no gross extraovarian dissemination has occurred. Climie and Heath reported only two deaths among 13 patients in whom the tumors met these criteria.

The treatment of benign cystic teratomas is surgical extirpation. Since a clear tissue plane exists between the cyst wall and normal ovary, ovarian conservation is readily accomplished. Because of the possibility of bilateral tumors, the contralateral ovary should be carefully scrutinized. If childbearing function is not a consideration most gynecologists as well as their patients prefer hysterectomy and either unilateral or bilateral salpingo-oophorectomy, depending on the proximity of anticipated menopause. In the event of intraperitoneal rupture, the gastrointestinal tract must be carefully inspected for potential areas of obstruction secondary to a granulomatous process or dense adhesions. Although this complication was associated with a high mortality in the past, Kistner (1953) has pointed out that the danger has been overexaggerated, and most patients treated for intraperitoneal rupture in recent years have survived. If malignant change has not precipitated the perforation and if intestinal obstruction does not supervene, the mortality associated with this complication need not be higher than that following any major laparotomy.

STRUMA OVARII.—On microscopic examination, 5% to 10% of benign cystic teratomas contain clusters of typical thyroid acini (Fig 7–43). Occasionally the thyroid tissue occupies all or most of the tumor, which is then designated a struma ovarii. Some pathologists, however, apply this diagnosis to cystic teratomas in which the thyroid tissue is recognizable grossly. The tumor is usually unilateral, measuring 6 to 8 cm in greatest diameter. The external surface is smooth and rounded and the cut surface has the glistening amber appearance of thyroid tissue. Microscopically, the tissue resembles that of the normal thyroid gland, with rounded follicles that are lined by cuboidal epithelium and contain periodic acid-Schiff (PAS)-positive colloid. Typically the colloid tends to retract from the epithelial cells and frequently is vacuolated. Scully has seen a number of typical strumas that imperceptibly merge with carcinoid tissue.

Six percent of patients with struma ovarii are thyrotoxic, but only about half of these have a disappearance of symptoms after excision of the neoplasm. Papillary or follicular thyroid carcinoma has developed in 5% of strumas, but only 17 of 45 reported cases have been associated with metastases. In the latter instance the treatment should be the same as that for metastatic thyroid carcinoma.

OVARIAN CARCINOID (ARGENTAFFINOMA).— Although the first ovarian carcinoid was reported in 1939, the prevalence and clinical significance of this neoplasm has been recognized generally only during the past 15 years. Most ovarian carcinoids are of the insular type comparable with those derived from the midgut (jejunum, ileum, appendix), but Robboy and associates (1976) have reported 18 trabecular carcinoids that are histologically identical to those of the foregut and hindgut. Insular and trabecular carcinoids are occasionally intermixed and either, particularly the latter,

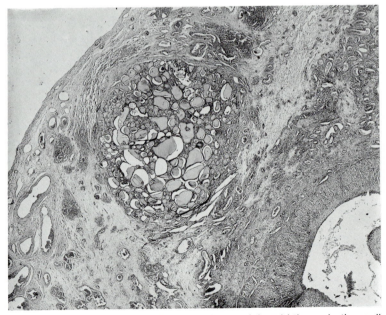

Fig 7–43.—Cystic teratoma showing a focus of thyroid tissue in the wall.

may be associated with a struma ovarii (strumal carcinoid). Since the ovaries are a frequent site of metastasis from gastrointestinal carcinoids, a careful differentiation must be made between primary and secondary carcinoids of the ovary.

In a review of 48 insular carcinoids Robboy and co-workers (1975) found that 60% clearly arose in benign cystic teratomas and 13% in mature solid teratomas. Four percent originated from the argentaffine cells of mucinous cystadenomas, and 23% occurred as pure carcinoid tumors. Most pathologists believe that the latter are examples of specialized monodermal teratomas in which other tissue elements have been overgrown. Sixteen of the 18 cases of trabecular carcinoid previously mentioned were associated with teratomatous elements. Curiously, the median ages of the patients with insular and trabecular carcinoids were 57 and 47 years, respectively, both well above the median age for benign cystic teratomas.

Grossly, these tumors have varied between 3 and 28 cm in diameter with a median of 10 cm. On section, the cavity of a dermoid cyst may be encountered and the carcinoid identified as a firm, yellow-tan, 3 to 4 cm projection into the cavity. The larger the carcinoid component, the more solid the tumor becomes, and persistent cystic cavities are lined by carcinoid tissue. Microscopically, insular carcinoids consist of discrete islands of cells that are arranged in solid or acinar structures and are separated by a dense fibrous stroma. The cells are polygonal with centrally placed, round nuclei containing clumped chromatin. The cytoplasm of peripheral cells contains argentaffine granules. Actual gland formation is common in functioning carcinoids and these consist of columnar cells in acinar arrangement with basal nuclei and abundant cytoplasm bordering on the central lumina. Microscopic examination of trabecular tumors reveals long wavy ribbons of epithelial cells separated by loose fibrous stroma. The ribbons consist of tall columnar cells with their long axes parallel to one another. The nuclei are oval and centrally placed with abundant cytoplasm at either pole. Argentaffine granules are found in only about one third of trabecular carcinoids.

One third of insular carcinoids produce sufficient 5-hydroxytryptamine (serotonin) to cause symptoms of the carcinoid syndrome. Hot flushes were described by 13 of the 16 patients with this syndrome reported by Robboy et al. Ten patients complained of diarrhea and six had pedal edema. Hypertension was noted in five patients and cardiac murmurs due to right heart valvular disease were discovered in six. Urinary levels of 5-hydroxyindoleacetic acid were elevated in all seven of the symptomatic patients in whom the determination was performed, and fell to normal after tumor excision. Symptoms regressed in all patients after removal of the tumor, although cardiac valvular damage in one patient was sufficient to induce cardiac failure three years later. Robboy and associates have related the onset of the carcinoid syndrome to the size of the tumor. Only one of 20 tumors (5%) in which the carcinoid component was 4 cm or less in diameter produced the syndrome, whereas six of 14 patients (43%) with tumors from 4 to 7 cm and nine of 13 patients (69%) with tumors greater than 7 cm experienced carcinoid symptoms. Carcinoids of the ovary, in contrast to those of the small bowel and appendix, may induce the syndrome in the absence of metastatic disease. This disparity is readily explained by the fact that serotonin from midgut tumors is carried by the portal system to the liver where it is metabolized. Serotonin from ovarian tumors obviously bypasses the liver. Trabecular carcinoid of the ovary has not been associated with the carcinoid syndrome.

If a diagnosis of carcinoid tumor is made at the time of operation and a teratomatous origin is not apparent, an attempt to exclude an ovarian metastasis must be made by thorough exploration of the gastrointestinal tract. Involvement of the opposite ovary or peritoneal spread strongly suggests a small bowel primary tumor, which may be difficult to find. If the tumor is unilateral or associated with a teratoma and extraovarian metastases are not visible, the carcinoid may be considered primary in the ovary. The optimal treatment is hysterectomy and bilateral salpingo-oophorectomy unless preservation of childbearing capacity or ovarian function is important. In this instance unilateral salpingo-oophorectomy is acceptable. The contralateral ovary must be biopsied to confirm the primary nature of the disease and to exclude contralateral dermoid cyst or cystoma, one of which was present in 16% of patients reported by Robboy et al.

The prognosis is good. Only two of the 48 patients with insular carcinoids had recurrence; both of them died. Only one of the 18 patients with trabecular carcinoids died from the disease.

Endodermal Sinus Tumor

Among the malignant neoplasms of the ovary occurring before the age of 20 years the endodermal sinus tumor ranks second in frequency to the dysgerminoma and is equally prevalent before the age of 15 years (Norris and Jenson). Furthermore, an associated fatality rate of 90% had placed the endodermal sinus tumor first as a cause of death from ovarian cancer in childhood and adolescence. Despite its significance in this age group, this tumor was largely ignored as a specific entity in the past because it was either included in

the teratoma group or was categorized as a mesonephric rest tumor on the basis of Schiller's original description in 1939 (see the section "Clear Cell Carcinoma"). In 1954, Teilum pointed out Schiller's error and suggested an extraembryonic germ cell origin for the tumor. By 1959, he had identified the tissue as proliferating yolk sac endoderm, and because of a marked resemblance to the normal endodermal sinuses of the rat placenta Teilum proposed that this term be applied. *Endodermal sinus tumor* has now been adopted by the WHO.

The largest series published is that of the AFIP (Kurman and Norris, 1976). The ages of the 71 patients ranged from 14 months to 45 years, with a median of 19 years. The most common presenting symptoms were abdominal pain in 77%, an abdominal mass in 27%, and fever in 24%. The virulence of this tumor was manifested by a brief interval from onset of symptoms to diagnosis, less than two weeks in two thirds of the patients. An acute onset of symptoms resulted from torsion or intraperitoneal rupture in seven patients.

The size of endodermal sinus tumors ranges from 6 to 30 cm in diameter, but the usual size is between 10 and 20 cm. These tumors are consistently unilateral unless gross metastases are apparent in other sites as well. The external surface is smooth and the cut surface is yellowish tan or gray, with areas of necrosis

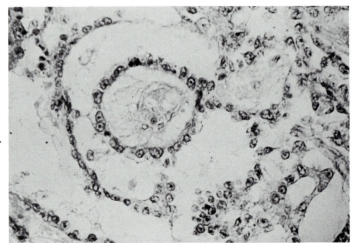

Fig 7–44.—Endodermal sinus tumor. Reticular pattern with a Schiller-Duval body in the center.

or hemorrhage occasionally present. Multiple small cystic structures may lend a Swiss-cheese appearance. Microscopically, the classic pattern has been termed *reticular* and consists of a network of sinusoidal spaces lined by cuboidal cells with scanty cytoplasm (Fig 7–44). The occasional hobnail appearance of the cells added to the confusion with Schiller's type 2 mesonephroma (clear cell carcinoma) in the past (see Fig 7–26,B). Schiller-Duval bodies, which consist of a mantle of yolk sac endoderm surrounding a capillary, are prominent (see Fig 7-44). Although Schiller-Duval bodies are diagnostic they were present in only 75% of the AFIP tumors. The authors point out the ubiquity of intracellular and intercellular hyaline droplets, which were present in 100%. Using an immunoperoxidase reaction, the authors showed that α-fetoprotein was present in all 15 tumors in which the histochemical analysis was carried out, and appeared to be concentrated in the hyaline droplets.

In the manner of most malignant ovarian neoplasms, endodermal sinus tumors disseminate by implantation on peritoneal surfaces. The frequent occurrence of metastases after removal of a well-encapsulated tumor is inexplicable. Lymph node metastases are common in autopsy series and occult nodal involvement by otherwise encapsulated tumors could account for subsequent peritoneal metastases as suggested by Kurman and Norris. In the terminal phase of the disease hematogenous dissemination is commonly manifested by intrahepatic and pulmonary metastases.

Only five of the 71 patients (13%) in the AFIP series survived, and the survival rate was little better when the tumor was confined to the ovary (16%). Three of five patients with tumors under 10 cm in diameter survived, but no other factors were of prognostic significance. Neither age, histologic pattern, mitotic activity, nor the integrity of the tumor capsule affected survival. Paradoxically, preoperative or intraoperative tumor rupture was associated with an 18% survival rate. As noted by others, all deaths occurred during the 30-month interval from diagnosis.

The surgical treatment of endodermal sinus tumors is unilateral salpingo-oophorectomy. No benefit is derived from hysterectomy and bilateral salpingo-oophorectomy unless this procedure is an integral part of a planned "debulking" operation prior to chemotherapy. Irradiation has been totally ineffective both as a surgical adjuvant with localized tumors and as palliation for advanced or recurrent disease. One of the more gratifying accomplishments of chemotherapy has been the combined effect of vincristine, dactinomycin (actinomycin D), and cyclophosphamide (VAC) on endodermal sinus tumors. Three of the four stage I patients in the AFIP series who received this drug combination survived. Similarly, Smith and Rutledge at the M. D. Anderson Hospital and Tumor Institute have reported a disease-free survival rate of 100% among seven stage I patients for periods of four to 47 months. More remarkably, eight of 13 patients with disseminated tumor were free of disease at the time of their report. Subsequent studies by Cangir et al. (1978), Creasman et al. (1979), and Gershenson et al. (1983) have confirmed the dramatic effectiveness of combination chemotherapy with endodermal sinus tumors. Clearly, all patients with endodermal sinus tumor should receive adjuvant chemotherapy with VAC, although the optimal duration of therapy is not yet defined. The presence of measurable serum levels of α-fetoprotein uniformly associated with yolk sac tumors provides a sensitive marker for assessment of therapeutic results and detection of early recurrence (Romero and Schwartz, 1981).

Choriocarcinoma

The choriocarcinoma is an extremely rare, but highly malignant, tumor that may be primary in the ovary or secondary to a uterine choriocarcinoma. During the childbearing years most of these tumors fall into the second category, even in the absence of a pregnancy history or a demonstrable uterine tumor. Occasionally associated placental villi establish both the primary nature of the tumor and its origin from an ovarian pregnancy. Almost all primary choriocarcinomas are represented as a component of mixed germ cell tumors. Six of the 30 mixed germ cell tumors reported by Kurman and Norris contained choriocarcinomatous elements, and in two this tissue predominated. Although choriocarcinomas rarely obliterate the other germ cell components, the hemorrhagic tendency of choriocarcinomas may obscure their identity. The diagnosis of a pure nongestational choriocarcinoma can only be made with certainty in prepubertal girls. Although several of these have been reported, the recent elucidation of ovarian embryonal carcinoma by Kurman and Norris has cast some doubt on their existence.

Ovarian choriocarcinomas are always unilateral. The tumor surface is nodular, and hemorrhagic tissue within a thin capsule imparts a red or purplish color. The tumor is extremely friable, consisting of spongy tissue infiltrated by blood. Areas of necrosis and cavitation may be apparent. The microscopic appearance is similar to that of the primary uterine choriocarcinoma. There are masses of syncytiotrophoblastic and cytotrophoblastic cells admixed in a plexiform pattern. Syncytiotrophoblastic tissue may line blood-filled spaces similar to the intervillous spaces of the placenta or it may cover islands of cytotrophoblast. The opposite ovary is frequently enlarged by theca-lutein cysts or shows marked stromal luteinization as a result of the chorionic gonadotropin secretion.

Primary choriocarcinoma is a tumor of childhood and early adolescence. A few that have been associated with other germ cell elements or benign cystic teratomas, however, have been reported in the 20s and early 30s. The symptoms are those of a rapidly enlarging tumor mass and are often aggravated by ascites. Rupture of the tumor with intraperitoneal hemorrhage is a common complication and represents an acute surgical emergency. Unless the tumor is large, the clinical picture simulates that of a ruptured ectopic pregnancy. The high gonadotropin level stimulates the ovarian stroma and induces precocious puberty in children. Similarly, irregular uterine bleeding and breast enlargement are common symptoms in the postpubertal woman.

Ovarian choriocarcinomas were uniformly fatal until the advent of adjuvant chemotherapy. The involved ovary must be removed and subjected to meticulous histologic examination to determine the origin of the tumor. The prognosis is good in the case of gestational trophoblastic disease, utilizing the chemotherapeutic program outlined in Chapter 12. Nongestational choriocarcinoma of the ovary has been considerably less sensitive to single-agent chemotherapy than its gestational counterpart. Triple-agent combination chemotherapy consisting of methotrexate, dactinomycin (actinomycin D), and cyclophosphamide (MAC) has greatly improved the outcome. In a recent report by Gerbie and associates at Northwestern University Medical School, four of eight patients were in remission for more than one year.

Embryonal Carcinoma

The embryonal carcinoma is a rare tumor that was first described in late 1976 by Kurman and Norris. As extraembryonic tumors, they are homologous to the testicular embryonal carcinomas but have previously been classified as endodermal sinus tumors or choriocarcinomas, to which they are closely related. The ages of the 15 patients reported by Kurman and Norris ranged from 4 to 28 years, with a median of 14 years. The tumor appears to afflict a younger age group than the other extraembryonic tumors, and 47% of the patients were prepubertal. Although the symptoms were similar to those associated with endodermal sinus tumors, abnormal hormonal manifestations were noted in 60% of patients. These consisted of precocious puberty and irregular bleeding or amenorrhea in the postpubertal patients. Pregnancy tests were positive in all nine patients in whom they were performed.

The tumors were unilateral and ranged from 10 to 25 cm in diameter. Externally they were smooth, and section revealed solid gray to yellow tissue with occasional cysts and areas of necrosis and hemorrhage. Microscopically, there were sheets or nests of large primitive pleomorphic cells with well-defined cell membranes and round vesicular nuclei containing prominent nucleoli. Syncytiotrophoblastic giant cells, identified by the immunoperoxidase reaction for HCG, were scattered at the periphery or throughout the stroma. Hyaline droplets characteristic of endodermal sinus tumors were found in 12 of the 15 tumors, and α-fetoprotein was demonstrated in these and in the mononuclear embryonal cells by the immunoperoxidase reaction. The overall microscopic appearance suggested a uniphasic overgrowth by cytotrophoblast with scattered isolated syncytiotrophoblastic cells. The admixture of both cell types in the plexiform pattern of choriocarcinoma was not observed.

The actuarial five-year survival rate was 39% for the entire group, and 50% for those with localized tumors. Treatment should consist of unilateral salpingo-oophorectomy and adjuvant chemotherapy. Although methotrexate alone appeared to benefit two patients, the optimal chemotherapeutic regimen has yet to be defined. The responsiveness of choriocarcinomas to the MAC regimen (methotrexate-actinomycin D-cyclophosphamide) and of endodermal sinus tumors to the VAC regimen suggests that this type of combination chemotherapy may be effective against embryonal carcinoma as well. Human chorionic gonadotropin determinations may provide an effective serum marker, and the histochemical demonstration of α-fetoprotein suggests that serum assays for this oncofetal protein may also be useful.

Nonintrinsic and Metastatic Tumors

Fibromas

Despite the inclusion of fibromas in a common category with thecomas in the WHO classification, we have preferred to retain them in the nonintrinsic tumor group proposed by Hertig and Gore. Admittedly, fibromas and thecomas may be impossible to differentiate histologically, and a practical approach to ovarian tumor classification would seem to militate against their separation. We believe, as suggested by Norris and Taylor, that a diagnosis of either a granulosa cell tumor or thecoma should be based on specific histologic criteria. Uncertainty in differentiating between the thecoma and fibroma after appropriate staining techniques should relegate the tumor to the fibroma category. Fibromas in contrast to thecomas are hormonally inert, and estrogenic activity associated with fibromas is the result of stimulation and luteinization of non-neoplastic theca. Although fibrous tissue is part of the adult ovarian stroma, it is not specialized ovarian tissue and enters the ovary with blood vessels during the stage of vascularization.

The incidence of these tumors varies considerably, depending on the care with which ovaries are studied histologically and whether microscopic fibromas are included. The relative frequency reported in the literature varies from 1.5% to 5.0%. At the Brigham and Women's Hospital, 740 fibromas were included among 2,530 ovarian tumors, a relative incidence of 29.2% (Kent and McKay). The apparently excessive prevalence of fibromas in this series resulted from the inclusion of microscopic lesions. Fibromas are most commonly seen during the late childbearing period, the median age being 48 years.

The average diameter approximates 6 cm, and about 5% exceed 20 cm. They are bilateral in 10% of cases, and multiple tumors are occasionally discovered within the same ovary. A fibroma is hard and homogeneous in consistency, but on occasion it may feel cystic because of marked edema. Although the cut surface is typically white with a whorled appearance, intrinsic hemorrhage may impart a multicolored appearance. Microscopically, the basic cell type is the fibroblast and when these spindle-shaped cells are closely approximated in individual bundles the tumor acquires a fasciculated appearance. Varying amounts of collagen are present. Some degree of calcification is present in 3% to 4% of tumors.

The symptoms associated with ovarian fibromas are related to their size and are identical to those produced by the other benign ovarian tumors. The weight of the tumor tends to elongate a pedicle, and torsion is a relatively frequent complication. Ovarian fibromas in conjunction with ascites and right hydrothorax constitute the Meigs' syndrome. Although the etiology of the serous effusions has not been well explained, partial torsion and occlusion of venous drainage may result in a large, edematous, weeping tumor. Undoubtedly, the right pleural effusion results from the permeation of serous fluid through the diaphragmatic lymphatics.

Simple excision is adequate therapy for an ovarian fibroma. If the patient is postmenopausal, the opposite ovary also should be removed to avoid a second fibroma. In this instance hysterectomy is advisable but by no means mandatory.

Fibrosarcomas

Fibrosarcomas are exceedingly rare, highly malignant tumors that most often occur in postmenopausal women. The tumor is usually lobulated and of moderate size, averaging 10 cm in diameter. The cut surface shows focal areas of necrosis and cystic degeneration. Microscopically, the tumor is of the spindle-cell type, but intermixture of smooth muscle cells is common. In this instance the tumor may be termed a leiomyosarcoma; if myxomatous tissue is identified it has been designated a myxosarcoma. Seven fibrosarcomas and leiomyosarcomas were included by Azoury and Woodruff among their 43 reported cases of ovarian sarcomas. These seven represented 50% of sarcomas arising from the ovarian stroma. Six of the seven patients died of their disease within eight years of diagnosis, and the final patient was lost to follow-up.

Lymphomas

Ovarian involvement by lymphomas has been discovered at autopsy in one fourth of women with intact reproductive organs who die from these diseases. On the other hand, a very small percentage of women have had ovarian involvement as the initial manifestation of their disease, and the AFIP study by Chorlton and associates reported only one in 500 women with lymphomas in the latter category. In general, lymphocytic lymphomas make up slightly more than half of these tumors, whereas one-third are histiocytic lymphomas and less than one-sixth are Hodgkin's lymphomas.

The 19 ovarian lymphomas in the AFIP series varied between 2 and 20 cm in greatest diameter, with a median diameter of 10 cm. Three of the stage I tumors were bilateral (stage Ib). The external surface is usually smooth and encapsulated, but the tumor may be nodular or lobulated. Section reveals a rubbery gray-tan or pink tissue, which often contains cystic cavities and areas of necrosis and hemorrhage. Microscopically, the lymphomatous tissue has a diffuse or nodular pattern and infiltrates the ovarian stroma without destroying the normal architecture. This unique characteristic aids in differentiating lymphomas from carcinomas. The diagnosis can usually be made on routine hematoxylin and eosin-stained sections, but occasionally reticulum or Giemsa stains are required to elucidate the diagnosis.

Ovarian lymphomas affect women at all stages of life. The median age in the AFIP series was 38 years, with a range from 7 to 59 years. The principal signs and symptoms are those of an enlarging pelvic mass. Abnormal vaginal bleeding occurs in 20% to 30%, but anemia is out of proportion to the amount of bleeding.

Although nearly 25% of all lymphomas arise at extranodal sites, it is not clear whether the ovary can be a primary site or is only the initial organ to be clinically involved in a generalized disease process. Nine of the 19 patients in the AFIP series had localized tumors, thus qualifying them as extranodal lymphomas, stage Ie (Ann Arbor staging). Only four of these, or 45%, survived one year; two (22%) survived five years. These figures are markedly worse than the 92% one-year survival and 68% five-year survival reported for stage Ie lymphomas by Peters et al. in 1968. Although the poor survival rate tends to negate the concept of the ovary as a site of origin, staging of the ovarian lymphomas was only visual in contrast to the complex staging programs currently in use for these neoplasms.

The treatment of ovarian lymphomas consists of surgical removal of the tumor. Careful intraperitoneal staging must be carried out in consultation with a medical oncologist. Enlarged retroperitoneal nodes as well as enlargement of the liver and spleen must be carefully noted. Postoperatively, radiation and/or chemotherapy is indicated.

Krukenberg's Tumor

The term *Krukenberg's tumor* should be reserved for those metastatic ovarian tumors with the characteristic histologic picture of mucin-laden, signet-ring cells infiltrating a hyperplastic ovarian stroma of spindle-shaped cells (Fig 7–45,A). Krukenberg in his original description in 1896 called his tumor a "fibrosarcoma mucocellulare carcinomatodes" and believed it to be a primary ovarian neoplasm. Subsequent studies revealed that it was metastatic, usually from carcinoma of the stomach (Holtz and Hart, 1982). Although colon, breast, and pancreatic carcinomas have produced the same histologic picture (Fig 7–45, B), most ovarian metastases from these sites do not.

These tumors are usually bilateral, of moderate size, and, curiously, the normal shape of the ovary is retained. The cut surface typically exhibits gelatinous necrosis and mucin-filled cystic cavities of variable size.

Symptoms of the primary tumor are often absent or unrecognized and the typical symptoms of a large pelvic mass supervene. With increasing size, ascites and peritoneal implants are often found. Since the ovarian tumor tends to grow more rapidly than the primary tumor, the surgeon may be confronted with an anatomic picture indistinguishable from primary ovarian carcinoma. Rapid histologic section may provide an intraoperative

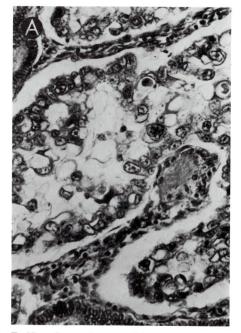 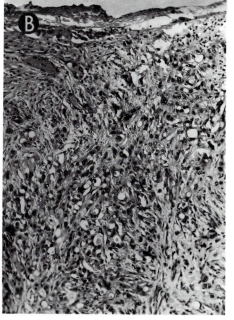

Fig 7–45.—A, carcinoma of the pancreas metastatic to the ovary. **B,** Krukenberg's tumor, showing rounded and polyhedral cells metastatic from a gastric cancer. Numerous "signet-ring" cells are seen.

diagnosis and permit a more thorough abdominal exploration if the primary tumor had been overlooked initially. Since many patients have survived for several years after diagnosis, the ovaries as well as the uterus should be removed. In their report of 48 cases in 1960, Woodruff and Novak described four patients who were living and well after five or more years.

Miscellaneous Metastatic Tumors

In 1962, Sternberg stated that "the ovaries present a congenial environment for the luxuriant growth of metastatic adenocarcinoma." Indeed the ovaries frequently appear to be the sole repository of metastatic tumor originating from a distant site. Certainly, occult metastases are present at other sites but the propensity for rapid growth within the ovary has never been explained. Equally puzzling is the route by which the tumor cells reach the ovary. Four possibilities have been suggested: (1) transport by peritoneal fluid with direct implantation on the ovarian surface; (2) lymphatic metastases; (3) hematogenous metastases; and (4) spread by direct contiguity with the primary cancer. Hertig and Gore believe that retrograde lymphatic spread best explains metastases from the gastrointestinal tract. The frequency with which carcinoma of the breast metastasizes to bones, lungs, and

abdominal viscera suggests that the bloodstream is the most likely route to the ovaries as well. Ovarian metastases from carcinoma of the endometrium probably result from both lymphatic spread and implantation of malignant cells on the ovarian surface following retrograde tubal transport.

In a series of 120 metastatic ovarian tumors (excluding Krukenberg's tumors) from the Emil Novak Ovarian Tumor Registry, Woodruff and associates found that 32% originated from the endometrium, 20% from the gastrointestinal tract, and 14% from the breast. In 16%, the primary site could not be determined; the remaining 19% were derived from tumors of the lung, thyroid, kidney, cervix, fallopian tube, central nervous system, and skin (melanoma).

More than 50% of metastatic ovarian tumors are bilateral. They have a smooth surface and a well-developed capsule, which does not become adherent to surrounding structures. The microscopic appearance is quite variable. The stroma may be hypercellular in certain areas while in others it is edematous or occasionally myxomatous. The epithelial elements may form acinar or glandular structures, and metastases from the gastrointestinal tract often simulate a mucinous cystadenocarcinoma or a malignant Brenner tumor. The individual cells that metastasize

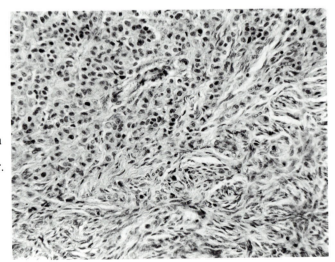

Fig 7–46.—Carcinoma of the breast metastatic to the ovary. The cells in the upper half of the photomicrograph resemble granulosa cells, and the architecture is also reminiscent of a granulosa cell tumor.

from a breast cancer may infiltrate the ovarian stroma in such a way as to resemble a granulosa-theca cell tumor (Fig 7–46).

Unless widespread tumor dissemination is evident, hysterectomy and bilateral salpingo-oophorectomy should be performed. This procedure is usually palliative but on occasion the primary tumor is susceptible to radiation or chemotherapy. In addition, a rare primary tumor that has been mistaken for metastatic disease will have been properly treated.

Carcinoma of the Ovary

Epidemiology

Carcinoma of the ovary is the fourth leading cause of cancer deaths among American women, following cancer of the breast, colon, and lung. Approximately 14,000 new cases are diagnosed each year, from which 11,000 deaths occur annually. According to current estimates, one of every 100 women in the United States is destined to die from this disease. Although the age-adjusted mortality rate from ovarian cancer more than doubled between 1930 and 1955, the incidence of the disease did not change significantly during the 22 years between the Second National Cancer Survey, 1947, and the Third National Cancer Survey, 1969–1971 (Cramer and Cutler). Age-specific mortality curves rise sharply after age 40 years and do not decline until after ages 65 and 80 years in nonwhites and whites, respectively. Consequently, it seems safe to conclude that increased longevity unmet by improvement in disease control is responsible for the continuing rise in crude mortality. Despite improvement in therapeutic modalities since 1950, only a minimal gain has been made in nationwide five-year survival rates—from 29% to 32% (Cutler et al., 1975).

Epidemiologic studies have failed to identify environmental or other predisposing factors to explain the geographic distribution of the disease. There are wide demographic differences in age-adjusted mortality rates ranging from a low of 1.69 in Japan to 11.02 in Denmark. Parallel differences in breast cancer mortality suggest a common endocrine background, and women with previously treated carcinomas of the breast or endometrium are more likely to develop second primary cancer in the ovary than at other sites. An environmental etiology may be inferred from the observation that Japanese women after immigrating to the United States incur a significantly greater risk of dying from ovarian cancer, which during middle life approaches that of white Americans (Wynder). An increased prevalence of ovarian cancer noted in nuns, other single women, and nulliparous married women suggests that incessant ovulation uninterrupted by pregnancy may be a predisposing factor. (It is of some interest that ovarian carcinoma is the most common epithelial tumor in the best known of incessant ovulators, the domestic fowl. In addition, the incidence of ovarian carcinoma in hens is greatly enhanced by constant environments designed to promote egg production [Fathalla].) Also, women who used oral contraceptives have a reduced risk of later developing epithelial ovarian cancer (Cramer et al. 1982).

Exposure to talc (asbestos) may also be related to the development of epithelial ovarian cancer. Graham and Graham (1967) were able to induce ovarian neoplasms with asbestos in guinea pigs. Cramer et al. (1982) observed that women who regularly dusted their perineum with talc and used talc on sanitary napkins had a threefold increased risk of developing ovarian cancer.

Prevention

Between 4% and 20% of reported patients with cancer of the ovary previously have undergone ablative pelvic operations with conservation of one or both ovaries. These percentages have led many surgeons to advocate the prophylactic removal of normal ovaries at the time of hysterectomy. Proponents of ovarian salvage argue that the risk of developing cancer in a residual ovary is negligible and is outweighed by the evils of early castration. There is no indication that the risk of ovarian cancer in women with residual ovaries differs from that of the general population or is reduced by removing only one ovary. Only about 6% of deaths from ovarian cancer will be prevented by prophylactic oophorectomy at the time of hysterectomy, but the risk to the individual is reduced from 1% to 0%.

Early Detection

The meager overall survival rate for all cases of ovarian cancer can be attributed to failure in early diagnosis. Between 1945 and 1949 only 27% of ovarian cancers were localized at diagnosis, and the corresponding figure for the years 1965 through 1969 was 28% (Cutler, 1976). The total failure to achieve earlier detection over a 20-year span reflects both the asymptomatic character of early ovarian cancer and the lack of a means whereby asymptomatic women can be screened for this disease. Despite earlier hopes, the increasingly prevalent annual pelvic examination and cervical cytologic smear have failed to increase the proportion of localized cases. In 1964, Graham and co-workers reported on the preclinical detection of ovarian cancer by the cytologic examination of peritoneal fluid obtained by transvaginal aspiration of the cul-de-sac. During the past decade McGowan has thoroughly explored this approach in both humans and experimental animals and has attained a high degree of accuracy by the concurrent use of cytologic and biochemical analysis of peritoneal aspirates. The value of a screening measure, however, is dependent on the prevalence of the disease as well as on the sensitivity of the technique employed. Despite its lethality, the incidence of ovarian cancer is sufficiently low that the detection of a single case would require screening of more than 5,000 women. The demonstration of tumor-associated antigens unique to epithelial ovarian cancers has raised the question of detecting immunoreactivity in women with these tumors. Knauf and Urbach (1980) have measured an ovarian tumor–associated antigen (OCA) in the serum of 78% of women with stage I epithelial ovarian cancer. Bast

and co-workers (1981) have developed a monoclonal antibody to human epithelial ovarian carcinoma. The development of radioimmunoassays for ovarian tumor–associated antigens may facilitate the early diagnosis of ovarian malignancy as well as monitoring the response to therapy.

Natural History

The primary mode of tumor dissemination consists of penetration of the tumor capsule by proliferating epithelium and subsequent implantation of clonogenic cells on peritoneal surfaces. Intraperitoneal spread follows the usual pathways by which peritoneal fluid and particulate matter are cleared from the cavity. The major route from the pelvis is cephalad along the right paracolic gutter to the undersurface of the right hemidiaphragm and then into the network of diaphragmatic lymphatics. Isolated diaphragmatic involvement has been noted with otherwise localized tumors, and obstruction of diaphragmatic lymphatics by tumor emboli may result in the early onset of ascites. The proximity to the pelvis of omentum, cecum, terminal ileum, and sigmoid colon makes these organs frequent sites of early implantation. In some instances, particularly in the presence of ascites, the surgeon may encounter widespread, 2 to 3 mm visceral and parietal peritoneal implantations resembling miliary tuberculosis. Para-aortic lymph nodes are frequently involved, even early in the course of the disease. Knapp and Friedman found positive aortic nodes in four of 22 women with stage I epithelial cancers who underwent para-aortic node dissections. In two patients involved nodes were not palpably enlarged, but all four women had poorly differentiated tumors. Extra-abdominal dissemination by the lymphatic route is slow, and hematogenous spread is usually a late manifestation. As a group, the epithelial carcinomas are relatively noninvasive, and destruction of vital organs is infrequent. With increasing tumor growth, however, there is a progressive mechanical interference with the function of abdominal organs. Disordered small bowel motility secondary to adhesions and interference with neural transmission through the myenteric plexus is a prominent feature and may simulate small-bowel obstruction (Fig 7–47). Actual bowel obstruction is not uncommon but usually occurs at multiple sites. The overall effect of interference with gastrointestinal function, the production of serous effusions, and the metabolic demands of an enlarging bulk of tumor tissue, leads to progressive inanition. In general, the proximity of death appears related to the volume of proliferating tumor within the peritoneal cavity.

There is no evidence that the patient's age in itself influences the biologic activity of ovarian carcinomas. A better prognosis noted among women under 40 years of age, in whom the disease is less frequent, apparently results from a greater proportion of both borderline tumors and those of low histologic grade. Although the incidence of ovarian cancer increases dramatically after age 40 years, neither the incidence nor the virulence of the disease is affected by the menopause. A relatively poor prognosis after age 60 years most likely results from later diagnosis and the prevalence of intercurrent disease.

Staging of Ovarian Carcinoma (FIGO)

Stage I. Growth limited to the ovaries.

Stage Ia. Growth limited to one ovary; no ascites

    i. No tumor on the external surface; capsule intact

    ii. Tumor present on the external surface or/and capsule ruptured

Stage Ib. Growth limited to both ovaries; no ascites

    i. No tumor on the external surface; capsule intact

    ii. Tumor present on the external surface or/and capsule(s) ruptured

Stage Ic. Tumor either Ia or stage Ib, but

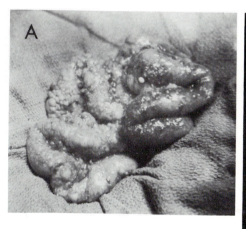

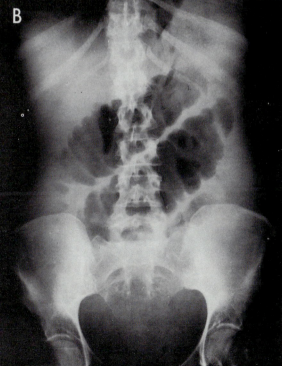

Fig 7–47.—A, densely implanted tumor nodules on terminal ileum to the left with less involved proximal ileum on the right. **B,** typical abdominal roentgenogram showing short, dilated segments of small bowel, which signify dense serosal involvement by tumor nodules.

with ascites present or positive peritoneal washings

Stage II.　Growth involving one or both ovaries with pelvic extension

Stage IIa.　Extension and/or metastases to the uterus and/or tubes

Stage IIb.　Extension to other pelvic tissues

Stage IIc.　Tumor either stage IIa or stage IIb, but with ascites present or positive peritoneal washings

Stage III.　Growth involving one or both ovaries with intraperitoneal metastases outside the pelvis and/or positive retroperitoneal nodes. Tumor limited to the true pelvis with histologically proved malignant extension to small bowel or omentum.

Stage IV.　Growth involving one or both ovaries with distant metastases. If pleural effusion is present there must be positive cytology to allot a case to stage IV. Parenchymal liver metastases equals stage IV.

Special category　Unexplored cases that are thought to be ovarian carcinoma.

The clinical stage or anatomic extent of tumor growth is considered the best indicator of prognosis. The staging classification proposed by FIGO has been adopted by WHO and the US End Results Group and is now the only acceptable staging system. Correlation between stage and five-year survival rates is demonstrated in Table 7–6 for a collected series of patients. Stage I substages relating to the status of the tumor capsule have only recently been added. In a study from the Mayo Clinic reported by Webb et al., the five-year survival rate of 111 patients in whom the tumor capsules were intact was 90%, whereas only 57% of 108 patients with capsular penetration or rupture survived.

Variation in survival within the major stages is in part determined by the histologic grade or degree of cellular differentiation which, in the epithelial cancers, operates independently as

TABLE 7–6.—RELATION OF STAGE TO PROGNOSIS*

STAGE	NO. OF PATIENTS	5-YR SURVIVAL, %
I	751	61
Ia	528	65
Ib	130	52
Ic	80	52
II	401	40
IIa	40	60
IIb	205	38
III	539	5
IV	101	3

*Collected series.

a prognostic factor. Of particular importance is the group of papillary tumors variously termed borderline, low-potential malignancy, or grade 0. If frank malignancy is evident there is further correlation of tumor grade (Broders or Ewing) with survival. Thus the five-year survival rate with grade 1 tumors may be two to four times that of grade 3 tumors within a given stage. The influence of histologic grade on the survival of patients with stage Ia and Ib epithelial carcinomas at the Mayo Clinic is illustrated in Figure 7–48 (Decker 1975). Borderline tumors are not separately considered, and one must assume that they are included in the grade 1 group, thereby influencing survival favorably. Although there is some interdependence of grade and histologic cell type, the latter appears to have little influence on prognosis independent of stage and histologic grade. In the evaluation of therapeutic results, particularly involving small numbers of patients, the histologic grade as well as the stage should be considered, lest differences in survival be erroneously attributed to therapy rather than to biologic differences in tumor growth.

Treatment

SURGICAL TREATMENT.—The initial abdominal operation is the keystone of ovarian cancer management, whatever the stage of disease. Implicit in this statement is the importance of a meticulous abdominal exploration and immediate annotation of the find-

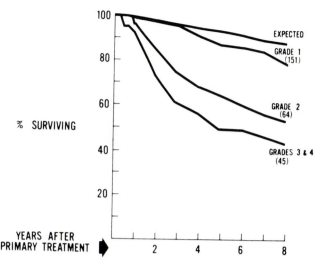

% SURVIVING

YEARS AFTER PRIMARY TREATMENT ▶

Fig 7–48.—Actuarial survival curves by grade for 260 patients with stages Ia and Ib ovarian carcinoma. (From Decker et al.: *Natl. Cancer Inst. Monogr.* 42:9, 1975.)

ings. Since 5% of malignant ovarian tumors are metastatic from occult primary cancers of the digestive tract, the stomach, colon, and pancreas must be carefully palpated. In the event that a curative procedure cannot be performed, both the selection and the efficacy of subsequent therapy are dependent on the observations and decisions made during the primary operation.

At the time of laparotomy gross criteria suggesting malignancy include hemorrhagic or solid areas within an ovarian cyst, tumor adherence to adjacent structures, papillary excrescences on the tumor surface, and the presence of ascites or peritoneal implantation. Despite the presence of one or more of these characteristics, the malignant nature of a tumor cannot be determined with certainty without excision and microscopic examination. As previously pointed out, irrevocable surgical decisions in the young nullipara must await an unequivocal histologic diagnosis of malignancy. The indications for conservative operations in young women have been discussed under the individual tumor headings.

When the tumor appears localized to one or both ovaries greater accuracy in staging will be achieved by thorough palpation of the diaphragm and biopsies of the distal omentum and aortic lymph nodes. Cytologic study of sa-

line irrigated through the peritoneal cavity is necessary for the current staging system. Hysterectomy and bilateral salpingo-oophorectomy are usually performed because of the frequency of synchronous or metachronous carcinomas in the contralateral ovary and endometrium as well as the possibility of occult metastases at these sites or on the uterine serosa. Opinion favoring the prophylactic removal of the omentum in stage I disease has waxed and waned for more than 40 years. Although small increments in survival have been demonstrated in a few series, this effect probably reflects the exclusion from the stage I category of patients with occult metastases discovered microscopically. An ample biopsy of the distal omentum should be equally effective in this regard, whereas the disadvantage of small bowel and transverse colon adherence to the anterior abdominal wall is avoided.

When tumor spread to the pelvic peritoneum has occurred (stage II), hysterectomy, bilateral salpingo-oophorectomy, and excision of all gross tumor is indicated. Rarely, segmental resection of bladder or rectum is necessary.

For more than 30 years a preponderance of expert opinion has favored the excision of as much tumor tissue as possible even when abdominal dissemination is encountered at primary operation. Although the removal of large masses may afford palliation there is little firm evidence that "debulking" procedures improve survival unless all or nearly all of the tumor is excised (Aure et al.; Griffiths). Apparently most important is the reduction in mass size to a point where subsequent chemotherapy or irradiation will exert a maximal effect. In two retrospective studies, improved survival of patients who received chemotherapy over those who did not was evident only when patients with minimal residual disease were compared (Griffiths et al., 1972). In a recent report, chemotherapy induced complete responses in 45% of patients with residual masses under 2 cm in diameter, whereas only 23% of patients with larger masses had complete responses (Young et al., 1976). Although these effects are clearly related to a small tumor volume, it can be argued that attainment of the latter depends more on limited or less invasive tumor growth than on extended surgical resection. In an attempt to answer this question Griffiths at the Brigham and Women's Hospital used a multiple linear regression equation with survival as the dependent variable to control simultaneously for multiple therapeutic and biologic variables.

TABLE 7–7.—SURVIVAL BY
DIAMETER OF LARGEST RESIDUAL
MASS

SIZE (CM)	NO. OF PATIENTS	MST* (MO)
0	29	39
0.3 ($\pm$0.2)	28	29
1.0 ($\pm$0.5)	16	18
>1.5	29	11†

*Median survival time.
†Mean survival 12.7 months (SE = 1.56 months).

Irrespective of other prognostic factors, survival was uniformly poor if the diameter of the largest residual tumor mass exceeded 1.0 ± 0.5 cm but increased in proportion to decrements in mass size below 1.5 cm (Table 7–7). Analysis of a subset of patients in whom a residual mass size of 1.5 cm or less was achieved by surgical excision of larger metastatic lesions indicated that this group fared as well as those whose largest metastatic lesions were below this size limit at the outset. These relationships are demonstrated in Figure 7–49.

Optimal operative procedures designed for the cure or palliation of patients with most solid tumors have evolved through the years. Carcinoma of the ovary is a notable exception.

Fig 7–49.—Relationship of survival to size of largest residual metastasis after primary operation for stage III ovarian carcinoma. The survival curve of patients whose mass size was reduced to 1.5 cm or less by excision of larger metastases was identical to that of *all* patients with a residual mass size below this limit. (From Griffiths C.T., Fuller A.F. Jr.: *Surg. Clin. North Am.* 58:131–142, 1978.)

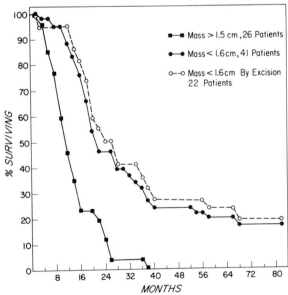

Admonitions such as "remove all you can" and purposeful terminology ("maximal surgical effort," "debulking procedures," "reductive surgery") hardly constitute guidelines for the safe performance of surgical procedures. Despite misconceptions to the contrary, tumor masses need not be transected since lines of cleavage between tumor-bearing peritoneum and normal tissue are usually found. Although limited bowel resection may be necessary, ovarian cancer masses can often be freed from the bowel muscularis by sharp dissection. Excision of all gross tumor in the pelvis is facilitated by a retroperitoneal dissection along the iliac vessels and ureters from the pelvic brim to the lower limit of tumor growth. By incising the bladder and rectal serosa, the entire tumor-bearing parietal and visceral pelvic peritoneum can be removed in continuity with the internal genitalia. The omentum, frequently laden with tumor, is removed from the greater curvature of the stomach following ligation of the gastroepiploic vessels. By exposing the lesser sac and transverse mesocolon, dissection of omental tumor from the transverse colon can be accomplished safely. Whatever procedures are necessary, an optimal operation is one that is carefully planned after thorough abdominal exploration and it cannot be supplanted by the indiscriminate excision of tumor bulk.

RADIATION THERAPY.—Traditionally, irradiation has held a favored position both as a surgical adjuvant with curative intent and as palliation in advanced cases. Despite these time-honored roles, insufficient supporting evidence has accumulated through the years to define clearly the place of radiation therapy in the management of epithelial ovarian cancers. As pointed out by Perez et al., adequate assessment of therapeutic efficacy has been hindered by a lack of uniformity in staging and histologic classifications, marked variability in both patient selection and radiation techniques, and, most important, the absence of controlled, let alone randomized, clinical studies. Although preoperative irradiation has

TABLE 7–8.—FIVE-YEAR SURVIVAL RATES*

| | — OPERATION ONLY — | | | OPERATION AND RADIATION | | |
	NO.	RANGE (%)	MEAN (%)	NO.	RANGE (%)	MEAN (%)
Stage I	319	49–91	66	333	53–80	59
Stage II	89	0–33	24	363	28–69	39
Stage III	268	0–11	5	811	2–17	10

*Collected series.

its proponents, radiotherapy has been used almost exclusively following primary operation. Collected five-year survival rates from eight series reported since 1960 in which FIGO staging is adaptable are listed in Table 7–8. Postoperative irradiation was employed in all eight series, and in five a group of nonirradiated patients was included for comparison.

Postoperative pelvic irradiation for stage 1 cancer has been used extensively without apparent improvement in five-year survival rates. Although irradiation has appeared to lessen stage I survival rates in several comparative studies, patients with poorly differentiated tumors or other adverse characteristics have tended to be those selected for adjuvant therapy (Webb et al.). It may be that pelvic or abdominal irradiation has improved survival among poor-risk stage I patients but without a controlled clinical trial no conclusions can be drawn.

The merit of postoperative external beam irradiation in stage II disease has been generally accepted, but the supporting data must be interpreted with caution. The apparent advantage conferred by irradiation (see Table 7–8) is dampened by the variability of results and small numbers in the control groups. Survival appeared to be dramatically improved by irradiation in some series, but the comparison was historical, and less extensive surgical procedures in the nonirradiated groups were implied. The adverse effect of residual tumor masses larger than 2 cm in diameter was evident in Delclos and Smith's series.

Most reported series have incorporated a mixture of patients treated by orthovoltage, cobalt, and megavoltage sources without correlative results. Results of megavoltage therapy recently reported are somewhat improved over earlier years, but higher dosage and extended radiation fields appear responsible rather than the energy source itself. Currently, pelvic irradiation for stage I and stage II tumors usually consists of 4,000 to 5,000 rads delivered to the midcoronal plane through single or opposing portals. For stage II and stage III disease the upper abdomen is also irradiated, usually as a separate field, to 3,000 rads. The danger of radiation nephritis and hepatitis when dosage exceeds 2,000 rads and 3,000 rads, respectively, has necessitated corresponding dose limitations to these organs. Consequently, "sanctuary" areas are provided at anatomic sites where metastatic tumor is most likely to lodge. Nevertheless, the importance of upper abdominal irradiation in controlling stage II cancers seems well established (Perez et al.; Delclos and Smith). Other variations for stage II and stage III tumors are single-field whole abdominal irradiation followed by a supplementary pelvic dose or whole abdominal irradiation by the moving strip technique. Proponents of the moving strip technique, in which only a small portion of the abdomen is irradiated at one time, have hoped for an improved therapeutic index. Unfortunately this hope has not been realized and 11 of the first 65 patients with ovarian cancer treated by this method at the M. D. Anderson Hospital succumbed to radiation hepatitis (Wharton et al.). In a subsequent randomized study by Fazekas and Maier comparing the strip technique to open-field abdominal irradiation, neither method demonstrated therapeutic superiority or significantly fewer side effects.

The efficacy of irradiation in the therapy of ovarian cancer was recently evaluated in a prospective, randomized study of 190 patients with stages IB, II, and III disease at the Princess Margaret Hospital (Dembo et al., 1979). Patients were randomized to receive either pelvic irradiation alone, pelvic irradiation and chlorambucil, or pelvic and abdominal irradiation. Patients with extensive tumor burdens had a poor prognosis regardless of the treatment strategy. The relapse-free survival in stage II patients with minimal residual disease was 79% in patients treated with pelvic and abdominal irradiation and only 46% in patients treated with pelvic irradiation alone. Pelvic and abdominal irradiation with no diaphragmatic shielding significantly improved patient survival and long-term control of occult or minimal upper abdominal disease. Furthermore, patients tolerated whole abdominal irradiation with minimal morbidity. Therefore, in patients with stages II and III ovarian cancer with minimal residual disease, pelvic and abdominal irradiation appears to be an appropriate therapeutic option with curative potential.

Recently interest has been reawakened in the intraperitoneal instillation of colloidal radioactive isotopes as a surgical adjuvant for stage I ovarian carcinoma. These agents, particularly ^{138}Au, were used extensively in the 1950s, but results were variable and complications significant. The superficial penetration of alpha and beta particles does not significantly affect tumor masses, but a lethal effect on superficial tumor cell aggregates might be anticipated. In two studies, one employing ^{138}Au and the other ^{32}P chromic phosphate, five-year survival rates of 83% and 93%, respectively, were obtained in stage Ia cases (Clark et al.). In a review by Decker et al. of experience at the Mayo Clinic with intraperitoneal ^{138}Au, only those patients with stage I disease in whom a malignant cyst had ruptured intraoperatively appeared to benefit from the treatment. Recently, ^{32}P chromic phosphate, a pure beta-emitter with a half-life of 14.2 days, has been favored over ^{138}Au (10% gamma emission, half-life 2.7 days) because of a near absence of intestinal complications.

CHEMOTHERAPY.—The observation in the early 1950s that nitrogen mustard could induce significant regression in the size of ovarian tumor masses has led to the widespread

use of alkylating agents in the management of this disease. The term *alkylating* refers to the ability of this class of drugs to bind a highly reactive alkyl group to metabolically important sites within the cell, rendering them incapable of functioning in their usual manner. Although mustard drugs react indiscriminately with a number of cellular components, the primary antitumor action is related to the ability of the chloroethyl arms to cross-link the helical strands of the DNA molecule in the manner of a grappling hook. This mechanism impedes DNA replication and explains the inability of the cell to undergo mitosis despite continuing cytoplasmic growth. Since these compounds directly attack the DNA molecule they are equally effective during any phase of the mitotic cycle and may inflict lethal chromosomal damage on noncycling cells. For these reasons alkylating agents have an immediate antitumor action and are effective against large tumors in which the growth fraction (percentage of cycling cells) is low, i.e., ovarian carcinoma. On the other hand, the cell renewal systems of the body—particularly the bone marrow and gastrointestinal epithelium—are equally affected. Consequently successful cancer chemotherapy is dependent on the ability of normal host tissue to recover more rapidly than tumor tissue. This differential in cell recovery time, which permits continuation of therapy prior to tumor regrowth, is essential to the achievement of a stepwise fractional reduction in tumor volume.

Because of the highly reactive and vesicant properties of nitrogen mustard, various modifications of the mustard molecule have been made in attempts to reduce toxicity, facilitate administration, or promote a selective action against the cancer cell. As a group, the substituted mustards have the advantage of oral administration and a relatively slow onset of action, which results in a wider margin of safety and minimal gastrointestinal side effects. Unfortunately myelosuppression, the major toxic and dose-limiting effect of nitrogen mustard, has not been sufficiently altered to improve the therapeutic index. The structural formulas of the substituted mustards commonly used in the management of ovarian cancer are shown in Figure 7–50. Chlorambucil with a phenylbutyric acid substitution is usually given in a divided daily dosage of 0.1 or 0.2 mg per kg. The higher dosage form is best given in four-week courses with an intervening period to allow for marrow recovery. The phenylalanine substituted mustard, melphalan, is the most widely used anticancer agent for ovarian cancer because of the virtual absence of gastrointestinal side effects and the convenience of oral administration in short courses. The drug is administered orally in courses at four- to five-week intervals at a dosage of 1 mg/kg divided over a five-day period. Unfortunately, prolonged use of either chlorambucil or melphalan is associated with a persistent and severely dose-limiting thrombocytopenia.

Cyclophosphamide (Cytoxan) is another example of the "Trojan horse" approach to tumor cell selectivity. Based on the studies of Gomorri and others, which demonstrated high levels of phosphatases and phosphamidases in tumor tissue, a cyclic phosphoramide

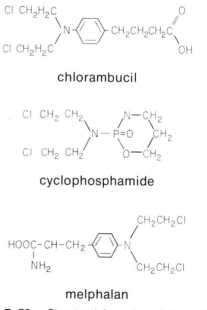

Fig 7–50.—Structural formulas of the substituted mustards.

was combined with the mustard moiety. Unlike the other alkylating agents, cyclophosphamide is inactive in vitro and active in vivo only after breakage of the phosphoramide ring. It now appears that this oxidative process takes place in the liver and is unrelated to phosphamidase hydrolysis. This drug seems to have a slightly wider spectrum of antitumor activity than the other mustards but its mechanism of action is the same. Its toxicity is somewhat different in that thrombocytopenia is uncommon at standard dosage. Countering the platelet-sparing advantage is a 25% incidence of alopecia and an occasional case of hemorrhagic cystitis. Hemorrhagic cystitis results from the exposure of the bladder mucosa to the active breakdown products and can be prevented by maintaining a high urine output.

The first alkylating agent used in a significant number of patients with ovarian cancer was triethylenethiophosphoramide (thiotepa). This agent is administered by the intravenous route and its toxicity is similar to that of the substituted mustards.

Table 7–9 lists the collected objective responses to the previously discussed agents obtained from a number of published reports. An objective response is defined as a reduction in tumor size by 50% or more, and a complete response signifies a complete disappearance of palpable tumor or tumor demonstrable on roentgenograms. Available evidence suggests that the alkylating agents have the same mechanism of cytotoxic action and about the same spectrum of antitumor activity. Certainly none of these drugs has demonstrated therapeutic superiority over the others in ovarian cancer. In general, tumors with de novo or acquired resistance to one alkylating agent have been resistant to other alkylating agents. Cisdichlorodiammineplatinum (cisplatin), a new agent, appears to be a notable exception and the 29% objective response rate reported by Wiltshaw and Kroner occurred in patients previously treated by other alkylating agents.

Responsiveness of ovarian carcinoma to

TABLE 7–9.—COLLECTED RESPONSES OF OVARIAN CARCINOMA TO ALKYLATING-AGENT CHEMOTHERAPY

DRUG	TOTAL NO. OF PATIENTS	% RESPONSES
Nitrogen mustard	25	36
Chlorambucil	388	51
Melphalan	541	47
Cyclophosphamide	371	45
Thiotepa	337	48
Cisplatin	31*	29

*Prior chemotherapy.

other classes of anticancer drugs has been disappointing (Table 7–10). The relative inactivity of other agents in comparison to those of the alkylating class has been attributed to their employment as "second-line" therapy. Stanhope et al., from the M. D. Anderson Hospital, reported a meager 6.1% response rate among 347 patients who received a second drug regimen irrespective of the response to initial chemotherapy. In most of the series included in Table 7–10, differentiation between previously treated and untreated patients was not made.

In contrast to the alkylating agents, which attack the DNA molecule directly, another class of chemotherapeutic agents, the antimetabolites, exerts an antitumor effect by inhibiting the synthesis of DNA. Since these drugs act primarily during the phase of DNA synthesis in the mitotic cycle (S phase) they are maximally effective against small tumor populations in which the growth fraction is high. A consistently low activity of fluorouracil and methotrexate is not surprising since ovarian carcinomas considered evaluable in

TABLE 7–10.—COLLECTED RESPONSES OF OVARIAN CARCINOMA TO NONALKYLATING-AGENT CHEMOTHERAPY

DRUG	TOTAL NO. OF PATIENTS	% RESPONSES
Fluorouracil	92	20
Methotrexate	33	25
Doxorubicin	108	20
Vincristine	22	0

clinical trials have palpable and therefore bulky tumor masses with a presumably low growth fraction. Even with previously untreated patients, only 21% have responded to fluorouracil. The value of either fluorouracil or methotrexate as consolidation therapy when minimal residual disease and a high growth fraction obtain is currently being investigated. Both fluorouracil and methotrexate are being used in drug combinations for the purpose of inhibiting the tumor cell's ability to repair DNA damage inflicted by alkylating agents.

Antibiotic chemotherapeutic agents intercalate with the DNA molecule but in contrast to alkylating agents they interfere with DNA function rather than with its structure. Dactinomycin, which has not been used as a single agent in ovarian cancer, has been included in drug combinations, particularly those that have been effective against malignant germ cell tumors. Although doxorubicin (Adriamycin) has been the most promising antineoplastic agent introduced in recent years, a meager 20% response rate was obtained in the collected series listed in Table 7–10. Nevertheless, in a randomized trial reported by dePalo and associates comparing Adriamycin and melphalan, seven of 14 previously untreated patients responded to Adriamycin, whereas only four of 16 responded to melphalan. Vincristine, a vinca alkaloid that interferes with mitotic spindle formation, has shown no activity in the epithelial ovarian cancers but is an important component of the VAC regimen for germ cell tumors.

Although combination chemotherapy of ovarian cancer was initiated by Greenspan's use of thiotepa and methotrexate in the early 1960s, evidence of superiority over single–alkylating-agent therapy has emerged only in recent years (Table 7–11).

Young et al., in 1978, reported the first study that demonstrated improved survival in advanced ovarian cancer with a combination drug regimen in a prospective comparison with an alkylating agent. Eighty previously untreated patients were randomized to receive either melphalan in conventional doses, or a combination of hexamethylmelamine, cyclophosphamide, methotrexate, and fluorouracil (Hexa-CAF). Treatment with the combination regimen attained a significantly increased overall response rate (75% vs. 54%), more complete responses (33% vs. 16%), and longer median survival (29 vs. 17 months). The combination regimen was most effective in patients with minimal residual disease. Patients achieving complete remission documented by operative restaging had a long survival and 60% of these women were free of disease for at least four years. Significant prolongation of survival depended on the attainment of a complete response.

At the Mayo Clinic (Edmonson et al., 1979), 111 patients with advanced ovarian cancer were randomized to receive either cyclophosphamide alone or cyclophosphamide and doxorubicin (Adriamycin). In patients with bulky disease, the two regimens had comparable response rates and survival rates. However, in patients with minimal residual

TABLE 7–11.—RESPONSE RATES OF ADVANCED OVARIAN CARCINOMA TO COMBINATION CHEMOTHERAPY

INVESTIGATORS	AGENTS*	NO. OF PATIENTS	% RESPONSES
Young et al., 1978	Hexa-CAF	40	75
Edmonson et al., 1979	A-C	99	45
Delgado et al., 1979	CHF	12	83
Parker et al., 1980	A-C	41	83

*Hexa-CAF indicates hexamethylmelamine, cyclophosphamide, methotrexate, and fluorouracil; A-C, Adriamycin and cyclophosphamide; and CHF, cyclophosphamide, hexamethylmelamine, and fluorouracil.

disease, the combination regimen achieved a significant increase in both response rate and duration of survival.

Parker et al. (1980) at the Brigham and Women's Hospital and Dana Farber Cancer Institute have also evaluated the role of combination chemotherapy (doxorubicin and cyclophosphamide) in advanced ovarian cancer. Objective response was noted in 34 of 41 (83%) patients without prior cytotoxic chemotherapy but in only two of 12 patients (17%) who had failed a single alkylating agent or radiotherapy. This study emphasizes the marked reduction of activity of any regimen used as second-line therapy in advanced ovarian cancer as well as the lack of success of initiating therapy with an alkylating agent and then later attempting to save patients suffering relapse with more aggressive combination drugs. It is important to note that complete responses were more frequently obtained when only minimal disease was present at the onset of therapy. Similarly, Griffiths and Fuller at the Brigham and Women's Hospital reported that nine of 11 stage III patients (82%) who had optimal operations achieved laparoscopic complete responses after doxorubicin-cyclophosphamide therapy.

Several recent studies have therefore consistently indicated that combination chemotherapy induces a higher response rate with prolonged survival as compared with single alkylating agents in the treatment of advanced ovarian cancer. However, the greater effectiveness of combination chemotherapy appears to be limited to patients with minimal residual disease at the onset of treatment.

Following chemotherapy, it is important to accurately determine if the patient has had a complete response. Clinical examination and radiographic studies have limited capabilities to detect small foci of persistent intraperitoneal disease. Laparoscopy has been shown to be both safe and reliable in assessing intraperitoneal disease in patients who have experienced a complete clinical response (Berek et al., 1981). Piver et al. (1980) documented by laparoscopy evidence of persistent tumor in

36% of patients who had a complete clinical response and thereby avoided laparotomy. However, if a laparoscopy yields negative or inadequate results, laparotomy should still be performed to definitively determine tumor status. Mangioni et al. (1979) found persistent ovarian cancer at laparotomy in six of 18 patients with negative laparoscopy findings.

Attempts have been made to evaluate the antitumor activity of potentially useful chemotherapeutic agents using in vitro screening techniques. An in vitro tumor colony assay has been recently developed that assesses clonogenic potential after exposure to chemotherapy (Hamburger et al., 1978). The tumor colony assay may aid in the selection of second-line agents active against a patient's particular tumor and in the screening and identification of new drugs appropriate for phase 2 trials in ovarian cancer.

IMMUNOTHERAPY.—The antigenicity of malignant ovarian tumors and the immunoreactivity of the host have been the subjects of recent investigation. Intensive efforts have been made during the past decade to identify ovarian tumor–associated antigens. Heteroantisera have usually been raised by injecting animals with human ovarian tumor, ovarian carcinoma cell lines, or crude antigen preparations obtained by sonication and centrifugation of tumor tissue (Bhattacharya and Barlow, 1973). Monoclonal antibodies have recently been prepared against cell surface determinants of human ovarian carcinoma (Bast et al., 1981). Host responsiveness to tumor-associated antigens has been identified by the demonstration of a prompt cytotoxic effect on allogeneic cell lines by both lymphocytes and serum obtained from patients with ovarian carcinoma (DiSaia et al.). Levin et al. (1975) investigated the ability of lymphocytes from patients with ovarian carcinoma to undergo specific blast transformation. This response was apparent only when effector cells were obtained from patients in remission.

Intraperitoneal immunotherapy has been demonstrated to be effective in the treatment

of a murine ovarian carcinoma model (Knapp and Berkowitz, 1977). Intraperitoneal injection of either the immunostimulant *Corynebacterium parvum* or specific rabbit heteroantiserum can cure mice bearing 10^5 tumor cells. A combination of *C. parvum* and specific heteroantiserum was more effective than either single agent against a larger tumor burden of 10^6 cells.

Recently, *C. parvum* has been administered intraperitoneally in patients with residual ovarian cancer, and five of 11 (45%) patients had a surgically confirmed tumor regression (Bast et al., 1983). The Southwest Oncology Group has conducted a randomized controlled trial in 121 patients with advanced ovarian cancer comparing chemotherapy with doxorubicin and cyclophosphamide to a combination of similar chemotherapy with BCG vaccine administered by scarification (Alberts and Moon, 1980). The median survival of patients treated with chemoimmunotherapy (22.3 months) was significantly prolonged when compared with that of patients treated with chemotherapy alone (13.7 months). Additional randomized, prospective studies must be performed to determine if immunotherapy has a practical role in the management of ovarian cancer.

SUPPORTIVE TREATMENT.—A major advance in the treatment of advanced ovarian carcinoma has been the development of safe and effective parenteral nutrition utilizing crystalline amino acids in a concentrated glucose solution. Intravenous hyperalimentation has enabled these nutritionally depleted patients with disordered gastrointestinal function to undergo the rigors of extensive operation and intensive chemotherapy. Short-term hyperalimentation may have a palliative effect in advanced cases but it must be used judiciously to avoid prolongation of a hopeless and miserable existence.

The natural history of ovarian cancer often results in a protracted terminal phase. The patient is beleaguered with frequent nausea and vomiting, discomfort from a distended abdomen, dyspnea due to pleural effusions, and intermittent bouts of partial bowel obstruction. Operation for presumed bowel obstruction should be avoided, since isolated points of obstruction are rare and the surgeon is faced with adherent bowel and mesentery laden with tumor masses. Intermittent gastric or intestinal intubation may afford temporary relief. Hypercalcemia is the most common paraendocrine disorder associated with ovarian neoplasms, particularly clear cell carcinomas, but often goes unrecognized amidst the gastrointestinal and metabolic disturbances of advanced disease.

The physician's interaction with the patient and her family is of the greatest importance. Empathy must be tempered with hope and encouragement, but the patient's complete trust in her physician cannot be sacrificed by patent untruths, however well-meaning.

BIBLIOGRAPHY

Embryology

Moore K.L.: *The Developing Human.* ed. 2. Philadelphia, W.B. Saunders Co., 1977.

Patten B.M.: *Human Embryology.* ed. 3. New York, Blakiston Division, McGraw-Hill Book Co., 1968.

Ovarian Tumors

Afridi M.A., Vongtama V., Tsukada Y., et al.: Dysgerminoma of the ovary: Radiation therapy for recurrence and metastases. *Am. J. Obstet. Gynecol.* 126:190, 1976.

Arey L.B.: The origin and form of the Brenner tumor. *Am. J. Obstet. Gynecol.* 81:743, 1961.

Asadourian L.A., Taylor H.B.: Dysgerminoma: An analysis of 105 cases. *Obstet. Gynecol.* 33:370, 1969.

Azoury R.S., Woodruff J.D.: Primary ovarian sarcomas. *Obstet. Gynecol.* 37:920, 1971.

Barber H.R.K., Graber E.A.: The PMPO syndrome (postmenopausal palpable ovary syndrome). *Obstet. Gynecol.* 38:921, 1971.

Bennington J.L., Ferguson B.C., Haber S.L.: Incidence and relative frequency of benign and malignant ovarian neoplasms. *Obstet. Gynecol.* 32:627, 1968.

Berg J.W., Baylor S.M.: The epidemiologic pathology of ovarian cancer. *Hum. Pathol.* 4:537, 1973.

Caruso P.A., Marsh M.R., Minkowitz S., et al.: An

intense clinicopathologic study of 305 teratomas of the ovary. *Cancer* 27:343, 1971.

Chorlton I., Norris H.J., King F.M.: Malignant reticuloendothelial disease involving the ovary as a primary manifestation: A series of 19 lymphomas and one granulocytic sarcoma. *Cancer* 34:397, 1974.

Climie A.R.W., Heath L.P.: Malignant degeneration of benign cystic teratomas of the ovary. *Cancer* 22:824, 1968.

Czernobilsky B., Borenstein R., Lancet M.: Cystadenofibroma of the ovary: A clinicopathologic study of 34 cases and comparison with serous cystadenoma. *Cancer* 34:1971, 1974.

Dehner L.P., Norris H.J., Taylor H.B.: Carcinosarcomas and mixed mesodermal tumors of the ovary. *Cancer* 27:207, 1971.

Fenoglio C.M., Ferenczy A., Richart R.M.: Mucinous tumors of the ovary: Ultrastructural studies of mucinous cystadenomas with histogenetic considerations. *Cancer* 36:1709, 1975.

Fox H., Agrawal K., Langley F.A.: A clinicopathologic study of 92 cases of granulosa cell tumor of the ovary with special reference to the factors influencing prognosis. *Cancer* 35:231, 1975.

Garcia-Bunuel R., Berek J.S., Woodruff J.D.: Luteomas of pregnancy. *Obstet. Gynecol.* 45:407, 1975.

Gerbie M.V., Brewer J.I., Tamimi H.: Primary choriocarcinoma of the ovary. *Obstet. Gynecol.* 46:720, 1975.

Hart W.R., Norris H.J.: Borderline and malignant mucinous tumors of the ovary. *Cancer* 31:1031, 1973.

Hernandez W., DiSaia P., Morrow C.P., et al.: Mixed mesodermal sarcoma of the ovary. *Obstet. Gynecol.* 49:595, 1977.

Hertig A.T., Gore H.M.: Tumors of the ovary and fallopian tube, in *Tumors of the Female Sex Organs: part 3, sec. IX, fasc. 33, Atlas of Tumor Pathology.* Washington D.C., Armed Forces Institute of Pathology, 1961.

Hughesdon P.E.: Ovarian lipoid and theca cell tumors; their origins and interrelations. *Obstet. Gynecol. Surv.* 21:245, 1966.

Ireland K., Woodruff J.D.: Masculinizing ovarian tumors. *Obstet. Gynecol. Surv.* 31:83, 1976.

Kent S.W., McKay D.G.: Primary cancer of the ovary. *Am. J. Obstet. Gynecol.* 80:430, 1960.

Kistner R.W.: Intraperitoneal rupture of benign cystic teratomas: A review of literature with report of two cases. *Obstet. Gynecol. Surv.* 7:603, 1952.

Kurman R.J., Craig J.M.: Endometrioid and clear cell carcinoma of the ovary. *Cancer* 29:1653, 1972.

Kurman R., Norris H.J.: Embryonal carcinoma of the ovary. *Cancer* 38:2420, 1976.

Kurman R., Norris H.J.: Malignant mixed germ cell tumors of the ovary. *Obstet. Gynecol.* 48:579, 1976.

Kurman R., Norris H.J.: Endodermal sinus tumor of the ovary: A clinical and pathologic analysis of 71 cases. *Cancer* 38:2404, 1976.

Lauchlan S.C.: The secondary müllerian system. *Obstet. Gynecol. Surv.* 27:133, 1972.

Limber G.K., King R.E., Silverberg S.G.: Pseudomyxoma peritonaei: A report of ten cases. *Ann. Surg.* 178:587, 1973.

Linder D., McCain B.K., Hecht F.: Parthenogenic origin of benign ovarian teratomas. *N. Engl. J. Med.* 292:63, 1975.

MacDonald P.C., Grodin J.M., Edman C.D., et al.: Origin of estrogen in a postmenopausal woman with a nonendocrine tumor of the ovary and endometrial hyperplasia. *Obstet. Gynecol.* 47:644, 1976.

McKay D.G.: The origins of ovarian tumors. *Clin. Obstet. Gynecol.* 5:1181, 1962.

Malkasian G.D., Symmonds R.E.: Treatment of unilateral encapsulated ovarian dysgerminoma. *Am. J. Obstet. Gynecol.* 90:379, 1964.

Miles P.A., Norris H.J.: Proliferative and malignant Brenner tumors of the ovary. *Cancer* 30:174, 172.

Norris H.J., Chorlton I.: Functioning tumors of the ovary. *Clin. Obstet. Gynecol.* 17:189, 1974.

Norris H.J., Jenson R.D.: Relative frequency of ovarian neoplasms in children and adolescents. *Cancer* 30:713, 1972.

Norris H.J., Taylor H.E.: Prognosis of granulosa-theca tumors of the ovary. *Cancer* 21:255, 1968.

Norris H.J., Zirkin H.J., Benson W.L.: Immature (malignant) teratoma of the ovary: A clinical and pathologic study of 58 cases. *Cancer* 37:2359, 1976.

Novak E.R., Kutchmeshgi J., Mupas R., et al.: Feminizing gonadal stromal tumors. *Obstet. Gynecol.* 38:701, 1971.

Pantoja E., Noy M.A., Axtmayer R.W., et al.: Ovarian dermoids and their complications: Comprehensive historical review. *Obstet. Gynecol. Surv.* 30;1, 1975.

Papadiki L., Beilby J.O.W.: Ovarian cystadenofibroma: A consideration of the role of estrogen in its pathogenesis. *Am. J. Obstet. Gynecol.* 121:501, 1975.

Piver M.S., Sinks L., Barlow J.J., et al.: Five-year remissions of metastatic solid teratoma of the ovary. *Cancer* 38:987, 1976.

Robboy S.J., Norris H.J., Scully R.E.: Insular car-

cinoid primary in the ovary. *Cancer* 36:404, 1975.

Robboy S.J., Scully R.E.: Ovarian teratoma with glial implants on the peritoneum. *Hum. Pathol.* 1:643, 1970.

Robboy S.J., Scully R.E., Norris H.J.: Primary trabecular carcinoid of the ovary. *Obstet. Gynecol.* 49:202, 1976.

Rogers L.W., Julian C.G., Woodruff J.D.: Mesonephroid carcinoma of the ovary: A study of 95 cases from the Emil Novak Tumor Registry. *Gynecol. Oncol.* 1:76, 1972.

Rome R.M., Laverty C.R., Brown J.B.: Ovarian tumours in postmenopausal women: Clinicopathological features and hormonal studies. *Br. J. Obstet. Gynecol.* 80:984, 1973.

Savard R., March J.M., Rice B.F.: Gonadotropins and ovarian steroidogenesis. *Recent Prog. Horm. Res.* 21:285, 1965.

Scully R.E.: Gonadoblastoma: A review of 74 cases. *Cancer* 25:1340, 1970.

Scully R.E.: Recent progress in ovarian cancer. *Hum. Pathol.* 1:73, 1970.

Serov S.F., Scully R.E.: *Histological Typing of Ovarian Tumors*, International Histological Typing of Tumors, no. 9. Geneva, World Health Organization, 1973.

Talerman A., Huyzinga W.T., Kupiers T.: Dysgerminoma: Clinicopathologic study of 22 cases. *Obstet. Gynecol.* 41:137, 1973.

Taylor H.B., Norris H.J.: Lipid cell tumors of the ovary. *Cancer* 20:1953, 1967.

Teilum G.: *Special Tumors of Ovary and Testis and Related Extragonadal Lesions.* Copenhagen, Munksgaard, 1971.

Thompson J.D.: Primary ovarian adenoacanthoma. *Obstet. Gynecol.* 9:403, 1957.

Woodruff J.D., Murthy Y.S., Bkaskar T.N., et al.: Metastatic ovarian tumors. *Am. J. Obstet. Gynecol.* 107:202, 1970.

Woodruff J.D., Telinde R.W.: The histology and histogenesis of ovarian neoplasia. *Cancer* 38:411, 1976.

Ovarian Cancer

Alberts D.S., Moon T.E. (eds.): Randomized trial of chemotherapy versus chemoimmunotherapy for advanced ovarian carcinoma: A preliminary report of the Southwest Oncology Group Study, in *NCI Second International Conference on Immunotherapy of Cancer: Present Status of Trials in Man.* New York, National Cancer Institute, 1980, p. 13.

Aure J.C., Hoeg K., Kolstad P.: Clinical and histologic studies of ovarian carcinoma. *Obstet. Gynecol.* 37:1, 1971.

Bast R.C. Jr., Berek J.S., Obrist R., et al.: Intra-peritoneal immunotherapy of human ovarian carcinoma with *Corynebacterium parvum. Cancer Res.* 43:1395, 1983.

Bast R.C. Jr., Feeney M., Lazarus H., et al.: Reactivity of a monoclonal antibody with human ovarian carcinoma. *J. Clin. Invest.* 68:1331, 1981.

Berek J.S., Griffiths C.T., Leventhal J.M.: Laparoscopy for second-look evaluation in ovarian cancer. *Obstet. Gynecol.* 58:192, 1981.

Bhattacharya M., Barlow J.: Immunologic studies of human serous cystadenocarcinoma of ovary: Demonstration of tumor associated antigens. *Cancer* 31:588, 1973.

Björkholm E., Silfverswärd C.: Prognostic factors in granulosa-cell tumors. *Gynecol. Oncol.* 11:261, 1981.

Cangir A., Smith J., Van Eys J.: Improved prognosis in children with ovarian cancers following modified VAC (vincristine sulfate, dactinomycin and cyclophosphamide) chemotherapy. *Cancer* 42:1234, 1978.

Clark D.G.C., Hilaris B., Roussis C., et al.: The role of radiation therapy (including isotopes) in the treatment of cancer of the ovary (results of 614 patients treated at Memorial Hospital, New York, N.Y.), in Ariel I.M. (ed.): *Progress in Clinical Cancer*, vol. 5. New York, Grune & Stratton, Inc., 1973.

Cramer D.W., Cutler S.J.: Incidence and histopathology of malignancies of the female genital organs in the United States. *Am. J. Obstet. Gynecol.* 118:443, 1974.

Cramer D.W., Hutchison G.B., Welch W.R. et al.: Factors affecting the association of oral contraceptives and ovarian cancer. *N. Engl. J. Med.* 307:1047, 1982.

Cramer D.W., Welch W.R., Scully R.E., et al.: Ovarian cancer and talc—a case-control study. *Cancer* 50:372, 1982.

Creasman W.T., Fetter B.F., Hammond C.B., et al.: Germ cell malignancies of the ovary. *Obstet. Gynecol.* 53:226, 1979.

Curry S.L., Smith J.P., and Gallagher H.S.: Malignant teratoma of the ovary: prognostic factors and treatment. *Am. J. Obstet. Gynecol.* 131:845, 1978.

Cutler S.J., Myers M.H., White P.C.: Who are we missing and why? *Cancer* 37:421, 1976.

Cutler S.J., Myers M.H., Green S.B.: Trends in survival rates of patients with cancer. *N. Engl. J. Med.* 293:122, 1975.

Decker D.G., Malkasian G.D., Taylor W.F.: Prognostic importance of histologic grading in ovarian carcinoma. *Natl. Cancer Inst. Monogr.* 42:9, 1975.

Decker D.G., Webb M.J., Holbrook M.: Radiogold treatment of epithelial cancer of the ovary: Late results. *Am. J. Obstet. Gynecol.* 115:751, 1973.

Delclos L., Smith J.P.: Tumors of the ovary, in Fletcher G. (ed.): *Textbook of Radiotherapy.* Philadelphia, Lea & Febiger, 1973.

Delgado G., Schein P., MacDonald J., et al.: L-PAM vs cyclophosphamide, hexamethylmelamine, and 5-fluorouracil (CHF) for advanced ovarian cancer. *Proc. Am. Assoc. Cancer Res.* 20:434, 1979.

DePalo G.M., DeLena M., DiRie F., et al.: Melphalan versus Adriamycin in the treatment of advanced carcinoma of the ovary. *Surg. Gynecol. Obstet.* 141:899, 1975.

Dembo A.J., Bush R.S., Beale F.A., et al.: Ovarian carcinoma: Improved survival following abdominopelvic irradiation in patients with a completed pelvic operation. *Am. J. Obstet. Gynecol.* 134:793, 1979.

DiSaia P.J., Sinkovics J.G., Rutledge F.M., et al.: Cell-mediated immunity to human malignant cells. *Am. J. Obstet. Gynecol.* 114:979, 1972.

DiSaia P.J., Nalick R.H., Townsend D.E.: Antibody cytotoxicity studies in ovarian and cervical malignancies. *Obstet. Gynecol.* 42:644, 1973.

Edmonson H.J., Fleming T.R., Decker D.G., et al.: Different chemotherapeutic sensitivities and host factors affecting prognosis in advanced ovarian carcinomas versus minimal residual disease. *Cancer Treat. Rep.* 63:241, 1979.

Fathalla M.F.: Factors in the causation and incidence of ovarian cancer. *Obstet. Gynecol. Surv.* 27:751, 1972.

Fazekas J.T., Maier J.G.: Irradiation of ovarian carcinomas: A prospective comparison of the open-field and moving-strip technique. *A.J.R.* 120:118, 1974.

Gershenson D.M., Del Junco G., Herson J., et al.: Endodermal sinus tumor of the ovary: The M.D. Anderson experience. *Obstet. Gynecol.* 61:94, 1983.

Gordon A., Lipton D., Woodruff J.D.: Dysgerminoma: A review of 158 cases from the Emil Novak Ovarian Tumor Registry. *Obstet. Gynecol.* 58:497, 1981.

Graham J., Graham R.: Ovarian cancer and asbestos. *Environ. Res.* 1:115, 1967.

Griffiths C.T.: Surgical resection of tumor bulk in the primary treatment of ovarian carcinoma. *Natl. Cancer Inst. Monogr.*, no. 42, 1975.

Griffiths C.T.: The ovary and fallopian tube, in Holland J.F., Frei E. III (eds.): *Cancer Medicine,* ed. 2. Philadelphia, Lea & Febiger, 1982.

Griffiths C.T., Grogan R.H., Hall T.C.: Advanced ovarian cancer: Primary treatment with surgery, radiotherapy and chemotherapy. *Cancer* 29:1, 1972.

Griffiths C.T., Fuller A.F. Jr.: Intensive surgical and chemotherapeutic management of advanced ovarian cancer. *Surg. Clin. North Am.* 58:131, 1978.

Hamburger A.W., Salmon S.E., Kim M.B., et al.: Direct cloning of human ovarian carcinoma cells in agar. *Cancer Res.* 38:3438, 1978.

Holtz F., Hart W.R.: Krukenberg tumors of the ovary—a clinicopathologic analysis of 27 cases. *Cancer* 50:2438, 1982.

Hreshchyshyn M.M.: Single-drug therapy in ovarian cancer: Factors influencing response. *Gynecol. Oncol.* 1:220, 1973.

Jacobs A.J., Deppe G., Cohen C.J.: Combination chemotherapy of ovarian granulosa cell tumor with cis-platinum and doxorubicin. *Gynecol. Oncol.* 14:294, 1982.

Javaheri G., Lifchez A., Valle J.: Pregnancy following removal of and long-term chemotherapy for ovarian malignant teratoma. *Obstet. Gynecol.* 61:8S, 1983.

Johnson C.E., Decker D.G., VanHerik M., et al.: Advanced ovarian cancer: Therapy with radiation and cyclophosphamide in a random series. *A.J.R.* 114:136, 1972.

Knapp R.C., Berkowitz R.S.: *Corynebacterium parvum* as an immunotherapeutic agent in an ovarian cancer model. *Am. J. Obstet. Gynecol.* 128:782, 1977.

Knapp R.C., Friedman E.A.: Aortic lymph node metastases in early ovarian cancer. *Am. J. Obstet. Gynecol.* 119:1013, 1974.

Knauf S., Urbach G.I.: A study of ovarian cancer patients using a radioimmunoassay for human ovarian tumor-associated antigen OCA. *Am. J. Obstet. Gynecol.* 138:1222, 1980.

Krepart G., Smith J.P., Rutledge F., et al.: The treatment for dysgerminoma of the ovary. *Cancer* 41:986, 1978.

Lele S.B., Piver M.S., Barlow J.J.: Chemotherapy in management of mixed mesodermal tumors of the ovary. *Gynecol. Oncol.* 10:298, 1980.

Levin L., McHardy J.E., Curling O.M., et al.: Tumour antigenicity in ovarian cancer. *Br. J. Cancer* 32:152, 1975.

Mangioni C., Bolis G., Molteni P., et al.: Indications, advantages and limitations of laparoscopy in ovarian cancer. *Gynecol. Oncol.* 7:47, 1979.

McGowan L.: Peritoneal fluid profiles. *Natl. Cancer Inst. Monogr.* 42:75, 1975.

Munnell E.W.: The changing prognosis and treatment in cancer of the ovary. *Am. J. Obstet. Gynecol.* 100:790, 1968.

Parker L.M., Griffiths C.T., Yankee R.A., et al.: Combination chemotherapy with Adriamycin-cyclophosphamide for advanced ovarian carcinoma. *Cancer* 46:669, 1980.

Perez C.A., Walz B.J., Jacobson P.L.: Radiation therapy in the management of carcinoma of the ovary. *Natl. Cancer Inst. Monogr.* 42:119, 1975.

Piver M.S., Lele S.B., Barlow J.J., et al.: Second-look laparoscopy prior to proposed second-look laparotomy. *Obstet. Gynecol.* 55:571, 1980.

Romero R., Schwartz P.E.: Alpha fetoprotein determinations in the management of endodermal sinus tumors and mixed germ cell tumors of the ovary. *Am. J. Obstet. Gynecol.* 141:126, 1981.

Santesson L., Kottmeier H.L.: General classification of ovarian tumors, in Gentil F., Junqueira A.C. (eds.): *Ovarian Cancer*, UICC monograph series, vol. 2. New York, Springer-Verlag, 1968.

Scully R.E., Barlow J.F.: 'Mesonephroma' of ovary: Tumor of müllerian nature related to the endometrioid carcinoma. *Cancer* 20:1405, 1967.

Smith J.P., Rutledge F., Wharton J.T.: Chemotherapy of ovarian cancer: New approaches to treatment. *Cancer* 30:1565, 1972.

Smith J.P., Rutledge F.: Advances in chemotherapy for gynecologic cancer. *Cancer* 36:669, 1975.

Stanhope C.R., Smith J.P., Rutledge F.N.: Second-trial drugs in ovarian cancer. *Gynecol. Oncol.* 5:51, 1977.

Stenwig J.T., Hazekamp J.T., Beecham J.B.: Granulosa cell tumors of the ovary: A clinico-pathological study of 118 cases with long-term follow-up. *Gynecol. Oncol.* 7:136, 1979.

Tobias J.S., Griffiths C.T.: Management of ovarian carcinoma: Current concepts and future prospects. *N. Engl. J. Med.* 294:818, 1976.

Webb M.J., Decker D.G., Mussey E.: Factors influencing survival in stage I ovarian cancer. *Am. J. Obstet. Gynecol.* 116:222, 1973.

Wharton J.T., Delclos L., Gallagher H.S.: Radiation hepatitis induced by abdominal irradiation. *A.J.R.* 117:73, 1973.

Wiltshaw E., Kroner T.: Phase II study of *cis*-dichlorodiammine platinum II in advanced adenocarcinoma of the ovary. *Cancer Chemother. Rep.* 60:55, 1976.

Wynder E.L., Dodo H., Barber H.R.: Epidemiology of cancer of the ovary. *Cancer* 23:352, 1969.

Young R.C., Chabner B.A., Hubbard S.P., et al.: Prospective trial of melphalan (L-PAM) versus combination chemotherapy (Hexa-CAF) in ovarian adenocarcinoma. *N. Engl. J. Med.* 199:1261, 1978.

CHAPTER EIGHT

The Breast

ROBERT L. SHIRLEY, M.D.

GENERAL CONSIDERATIONS

THE CHARACTERISTICS that separate human beings from the lampreys, sharks, fishes, frogs, lizards, and birds are mammary glands. Officially, subphylum Vertebrata, class Mammalia includes those vertebrates that have breast and hair development.

The human breast is as central to the psychological core of *Homo sapiens* as any physical structure. The breast-offered–breast-received, nursing-suckling interrelationship is the subject of numerous treatises on psychodynamics. The female human breast has recently become the center of literary and commercial emphasis because of exaggerated emphasis on sexual social behavior.

The breast is a challenge to the gynecologist in the continuous struggle to secure early cancer detection. Unfortunately, many gynecologists do not examine the breasts as part of a routine physical examination. This group of subspecialists may consider themselves "pelvicologists" instead of recognizing that the Greek root *gyne* refers to the whole woman.

DEVELOPMENT AND PHYSIOLOGIC ALTERATIONS

Growth and development of the embryonic skin lead to the formation of specialized skin appendages. Specific sweat glands develop a specialized function, e.g., lacrimal and scent; but the most elaborate pattern is exemplified in the mammary glands. These develop along the milk line extending obliquely from each axilla to the homolateral pubic mons. In the human, the mammary glands differentiate on the ventral surface of the chest centered in the fourth thoracic segment slightly lateral to the midclavicular line.

Approximately 15 sweat glands bud inward in the region of each nipple, with an early branching that forms the anlage of future growth. Surrounding these primary papillae is another group of sudoriferous glands surrounding the nipple. They, in turn, develop into mammarylike areolar glands (the follicles of Montgomery).

At thelarche, usually age 9 to 11 years, the breast ducts enter a second growth phase with further extension of the duct systems. This coincides with pubic and axillary hair growth, stimulated by the increased secretion of estrogens and growth hormone. Menarche follows one or two years later. The expanding growth center of the breast may form a temporary round firm mass, which resembles a fibroadenoma. This usually appears in the superolateral portion of the subareolar region. This temporary condensation disappears gradually in about three months.

The breast duct systems further elongate and branch during the pubertal phase and form the final adult breast. The cyclic menstrual changes in breast tissue are often quite marked during the third, fourth, and fifth decades. A concerted effect of estrogen, progesterone, and prolactin induces epithelial and stromal cell hypertrophy as well as intracellular edema. These changes occur during the luteal phase and often peak at ovulation and menstruation.

The changes of pregnancy represent the final chapter of breast growth and development. Acinar development at the distal end of each terminal duct occurs under the influence of increasing levels of progesterone, estriol, other estrogens, and prolactin. The production and release of milk are finally realized with the release of prolactin and oxytocin at the time of parturition.

During the postmenopausal years the breast epithelium becomes atrophic and the previously dense stroma is replaced by fat. This fatty metamorphosis is a progressive process throughout old age.

ANATOMY

The paired hemispheres of breast tissue are attached on their planoconcave surface against the fascia of the ventral chest wall from the parasternal to the anterior axillary line covering the second through seventh ribs. Vascular supply is from the axillary vessels through the upper outer quadrants and through the perforating internal mammary vessels via the parasternal and intercostal spaces.

The innervation of the breast enters the breast skin and the substance from the lateral segmental sensory nerves of the second through sixth thoracic segments. Hyperextension injuries of the neck will commonly irritate one or more of these nerves, causing a patient to complain of breast pain.

The functional unit of the mammary gland is the lactiferous lobe. The distal end of each lobe empties through the nipple where it is firmly supported by dense connective tissue. Just below the nipple the lactiferous duct is wider for 1.5 to 2.0 cm. This preterminal dilatation is named the lactiferous sinus and represents a milk reservoir for the lactating breast. Associated with the distensibility of the subareolar duct system is a reduction in the supporting connective tissue. This makes the subareolar portion of the breast much sof-

ter than the more peripheral breast tissue. In many cases palpation of the subareolar area reveals a cuplike depression, which is surrounded by a ring of nodular peripheral breast tissue of a more dense nature. This can simulate the apex of a volcano mountain.

The distribution of lobes throughout the breast is quite asymmetric. Fewer than 20% of the ducts are formed in the medial half of the breast. Approximately 30% extend deep below the areolar region in the central portion of the breast. More than 50% of the ducts branch laterally, mostly upward in the tail of Spence toward the axilla extending over and under the pectoralis muscle group.

The supporting structures of the breast are fascial. The breast is contained in a fascial envelope, its superficial layer being subcutaneous and its deep layer adjacent to the fascia of the chest wall muscles. Fascial septa separate each lactiferous lobe into a separate entity. These fascial partitions extend from the deep to the superficial fascial envelope. In the superior aspect of the breast these fascial supports are thickest, presumably because of gravity traction, and are called Cooper's ligaments. This area presents a dense sensation to palpation in many larger breasts, called by some "Cooper's thickening."

The fat of the breast composes a significant proportion of the breast volume. It occurs as a 1 to 3 cm layer between the skin and the superficial fascia. With age, as atrophic changes affect the ductal and stromal elements, replacement by fatty metamorphosis characterizes the senile breast. The fatty tissue in the most dependent portion of the breast often becomes edematous and indurated as a function of gravity and dependency. This indurated area is known as the inframammary ridge. It is quite dense in some older women and its medialmost portion can mimic a tumor.

The lymphatics of the breast drain mostly to the axilla and then medially along the axillary vein. Most of these lymphatics drain around and under the pectoral muscles although some pathways do exist through and between the musculature (Rotter's nodes). The medial and centromedial areas of the breast contain lymphatics that course toward the sternum, perforate the intercostal spaces, and drain into the internal mammary chain inside the thorax. Lesser pathways of drainage include epigastric, supraclavicular, and anterior cervical lymphatics.

DISEASES OF THE BREAST

Inflammation

Inflammation in the breast most frequently occurs during the puerperium. Although maceration and traumatic dermatitis of the areolar skin occur with suckling, these are usually mild. Obstruction of the outflow of milk in the lactiferous duct occurs occasionally, usually in the nipple itself. With continued milk production behind the obstructed area, increased pressure develops within all branches of the obstructed lobe. This fullness and pain represent a "caked" segment of breast tissue. Proper treatment of this condition includes efforts to relieve the obstruction with manual expression of milk and/or suckling along with reduction in the luminal pressure of the lactiferous system by the local application of cold compresses or ice packs. This reduces the breast metabolism and thereby inhibits milk production. Conversely, application of heat to the engorged lactating breast will increase milk production and induce further intraluminal pressure increase.

Continuing congestion of a lactiferous unit will lead to segmental mastitis with increased pain and systemic manifestations. When fever appears with mastitis and there is no evidence of abscess formation, resolution will usually follow the addition of broad-spectrum antibiotics to the ice and drainage program.

After approximately one week of continued mastitis, abscess formation may occur. This requires drainage by large-needle aspiration or surgical incision. Radial incisions should be avoided because of resulting unsightly scars. Appropriate antibiotics should be instituted after specific bacteriologic sensitivity studies.

Cultures of puerperal breast abscesses usually show staphylococci or streptococci.

Nonseptic inflammation can occur at any time following trauma or spontaneous rupture of macrocystic disease into the breast tissue. These inflammatory reactions are often prolonged in resolution. If continued improvement occurs and there are no signs of malignancy, conservative therapy is indicated. However, in many cases biopsies must be carried out to exclude inflammatory carcinoma. Aspiration for culture and cytologic examination can be very helpful in supporting a plan either for conservative or for operative treatment.

Breast Discharges

After "priming" effects of more than five months of pregnancy, with elevated production of estrogens, progesterone, and placental lactogen, the onset of breast milk secretion is stimulated by an intense pituitary prolactin release. The breast acini and lobular epithelium respond by milk production in the presence of proper nutrition and cell energy levels. This requires caloric energy, rest, hydration, insulin, cortisol, and thyroxin support.

In addition to epithelial secretion, the breast duct systems require oxytocin stimulation of their musculature to effect the milk let-down or excretory phase of lactation. Oxytocin release as a reflex response follows stimulation of the cervix or chest wall structures.

Coincident with the onset of lactation, the supporting stroma of the breast undergoes an edematous phase or breast engorgement. This engorgement can be delayed or suppressed by exogenous sex steroid administration at the time of delivery.

After experiencing lactation, the breast may maintain a low-grade secretory activity throughout life. Therefore, it is not unusual to find a pigmented nipple secretion from both breasts of a multiparous patient. The source of this pigment is not clear. Normal breast secretions do not contain blood. Tests for occult blood are therefore helpful in evaluating a green or brown discharge from the nipple.

Bilateral secretory activity will occur after the use of oral contraceptives as well as following chest trauma or chest wall surgery. Relatively uncommon endocrine syndromes and hypothalamic and pituitary tumors as well as drugs that affect the central nervous system may stimulate innocuous secretory activity. In these cases the breasts are innocent receptors of endocrine stimulation (prolactin and others) and secretory activity is not a cause of concern.

Unilateral discharge that is clear and sticky or that contains blood requires further evaluation. Cytologic study of this fluid is of some value. The first fluid expressed is usually hypocellular and yields little cytologic information. Breast material prepared for cytologic examination must be placed on a slide with some special features for adherence. A thin coating of albumin or a totally frosted slide will suffice. Serial smears will demonstrate increased cytologic material since the fluid from the higher levels of the lactiferous system contain more cells. A persistent, bloody discharge is an indication for segmental resection of the involved lobe.

Technique of Nipple Flap Duct Resection

Careful inspection of the location of the duct within the nipple helps locate the lobe involved. Confirmatory evidence is obtained by milking the segment suspected and demonstrating further discharge. A periareolar incision is performed in the appropriate quadrant, and undermining of the skin centrally and peripherally permits sufficient retraction of the areolar skin to expose the lactiferous ducts. A meticulous dissection is necessary under the nipple to avoid disruption of the thin-walled lactiferous sinuses. Duct ectasia, if present, will be apparent grossly at this point in the dissection. Gentle occlusion of the suspected duct when identified should be followed by further milking action to confirm its positive identity. When the involved duct or ducts are identified, they are transected.

With gentle traction on the transected ducts, segmental dissection and removal of the involved lobe can be completed. Extensive branching of the duct system is found early in the dissection, and the lactiferous lobe broadens quickly. A gradually tapering dissection will not include the entire lobe.

Indolent drainage or crusting may occur with any skin disease of the nipple. Nevertheless, because Paget's disease may appear as a benign, inflammatory process, the gynecologist should be suspicious of this disease whenever the nipple appears abnormal. Unfortunately, this malignant ulceration of the nipple has been treated frequently as eczema for weeks or months before diagnosis. If the biopsy reveals Paget's disease and no masses are detectable in the breast, the cure rate by modified radical mastectomy approximates 90%. The glass slide contact smear for cytologic study will often expedite the diagnosis of Paget's disease.

Breast Pain

Pain in one or both breasts is a common complaint. Frequently this symptom does not represent breast disease but is referred to the breast from other regional disorders. Neck injuries are commonly followed by cervical and thoracic nerve root radiculitis. If the radicles involved include the upper thoracic segments, breast pain may be the only complaint. Similarly, pain arising from the rib and costal cartilages will often present as breast pain. Local palpation with rib compression will localize the pain to its musculoskeletal source. The diffuse anterior thoracic attachment of the pectoral muscles makes them a common source of breast-related pain. Active adduction of the arm by the patient will exacerbate this pain and clearly localize it to the muscle.

Painful engorgement and edema of the breast during the luteal phase of the menstrual cycle is a difficult problem. Dietary salt restriction may be helpful.

Suppression of the biphasic fluctuations of estrogen and progesterone associated with the normal menstrual cycle may reduce breast discomfort. This may be accomplished by the use of an oral contraceptive with low estrogen content (e.g., a combination of norethindrone acetate, 2.5 mg, and ethinyl estradiol, 50 μg [Norlestrin]). Similar suppression may be obtained by continuous administration of progestins such as medroxyprogesterone acetate in a dose of 20 mg daily. Methyltestosterone exerts an antiestrogenic effect on the breast and is usually given as a 10-mg sublingual tablet one or two times daily. If, however, the monthly dose exceeds 300 mg, some patients may note acne, hoarseness, or increased facial hair growth. Danazol and tamoxifen as potent antiestrogens, although quite expensive, have been successful in controlling difficult cases of mastodynia.

A host of other therapies that are less disturbing to the patient's metabolism have traditionally been offered to women suffering from pain associated with benign cyclic breast changes. Vitamin E therapy (400 to 600 units/day) has been associated with improved symptoms in 85% of patients treated. This apparently is associated with an antiestrogenic effect of increased mildly androgenic adrenal steroids. Elimination of cigarettes, caffeine, and other methylxanthines, and reduction of stress factors has been proposed by Minton to quiet the overactive cyclic adenosine monophosphate (AMP)-guanosine monophosphate (GMP) associated with hyperplastic fibrocystic breasts. In our experience, this seems very effective. Administration of vitamins A, B-complex, and C, as well as iodine and selenium, have also been recommended.

Inflammatory conditions in the breast usually produce pain. The comforting admonition that pain is not a sign of serious trouble is often relayed to patients complaining of breast pain. It must be remembered that approximately 20% of patients with breast cancer complain of pain in the area of their tumor. Of course the vast majority of those with inflammatory breast cancer complain of pain. Immediate aspiration, cytologic examination and bacteriologic cultures will help expedite the differential diagnosis and distinguish between inflammation and tumor.

LUMPS IN THE BREAST

Carcinoma

Carcinoma of the breast most often presents as a lump. Careful evaluation of breast lumps with maximum acuity is a significant contribution to patient care. Appropriate and rapid use of ancillary procedures assures maximum diagnostic evaluation.

Conditions that present as a dominant lump include carcinoma, fibrocystic disease, fibroadenomata, giant fibroadenomas or sarcomas, fat necrosis, and other uncommon breast lesions. These include galactoceles, sebaceous cysts, histiocytomas, leiomyomas, lipomas, adenolipomas, granular cell tumors, neurofibromas, sarcoidosis, and tuberculosis.

Carcinoma usually presents as a painless, firm, and deep-seated mass. Local infiltration may cause fixation of the tumor to the chest wall. This is elicted by adduction of the arm to set the pectoral muscles and fascia. Fixation or edema of the skin are other signs of advancing malignancy. Altered vascularity and increased metabolism of the tumor produce increased heat as measured by thermography or skin erythema after alcohol applications. The characteristic palpable mass that exhibits density contrast on mammograms and the gritty sensation of the needle tip at the time of aspiration are due to the very dense reaction in the stroma adjacent to the tumor, the desmoplastic response. Cytologic findings of the needle aspirate are suspicious or positive for malignancy in 95% of cases. Needle, incisional, or excisional biopsy is necessary to confirm the diagnosis. Ulceration of the skin and satellite-tumor nodules in the same breast indicate advanced disease.

Mirror-image biopsy of the opposite breast or upper outer quadrant site is recommended at the time of definitive surgery. Screening for evidence of metastatic disease by radioactive bone scanning and by measurement of liver and bone enzymes should precede therapy. At the time of original diagnosis and workup it is wise to register the status of tumor markers from the same blood sampling. These levels may be valuable in general prognosis and in assessing further therapy. The carcinoembryonic antigen (CEA) and the gross cystic disease protein (GCDP) are being used for this purpose. TNM (tumor, node, metastases) staging is shown in Table 8–1.

Proper treatment for breast cancer is undergoing reevaluation at this time. Two characteristics of the disease make it difficult to plan therapeutic stratagems. First is the multifocal nature of the process. Careful examination of cancerous breasts by Gall and later by Gallagher have revealed multiple foci of cancer origin in up to 50% of cases. Random biopsies of the opposite breast show bilateral disease in up to 20% of cases both in Urban's experience and in our own. The second problem in breast cancer treatment lies in the fact that up to 70% of the patients have disseminated disease at the time of diagnosis. At this time, programs of castration, antiestrogenic treatment, and chemotherapy given as adjuvant therapy have not made impressive inroads on ultimate recurrence. The possibility that adjuvant immunotherapy might make an important difference should be explored.

Either total mastectomy with axillary lymph node sampling or removal of the tumor followed by total breast tangential radiation with 5,000 to 6,000 rads and axillary node sampling seem interchangeably adequate for local control. Treatment of metastatic disease is diverse and depends on the estrogen and progesterone receptor assays of the tumor, as well as on the clinical setting within which the metastases arise. Probably the discovery of effective preventive measures and improvements in early detection are the only real hopes for improvement in breast cancer survival.

Fibrocystic Disease

Dominant lumps due to fibrocystic disease are common. Large cysts, 1 to 10 cm in diameter, are easily evacuated by aspiration.

TABLE 8–1.—STAGING SYSTEM FOR CANCER OF THE BREAST

T	Primary tumor measurement, preoperative (rule or caliper, xeromammography)
TO	No tumor
TIS	Preinvasive carcinoma (CIS), noninfiltrating intraductal carcinoma or Paget's disease of nipple and no demonstrable tumor
T1	Tumor size 2 cm or less
T1a	No fixation to pectoral fascia and/or muscle
T1b	Fixation to pectoral fascia and/or muscle
T2	Tumor size 2 to 5 cm
T2a	No fixation to pectoral fascia and/or muscle
T2b	Fixation to pectoral fascia and/or muscle
T3	Tumor size more than 5 cm
T3a	No fixation to pectoral fascia and/or muscle
T3b	Fixation to pectoral fascia and/or muscle
T4	Tumor of any size with direct extension to chest wall or skin (not including skin dimpling or nipple retraction)
T4a	Fixation to chest wall
T4b	Edema, infiltration or ulceration of skin (including peau d'orange), or satellite nodules confined to the same breast
T4c	Both (T4a and T4b)
N	Regional lymph nodes
N0	No palpable homolateral axillary nodes
N1	Movable homolateral axillary nodes
N1a	Metastasis not suspected
N1b	Metastasis suspected
N2	Fixed homolateral axillary nodes
N3	Homolateral supraclavicular or infraclavicular nodes or edema of the arm
M	Distant metastases
M0	No evidence of distant metastases
M1	Distant metastases present, including skin involvement beyond the breast area

STAGE-GROUPING

TIS	Carcinoma in situ				
Invasive carcinoma					
Stage I	T1a	N0	or N1a	M0	
	T1b	N0	or N1a	M0	
Stage II	T0	N1b			
	T1a	N1b			
	T1b	N1b			
	T2a	N0	or N1a	M0	
	T2b	N0	or N1a		
	T2a	N1b			
	T2b	N1b			
Stage III	Any T3	with any N			
	Any T4	with any N		M0	
	Any T	with	N2		
	Any T	with	N3		
Stage IV	Any T		Any N	with M1	

Up to 30 ml of cyst fluid may be removed. This fluid may be spread on a slide for cytologic study or mixed with 50% alcohol for cell-block histologic study. If aspiration-evacuation of a cyst returns the breast to normal, follow-up examination in three or four weeks is suggested.

Further subdivisions of fibrocystic disease are found on histologic study. These include apocrine metaplasia, mastitis, sclerosing adenosis, fibrosis, and blunt duct adenosis. These benign variations of fibrocystic disease have no premalignant potential. Those subdivisions of fibrocystic disease that demonstrate epithelial unrest, however, are considered to be premalignant. Patients whose biopsies reveal intraductal papillomas, papillomatosis, intraductal hyperplasia, and lobular hyperplasia have an increased possibility of subsequent malignancy in the breast (Fig 8–1). Furthermore, intraductal hyperplasia with almost complete occlusion of the ductal lumen, the so-called cribriform pattern, is even more foreboding to pathologists. Similarities and coexistence with intraductal carcinoma suggest that this is a premalignant lesion.

Comparison of breast hyperplasia to atypical hyperplasia of the endometrium is tempting. Similar age groups and hormonal influences are shared by the two conditions. The progression from atypical hyperplasia to carcinoma in situ to carcinoma, however, is better established in the endometrium.

Recurrent discomfort, cysts, and tumor formation are common in some women. Attempts at therapy similar to that for cyclic congestion symptoms are occasionally successful but, unfortunately, a few patients in their fourth decade are plagued by relentless and progressive fibrocystic disease.

Fibroadenomas

Fibroadenomas usually present as characteristic firm, round, nontender mobile masses, which commonly occur in young women. Their subcutaneous location has led to the term *poppability,* which describes their unusual mobility. During attempted aspiration they "bite" the needle with a rubbery tenacity that makes smooth withdrawal difficult. The aspirate usually reveals scant cellular material with benign duct cells and fibroblasts on cytologic examination.

Although the diagnosis of fibroadenoma is usually obvious in most cases, removal is still recommended. A carcinoma does occasionally masquerade as a fibroadenoma, and mammography may not be helpful in detecting early malignancy. Furthermore, a few fibroadenomas possess unusual growth potential and may progress to the "giant" fibroadenoma or cystosarcoma phyllodes. Existing fibroadenomas grow dramatically under the influence of high levels of estrogen. This may occur during pregnancy, and the very rapid growth may suggest a malignant lesion. The mass should be excised under local anesthesia as soon as it is detected.

Fat Necrosis

Fat necrosis has been mentioned previously in the discussion of inflammatory processes. Unfortunately, this lesion may look and feel exactly the same as carcinoma. Therefore, it is important to use all of the adjunctive diagnostic procedures before proceeding to surgery. Aspiration is usually less gritty than with cancer and the cytologic examination is characterized by inflammatory cells. Mammography is not always helpful in making a precise diagnosis.

Other Lumps

Adolescent breast buds, prominent subareolar lactiferous sinuses, thickenings of Cooper's ligament, prominent inframammary ridges, and the more prominent tail of Spence have been described. Both breasts should be examined and compared in order to determine the normality of lumplike findings. Fat lobules and hormonally stimulated breast lobules may seem to be dominant lumps if the patient is examined during the luteal phase. Reexamination on day 5, 6, or 7 of the next menstrual cycle will reveal the temporary and cyclic nature of these masses.

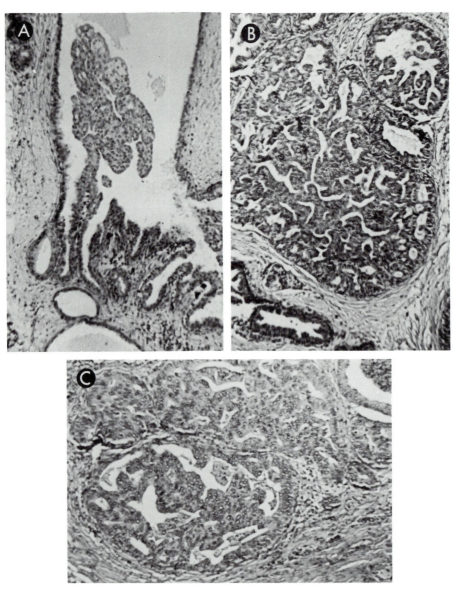

Fig 8–1.—Examples of breast epithelial hyperplasia. **A,** intraductal papilloma: benign overgrowth in the duct lumen. **B,** intraductal hyperpla-sia: benign overgrowth fills ducts. **C,** intraductal carcinoma: necrotic areas are evident. Cellular atypia may be mild. *(Continued)*

TECHNIQUES OF EVALUATING BREAST LUMPS

Friction-Free Examination

The breast skin can be rendered friction free by the use of powder, thin lubricating jelly, or warm soap and water, thus improving an appreciation of breast structures by palpa-tion. Previous biopsy sites are better delinea-ted as saucerized defects or linear suture-line densities. Subareolar prominences can be dis-tinguished as a circular ring of uniform struc-tures. Improved delineation of questionable areas in the breast by this simple approach will reduce the incidence of unnecessary breast resections and, perhaps more impor-

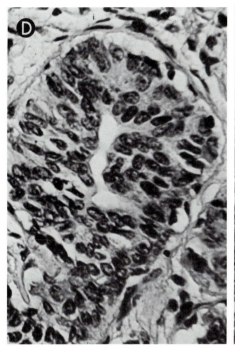 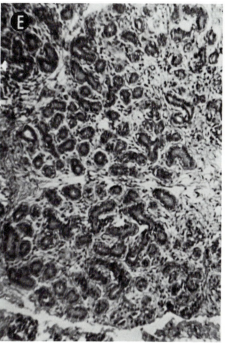

Fig 8–1 (cont.).—D, atypical blunt duct adenosis: benign acting, but may appear wild. **E,** lob-ular hyperplasia: active lobule may precede lob-ular carcinoma in situ and carcinoma simplex.

tant, will increase the incidence of patients having early malignancy detected.

Aspiration Cytology

Needle aspiration of the breast is a simple procedure. The mass or area of suspicion is held between two fingers of the left hand. Cutaneous spray with ethyl chloride until the skin is blanched provides adequate anesthesia for this puncture. A 20-gauge needle attached to a 10-ml syringe is quickly thrust into the center of the area. This syringe and needle are previously prepared by aspirating a small amount of normal saline into the dead space of the syringe and needle lumen. When the saline is expressed, approximately 0.05 ml of saline remains in the lumen of the needle and syringe tip. After insertion of the needle, vigorous suction is applied to the syringe while multiple small tracts are made in the breast tissue.

Aspirated cyst fluid is spread thinly on an albumin-coated or totally frosted slide and sprayed with cytologic fixative and submitted

as a Papanicolaou smear. If no cyst fluid is obtained, the contents of the needle are expressed onto a similar slide and it is rocked to and fro until the vehicular saline is evaporated. It is then sprayed with the cytologic fixative (Fig 8–2).

Mammography

Mammography has become an acceptable diagnostic procedure for the detection of breast cancer. The procedure is of major assistance in screening high-risk and difficult-to-examine patients. This technique is not only accurate in predicting a diagnosis but it scans the remainder of the breast tissue for non-palpable disease. Mammograms cannot, repeat NOT, be substituted for biopsy of a dominant mass in the breast. Densities and fine-speckled calcifications are suspicious findings that are due to the dense stromal reaction around a breast malignancy. Spiculation, or radiating lines, and the skin changes of thickening or retraction are suspicious findings presumably due to adjacent infiltration by

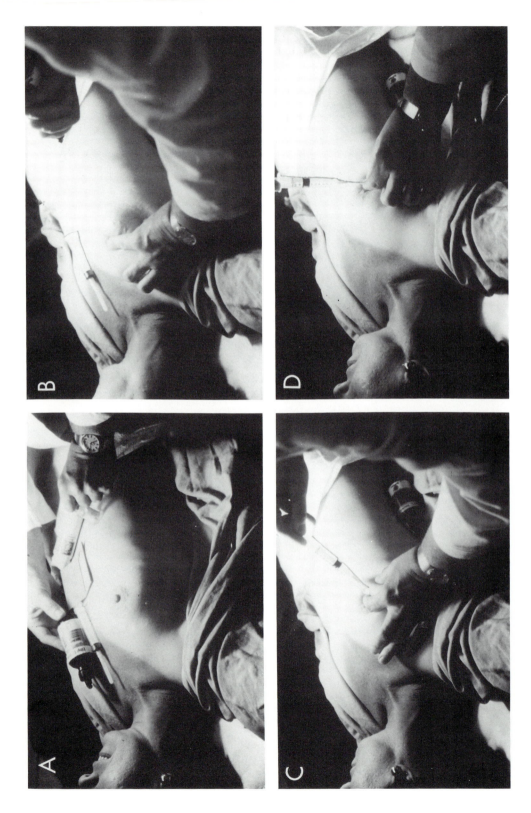

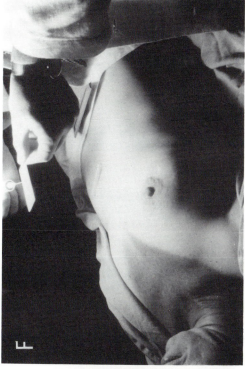

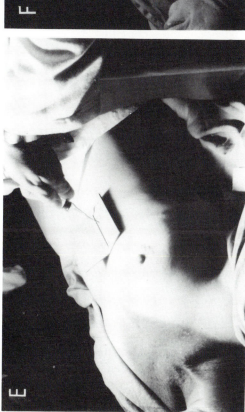

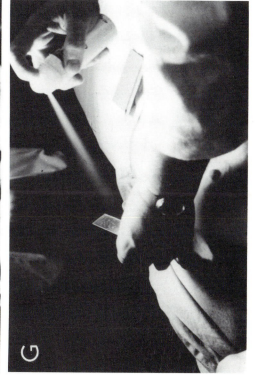

Fig 8–2.—Fine-needle aspiration of the breast for cytologic study. **A,** necessary equipment is shown: syringe (10 cc) and needle (20 gauge), ethyl chloride, cytology spray fixative, and totally frosted slide. **B,** appropriate area of breast is sprayed to an ice spot with ethyl chloride. **C,** puncture of area with syringe-needle combination premoistened with normal saline is followed by firm suction traction on the syringe. **D,** multiple-tract aspiration of the area is facilitated by pinching the skin up with the needle when backing up to start a new tract. **E,** the dead-space saline and cellular material are sprayed on the totally frosted glass slide. **F,** the cellular material is gently and evenly spread out. **G,** the still-moist (slightly) smear is sprayed with cytology fixative.

carcinoma. Despite the excellent diagnostic aid provided by mammography, 5% to 15% of cancers do not show characteristics that permit a diagnosis of malignancy. Obviously, then, biopsy must be performed when a persistent dominant mass is detected.

Another inadequacy of mammography is the impervious density of the breast tissue in young women. Mammography will detect an increasing number of breast cancers after the age of 40 years since, as breast tissue is replaced by fat, radiation detectability improves.

The hazards of radiation-induced breast cancer must be considered in critically evaluating mammography. The incidence of breast cancer has been reported to be increased in atomic bomb victims, following repeated fluoroscopy, and in patients irradiated for postpartum mastitis. Since the evidence that radiation can induce breast cancer in the human female seems incontrovertible, diagnostic procedures that utilize radiation modalities should be used with caution. Perhaps five to ten mammographic studies in a lifetime should be the upper limit of radiation exposure. Those women at high risk for breast cancer may be the ones who are most susceptible to a radiation oncogenesis.

Thermography

Continued research may ultimately improve the techniques and interpretation of thermographic mammometry. The wide variety of heat distribution in various breast diseases markedly reduces the precision of thermographic diagnosis. Thermography is seldom employed at the Boston Hospital for Women division of the Brigham and Women's Hospital.

Ultrasound

Although diagnostic ultrasound seems totally safe, its applicability to breast imaging is limited. Both contact and immersion ultrasonography are able to document that a dominant mass is fluid-filled or solid. Of course,

fine-needle aspiration can obtain this information more directly.

Breast Biopsy

A complete evaluation of any lump in the breast is possible only by excisional biopsy and histologic examination of the tissue. In women over the age of 50 years, any dominant breast lump is an indication for immediate excision. In younger patients, especially if menstruation is still occurring, reexamination should be scheduled after the next menstrual period and excision performed if the mass remains or becomes larger.

Technique of Breast Biopsy

There are three major considerations that affect the choice of the incision for biopsy. First, a relatively central location is desirable so that the subsequent mastectomy incision will not be compromised. Second, the cosmetic appearance of the scar is usually excellent if the skin incision is areolar or periareolar. Langer's lines in the skin of the breast are generally circumferential around the breast globe. Last, radial incisions should *never* be made in the breast skin. Within the substance of the breast, however, radial or elliptical incisions should be used in young women to preserve potential lactational function. Extensive skin undermining is sometimes necessary to reach the tumor or to ensure adequate exposure for proper dissection and closure of the breast excision site.

Incision within the breast to achieve removal of the lesion with a margin of normal breast tissue and a properly elliptical biopsy defect can be confusing if the breast is distorted with traction by hooks, clamps, or forceps. A freehand scalpel incision is usually preferred. This scalpel blade should be small to avoid cutting the retracted skin edges.

Hemostasis is best achieved after the biopsy specimen has been removed. The wound is packed tightly with sponges and then a search for significant "bleeders" will systematically reveal the vessels to be sutured, ligated, or coagulated. Compression suture-ligatures may be necessary if the vessel is detected in dense breast tissue. Minor oozing from the cut edge of the breast tissue can be controlled by compression approximation of the cut edges. The breast-closing sutures should all be held as an entire row of sutures to assure a smooth closure. Premature tying of one suture will make subsequent suture placement difficult and lead to a distorted lumplike biopsy site that will falsely alarm future examiners.

Compression dressing for six hours can be changed to a light dressing before discharge of the patient on the night of biopsy. Firm support with few limitations in activity are the general rules of postoperative care. Subcutaneous cuticular closure of the skin with polyglycolic acid suture material allows for the most trouble-free recovery.

Biopsy to investigate mammographic abnormalities is a special problem. By careful measurements of the x-rays and the patient's breast, an accurate estimation of the location is possible. Calcific densities may be verified by radiographic study of the biopsy specimen. Partial slicing or "bread-loafing" of the specimen before x-ray will help the pathologist find the calcific area.

Areas of density or radiating lines of spiculation cannot be verified by specimen radiology because their appearance depends on relative density within the breast tissue. Biopsy of a nonpalpable mammogram abnormality requires preoperative localization by placement of a Kopan's wire or other similar radiopaque marker in the vicinity of the designated area. Repeat mammography then pinpoints the area to be resected and allows a clear diagnostic evaluation with minimal breast tissue removal. This system has been quite helpful in avoiding the embarrassing nuisance of missing the target shadow.

Positive biopsy material should be submitted in ice for determination of estrogen and progesterone-binding protein of the tumor. A fresh portion of tumor, $1 \times 1 \times 1$ cm, shipped in dry ice should be rushed to a laboratory equipped to perform these assays.

EARLY DETECTION OF BREAST CANCER

With judicious use of the aforementioned tools and biopsy of all dominant masses, the detection of breast cancer before the stage of regional or distant metastases should be relatively more common. The grouping of patients at especially high risk for the development of breast cancer allows the focus of special attention on them for early detection. Identifiable patients for inclusion in this type of diagnostic breast clinic include:

1. Patients with previous unilateral breast cancer.
2. Patients whose previous biopsies have revealed epithelial abnormalities with premalignant potential, such as intraductal hyperplasia, papillomatosis, lobular neoplasia, or carcinoma in situ (Fig 8–2).
3. Patients with two epidemiologic risk factors from the following:
   a. Mother, sister, or daughter with breast cancer.
   b. Blood relatives with premenopausal breast cancer.
   c. Blood relatives with bilateral breast cancer.
   d. Nulliparous patients or patients whose first pregnancy was after the age of 30 years.

Another helpful adjuvant to encourage early diagnosis is to lower the threshold for biopsy. Patients who are not suspicious for

TABLE 8–2.—STAGE I RATES OF BREAST CANCER AT THE BRIGHAM AND WOMEN'S HOSPITAL

PERIOD	STAGE I RATE (%)
1905–1946	36
1947–1961	42
1964–1967	52
1971	54
1972	67
1973	64
1974	50
1975	81

malignancy may be biopsied as outpatients or day-service patients and discharged the same day. If the patient knows that no provisions for immediate mastectomy have been made, her breast sampling process will be much less of an ordeal.

Success in early breast cancer detection is manifested by a significant percentage of the patients having negative lymph nodes at the time of treatment. Improvement in the stage I rate of breast cancer cases at the Brigham and Women's Hospital is depicted in Table 8–2.

BIBLIOGRAPHY

Abele J.S., Miller T.R., Goodson W.H., et al.: Fine-needle aspiration of palpable breast masses. *Arch. Surg.* 118:859, 1983.

Bell D.A., et al.: Role of aspiration cytology in the diagnosis and management of mammary lesions in office practice. *Cancer* 51:1182–1189, 1983.

Brooks P.G., Gart S., Heldfond A.J., et al.: Measuring the effect of caffeine restriction of fibrocystic disease. *J. Reprod. Med.* 26:279, 1981.

Chaudary M.A., et al.: Nipple discharge: The diagnostic value of testing for occult blood. *Ann. Surg.* 196:651, 1982.

Cole P., MacMahon B.: Epidemiology of breast cancer. *J. Natl. Cancer Inst.* 51:21, 1973.

Haagensen C.D.: *Diseases of the Breast.* Philadelphia, W.B. Saunders Co., 1971.

Leis H.P. Jr., Pilnik S.: Nipple discharge. *Hospital Medicine,* November 1970, p. 29.

Minton J.P., Foecking M.K., Webster D.J.I., et al.: Caffeine, cyclic nucleotides, and breast disease. *Surgery* 86:105, 1979.

Reid D.E., Christian C.D.: *Controversy in Obstetrics and Gynecology,* ed. 2. Philadelphia, W.B. Saunders Co., 1974.

Urban, J.A.: Biopsy of the "normal breast" in treating breast cancer. *Surg. Clin. North. Am.* 49:291–301, 1969.

CHAPTER NINE

Endometriosis

ROBERT BARBIERI, M.D.
ROBERT W. KISTNER, M.D.

ALTHOUGH ENDOMETRIOSIS WAS DESCRIBED in detail more than a century ago, it continues to be one of the unsolved, enigmatic diseases affecting the female. The first known report was written by Rokitansky in 1860, but following this only a few scattered reports appeared until about 1900, when Cullen and Meyer published extensive descriptions of their findings. Yet Cattell and Swinton were able to find fewer than 20 reports concerning endometriosis in the world literature prior to 1921.

In 1921, Sampson published the first of his series of reports, recording for posterity his theory of implantation as the causative factor in the disease. His articles awakened wide interest, even controversy, in the subject, and today his theory kindles as much heated argument among physicians as it did after publication of his first reports.

DEFINITIONS.—*Endometriosis* may be defined as the presence of functioning endometrial tissue outside of its normal situation, but usually confined to the pelvis in the region of the ovaries, uterosacral ligaments, cul-de-sac, and uterovesical peritoneum. The development and extension of endometrial tissue into the myometrium is termed *adenomyosis*. This disease entity seems unrelated histogenetically and is characterized by an entirely different clinical situation. Furthermore, the pelvic examination presents none of the characteristics of endometriosis. It should be re-

iterated that the term endometriosis implies *proliferating growth and function* (usually bleeding) in an extrauterine site. An *endometrioma* may be defined as an area of endometriosis, usually in the ovary, that has enlarged sufficiently to be classified as a tumor. When the endometrioma is filled with old blood, resembling tarry or chocolate-colored syrupy fluid, it is commonly known as a "chocolate cyst." It should be remembered, however, that a corpus luteum hematoma may have an identical gross appearance, so that all chocolate cysts should not be considered to be caused by endometriosis. Even in bona fide endometriomas the histologic picture may be confusing, since endometrial glands and stroma may become compressed by the pressure of the trapped blood and the pathologist is unable to make a specific diagnosis. If the endometriosis is not completely "burned out," close examination of the wall usually reveals numerous hemosiderin-laden macrophages, lymphocytes, and patches of condensed endometrial stroma without glands.

ETIOLOGY

The two most popular theories of histogenesis are the *transport theory* and the *coelomic metaplasia theory*.

The transport theory states that viable fragments of endometrium are carried to intraperitoneal sites by retrograde regurgitation through the oviducts or by transport via lymphatics or vascular channels. In support of the transport theory are the following observations: (1) during menstruation, retrograde regurgitation of desquamated endometrium commonly occurs, (2) some desquamated menstrual endometrium is viable and can seed and grow in intraperitoneal locations, and (3) endometrium can be found in pelvic lymphatic channels. The transport theory provides a possible explanation for the presence of endometriosis in old laparotomy or laparoscopy sites and for the presence of endometriosis in such distant sites as the lung, pleura, arm, thigh, and pelvic lymph nodes.

The coelomic metaplasia theory states that the ovarian epithelium and pelvic peritoneal mesothelium are capable of differentiating into müllerian elements such as endometrium. The stimuli that cause the transformation of these epithelial elements into endometrium are poorly characterized. However, inflammatory processes, such as the irritation of the pelvic peritoneum by regurgitated menstrual blood, may be important stimuli for metaplasia. It is likely that both retrograde transportation and coelomic metaplasia are important factors in the pathogenesis of endometriosis.

A key concept is that *hormonal factors are of central importance in the pathogenesis of endometriosis.* The importance of hormonal factors is highlighted by the following clinical observations: (1) endometriosis is uncommon prior to the menarche and occurs infrequently after the menopause, (2) ovarian ablation usually results in complete and prompt regression of ectopically located endometrial glands and stroma (although scar tissue may persist), (3) endometriosis is rarely observed in amenorrheic women but is common in women with uninterrupted cyclic menstruation for more than five years, (4) endometriosis improves or stabilizes during episodes of physiologically induced (pregnancy) or artificially induced (hormones) amenorrhea, and (5) frequent pregnancies, if initiated early in reproductive life, appear to prevent the development of endometriosis. The hormonal requirements of endometriotic implants are discussed below.

Little experimental evidence is available concerning the hormonal requirements of the endometrial implants of endometriosis. However, it is known that normal endometrium and the implants of endometriosis contain estrogen, androgen, and progesterone receptors. It is likely that the endometriotic implants retain patterns of hormonal responsiveness similar to those of normal endometrial cells. The following are true in normal endometrium: (1) estrogen in physiologic doses stimulates endometrial hyperplasia in a dose-dependent fashion if unopposed by progesterone, (2) androgens produce atrophy of the endometrium, (3) physiologic doses of progesterone support endometrial growth and secretory changes, and (4) pharmacologic doses of progestational agents produce a decidual reaction when adequate estrogen is present and atrophy when a hypoestrogenic environment exists (Table 9–1). To test the hypothesis that implants of endometriosis retain hormonal responses similar to those of normal endometrium, DiZerega studied the effects of estrogen, progesterone, or no hormonal replacement on the growth of peritoneal endometriotic implants in castrated monkeys. Estrogen alone was able to support the growth of the endometriotic tissue in the peritoneal cavity. In a hypoestrogenic, hypoprogestational environment the endometriotic tissue atrophied. Progesterone alone was also able to support the growth of the endometriotic tissue. These hormonal responses of

TABLE 9–1.—THE EFFECTS OF ESTROGENS, ANDROGENS, AND PROGESTINS ON ENDOMETRIAL TISSUE

	PHYSIOLOGIC DOSES	PHARMACOLOGIC DOSES
Estrogens	Growth	Hyperplasia
Androgens	. . .	Atrophy
Progestins	Secretory changes	Decidual reaction or atrophy

endometriotic tissue are the basis for tailoring effective hormonal therapy.

Unfortunately, the ectopic endometrium in endometriosis does not always respond to progestin stimulation to the same degree as the normally situated endometrium. Endometriotic implants frequently do not exhibit a secretory response to progesterone during the luteal phase of the cycle. This refractory behavior to progesterone suggests that the displaced endometrium is immature or is incapable of complete differentiation.

PATHOLOGY

The four basic structures seen microscopically in endometriosis are endometrial epithelium, glands or glandlike structures, stroma, and hemorrhage (Fig 9–1). Continuing function in areas of endometriosis tends to destroy its microscopic characteristics; thus Hertig's observation, "the more advanced the lesion clinically, the poorer the histologic detail" is the most descriptive. Early lesions, particularly those of the cul-de-sac, if excised in toto and properly oriented for the pathologist, usually demonstrate classic histology, whereas the large endometrial cyst of the ovary, obvious to the gynecologist at the operating table, may show only hemosiderin-laden macrophages with varying amounts of fibrous connective tissue and inflammatory cells. It is important, however, to remember that it is the endometrial stroma that is responsible for bleeding in endometriosis, not the glands or epithelium. The presence of stroma alone is diagnostic of the disease, and the experienced gynecologic pathologist usually makes the diagnosis of endometriosis without difficulty. The presence of a decidual reaction or a typical "naked-nuclei" cellular pattern surrounded by a delicate reticulum or spiral arterioles with adjacent predecidua, either with or without old or recent hemorrhage, is sufficient to permit the diagnosis to be made without glands.

Malignancy in endometriosis is rare. Criteria for the diagnosis of carcinoma arising in endometriosis were outlined by Sampson in 1925 and are still acceptable. They are: (1) the ovary must be the site of benign endometriosis, (2) there must be a genuine adenocarcinoma, and (3) a transition from benign to malignant areas must be demonstrated. Of

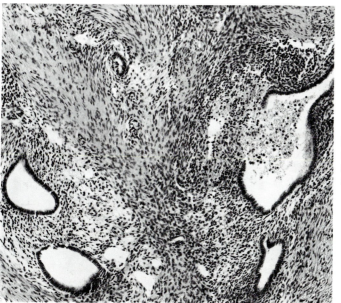

Fig 9–1.—Endometriosis of uterosacral ligament. Typical endometrial glands and stroma are evident in the fibrous connective tissue of the ligament.

interest is the observation that many cases of clear cell carcinoma of the ovary are associated with endometriosis.

The commonest site of endometriosis is the ovary, and in about 50% of patients both ovaries are involved. Other areas and organs affected (in order of incidence) are: uterosacral ligaments and rectovaginal septum, sigmoid colon, lower genital tract (cervix, vulva, and vagina), round ligaments, pelvic peritoneum, small intestine, umbilicus and laparotomy scars, bladder and ureter, breast, arm, leg, pleura, and lung (Fig 9–2). Early endometriosis may occur either as small, bluish, punctate or hemorrhagic areas on the surface of the ovary or uterosacral ligaments or as small cysts or foci of pink tissue lying beneath the surface epithelium or within the ovarian cortical stroma. The benign endometrial cyst of the ovary varies from microscopic size to a mass 8 to 10 cm in diameter. The cysts may be multiple in the early stages but subsequently coalesce into a single large cyst. During the early stage of development, endometriotic cysts are usually free and have smooth surfaces. As growth progresses, however, and there is surface bleeding, the cyst becomes densely adherent to surrounding structures, particularly the serosa of the sigmoid colon. The convex border (lateral aspect) of the ovary is more often involved and may become adherent to the ileum or lateral pelvic peritoneum. Frequently the ovary shows multiple areas resembling "powder burns" as a result of changes in blood pigments. Minute red or blue cystic areas (raspberry or blueberry spots) with adjacent puckering may be identified on the ovarian surface but are noted more often on the uterosacral ligaments or pelvic peritoneum. The lining of the endometrial cyst varies from red to dark brown, depending on the extent and duration of bleeding. It may be thin and smooth or thick and velvety, depending on the preponderance of fibrous tissue or functioning endometrium. If discrete papillary or polypoid lesions

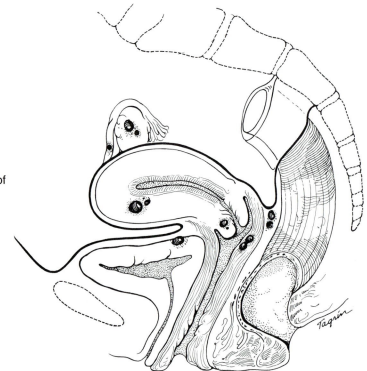

Fig 9–2.—Common sites of pelvic endometriosis.

are found in the cyst cavity, the possibility of malignancy should be considered. The contents of the cyst are usually thick, resembling chocolate syrup or tar.

The uterosacral ligaments or rectovaginal peritoneum may be involved separately or there may be a fused mass incorporating both structures (Fig 9–3). The discovery of bluish red or brown nodules with surrounding areas of puckering on the uterosacral ligaments, adjacent cul-de-sac, peritoneum, or serosa of the sigmoid is a characteristic finding, and if these reach adequate size, they may be palpated easily on rectovaginal examination. Eventually an intensive fibrous connective tissue reaction occurs, with fusion of the rectosigmoid to the back of the cervix and vagina. Masses of this type may become so firm that malignancy is suspected. Since bilateral oophorectomy will bring about permanent arrest of the disease, this procedure should be performed in preference to extensive bowel resection.

The lower genital tract may occasionally be the site of endometriosis; lesions of the cervix, vagina, and vulva have been reported. Usually there is a history of antecedent trauma, such as cervical cauterization or conization, vulvar surgery, or episiotomy. Surface endometriosis of this variety is almost certainly derived from implantation of viable endometrium and, in general, responds actively to estrogen and progesterone. When endometriosis involves the portio vaginalis of the cervix, the gross examination is usually pathognomonic, with blue-black, elevated nodules, either discrete or confluent, being evident by speculum examination.

The round ligament is occasionally the site of endometriosis, and if the lesion exceeds 0.5 cm in diameter, it can usually be palpated by examination of the inguinal areas. Subjective complaints in the region of the internal ring and/or canal of Nuck are frequently cyclic in nature and may be correlated with the menses.

Small bowel involvement is rare (about 0.1% to 0.2%) but may lead to an erroneous preoperative diagnosis. There is usually twisting or coiling about the lesion with resultant symptoms of nausea and crampy midabdominal or periumbilical pain. Grossly, the mu-

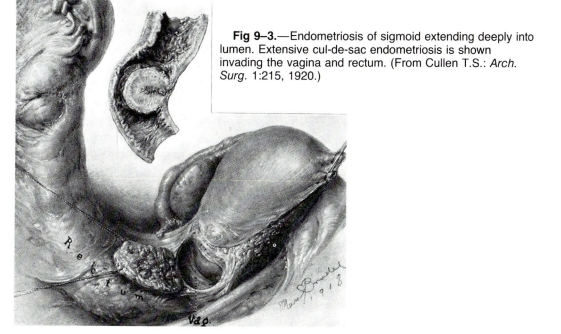

Fig 9–3.—Endometriosis of sigmoid extending deeply into lumen. Extensive cul-de-sac endometriosis is shown invading the vagina and rectum. (From Cullen T.S.: *Arch. Surg.* 1:215, 1920.)

cosal surface is usually smooth with subjacent fibrosis and scarring. In extensive pelvic endometriosis, several loops of ileum may be involved by contiguity so that resection of the areas is necessary. Similarly, the serosa of the appendix is often involved.

Endometriosis of the umbilicus and of laparotomy scars has been reported rather frequently. Although the theory of coelomic metaplasia is usually invoked to explain these lesions, Scott has suggested that various lymphatics situated along the obliterated hypogastric vessels might function as the route of transmission. Discomfort in the region of the umbilicus with cyclic nodularity and swelling or even gross bleeding serve to alert the clinician to the probability of endometriosis.

Urinary tract endometriosis is not common but probably occurs more often than is reported in the literature. The involvement of the serosal surface of the bladder is seen rather frequently but is usually asymptomatic. By the time the muscularis or mucosa is involved, the patient usually has noted cyclic hematuria and pain. Cystoscopy may show typical bluish "mulberry" lesions, and endoscopic biopsy confirms the diagnosis. Ureteral involvement has been reported and probably explains many cases of idiopathic, unilateral hydronephrosis (Fig 9–4). Cyclic flank pain, fever, and pyuria may occur as a result of intermittent ureteral obstruction. The excretory urogram may show beginning ureteral dilatation if obtained at the optimum time in the cycle. A tentative diagnosis may be confirmed by noting cessation of symptoms and improvement in the urogram following prolonged periods of induced anovulation (see the section entitled "Treatment").

Several cases are now on record of biopsy-proved pleural and pulmonary endometriosis in which a hematogenous mode of dissemination must be postulated.

In summary, the pathologic process of endometriosis, although microscopically benign, produces extensive havoc in the pelvis as important structures are gradually involved. The process is unique in that it spreads in a can-

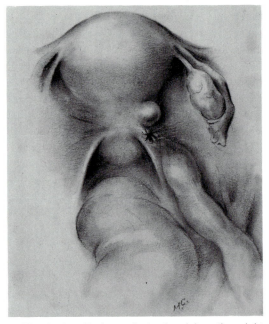

Fig 9–4.—Endometriosis involving the right uterosacral ligament, with fibrosis producing marked right hydroureter. (Courtesy of Dr. Thomas Leavitt.)

cerlike manner, which is frequently terminated by fibrosis and scarring. The end result may be ovarian destruction, oviduct deformity, bladder dysfunction, large bowel obstruction, and ureteral constriction.

CLINICAL FEATURES

Incidence

Endometriosis is exceedingly common. At the Brigham and Women's Hospital it is the most common "benign" gynecologic condition requiring hospitalization. It is present in 5% to 15% of women 25 to 35 years of age undergoing laparotomy on a general surgical service. Approximately 30% of patients undergoing laparoscopy for infertility have endometriosis. In general, mild and moderate stages of the disease are more common than severe stages of the disease. The epidemiology of endometriosis is controversial. The median age of patients at the time of diagnosis is approximately 30 years. It is likely that endometriosis is more common in upper–middle-class professional women. Delayed and infrequent pregnancies may account for this association.

Symptoms

The characteristic symptoms associated with this disease are: (1) progressive, acquired, severe pain associated with or occurring just prior to menstruation; (2) dyspareunia; (3) painful defecation; (4) premenstrual staining and hypermenorrhea; (5) suprapubic pain, dysuria, and hematuria; and (6) infertility (Table 9–2). Some patients do not have "acquired" dysmenorrhea but state that they have always had painful periods. Most will admit, however, to a recent increase in severity. In many patients the pain cannot be classified as dysmenorrhea but is actually premenstrual and varies from mild discomfort to severe pain that is characteristically in the lower abdomen, usually bilateral and associated with a sense of rectal pressure. A constant soreness in the lower abdomen or pelvis throughout the month that is aggravated just before the menses or during coitus may be the only complaint. The pain in endometriosis is of unknown cause but is probably related to the development of secretory changes, with subsequent miniature menstruation and bleeding in areas that are totally or partially encapsulated by fibrous tissue. That this is due to intermittent stimulation and withdrawal of progesterone is substantiated by the fact that dysmenorrhea is not evident if ovulation is prevented.

Pain is not always associated with endometriosis even when the disease is extensive. Bilateral, large ovarian endometriomas frequently are not symptomatic unless rupture occurs. On the other hand, incapacitating pelvic discomfort may be associated with minimal amounts of active endometriosis. Often there are only puckering and scarring of the posterior cul-de-sac with an adherent rectosigmoid to account for the multiplicity of symptoms.

Correlation With Infertility

There exists a definite correlation between infertility and endometriosis. The expectation of pregnancy when this disease is present is about half that in the general population. Therefore, compared with a natural prevalence of infertility approximating 15%, in patients with endometriosis the sterility prevalence is 30% to 40%. The pathophysiologic mechanisms that link advanced endometriosis and infertility have not been fully delineated. Although infertility may cause endometriosis (by chronic uninterrupted menstrual cycles), most investigators have studied how endometriosis causes infertility. In cases of endometriosis in which severe tubal or ovarian pathologic findings are present, *structural* problems in ovum release and tubal transport are the likely causes of infertility. However, in more mild cases of endometriosis the link between the disease and infertility is unclear. Some investigators have proposed that *functional* problems in tubo-ovarian action are the cause of infertility in these patients. The proposed functional disorders include: (1) increased levels of prostaglandins, (2) inadequate luteal phase, (3) premature luteinization of the follicle, (4) hyperprolactinemia, and (5) autoimmune mechanisms. However, to date, none of these hypotheses have been clearly documented.

Diagnosis and Staging

Although *the diagnosis of endometriosis* may be suggested by the history and physical examination, it *can only be made definitively by laparoscopy or laparotomy.*

In patients with endometriosis, the physical

TABLE 9–2.—SYMPTOMS
AND SIGNS OF ENDOMETRIOSIS

Symptoms
  Progressive dysmenorrhea
  Dyspareunia
  Infertility
  Premenstrual staining
  Painful defecation
Signs
  Cul-de-sac induration
  Uterosacral ligament nodularity
  Fixed ovarian masses

examination often reveals nodular uterosacral ligaments in conjunction with a fixed, retro-verted uterus. Palpable ovarian masses are present in approximately 20% of patients with endometriosis. The ovaries are often fixed in the cul-de-sac, and can only be palpated by rectovaginal examination.

In patients with mild to moderate endo-metriosis laparoscopy reveals the classic "powder-burn" lesions, which consists of small (less than 2 mm) purple spots visible on the pelvic peritoneum. Scarring and adhe-sions are commonly seen in association with cases of moderate to severe endometriosis. Evaluation of ovarian masses by laparoscopy is difficult and the diagnosis of ovarian en-dometrioma should not be made by laparo-scopic evaluation. Biopsy of small endome-triotic lesions via the laparoscope can be

helpful to confirm the diagnosis. However, it should be remembered that some endome-triotic implants may contain only stroma with hemorrhage, thus making the diagnosis diffi-cult for the pathologist.

A critical concept is that endometriosis is a heterogeneous disease. Therefore, surgical-pathologic staging is of utmost importance. Three major staging systems have been pro-posed by (1) Acosta, (2) Kistner, and (3) the American Fertility Society (AFS). The Acosta system is outlined in Table 9–3. The Kistner system is outlined in Table 9–4 and Figure 9–5. The AFS system is outlined in Figure 9–6. Every gynecologist should carefully stage every case of endometriosis by one of the available systems. The Acosta and Kistner systems are easy to use but occasional cases occur that are difficult to stage reliably. The AFS system is more difficult to use but is an excellent system for clinical research because it lends itself to computerized data analysis. Careful staging is important for planning ther-apy, determining a prognosis, following the

TABLE 9–3.—A PROPOSED CLASSIFICATION
OF PELVIC ENDOMETRIOSIS*

Mild
  Scattered, fresh lesions (i.e., implants not associated with scarring or retraction of the peritoneum) in the anterior or posterior cul-de-sac or pelvic peritoneum
  Rare surface implant on ovary, with no endometrioma, without surface scarring and retraction, and without periovarian adhesions
  No peritubal adhesions
Moderate
  Endometriosis involving one or both ovaries with several surface lesions, with scarring and retraction or small endometriomas
  Minimal periovarian adhesions associated with the ovarian lesions
  Superficial implants in the anterior or posterior cul-de-sac, or both, with scarring and retraction. Some adhesions, but no sigmoid invasion
Severe
  Endometriosis involving one or both ovaries with endometriomas over 2 × 2 cm
  One or both ovaries bound down by adhesions associated with endometriosis, with or without tubal adhesions to ovaries
  One or both tubes bound down or obstructed by endometriosis, with associated adhesions or lesions
  Obliteration of the cul-de-sac by adhesions or lesions, associated with endometriosis
  Thickening of the uterosacral ligaments and cul-de-sac lesions from invasive endometriosis, with obliteration of the cul-de-sac
  Significant bowel or urinary tract involvement

*From Acosta et al.: *Obstet. Gynecol.* 42:19, 1973.

TABLE 9–4.—CLASSIFICATION
OF ENDOMETRIOSIS*

STAGE I
Pelvic or adnexal adhesions are minimal. No tubo-ovarian distortion or adenxal fixation. Implants are limited to 5 mm or less on the pelvic peritoneum (i.e., cul-de-sac, uterosacral ligaments) but not the ovary
STAGE II
A. Endometriomas of one or both ovaries, but the remainder of the pelvis is free of adhesions or tubal disease
B. Moderate number of adhesions in the pelvis or periadnexal area with tubo-ovarian distortion, but the fimbria are free and the tubes are patent. The ovaries are fixed to the posterior leaf of the broad ligament, but the involvement with endometriosis is less than 2 cm
STAGE III
Pelvic or adnexal adhesions are dense with distortion of the tubes and ovaries, with the tubes covered by adhesions and requiring fimbrioplasty to recover identifiable fimbria. Ovarian fixation to the posterior leaf of the broad ligament is present.
STAGE IV
Extragenital involvement of either bladder, intestines, lungs, etc
The staging is made only at the time of the first or initial operative intervention

*From Kistner et al.: *Fertil. Steril.* 28:1008, 1977.

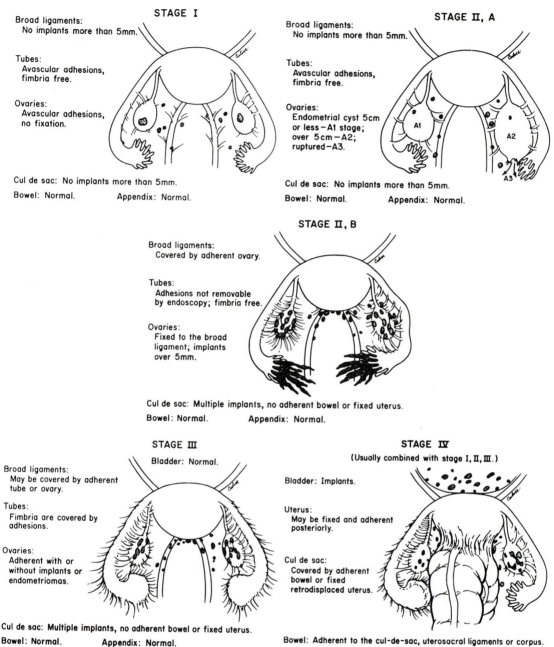

STAGE I

Broad ligaments:
  No implants more than 5mm.

Tubes:
  Avascular adhesions,
  fimbria free.

Ovaries:
  Avascular adhesions,
  no fixation.

Cul de sac: No implants more than 5mm.
Bowel: Normal.   Appendix: Normal.

STAGE II, A

Broad ligaments:
  No implants more than 5mm.

Tubes:
  Avascular adhesions,
  fimbria free.

Ovaries:
  Endometrial cyst 5cm
  or less—A1 stage;
  over 5cm—A2;
  ruptured—A3.

Cul de sac: No implants more than 5mm.
Bowel: Normal.   Appendix: Normal.

STAGE II, B

Broad ligaments:
  Covered by adherent ovary.

Tubes:
  Adhesions not removable
  by endoscopy; fimbria free.

Ovaries:
  Fixed to the broad
  ligament; implants
  over 5mm.

Cul de sac: Multiple implants, no adherent bowel or fixed uterus.
Bowel: Normal.   Appendix: Normal.

STAGE III

Bladder: Normal.

Broad ligaments:
  May be covered by adherent
  tube or ovary.

Tubes:
  Fimbria are covered by
  adhesions.

Ovaries:
  Adherent with or
  without implants or
  endometriomas.

Cul de sac: Multiple implants, no adherent bowel or fixed uterus.
Bowel: Normal.   Appendix: Normal.

STAGE IV
(Usually combined with stage I, II, III.)

Bladder: Implants.

Uterus:
  May be fixed and adherent
  posteriorly.

Cul de sac:
  Covered by adherent
  bowel or fixed
  retrodisplaced uterus.

Bowel: Adherent to the cul-de-sac, uterosacral ligaments or corpus.
Appendix: May be involved.

Fig 9–5.—Classification of endometriosis.

course of disease, and communicating with other care providers. The importance of staging endometriosis is highlighted by recent reports that most patients with untreated stage I (Kistner system) endometriosis have a fecundity potential no different than that of the general population. This observation indicates that stage I endometriosis has a prognosis quite different than stage II, III, or IV endometriosis.

AMERICAN FERTILITY SOCIETY CLASSIFICATION OF ENDOMETRIOSIS

Patient's name _____

Stage I	(Mild)	1–5
Stage II	(Moderate)	6–15
Stage III	(Severe)	16–30
Stage IV	(Extensive)	31–54

Total _____

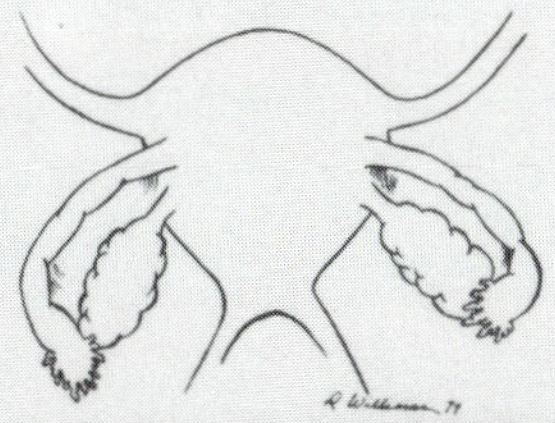

			<1 cm	1–3 cm	> 3 cm
PERITONEUM	ENDOMETRIOSIS		<1 cm	1–3 cm	> 3 cm
			1	2	3
	ADHESIONS		filmy	dense w/ partial cul-de-sac obliteration	dense w/ complete cul-de-sac obliteration
			1	2	3
OVARY	ENDOMETRIOSIS		<1 cm	1–3 cm	> 3 cm or ruptured endometrioma
		R	2	4	6
		L	2	4	6
	ADHESIONS		filmy	dense w/ partial ovarian enclosure	dense w/ complete ovarian enclosure
		R	2	4	6
		L	2	4	6
TUBE	ENDOMETRIOSIS		<1 cm	> 1 cm	tubal occlusion
		R	2	4	6
		L	2	4	6
	ADHESIONS		filmy	dense w/ tubal distortion	dense w/ tubal enclosure
		R	2	4	6
		L	2	4	6

Fig 9–6.—American Fertility Society classification of endometriosis.

TREATMENT

Patients with endometriosis typically present with complaints of pelvic pain and/or infertility. Therapeutic interventions should be designed to adequately address these two issues. Therapy will be discussed under five headings: (1) prophylaxis, (2) observation and analgesia, (3) hormonal therapy, (4) conservative operation, and (5) extirpative operation.

Prophylaxis

Manipulations that produce amenorrhea or cause endometrial atrophy are likely to decrease the chance of developing endometriosis. Early and frequent pregnancies appear to effectively decrease the frequency of endometriosis, but this therapeutic strategy is incompatible with the life plans of most patients. Exercise-induced amenorrhea may prove to be an effective prophylactic modality.

There is suggestive evidence that women who have been taking oral contraceptives for prolonged periods of time, especially those with a potent progestin and a minimal amount of estrogen, may have a diminished chance of developing endometriosis. This is based on the observation that these agents produce endometrial atrophy and lessen menstrual flow, thus preventing tubal reflux of menstrual detritus into the peritoneal cavity.

Observation and Analgesia

Observation as a form of treatment is often rewarding since many patients either "out-

grow" their endometriosis or become pregnant and remain asymptomatic indefinitely. Expectant treatment is worthwhile for the patients who have only minimal symptoms and pelvic findings. For these patients, reassurance and mild analgesics are often effective. Since excessive production of prostaglandins may account for the pain associated with endometriosis, antiprostaglandin agents may be the analgesics of first choice.

Hormonal Therapy

The hormonal management of endometriosis has undergone a significant evolution during the past three decades. High-dose diethylstilbestrol therapy and methyltestosterone therapy both achieved moderate degrees of success in providing relief from the symptoms of endometriosis. However, the high percentage of disturbing side effects produced by these two hormonal regimens precluded their widespread use. In the late 1950s the introduction of "progestin-only" and pseudopregnancy regimens resulted in a marked improvement in the medical management of endometriosis. In the mid-1970s the synthetic androgen danazol was introduced as yet another option in the medical management of endometriosis. Guidelines to the use of a pseudopregnancy regimen or danazol in the treatment of endometriosis are reviewed below.

Pseudopregnancy Regimens

In response to chronic, noncyclic stimulation by both estrogen and progesterone the endometrium becomes inactive and demonstrates decidualization. Figure 9–7 illustrates this phenomenon. This observation is the basis for the use of uninterrupted combined estrogen-progestogen agents in the treatment of endometriosis. Figures 9–8 through 9–10 demonstrate the decidual changes induced in implants of endometriosis by combined estrogen-progestogen therapy. There is no evidence that any one preparation of estrogen-progestogen pill is uniquely effective in the treatment of endometriosis. Therefore, any combined estrogen-progestogen preparation may be employed. A standard regimen would employ ethinyl estradiol 0.03 mg with norgestrel 0.3 mg, daily (Lo/Ovral). When breakthrough bleeding occurred, the patient could be instructed to start ethinyl estradiol 0.05 mg with norgestrel 0.5 mg, daily (Ovral). With the next episode of breakthrough bleeding the dose would be increased to ethinyl estradiol 0.08 mg with norgestrel 0.8 mg, daily (one Lo/Ovral plus one Ovral).

A pseudopregnancy regimen should only be used in a patient with endometriosis proved by laparoscopy. The side effects are dose related and are those commonly associ-

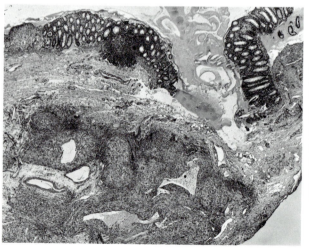

Fig 9–7.—Biopsy of a mass in the rectovaginal septum during the 14th week of pregnancy. Rectal mucosa is seen at the top of the section. Approximately two thirds of the rectal wall has been replaced by endometriotic tissue made up of inactive glands and decidua. The endometrial stroma (as decidua) is packed in whorl-like accumulations (magnification, × 40). (From Kistner R.W.: *Clin. Pharmacol. Ther.* 1:525, 1960.)

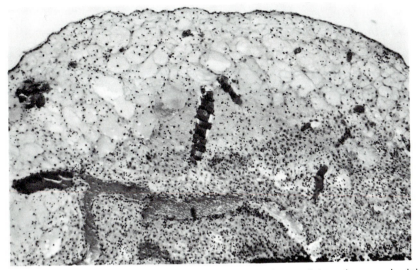

Fig 9–8.—Endometrial biopsy after 15 weeks of increasing doses of norethynodrel with ethinyl estradiol. There is a variation in response in the separate levels of the endometrium. Note the pronounced edema and decidual necrosis under the surface epithelium. In the midzone there are moderate intercellular edema and minimal necrosis of decidual cells. The basalis is made up of compact, well-preserved decidual cells (magnification, × 50). (From Kistner R.W.: *Clin. Obstet. Gynecol.* 2:884, 1959.)

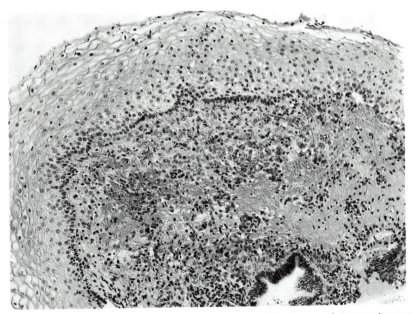

Fig 9–9.—Biopsy of vaginal mucosa during stage of premenstrual staining. Typical endometriosis in a menstrual phase is evident. Note hemorrhage into stroma, inflammatory cells and an endometrial gland in the lower portion. (From Kistner R.W.: *Fertil. Steril.* 10:547, 1959.)

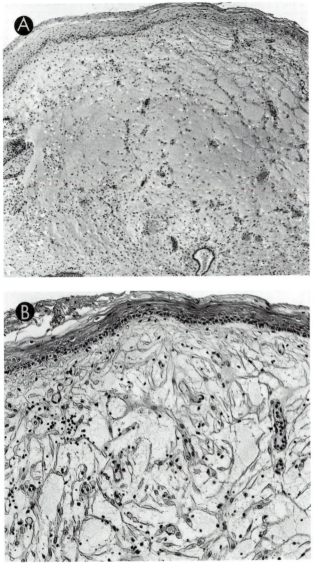

Fig 9–10.—Biopsy of an area of vaginal endometriosis after 12 weeks of continuous norethynodrel with ethinyl estradiol therapy. **A,** there is evidence of a marked generalized edema throughout the endometriosis. Under the vaginal epithelium the decidua is well maintained but most of it is undergoing necrosis. **B,** high-power view of an area in **A.** An unusual pattern of decidual change is evident. Most decidual cells remain as "naked nuclei" or a cytoplasmic strand in an edematous stroma. A few lymphocytes and macrophages are present and suggest an absorptive process of the necrotic endometriosis. (From Kistner R.W.: *Fertil. Steril.* 10:549, 1959.)

ated with oral contraceptives (see Chapter 16). Use of pseudopregnancy regimens prior to conservative laparotomy will often cause areas of endometriosis to enlarge and appear hemorrhagic, making identification, excision, and fulguration simpler and more complete.

Danazol

The medical management of endometriosis has been significantly advanced by the intro-duction of the synthetic steroid danazol. Danazol (Fig 9–11) has at least four pharmacologic properties that could account for its therapeutic efficacy in the treatment of endometriosis: (1) suppression of gonadotropin-releasing hormone and/or gonadotropin secretion; (2) direct interaction with endometrial androgen and progesterone receptors; (3) direct inhibition of ovarian steroidogenesis; and (4) increased metabolic clearance of estradiol

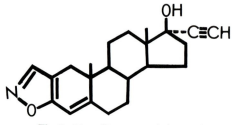

Fig 9–11.—Structure of danazol.

and progesterone. These properties of danazol produce an endocrine environment that inhibits the growth of endometrial tissue. By a direct androgenic and antiprogestational action on the endometrial implants of endometriosis, danazol produces atrophy of this tissue. In addition, danazol blocks ovarian follicular growth by direct actions on the hypothalamic-pituitary axis and the ovary. The lack of ovarian follicular activity results in a hypoestrogenic-hypoprogestational environment that also inhibits endometrial growth. Finally, by producing amenorrhea, danazol prevents the peritoneal "reseeding" of endometrial tissue that could occur during the menses. Given these pharmacologic properties of danazol, it is not surprising that danazol therapy results in a significant degree of symptomatic and objective improvement in patients with endometriosis.

Guidelines concerning the use of danazol continue to evolve. The following discussion highlights the areas of consensus and the breadth of disagreement concerning the use of danazol.

SELECTION OF PATIENTS FOR THERAPY.— Most clinicians agree that patients with a suspected diagnosis of endometriosis must have confirmation of the diagnosis by laparoscopy or laparotomy prior to initiation of therapy. Other than this one caveat, the indications for danazol therapy are controversial; following is a discussion in greater detail.

INITIATON OF THERAPY.—When administered to pregnant women, danazol and related isoxazole compounds can produce urogenital abnormalities in the offspring. Consequently, great care must be taken to ensure that patients initiating danazol therapy are not pregnant. In most cases, therapy with danazol should be initiated during menstruation. Otherwise, appropriate tests should be done to demonstrate that the patient is not pregnant. In patients with poor drug compliance, on a regimen of low doses of danazol, careful monitoring of the patient for a possible unsuspected intervening pregnancy must be maintained.

DOSAGE.—The patient package insert for danazol suggests a dose of 800 mg/day. However, many experienced clinicians now suggest that all patients start on a dose of 400 mg/day. In most patients this dose produces rapid relief of symptoms, cessation of menses, and objective regression of disease. In those patients who do not respond to 400 mg/day of danazol, the dose can be increased to 600 or 800 mg/day. In those patients requiring 600 or 800 mg/day of danazol to obtain a clinical response, the dosage can often be reduced after two to three months of therapy without precipitating a return of symptoms and physical findings. Doses of danazol below 400 mg are associated with a significant incidence of ovulation. Therefore, in general, doses below 400 mg should not be prescribed.

DURATION OF THERAPY.—Initial trials investigating the efficacy of danazol evaluated a six-month therapy regimen. This therapy interval need not be followed rigidly. Individualization of care is important when danazol is used to treat endometriosis. For example, in the patient with advanced endometriosis who is scheduled for conservative laparotomy, a 12- to 24-week preoperative course of danazol might be appropriate. For the patient with painful endometriosis who does not desire pregnancy and who is adamantly opposed to surgery, a 52- to 78-week course of danazol is not unreasonable if side effects are carefully monitored.

SIDE EFFECTS.—The major side effects seen with danazol therapy are (in decreasing order of frequency): weight gain, edema, decreased breast size, acne, oily skin, hirsutism, deepening of voice, headache, hot flashes, changes in libido, and muscle cramps. Significant weight gain (2 to 10 kg) is not uncommon. In our experience, more than three quarters of patients receiving danazol will complain of one or more side effects; however, discontinuation of the drug because of side effects is uncommon.

CONTRAINDICATIONS.—In the nonpregnant, non–breast-feeding patients with documented endometriosis, relatively few absolute contraindications to danazol therapy exist. Danazol is metabolized largely via hepatic mechanisms and has been reported to produce mild to moderate hepatocellular damage in some patients (elevated serum glutamic oxaloacetic transaminase and serum glutamic pyruvic transaminase levels). Therefore, in patients with hepatic dysfunction, danazol is relatively contraindicated. Since danazol can induce marked fluid retention, patients with severe hypertension, congestive heart failure, or borderline renal function may experience deterioration of their medical condition after danazol therapy is begun.

TIMING OF ATTEMPTS AT CONCEPTION AFTER COMPLETION OF THERAPY.—Dmowski and Cohen have reported a high number of second- and third-trimester intrauterine fetal deaths in patients who conceived within the first three cycles after discontinuation of danazol. They suggest that this degree of fetal wastage may be secondary to implantation in an atrophic endometrium and that following a course of danazol one full menstrual cycle of normal flow and duration be observed prior to any attempts to conceive. In contrast to these observations, Daniell and Christianson observed no increase in fetal wastage in patients conceiving within three months of completing a course of danazol. Barbieri, Evans, and Kistner confirmed that danazol therapy was not associated with increased fetal wastage. Further information is needed to resolve these discrepancies.

USE WITHOUT SURGERY IN THE TREATMENT OF THE INFERTILITY OF ENDOMETRIOSIS.—Endometriosis is a heterogeneous disease and the stage of the disease is one of the most important factors in planning therapy. Patients with infertility and severe endometriosis with marked anatomic abnormalities of the fallopian tubes, ovaries, and cul-de-sac will usually require surgery to enhance fertility. However, patients with infertility and mild endometriosis often have no major anatomic abnormalities. Recent studies suggest that *a course of danazol alone* might be able to enhance fertility in patients with mild endometriosis. Van Zyl and associates studied 20 infertility patients with mild to moderate endometriosis (staging system of Acosta and associates), and eight conceptions were obtained by using danazol without surgery. In 38 infertility patients with stage I and stage II endometriosis (staging system of Kistner), a course of danazol without surgery resulted in a 50% uncorrected fertility rate. These findings must be tempered by the report of Seibel that most cases of stage I (Kistner) endometriosis are not associated with infertility.

USE OF DANAZOL WITH SURGERY IN THE TREATMENT OF THE INFERTILITY OF ENDOMETRIOSIS.—In patients with infertility and advanced stages of endometriosis, surgery is usually necessary to repair anatomic abnormalities and to remove implants of endometriosis. Little experimental data are available concerning the value of danazol in the preoperative or postoperative management of endometriosis. Some experienced clinicians suggest that danazol has little value in the preoperative management of endometriosis. Others believe that danazol may improve the prognosis for infertile women with endometriosis by decreasing the number and size of endometriotic areas, thereby minimizing the extent of surgery. In addition, the preoperative use of danazol eliminates the chance of traumatizing a corpus luteum. Use of danazol in the postoperative management of the infertile patient with endometriosis is even more controversial. Most conceptions following surgical therapy occur within the first six months after surgery. Therefore, by treating the surgical patients with danazol for a prolonged period postoperatively, the time interval with the highest fertility potential will be passed over. It is our belief that danazol should be used in most patients preoperatively but that postoperative danazol therapy in infertility patients should be minimized.

USE IN THE TREATMENT OF ENDOMETRIOSIS IN PATIENTS NOT DESIRING FERTILITY.—For the patient older than 40 years with symptomatic endometriosis who has completed her family, the definitive therapy is total abdominal hysterectomy and bilateral oophorectomy. However, some patients may want to postpone or avoid major surgery. For these patients a trial of danazol may be reasonable. For the young symptomatic patient with endometriosis who intends to delay pregnancy, danazol therapy is highly effective in relieving symptoms and physical findings.

TREATMENT OF ENDOMETRIOMAS.—No systematic study assessing the effect of danazol on endometriomas has been reported. Clinical experience suggests that danazol can often reduce the size of endometriomas, but that it is unusual for danazol to cause complete regression of an endometrioma. In general, danazol is more effective in causing regression of peritoneal endometriotic implants of small diameter.

USE IN METASTATIC ENDOMETRIOSIS.—For the majority of patients with endometriosis involving organs outside the pelvis, total abdominal hysterectomy and bilateral oophorectomy are necessary. However, certain patients will refuse surgery and others are extremely poor operative risks. In these patients, danazol therapy is an alternative of last report. Danazol has been successful in the treatment of pulmonary endometriosis, bowel obstruction, and ureteral obstruction caused by endometriosis.

RECURRENCE RATES AFTER THERAPY FOR ENDOMETRIOSIS.—A major problem in the treatment of endometriosis is that the disease tends to recur unless definitive surgical therapy is performed. Following a course of danazol therapy the recurrence of symptoms and physical findings is approximately 5% to 20% per year. A second course of danazol therapy is often successful in inducing a remission of disease symptoms and physical findings. An important point to emphasize is that in no clinical study examining the efficacy of danazol have the investigators routinely performed repeated laparoscopy of all patients with recurrence of symptoms and/or physical findings. It has been our experience that a few patients who have completed a course of danazol and have recurrence of symptoms and physical findings have no evident endometriosis on a "third-look" laparoscopy. It is possible that microscopic endometriosis is present and cannot be identified by gross examination. Alternatively, other causes of the symptoms may be present.

DANAZOL VS. PSEUDOPREGNANCY.—Very little data are available that directly compare the efficacy of danazol vs. a pseudopregnancy regimen in the treatment of endometriosis. The results of one small, prospective, randomized trial of danazol vs. a combination of mestranol and norethynodrel have been reported by Noble and Letchworth. A total of 86% of the patients treated with danazol reported improvement in their symptoms. Only 30% of the pseudopregnancy group reported symptomatic improvement. Improvement in objective findings was demonstrated in 84% of patients treated with danazol compared to only 18% of patients on the pseudopregnancy regimen. Side effects were a major problem for patients receiving both therapeutic regimens. Only 4% of the danazol group but 41% of the pseudopregnancy group discontinued therapy because of side effects. In a retrospective study of 438 patients, Mettler and Semm found that patients with endometriosis treated medically had a higher fertility rate when treated with danazol (45%) than when treated with lynestrenol (32%). However, it is difficult to assess the validity of the results of either study because of several deficiencies in design. The clinical impression of those who have used danazol extensively is that it is more effective than pseudopregnancy in the treatment of endometriosis. The major factor that has inhibited the widespread use of danazol is its high cost (approximately $1.00 per 200 mg).

An area of continuing controversy is the role of hormonal vs. surgical therapy. In general, those patients interested in only pain relief should be first treated with hormonal regimens unless they are near the menopause and have completed their families. If the hormonal regimen fails, then surgery can be planned. For the patient with advanced endometriosis and infertility, surgery will almost always be required. Table 9–5 summarizes therapeutic approaches to endometriosis.

The success rates of various hormonal and surgical approaches to endometriosis are summarized in Table 9–6.

Surgical Treatment

In contemplating surgical treatment of endometriosis, one should always bear in mind that functioning ovarian tissue is necessary for the continued activity of the disease. Therefore, the successful treatment of endometriosis depends on a knowledge of when it is rea-

TABLE 9–6.—PREGNANCY RATES IN PATIENTS TREATED FOR ENDOMETRIOSIS AT THE BRIGHAM AND WOMEN'S HOSPITAL

THERAPY	NO. OF PATIENTS	UNCORRECTED % PREGNANCY
Pseudopregnancy	186	51
Danazol	100	46
Surgery		
No adhesions	232	76
Adhesions	106	38

sonably safe or desirable to maintain ovarian function and when it is necessary to destroy it. It is quite obvious that ovarian function should be conserved in treating the very early and, perhaps, symptomless lesions, and destroyed when the pelvic organs are hopelessly invaded by endometriosis. Unfortunately, from the standpoint of definite surgical indications, the majority of cases will fall between these two extremes and may present problems in surgical judgment seldom encountered in any other pelvic disease. As our knowledge of the life history of endometriosis has increased, there has been a definite tendency to become more conservative, particularly in the treatment of the early and borderline cases. In general it is believed that one should err on the side of conservatism; this belief is based on the fact that endometriosis (1) usually progresses slowly over a period of years; (2) is not, and rarely becomes, malignant; and (3) regresses at the menopause.

TABLE 9–5.—MANAGEMENT STRATEGIES IN THE TREATMENT OF ENDOMETRIOSIS

	PRESENTING COMPLAINT		
	PELVIC PAIN (FERTILITY NOT AN IMMEDIATE ISSUE)		
STAGE	FAMILY NOT COMPLETED	FAMILY COMPLETED	INFERTILITY
I	Hormonal therapy	Hormonal therapy	Hormonal therapy
II, III	Hormonal therapy	Hormonal therapy or surgery	Hormonal therapy followed by surgery
IV	(1) Hormonal therapy; (2) surgery if hormonal therapy unsuccessful	Hormonal therapy followed by definitive surgery	Hormonal therapy followed by surgery

Early implantations on the surface of the peritoneum, wherever they are located, may be ignored, excised, or destroyed with a cautery. Small endometrial cysts on the ovary may be excised or a major portion of one or both ovaries may be resected. Small endometrial implants on the intestines should be excised. Conservative operations should also be accompanied by correction of uterine displacements, relief of cervical obstruction, and removal of any other concomitant pelvic pathologic lesions to aid in the prevention of a recurrence of the condition. Endometriosis coexisting with uterine myomas, ovarian cysts, or other pelvic pathologic lesions may be insignificant but, on the other hand, the extent or location may be such as to make conservative surgery hazardous.

CONSERVATIVE SURGERY TECHNIQUE.—If childbearing function is to be preserved, operative procedures should be as conservative as possible. All surgical procedures should be preceded by a thorough curettage and every patient should have had vaginal cytologic examination to exclude possible malignancy of the cervix.

The approach should usually be through a suprapubic transverse incision. Thorough exploration of the pelvic and abdominal organs should be performed routinely and the decision reached as to whether conservative or radical surgery is feasible. The uterus is frequently found to be adherent to the rectosigmoid. These adhesions are separated by either blunt or sharp dissection in the midline and the uterus is brought forward. Traction sutures of 1-0 Mersilene are then placed around the round ligaments to lift the corpus forward and out of the cul-de-sac (Fig 9–12,A). With the uterus held forward, further adhesions may then be separated under direct vision. As previously mentioned, the use of progestational agents for six to 12 weeks preoperatively greatly softens the adhesions and makes the posterior dissection relatively easy. Danazol produces a similar effect. Endometrial implants on the uterosacral ligaments or

cul-de-sac are excised. Similar excision of implants on the serosa of the rectosigmoid is then carried out (Fig 9–12,B). If the bowel lumen is entered, a layered closure of submucosa and seromuscular layers is done in the usual manner. After all areas of endometriosis have been removed, the edges of available peritoneum are closed with fine Vicryl. Occasionally the posterior aspect of the uterus may have to be approximated to the serosa of the rectosigmoid, thus obliterating the cul-de-sac, to secure adequate peritonization of the pelvis.

Endometrial cysts of the ovary are excised (Fig 9–12,C and D). These cysts are usually adherent and do not separate freely as do corpus luteum or follicular cysts. After as much of the cyst as possible has been removed, the walls of the ovary are approximated with several mattress sutures of fine catgut and the surface closed with a running, locked suture of 3-0 Vicryl. Occasionally all ovarian tissue is destroyed and oophorectomy is necessary. Nevertheless, it is remarkable how frequently an ovarian cyst can be enucleated and a fairly thick capsule of cortical tissue left in situ. We have had the experience of performing unilateral oophorectomy and resection of 90% of the remaining ovary and of being rewarded by subsequent ovulation and pregnancy. This is not always the case, however; some patients have premature menopause following such surgery.

If reproduction is not a prime factor or if there is evidence of extensive involvement of other pelvic structures, such as bowel or ureter, a hysterectomy and bilateral oophorectomy should be done.

Since leiomyomas of the uterus are found in about 15% of the patients with endometriosis, single or multiple myomectomy should be carried out as part of the conservative approach. It has been our practice to do a presacral neurectomy if the location of endometriotic areas is in the midline. Even if the patient has not had dysmenorrhea or pelvic pain preceding surgery, these symptoms may develop postoperatively. The presacral pro-

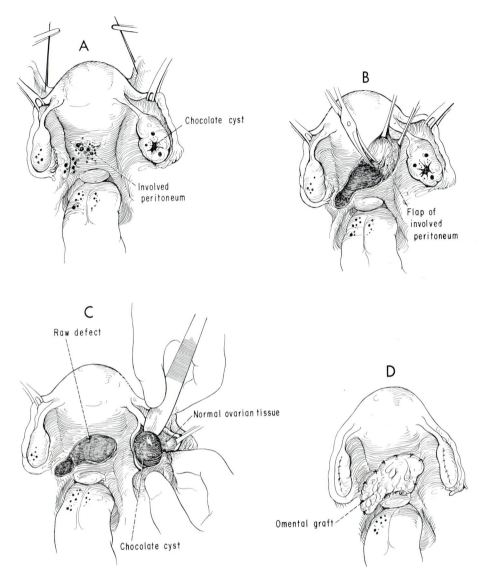

Fig 9–12.—A, traction sutures placed around the round ligaments and the uterus are drawn forward; areas of endometriosis are shown on the ovaries, posterior aspect of the uterus and anterior surface of sigmoid colon. **B,** serosa of posterior aspect of uterus involved by endometriosis is excised. **C,** endometrioma of the right ovary is excised preserving as much normal ovarian cortex as possible. **D,** defects in both ovaries are corrected using fine catgut; a free omental graft is placed over the defect in the uterine serosa.

cedure should be rather extensive, all nerve tissue between the right ureter and the superior hemorrhoidal vessels being excised. In addition, we usually remove a part of the uterosacral ligaments just at their insertion into the uterus, thus accomplishing a "pelvic denervation."

An appendectomy is performed at the time of surgery, and we have been surprised to see functioning endometriosis of the appendiceal serosa in many patients. Endometriosis of the terminal ileum is seen only rarely and may be treated by superficial excision. If the muscularis and mucosa are involved, adequate resection and end-to-end anastomosis should be performed. A uterine suspension is performed routinely and the uterosacral ligaments are plicated in the midline. This accomplishes forward fixation of the uterus, and the shortened uterosacral ligaments produce a backward pull on the cervix, effecting a more normal anatomic attitude. Pseudopregnancy is induced or danazol is given for a minimum of three months after operation if all areas of endometriosis cannot be excised; then concerted efforts toward conception are made. About 50% of women so treated will become pregnant if no other cause for infertility exists. One author has reported the incidence of pregnancy to be as high as 90% following conservative surgery, but this seems to be an exceptionally high success rate and may depend on patient selection.

It has been our policy to perform a careful peritoneal toilet and irrigate the pelvis with warm isotonic saline at the conclusion of the surgical procedure. Since it is almost impossible to remove an endometrioma intact without spillage, removal of the cellular debris and thick fluid contents is advised. In an effort to reduce the incidence of postoperative adhesions we have, since 1966, utilized dexamethasone and promethazine preoperatively, intraperitoneally before closure, and postoperatively (20 mg of dexamethasone and 25 mg of promethazine two hours prior to surgery and then every four hours for 12 doses postoperatively; the same amount is placed in the cul-de-sac through a small catheter).

The incidence of pregnancy following conservative surgery varies widely and is dependent on such factors as extent of the disease, age of the patient and husband, frequency of coitus, previous parity, and the presence of other pelvic pathologic lesions (leiomyomas, tubal disease, or adhesions) at the time of surgery. It seems reasonable to expect that approximately 40% to 70% of patients who are desirous of childbearing will become pregnant after conservative surgical treatment for endometriosis (see Table 9–6). Most pregnancies will occur within the first 12 months after conservative surgery.

EXTIRPATIVE SURGERY.—The treatment of choice for extensive endometriosis in women who no longer desire pregnancy is total hysterectomy and bilateral salpingo-oophorectomy. It has not seemed reasonable to us to leave the ovaries in situ if the uterus is removed for this disease, since ovulation continues in cyclic fashion and remaining areas of endometriosis may be stimulated to grow by endogenous estrogen and progesterone. In experimental endometriosis in monkeys, the most extensive growth has been obtained by the cyclic administration and withdrawal of estrogen and progesterone. This is exactly the situation that exists when functioning, ovulating ovaries are left in situ. When there is extensive bladder, bowel, or ureteral endometriosis, hysterectomy and bilateral oophorectomy will effect a cure.

Large bilateral ovarian endometrial cysts with extensive peritoneal endometriosis and numerous pelvic adhesions or with marked invasion of the rectosigmoid and rectovaginal space constitute the most urgent indications for radical removal of all the pelvic organs, regardless of the age of the patient. *Failure to castrate in the presence of marked endometriosis of the bowel is undoubtedly the most hazardous of all attempts at conservative surgery because of the dangers of subsequent intestinal obstruction.*

From the operative standpoint, early or moderately advanced endometriosis offers no unusual difficulties, but extensive endometriosis may present many technical problems. Endometriosis, in contrast to pelvic inflammatory disease (particularly that due to gonorrheal infection), produces an extremely dense type of pelvic adhesions with almost complete absence of planes of cleavage. Therefore, much of the dissection must be done with sharp instruments, and the dangers of damage to adherent structures are thereby increased. This hazard may be diminished by the use of preoperative pseudopregnancy or danazol. The ureters should be identified and followed to the level of the uterine vessels. These vessels should be ligated lateral to the ureter.

A hysterectomy and bilateral salpingo-oophorectomy can usually be done on patients with large ovarian endometrial cysts and extensive pelvic adhesions and even on those with marked invasion of the rectovaginal septum. This may be facilitated by incising the posterior peritoneum above the insertion of the uterosacral ligaments. The endopelvic fascia and rectosigmoid may then be reflected and the danger of fistula is minimized. It may, at times, be necessary to leave a considerable portion of the growth attached to the bowel or other pelvic structures, but these remnants will regress along with other müllerian tissue in the pelvis following ablation of the ovaries, a fact of great importance in the treatment of this disease.

A few cases have been reported where this atrophy did not occur; one may suspect, however, that all ovarian tissue was not completely removed in some of these cases.

It is frequently impossible to remove an adherent ovarian endometrial (chocolate) cyst without rupturing it and soiling the field of operation with its grumous contents. While this material is usually sterile, it is irritating to the peritoneum and it is good practice in these cases to insert a drain through the vaginal vault to prevent postoperative accumulations in the pelvis. Peritonization is often difficult following removal of extensive lesions, and areas that cannot be covered should be protected by some type of drainage, for it has been observed that postoperative ileus and partial intestinal obstruction are more common following operations on extensive endometriosis than on any other ordinary pelvic condition. Although the postoperative morbidity is high, the mortality has been very low, probably because of the age and generally good condition of the patients, the nature

of the disease, and the absence of malignancy and infection.

There is no contraindication to the continuous administration of estrogen in small doses following hysterectomy and bilateral salpingo-oophorectomy. We have given ethinyl estradiol (Estinyl), 0.625 mg; or conjugated estrogens (Premarin), 1.25 mg, daily for indefinite periods to control untoward symptoms following surgical castration. Administration of these estrogens may gradually be diminished both in quantity and frequency over a period of years. In some patients a study of vaginal cytology will reveal the presence of adequate endogenous estrogen, presumably of adrenal origin, years after surgical castration. Exogenous estrogens need not be given to these patients. I have not seen endometriosis aggravated or "rekindled" by the use of estrogens after hysterectomy and bilateral salpingo-oophorectomy if the dose is as just indicated.

The use of estrogen-progestin combinations given in 20-day cycles or sequential estrogen-progestin preparations, however, has been shown to reactivate endometriosis. These preparations should never be used in a patient who has had a hysterectomy and bilateral salpingo-oophorectomy for endometriosis. Similarly, they should not be given to postmenopausal women for relief of menstrual symptoms if the past history suggests that endometriosis might be present.

The use of x-ray or radium for nonmalignant pelvic conditions has been discontinued at the Brigham and Women's Hospital. This includes x-ray castration for endometriosis. Besides the possibility of a subsequent carcinoma of the cervix, endometrium, or ovary, serious large and small bowel injuries may occur as late sequelae. Some gynecologists do employ x-ray castration to relieve intolerable pelvic pain in the immediately premenopausal woman who has already undergone one or more operations for the disease, but ovarian function may be markedly diminished in a far simpler fashion, e.g., by administering medroxyprogesterone acetate (Depo-Provera), 200 mg every two weeks for four doses, then

400 mg every month for one year. Measurements of ovarian steroids in urine have shown a diminution to postmenopausal levels within ten days of the first injection. Furthermore, the action of this progestin is so prolonged that subsequent ovulation will not occur for at least one year subsequent to the conclusion of treatment.

BIBLIOGRAPHY

Acosta A.A., Buttram V.C., Besch P.K., et al.: A proposed classification of endometriosis. *Obstet. Gynecol.* 42:19, 1973.

American Fertility Society: Classification of endometriosis. *Fertil. Steril.* 32:633, 1979.

Barbieri R.L., Canick J.A., Makris A., et al.: Danazol inhibits steroidogenesis. *Fertil. Steril.* 28:809, 1977.

Barbieri R.L., Lee H., Ryan K.J.: Danazol binding to rat androgen, glucocorticoid, progesterone, and estrogen receptors. *Fertil. Steril.* 31:185, 1979.

Barbieri R.L., Ryan K.J.: Danazol: Endocrine pharmacology and therapeutic applications. *Am. J. Obstet. Gynecol.* 141:453, 1981.

Barbieri R.L., Evans S., Kistner R.W.: Danazol in the treatment of endometriosis: Analysis of 100 cases with a four-year follow-up. *Fertil. Steril.* 37:737, 1982.

Buttram V.C.: Conservative surgery for endometriosis. *Fertil. Steril.* 31:117, 1979.

Daniell J.F., Christianson C.: Combined laparoscopic surgery and danazol therapy for pelvic endometriosis. *Fertil. Steril.* 35:521, 1981.

DiZerega G.S., Barber D.L., Hodgen G.D.: Endometriosis: Role of ovarian steroids in initiation, maintenance and suppression. *Fertil. Steril.* 33:649, 1980.

Dmowski W.P., Cohen M.R.: Antigonadotropin (danazol) in the treatment of endometriosis. *Am. J. Obstet. Gynecol.* 130:41, 1978.

Hammond M.G., Hammond C.B., Parker R.T.: Conservative treatment of endometriosis externa: The effect of methyltestosterone therapy. *Fertil. Steril.* 29:651, 1978.

Hertig A.T., Gore H.: Tumors of the female sex organs: part 3. Tumors of the ovary and fallopian tube. sec., IX, fasc., 33, *Atlas of Tumor Pathology.* Washington, D.C., Armed Forces Institute of Pathology, 1961.

Kistner R.W.: The use of newer progestins in the treatment of endometriosis. *Am. J. Obstet. Gynecol.* 75:264, 1958.

Kistner R.W.: The use of steroidal substances in endometriosis. *Clin. Pharmacol. Ther.* 1:525, 1960.

Kistner R.W., Siegler A.M., Behrman S.J.: Suggested classification for endometriosis: Relationship to infertility. *Fertil. Steril.* 28:1008, 1977.

Kistner R.W.: Management of endometriosis in the infertile patient. *Fertil. Steril.* 31:117, 1979.

Meigs J.V.: Endometriosis. Etiologic role of marriage, age and parity: Conservative treatment. *Obstet. Gynecol.* 2:46, 1953.

Mettler L., Semm K.: Clinical and biochemical experiences with danazol in the treatment of endometriosis in cases with infertility. *Postgrad. Med. J.* 55(suppl. 5):27, 1979.

Mostoufizadeh M., Scully R.E.: Malignant tumors arising in endometriosis. *Clin. Obstet. Gynecol.* 23:951, 1980.

Muse K.N., Wilson E.A.: How does mild endometriosis cause infertility? *Fertil. Steril.* 38:145, 1982.

Noble A.D., Letchworth A.T.: Medical treatment of endometriosis: A comparative trial. *Postgrad. Med. J.* 55(suppl. 5):37, 1979.

Ranney B.: The prevention, inhibition, palliation, and treatment of endometriosis. *Am. J. Obstet. Gynecol.* 123:778, 1975.

Sampson J.A.: Intestinal adenomas of endometrial type: Their importance and their relation to ovarian hematomas of endometrial type. *Arch. Surg.* 5:217, 1922.

Seibel M.M., Berger M.J., Weinstein F.G., et al.: The effectiveness of danazol on subsequent fertility in minimal endometriosis. *Fertil. Steril.* 38:534, 1982.

Scully R.E., Richardson G.S., Barlow J.F.: The development of malignancy in endometriosis. *Clin. Obstet. Gynecol.* 9:384, 1966.

Telinde R.W., Wharton L.R. Jr.: Further studies on experimental endometriosis. *Am. J. Obstet. Gynecol.* 66:1082, 1953.

Williams T.J.: The role of surgery in the management of endometriosis. *Mayo Clin. Proc.* 50:198, 1975.

Van Zyl J.A., Muller M.S., Van Niekerk W.A.: Danazol in the treatment of endometriosis externa. *S. Afr. Med. J.* 58:591, 1980.

CHAPTER TEN

Infertility

STEPHEN EVANS, M.D.
ROBERT W. KISTNER, M.D.

GENERAL CONSIDERATIONS

CURRENT INFORMATION indicates that for every 85 married couples producing one or more offspring there are still 15 couples in this country who are unable to conceive. As physicians, we must concern ourselves with the challenge of helping more than 3 million involuntarily childless couples in the United States. Certain geographic and socioeconomic variations must be considered before broad statements are made regarding etiologic factors. Thus, in France there is a high incidence of oviduct closure; in Israel and in Scotland genital tuberculosis is a major cause of infertility in women. In this country, gynecologic clinics affiliated with large metropolitan hospitals are frequented by indigent patients or patients in the lower-income brackets. Pelvic inflammatory disease (gonococcal and enterococcal) is the major cause of tubal closure in these patients; endometriosis and hormonal abnormalities are rarely seen. The major causes of infertility are: cervical factor, 10%; tubal factor, 30% to 35%; male factor, 30% to 35%; hormonal factor, 25%.

Current aspects of research in human reproduction do not, at the moment, hold the promise of immediate aid to the physician in his ultimate goal. Fortunately, the intricate processes involved do not demand meticulous control or perfected performance, since in most people there is a helpful range of variation. There remain, however, a small number of apparently healthy, regularly copulating couples who fail to reproduce. In this specific failure group, a knowledge of reproductive physiology is necessary for success.

Certain demographic correlates pertaining to fecundability bear discussion. According to the *United Nations Multilingual Demographic Dictionary*, the term *fecundity* is the capacity of a man, a woman, or a couple to participate in the production of a live child. As we are interested in the probability of conception in the absence of contraception, the term *fecundability* is preferable. Generally speaking, then, four factors affecting the chances of fertility or fecundability emerge: (1) age of the wife, (2) age of the husband, (3) the rate of intercourse, and (4) the length of exposure.

Fecundability is maximal in the female around the age of 24 years, after which it gradually tapers down to the age of 30 years and rapidly declines thereafter. A multicenter study in France was recently completed using 2,193 patients with azospermic husbands, who underwent artificial donor insemination. The cumulative success rate after 12 cycles of insemination was 73% for women younger than 25 years, 74.1% for those 26 to 30 years of age, 61.5% for those 31 to 35 years of age, and only 53.6% for women over the age of 35 years. Similarly, fecundability in the male is maximal around age 24 to 25 years, conceptions occurring in 75% of couples in less than

415

six months. In males over age 40 years, only 22% of couples become pregnant in six months or less.

MacLeod's 1953 study indicates that at almost any age level the proportion of conceptions achieved in less than six months rises with frequency of intercourse. He points out that the most important aspect of the semen in respect to ease of conception, i.e., the degree and quality of motility, is enhanced by frequent ejaculation. He states that from the single criterion of achievement of pregnancy the average of intercourse two times weekly reported by most married couples is by no means best, four times or more weekly being ideal to assure impregnation at all ages.

Observed and estimated studies on the number of months required for conception in the absence of use of contraception clearly indicate that 25% of women will be pregnant within the first month, 63% in six months, 75% in nine months, 80% in a year, and 90% in 18 months. Thereafter, irrespective of the age of wife or husband or the frequency of coital exposure, the longer the couple have been married the greater the progressive decline in conception rate. Almost certainly, in these later cases, other undiscovered medical factors exist.

The newly married couple thus has a predictable chance of conception depending on the age of the wife, the age of the husband, coital exposure, and duration of marriage, further modified by whatever other physical, physiological, or psychological medical factors pertain. These are the cases that will benefit from a complete investigation by the fertility specialist. It has been variously estimated that at least 10% of them will be aided by such an evaluation, but with the advent of the newer ovulating agents (e.g., clomiphene and human menopausal gonadotropin) management of hormonal deficiencies of the corpus luteum, improved surgical techniques for tubal reconstruction and uterine defects, therapy for immunological incompatibilty, increased use of artificial insemination, and improved diagnostic techniques such as laparoscopy and

hysteroscopy, it can be safely said that the eventual percentage of patients that can be helped is considerably higher.

Despite this apparent progress in infertility management, there remains an approximate 5% to 10% of all married couples who are medically healthy and in whom no cause for barrenness can be determined. This group must be the focal point of future research and investigation and is, in fact, the background of the current tremendous interest in basic reproductive physiology as well as the purpose of this chapter.

The so-called normal infertile couples obviously are *not* normal or they would not have an infertility problem, yet they are the most poorly managed patients. They must, then, *not be allowed to leave the office with the impression that they are normal.* Perhaps the significance of this problem has best been stated by Jones and Baramki: "frequently unless a special effort is made to make them realize that they must have a factor which cannot be detected by current medical methods, such a couple is apt to leave your office with false impressions and unfounded high hopes. Actually, far from being a good prognosis, this factor offers a poor prognosis. In a group of 315 patients between the ages of 20 and 35 years, studied for infertility and completely investigated, and adequately treated we found a 46% pregnancy rate, while in 15 patients in these series who were investigated with no factor found, only three pregnancies occurred."

Another serious and frustrating deterrent to an adequate diagnostic evaluation of the infertile couple is the indifference of the physician. Equally distressing is the lack of cooperation of the male partner. Too often the wife has accepted the responsibility for childlessness when, in fact, the husband may have been exposed to radiation or to heavy metal poisoning or is oligospermic as a result of chronic alcoholism or nicotine intoxication. It is therefore imperative that both marital partners share the responsibility in the planned investigation and subsequent treatment. Therapeutic nihilism and pessimistic abnegations are fruitless and, although the ultimate aim of the investigation is to enable the couple to bear a child, the ancillary purpose of prognosis is also served.

In summary, then, a thorough infertility investigation by an interested individual knowledgeable in the field of infertility has three important purposes: (1) It offers an explanation for the infertility; (2) it furnishes a prognosis that in itself is important to the psychological well-being of the couple; and (3) it may well afford a basis for therapy.

CLINICAL MANAGEMENT

An infertility study should have a definite plan with a predictable end point. Such a standardized regimen usually can be concluded in three or four office visits spaced at approximately one-month intervals, and the couple should be so informed at the first visit. Today more and more infertile couples are seeking help in achieving conception and, perhaps because they are marrying early, they seem to be coming for help earlier. In this situation I believe that traditional injunctions to "wait and see" should give way to the concept that any couple who have cohabited normally and have not conceived within a year are entitled to a full infertility workup. On the premise that infertility is often a syndrome of multiple origin, an adequate investigation therefore requires study of all reasonable etiologies in *both* husband and wife. Thus, the finding of a single causative factor—such as cervicitis in the wife—does not rule out the possibility of other causes as well—such as oligospermia in the husband. Nor does it rule out the possibility that more than one factor is operative in one or both partners. Although statistical data are only approximate, there is evidence that fully 35% of all infertility problems are of multiple origin. The variety of possible causes (Table 10–1) underscores the need for systematic investigation in both husband and wife, and only on

TABLE 10–1.—ETIOLOGIC INTERPRETATION OF CAUSE OF INFERTILITY AS RELATED TO HUSBAND, WIFE, AND THE COUPLE AS A UNIT

FEMALE FACTORS	MALE FACTORS
General	General
Dietary disturbances	Fatigue
Severe anemias	Excess smoking,
Anxiety, fear, etc.	alcohol
(hypothalamus)	Excess coitus
	Fear, impotence, etc.
Developmental	Developmental
Uterine absence,	Undescended testis
hypoplasia	Testicular germinal
Uterine anomalies	aplasia
Gonadal dysgenesis	Hypospadias
	Klinefelter's syndrome
Endocrine	Endocrine
Pituitary failure	Pituitary failure
Thyroid disturbances	Thyroid deficiency
Adrenal hyperplasia	Adrenal hyperplasia
Ovarian failure,	Hyperprolactinemia
polycystic disease	
Hyperprolactinemia	
Genital disease	Genital disease
Pelvic inflammation,	Orchitis, mumps
tuberculosis	Venereal disease
Tubal obstructions	Prostatitis
Endometriosis	
Myomas and polyps	
Cervicitis	
Vaginitis	

MALE-FEMALE FACTORS

Marital maladjustments
Sex problems
Ignorance (timing, douching, sperm leakage, etc.)
Low fertility index
Immunologic incompatibility

this basis can therapy be undertaken with maximum expectation of success.

With the proper balance between the resources of his private office and of the hospital, a lead to the answers can often be obtained in short order. Since an expensive, time-consuming study of the woman serves no useful purpose if the male partner is azoospermic, the essentials necessary for adequate evaluation of the man will be outlined first.

Study of the Male Partner

If the husband is unwilling to cooperate fully, it is futile to study the wife unless her complaint is one of complete amenorrhea or it is known without doubt that tubal closure is present. An outline of diagnostic procedures for the husband is given in Table 10–2; regardless of whether these procedures are performed by the so-called generalist or by the specialist, a systematic approach must be adopted.

The physician should question the patient specifically regarding certain illnesses (mumps, orchitis, childhood diabetes), occupational hazards (exposure to roentgen rays or to other radioactive substances), sexual habits (impotence, infrequent coitus), social habits (excessive smoking and alcoholism), and the use of precoital lubricants. The husband also should be questioned regarding coital positioning, premature ejaculation, and his knowledge of vaginal entrance (we have seen several "infertility" patients with practically intact, rigid hymenal membranes through which, unknown to both partners, intromission had never occurred).

TABLE 10–2.—DIAGNOSTIC PROCEDURES—
MALE PARTNER

1. History and physical examination
2. Laboratory studies
   Blood cell count and sedimentation rate
   Urinalysis
   Prostatic secretion
3. Thyroxine (T_4) and thyroid-stimulating hormone (TSH) assays, thyroxine-binding globulin (TBG) index
4. Prolactin assay
5. Semen examination
6. Sperm penetration assay
7. *Mycoplasma* culture

STANDARDIZED NOMENCLATURE FOR SEMEN ANALYSIS*

-spermia: Referring to semen volume
Aspermia: No semen
Hypospermia: Volume less than 2 ml
Hyperspermia: Volume greater than 6 ml
-zoospermia: Referring to spermatozoa in semen
Azoospermia: No spermatozoa in semen
Oligozoospermia: Less than 40 million spermatozoa per milliliter
Normozoospermia: 100 to 200 million spermatozoa per milliliter
Polyzoospermia: More than 250 million spermatozoa per milliliter
Asthenozoospermia: Decreased motility of spermatozoa
Teratozoospermia: More than 40% abnormal spermatozoa

*Modified from *Andrologia* 6:100, 1974 and *Biol. Reprod.* 1:3–28, 1973.

Occupations associated with the use of certain metals (lead, iron, zinc, copper), such as painting, plumbing, or printing, may affect the male fertility potential deleteriously. Prolonged periods spent behind the wheel of an overheated automobile with exposure to gasoline fumes and carbon monoxide may be undetected but important etiologic factors. The associated fact that heat affects spermatogenesis adversely is important, since most truck and taxi drivers may have excessive heat surrounding the scrotal area. Persons who lead sedentary, indoor lives, who are markedly obese, or who wear tight underclothing may have abnormal spermatogenesis due to interference with the thermoregulatory mechanism of the scrotum.

The family history and the couple's attitude toward parenthood should be reviewed. Details of surgical procedures, congenital defects, and accidents should be obtained. The examiner should not overlook the importance of the effects of emotional and physical stress, dietary irregularities, weight loss or gain, and the availability of periods of rest, relaxation, and diversion.

A complete physical examination of the male partner is mandatory, and particular attention should be given to certain secondary male characteristics and to evidence of endocrinopathy. Congenital abnormalities such as hypospadias, cryptorchidism, and absence of the vas deferens are of obvious importance. Testicular atrophy, marked varicocele, or prostatoseminal vesiculitis may indicate the need for subsequent definitive therapy. Excess or absence of hair, unusual fat deposits, or evidence of malnutrition should be searched for. The examiner should gain a definite impression concerning the overall habitus and general muscular development.

Table 10–2 lists all of the laboratory procedures that can be performed as part of the male survey. The most important procedure is the analysis of the semen. Any physician can do a preliminary semen analysis that is adequate to determine whether the aid of a specialist is indicated if he will observe the following simple rules. Before a final conclusion is made, at least two specimens obtained at intervals of two to four weeks should be examined.

1. The patient should observe approximately two days (or more) of sexual abstinence prior to examination.

2. The specimen should be collected in a clean, dry, glass container (not a condom or plastic jar; the alkaline pH of the semen should be preserved).

3. Examination for motility should be made within two to four hours.

4. An accurate sperm count should be made.

5. Sperm morphology by stained smear should be studied.

6. The semen study should be correlated with the past and recent history as well as with the physical examination of the husband (wide fluctuations in normal and abnormal spermatogenic behavior are common; a single specimen should never be interpreted as a true representation of total potential).

Certain normal variations in specific sperm characteristics should be recognized. Although normal semen is said to have a minimum volume of 3 ml with 60% motile spermatozoa after two hours, 60 million sperm/ml and 60% normal morphology, this "rule of the 60s" is not absolute. Furthermore, it has been suggested that too great a volume (over 6 ml) is just as undesirable as too little (under 2.5 ml). Clinical examination of sperm motility should include the character of motility and the number of motile sperm related to the time since ejaculation. Although a count of 60 million sperm per milliliter is generally desirable, it has been shown that the count is frequently as low as 20 million in normally fertile men. It should be remembered that the sperm count is the result of spermatogenesis that occurred three weeks previously. Close attention to previous illnesses is imperative. A Gram stain of the semen specimen may reveal leukocytes and bacteria, both of which may be regarded as potential contributing factors in male infertility. Certain bacteria may

affect the fertilizing capacity of spermatozoa without affecting sperm count, morphology, or motility. Also, the stained spermatozoa may show an increased number of abnormal forms (macrocephalic, microcephalic, tapered) that are incapable of fertilization.

If the semen specimen, examined according to the foregoing requirements, shows on more than one test a sperm count of less than 10 million/ml, other tests of endocrine function should be done. Since these procedures are usually under the direction of a urologist or an infertility specialist, they will merely be mentioned here. They include determinations of prolactin, testosterone, pituitary gonadotropins, and triiodothyronine (T_3)-thyroxine (T_4). Testicular biopsies are suggested in azoospermia, in clinically demonstrable endocrine disorders, and in severe oligospermia when the patients desire that every diagnostic procedure be completed. Occasionally, other diagnostic studies, such as a chest roentgenogram, intravenous urogram, catheterization of the ejaculatory ducts, seminal vesiculography, and urethrography, may reveal a specific clinical entity responsible for the infertile state. *Mycoplasma* cultures can also be performed, with positive cultures having some correlation with poor sperm motility (as discussed later in the chapter). The sperm penetration assay is currently being employed in patients with unexplained infertility, with no obvious male or female factors. The test is performed using zona-free hamster eggs, obtained by superovulating hamsters and using protease enzymes to remove the species-specific zona pellucida. The ova are then observed for penetration by sperm from the patient. A control group of ova using documented fertile sperm from a donor are also used. A penetration of 10% or less of the ova appears to correlate with inability to fertilize. Rogers examined 6,266 eggs and found an average fertilization rate of 56.3% in fertile men and an average rate of only 3.1% in infertile men with documented fertile partners. At present, the test is still in its refinement stage and is quite expensive, but will hopefully be able to delineate criteria for suitability of donor insemination candidates.

Therapy in male infertility remains controversial. With few exceptions, no specific treatment for oligospermia or azoospermia is currently available. The rebound phenomenon associated with the administration of testosterone has been found ineffective by most investigators, and this use of testosterone is not advised. The various vitamin compounds and mixtures of vitamins and hormones have also proved disappointing. The use of desiccated thyroid or liothyronine (Cytomel), even in euthyroid persons, has enjoyed widespread acceptance, but the effects of thyroid hormones are of limited value. Radiation therapy to the testes or pituitary gland has not effectively corrected abnormal spermatogenesis.

Clomiphene citrate has been used to treat patients with oligospermia and with decreased motility, but results have been dubious. Elevated counts and increased motility appear only transiently, and improved fertility has yet to be documented. Human chorionic gonadotropin has also been used to increase sperm motility, but again, there is no clear evidence for its clinical effectiveness. The treatment of oligospermia or azoospermia secondary to hyperprolactinemia has been very successful with bromocriptine, using the same dosage regimen as in amenorrheic-galactorrheic patients (see Chapter 13).

What then can be offered to the husband in the way of positive therapy? Even if the semen analysis is normal, the following suggestions are frequently of value.

1. Avoidance of excesses of alcohol, tobacco, caffeine, and coitus.

2. Regular hours of sleep, exercise, and work.

3. A diet with adequate protein and vitamin constituents, and a weight-reduction diet for the obese patient.

4. Adequate vacations from business and social responsibility.

5. Adjustment of the local environment so that excessive and prolonged heat does not interfere with the thermoregulatory mechanism of the scrotum.

6. Correction of hypothyroidism by appropriate medication.

7. Administration of chorionic gonadotropin *only* to those patients who have a demonstrated deficiency in gonadotropins and who have an immature testis revealed by biopsy.

8. Elimination of chronic sources of infection resulting in prostatitis and seminal vesiculitis.

9. Coitus at regular intervals—every two to three days. Prolonged continence may increase the total count but will diminish sperm motility.

Although surgical measures by themselves cannot correct abnormal spermatogenic activity, they are indicated when congenital abnormalities or obstruction prevents normal passage of spermatozoa. Correction of penile-scrotal hypospadias or epididymal obstruction by plastic procedures is associated with a high percentage of subsequent pregnancies. Varicocelectomy has been suggested as a wise prophylactic measure in prepubertal boys who have marked venous distortion, but it is doubtful that the operation will cure testicular atrophy. This, however, should be an individual problem worked out with each patient with the realization that there may be a delay of one or two years after operation before maximum spermatogenesis or fertility appears. Varicocelectomy may prove beneficial in elevating sperm count and increasing motility, and we have found this to be of value in numerous patients. Testicular cooling has been suggested as a therapeutic measure but its value is yet to be determined. From the viewpoint of prophylaxis, the early correction of cryptorchidism is of major importance. Recent evidence strongly favors orchiopexy before age 3 years and certainly before age 5 years. For those patients with irreversible oligospermia or azoospermia, artificial insemination with donor semen (AID) serves as a good alternative. Success rates approach 80%, with over 90% of all pregnancies occurring in the first six cycles. Timing for insemination relies on the patient's basal body temperature charts. If there is considerable variability in the duration of their cycles, then clomiphene is used to regulate their ovulation and maximize results. Artificial insemination with husband serum (artificial insemination, homologous [AIH]) is useful in couples with severe vaginismus, hypospadias, or problems related to depositing sperm intravaginally. When AIH is performed in conjunction with using split-ejaculate or pooling (to attempt increasing sperm counts), then results are no greater than a 20% pregnancy rate.

Study of the Female Partner

The routine minimal diagnostic procedures for the evaluation of female infertility are given in Table 10–3. A detailed historical summary should, in particular, outline the menstrual pattern, including age of onset, duration and frequency of flow, amount of bleeding, presence or absence of pain, and any gross irregularities. In addition, the physician should inquire about premarital and postmarital coitus, especially with relation to frequency and timing with ovulation. Other points of importance include use or disuse of

TABLE 10–3.—Diagnostic Procedures—
Female Partner

1. History and physical examination
2. Laboratory studies
   Blood cell count and sedimentation rate
   Urinalysis
3. Postcoital test
4. Endometrial biopsy
5. Hysterosalpingogram
6. Diagnostic laparoscopy and lavage
7. Assays of LH, FSH, DHEA, DHEA-S, testosterone (free and bound), and androstenedione (Δ^4-androstene)
8. T_4 and TSH assays, TBG index
9. Serum progesterone determination
10. Serum prolactin determination
11. Miscellaneous
    Papanicolaou's stain
    Fern test—spinnbarkeit
    Schiller's test—cervical smear
    Hanging-drop test for Candida (Monilia) and Trichomonas
    Incompatibility test—cervical mucus and semen

contraceptives, present and past occupations, history of pelvic infections, use of cigarettes and alcohol, past surgery, accidents or illnesses, and the use of intravaginal lubricants or douches.

When previous abdominal operations have been performed, it is advantageous to secure copies of the operative notes and the pathology reports. Surgery performed during childhood for a ruptured appendix suggests peritubal adhesions as a possible etiologic factor. Often an operation described by the patient as "conservative" has, in fact, been a bilateral salpingectomy. Extensive (and expensive) investigation is thus immediately avoided.

During the physical examination the physician should pay particular attention to external body contour, hair distribution, fat deposits, and breast development. Hyperpigmentation consistent with acanthosis nigricans should be documented because of its newly found association with polycystic ovarian disease. The breasts should be thoroughly examined for nipple abnormality or dominant lumps (we have seen early breast carcinomas in two patients referred for endocrine infertility). Galactorrhea should be screened for an examination in all patients to identify those patients with hyperprolactinemia.

Stigmata of hypothyroidism should be looked for. A thorough pelvic examination should be conducted, in which the size, shape, and position of the internal and external genitalia are noted and particular search made for infections. An enlarged clitoris and male distribution of pubic hair should warn the examiner to look for other evidence of masculinization due to adrenal or ovarian tumors. If purulent material can be expressed from the urethral meatus or periurethral glands, it should be stained and cultured for gonococci. Specific vaginal infections, such as those caused by *Trichomonas* and *Candida* (*Monilia*), may be important factors in infertility because the severe dyspareunia they cause may prevent normal frequency of coitus. The finding of a vaginal septum or double cervix demands that the uterus, oviducts, and upper urinary tract be investigated radiologically for other congenital abnormalities. An intravenous urogram should also be performed because of the increased incidence of congenital abnormalities of the urinary tract.

Although the importance of the cervical factor will be considered separately, much can be gained at the first visit if (1) a cervical aspiration for cytologic examination is obtained (two slides may be made, one for Papanicolaou's stain to determine malignancy and one for the Harris-Shorr stain to determine estrogen effect); (2) Schiller's test is performed routinely; and (3) biopsies are taken of all nonstaining areas and of obvious cervical erosions. Although the infertile patient statistically is less likely to have carcinoma in situ of the cervix than is her multiparous counterpart, she should not be denied a complete diagnostic survey.

The laboratory procedures advocated are: (1) complete blood cell count and erythrocyte sedimentation rate; (2) urinalysis; (3) luteinizing hormone (LH), follicle-stimulating hormone (FSH), dehydroepiandrosterone (DHEA), dehydroepiandrosterone sulfate (DHEA-S), testosterone, and androstenedione determinations, if any endocrine abnormalities are noted (especially anovulation, or oligo-ovulation); (4) T_4 and TSH assays and TBG index, for anyone with evidence of thyroid dysfunction and probably for those couples with negative results of workup and unexplained infertility; (5) serum progesterone determination to document ovulation and/or luteal-phase dysfunction; and (6) serum prolactin determination.

It has been mentioned that the various diagnostic procedures can be completed in approximately three or four visits, and prognostic advice may then be given the couple (Fig 10–1). The procedures require proper timing and interpretation, and each will now be discussed in some detail. Finally, certain specific factors causing infertility (cervical, uterine, tubal, ovarian) will be evaluated with particular reference to therapy.

Postcoital Test

The postcoital test is optimally performed at the time of ovulation, and, since experience with donor insemination has shown that conception occurs most frequently within the 48 hours just preceding the rise in basal body temperature (BBT), postcoital tests planned for 15 to 16 days before an expected menstrual period are often therapeutic. The interval between coitus and examination may vary, but a minimum of at least two to four hours (maximum, 16 hours) is desirable for the study of sperm survival. No douches or intravaginal medication should be used during the 48 hours preceding the test.

TECHNIQUE.—Figure 10–2 illustrates a long, narrow, dressing forceps with a small oval aperture at the tip. With this instrument a sample of mucus is easily obtained from high in the endocervical canal where sperm motility and survival are maximum. If the cervical os is too small to admit a metal instrument, a polymeric silicone (Silastic) tubule may be inserted through the external os into the endocervix. A syringe may then be attached to the tubule, and gentle suction will obtain an adequate specimen. If the mucus is clear, abundant, and watery, with good elasticity, it is suitable for evaluation of sperm penetration. At the time of ovulation, the mucus forms a thin, continuous thread as it is pulled apart—a phenomenon called *spinnbarkeit*. This physical characteristic is a function of increasing levels of estrogen and disappears after the appearance of progesterone. Such mucus, when allowed to dry on a slide, crystallizes into a fernlike pattern, the "arborization phenomenon" (see Chapter 4). This phenomenon also disappears after ovulation as a result of progesterone secretion. When the cervical mucus is examined under the high-dry magnification, the number of cellular elements (leukocytes) and spermatozoa per high-power field are noted. The motility and quality of progression of the spermatozoa are similarly observed.

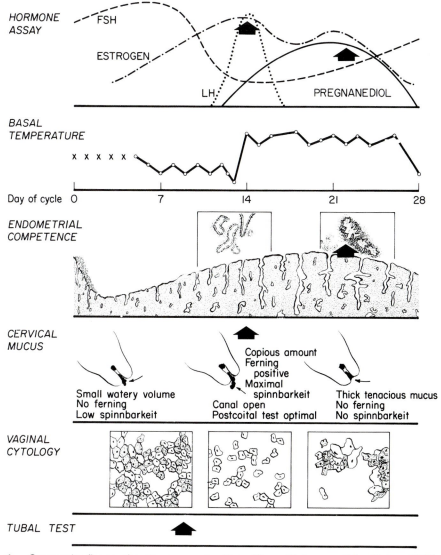

HORMONE ASSAY

FSH

ESTROGEN

L.H.   PREGNANEDIOL

BASAL TEMPERATURE

x x x x x

Day of cycle   0   7   14   21   28

ENDOMETRIAL COMPETENCE

CERVICAL MUCUS

Small watery volume
No ferning
Low spinnbarkeit

Copious amount
Ferning
positive
Maximal
spinnbarkeit
Canal open
Postcoital test optimal

Thick tenacious mucus
No ferning
No spinnbarkeit

VAGINAL CYTOLOGY

TUBAL TEST

Fig 10–1.—Composite figure of major areas of investigation in cases of infertility. Large arrows indicate optimal day for each specific investiga-tion. (From Behrman S.J., Kistner R.W. (eds.): *Progress in Infertility,* ed. 2. Boston, Little, Brown & Co., 1975.)

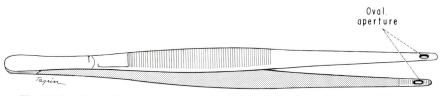

Oval aperture

Fig 10–2.—Long dressing forceps adapted for collection of seminal fluid from the endocervical canal.

INTERPRETATION.—No normal value may be assigned to this test, but in general the pregnancy rate is significantly higher if good mucus is associated with the finding of several actively motile spermatozoa per high-power field than if rare or inactive spermatozoa are observed. Spermatozoa are rarely seen in poor mucus, and therefore such a result on a *single* observation is of no prognostic value. The physician should remember that this test reflects not only the cervical environment of spermatozoa but also the ovarian function controlling it. As such, it is of extremely great value. Furthermore, since the greatest number of conceptions in an infertile population occur within the menstrual cycle following the first consultation, a well-timed postcoital test is a most useful therapeutic contribution. Davajan and Nakamura have described a fractional in vivo and in vitro examination of postcoital cervical mucus, and details of this technique are given in their chapter, "The Cervical Factor," in Behrman and Kistner's *Progress in Infertility*, ed. 2. Boston, Little, Brown & Co., 1975.

Endometrial Biopsy

The endometrial biopsy is a convenient office procedure that causes only minor discomfort and does not require local or general anesthesia. Although the test is usually employed as a test for ovulation, the finding of secretory changes in the endometrium is only *presumptive* evidence of ovulation (luteinized follicles may occasionally produce the same changes). Since the incidence of anovular cycles in infertile women is between 5% and 10%, the significance of the test is obvious. The timing of the procedure is important, the optimum time being the first day of the menses. The bleeding may then be correctly interpreted as being menstrual or anovular in type, and the chances of disrupting a normal pregnancy are minimal. Some pathologists prefer the well-maintained late secretory endometrium of day 27 or 28 to the fragmented tissue obtained after menstruation has begun. In women with regular cycles this can be timed rather precisely but the patient is warned not to have coitus at the time of ovulation during that cycle. Biopsies at the time of menstruation have the added advantage of occasionally revealing tuberculous endometritis. Unfortunately, biopsy at this time is not always a practical arrangement, and an alternate method is to perform the biopsy on or before the sixth postovulatory day as estimated from the menstrual history. At this time the ovum is either in the oviduct or in the uterine fluid, since implantation does not occur until the fifth to eighth postovulatory day. If coitus is avoided during a given month, the biopsy specimen may be obtained at the theoretical apex of progesterone activity (i.e., day 22 or 23 of a 28-day cycle). This may be of particular importance in patients with an "insufficient luteal phase" when exacting studies of glandular and stromal changes in the endometrium are necessary.

TECHNIQUE.—A pelvic examination should precede the biopsy so that the position and size of the uterus can be ascertained. The cervix is exposed with a speculum and cleansed with an alkaline astringent solution (Alkalol) or tyloxapol (Alevaire). Slight traction is placed on the cervix with a tenaculum. Although we prefer the Duncan curet (Fig 10–3,A) because of its smaller size, any of the various types will give adequate samples. It has been our routine to obtain tissue from both the anterior and posterior surfaces of the endometrial cavity, using a firm but gentle stroke from the fundus to the cervix (Fig 10–3,B). The most representative samples are obtained from high in the corpus. The tissue is immediately fixed in Bouin's fluid. Care should be taken not to traumatize the tissue in transferring it from the curet to the fixative.

INTERPRETATION.—Although exact dating of the endometrium during the secretory phase of the cycle is practiced by gynecologic pathologists, it is not absolutely necessary, and adequate interpretation or presumption of ovulation may be made in most patients. If

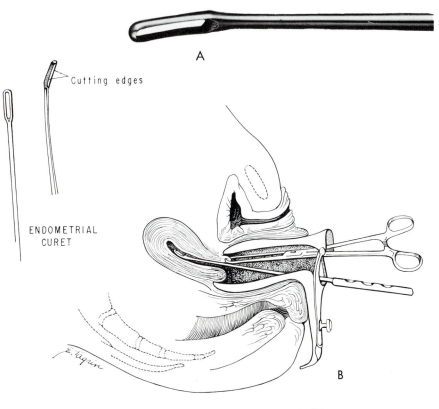

A

Cutting edges

ENDOMETRIAL
CURET

ENDOMETRIAL BIOPSY

B

Fig 10–3.—A, cutting edge of Duncan curet. This instrument can be introduced easily through an undilated, nulliparous cervical os without undue discomfort. **B,** proper technique of endometrial biopsy with the Duncan curet.

the endometrial biopsy reveals abnormal tissue of any variety, a thorough curettage should be done for adequate diagnosis and to rule out malignancy.

Noyes has suggested certain essentials for obtaining and interpreting the endometrial biopsy. (1) Chart the basal body temperature (BBT) and perform the biopsy during a BBT cycle. (2) Biopsy after two or three BBT cycles have been charted and biopsy at least during two cycles. (3) Biopsy on the sixth and ninth postovulatory days; be certain to get fundal surfaces. (4) Try to obtain superficial endometrium—do not go too deep. (5) Fix the tissue in Bouin's solution. (6) Date the endometrium, but date the most advanced area. (7) Look at your own slides.

Hysterosalpingography

Hysterosalpingography (HSG) and tubal lavage have virtually eliminated the need for using tubal insufflation. Rubin's ingenious test has now become of historical significance only primarily due to the added information gained from HSGs. The HSG can outline the uterine cavity and detect anomalies such as septa, intrauterine synechiae, and submucosal fibroids, in addition to identifying tubal patency (with a much lower false-positive and false-negative rate than tubal insufflation). Unfortunately, the ideal fluid for instillation is not as yet available. Theoretically, it should be water soluble, painless when injected, and harmless, and it should afford adequate contrast on roentgenograms and remain visible

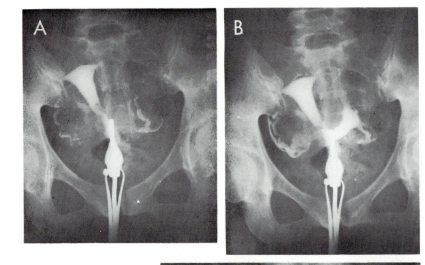

Fig 10–4.—Hysterosalpingograms. **A,** visualization of uterus and both oviducts in a normal patient. **B,** second film, showing free passage of the dye from the oviduct into the peritoneal cavity. **C,** patient with chronic pelvic inflammatory disease and bilateral hydrosalpinges. Note the dilated and convoluted tube on the right and the accumulation of dye in sacculations at the tubal fimbria.

for a number of days after instillation. Figure 10–4 shows the normal findings obtained by tubograms and the findings seen in chronic pelvic inflammatory disease. Viscous oils, such as iodized poppy-seed oil (Lipiodol), remain in the pelvic cavity for long periods and may cause oil granulomas. Iodine-oil preparations are no longer used in our unit because of the high incidence of oil granulomas we have encountered. Nonviscous oils are quickly absorbed from the peritoneum but

also remain in the pelvic cavity too long. Water-soluble media may cause abdominal cramps, and a 24-hour follow-up film is not possible because of rapid absorption. Many authorities still prefer the use of the opaque oils with a 24-hour film or special positioning of the patient after injection of 3 to 6 ml of oil to fill the uterine cavity and oviducts. Thus the patient may be placed on the right side, the left side, and then in lithotomy position so that spill through the pelvis can be demonstrated on the initial visit. The procedure of cinefluoroscopy for evaluation of tubal motility and patency has been adopted in many clinics but its advantages over endoscopy and indigo carmine lavage of the tubes remains to be proved. Currently we are using a water-soluble contrast media, Renografin-60, and obtain excellent uterine and tubal roentgenograms. Candidates for the HSG should not have any previous history of pelvic inflammatory disease, tubal surgery, or ectopic pregnancy. These patients are at much higher risk for having an acute flare-up of salpingitis after the procedure and should undergo laparoscopy and tubal lavage to document patency. We currently give prophylaxis to all of our patients undergoing HSG with a broad-spectrum antibiotic, and premedicate with an antiprostaglandin agent to prevent uterine cramping.

The following summary by Parekh and Arronet indicates the most common causes of false-positive and false-negative findings with hysterosalpingography.

1. Causes of false-positive findings (open tubes):
   a. Foley catheter blocking uterine cavity or tip of cannula impinging on myometrium (avoidable).
   b. Widening of cervical canal with stenosis of internal os (unavoidable).
   c. Admixture of air or blood with the dye, producing spasm (avoidable).
   d. Cornual spasm due to procedure (avoidable).
   e. Localized uterine contraction or synechiae (unavoidable).
   f. Differences in tubal diameter or structure producing apparent unilateral closure (unavoidable).
   g. Too little contrast medium or omission of delayed film (avoidable).
   h. Large uterine cavity (avoidable).
   i. Extravasation of dye into myometrium (unavoidable).
   j. Peritubal adhesions or narrow fimbrial opening (unavoidable).
   k. Pocketed spill near fimbriae that may

be mistaken for hydrosalpinx, or vice versa.
   l. In tuberculous salpingitis, the tobacco-pouch appearance of the fimbriae that may give the impression of pocketed spill.
2. Causes of false-negative findings (closed or phimotic tubes):
   a. Free spillage from a pinpoint opening of an otherwise phimotic fimbria may suggest normal fimbrial function.
   b. Extravasation of dye through uterine or ovarian vasculature may be misinterpreted as tubal patency.
   c. Localized constriction in a tortuous hydrosalpinx may suggest pocketed spill.
   d. Free pelvic dissemination of dye from a unilateral phimotic tube may give the impression of bilateral spill.

Laparoscopy

Laparoscopy has almost completely eliminated the use of culdoscopy at most institutions, to the extent that culdoscopy is of historical significance only (Fig 10–5). From an operative point of view, laparoscopy is far superior in lysing adhesions, fulgurating endometriosis, or for performing ovarian biopsies. At the same time as the laparoscopy is being done, tubal lavage is performed using an intrauterine cannula and indigo carmine. Laparoscopy and hysterosalpingography (HSG) are commonly compared for their diagnostic capabilities. El-Minawi studied 352 cases of infertility in which both laparoscopy and HSG were performed. There was complete agreement in findings in 56.7% of the cases. Pelvic adhesions were suggested by HSG in 76 cases compared to 151 cases documented by laparoscopy. Of major significance is that laparoscopy found pathologic lesions (i.e., pelvic adhesions and endometriosis) in 57.14% of patients with unexplained infertility. This reconfirms that the HSG has a specific role in the infertility workup, namely, allowing diagnosis of intrauterine malformations, adhesions, and

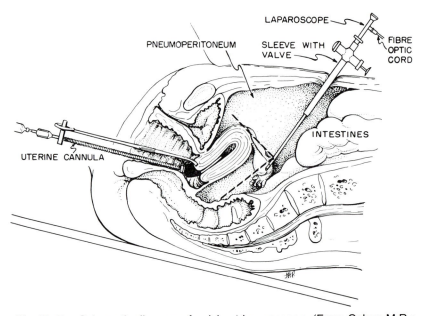

Fig 10–5.—Schematic diagram of pelvis at laparoscopy. (From Cohen M.R.: *Laparoscopy, Culdoscopy, and Gynecography.* Philadelphia, W.B. Saunders Co., 1970.)

fibroids (submucosal) and confirming tubal patency. With patients who are suspected of having tubal disease, endometriosis, or any other pelvic pathologic condition, then the obvious workup should bypass HSG and go straight to laparoscopy and tubal lavage.

A methodical approach to the infertile couple is extremely important. If after a detailed history and physical examination of both partners there are no obvious etiologies, then semen analysis, postcoital test, and serum progesterone assay (days 19, 21, and 23) are all performed within the first month. This supplies a good initial screening to identify obvious problems with the male factor, ovulatory dysfunction, cervical factor, and immunologic incompatibility. If ovulatory dysfunction is apparent, then hormonal analysis is necessary, including assays of LH, FSH, DHEA, DHEA-S, testosterone, free testosterone, prolactin, and Δ^4-androstenedione. Tubal patency should be documented with histories suggestive of mechanical obstruction. Clearly outlined documentation of each of these tests should be kept in each couple's chart to define what has and has not

been eliminated as a possible cause of their infertility. Only with this approach can the physician expect to isolate the specific factor or factors accounting for their inability to conceive. A detailed look at each of the individual factors will help in deciding the appropriate management.

THE CERVICAL FACTOR

The importance of the postcoital test has already been emphasized. The endocervical canal is lined by racemose glands composed of mucus-containing columnar cells. These cells produce a cervical mucus that contains a variety of sugars and amino acids and, although the effects of these substances on sperm metabolism and migration are not completely known, spermatozoa maintain motility longer in favorable cervical mucus than in seminal fluid.

Hormonal, anatomic, and infectious aspects of the cervical factor are important. Stated simply, estrogen stimulates the secretory activity of the endocervical glands, and progesterone inhibits this activity. The estrogen effect may be assayed by microscopic examination of the mucus, which demonstrates the fern pattern, and by gross inspection, which reveals the formation of spinnbarkeit. Furthermore, estrogen produces specific anatomic changes in the isthmic canal. Two days before ovulation this area assumes a funnel shape due to relaxation of the sphincteric construction, and it becomes shorter and wider. After ovulation the canal becomes longer and narrower. If estrogen deficiency is detected, exogenous estrogen may be administered, but care must be taken to keep the dose low enough so that ovulation is not inhibited. Ethinyl estradiol (Estinyl), 0.02 mg, may be given daily for several months under these circumstances.

Anatomic variations in the position of the cervix do not seem to be as important as previously suggested by various observers. Spermatozoa seem to enter the anteriorly directed cervix associated with a third-degree retroversion as readily as they enter the cervix directed into the mythical seminal pool. The cervix that is prolapsed beyond the introitus, however, is poorly conditioned to accept the seminal fluid. Correction of the prolapse by pessaries, cervical cups, or operation is frequently followed by pregnancy. Although the size and shape of the cervix may not be related to infertility, the hypoplastic cervix may be a predisposing factor because of scant mucus. Similarly, a small, tight endocervical canal and a tight internal os may be benefited by careful, but not overzealous, dilatation. As a matter of fact, in several articles the authors suggest that the passage of sounds or dilators through the cervix is attended by a large measure of success in overcoming infertility. Such success cannot be assigned to the process of dilatation alone. Thus, hypothalamic and other stimuli might have had more effect than the cervical dilatation. If one chooses to follow this advice, care should be taken not to traumatize the endocervix by use of large dilators and perhaps predispose the patient to subsequent midtrimester abortion because of cervical incompetence.

Specific cervical lesions and infections demand careful and individual attention. If biopsy reveals invasive carcinoma, the indicated treatment immediately ends the reproductive potential. If carcinoma in situ is found, conservative therapy may allow further childbearing if the patient agrees to close follow-up supervision. Large endocervical polyps should be excised and the base lightly cauterized. Although cervical erosions and eversions are commonly found in infertile patients, their etiologic significance has been overemphasized. Nevertheless, erosions and eversions should be corrected by thorough electrocauterization or cryosurgery, but care should be taken not to destroy the endocervical mucosa. Gentle passage of a uterine sound should be performed after complete healing of the cauterized areas in order to prevent stenosis. Severely lacerated and distorted cervices occasionally may be improved by meticulous plastic surgery, comprising excision of the scar and restoration of as much of the normal anatomy of the portio vaginalis as possible. Conization (unless performed as a therapeutic measure in carcinoma in situ) is not advised as a procedure to increase the fertility potential.

Acute cervicitis should be treated by the antibiotics or sulfonamides indicated by cultures and the sensitivities of the responsible organism. At a later date, chronic foci of infection in the cervix should be obliterated by cauterization or by the use of topically or systemically administered antibiotics, or both. Enzymatic debridement with fibrinogen-deoxyribonuclease preparations may be less traumatic to the cervix than cautery. In certain instances the anatomic or physiologic insufficiency of the cervix may be overcome by artificial insemination with the husband's semen. The use of polyethylene cups that can be trimmed to fit the contours of the grossly abnormal cervix has simplified the technique of this procedure.

Various diagnostic tests have been designed to test the cervical factor in infertility. These are: (1) evaluation of cervical mucus for arborization and spinnbarkeit (described in Chapter 4), (2) the postcoital test (identification of very poor motility or sperm agglutination on postcoital test after a normal semen analysis should make one suspect an immunologic etiology. Further workup in this area is discussed later in the chapter), (3) an in vitro test of mucus penetration by spermatozoa, (4) pH of cervical mucus, (5) tests of cervical glucose, (6) test of cervical mucus chloride, (7) changes in cervical mucus proteins, and (8) cultures of the cervix.

The reader is referred to the chapter entitled "The Cervical Factor" by Davajan and Nakamura in *Progress in Infertility*, ed. 2, for a complete review of the subject.

THE UTERINE FACTOR

The importance of an adequately developed, receptive endometrium was mentioned in the section on endometrial biopsy. If luteal activity is believed to be deficient and if the endometrial biopsy reveals evidence of progestational insufficiency, improvement may be expected with the use of a progestational substance. We have used progesterone vaginal suppositories in a dose of 25 mg twice daily from day 15 through day 25 of a 28-day cycle.

Therapy should not be started too soon after ovulation, nor should the dose be excessive, since glandular and stromal abnormalities occur that may affect implantation deleteriously. Noyes has suggested that the endometrium may be either "overdeveloped" or "underdeveloped." If the latter, he prefers to administer human chorionic gonadotropin (to stimulate the corpus luteum) than to give exogenous progesterone. If the endometrium is "overdeveloped," he gives ethinyl estradiol, 0.05 mg, from the low point on the BBT cycle for eight consecutive days. Infertility resulting from endocrine abnormalities affecting the endometrium will be discussed in Chapter 11.

The presence of large submucous leiomyomas may be verified by diagnostic curettage and hysterography. Their importance in infertility and repetitive abortion has been established, and myomectomy (see Chapter 5) is indicated if tubal patency is assured and study of the male partner is adequate.

We have currently been confirming the presence of submucous fibroids by using the hysteroscope, and have actually removed a very limited number of fibroids via the operating hysteroscope. On abdominal myomectomies, both tourniquets around the uterine vessels and bulldog clamps on the ovarian vessels are used to minimize blood loss. Prophylactic antibiotics are always used in the perioperative period. Malone and Ingersoll and others have described the poor outcome for the infertility myomectomy in patients older than 35 years. Results are also quite bleak when myomectomy is performed on patients with unexplained infertility.

Uterine retroversions should be corrected by manual replacement and the insertion of a Smith-Hodge pessary (see Fig. 5–22). If pregnancy occurs, the pessary should be left in place until the 12th week of gestation. Suspension of the retroverted uterus as a primary procedure for infertility is not warranted unless more conservative measures have failed. As previously mentioned, suspension is not necessary to place the cervix in a more favorable position for the reception of semen. In certain patients the uterus cannot be replaced manually even under anesthesia. In such cases, provided that results of all other studies are normal and that the patients have been observed during a 12-month period of involuntary sterility, endoscopy is performed. Laparotomy and suspension are suggested if specific etiologic factors are discovered. Endometriosis or pelvic adhesions will be found to be the cause of uterine retroversion in most of these women. Congenital abnormalities of the uterus (bicornuate or septate uterus, etc.) may be diagnosed by hysterography and should be corrected surgically if they are associated with infertility or repetitive abortion (Chapter 11, "Habitual Abortion").

Postpartum curettage will occasionally result in permanent intrauterine damage with destruction of the endometrium (Asherman's syndrome). The possibility of restoring fertility by surgery in these patients is small, although transplantation of endosalpingeal mucosa has been attempted. Spontaneous regeneration occurs but may take four to five years. Prognosis for subsequent pregnancy is poor. Louros has suggested the use of an intrauterine device immediately following a curettage to break up the adhesions. The uterine walls are thus prevented from coapting and an estrogen-progestin pseudopregnancy is started in the patient. Results from this method of therapy seem encouraging, with March and Israel reporting pregnancies after the use of this method. Their current use of the operating hysteroscope to treat intrauterine adhesions has been very successful. Small scissors are used in the uterine cavity to lyse the synechiae under direct visualization. Of 27 patients who presented with infertility and intrauterine adhesions, ten achieved successful pregnancies. We are also using hysteroscopy (with dextran 70 as the contrast medium) for this purpose as well as for detecting endometrial polyps, intrauterine malformations, and localizing embedded intrauterine devices. Some institutions are actually using the operating hysteroscope for correcting septate uteri, but results are too preliminary to draw any conclusions.

Inflammatory lesions of the endometrium are known causes of infertility. Moyer has suggested six general categories:

1. Endometrial infections may follow procedures that destroy or alter the usual protective role of the cervical secretions. Bacteria are normally present in the vagina and lower cervical fluids but are absent in the upper endocervical canal. When the normal secretion of the endocervical glands is altered, bacteria may find their way into the endometrial cavity. Procedures at fault include extensive biopsy, conization, and cauterization of the cervix.

2. Endometrial infections may result when the normally contaminated cervical mucus is pushed up into the endometrial cavity by instrumentation. Endometrial biopsy, hysterosalpingography, and tubal insufflation procedures, as well as therapeutic abortions, use of the stem pessary for dysmenorrhea, and insertion of gauze or radium into the uterine cavity may be the cause of infection.

3. Uterine infections are more likely to occur when the bacteriostatic environment of the endometrium is altered, as during the parturitional period when the endometrium is atrophic and quiescent. At this time the tissues are not stimulated by estrogen, so that marked changes in the secretion of uterine fluid and alteration of the phagocytic system take place.

4. Ascending infection of organisms having the ability to penetrate the usual bacteriostatic mechanisms of the cervix, such as *Neisseria gonorrhoeae*, may produce infections of the uterine lining.

5. Infections may be borne to the endometrium by the blood.

6. Drainage of purulent material from chronically infected fallopian tubes may produce endometritis. This mechanism occurs rarely, and may take place early in the course of chronic salpingitis, because the longer the tubes remain infected, the greater the possibility of occlusion of the isthmus.

THE TUBAL FACTOR

The fact that blocked tubes can be opened—by time, sexual rest, and antispasmodics—has been well documented. Some investigators have advocated repeated tubal insufflations with pressures as high as 300 mg together with pelvic heat and sexual abstinence as a method superior to tubal surgery. Unfortunately, the two methods utilized to evaluate tubal factors in infertility demonstrate only passage or nonpassage of the medium through the oviduct and are not significant in evaluating details of tubal anatomy, physiology, or pathology. The clinician should remember that the fertilized ovum remains in the oviduct for three or four days before reaching the endometrial cavity. Research in tubal physiology is scant, but the data suggest that the oviduct is more than just a transporting organ (e.g., certain mammalian ova, transferred from the oviduct to the uterus within 20 hours of fertilization, do not implant). The effects of steroid hormones on tubal physiology and ovum transport are definite and measurable, but clinical application must await more extensive study.

Studies of patients with pelvic inflammatory disease have negated the generally accepted opinion that most salpingitis is due to the gonococcus. Cultures obtained from pyosalpinges frequently reveal that the etiologic organisms are mixed flora of aerobes and anaerobes. Therefore, therapy for the acute episodes should be initiated with broad-spectrum antibiotics effective against this polymicrobial infection in order to preserve the function of the endosalpinx. Several types of tubo-ovarian disease producing infertility are shown in Figure 10–6.

Surgical treatment for a closed oviduct occasionally may be indicated when the husband is normal and all studies in the female indicate normal function except for nonpatency of the tubes on *repeated examinations* with both lavage and hysterosalpingography.

If the oviducts are apparently closed on the basis of salpingography, I insist on lavage of the oviducts by endoscopy before proceeding to tuboplasty. Then, even before beginning the tubal surgery, I attempt transuterine lavage with indigo carmine dye. This is easily accomplished by occluding the cervix with a special clamp, then inserting an 18-gauge needle into the uterine cavity via the fundus. I have been pleasantly surprised on numerous occasions to see an easy efflux of dye from the fimbriated portions of the oviducts when previous testing by x-ray and endoscopy indicated bilateral closure. Undoubtedly the false impression had been due to tubal spasm or improper technique.

Many surgeons view the surgical treatment of tubal closure as being quite simple. Nothing could be further from the truth. While a radical hysterectomy may be more daring and may even thrill the observer, the judgment, skill and patience of the surgeon doing reconstructive work is usually less well appreciated. There is no doubt that the inexperience of the operator will lead to poor results, and therefore analysis of published reports must be viewed critically. Shirodkar has suggested that the three basic reasons for poor results are: (1) inexperience of the surgeon, (2) improper selections of cases, and (3) poor techniques. Garcia has suggested that consistently good results can be obtained by meticulous handling of tissues, guided by the judgment that can be gained only with practice. Skill can be achieved by years of critical appraisal of many cases, or more effectively after individual tutelage by assisting someone with wide experience. But without a knowledge of reproductive physiology even the most skillful surgeon will fail.

Although all reconstructive surgery performed on the oviduct is referred to as a *tuboplasty*, this overall term is misleading since certain procedures have a fairly good prognosis for eventual pregnancy and others do not. A classification suggested by Moore-White is as follows: (1) Salpingolysis—the separation of peritubal adhesions usually secondary to an infectious perisalpingitis or endometriosis. (2) Salpingoplasty—opening of the totally occluded distal end of the tube, as in a hydrosalpinx, either by a linear salpingostomy, removal of a wedge of tissue producing a fish-mouth eversion, or by the more popular distal resection creating a new ostium and fimbrial cuff. (3) Midsegment reconstruction—removal of a segment of occluded oviduct due either to previous salpingitis or surgical ligation. (4) Cornual or interstitial resection and reimplantation.

The physician should present all of the available data to the couple and permit them to decide if surgery is desirable. The operation for tubal reimplantation is shown in Figure 10–7. Roland has devised a spiral Teflon stent to be used after salpingoplasty. It may

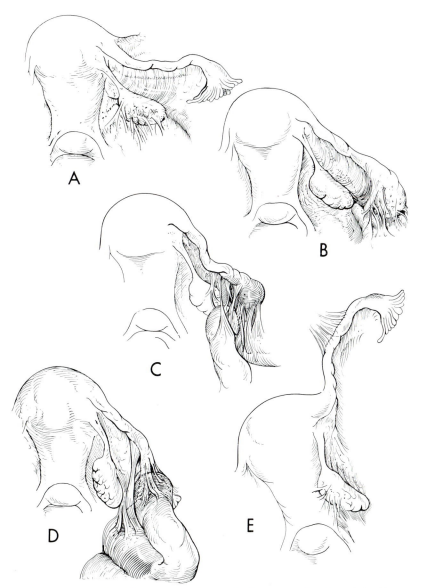

Fig 10–6.—Tubo-ovarian distortion produced by adhesions. **A,** periovarian adhesions producing ovarian fixation following ovarian cystectomy. **B,** fimbrial occlusion without tubal disease due to prior peritonitis. **C,** cecal tubo-ovarian adhesions following a ruptured appendix. **D,** occlusion of tubal fimbriae by adhesions between the cecum and tube secondary to salpingitis, previous tubal surgery, or pelvic hematoma. **E,** abnormal fixation of tube due to adhesions following appendectomy. The ovary is similarly involved by adhesions. (From Kistner R.W., Patton G.W.: *Atlas of Infertility Surgery.* Boston, Little, Brown & Co., 1975.)

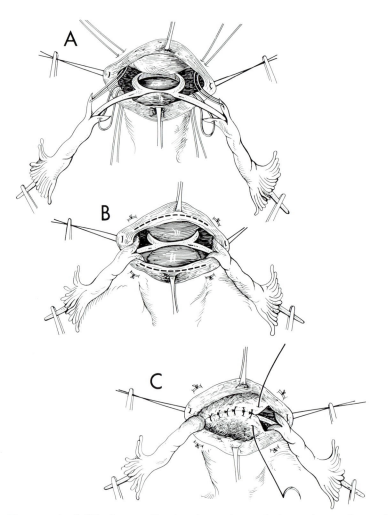

Fig 10–7.—Placement of Silastic prosthesis for bilateral tubal implantation. **A,** the prosthesis is seated in the endometrial cavity with both limbs extending from the fimbriated ends of the tubes. Sutures have been placed through the lower angle of the cornual incision to occlude the ascending branch of the uterine artery. **B,** position of the fish-mouthed tubes after the Mersilene sutures have been tied on the surface of the uterus. Transverse incisions are then made in the anterior and posterior myometrium to facilitate closure of the uterus in two layers. **C,** the deep myometrial layer is closed with interrupted sutures of 2–0 chromic catgut or polyglycolic acid (Dexon). *(Continued)*

be removed from its abdominal wall attachment without a second laparotomy. We are currently not using the hood prosthesis for corrective salpingoplasty, but rather are relying on microsurgical technique using fine nylon suture, such as 6-0 Prolene. The reader is referred to a review of these surgical techniques in the chapter "Surgical Reconstruction of the Oviduct," *Atlas of Infertility Surgery* by Kistner and Patton.

Since the physician is dealing with a malformed or diseased organ, the increased incidence of tubal ectopic pregnancy subsequent to operation is not surprising. Also, smoldering pelvic inflammatory disease may be reactivated at the time of salpingoplasty; this in-

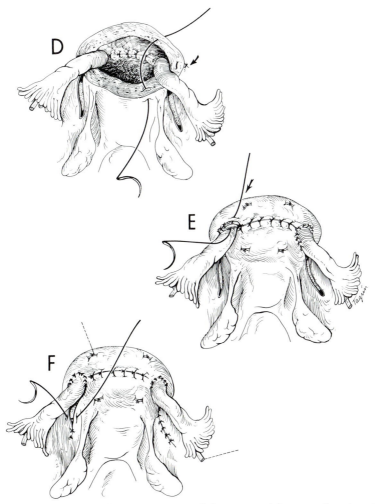

Fig 10–7 (cont).—D, the superficial myometrial layer and serosa are similarly closed. Arrow shows the angle suture-tied. **E,** the fundal incision is closed and the tubal and uterine serosa is approximated with interrupted sutures of 3-0 chromic catgut or Dexon. **F,** the peritoneal leaves of the mesosalpinx are closed and the upper angle is sutured to the uterine serosa for additional support. An omental graft is placed over the suture line. (From Kistner R.W., Patton G.W.: *Atlas of Infertility Surgery.* Boston, Little, Brown & Co., 1975.)

flammatory reaction may be extensive enough to necessitate hysterectomy and bilateral salpingo-oophorectomy. The selection of patients for oviduct surgery and the choice of a surgeon to perform such an operation should be made on specific and stringent criteria.

The incidence of pregnancy after salpingolysis varies from 20% to 60%, and the overall salvage rate is 38%. The number of pregnancies subsequent to fimbrioplasty varies from 5% to 50%. In 868 cases the incidence of pregnancy was 18%. The wide discrepancy obviously reflects patient selection and the degree of tubal destruction. Garcia has reported a gross pregnancy rate of 52.6% in patients with bilateral hydrosalpinges whose tubes remained patent subsequent to surgery. The live birthrate corrected for ectopic pregnancy and abortion was 36.8%. Grant reported a pregnancy rate of 32% when tubal splints or hoods were used, whereas 35% of women became pregnant without splints. He increased the latter figure to 43% by the use of hydrocortisone transtubation every three days during the first two weeks after surgery, followed by chymotrypsin transtubation later.

The overall incidence of pregnancy in surgery for interstitial occlusion of the oviduct was 30% in 583 patients reported by 17 authors. Horne reported a gross pregnancy rate of 64% and a term pregnancy rate of 46% using a ring splint with dexamethasone and promethazine. Unfortunately many reports give pregnancy results on the basis of patients with patent tubes after surgery, not on the overall number of patients treated. Most reports list the gross number of pregnancies that occurred without correcting for abortion, ectopic pregnancies, and perinatal deaths. Ectopic pregnancies occur in from 15 to 20% of women subjected to tubal surgery. Finally, many reports of tuboplasties do not indicate that they correct for patients in whom the contralateral tube was patent.

There is no doubt that one of the major reasons for failure to accomplish pregnancy following tuboplasty is the formation or repeated formation of adhesions with resultant tubo-ovarian malfunction. The rationale for using the combination of dexamethasone and promethazine is based on the work of Replogle et al. who showed that these compounds tended to minimize postoperative adhesions in dogs after deliberate abrasion of the bowel. The promethazine presumably acts to block the action of histamine and to enhance vascular integrity at the site of trauma and to minimize the early formation of a fibrinous exudate. The dexamethasone acts to inhibit local fibroblastic proliferation necessary for the formation of collagenous connective tissue.

Horne published results using a protocol of dexamethasone, 20 mg, and promethazine, 25 mg, given two hours prior to surgery then repeated intraperitoneally, and then intramuscularly every four hours for 12 doses. Of 219 patients with infertility laparotomies studied, 99 (45%) became pregnant and 70 (32%) went to term (excluding ectopic pregnancies and miscarriages). Eight patients had their pelvis reinspected, and in only one of these were significant adhesions present. Unfortunately, this study as most others dealing with surgical adjuvants for adhesion prevention, are not adequately controlled. In fact, only Swolin's study with glucocorticoids is adequately controlled, in which he instilled intraperitoneal hydrocortisone (2 gm) to every other woman undergoing surgery for tubal gestations. Laparoscopy was performed in all patients three months after surgery and clearly identified fewer adhesions in the hydrocortisone-treated group.

Dextran has also received wide attention as a surgical adjunct in recent years. When instilled intraperitoneally, dextran creates an osmotically induced transudate from all surfaces, which should theoretically allow for surface separation. It also covers all surfaces with a thin, filmy layer, which may also suppress adhesion formation. Seitz et al. performed a double-blind prospective study in monkeys comparing low molecular weight dextran and saline and found no difference in adhesion formation. There are other data in animal models that seem to contradict these results. There is currently a multicenter study being done comparing glucocorticoids with antihistamines to dextran with a control group. This will hopefully help to sort out which agent is more effective in prevention of postoperative adhesions.

Because of the depressingly low pregnancy rates in tubal reconstruction, much research has been done to find an alternative route. In vitro fertilization (IVF) has erupted as the largest single breakthrough in infertility and reproductive biology in the last decade. Because it is in its infancy, the technical aspects of the procedure are changing as rapidly as the success rates. However, we can merely outline the routine steps in performing IVF, quote some success rates, and identify needed areas of improvement.

All patients are screened medically and psychologically prior to being chosen as candidates for IVF. Currently we are taking only those patients with tubal disease, proved to be surgical failures. We are sure this will expand to include those with unexplained infertility as well in the future. The basic steps of IVF include induction of superovulation with either clomiphene or human menopausal gonadotropin, followed by human chorionic gonadotropin. Ovulation induction is monitored with daily serum estradiol determinations and ultrasound examinations. Harvesting of the eggs (at least two or three) is performed via the operating laparoscope with aspiration of each follicle separately. This is then followed by isolation of the ova in medium, sperm capacitation, fertilization, and reimplantation using embryo transfer pipettes into the uterine cavity. Current success rates vary anywhere from 15% to 40%. The current stumbling block is not with obtaining fertilization, but rather with reimplantation into a hostile endometrium secondary to the ovulation-induction agents. As the success rates increase with IVF, so will its implementation increase as an alternative to tubal surgery.

THE OVARIAN FACTOR

The major abnormalities concerning the ovary are those involving the process of ovulation and the anatomic and functional changes following endometriosis. Several presumptive clinical methods for the determination of ovulation have already been given (endometrial biopsy, serum progesterone determination). In addition, the patient may be asked to chart her basal body temperature (BBT) for a period of three or four months so that some idea of the average point of ovulation and the thermogenic response to the secretion of progesterone may be gained. It is useless, however, to indicate *a fertile day* to the patient, and prolonged observation of the BBT probably does more harm than good. This soon becomes a fetish, and what should be an enjoyable communal act becomes stilted as a result of prearrangement. The best advice is to recommend coitus during days 11, 13, and 15 or days 12, 14, and 16 of a 28-day cycle. It is not necessary for the couple to abstain prior to these days to increase the sperm count, since present evidence indicates that although the count may be increased by this arrangement, sperm motility is diminished. Men who have intercourse four or more times weekly have somewhat lower sperm counts on each occasion, but it has been shown that the rate of conception is higher.

Polycystic Ovarian Disease

In 1935 Stein and Leventhal called attention to a particular syndrome that has been considered by clinicians to be a singular disease process. As more basic research is accomplished, particularly in the field of steroid synthesis of the ovary, it is becoming apparent that this so-called disease syndrome may actually embrace many diseases of the endocrine system that result in persistent lack of ovulation.

As originally described, the syndrome was characterized by menstrual abnormalities, usually oligomenorrhea or amenorrhea, obesity, a tendency toward virilization (with hirsutism in about one-half the patients), and infertility. The ovaries are large, frequently each ovary being larger than the uterus, and the surface of the ovary appears thickened, pale, and smooth (Fig 10–8,A). They have been described as similar to large oysters in appearance. When the ovary is bisected (Fig 10–8,B), numerous cystic follicles may be identified beneath the capsule. These measure 5 to 7 mm in diameter and contain clear fluid. Microscopically, there is fibrosis of the cortical stroma with areas of hyalinization (Fig 10–9). Examination of the cystic follicles reveals an unusual activity of the theca-interna cells with luteinization. Corpora albicantia and corpora lutea are usually absent, but on occasion one or more may be identified. Although at one time this microscopic picture

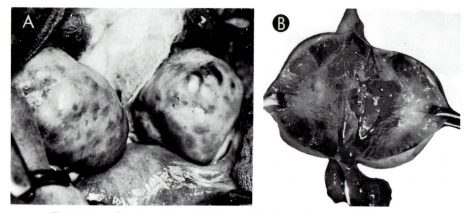

Fig 10–8.—Ovaries of the Stein-Leventhal type. **A,** gross appearance. (From Ingersoll F.M.: *Clin. Obstet. Gynecol.* 4:814, 1961.) **B,** on bisection.

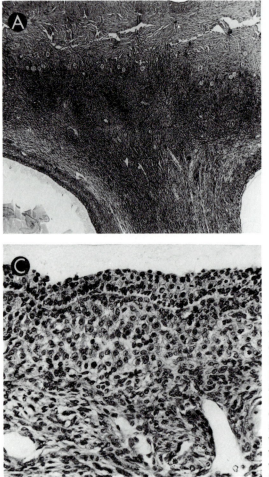

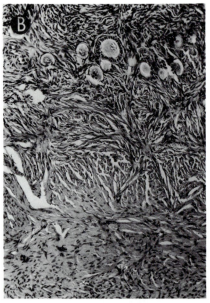

Fig 10–9.—Ovary in Stein-Leventhal syndrome. **A,** low-power view. Note cystic follicles and collagenous character of the cortex. **B,** higher-power view. Numerous primordial follicles are seen in the zone between the normal cortex below and the hyperplastic fibrotic cortex above. **C,** high-power view, showing the wall of a cystic follicle with a narrow layer of granulosa cells toward the lumen of the cyst and a wide layer of luteinized theca cells below.

was thought to be pathognomonic of Stein-Leventhal syndrome, present evidence suggests that it is merely representative of prolonged periods of anovulation from various causes. Scott and Wharton produced a similar appearance in the ovary by the administration of testosterone to monkeys in an attempt to eradicate areas of implanted endometriosis. A similar, though not identical, picture in the ovary has been described in association with abnormal adrenocortical function, adenomas of the pituitary, Cushing's disease, and other syndromes in which amenorrhea is secondary. The uterus is usually of normal size in Stein-Leventhal syndrome and the endometrium shows varying degrees of proliferation, including hyperplasia. A few patients with concomitant endometrial carcinoma have been reported. Although research activity in this disease has yielded several significant findings, the precise etiology remains obscure and its pathogenesis is unknown. Fechner and Kaufman described endometrium indistinguishable from well-differentiated adenocarcinoma in four women with sclerocystic ovaries. They suggest a conservative approach in such patients since the lesion may be reversible when treated by curettage, wedge resection, or induction of ovulation with clomiphene citrate.

Leventhal has reported observations of ovaries and adrenal glands in patients with Stein-Leventhal syndrome. Examination of the adrenal glands in two hirsute patients with typical Stein-Leventhal syndrome disclosed no histologic evidence of hyperfunction. Furthermore, a study of ovarian tissue showed the hilus to be normal in each individual. The really significant anatomic finding was the unusual hyperplasia of the theca cells. This report agreed with the previous findings of Benedict as well as those of Sommers, both of whom described normal adrenal morphology in patients with Stein-Leventhal syndrome. Sommers described autopsy findings in 11 patients and, aside from the polycystic ovaries, the only endocrine pathologic finding was a diffuse basophilia of the pituitary gland.

Jones, however, in discussing the report of Leventhal, contended that in approximately 25% of cases there is an association between bilateral polycystic ovaries and adrenal function. Jones also felt that the primary site of pathologic disorder in this disease process might well be in the hypothalamus.

In a few patients the menstrual history before the development of oligomenorrhea or amenorrhea may have been perfectly normal. Usually, however, the menstrual history reveals a rather marked irregularity since the menarche. Breast development may be normal or may be slightly deficient in some patients.

Etiology

The basic etiology of the polycystic ovarian syndrome is unknown. Until 1956 it was theorized by many pathologists and clinicians that the cause of anovulation was the thickened cortex that trapped the ova beneath the hyalinized tunica, preventing their escape. This concept is no longer tenable. Greenblatt observed ovulation in a patient with Stein-Leventhal syndrome following simple extirpation of one ovary. Ovulation promptly occurred through the thickened cortex of the remaining ovary. Similarly, patients with borderline adrenocortical malfunction, in whom a moderate elevation of the serum DHEA-S level is found, will readily ovulate through the thickened cortex on the administration of small doses of cortisone. In these patients the lack of ovulation is thought to be due to abnormal adrenocortical function, with formation of excess adrenal androgens instead of cortisone. The elevated androgen level apparently prevents ovulation, but when this process is interrupted by the administration of cortisone, ovulation promptly ensues.

Other theories of etiology have included abnormalities of gonadotropic function. Thus, many of the ovaries appear pathologically similar to the ovary of the adolescent female except for the multiple cystic follicles. It has been suggested that these multiple follicle cysts and thickened cortex are the result of overproduction of FSH. A persistent elevation of FSH secretion, however, has not been demonstrated in these patients.

Using the standard mouse uterine weight assay for "total" (FSH and LH) urinary gonadotropins, normal levels have been reported in numerous studies. Normal levels of FSH in urine have also been noted by the ovarian augmentation assay method. Another evidence in favor of the pituitary as an integral factor in the disease has been an irregular fluctuation of LH excretion as measured in urine using the ventral prostate assay method. Mishell has demonstrated this irregular, somewhat elevated LH activity in patients with this syndrome by the immunoassay method. In such a situation it might be possible that the burst of LH activity necessary to produce ovulation is lacking. Mishell, using immunoassay, has clearly shown a marked rise in LH, similar to that seen at the time of ovulation in the normal cycle, subsequent to the administration of clomiphene. This was followed by a rise in the basal body temperature and other indices of apparent ovulation.

Another theory of etiology suggests that the ovary in the polycystic syndrome is excessively sensitive to the stimulus of gonadotropic substances. Thus, the ovary responds by growth of numerous follicles, which develop only partially and subsequently become cystic. Secondarily, hyperplasia of the stroma and luteinization of the theca develop as a result of the irregular but constant LH stimulation. An increased ovarian response to exogenous FSH has been demonstrated in patients with this syndrome and the response to clomiphene citrate seems equally labile.

Lloyd, Goldzieher, and others have suggested that the basic derangement in the Stein-Leventhal syndrome lies in the hypothalamus. They postulate that the median eminence nuclei produce a *tonic* rather than a rhythmic discharge of releasing factors. This hypothesis of a constant, low-level gonadotropin discharge, chronically stimulated by estrogen, is consistent with the clinical findings.

The polycystic ovary has the histologic and functional behavior of an overstimulated organ and persistent estrogen production has been documented.

Kahn and et al. identified two groups of women in 1976 who showed hyperinsulinemia and acanthosis nigricans. The type A insulin resistance was in young women with signs of virilization. The type B resistance was in older women with evidence of immunologic disease. Since 1976, considerable investigation has gone into this type A syndrome of insulin resistance. Burghen et al. were able to identify a solid correlation between hyperinsulinism and hyperandrogenism in patients with polycystic ovarian disease. Hyperinsulinism in itself may act as the stimulus to increase androgen production in the ovary, which would subsequently lead to chronic anovulation and polycystic ovarian disease. Continued research in this area will hopefully lead to the etiology of this most complexing problem.

Studies of Steroid Biosynthesis

Prior to 1960, laboratory assays in patients with the sclerocystic ovarian syndrome were of no particular diagnostic value. The usual evaluation of the patient revealed normal values for total neutral 17-ketosteroids, FSH, T_3 and T_4, and ketogenic steroids. The x-ray of the sella turcica was also normal. If all of these parameters were within normal range and the ovaries were thought to be enlarged, the most probable diagnosis, by exclusion, was a primary ovarian disorder of the Stein-Leventhal type. Refinements in the techniques of laboratory assays for steroids in blood and urine have revealed the fallacy of this particular conclusion.

Two major ovarian steroidogenic abnormalities have been identified: (1) a deficiency in *aromatization*, i.e., in the conversion of 19-oxygenated androgens to estrogen with an accumulation of 19-oxoandrogens, and (2) a deficiency in 3β-ol-dehydrogenase, i.e., in the conversion of Δ^5-3β-ol to Δ^4-3-keto compounds. These inadequacies are due to an in-

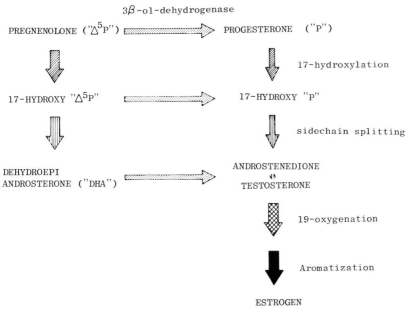

Fig 10–10.—Enzymatic sequences in ovarian steroidogenesis. (From Goldzieher J.W., in Behrman S.J., Kistner R.W. (eds.): *Progress in Infertility,* ed. 2. Boston, Little, Brown & Co., 1975.)

sufficiency of specific enzymes, as noted in Figure 10–10.

Dorfman pubished the results of determinations of testosterone in human plasma obtained from normal men, normal women, hirsute women of the Stein-Leventhal type, and hirsute women with diagnosis not established. The mean testosterone level in nine normal men was 0.56 μg/dl, whereas the mean level in ten normal women was 0.12 μg/dl. Six hirsute women who had polycystic ovaries of the Stein-Leventhal type were studied and were found to have mean testosterone levels ranging from 0.25 to 0.42 μg/dl. The average for these individuals was 0.33 μg/dl. Four hirsute women with a diagnosis not established were studied in a similar manner, and the range was found to be 0.11 to 0.32 μg/dl of testosterone, with a mean of 0.25 μg/dl. The total 17-ketosteroids excreted per day in urine in these two groups was, however, only 12.2 mg/24 hours in patients with Stein-Leventhal syndrome, and 13.7 in hirsute women with unestablished diagnosis. Dorfman also reported studies on five virilized women with

polycystic ovaries of the Stein-Leventhal type; the range for testosterone was 0.30 to 0.74 μg/dl, with a mean of 0.49 μg/dl. In this group the 17-ketosteroids ranged from 6.4 to 20.0 mg/24 hours—certainly not a high level in most laboratories. Bilateral ovarian wedge resection was performed in three hirsute women, and reductions of plasma testosterone levels were seen in each patient. The mean testosterone levels before wedge resection in these three patients were 0.53, 0.77, and 0.58 μg/dl. All of these values approached that seen in the normal male. After wedge resection these values were 0.11, 0.34, and 0.22 μg/dl, respectively. Oophorectomy in five hirsute women with high mean testosterone values before surgery was followed by a mean value of 0.11 μg/dl.

DeVane and associates measured serum gonadotropins, estrogen, and androgen levels in 19 patients with polycystic ovarian disease and ten normal women during the early proliferative phase of the cycle. In patients with polycystic ovarian disease the mean concentration of LH was significantly higher (35 mIU) than that of normal females (12.7 mIU). Levels of FSH were not significantly different (10.3 mIU in women with polycystic ovarian disease; 8.7 mIU in normal females). Estrone levels were higher in patients with polycystic ovarian disease (92 mIU) than in the controls (52 mIU). Estradiol levels were comparable in both groups but testosterone, androstenedione, and dehydroepiandrosterone were significantly increased in patients with polycystic ovarian disease over controls. Although both dehydroepiandrosterone and dehydroepiandrosterone sulfate may be produced by the ovary, these hormones are principally secreted by the adrenal glands. This suggests that both the adrenal glands and the ovaries may be involved in increased androgen metabolism in polycystic ovarian disease. All of these observations are acceptable evidence in favor of the concept that the Stein-Leventhal syndrome is not in itself a specific entity but is merely a part of a progressive and probably polyglandular endocrinopathy.

Diagnostic Measures

To make the diagnosis of polycystic ovarian disease, certain hormonal assays are necessary. These include LH, FSH, testosterone (free and bound), androstenedione, DHEA, and DHEA-S. If DHEA-S levels are elevated, then serum 17 α-hydroxyprogesterone and 11-desoxycortisol should be measured to rule out an adult-onset congenital adrenal hyperplasia.

A clinical diagnosis of polycystic ovarian disease may be made when there are bilaterally enlarged ovaries and signs and symptoms compatible with the disorder. If, however, reliance is placed on the presence of enlarged ovaries to make the diagnosis, the disorder will be missed in a significant number of women. Approximately one third of women with polycystic ovarian disease do not have enlarged ovaries.

A nonsurgical diagnosis is a real challenge and may be impossible when the ovaries are not enlarged. There is usually hyperandrogenism and deranged LH and FSH secretion

even though the ovaries are not enlarged. Approximately 85% of the women we have seen with proved polycystic ovarian disease have elevated levels of androstenedione, testosterone, or both, and an abnormally high LH/FSH ratio in the plasma. The presence of hyperandrogenism, however, does not differentiate polycystic ovarian disease from congenital adrenal hyperplasia.

The differential diagnosis between polycystic ovarian disease and mild congenital adrenal hyperplasia is particularly troublesome in hirsute women with normal-sized ovaries. In this situation we have found the family history to be helpful. A high incidence of oligomenorrhea or hirsutism or both in the female kin usually suggests polycystic ovarian disease, since it can occur as a dominantly inherited disorder. Congenital adrenal hyperplasia, on the other hand, is a recessively inherited disorder. Because of this difference in the mode of inheritance, our experience has been that the odds are 10:1 that the obese, hirsute, oligomenorrheic women will have polycystic ovarian disease rather than congenital adrenal hyperplasia. How useful a high ratio of LH to FSH is in differentiating the two conditions remains to be determined.

Adrenocortical and Ovarian Suppression Studies

In 1951 Sohval and Soffer showed that administration of cortisone caused an immediate increase in gonadotropins in urine in a few patients with polycystic ovaries; an increase in total gonadotropins in normal women after cortisone or dexamethasone has been reported by Barlow. Mahesh and Greenblatt showed a reduction in urinary dehydroepiandrosterone, androsterone, and etiocholanolone after adrenal suppression in some patients with Stein-Leventhal syndrome, but in others these metabolites remained elevated even after adrenal suppression. Subsequently, they were able to suppress the elevated 11-deoxycorticosterone (after dexamethasone) by diethylstilbestrol, suggesting an ovarian origin of these steroids.

Barlow noted an increase in urinary estrogens when dexamethasone was given to normal women during the follicular phase of the cycle but not during the luteal phase, and Netter noted an increase in urinary estrogens in patients with polycystic ovaries during dexamethasone suppression.

A further refinement in differential testing has been to superimpose stimulation of the ovaries by gonadotropin on the suppression of the adrenals with corticosteroids. On the basis of increased or decreased excretion of 17-ketosteroids after human chorionic gonadotropin (HCG) stimulation, some observers felt that it was possible to differentiate adrenal and ovarian components. This interpretation depends on two assumptions: (1) that corticosteroids have a reproducible effect on the adrenal but none on the ovary and (2) that HCG affects the ovary but not the adrenal. There is substantial evidence that both of these assumptions are false. For example, corticosteroids increase the excretion of gonadotropins in urine and HCG evokes an adrenal response in certain patients.

In any patient who presents with oligo-ovulation or anovulation and evidence of virilization, we are currently doing overnight dexamethasone (2 mg) suppression and measuring an 8 A.M. plasma cortisol level to rule out Cushing's syndrome. If the level does not exceed 5 μg/dl, then we proceed with a four-day dexamethasone suppression test, 2 mg/day in four divided doses. The morning of the fifth day, DHEA, DHEA-S, testosterone (free and bound), and androstenedione are remeasured. A functional adrenal contribution will show adequate suppression of DHEA-S. If there is not suppression, then an androgen-secreting adrenal tumor should be considered.

Adrenocortical and Ovarian Stimulation Tests

Lanthier showed an increased urinary excretion of androsterone and etiocholanolone after HCG, but the degree of increase was no greater than that seen in normal subjects.

HCG did not affect the excretion of pregnanediol or pregnanetriol in urine. Dignam showed an increase in plasma testosterone in some patients with polycystic ovaries after HCG administration.

The administration of homologous or heterologous FSH to women with polycystic ovaries results in gross ovarian enlargement, but the steroid consequences of such stimulation are variable. Gemzell and Crooke noted a marked increase in estrogens in urine after such stimulation and Shearman noted a marked increase in estrogens plus urinary pregnanetriol and Δ^5-pregnenetriol. Mahesh and Greenblatt, however, noted an increase in urinary 17-ketosteroids, pregnanetriol, and Δ^5-pregnenetriol, but no increase in estrogens.

Adrenocorticotropin (ACTH) stimulation results in a greater increase in 17-ketosteroids, androsterone, and etiocholanolone in women with polycystic ovaries than in controls. Mahesh also found an increase in pregnanetriol, Δ^5-pregnenetriol, tetrahydrocorticoids, and 11-oxygenated 17-ketosteroids.

Although an exaggerated rise in DHEA-S after ACTH stimulation is commonly found in hyperandrogenic states of adrenocortical origin, this response is not a consistently reliable test. An elevation of 17α-hydroxyprogesterone would suggest a biochemical adrenal defect similar to that found in congenital adrenal hyperplasia. A rise in DHEA-S after ACTH in the Stein-Leventhal syndrome and suppression of the DHEA-S by a corticosteroid would point to an important adrenocortical factor. Confusion regarding the pathogenesis of Stein-Leventhal syndrome has not been dispelled, but a trial of corticosteroid suppression of a potential adrenal component has come to be an integral therapeutic maneuver.

Treatment

Stein and Leventhal suggested the original effective treatment of bilateral wedge resection in 1935. In their series, menstrual cycles returned to normal in about 95% of the patients, and approximately 85% of the infertile patients became pregnant within a short time after surgery. Since that time, wedge resection has been extensively practiced and has been overused.

The use of wedge resection in treatment of this disease process should be the *last,* not the first method employed. Nevertheless, since curettage in some of these patients has revealed atypical endometrial hyperplasia, every avenue of therapy to produce ovulation should be explored.

The optimum therapy to be used initially, if the DHEA-S level is elevated to greater than 4 µg/ml, is that of cortisone or prednisone. Forchielli and associates found a rather decided drop in mean testosterone levels after administration of 10 to 20 mg of prednisone daily. Whereas the surgical procedure of bilateral wedge resection caused a net decrease of 0.41 µg/dl of plasma (from a mean of 0.63 to 0.22 µg/dl), prednisone effected a change from 0.34 to 0.07 µg/dl, a net decrease of 0.27 µg/dl of plasma testosterone. If the basal body temperature graph does not reveal apparent ovulation within six months of the initiation of cortisone therapy, a complete reevaluation of the patient's condition should be undertaken. We have employed doses of hydrocortisone of 30 mg daily, and if ovulation occurs therapy is continued for nine to 12 months. The medication is then withdrawn and the patient followed carefully to evaluate whether or not spontaneous ovulation occurs.

If the DHEA-S level is normal, clomiphene citrate is given as primary therapy. In 1959, Smith and Kistner reported induction of ovulation with a nonsteroidal estrogen antagonist, MER-25. Tyler reported similar results in 1962. Since this compound had certain toxic effects, a similar preparation known as clomiphene citrate, was substituted. The ovarian response to clomiphene was more striking but less physiologic than that demonstrated with MER-25. Clomiphene citrate seemed to be effective in the patient who had an arrest in the maturation of follicles but in whom adequate estrogen was present. This

was particularly true of patients with Stein-Leventhal syndrome; in these patients the follicles seemed ready to extrude their ova, but a burst of LH activity was apparently lacking.

In a composite study, 359 of 436 patients classified as having the Stein-Leventhal syndrome apparently ovulated after the first course of clomiphene, and an additional 58 did so after two or more courses of prolonged use. This incidence of effectiveness of 95% is precisely equivalent to that reported by Stein and Leventhal as a result of ovarian wedge resection. The incidence of pregnancy subsequent to the use of clomiphene does not, however, approach the 85% pregnancy rate reported for surgical intervention by Stein and Leventhal.

Effects of Clomiphene

The mechanism of action may be directly on the ovary or on the hypothalamus (Fig 10–11). Greenblatt and co-workers found an initial rise in FSH excretion, followed by an increase in estrogen secretion and then a rise in LH. This LH peak was followed by a further rise in estrogen excretion and an increase in pregnanediol. The increase in estrogens was accompanied by a rise in urinary 17-ketosteroids and tetrahydrocorticoids. The changes in FSH and LH subsequent to clomiphene administration in women with polycystic ovaries have now been studied using immunoassay methods and, in general, parallel the pattern just described. Figure 10–12 illustrates the effect of clomiphene citrate on serum LH and FSH in a patient with Stein-Leventhal syndrome. In our original report only 38% of patients became pregnant. There are numerous reasons that negate the validity of a direct comparison of results of surgery vs. clomiphene:

1. Wedge resection is usually reserved for patients who are married and desirous of pregnancy, and usually is not performed until the male has demonstrated normal seminal fluid analyses; clomiphene, however, has been administered to numerous patients with the Stein-Leventhal syndrome who are un-

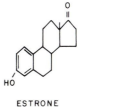

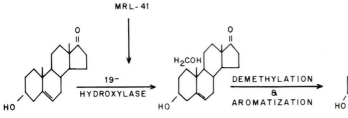

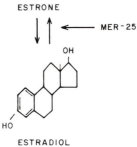

Fig 10–11.—Graphic representation of possible sites of action of clomiphene citrate (MRL-41) and MER-25 on ovarian steroidogenesis.

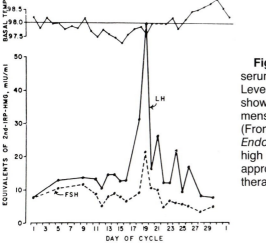

Fig 10–12.—Effect of clomiphene citrate on serum FSH and LH in a patient with Stein-Leventhal syndrome. **A,** graphic illustration showing variations of LH and FSH during the menstrual cycle in a normally ovulating woman. (From Midgley A.R., Jaffe R.B.: *J. Clin. Endocrinol. Metab.* 33:962, 1971.) **B,** note the high baseline levels of LH and the "burst" of LH approximately four days after the last day of therapy. (Courtesy of Dr. Daniel Mishell.)

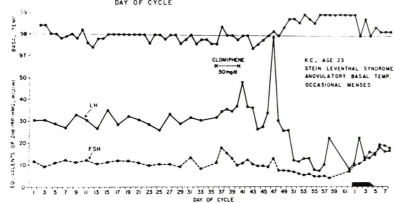

married, or married but not desirous of pregnancy, and without complete study of the male.

2. The length of follow-up of patients treated with clomiphene is not as long as surgically treated patients, since reports have frequently been submitted after three or four treatment cycles.

3. Many clomiphene-treated patients have not had a complete evaluation of tubal patency, whereas most of those treated surgically had tubal patency demonstrated either before or at the time of surgery.

Whereas clomiphene has been used in the Stein-Leventhal syndrome for the control of abnormal menses, wedge resection is usually reserved for infertility due to anovulation. If the permanency of ovulation following wedge resection approximated the 95% reported by Stein and Leventhal, this certainly would be the procedure of choice. In numerous reports compiled by Goldzieher, however, for a total of 1,079 patients the incidence of ovulation approximated 80% (with a range from 6% to 95%) and a high rate of recurrence of oligo-ovulation was noted. The mean incidence of pregnancy was 63% with a range of 13% to 89%. Furthermore, we have been impressed with the number of patients referred to us because of recurrent amenorrhea or oligo-ovulation subsequent to wedge resection who have demonstrated extensive peritubal and periovarian adhesions by endoscopy. Not only was the primary surgical procedure inadequate for the consistent regulation of ovulation, but it was responsible also for tubal adhesions of such severity that pregnancy was virtually impossible. None of these patients have become pregnant even though regular ovulatory cycles were established with clomiphene, and subsequent reparative tuboplasty undoubtedly will be necessary for restoration of normal tubal mobility and ovum pickup. Buttram and Vaquero reviewed the results of 173 patients who were followed up for one year after ovarian wedge resection and they found by endoscopy that adhesions were present in 59 of 111 patients not lost to follow-up.

Forty-three patients who desired conception did not conceive; 40 of these had developed postoperative adhesions. The investigators concluded that hormonal therapy for polycystic ovarian disease offered results comparable to those of surgery and eliminated the risk of adhesions.

In the young, unmarried patient with oligo-ovulation or secondary amenorrhea due to the Stein-Leventhal syndrome, it is obviously not necessary to secure recurrent ovulation with clomiphene, since prolonged treatment may be necessary for the restoration of normal cycles. But neither is it advisable to perform major surgery with the possibility of recurrent ovulatory insufficiency and tubal malfunction. Adequate, although temporary, therapy may be utilized in the form of cyclic estrogen-progestin combinations. These preparations will suppress the constant, irregular stimulation of the ovary by follicle-stimulating and luteinizing hormones. Since the histologic features of the ovary (hypertrophy, hyperplasia of the cortex, increased number and size of follicles) undoubtedly represent chronic stimulation by gonadotropic hormones, suppression of these stimuli should prevent the progressive changes noted in the ovary. The excessive androgen production will thus be reduced and hirsutism diminished. Finally, the tendency toward endometrial hyperplasia will be corrected by the progestin and regular withdrawal flow will occur.

There are a very small number of patients with Stein-Leventhal syndrome who apparently ovulate subsequent to the administration of clomiphene but in whom pregnancy does not occur. Leventhal has suggested that the ovarian cortex in these patients is excessively thickened and the indirect indices of ovulation, i.e., progesterone production, may be due to intraovarian ovulation without ovum release. In this small group of patients, wedge resection is advised. But this surgical approach should be the *last*, not the first therapeutic measure.

We presently use clomiphene citrate as primary therapy for polycystic ovarian disease

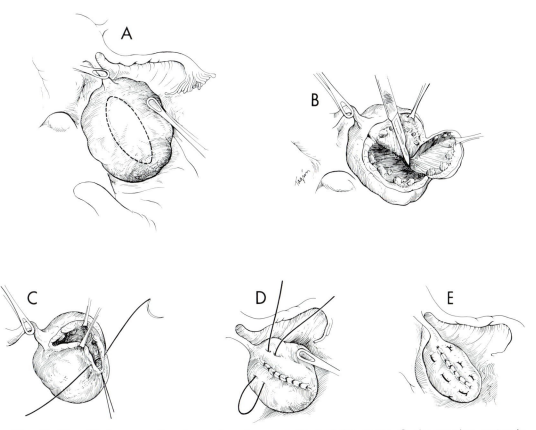

Fig 10–13.—Wedge resection for polycystic ovarian syndrome. **A,** William clamps are placed on the utero-ovarian ligament and the cephalad portion of the ovary near the infundibulopelvic ligament. Ovary is held in left hand of the operator, and two incisions are made over the convexity of the ovary about 2 cm apart. **B,** a wedge-shaped segment of ovarian cortex is excised. Care should be taken to avoid the ovarian hilus. The pie-shaped segment may approximate almost one third of the ovary. **C,** the ovarian cortex is approximated with interrupted sutures of 3-0 Dexon. Care is taken to secure close proximity of cortical edges so that stroma does not bulge through the surface. **D,** an inverted mattress suture is placed through the ovary above the hilus to reduce dead space and improve hemostasis. **E,** the reconstructed ovary. (From Patton G.W., Kistner R.W.: *Atlas of Infertility Surgery,* ed. 2. Boston, Little, Brown & Co., 1984.)

and if, after six to eight cycles, there is failure to ovulate (at a dose of 250 mg in addition to administration of HCG), then we proceed with administration of human menopausal gonadotropin (HMG). Only after failure to ovulate with HMG-HCG will we proceed with bilateral ovarian wedge resection (Fig 10–13).

Ovarian Wedge Resection

The technique for wedge resection of the ovary used at the Brigham and Women's Hospital (Fig 10–13) has been essentially that described by Stein and Leventhal in their original paper. A "generous" segment of ovarian tissue is excised from the antimesenteric border, the surface being about 3 to 5 mm in width. We have not adopted medullary resection of the ovary since we did not wish to interfere with the ovarian blood supply and since, in view of the studies of Salhanick and Warren, the actual source of the androgenic hormone seemed conclusively to be in the cortex and not in the medulla. After the segment has been excised, the surfaces are approximated with interrupted sutures of 3-0 Dexon or chromic catgut. A single suture of inverted mattress type is then placed through the approximated edges to eliminate dead space and the accumulation of blood or fluid in this area. Meticulous hemostasis is imperative to prevent subsequent tubo-ovarian adhesions. Despite the importance and obvious success of ovarian wedge resection in patients with Stein-Leventhal syndrome, it now appears that the use of clomiphene citrate in this syndrome will relegate the surgical approach to a very minor position.

Induction of Ovulation

A major difficulty confronting the clinician in the field of infertility is that of oligo-ovulation or anovulation. Not only is it difficult to evoke release of an ovum from a recalcitrant follicle, but the capricious occurrence of isolated spontaneous ovulation makes evaluation of specific therapeutic measures extremely difficult. Various investigations have suggested a lack of specificity of most therapeutic schemes. Thus the effects of estrogens alone or combined with synthetic progestins, of synthetic progestins alone, and of progester-

one alone or preceded by FSH priming have been critically observed and have been found inadequate. Since lack of the ovulatory process, however, may merely represent deficiencies in other endocrine organs, a systematized investigation is mandatory. An effort should be made to localize the cause as being of pituitary, thyroid, adrenal, or ovarian origin.

Clomiphene

In 1960, Kistner and Smith reported successful induction of ovulation and pregnancies after administration of a nonsteroidal estrogen antagonist, MER-25 (ethamoxytriphetol) in four patients with Stein-Leventhal syndrome. MER-25 and Clomid are closely related compounds and their similarity in structural formulas is illustrated in Figure 10–14.

The clinical uses of clomiphene are based on several biologic actions in the anovular patients. If follicular maturation in the ovary is adequate, ovulation occurs as a result of release of increased amounts of FSH and LH, the exact ratio of increase being unknown. Progesterone is subsequently secreted by the corpus luteum in amounts large enough to

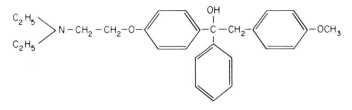

1-(*p*-2-diethylaminoethoxy phenyl)-1-phenyl-2-*p*-anisylethanol

MER – 25

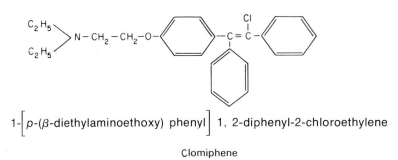

1-[*p*-(β-diethylaminoethoxy) phenyl] 1, 2-diphenyl-2-chloroethylene

Clomiphene

Fig 10–14.—Structural formulas for MER-25 and clomiphene.

prepare the endometrium for nidation and to maintain the conceptus until chorionic estrogen and progesterone assume this role. In certain instances clomiphene may result in luteinization of cystic follicles, without ovulation, with subsequent secretion of progesterone from the luteinized cells. This will, of course, produce a sustained rise in the basal body temperature that might be mistaken for ovulation.

Clomiphene is indicated for the anovular patient who shows evidence of follicular function and adequate endogenous estrogen but who lacks adequate and cyclic stimulation by pituitary gonadotropic function. The typical patient usually has normal or slightly elevated levels of DHEA-S, normal thyroid function, and normal or slightly diminished levels of pituitary gonadotropins. Evidence of adequate

endogenous estrogen production by vaginal smear, endometrial biopsy, assay of urinary estrogen, or bleeding in response to progesterone gives a favorable prognosis for treatment. Although a reduced estrogen level affords a less favorable prognosis for subsequent ovulation, it does not always preclude successful therapy. Most patients with polycystic ovarian syndrome (Stein-Leventhal syndrome) exhibit an ovulatory response to clomiphene, but only about 40% have become pregnant (Fig 10–15).

Dosage and administration.—The precise dose of clomiphene citrate cannot be stated since it will depend on the type of patient being treated and on the sensitivity of the ovary. The usually recommended dose is 50 mg/day (one 50-mg tablet) for five days of

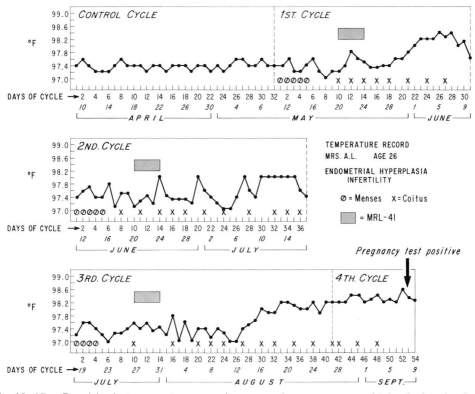

Fig 10–15.—Basal body temperature records of a 26-year-old patient with a history of three curettages for endometrial hyperplasia. The last endometrial tissue revealed carcinoma in situ, and hysterectomy was advised. Ovulatory cycles with normal menses were obtained after the first two clomiphene cycles, and the patient became pregnant about 12 days after the third clomiphene treatment.

the menstrual cycle, usually days 5 through 9. The patient should then be reevaluated after the first cycle regarding symptoms. If there is no ovulation on this dose after one cycle, then the dose should be increased to 100 mg in the following cycle. If ovulation is still not achieved then the dose should be increased monthly to 150 mg, 200 mg, and, finally, 250 mg. If ovulation is documented at any of these doses, then that dose should be maintained monthly. Gorlitsky et al. have achieved an additional 15% pregnancy rate at the 150-mg dose and higher. Basal body temperature charts should be kept monthly to document ovulation. Spontaneous menstruation does not necessarily confirm ovulation since it may be estrogen-withdrawal bleeding. If there is no success with the 250-mg dose, then we add 10,000 units of HCG as a single dose on the seventh day after the clomiphene administration is completed. Prior to the HCG, ultrasound is performed to document and confirm adequate follicular ripening.

Since the safety of long-term administration of clomiphene has not yet been conclusively demonstrated, this preparation cannot be recommended as "maintenance" therapy for the patient whose ovulatory defect recurs promptly when treatment is discontinued. Although we originally recommended estrogen-priming in patients whose endometrial biopsies were classified as atrophic, we no longer feel that this is a necessary part of treatment. Clomiphene should not be given if there is an ovarian cyst, but this contraindication does not apply to the moderate bilateral ovarian enlargement that occurs in patients with polycystic ovarian disease.

Ovulation may be expected to occur in approximately 70% of women with secondary amenorrhea. The diagnosis of apparent ovulation is based on the finding of menstrual or secretory endometrium by biopsy, by basal body temperature graphs, or by increase in the assay of serum progesterone.

Some patients respond regularly to each course of clomiphene therapy; others respond to some but not all courses of treatment. It should be pointed out that patients with severe panhypopituitarism (Simmonds' disease) have not responded even though other hormonal deficiencies have been completely corrected. Patients with complete ovarian insufficiency, such as gonadal dysgenesis (Turner's syndrome) or premature menopause, have not responded to clomiphene.

Pregnancy has been reported in approximately 40% of women who ovulate subsequent to the use of clomiphene. But this proportion is not a reflection of clomiphene failure since 10% of women treated were single and other married patients were not immediately desirous of pregnancy. Furthermore, many patients were treated for only one or two cycles, and in others tubal factors or male insufficiency predisposed to the infertility status.

There is an increased incidence of multiple pregnancy in patients conceiving immediately following clomiphene therapy: one in every 16. (The incidence of twins in the general population is one in 80.) The increased incidence of multiple pregnancy is undoubtedly due to fraternal twinning consistent with observation of superovulation after clomiphene therapy. The incidence of spontaneous abortion is not increased.

The most striking side effect of clomiphene is ovarian enlargement due to the enlargement of cystic follicles, cystic corpora lutea, or other physiologic cystic structures. Such cystic enlargement is perhaps the most convincing evidence that clomiphene is capable of stimulating ovarian secretory activity in the human female. Microscopic study of ovarian cysts and the associated endometrium has indicated that these structures are indeed of functional nature.

Experience has shown that these physiologic cysts regress spontaneously within seven to 28 days following cessation of therapy. They should always be managed conservatively unless there is a specific indication for surgical intervention. Clomiphene therapy should be initiated subsequently only after the ovaries have returned to pretreatment size. If marked enlargement occurs during any course of therapy, the dose or duration of the subsequent course should be reduced. *Clomiphene should never be given in the presence of an ovarian cyst.*

Before initiating therapy with clomiphene in patients with prolonged secondary amenorrhea, certain endocrinological studies should be performed: DHEA-S, T_3 and T_4, serum FSH and LH, and serum prolactin levels should be determined. A thorough evaluation of this type will materially reduce the incidence of patients who fail to respond to clomiphene. If, however, the patient is infertile because of irregular ovulation, but has not experienced prolonged amenorrhea, trials of clomiphene may be initiated without a detailed endocrine survey. If the response, as measured by the basal body temperature or endometrial biopsy, is unfavorable, the various parameters previously evaluated must be rechecked. The patient may be amenorrheic because of premature menopause, and it is important that a repeat determination of serum FSH and LH be obtained. Endoscopy will permit making a diagnosis of ovarian agenesis, and this may be aided by a karyotype of the patient. Every patient with primary amenorrhea should have a chromosomal study performed. Patients with secondary amenorrhea should be questioned carefully regarding the presence of headaches or visual abnormalities in order that a pituitary or extrasellar tumor will not be missed.

In patients having low levels of gonadotropins, both FSH and LH, low levels of estrogen, small ovaries by endoscopy, and atrophic endometrium, ovulation may be very difficult to achieve, even with maximum doses of clomiphene in conjunction with HCG. These patients should then begin HMG-HCG therapy.

Clomiphene is apparently more effective in stimulating the release of follicle-stimulating releasing hormone from the hypothalamus than in stimulating release of luteinizing hormone releasing factor in such patients since it will not uniformly induce ovulation after follicular development has been produced with

human menopausal gonadotropin, HMG (Pergonal). Clomiphene acts in a similar fashion to HMG in effecting development of the follicle, but the precise LH action of sequential HCG is necessary to rupture the mature follicle.

For clomiphene and HCG to be effective, a responsive pituitary and ovary must be present. Human pituitary FSH and HMG plus HCG will result in ovulation if total gonadotropins are absent (e.g., after hypophysectomy) or are extremely low. In either case, however, the ovary must be capable of follicular development, maturation, and ovum release.

Human Menopausal Gonadotropin

In 1958 a new era in therapy for the infertile female was initiated by Gemzell in Sweden when he described the use of FSH derived from human pituitary glands. When this substance was followed in sequence with human chorionic gonadotropin, basically luteotrophic in action, ovulation was induced in a large percentage of infertile and amenorrheic women. The supply of this substance is limited, and therefore search for another source was begun. Lunenfeld, in Israel, and Rosemberg, in the United States, succeeded in isolating gonadotropic substances from the urine of postmenopausal females that, when followed sequentially with HCG, were capable of inducing ovulation. Menopausal gonadotropin is available as Pergonal.*

The FSH content of Pergonal has varied from 76 to 103 international units (IU) per ampule. At the present time each ampule contains 75 IU of FSH and 75 IU of LH plus 10 mg of lactose in the lyophilized form.

Infertility due to lack of ovulation is the chief indication for therapy with HMG. Patients having persistently low or absent gonadotropins may be treated if pituitary or hypothalamic tumors and cysts have been ruled out. Patients demonstrating primary gonadotropin insufficiency, hypothalamic amenorrhea, Sheehan's syndrome, or an arrested pi-

_____
*Serono Laboratories

tuitary tumor or cyst usually respond promptly to HMG-HCG therapy.

The etiologic factors causing many cases of secondary amenorrhea with normal gonadotropin levels remain obscure, yet ultimately many of these may respond to gonadotropin administration. All patients with normal gonadotropin levels should be given at least eight courses of clomiphene therapy before resorting to menopausal gonadotropin treatment. Certain patients who fail to ovulate with clomiphene alone may do so with clomiphene-HCG sequential therapy or with HMG (Pergonal)-HCG sequential therapy.

Patients with persistent anovular cycles who fail to respond to clomiphene or clomiphene-HCG will usually respond to Pergonal if the ovary has not been depleted of follicles. Patients with marked elevation of endogenous gonadotropins will not respond to exogenous gonadotropins.

The combination of FSH and LH in menopausal gonadotropin stimulates the development of ovarian follicles and the subsequent secretion of estrogen. A direct chemical measurement of estrogen is the most accurate assessment of follicular activity. Following the administration of Pergonal, total estrogen levels have been noted to rise as high as 1,000 μg per 24 hours (normal 20 to 60 μg). This marked rise undoubtedly represents follicular overstimulation. Elevated estrogen levels have been correlated with multiple pregnancies and with the occurrence of ovarian enlargement and ascites. It is important, therefore, to determine the extent of follicular activity in order to prevent excessive ovarian stimulation. This can be accomplished by monitoring levels of serum estradiol.

Before treatment with Pergonal is instituted, a thorough gynecologic and endocrinologic evaluation must be performed. This should include a hysterosalpingogram or endoscopy and tubal lavage to exclude uterine and tubal pathologic conditions and documentation of anovulation by means of basal body temperature, serial vaginal smears, examination of cervical mucus, determination of serum progesterone, and endometrial biopsy. Evaluation of the husband's seminal fluid should be completed prior to Pergonal therapy. Primary ovarian failure should be excluded by the determination of serum FSH or LH. Careful examination should be made to rule out the presence of an early pregnancy. Uterine curettage should also always be done before starting Pergonal therapy if there has been a past history of abnormal bleeding or previous endometrial hyperplasia. Finally, clomiphene citrate alone or followed by HCG should have been tried if the diagnosis indicates a possibility of response to these agents.

DOSAGE AND ADMINISTRATION.—The current therapy at the Brigham and Women's Hospital for Pergonal is individualized for each patient. Each patient is initially begun on two ampules (150 IU of FSH and LH) for the first four days, then the dosage is varied pending each daily serum estradiol determination. Serum esteradiol levels are plotted and Pergonal is increased appropriately to assure an accelerated rise. After the serum estradiol level is greater than 600 pg/ml, then monitoring of follicular growth is aided by daily or every other day ultrasounds. Once adequate follicular growth is observed, then 10,000 IU of HCG are given 24 to 36 hours after the last dose of Pergonal. Pelvic examination is always performed prior to the administration of HCG to reduce the incidence of hyperstimulation. Ultrasound should be performed prior to HCG administration to determine the number and size of follicles.

During short-course treatment with both Pergonal and HCG and during a two-week posttreatment period, patients should be examined for signs of excessive ovarian stimulation. It is recommended that Pergonal administration be stopped if the ovaries become significantly enlarged or abdominal pain occurs. Ovarian hyperstimulation occurs after treatment has been discontinued and reaches its maximum at about seven to ten days postovulation. Patients should be followed up for at least two weeks after HCG administration.

The couple should be encouraged to have intercourse daily, beginning on the day prior to the administration of HCG until ovulation becomes apparent from the usual indices. Care should be taken to insure insemination.

The contraindications for the use of Pergonal-HCG are:

1. A high level of endogenous gonadotropin indicating primary ovarian failure.

2. The presence of overt thyroid and adrenal dysfunction.

3. An organic intracranial lesion such as a pituitary tumor.

4. The presence of any cause of infertility other than anovulation.

5. Abnormal bleeding of undetermined origin.

Pergonal is a potent gonadotropic substance capable of causing mild to severe adverse reactions. It must be used with caution.

Pergonal does not appear to influence the incidence of abortion in the subfertile individual. The abortion rate for the subfertile individual is reported to be approximately 20% in patients with primary infertility and 30% in secondary infertility. The abortion rate following Pergonal-HCG therapy has been 25%.

Multiple births occur frequently following treatment with Pergonal-HCG, the incidence being approximately 20%, and four out of five multiple pregnancies being twins.

Taymor reached the following conclusions after extensive and detailed studies:

1. HMG combined with or followed by HCG provides a potent method of ovulation stimulation.

2. This combination can be used as primary therapy in amenorrheic patients with absent gonadotropins. In patients with secondary amenorrhea associated with low or normal gonadotropin levels or with anovular cycles, its use should be postponed until other therapeutic measures have proved unsuccessful (e.g., clomiphene).

3. Each patient responds individually, and close observation is mandatory. Patients who have secondary amenorrhea associated with normal gonadotropins as well as those with polycystic ovarian disease appear more sensitive. Thorough pretreatment workup is necessary to avoid specific and known complications.

4. The amount and duration of administration of HMG may be increased slowly in subsequent cycles.

5. HCG may be administered as 8,000 to 12,000 units in a single dose.

In an effort to diminish the incidence of multiple pregnancy, ovarian hyperstimulation syndrome, and the excessive cost of HMG administration, we tried a sequence of clomiphene-HMG-HCG in 80 patients with infertility due to prolonged amenorrhea. Criteria for this therapeutic regimen were: (1) normal seminal fluid analysis and postcoital test; (2) lack of withdrawal bleeding from progesterone following amenorrhea of more than six months' duration; (3) normal x-ray of the sella turcica and visual fields; (4) low serum FSH and LH levels; (5) normal results of endoscopic examination; and (6) lack of response to clomiphene in excessive doses (200 mg daily for five days) or prolonged doses (100 mg daily for ten days) with or without HCG, or apparent ovulatory response to this clomiphene-HCG sequence for five or six consecutive cycles without pregnancy.

Clomiphene was administered in a dose of 100 mg daily for seven days. Human menopausal gonadotropin was then given in the following manner: two ampules daily for four days, then one ampule daily for two days. After a 24-hour interval without treatment, 10,000 IU of HCG were given; 2,000 IU of HCG were given four days later.

Twenty-three pregnancies occurred in 80 patients. Fifteen of the first 25 patients became pregnant, but in these women the only previous abnormality noted was lack of ovulation. Six additional pregnancies occurred subsequent to one or more unsuccessful cycles. Multiple pregnancies occurred in only two patients (twins delivered at 32 weeks in one and an abortion of five fetuses at 20 weeks in another). Multiple pregnancy occurred in only one additional patient whose urinary estrogen level was monitored and in whom the level was 100 μg or less when the HCG was given. The ovarian hyperstimulation syndrome did not occur in any patient.

6. A pregnancy rate of 50% within the first two treatment cycles may be expected to occur if no other causes for infertility exist.

7. Close adherence to precautionary measures will enable the physician to secure a reasonable conception rate in patients for whom no satisfactory treatment previously existed. Furthermore, most severe adverse reactions or multiple pregnancies beyond twins will be avoided. Undoubtedly, complications will occur, but they will be less frequent if a slight undertreatment is utilized during the initial cycle.

Bromocriptine

Hyperprolactinemia can alter normal ovulatory mechanisms and lead to an entire spectrum of clinical presentations. With a prolactin concentration above 25 ng/ml in granulosa cell tissue cultures, McNatty was able to show a decline in progesterone production in the setting of adequate gonadotropin stimulation. Prolactin has also been shown to alter the tonic release of gonadotropins and to diminish the pulsatile secretion of gonadotropin-releasing hormone.

Bromocriptine (2-bromo-α-ergocryptine), an ergot alkaloid, works directly at the level of the pituitary to suppress the release of prolactin. Being a dopamine agonist, it also probably works on the hypothalamus to alter prolactin secretion. When administered to patients who are anovulatory on the basis of elevated prolactin levels, bromocriptine induces ovulation in over 80% of patients. High-resolution computed tomographic (CT) scans of the pituitary should be performed in all patients prior to initiating treatment.

DOSAGE AND ADMINISTRATION.—Because of bromocriptine's dopaminergic actions, it has many side effects, which must be described to the patient prior to therapy. Nausea, vomiting, fatigue, and headache are commonly experienced. Syncope has been noted in a very small number of patients after their first dose. Because of the above, we begin our patients on 1.25 mg at bedtime for five to seven days then, if tolerated, increase their dosage to 2.5 mg with dinner. If a further dose increase is necessary, then increments of 2.5 mg should be added progressively at each meal. Basal body temperature charts should be monitored closely, and at the earliest signs of pregnancy the medication should be stopped. Griffith et al. showed no adverse outcome with mothers on bromocriptine, but care should be taken in following these patients. We feel there is no role for bromocriptine in patients who are euprolactinemic with unexplained infertility.

ENDOMETRIOSIS

Endometriosis has been definitely correlated with infertility, and it has been estimated that the expectation of pregnancy in this disease is about half that of the general population. Thus, with a natural incidence of infertility approximating 15%, it is safe to say that in the presence of endometriosis the sterility incidence approaches 30% to 40%. If the studies of the patient show that ovulation is occurring regularly, that the oviducts are patent, the endometrium normal, and the postcoital test adequate, the presence of endometriosis should be considered. Diagnosis may be suggested by the history, corroborated by the pelvic examination and verified by biopsy or endoscopy. Treatment may be varied, utilizing analgesics and expectation, operation, hormones, or combinations of these (see Chapter 9, "Endometriosis").

If childbearing function is to be preserved, operative procedures should be as conservative as possible. The optimum treatment for endometriosis is pregnancy. In the past we have suggested the use of a pseudopregnancy in the infertile patient, utilizing increasing doses of estrogen and progestins for six to nine months. A decidual reaction is produced in the areas of endometriosis; these areas subsequently undergo degeneration and necrosis. Much of the endometriotic tissue may be absorbed so that subsequent fertility is improved. We currently use danazol as the primary medical therapy for endometriosis. Its pharmacology and efficacy are discussed in Chapter 9.

IMMUNOLOGIC FACTOR

The immunology of the reproductive tract is quite complex and has become a considerable challenge to investigators attempting to identify its role in infertility. Most studies to date lack adequate controls so interpretation of results is rather difficult. A look at the tests currently available, their interpretation and significance, and available therapies may help to clarify this somewhat confusing area of infertility.

Tests used to detect antibodies to human spermatozoa in serum can be placed into four categories: microagglutination, macroagglutination, immobilization, and immunofluorescence. Franklin and Dukes developed their microagglutination test in 1963 and found 78.9% of unexplained infertility patients and 11.8% of known fertile patients to have circulating antispermatozoal antibodies. Since the original study, the percent incidence of antibodies in the control fertile population has been as high as 45.8%. Kibrick et al. published their macroagglutination test in 1952 and a summary of the results of this test in the last ten years shows a 14% incidence of antibodies in unexplained infertility and a 21.4% incidence in pregnant patients. It is obvious from the above two test results that the significance of sperm agglutination to infertility is unclear.

Isojima et al. developed the sperm immobilization assay in 1968 and it appears to have a better specificity than the sperm agglutination tests. A summary of the test results over the last ten years shows an 8.95% incidence of antibodies in unexplained infertility and 0% incidence in pregnant patients. Because of its apparent specificity, it may lack adequate sensitivity when compared with the Kibrick and Franklin-Dukes tests.

The most recent tests developed are the immunofluorescent assays. Although the abil-

ity of these tests to define specific antigen response is excellent, their correlation to other relatively proved tests and to infertile populations is unclear. Haas et al. have recently developed a quite specific radiolabeled antiglobulin test for antisperm antibody, which is not found in fertile controls. Their study involves small numbers but the results are promising.

All of the aforementioned tests are looking at the systemic response to human spermatozoa, but considerable work is going on to identify the local immune response. The technical aspects of studying endometrial cavity fluids and cervical mucus are obvious. Given that, however, the correlation between local and systemic antibody activity is very poor. Levels of IgA are much higher in local secretion and IgG levels much lower as compared with serum levels. Cell-mediated immunity is also very active in the reproductive tract and studies are currently under way looking at local T-cell and macrophage activity toward spermatozoa.

Available therapy offers three current modalities, all of which are open to criticism. Occlusive or condom therapy has been widely used for many years with considerable variation in outcome. Decreasing the antigenic exposure should lead to a decreased immune response, but some patients appear to become pregnant in spite of high antibody titers, with or without condom therapy. Shulman has performed intrauterine inseminations using washed sperm (to remove antigens and to circumvent interaction with cervical mucus), but the current number of treated patients is limited. In addition, the endometrial cavity can mount an antigenic response, so washing may only aid in removing prostaglandin to make intrauterine insemination feasible. Lastly, use of high-dose glucocorticoids (methylprednisolone, 96 mg/day for seven days) has shown moderate success, but patient selection must be done with extreme scrutiny. There are considerable side effects involved and one serious complication reported (bilateral aseptic necrosis of the femoral heads).

We currently rely on at least two or more

of the available tests to confirm an immunologic factor (greater than 1:16 titer). If confirmation is obtained, then patients are placed on high-dose methylprednisolone, according to Shulman's protocol. These patients are followed very closely and there is a low threshold for stopping therapy if any adverse reactions occur.

MYCOPLASMA AND CHLAMYDIA

Ureaplasma urealyticum and *Chlamydia trachomatis* have been the subject of considerable investigation in recent years. It is unfortunate that many of the studies were of such small numbers or without adequate controls, making interpretation difficult. There is information available, however, that does help define what role *Mycoplasma* and *Chlamydia* play in infertility.

Isolation rates of *U. urealyticum* vary depending on a number of socioeconomic factors, but whether there is a significant difference between infertile and fertile populations has been quite controversial. Stray-Pedersen et al. showed no difference in *U. urealyticum* colonization of the cervix in fertile or infertile patients, but did show a difference in endometrial colonization (27% to 50% in infertility patients and only 6% to 7% in fertile patients). However, when cervical contamination was prevented, Cassell et al. showed no difference in endometrial colonization in the two groups. In fact, they were only able to find one specific subpopulation of infertile patients in which *Ureaplasma* was isolated more frequently, namely, that group of women identified with infertility on the basis of a male factor. This subpopulation isolated *Ureaplasma* more than twice that in all other infertile groups, and also more than twice that in the fertile controls. At the present time, available studies are unable to show any direct correlation between *Ureaplasma* colonization and infertility on the basis of the female factor alone.

The effect of *U. urealyticum* on spermatogenesis and sperm motility have been well studied by Fowlkes and others, and it appears that there is definitely a decrease in sperm motility. Appropriate treatment will almost always show improvement in motility. However, what effect this has on fertility is somewhat unclear. Toth et al. studied the follow-up of 161 couples seen in their infertility unit with positive *Mycoplasma* cultures in seminal fluid. All couples were treated appropriately with doxycycline. Of 129 men treated successfully (follow-up culture negative), the three-year rate of successful pregnancies was 60%. Of 32 men with persistently positive cultures, the three-year rate of successful pregnancies was only 5%. There were obviously multiple causes of infertility in all the couples studied, but this does lead one to believe that *Mycoplasma* is a contributory factor to infertility (with its primary effect on male infertility). To date, only two studies have been done in a double-blind, randomized, controlled fashion looking at outcome after treatment with doxycycline. Harrison's study showed no effect on the rate of conception in the doxycycline-treated population with *Mycoplasma* infection as compared to controls. This is in contrast to the study by Hinton et al., which did show a difference in the two groups. These conflicting reports are, in part, due to the small numbers involved, and possibly from the lack of follow-up cultures obtained. We currently do *Mycoplasma* cultures of both partners in cases of habitual abortion and in unexplained infertility. There is no role for the empiric treatment with doxycycline in all couples presenting with infertility.

Chlamydia trachomatis has been shown to be a major pathogen in acute salpingitis. Both Scandinavian and U.S. studies show at least 20% of acute salpingitis cases associated with chlamydial infection. Attempts have been made to isolate *C. trachomatis* in infertility patients and identify it as a marker for asymptomatic tubal disease. Moore et al. performed serologic testing of *C. trachomatis* antibodies in fertility patients and found that 73% of women with tubal obstruction and 21% with peritubal adhesions had antibodies present.

Jones et al. repeated similar testing and found a small population of patients without any history of pelvic infection, with elevated antichlamydial antibodies, and subsequent evidence of tubal factor as the cause for their infertility.

From a practical point of view, we currently do *Chlamydia* cultures in both partners only in the setting of unexplained infertility (and even here, all patients have had or will have laparoscopy performed) and in patients with a question of a chronic salpingitis, in order to initiate antibiotic treatment.

THE ADRENAL FACTORS

Certain disorders of the adrenal may lead to oligo-ovulation, anovulation, amenorrhea, and infertility. Adrenal insufficiency, however, does not interfere with menstrual function. The most common type of disorder, congenital adrenogenital syndrome, is discussed in Chapter 13 ("Endocrine Disorders"). Hyperfunction of the adrenal cortex associated with either Cushing's syndrome or adrenogenital syndrome, may produce irregular menses and infertility. Cushing's syndrome is characterized by an overproduction of glucocorticoids and may be due to either bilateral adrenal hyperplasia, adenoma of the adrenal gland, adrenal carcinoma, or a nonadrenal tumor. Cushing's syndrome is also discussed in Chapter 13.

But there are many patients who have an intermediate degree of adrenal abnormality who do not have Cushing's syndrome, or a virilizing adrenal tumor, or adrenogenital syndrome. They are neither virilized nor obese. As a matter of fact, they appear to be normal individuals. Some patients may have a variant of the Stein-Leventhal syndrome; others may have slight degrees of adrenal hyperplasia. But they are infertile, and the infertility is usually due to irregular, or totally absent, ovulation. The endocrine survey reveals only two abnormalities: (1) a slight elevation in the DHEA-S level, and (2) a deficiency in the midcycle burst of LH. The precise mechanism by which the hypothalamus fails to elaborate LH-releasing factor is unknown, but the disturbed physiologic mechanism is corrected by the administration of hydrocortisone in a dose of 10 mg, three times daily. If the patient subsequently ovulates and becomes pregnant it is important that the hydrocortisone be continued until fetal organ development is complete. A recurrence of the elevated androgen levels could produce masculinization of the external genitalia of a female fetus.

The diagnosis of this "gray-zone" adrenal hyperactivity may be aided by testing with metyrapone, an 11β-hydroxylase inhibitor, since this compound causes an excessive increase in 17-ketosteroids and pregnanetriol in urinary assays of patients with this disorder. A similar variation has been described in a few patients who noted irregular menses, slight virilization, and infertility. Although the DHEA-S level is elevated, the patients do not have Cushing's syndrome. Chromatographic fractionation of the 17-hydroxysteroids showed that the elevation is due to deoxycortisol. This finding led to the diagnosis of an 11β-hydroxylase deficiency producing this type of the adrenogenital syndrome.

THE THYROID FACTOR

Thyroid hormone has a narrow but specific application in the management of anovulation and subsequent infertility. Overt hypothyroidism may cause lack of ovulation and amenorrhea in the female and inadequate spermatogenesis in the male. Untreated thyrotoxicosis is associated with excessive fetal loss. These facts are well documented and therapy is available to restore normality to these processes. But the "thyroid myth" persists, perhaps because it was the first hormone to be used in the treatment of irregular menses and infertility. Because of its seniority, therefore, clinicians have been loath to discard this medication.

Testimonials for the efficacy of thyroid extract in the management of every phase of reproductive behavior are quite easy to obtain—mostly on the basis of uncritical clinical experience, not from carefully controlled and properly designed experiments. Its magic has been extolled for the stimulation of sexual activity, improvement of fertility, prevention of habitual abortion, and the reduction of pregnancy complications.

Both hypothyroidism and thyrotoxicosis may be associated with abnormalities in sexual interest and activity. In myxedema, diminished sex interest and impotence have been noted. Undoubtedly this is related to the effect of thyroid dysfunction on the secretion, metabolism, and end-organ responsiveness of gonadal steroids. But this should be evaluated in the light of the old cliché that 10% of libido is derived from structures below the level of the sella turcica and 90% arises above this area. Despite the extensive derangement in ovarian steroidal patterns in myxedema, the diminished sexual activity is probably more often due to lack of vigor, tiredness, and apathy.

Sexual activity is altered more profoundly in thyrotoxicosis than in myxedema, and while increased libido has been reported in this disease, the extreme degree of mental and physical exhaustion frequently causes complete lack of sexual interest. From the therapeutic aspect, the clinician may assure the patient that those abnormalities in sexual behavior that are due to thyroid dysfunction will be corrected when a euthyroid state is effected. But those disturbances in sexual patterns that are brought about by emotional conflict will remain, and will necessitate specific treatment.

Thyroid deficiency may be classified into three distinct syndromes: (1) myxedema, (2) hypothyroidism, and (3) pituitary myxedema. Impaired ovulation, irregular menstruation, and infertility are frequently associated with both myxedema and hypothyroidism. In pituitary myxedema the absence of other trophic hormones regulating the adrenal and ovary accounts for total amenorrhea and infertility. The establishment and continuation of pregnancy in the patient with myxedema are rare, and the reasons for the infertility are quite obvious. Only 17 documented cases of pregnancy in myxedema have been reported, one woman bearing six children during 15 years. In mildly hypothyroid patients, however, the anovular process is frequently interrupted by spontaneous ovulation and an occasional pregnancy. Present evidence suggests that in myxedema there is adequate formation and secretion of FSH but diminished or ineffective LH secretion. Most of these studies have utilized bioassay methods and when these patients are restudied using radioimmunoassay or gonadotropins, the basic inadequacy may be just the burst of LH needed at midcycle.

Hamolsky has summarized interrelationships as follows:

1. Thyroid hormone has a direct action on gonadal function, either:
   a. On specific biochemical mechanisms within the ovary or testis.
   b. Via a fundamental energy-controlling process in all tissues, or
   c. By indirect modulation of gonadal sensitivity to FSH and LH.
2. Thyroid-releasing hormone (TRH) stimulates the release of prolactin, and in cases of moderate to severe hypothyroidism, can lead to hyperprolactinemia and anovulation.
3. Thyroid exercises an indirect effect on the gonads via a stimulatory or inhibitory effect on hypothalamic releasing factors.
4. Thyroid has an indirect effect on gonadal function by way of alterations produced in the adrenals.
5. The gonads have a primary role in determining thyroid function.

Feldman has explained the conflicting reports that (1) ovarian hormones depress thyroid function, (2) ovarian hormones increase thyroid activity, and (3) estrogens can both stimulate and depress thyroid function. Apparently estrogen has all of these functions, the ultimate effect depending on the dose of estrogen and its length of administration.

The controversial aspect of the thyroid problem as it relates to infertility centers on the diagnosis and treatment of an entity that may or may not exist. The syndrome is known as "subclinical hypothyroidism" and the diagnosis implies a mild but measurable degree of thyroid insufficiency that even protagonists are unable to demonstrate by objective criteria. If a patient is infertile or has irregular menses and all parameters of thyroid function are normal, the clinician may still give a "small amount of thyroid" and even a "small amount of estrogen." Should pregnancy ensue, the conclusion is obvious. The patient has "subclinical hypothyroidism" and even subclinical hypoestrinism." Such concepts persist and no amount of logical or scientific information will change them. Needless to

say, I do not advise treatment of the euthyroid patient in small, large, or intermediate doses of thyroid replacement.

Therapy for thyroid dysfunction will be discussed in Chapter 11 ("Habitual Abortion"). It should be remembered, however, that the normally functioning thyroid gland secretes daily the calorigenic equivalent of about 120 to 180 mg of a potent preparation of desiccated thyroid. Therefore, in the absence of significant endogenous thyroid secretions, this is the usual maintenance dose. If this dosage does not correct fully all the signs and symptoms attributable to thyroid insufficiency, other causes of the symptoms should be sought. In patients with pituitary myxedema, it is imperative that the adrenal insufficiency be corrected before beginning treatment with thyroid extract. Not to do so might precipitate fatal adrenal insufficiency.

BIBLIOGRAPHY

General Considerations

Behrman S.J., et al.: ABO (H) blood incompatibility as a cause of infertility. *Am. J. Obstet. Gynecol.* 79:847, 1960.

Bergman P.: Treatment of sterility of intrauterine origin. *Clin. Obstet. Gynecol.* 2:852, 1959.

Buxton C.L., Herrman W.: Induction of ovulation in the human with human gonadotropins. *Am. J. Obstet. Gynecol.* 81:584, 1961.

Buxton C.L., Mastroianni L.: Evaluation of tubal function. *Fertil. Steril.* 8:561, 1957.

Buxton C.L., Southam A.L.: *Human Infertility.* New York, Paul B. Hoeber, Inc., 1958.

Buxton C.L., Kase N., Van Orden D.: Effect of human FSH and HCG on the anovulatory ovary. *Am. J. Obstet. Gynecol.* 87:773, 1963.

Charny C.W., Wolgin W.: *Cryptorchism.* New York, Paul B. Hoeber, Inc., 1957, pp. 78, 124.

Davajan V., Kunitake G.M.: Fractional in vivo or in vitro examination of postcoital cervical mucus in the human. *Fertil. Steril.* 20:197, 1969.

Davajan V., Nakamura R.M.: The cervical factor, in Behrman S.J., Kistner R.W. (eds.): *Progress in Infertility*, ed. 2. Boston, Little Brown & Co., 1975.

Federation CECOS, Schwartz D., Mayanx M.J.: Female fecundity as a function of age. *N. Engl. J. Med.* 306:404, 1982.

Getzoff P.L.: Principles of management of the in-

fertile male. *Clin. Obstet. Gynecol.* 2:752, 1959.

Grant A.: Evaluation of the tubal factor in infertility. *Clin. Obstet. Gynecol.* 2:777, 1959.

Grant A.: The Fred A. Simmons Memorial Address: Experience, experiment and error in sterility. *Fertil. Steril.* 11:1, 1960.

Greenblatt R.B., et al.: Induction of ovulation with MRL-41. *J.A.M.A.* 178, 101, 1961.

Hamolsky M.: Thyroid factors, in Behrman S.J., Kistner R.W. (eds.): *Progress in Infertility*, ed. 2. Boston, Little Brown & Co., 1975.

Horne H.W., Hertig A.T., Kundsin R.B., et al.: Sub-clinical endometrial inflammation. T-mycoplasma: A possible cause of human reproductive failure. *Int. J. Fertil.* 18:226, 1973.

Horne H.W., Clyman M., Debrovner C., et al.: The prevention of postoperative pelvic adhesions following conservative operative treatment for human infertility. *Int. J. Fertil.* 18:109, 1973.

Jefferies W.M.: Further experience with small doses of cortisone and related steroids in infertility associated with ovarian dysfunction. *Fertil. Steril.* 11:100, 1960.

Jones H.L. Jr., Baramki T.A.: Congenital anomalies, in Behrman S.J., Kistner R.W. (eds.): *Progress in Infertility*, ed. 2. Boston, Little Brown & Co., 1975.

Kelly J.V., Rock J.: Culdoscopy for diagnosis in infertility. *Am. J. Obstet. Gynecol.* 72;523, 1956.

Kistner R.W.: Endometriosis and infertility. *Clin. Obstet. Gynecol.* 2:877, 1959.

Kistner R.W.: Infertility with endometriosis: A plan of therapy. *Fertil. Steril.* 13:237, 1962.

Kistner R.W., Smith O.W.: Observations on the use of a non-steroidal estrogen antagonist: MER-25. *Surg. Forum* 10:725, 1959; *Fertil. Steril.* 12:121, 1961.

Kistner R.W., Patton G.W.: *Atlas of Infertility Surgery.* Boston, Little Brown & Co., 1975.

Kundsin R.B., Driscoll S.G.: Mycoplasmas and human reproductive failure. *Surg. Gynecol. Obstet.* 131:89, 1970.

Kundsin R.B., Driscoll S.G., Ming P.L.: Strain of *Mycoplasma* associated with human reproductive failure. *Science* 157:1573, 1967.

Kunitake G.M., Davajan V.: A new method of evaluating infertility due to cervical mucus-spermatozoa incompatibility. *Fertil. Steril.* 21:706, 1970.

Kupperman H.S.: Treatment of endocrine causes of sterility in the female. *Clin. Obstet. Gynecol.* 2:808, 1959.

Leventhal J.M.: The place of culdoscopy and laparoscopy in diagnosis and patient management, in Reid D.E., Christian D.W. (eds.): *Controversies in Obstetrics and Gynecology.* Philadelphia, W.B. Saunders Co., 1974.

McElin T.W., Danforth D.N., Young I.J.: Study of infertility in the private practice of obstetrics and gynecology. *Fertil. Steril.* 11:135, 1960.

MacLeod J., Gold R.Z.: The male factor in fertility and infertility: VIII. A study of variation in semen quality. *Fertil. Steril.* 7:387, 1956.

MacLeod J., Gold R.Z.: An analysis of human male infertility. *Int. J. Fertil.* 3:382, 1958.

Moore-White M.: Evaluation of tubal plastic operations. *Int. J. Fertil.* 5:237, 1960.

Moyer D.L.: Endometrial diseases in infertility, in Behrman S.J., Kistner R.W. (eds): *Progress in Infertility,* ed. 2. Boston, Little Brown & Co., 1975.

Noyes R.W.: Uniformity of secretory endometrium. *Fertil. Steril.* 7:103, 1956.

Noyes R.W., Hertig A.T., Rock J.: Dating the endometrial biopsy. *Fertil. Steril.* 1:3, 1950.

O'Brien J.R., Arronet G.H.: Operative treatment of fallopian tube pathology in human infertility. *Am. J. Obstet. Gynecol.* 103:520, 1969.

Parekh M.C., Arronet G.H.: Diagnostic procedures and methods in the assessment of female pelvic organs, with special reference to infertility. *Clin. Obstet. Gynecol.* 15:1, 1972.

Patton G.W., Kistner R.W.: Surgical reconstruction of the oviduct, in Behrman S.J., Kistner R.W. (eds.): *Progress in Infertility,* ed. 2. Boston, Little Brown & Co., 1975.

Raymont A., Arronet G.H., Arrata W.S.M.: Review of 500 cases of infertility. *Int. J. Fertil.* 14:141, 1969.

Riva H.L., Hatch R.B., Breen J.L.: Culdoscopy for infertility: An analysis of 203 cases. *Am. J. Obstet. Gynecol.* 78:1304, 1959.

Rubin I.C., *Uterotubal Insufflation.* St. Louis, C.V. Mosby Co., 1947.

Schneeberg N.G.: The thyroid gland and infertility. *Clin. Obstet. Gynecol.* 2:826, 1959.

Siegler A.M.: *Hysterosalpingography.* New York, Harper & Row, 1967.

Siegler A.M.: Dangers of hysterosalpingography. *Obstet. Gynecol. Surv.* 22:284, 1967.

Siegler A.M., Perez R.J.: Reconstruction of fallopian tubes in previously sterilized patients. *Fertil. Steril.* 26:383, 1975.

Siegler A.M., Hellman L.M.: Tubal plastic surgery: Report of a survey. *Fertil. Steril.* 7:170, 1956.

Southam A.L.: Evaluation of cervical factors in infertility. *Clin. Obstet. Gynecol.* 2:763, 1959.

Southam A.L.: What to do with the "normal" infertile couple. *Fertil. Steril.* 11:543, 1960.

Southam A.L., Buxton L.: Seventy postcoital tests made during the conception cycle. *Fertil. Steril.* 7:133, 1956.

Stein I.F.: The management of bilateral polycystic ovaries. *Fertil. Steril.* 6:190, 1948.

Stein I.F., Leventhal M.L.: Amenorrhea associated with bilateral polycystic ovaries. *Am. J. Obstet. Gynecol.* 29:18, 1935.

Sweeney W.J.: Pitfalls in present day methods of evaluating tubal function: I. Tubal insufflation; II. Hysterosalpingography. *Fertil. Steril.* 13:124, 1962.

Tyler E.T.: The thyroid myth in infertility. *Fertil. Steril.* 4:218, 1953.

Tyler E.T.: *Sterility: Office Management of the Infertile Couple.* New York, McGraw-Hill Book Co., Inc., 1961.

Clinical Management

Charny C.W.: Clomiphene therapy in male infertility: A negative report. *Fertil. Steril.* 32:551, 1980.

El-Minawi M.F., et al.: Comparative evaluation of laparoscopy and hysterosalpingography in infertile patients. *Obstet. Gynecol.* 51:29, 1978.

March C.M., Israel R.: Hysteroscopic management of intrauterine adhesions. *Am. J. Obstet. Gynecol.* 130:653, 1978.

Nachtigall R.D., et al.: Artificial insemination of husband's sperm. *Fertil. Steril.* 32:141, 1979.

Overstreet J.W., et al.: Penetration of human spermatozoa into the human zona pellucida and the zona-free hamster egg: A study of fertile donors and infertile patients. *Fertil. Steril.* 32:41, 1979.

Rogers B.J., et al.: Analysis of human spermatozoal fertilizing ability using zona-free ova. *Fertil. Steril.* 32:556, 1979.

Segal S., et al.: Male hyperprolactinemia: Effects on fertility. *Fertil. Steril.* 32:556, 1979.

Segal S., et al.: Prolactin in seminal plasma of infertile men. *Arch. Androl.* 1:49, 1978.

Tyson J., et al.: Inhibition of cyclic gonadotropin secretion by endogenous human prolactin. *Am. J. Obstet. Gynecol.* 121:374, 1975.

The Uterine Factor

Malone M.J., Ingersoll F.M.: Myomectomy in infertility, in Behrman S.J., Kistner R.W. (eds.): *Progress in Infertility*, ed. 2. Boston, Little Brown & Co., 1975.

The Tubal Factor

Garcia C.R.: Surgical reconstruction of the oviduct in the infertile patient, in Behrman S.J., Kistner R.W. (eds.): *Progress in Infertility*. Boston, Little Brown & Co., 1968.

Green-Armitage V.B.: Tubouterine implantation. *Br. Med. J.* 1:1222, 1952, *Br. J. Obstet. Gynaecol.* 64:47, 1957.

Hanton E.M., Pratt J.H., Banner E.A.: Tubal plastic surgery at the Mayo Clinic. *Am. J. Obstet. Gynecol.* 89:934, 1964.

Hayashi M.: *Tubal Factor in Sterility*, proceedings of Third Asiatic Congress of Obstetrics and Gynecology, 1965, p. 361.

Horne H.W.: Conservative laparotomy for infertility: A five year follow-up. *Int. J. Fertil.* 9:391, 1964.

Malkin H.J.: Discussion on modern methods of salpingostomy. *Proc. R. Soc. Med.* 53:358, 1960.

Moore-White M.: Techniques of tubal plastic operations. *Ann. Ostet. Ginecol.* 81:90, 1959.

Moore-White M.: Evaluation of tubal plastic operations. *Int. J. Fertil.* 5:237, 1960.

Mutch M.G. Jr.: Sterility and tuboplasties: Critical analysis of 42 cases. *Fertil. Steril.* 10:240, 1959.

Palmer R.: Salpingostomy—a critical study of 396 personal cases operated upon without polythene tubing. *Proc. R. Soc. Med.* 53:357, 1960.

Replogle R.L., et al.: Studies on the prevention of postoperative intestinal adhesions. *Ann. Surg.* 163:580, 1966.

Shirodkar V.N.: *Contributions to Obstetrics and Gynecology*. Edinburgh, Livingstone, 1960, p. 65.

Shirodkar V.N.: Plastic surgery of fallopian tubes. *West. J. Surg.* 69:253, 1961.

Seitz H.M., et al.: Postoperative intraperitoneal adhesions: A double-blind assessment of their prevention in the monkey. *Fertil. Steril.* 24:935, 1973.

Siegler A.M.: Tubal plastic surgery, the past, the present and the future. *Obstet. Gynecol. Surv.* 15:680, 1960.

Siegler A.M.: Tuboplasty. *Clin. Obstet. Gynecol.* 5:820, 1962.

Siegler A.M., Hellman L.M.: Tubal plastic surgery: Report of a survey. *Fertil. Steril.* 7:170, 1956.

Swolin K.: Die Einwirkung von grossen, intraperitonealen dosen Glukokortikoid auf die bildung von postoperativen Adhasionen. *Acta Obstet. Gynecol. Scand.* 46:204, 1967.

Young P.E., Egan J.E., Barlow J.J., et al.: Reconstructive surgery for infertility at the Boston Hospital for Women. *Am. J. Obstet. Gynecol.* 108:1092, 1970.

The Ovarian Factor

Adashi E.Y., et al.: Fertility following bilateral ovarian wedge resection: A critical analysis of 90 consecutive cases of polycystic ovary syndrome. *Fertil. Steril.* 36:320, 1981.

Andrews W.C., Andrews M.C.: Stein-Leventhal syndrome with associated adenocarcinoma of the endometrium. *Am. J. Obstet. Gynecol.* 80:632, 1960.

Barbieri R.L., Ryan K.J.; Bromocriptine: Endocrine pharmacology and therapeutic applications. *Fertil. Steril.* 39:727, 1983.

Benedict P.H., et al.: Ovarian and adrenal morphology in cases of hirsutism or virilism and Stein-Leventhal syndrome. *Fertil. Steril.* 13:380, 1962.

Burghen G.A., et al.: Correlation of hyperandrogenism with hyperinsulinism in polycystic ovarian disease. *J. Clin. Endocrinol. Metab.* 50:113, 1980.

Buttram V.C., Vaquero C.: Post-ovarian wedge resection adhesive disease. *Fertil. Steril.* 26:874, 1975.

Charles D.: MRL-41 in treatment of secondary amenorrhea and endometrial hyperplasia. *Lancet* 2:278, 1962.

Charles D., Barr W., McEwan H.P.: The use of clomiphene in dysfunctional bleeding due to endometrial hyperplasia. *Br. J. Gynaecol.* 71:66, 1964.

Charles D., Loraine J.A., Bell E.T., et al.: The mechanism of action of clomiphene, in *Fertility and Sterility*, proceedings of Fifth World Congress on Fertility and Sterility, Stockholm, 1966. Amsterdam, Excerpta Medica, 1967, p. 92.

DeVane G.W., Czekala N.M., Judd H.L., et al.: Circulating gonadotropins, estrogens and androgens in polycystic ovarian disease. *Am. J. Obstet. Gynecol.* 121:496, 1975.

Dorfman R.I.: A review, steroid hormones in gynecology. *Obstet. Gynecol. Surv.* 18:65, 1963.

Evans T.N., Riley G.M.: Polycystic ovarian disease, a clinical and experimental study. *Am. J. Obstet. Gynecol.* 80:873, 1960.

Fechner R.E., Kaufman R.H.; Endometrial adenocarcinoma in Stein-Leventhal syndrome. *Cancer* 34:444, 1974.

Forchielli E., et al.: Testosterone in human plasma. *Anal. Biochem.* 5:416, 1963.

Gemzell C.A.: Multiple births following treatment with human gonadotropins, in *Fertility and Sterility*, proceedings of the Fifth World Congress on Fertility and Sterility, Stockholm, 1966. Amsterdam, Excerpta Medica, 1967, p. 92.

Gold J.J., Frank R.: The borderline adrenogenital syndrome: An intermediate entity. *Am. J. Obstet. Gynecol.* 75:1034, 1958.

Goldfarb A.F., Groll M., Rakoff A.E.: Experience in the induction of ovulation with sequential Clomid-menotropin therapy, in Rosenberg E. (ed.): *Gonadotropin in Female Infertility*, International Congress Series no. 226. Amsterdam, Excerpta Medica, 1974.

Goldzieher J.W.: Polycystic ovarian disease, in Marcus S.L., Marcus C.C. (eds.): *Advances in Obstetrics and Gynecology,* vol. 1. Baltimore, Williams & Wilkins Co., 1967.

Goldzieher J.W.: Polycystic ovarian disease, in Behrman S.J., Kistner R.W. (eds.): *Progress in Infertility*, ed. 2. Boston, Little Brown & Co., 1975.

Goldzieher J.W., Axelrod L.R.: Clinical and biochemical features of polycystic ovarian disease. *Fertil. Steril.* 14:631, 1963.

Goldzieher J.W., Axelrod L.R.: The polycystic ovary, in Rashad M.N., Morton W.R.M. (eds.): *The Genital System.* Springfield, Ill., Charles C Thomas, Publisher, 1966.

Goldzieher J.W., Axelrod L.R.: The polycystic ovary: II. Urinary steroid excretion. *J. Clin. Endocrinol. Metab.* 22:425, 1962.

Goldzieher J.W., Green J.A.: The polycystic ovary: I. Clinical and histological features. *J. Clin. Endocrinol. Metab.* 22:325, 1962.

Gorlitsky G.A., et al.: Ovulation and pregnancy rates with clomiphene citrate. *Obstet. Gynecol.* 51:265, 1978.

Greenblatt R.B.: The syndrome of large, pale ovaries and its differentiation from adrenogenital syndrome and Cushing's disease. *Postgrad. Med.* 9:492, 1951.

Greenblatt R.B.: The polycystic ovary syndrome. *Md. State Med. J.*, March 1961, p. 1.

Greenblatt R.B., Baldwin K.R.: The polycystic ovary syndrome (Stein-Leventhal syndrome). *J. Clin. Endocrinol. Metab.* 1:498, 1960.

Greenblatt R.B., Barfield W.E., Lampros C.T.: Cortisone in the treatment of infertility. *Fertil. Steril.* 7:203, 1956.

Greenblatt R.B., Barfield W.E., Jungck E.C., et al.: Induction of ovulation with MRL-41. *J.A.M.A.* 178:101, 1961.

Greenblatt R.B., Roy S., Mahesh V.B.: Induction of ovulation. *Am. J. Obstet. Gynecol.* 84:900, 1962.

Griffith R.W., et al.: Outcome of pregnancy in mothers given bromocriptine. *Br. J. Clin. Pharmacol.* 5:227, 1978.

Holtkamp D.E., Greslin J.G., Root C.A., et al.: Gonadotropin inhibiting and antifecundity effects of clomiphene. *Proc. Soc. Exp. Biol. Med.* 105:197, 1960.

Huang K.E.: The induction of ovulation in amenorrheic patients with synthetic luteinizing hormone-releasing hormone: The significance of pituitary responsiveness. *Fertil. Steril.* 27:65, 1976.

Huang K.E., et al.: Induction of ovulation with MRL-41. *J.A.M.A.* 178:101, 1961.

Ingersoll F.M., McArthur J.W.: Longitudinal studies of gonadotropin excretion in the Stein-Leventhal syndrome. *Am. J. Obstet. Gynecol.* 77:795, 1959.

Huang K.E., McDermott W.M. Jr.: Bilateral polycystic ovaries, Stein-Leventhal syndrome. *Am. J. Obstet. Gynecol.* 60:117, 1950.

Jackson R.L., Dockerty M.B.: The Stein-Leventhal syndrome: Analysis of 43 cases with special reference to association with endometrial carcinoma. *Am. J. Obstet. Gynecol.* 73:161, 1957.

Jeffries W.M.: Effect of small doses of cortisone upon urinary 17-ketosteroid fraction in patients with ovarian dysfunction. *J. Clin. Endocrinol. Metab.* 22:255, 1962.

Jewelewicz R.: Management of infertility resulting from anovulation. *Am. J. Obstet. Gynecol.* 122:909, 1975.

Johnson J.E. Jr.: Outcome of pregnancies following clomiphene citrate therapy, in *Fertility and Sterility*, Proceedings of Fifth World Congress on Fertility and Sterility, Stockholm, 1966. Amsterdam, Excerpta Medica, 1967, p. 101.

Jones H.W., Jones G.S.: Editors note. *Obstet. Gynecol. Surv.* 18:126, 1963.

Kahn C.R., et al.: The syndromes of insulin resistance and acanthosis nigricans. *N. Engl. J. Med.* 294:739, 1976.

Kase N.: Steroid synthesis in abnormal ovaries. III. Polycystic ovaries. *Am. J. Obstet. Gynecol.* 90:1268, 1964.

Kase N., Forchielli E., Dorfman R.I.: Biosynthesis of testosterone and androst-4-ene-3, 17-dione in patients with polycystic ovaries. *Acta Endocrinol.* 44:8, 1963.

Kase N., Kowal J., Perloff W., et al.: In vitro production of androgens by virilizing adrenal adenoma and associated polycystic ovaries. *Acta Endocrinol.* 44:15, 1963.

Kase N., Kowal J., Soffer L.J.: In vitro production of testosterone and androstenedione in normal and Stein-Leventhal ovaries. *Acta Endocrinol.* 44:8, 1963.

Kaufman R.M., Abbott J.P., Wall J.A.: The endometrium before and after wedge resection of the ovaries in the Stein-Leventhal syndrome. *Am. J. Obstet. Gynecol.* 77:1271, 1959.

Keettel W.C., Bradbury J.T., Stoddard F.J.: Observations on the polycystic ovary syndrome. *Am. J. Obstet. Gynecol.* 73:954, 1957.

Kistner R.W.: Further observations on the effects of clomiphene citrate (Clomid) in anovulatory females. *Am. J. Obstet. Gynecol.* 92:380, 1965.

Kistner R.W.: Induction of ovulation with clomiphene citrate (Clomid). *S. Afr. J. Obstet. Gynaecol.* 5:25, 1967.

Kistner R.W.: Induction of ovulation with clomiphene citrate, in Behrman S.J., Kistner R.W. (eds.): *Progress in Infertility*, ed. 2. Boston, Little Brown & Co., 1975.

Kistner R.W.: Peritubal and periovarian adhesions subsequent to wedge resection of the ovaries. *Fertil. Steril.* 20:35, 1969.

Kistner R.W.: Use of clomiphene citrate, human chorionic gonadotropin, and human menopausal gonadotropin for induction of ovulation in the human female. *Fertil. Steril.* 17:569, 1966.

Kistner R.W.: Sequential use of clomiphene citrate and human menopausal gonadotropin in ovulation induction. *Fertil. Steril.* 27:72, 1976.

Kistner R.W., Lewis J.L., Steiner G.J.: Effects of clomiphene citrate on endometrial hyperplasia in the premenopausal female. *Cancer* 19:115, 1966.

Kistner R.W., Smith O.W.: Observations of use of non-steroidal estrogen antagonist: MER 25. *Surg. Forum* 10:725, 1960.

Kistner R.W., Smith O.W.: Observations on use of non-steroidal estrogen antagonist: MER 25. II. Effects in endometrial hyperplasia and Stein-Leventhal syndrome. *Fertil. Steril.* 12:121, 1961.

Lanthier A.: Urinary 17-ketosteroids in the syndrome of polycystic ovaries and hyperthecosis. *J. Clin. Endocrinol. Metab.* 20:1587, 1960.

Lanthier A., Sandor T.: The urinary excretion of pregnanediol and pregnanetriol in the polycystic ovary (Stein-Leventhal) syndrome. *Acta Endocrinol.* 46:245, 1964.

Lerner L.J., Holthaus F.J., Thomson C.R.: A nonsteroidal estrogen antagonist 1-(p-2-diethylaminoethoxy-phenyl)-1-phenyl-2-p-methoxy-phenyl ethanol. *Endocrinology* 63:295, 1958.

Leventhal M.L.: Functional and morphologic studies of the ovaries and suprarenal glands in the Stein-Leventhal syndrome. *Am. J. Obstet. Gynecol.* 84:154, 1962.

Lloyd C.W., Weisz J.: Hypothalamus and anterior pituitary, in Behrman S.J., Kistner R.W. (eds.): *Progress in Infertility*. Boston, Little Brown & Co., 1968.

McArthur J.W., Ingersoll F.M., Worcester J.: The urinary excretion of interstitial cell and follicle stimulating hormone activity by women with diseases of the reproductive system. *J. Clin. Endocrinol. Metab.* 18:1202, 1958.

McNatty K., et al.: A possible role of prolactin in control of steroid secretion by the human graafian follicle. *Nature* 250:653, 1974.

Mahesh V.B., Greenblatt R.B.: Isolation of dehydroepiandrosterone and 17-alpha-hydroxy-delta-^{5}-pregnenolone from the polycystic ovaries of the Stein-Leventhal syndrome. *J. Clin. Endocrinol. Metab.* 22:441, 1962.

Mahesh V.B., Greenblatt R.B.: Secretion of androgens by the polycystic ovary and its significance. *Fertil. Steril.* 13:513, 1962.

Mahesh V.B., Greenblatt R.B.: Steroid secretions of the normal and polycystic ovary. *Recent Prog. Horm. Res.* 20:341, 1964.

March C.M., Treadway D.R., Mishell D.R.: Effect of pretreatment with clomiphene citrate upon human menopausal gonadotropin therapy for anovulation. *Fertil. Steril.* 26:191, 1975.

Marshall J.R.: Human menopausal gonadotropin, in Behrman S.J., Kistner R.W. (eds.): *Progress in Infertility*, ed. 2. Boston, Little Brown & Co., 1975.

Mellinger R.C., Thompson R.J., Mansour J.A.: Pituitary-gonadal stimulating effect of clomiphene. *Clin. Res.* 11:224, 1963.

Mishell D.R.: Daily immunoassay of luteinizing hormone excretion in patients receiving clomiphene citrate. *Fertil. Steril.* 18:102, 1967.

Naville A.H., Kistner R.W., Wheatley E.R., et al.: Induction of ovulation with clomiphene citrate. *Fertil. Steril.* 15:290, 1964.

Parkes D.: Bromocriptine. *N. Engl. J. Med.* 301:873, 1979.

Paulsen C.A.: Biologic activities of synthetic progestins and a new nonsteroidal compound, in Goldfarb A.F. (ed.): *Advances in the Treatment of Menstrual Dysfunction*. Philadelphia, Lea & Febiger, 1964, p. 55.

Riley G.M., Evans T.N.: Effects of clomiphene citrate on anovulatory function. *Am. J. Obstet. Gynecol.* 89:97, 1964.

Roy S., Greenblatt R.B., Mahesh V.B., et al.: Clomiphene citrate: Further observations on its use in the induction of ovulation in the human and on its mode of action. *Fertil. Steril.* 14:575, 1963.

Rust L.A., Israel R., Mishell D.R.: An individualized graduated therapeutic regimen for clomiphene citrate. *Am. J. Obstet. Gynecol.* 120:785, 1974.

Ryan K.J.: Biological aromatization of steroids. *J. Biol. Chem.* 234:268, 1959.

Ryan K.J., Smith O.W.: Biogenesis of estrogens by human ovary: I. Conversion of acetate-1-C-14 to estrone and estradiol. *J. Biol. Chem.* 236:705, 1961.

Scott R.B., Wharton L.R.: Effect of testosterone on experimental endometriosis in Rhesus monkeys. *Am. J. Obstet. Gynecol.* 78:1020, 1959.

Shearman R.P.: The enigmatic polycystic ovary. *Obstet. Gynecol. Surv.* 21:1, 1966.

Shearman R.P.: Induction of ovulation. *Australas. Ann. Med.* 15:266, 1966.

Shearman R.P., Cox R.I.: Clinical and chemical correlations in the Stein-Leventhal syndrome. *Am. J. Obstet. Gynecol.* 92:747, 1965.

Shearman R.P., Cox R.I.: The enigmatic polycystic ovary. *Obstet. Gynecol. Surv.* 21:1, 1966.

Shearman R.P., Cox R.I., Gannon A.; Urinary pregnanetriolone in the diagnosis of Stein-Leventhal syndrome. *Lancet* 1:260, 1961.

Short R.V.: Further observations on the defective synthesis of ovarian steroids in the Stein-Leventhal syndrome. *J. Endocrinol.* 24:359, 1962.

Short R.V., London D.R.: Defective biosynthesis of ovarian steroids in the Stein-Leventhal syndrome. *Br. Med. J.* 5241:1724, 1961.

Smith O.W.: Chemical induction of ovulation. *J.A.M.A.* 179:99, 1962.

Smith O.W., Day C.F.: Effect of clomiphene on aromatization of steroids by the human placenta in vitro. *Acta Endocrinol.* 44:519, 1963.

Smith O.W., Ryan K.J.: Estrogen in the human ovary. *Am. J. Obstet. Gynecol.* 84:141, 1962.

Smith O.W., Smith G.V., Kistner R.W.: Action of MER-25 and clomiphene on the human ovary. *J.A.M.A.* 184:878, 1963.

Smith O.W., Smith G.V., Kistner R.W.: Action of gonadotropin (ICSH)-inhibiting substance in Stein-Leventhal syndrome. *J. Clin. Endocrinol. Metab.* 24:656, 1964.

Sohval A.R., Soffer L.J.: The influence of cortisone and adrenocorticotropin in urinary gonadotropin excretion. *J. Clin. Endocrinol. Metab.* 11:677, 1951.

Sommers S.C.: Pituitary cell relations to body states. *Lab. Invest.* 8:588, 1959.

Sommers S.C., Meissner W.A.: Endocrine abnormalities accompanying human endometrial cancer. *Cancer* 10:516, 1957.

Sommers S.C., Wadman P.J.: Pathogenesis of polycystic ovaries. *Am. J. Obstet. Gynecol.* 72:160, 1956.

Southam A.L., Janovski N.A.: Massive ovarian hyperstimulation with clomiphene citrate. *J.A.M.A.* 181:443, 1962.

Stein I.F.: The Stein-Leventhal syndrome: A curable form of sterility. *N. Engl. J. Med.* 259:420, 1958.

Stein I.F., Leventhal M.L.: Amenorrhea associated with bilateral polycystic ovaries. *Am. J. Obstet. Gynecol.* 29:181, 1935.

Taymor M.L., Barnard R.: Luteinizing hormone excretion in polycystic ovary syndrome. *Fertil. Steril.* 13:501, 1962.

Taymor M.L., Berger M.J., Nademberg F.: The combined use of clomiphene citrate and human menopausal gonadotropin in ovulation induction, in *Fertility and Sterility*, proceedings of Seventh World Congress on Fertility and Sterility. International Congress Series no. 278. Amsterdam, Excerpta Medica, 1973.

Taymor M.L., Clark B.J., Sturgis S.H.: The polycystic ovary: A clinical and laboratory study. *Am. J. Obstet. Gynecol.* 86:188, 1963.

Townsend S.L., Brown J.B., Johnstone J.W., et al.: Induction of ovulation. *Br. J. Obstet. Gynaecol.* 73:529, 1966.

Tyler E.T., Winer J., Gotlib M., et al.: Effects of MRL-41 in human male and female fertility studies. *Clin. Res.* 10:119, 1962.

Vorys N., Gantt C.L., Hamwi G.J., et al.: Clinical utility of chemical induction of ovulation. *Am. J. Obstet. Gynecol.* 88:425, 1964.

Warren J.C., Salhanick H.A.: Steroid biosynthesis in the human ovary. *J. Clin. Endocrinol. Metab.* 21:1218, 1961.

The Immunologic Factor

Beer A.E., Neaves W.B.: Antigenic status of semen from the viewpoints of the female and male. *Fertil. Steril.* 29:3, 1978.

Franklin R.R., Dukes C.D.: Antispermatozoal antibody and unexplained infertility. *Am. J. Obstet. Gynecol.* 89:6, 1964.

Haas G.G., et al.: Immunologic infertility: Identification of patients with antisperm antibody. *N. Engl. J. Med.* 303:722, 1980.

Isojima S., et al.: Immunologic analysis of sperm immobilizing factor found in sera of women with unexplained sterility. *Am. J. Obstet. Gynecol.* 101:677, 1968.

Kibrick S., et al.; Methods for the detection of antibodies against mammalian spermatozoa. *Fertil. Steril.* 3:430, 1952.

Shulman S., et al.: Immune infertility and new approaches to treatment. *Fertil. Steril.* 29:309, 1978.

Shulman J.F., Shulman S.: Methyl-prednisolone treatment of immunologic infertility in the male. *Fertil. Steril.* 38:591, 1982.

Mycoplasma *and* Chlamydia

Cassell G.H., et al.: Microbiologic study of infertile women at the time of diagnostic laparoscopy. *N. Engl. J. Med.* 308:502, 1983.

Cassell G.H., Cole B.C.: Mycoplasmas as agents of human disease. *N. Engl. J. Med.* 304:80, 1981.

Fowlkes D.M., et al.: T-mycoplasmas and human infertility: Correlation of infection with alterations in seminal parameters. *Fertil. Steril.* 26:1212, 1975.

Harrison R.F., et al.: Doxycycline treatment and human infertility. *Lancet* 1:605, 1975.

Hinton R.A., et al.: A double-blind cross-over study of the effect of doxycycline on mycoplasma infection and infertility. *Br. J. Obstet. Gynecol.* 86:379, 1979.

Jones R.B., et al.: Correlation between serum antichlamydial antibodies and tubal factor as a cause of infertility. *Fertil. Steril.* 38:553, 1982.

Mardh P.A., et al.: *Chlamydia trachomatis* infections in patients with salpingitis. *N. Engl. J. Med.* 296:1377, 1977.

Moore D.F., et al.: Increased frequency of serum antibodies to *Chlamydia trachomatis* in infertility due to distal tubal disease. *Lancet* 2:574, 1982.

Taylor-Robinson D., McCormick W.M.: The genital mycoplasmas. *N. Engl. J. Med.* 302:1003, 1063, 1980.

Toth A., et al.: Subsequent pregnancies among 161 couples treated for T-mycoplasma genital-tract infection. *N. Engl. J. Med.* 308:505, 1983.

CHAPTER ELEVEN

Habitual Abortion

VERONICA A. RAVNIKAR, M.D.

HABITUAL ABORTION is usually defined as a sequence of three or more consecutive failures of pregnancy prior to the 28th week of gestation. In order to encompass all of the studies that have attempted to define the etiologies for habitual miscarriage in this chapter, this definition should be broadened to include women who have had term births, especially stillbirths or anomalous live infants, and/or two consecutive spontaneous miscarriages.

In this chapter, attention will first be given to causes of abortion intrinsic to the developing fetus itself, that is, genetic abnormalities that result in pathologic ova. In fact, it must be emphasized that chromosomal aberrations either in the aborters or the abortuses remain the only proved cause for spontaneous fetal loss. A description of factors exogenous to the fetus will also be given. For example, the hormonal, anatomic, environmental, and immunologic factors that may cause abortion will be analyzed. Since many of these factors have not themselves been tested in a double-blind, randomized fashion to prove a causative relationship to abortions, we must be careful in the interpretation of some of these newer speculations. However, abnormalities of the environment or intrinsic hormonal aberrations may reasonably result in pathologic ova or in abnormal endomyometrial function. Therefore, there is justification in looking at all of the diverse causes of miscarriage that we have been able to decipher to date.

GENERAL INCIDENCE

Preclinical Losses

To establish the true incidence of preclinical pregnancy losses in humans is extremely difficult. A preclinical pregnancy loss is one that occurs prior to the actual missed menstrual period.

A classic study performed by Hertig et al. in 1959 described morphologic abnormalities in the preimplantation embryo. Thirty-four fertilized human ova were recovered during the first 17 days of development from 210 women who had proved fertility and who were considered optimal for the probability of early conception. On histologic analysis, only 24 of the 34 eggs were considered normal. The remaining ten showed growth disorganization. An analysis of the data according to times postovulation (deduced by basal body temperature charts and coital times) revealed the greatest ovular loss occurred prior to day 20 of the menstrual cycle—the preimplantation stage.

More recently, Jones and the Norfolk In Vitro Fertilization Group compared their statistics for early pregnancy loss to that which occurs in natural fertilization. In 190 consecutive cycles, a 33% preclinical and clinical abortion rate was detected, which was lower than that reported by others. They, however, were all Pergonal-human chorionic gonadotropin (HCG) cycles with multiple egg transfers. Assays of β-HCG were used to monitor

467

losses when they became clinically accurate (which is ten days after conception). They hypothesized that multiple egg transfers and the actual techniques of in vitro fertilization preselect against bad embryos. In Melbourne, Australia Lopata et al., 1983, in an analysis of their 1982 in vitro data, found that 655 fertilized ova transferred into 272 patients yielded only 55 pregnancies with 30 ongoing. How much of this fetal wastage is true embryo loss or in vitro technique is a major question. However, with the availability of in vitro fertilization today we may better be able to study the factors due to nature with genetic probes (i.e., cytogenetic defects) or those due to nurture (i.e., endogenous maternal endocrinologic problems or environmental influences) that account for these early preclinical pregnancy losses.

Determining β-HCG levels can only detect postimplantation, preclinical pregnancy losses (occurring ten days after conception onward) (Batzer, 1980). Secretory trophoblast is necessary for the production of HCG. Measuring β-subunit HCG assays in cycles of normal women or a population of infertile women demonstrates the high incidence of subclinical abortions (Edmonds et al., 1982; Chartier et al., 1979). An estimate of 61.9% of the concepti detected by β-subunit HCG assays in 207 cycles were lost prior to 12 weeks and the majority of these losses occurred without the mother's knowledge. This is not unlike the data from in vitro programs.

A major area of current research is elaborating on other factors that may be detected in the maternal serum after conception but prior to implantation of the embryo. The study of serum relaxin (Quagliarello et al., 1981), progestogen-associated endometrial protein (Joshi et al., 1982), Schwanzgerschaftsprotein I (SPI), and pregnancy-associated plasma protein A (PAPP-A) (Masson et al., 1983), pregnancy zone protein (Damber et al., 1978) and early pregnancy factor (Rolfe, 1982; Smart et al., 1981) are being investigated for their specificity and sensitivity in detecting preclinical preimplantation losses.

In fact, the latter, early pregnancy factor has led to a number of studies that implicate it as the blocking factor that prevents maternal rejection of the fetal allograft. Its detection via an in vitro rosette inhibition assay requires standardization. Nevertheless, it is very specific in detecting pregnancy immediately after fertilization and it disappears immediately after a pregnancy becomes nonviable. This is in contrast to the need for implantation prior to the detection of HCG in the serum and its long half-life after the pregnancy actually is lost (up to two weeks) (Batzer, 1980).

Clinical Pregnancy Loss

A spontaneous miscarriage will present the following physical signs: severe pelvic cramping, bleeding, and the passage of clots and/or fetal tissue. On physical examination of such individuals, note should be made of vital signs, uterine size on bimanual examination (along with the presence or absence of any adnexal masses), and dilatation of the cervix with or without the presence of tissue at the os. A hematocrit reading and blood typing for ABO and Rh subgroups is required. The bleeding from the miscarriage may be profound, requiring transfusion. RhoGAM (Rh$_0$ [D] immune globulin [human]) should be administered in the Rh-negative mother. On further evaluation, note should be made of the passage of fetal tissue spontaneously and/or the presence of villi on the curetted specimen. An ectopic pregnancy can at times mask itself as a spontaneous miscarriage.

A spontaneous abortion may be further classified as complete or incomplete. In the latter case a dilatation and evacuation may be needed to remove the remaining tissue. A missed abortion is a pregnancy loss detected by the failure of appropriate uterine growth or fetal growth (by scan), an empty gestational sac (by scan), lack of fetal heart tones (by Doppler ultrasound or scan when appropriate).

A threatened abortion is one that presents with bleeding and cramping in the first half of pregnancy. Approximately half of these will abort.

In order to do chromosomal karyotyping on the fetal specimen it is important that the specimen is handled in a sterile fashion and placed in saline by the patient (if passed at home) or by the physician (after dilation and curettage of uterus). Ironically, it is the abnormal concepti that are macerated (especially after a missed abortion) that grow poorly in tissue culture. The advent of biopsies of the chorionic villi may in the future be helpful in detecting abnormal concepti. Once an abnormal pregnancy is identified or once a pregnancy is identified in a high-risk habitual aborter, a quick karyotypic analysis can be made (Cadkin and Sabbagha, 1980).

The routine biophysical and biochemical profile used to monitor pregnancies today is that of real-time ultrasonic imaging of the fetal crown-rump length, the gestational sac, and the fetal heart beat. The sac can be visualized by five to six weeks gestation (menstrual dates), and by eight weeks fetal echoes can be definitely determined within the sac. The absence of fetal echoes by seven to eight weeks gestational age is consistent with a blighted ovum. For an ultrasonic demonstration of a normal intrauterine fetus and a blighted ovum refer to Figures 11–1 and 11–2.

The majority of first-trimester abortuses are chromosomally abnormal (triploidy, etc.). Morphologically, the tissue recovered will either appear as a macerated fetus, an intact empty sac, or an empty sac with or without a cord stump. On ultrasonographic evaluation they appear as empty gestational sacs or fetuses with crown-rump lengths that lag behind the norm for the developmental stage. In defining the phenotypic expressions of triploidy in 40 spontaneous abortions (Harris et al., 1981), the following characteristics predominated on gross specimen analysis: cystic placental villi (short of molar degeneration), limb and facial developmental defects, and anachronistic development of retinal pigment. Therefore, it is advisable to detail the phenotype of such pregnancies via morphologic analysis and ultrasonography, since it may be difficult to determine the genotype of such specimens by conventional chromosomal analysis.

Serial trends in the patient's hormonal pro-

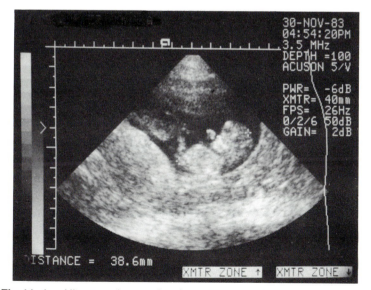

Fig 11–1.—Ultrasound scan showing a 10-week, 5-day-old intrauterine fetal gestation (crown-rump length, 38.6 mm; Acuson 128 imaging; 3-MHz transducer). (Courtesy of Dr. Beryl Benacerraf.)

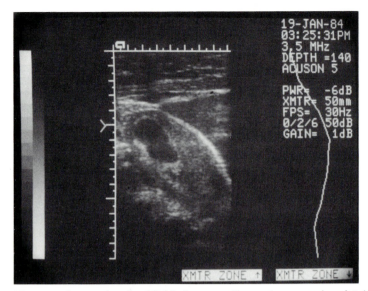

Fig 11–2.—Ultrasound scan showing blighted ovum with empty sac and no fetal heartbeat (Acuson 128 imaging; 3-MHz transducer). (Courtesy of Dr. Beryl Benacerraf.)

files can be evaluated. There is a predictable rise of HCG in the first trimester of pregnancy (Batzer, 1980; Chartier et al., 1979; Vaitukaitis et al., 1972; Saxena and Landesman, 1978; Lagrew et al., 1983). With knowledge of menstrual dating, serial low levels of HCG prior to the first 60 days of pregnancy may predict poor fetal outcome. The exponential linear rise in peripheral β-HCG titers detected by radioimmunoassay is depicted in Figure 11–3. A doubling time of HCG plasma concentration compatible with normal, early gestational growth has been reported as 1.4 to 2.0 days. The trend of serial HCG titers and plasma 17β-estradiol levels along with ultrasonographic imaging of the fetus provide the best assessment of fetal viability in early pregnancy (Jovanovic et al., 1978; Schweditsch et al., 1979). In the future, chorionic villi biopsies may also serve as an important clinical tool in determining the genotype of embryos in patients who have habitual miscarriage.

INCIDENCE OF SPONTANEOUS ABORTION

The incidence of spontaneous abortion and its recurrence risks have been analyzed both retrospectively and prospectively in large population studies. An evaluation of these statistics is mandatory since the more pessimistic the figures, the more optimistic any mode of therapy for spontaneous losses will appear.

In dealing with the recurrence frequency of clinically apparent abortions, Malpas in 1938 devised a mathematical model (later revised by Eastman) to estimate the risk of abortion recurrence after a prior miscarriage (or loss). A critique of these data was performed by Warburton and Fraser. According to Malpas, the risk of abortion with the first pregnancy was estimated as 18%; according to the mathematical model, the risk increased to 84% after three consecutive abortions. Warburton and Fraser point out that the initial incidence of 18% was derived from the abortion frequency in 11,430 pregnancies in 3,000 women compiled in 1929; it is not the true incidence of a first miscarriage. The risk of miscarriage for a recurrent cause was set at 1%, which is fallacious since different etiologies for miscarriage have different rates of recurrence.

Subsequently, Warburton and Fraser retrospectively studied 2,134 families in which every woman interviewed had at least one liv-

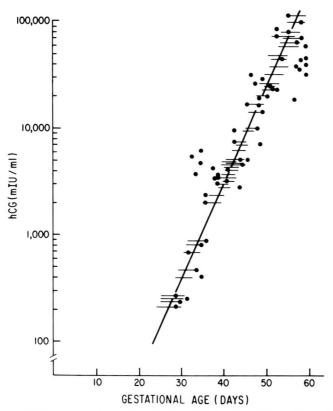

Fig 11–3.—Exponential increase in maternal serum human chorionic gonadotropin (HCG) concentrations during the first 60 days' gestation. Regression equation: Day of test = 5.073 Ln (HCG concentrations) − 0.1322, r^2 = .8263, F = 275.9, P<.0001. After 60 days' gestation, there is a wide individual variation in HCG values. (From Lagrew D., et al.: *Obstet. Gynecol.* 62:37–40, 1983.)

ing child. The abortion rate as a whole was 14.7% ± 0.4%. The subsequent rates were as follows: 12.3% with no history of previous miscarriage, 23.7% with one previous abortion, 26.2% with two previous losses, 32.2% with three, and 25.9% with four prior losses. In conclusion, a woman with one previous abortion has a 25% to 30% chance of aborting in each successive pregnancy providing she has had one live proband. These data may, therefore, not apply to women who have never had a living child.

Poland et al., in a prospective analysis of 472 patients and 638 pregnancies, determined a higher overall rate of 22.1% if there was no live proband. After one spontaneous abortion there was a 19% chance of recurrence; the rate increased to 47% after three spontaneous abortions. This work justifies an investigation for the cause of repetitive abortion after the second one, if there is no live proband.

Age and gravidity may have a role in abortion recurrence risk. Naylor and Warburton, in a retrospective analysis, determined a sizable increase in risk associated with maternal gravidity but not with age, which corroborated previous results. However, their sample size included few women over the age of 35 years.

Chromosomal studies from embryos from induced abortions in pregnant women aged 35 years and over show an increased risk of chromosomal anomalies in the abortal specimens (Tsuji and Nakano, 1978). Trisomy is the most frequent chromosomal anomaly found in abortal specimens, especially trisomy

16. There is an epidemiologic relationship between increased maternal age and trisomic abortuses. However, a woman who has an abortus with monosomy X is younger on the average (Stein, 1983) than a woman who has a live birth or a woman who has an abortion without an anomaly. This suggests an environmental determinant predisposing to such an anomaly.

The effect of maternal age on the incidence of abortion shows an increased risk of 23% at ages 30 to 34 years, increasing to 48% at ages 35 to 39 years. Paternal age does not appear to be a major factor in the risk of miscarriage with chromosomally abnormal abortuses. However, it has been implicated in inducing new dominant mutations (Freedman, 1981).

Increasing maternal age and a proximate history of previous abortion, especially without a live proband, are therefore the two main factors increasing the subsequent abortion risk in a female.

Neural tube defects are the only known multifactorial genetic disorders associated with recurrent abortion in maternal history. Anencephaly is the predominant feature and most of these infants are female. Abortion risk is not otherwise increased in mothers who have live-born infants with a wide variety of defects of a multifactorial nature (Warburton and Fraser, 1964).

A statistically significant association between ectopic pregnancies and prior spontaneous abortion has been implicated. However, a higher rate of chromosomal anomalies in the ectopic pregnancies beyond that expected for gestational age has not been demonstrated to date (Elias et al., 1981).

Previous induced abortions were thought to statistically increase the chance of subsequent pregnancy failure (Madore et al., 1981). These data were challenged by the results of a large series published from the Brigham and Women's Hospital. A review of 5,003 records of consecutive deliveries between 1975 and 1976 reported no increased risk for poor pregnancy outcome in women with a single prior induced abortion. However, offspring of secundigravida women with a proximate spontaneous abortion had an increased frequency of short gestations, low birth weights, low Apgar scores, and congenital malformations.

Jansen comprehensively analyzed the published series on pregnancies after infertility treatment. Ovulation induction with bromocriptine in hyperprolactinemic anovulation, artificial insemination with donor semen for azoospermia, and operation for endometriosis had an abortion incidence that approached the norm for the general population. Abortion incidences accompanying other modes of therapy were found to be higher. Induction of ovulation with Clomid (clomiphene) and Pergonal (human menopausal gonadotropin) is associated with a higher rate of miscarriage (19.3% and 22.7%, respectively). Artificial insemination with husband's semen and salpingostomy for distal tube occlusion were also associated with higher than normal abortion rates (24.3% and 26.7%). The reasons for such, presented by Jansen, may be postovulatory aging of the secondary oocyte, polyspermy, sperm selection at a normal tubal isthmus, and delayed or accelerated ovum transport due to pharmacologically induced steroid hormone levels that are in excess of the norm.

In conclusion, it is important to consider all of these factors in a patient's history when evaluating a couple for recurrent abortion (Table 11–1). A knowledge of these studies offers the appropriate incidence figures in counseling patients.

ETIOLOGIC FACTORS

Concepti tend to abort at the same developmental state in consecutive pregnancies (Poland et al., 1977). A conceptus in an early pregnancy loss is more likely to have a cytogenetic abnormality whereas a late abortion is generally due to maternal or environmental factors.

Cytogenetic Etiology

Karyotypic analysis of 1,498 abortuses of less than 12 weeks' gestation revealed 38.52%

TABLE 11–1.—EVALUATION PROCEDURE
FOR RECURRENT ABORTION

TABLE 11–1.—EVALUATION PROCEDURE
FOR RECURRENT ABORTION

Obstetric history
  No. of miscarriages
  Timing of events: first or second trimester
  Symptoms of miscarriage: cramping, bleeding, no
    symptoms
  Previous premature or anomalous births (especially
    anencephaly)
Gynecologic history
  Previous dilation and curettage procedures
  Previous missed abortion with infection
  Abnormal finding on pelvic examination (or further
    documentation): endometriosis, leiomyomas,
    uterine septum
  History of amenorrhea
  History of maternal DES exposure
  History of shortened luteal phase on basal body
    temperature recording
  History of infertility
  History of tubal surgery or use of ovulation inducing
    agents
Medical history
  Systemic lupus erythematosus
  Diabetes mellitus
  Alcohol and cigarette consumption
Abnormal family pedigree
  Possible müllerian defects
  Relatives with Down's syndrome, repeated
    miscarriage, etc.
Physical examination
  Size and shape of uterus
  Dilatation, laceration of cervix
  Stigmata of DES exposure
Diagnostic tests
  Karyotype of abortus
  Karyotype of parents
  Tubogram
  Mycoplasma cultures

to be normal and 61.48% to be abnormal. The most frequent aneuploid karyotype found was trisomy (52%) followed by monosomy (15.3%) (Boue et al., 1973). More specific staining techniques highlighting certain areas of the chromosomes (Q banding) can delineate deletions of chromosomal complements that can later be traced to a parental source for the structural rearrangement. A cytogenetic study of 27 spontaneous abortions analyzed by this technique revealed 59% with a chromosomal anomaly (McConnell and Carr, 1975). Trisomy was found in nine of 16; the chromosomes involved were no. 2, 8, 14, 16, and 22. The frequency of these different trisomic forms among abortuses is different from those

at birth. Trisomy 16 compromises nearly one third of all anomalies seen in every series, yet this malformation rarely proceeds to the stage of a recognizable embryo (Stein, 1983).

Presumably, sporadic problems during gametogenesis, namely, anaphase lag and nondisjunction during meiosis, are causative for the development of these abnormal embryos. However, a small percentage of these will be due to a parental carrier state of a cytogenetic abnormality. In fact, the incidence of significant chromosomal rearrangements is higher in persons with histories of repetitive miscarriage.

Khudr, in his review of the cytogenetics of habitual abortion until 1973, found an average overall incidence of parental balanced translocation carriers of 6.2%; the average for the population at large is less than 1%.

Structural chromosomal variations of the reciprocal (between metacentric or submetacentric chromosomes) or robertsonian (between acrocentric chromosomes) variety are found more frequently in the woman with a history of repetitive fetal wastage. In 24 of 41 women with translocations, 16 of the 24 were of the D/D variety. This has been corroborated by succeeding authors; 31.2% of 16 couples with habitual abortion had balanced translocations in the female partner (Tho et al., 1982; Heritage et al., 1978).

Tho et al. tabulated data for 110 couples with reproductive failure and found 17% to have chromosomal anomalies. They subclassified these as chromosomal variants and major chromosomal rearrangements. Chromosomal variants found in 13 couples (12%) resulted from duplication, deficiency, or pericentric inversion of heterochromatin. Major chromosomal rearrangements found in six (5.4%) of the couples included balanced chromosomal translocations and pericentric inversions involving a large chromosomal segment (the latter abnormality was associated with the poorest reproductive outcome). A pericentric inversion is one in which the centromere of the particular chromosome is involved. A paracentric inversion (one in which the inverted segment is within one arm of the chromosome) was recently reported in two generations of a couple with three consecutive abortions. It has also been suggested that the length of the Y chromosome may be related to reproductive performance (Khudr, 1974; Verma et al., 1983; Verp et al., 1983). Female sex chromosome mosaicism (46 XX/47 XXX) has also been implicated in poor reproductive performance (Singh et al., 1980).

When analyzing the pedigree of a couple with fetal loss, it is important to clarify all previous obstetric outcomes. The risk of parental translocation is higher if there is a history of abortions only and no term live births. The yield on chromosomal analysis of parents is higher if abortion histories interspersed with stillbirths and live-born infants with congenital anomalies. Two hundred couples with two or more spontaneous miscarriages and a mixed obstetric history were found to have a 3.7% incidence of balanced translocation in either parent. Forty-eight of these had two or more abortions with an 8.4% incidence of balanced translocations. With four miscarriages, the risk increased to 10% (Michels et al., 1982). Studies from other centers, however, may dispute these high figures. One recent report by Fitzsimmons et al. at Thomas Jefferson University in Philadelphia detailed significant chromosomal anomalies in only 1.8% of persons with two or more abortions; the incidence went up to 2.3% with three or more losses. The incidence figures appear to vary depending on the type of referrals made to these genetic units in large medical centers.

After a history of two or more abortions, especially in the absence of a live birth, it is reasonable to obtain parental chromosomal analysis, looking specifically for structural rearrangements, deletions, and inversions of chromosomes. If a balanced translocation is detected in the woman, no therapy is currently available. Donor embryo transfer may be applicable in the future. If the male is the carrier, artificial donor insemination may be offered. If an affected couple succeeds in carrying a pregnancy beyond 12 weeks, then a second trimester amniocentesis should be offered.

There is a subgroup of patients who are karyotypically normal but who still suffer repeated pregnancy wastage with recurrent aneuploidy in fetal specimens (Boue et al., 1973). In studying a subgroup of women (30 of 473) who had karyotyped abortuses, there was an increased incidence of an abnormal abortus if the previous one was abnormal despite normal parental chromosomal analyses. If the previous abortus was normal, however, there was a greater likelihood that the second would be normal also. Furthermore, in an analysis of 1,384 abortal specimens, the mothers who delivered a chromosomally normal abortus more often had a history of repeated abortion. Those in whom a chromosomally abnormal abortus was miscarried tended to have fewer repeated abortions but had an increased incidence of premature births of children with Down's syndrome. It is hypothesized that these women who have multiple miscarriages but who have normal chromosomal complements undergo repeated nondisjunctional events in their gametes. Therefore, persons with repeat trisomic abortuses and repeated multiple nonkaryotyped miscarriages should undergo second trimester amniocentesis if a subsequent pregnancy proceeds past 12 weeks' gestation, to exclude the possibility of trisomy.

Anatomic Causes

Anatomic causes for spontaneous abortion are embryonic müllerian defects, incompetent cervical os, uterine synechiae, and pelvic endometriosis. Women with diethylstilbestrol exposure in utero also have a greater incidence of abnormally developed uteri and cervices. Generally, these causative factors induce a miscarriage in the second trimester and manifest themselves with cramping and bleeding. If the symptoms occur in the latter part of the second trimester when fetal viability is assumed, then the presentation is that of premature labor, and tocolysis may be instituted. Cervical incompetence classically manifests itself only after the cervix has painlessly dilated; the only prospective clue may be the occurrence of excessive mucoid discharge and vaginal pressure. Uterine synechiae (Asherman's) may present as a missed abortion.

These anatomic defects may be described using techniques of hysterosalpingography and hysteroscopy (combined, when appropriate, with laparoscopy) (Kistner and Patton, 1975; Sanfilippo et al., 1978; Barbot et al., 1980; Siegler, 1983; March, 1983; Valle and Sciarra, 1979; Taylor and Hamon, 1983).

MÜLLERIAN ANOMALIES.—Failure of fusion of the müllerian ducts in the female embryo can result in many distinct abnormalities of uterine development (Fig 11–4) (see Kistner R.W., Patton G.W. (eds.): *Atlas of Infertility Surgery*. Boston, Little Brown & Co., 1975, chap. 5). These abnormalities of fusion

have been classically divided into two categories (Semmens classification): Group 1 consists of uteri of *single* müllerian origin: the didelphic uterus, the unicornuate uterus, and the bicornuate uterus with one rudimentary horn. Group 2 consists of uteri of *dual* müllerian origin: the bicornuate uterus, septate uterus, and the arcuate uterus. Recently, Buttram proposed a broader classification, which follows:

Class 1. Müllerian agenesis
Class 2. Unicornuate uterus
Class 3. Uterine didelphys
Class 4. Uterus bicornuis
    A.   Complete
    B.   Partial
    C.   Arcuate
Class 5. Septate uterus
    A.   Complete
    B.   Partial
Class 6. Diethystilbestrol anomalies

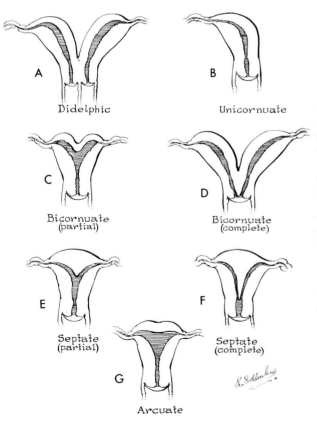

A, Didelphic
B, Unicornuate
C, Bicornuate (partial)
D, Bicornuate (complete)
E, Septate (partial)
F, Septate (complete)
G, Arcuate

Fig 11–4.—Nonobstructive maldevelopment of the uterus. **A,** uterus didelphys. **B,** unicornuate uterus. **C,** a partial bicornuate uterus as evidenced by the external configuration. **D,** a complete bicornuate uterus as evidenced by the external configuration and a double cervix. **E** and **F,** septate uterus, partial and complete, as evidenced by a normal external configuration of the uterus and the septum, which can be diagnosed only by radiographic means. **G,** arcuate uterus, which is the mildest form of malformation and seldom associated with reproductive difficulties. (From Jones H.W., Jones G.S.: *Am. J. Obstet. Gynecol.* 65:325, 1953.)

This may well be the future classification to use in tabulating reproductive histories of women with uterine anomalies.

Patients with a hemiuterus (Semmens group 1 and Buttram classes 2 and 3) have better reproductive function than those with a double uterus (Semmens group 2 and Buttram classes 4, 5, and 6) the overall rate of late abortion being 17.3% and 34.7% respectively. Nevertheless, both anomalies are manifested by repetitive pregnancy loss, usually in the second trimester or with premature delivery. Again, since some of these are found initially at delivery it is mandated that a *complete* workup to exclude other causes of abortion be performed prior to surgical correction of the defect for the purpose of alleviating habitual abortion. Depending on clinical suspicion of a uterine defect, the incidence has been variously reported as 0.06% to 0.48% in the general population (Green and Harris, 1976). The etiology of müllerian defects is unknown; familial aggregates have been reported. The mode of inheritance may be polygenic or multifactorial, although an autosomal recessive pattern had been implicated (Verp et al., 1983). It is also important to exclude renal abnormalities (by intravenous pyelogram or ultrasound) in patients with uterine anomalies (Marshall and Beisel, 1978).

The different surgical corrective procedures used are the Jones technique (the excision of a wedge of fundal uterus), the Strassman technique (first performed on, and still mainly applicable to bicornuate uteri), and the Tompkins technique for unification of a subseptate uterus (Jones, 1981; Barnes et al., 1980).

Rock and Jones, reporting from an updated series in their institution from 1964 through 1975, found that only one in five patients with uterine malformations (mainly the septate variety) had reproductive difficulties. The actual cause for reproductive losses in septate or bicornuate uteri has been postulated to be due to vascular insufficiency and inadequate endometrial development, which result in an abnormal placentation. Once the diagnosis is made by laparoscopy and hysteroscopy, surgical correction can be achieved. A recent, small series showed that of 49 patients, there was an 85% to 90% incidence of wastage in the presence of bicornuate or septate uteri. Twenty-one patients who successfully underwent a metroplasty (uterine repair) had a 75% incidence of successful pregnancy (Musich and Behrman, 1978). In a series reported from the Brigham and Women's Hospital using the Tompkin's technique for uterine septum, 71% of 20 patients had successful term pregnancies, with 86% conceiving in 11 months (McShane et al., 1983). This is not unlike the 77% success rate reported at Johns Hopkins University, Baltimore, with the wedge technique (Rock and Jones, 1977). Recently, hysteroscopic resection of uterine septa has also been described (Daly et al., 1983). This would obviate the necessity of a cesarean section, which is usually required after a traditional metroplasty. Both cervical incompetence and uterine synechiae are potential complications of metroplasty.

Ironically, women who took the nonsteroidal estrogen diethylstilbestrol (DES) due to their own poor reproductive performance produced daughters with anatomic abnormalities that may lead to increased pregnancy wastage. There is interest in the variety of ways that DES can cause reproductive difficulties, since the majority of these women are now in the childbearing age group. Many studies have concentrated on the reproductive performance of DES daughters and show different incidences of spontaneous abortion. The majority of these correlate with a higher incidence of the latter if severe uterine and/or cervical structural changes were produced by the DES. Only a few of these studies will be elaborated herein. The reader is referred to Stillman's excellent review of this subject (Stillman, 1982).

Kaufman et al. reported on 267 DES-exposed offspring, of whom 69% demonstrated a uterine abnormality that was associated with poor pregnancy outcome. The spontaneous abortion rate in his series (both first and second trimester) was 32%. The most common roentgenographic finding in this series was a T-shaped uterus with a cavity less than 2.5 cm in length (measured by planimetry). Thirty-nine percent of women with an abnormal tubogram had a spontaneous abortion. Of 119 pregnancies in 93 women, only 45% resulted in a term delivery (Kaufman et al., 1983). Herbst and associates noted that the presence of cervicovaginal ridges increased the incidence of abortion; in his series, this included a 27% abortion rate compared with 16% in controls. A study was also reported by Schmidt et al. at the University of North Carolina in 276 female offspring of women who had taken DES during pregnancy. Of 106 female offspring who attempted pregnancy there were 129 conceptions and 58 live births. The fetal wastage was 43% for the first pregnancy and 37% for all pregnancies; 25% were due to spontaneous abortions.

Barnes et al., in the series from the National Cooperative Diethylstilbestrol Adenosis (DESAD) Project, disagreed with these findings. They reported an increased risk ratio of any unfavorable outcome of pregnancy among DES-exposed daughters as 1.69 (P < .01), and the risk ratio of abortion was 1.61. Ironically, 36 women with structural uterine defects had a 16.7% miscarriage rate, whereas

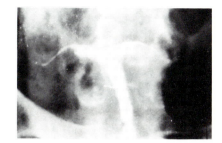

Fig 11–5.—Tubogram of patient exposed to diethylstilbestrol in utero during mother's first trimester of pregnancy. Note T-shaped uterus.

the 184 who did not have a noted structural defect had a rate of 27.7%.

Furthermore, no suitable corrective procedure has been described or recommended for a typical T-shaped DES uterus (Fig 11–5). It is suggested that DES daughters, nevertheless, should be checked frequently in the late first and second trimesters for cervical dilatation. Only then is surgical correction of an incompetent cervix recommended.

CERVICAL INCOMPETENCE.—Classically, the diagnosis of an incompetent cervix (Fig 11–6) is made by history: painless dilatation between the 16th and 28th week of pregnancy with symptoms of pelvic pressure and increased mucoid discharge. If a no. 18 cervical dilator can be inserted into the cervix in the

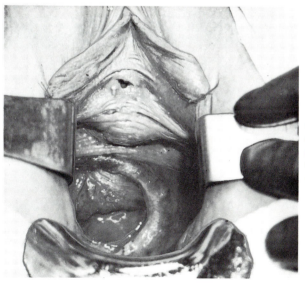

Fig 11–6.—Incompetent cervical os seen during the 32nd week of gestation. The cervix is widely patulous and the membranes clearly visible. (From Easterday C.L., Reid D.E.: *N. Engl. J. Med.* 260:687, 1959.)

nonpregnant state and a typical obstetric history is elicited, then a diagnosis of incompetence is made. A tubogram can also aid the diagnosis. Quite typically, in the absence of obstructed tubes, there is backflow of the dye through the cervix; the cervical isthmus is also widened to greater than 1 cm.

The causes of cervical incompetence are either traumatic (i.e., multiple dilation and curettage procedures and wide conization of the cervix) or anatomic (congenital) (i.e., a history of DES exposure in utero). The frequency of pregnancy wastage ascribed to an incompetent cervix varies greatly. However, it is generally believed to be ascribed as the causative factor in about one of five midtrimester losses. A preconceptual (Lash) procedure or a postconceptual suture (Shirodkar or MacDonald) around the incompetent cervix can be used (the latter is the most frequently used.

The following criteria for operability are rigid and should not be violated: The patient should have had two or more spontaneous miscarriages; repeated pelvic examination after 12 weeks' gestation should reveal progressive cervical dilatation if the past history of miscarriage is not classic. The procedure should not be done before the 12th week of pregnancy to avoid "securing a blighted ovum." In the presence of cervicitis, vaginal infection, or rupture of membranes, the operation is contraindicated. The best results with postconceptual suture are achieved if minimal cervical dilatation is achieved. As soon as such is detected, the procedure should be performed. If not, the prognosis for success is much poorer if membranes are bulging through a dilated cervix.

Harger's series from Magee Women's Hospital, Pittsburgh (1971 through 1978) drew from a retrospective analysis of 251 cerclage procedures (Shirodkar or MacDonald) in 105 selected women for the procedure. Fetal survival was markedly improved from 20% to 80% in elective cases and reached an average of 60% if the procedure was performed in an emergent situation. Morbidity attributed to the cerclage procedure consisted of chorioamnionitis in 1.2% of the individuals; the remainder was due to cervical lacerations. Cervical scarring and elective cesarean section rates increased significantly to 16% to 25%. Furthermore, it has been suggested that the cerclage procedure be performed as soon as the diagnosis of cervical incompetence is made. The risk of chorioamnionitis is increased 2.6-fold and premature rupture of the membranes prior to the 32nd week may occur if the procedure is delayed or done under emergent conditions (Charles and Edwards, 1981).

UTERINE LEIOMYOMAS ("FIBROIDS").—Submucous leiomyomas may disturb endometrial function or encroach on the cavity of the uterus to such a degree that implantation is prevented. Large intramural leiomyomas may produce hyperirritability or dysfunction of the endometrium, resulting in abortion. The location of the fibroid appears to be more important than its overall size. Fibroids grow to larger dimensions during pregnancy due to the increases in estrogen and progesterone secretion. In this way, they can create a greater problem during pregnancy than that which would be predicted by their size prior to pregnancy. Surgical correction via myomectomy is indicated in patients who have experienced repetitive miscarriage when no other cause for abortion is found. If the uterine cavity is entered during myomectomy, a cesarean section is indicated at delivery of a subsequent term birth. An excellent review of the subject of myomas in general has been written by Buttram and Reeter (1981).

Recently, excision of uterine leiomyomas under hysteroscopic control has been described (Neuwirth, 1983). With hysteroscopic and laparoscopic control, morcellation of causative submucous leiomyomas can be performed using diathermic cautery. The pedunculated myomas with a distinct stalk are most conducive to removal by such a procedure. There are no large series to date to compare overall morbidity figures. However, such hysteroscopic resection, even if limited only to the pedunculated type of myomas, decreases morbidity, since it negates the need for a laparotomy for myomectomy and a subsequent cesarean section for delivery. These procedures, however, should be performed only by surgeons skilled in hysteroscopy. The patient must be prepared for laparotomy in the event of uncontrollable bleeding.

UTERINE SYNECHIAE.—Intrauterine adhesions are generally caused by iatrogenic means—traumatic curettage after a delivery and, especially, a missed abortion. A metroplasty and extensive excision or cautery of submucous myomas can also cause such adhesions. Another infrequent cause is genital tuberculosis. The eponym for this condition is Asherman's syndrome (Joaff and Ballas, 1978). Clinically, the diagnosis is suspected in an individual with postcurettage or postsurgical amenorrhea who has biphasic basal body temperatures and luteal serum progesterones, yet does not respond to estrogen-progesterone administration with withdrawal menstrual flow. Suspicion is heightened if filling defects are demonstrated on a hysterosalpingogram, but the diagnosis is made more accurately by hysteroscopy. The latter is both a diagnostic and therapeutic modality, since these adhesions can be graded and cut during hysteroscopy. The degree of intrauterine scarring is most closely correlated with the menstrual pattern, i.e., the more severe cases have complete amenorrhea. In a combined series (Schenker and Margalioth, 1982), 40% of women with untreated Asherman's syndrome suffered habitual or missed abortions. When such persons are treated with hysteroscopic lysis of adhesions, with insertion of an IUD for four to eight weeks followed by oral conjugated estrogen administration (treatment length and doses vary) for one month, the abortion rate decreased to 25%. More specifically, March and Israel were able to show that in 84 pregnancies in women with intrauterine adhesions, only 16.7% resulted in the delivery of a viable infant. Following treatment, 39 pregnancies resulted in a term gestation in 87.2%.

In conclusion, a sequela of intrauterine adhesion formation is poor reproductive performance. The ability to diagnose and treat such with hysteroscopy has aided our therapy in this syndrome. No standardized regimen of hormonal or antibiotic therapy exists. Nevertheless, most series report beneficial results with combined use of an intrauterine device (or Foley catheter) and hormonal therapy (Premarin, 2.5 mg/day for one month) to regenerate the endometrial lining.

PELVIC ENDOMETRIOSIS.—The frequency of miscarriage appears to be inversely related to the severity of documented endometriosis in an affected individual. A recent survey tabulated 34% of 226 pregnancies ending in a first trimester spontaneous abortion prior to conservative surgical treatment of the disease. This was compared to an incidence of 13% of pregnancies in control, primary infertility patients (n = 128). Mild endometriosis was associated with a greater incidence of miscarriage (49% in 87 patients) compared to 24% in severely afflicted patients (n = 107). Rock et al. found a 49% abortion risk in women with endometriosis; the figure was reduced to 20% if conservative surgery was chosen. Dmowski and Cohen also indicated an increased incidence of second- and third-trimester intrauterine fetal deaths in conceptions occurring within three cycles of discontinuation of danazol (Danocrine) pseudopregnancy therapy for endometriosis. This was not found in a four-year study performed in Kistner's practice in which, after Danocrine therapy for endometriosis, there was no increase in the miscarriage rate (Barbieri et al., 1982). These individuals, however, were advised not to conceive immediately after stopping Danocrine therapy.

What exactly causes miscarriages associated with endometriosis is speculative at this time. It may be related to the increased levels of peritoneal fluid prostaglandinlike compounds (thromboxane B_2 and 6-keto-prostaglandin

$F_{1\alpha}$) (Drake et al., 1981) or it may be related to poor luteal function.

To conclude from this discussion that endometriosis is directly causative of abortion and that conservative surgery is a better mode of therapy for achieving a full-term pregnancy is not accurate.

Hormonal Causes

Luteal-phase defects are broadly defined as defects in the functioning of the corpus luteum, which create problems in progesterone production. These deficiencies in luteal progesterone secretion are felt to be a cause of early first-trimester reproductive failure. Such defects were found to occur spontaneously in 3.5% of patients with primary infertility but in 25.0% of patients with repeated miscarriages. Recent reports estimate the incidence to be higher among the population of infertile patients with Rosenberg et al. reporting an incidence of 8.1%; Wentz, 19%; and Wentz and Seeger-Jones et al., 29.5% (the latter figure also includes the incidence in women receiving clomiphene citrate therapy).

In order to make the diagnosis of a defective luteal phase, a patient must demonstrate an aberrant thermal response per basal body temperature recordings and a midluteal progesterone level of less than 10 ng/ml. If these are suggestive of a defect, then the diagnosis is made by two consecutive-month, well-timed endometrial biopsies in the late luteal phase, two days out of phase in the expected secretory pattern defined by Noyes et al. The specific criteria for diagnosis are still very controversial, as is the exact treatment modality. The reader is referred to an excellent recent review on the subject by Andrews.

It is suggested that luteal phase defects may be due to a variety of central and/or an ovarian defect. DiZerega and Hodgen have described "luteal-phase dysfunction as a sequence of aberrant folliculogenesis." Their work in the primate model demonstrates aberrations in follicle-stimulating hormone (FSH) secretion and, hence, a central defect causing defective corpus luteum progesterone produc-

tion, which can be overcome by treatment with human menopausal gonadotropin. In fact these defects in follicular development can be caused by central defects in FSH and luteinizing hormone (LH) secretion that are spontaneous or pharmacologically induced (i.e., with Clomid or Pergonal treatment) or by a hyperprolactinemic state (St. Michel and DiZerega, 1983). An ovarian defect causing poor progesterone output can be due to deficiencies of low-density lipoprotein synthesis (i.e., individuals with abetalipoproteinemia) or low-density lipoprotein delivery to the corpus luteum (possibly due to defective vascularization of the corpus luteum) (Carr et al., 1982). A very rare defect creating absence of stromal cytosol receptors for progesterone, which is clinically demonstrated by absence of secretory endometrial changes, has also been documented (Keller et al., 1979). Much more work is needed in deciphering the actual causes of poor luteal functioning. In the past this entity has been treated empirically in all cases with exogenous progesterone. This is still a subject of great controversy.

When subjected to strict randomized double-blind procedure with placebo, the use of progesterone did not increase the salvage rate in a small group of habitual aborters (Goldzieher, 1964). Despite the fact that Clomid as an ovulatory-induction agent has itself been associated with luteal-phase defects, it has been favored as a treatment modality for inadequate luteal-phase progesterone production (Quagliarello and Weiss, 1981; Soules et al., 1981; Hammond and Talbert, 1982). Again, these studies did not decipher the cause for poor luteal progesterone production. In fact, when hyperprolactinemia is identified as a probable contributing factor to poor luteal progesterone production, bromocriptine (Parlodel) successfully reverses the defect.

The successful use of supplemental progesterone, either intramuscular (12.5 mg of progesterone in oil) or by vaginal suppositories (25 mg, twice a day), has been ascertained by some although these studies were not all performed in a double-blind fashion (Rosenberg et al., 1980; Soules et al., 1981). The use of progesterone supplementation in pregnancy has not been acknowledged as efficacious by the Food and Drug Administration. In fact, their use has been implicated with an increase in the incidence of congenital heart defects (Heinonen et al., 1977) although this is a subject of continuing debate (Chez, 1978). In fact, in patients who may have a poorly vascularized corpus luteum, exogenous progesterone supplementation may be the treatment of choice. In all such cases patients must be fully cognizant of the potential teratogenic effects of the use of such steroids in pregnancy. Currently, many in vitro programs are employing the use of progesterone supplementation after follicle aspiration for ovum recovery.

Infectious Etiology

Mycoplasma hominis and *Ureaplasma urealyticum* (*T mycoplasma* or T strains) can be isolated frequently from the female genital tract. The latter, the T strains, have been associated with early fetal wastage. In fact, T mycoplasma was first identified and described in abortal specimens from a spontaneous miscarriage (Kundsin et al., 1967). Much of this work was done by Driscoll, Kundsin, and Horne at the Boston Hospital for Women. The issue of whether or not the infection is caused by the abortal process itself has been raised. Large-scale randomized studies proving the fact that repeated miscarriages are due solely to *Mycoplasma* infestation are needed. Also, the exact relationship between an infectious agent and poor embryonic development requires elucidation.

There have been many studies detailing improved pregnancy outcome in women treated for such *T mycoplasma* infestation, although these again do not demonstrate a direct causal effect and have been disputed by others. *T mycoplasma* may be an opportunistic infection in an individual who has had multiple miscarriages; it still is more prudent to culture and treat such individuals. *T mycoplasma* is very sensitive to tetracyclines. It

is important not to treat habitual aborters empirically with tetracyclines, but rather to obtain antibiotic susceptibility testing pretreatment. The usual course of therapy in both partners is 100 mg of doxycycline twice daily for ten days. The woman is treated in the follicular phase.

Part of the difficulties in obtaining reliable results may be in the collection of specimens for *T mycoplasma*. Kundsin suggests that a cotton swab on a nonwooden stick be used to culture the endocervix of the female. Urine should be cultured simultaneously to increase the detection rate of the organism. In the male, the semen is a better source of culture than urine or urethral swabbings.

Uterine toxoplasmosis infections in developing countries have also been implicated as causative factors in habitual miscarriage (Stray-Pederson and Lorentzyn-Styr, 1977). However, these organisms were found only in the endometrium of postabortal women and did not appear in the serologic screening of patients. The colonization with the organism, therefore, could be a result of ascending infection rather than the cause of the miscarriage. Further work in the other microbiologic factors causing repeated fetal wastage is needed.

Immunologic

A possible predisposition to abortion is an immunization of the mother to fetuses of certain genotypes. Major blood incompatibilities (ABO) have been implicated, but this does not seem to represent a major causative factor for habitual abortion.

In fact, a newer line of research is investigating the exact opposite line of reasoning. It is now thought that a deficient maternal immune response may cause miscarriage or rejection by the mother of her fetus. This may be directly related to a greater antigenic similarity between the husband and wife. The hypothesis, therefore, would be that reproductive efficiency is decreased when antigenic similarity between the husband and wife is greater.

A normal pregnancy produces circulating

maternal lymphocytes that are sensitized against fetal antigens and that produce a lymphokine that prevents the migration of macrophages (macrophage-inhibiting factor [MIF]). Blocking antibodies (IgG) prevent the release of MIF from these sensitized lymphocytes and thereby secure a pregnancy. In a study done at the Brigham and Women's Hospital, it was noted that women who experienced idiopathic spontaneous abortions (three or more) produce lymphocyte migration inhibitory factor to paternal alloantigens, but their serums lack the blocking factor (an IgG antibody) (Rocklin et al., 1976).

Chance histocompatibility for HLA antigens may be a possible explanation for the lack of this specific IgG blocking factor's formation. The genomes within the major histocompatibility locus code for all surface molecules present on all nucleated cells of the body. Women with spontaneous, recurrent abortions of unknown etiology have a significantly increased frequency of sharing HLA antigens at the A, B, C, and D/DR loci. This is in comparison to control groups in which no more than one antigen is shared between spouses (Beer et al., 1982, 1981). Recent studies, nevertheless, have not all clearly demonstrated a cause-and-effect relationship between antigenic similarity and multiple miscarriages, or unexplained infertility (Grenier et al., 1979; Oksenberg et al., 1983; Caudle et al., 1983; Nordlander et al., 1983). This is especially important since the proposed treatment, infusing afflicted women with repeated leukocyte transfusions from different donors or by immunizing them with peripheral blood lymphocytes harvested from their husbands, is potentially dangerous (Taylor and Faulk, 1981). The need for further investigation in this area has been proposed by Scott who has addressed the following needed data: (1) the rate of normal pregnancies with a high rate of histocompatibility between husband and wife, (2) the results of large, prospective, double-blind placebo trials to ascertain the effectiveness of no treatment in histocompatible couples with spontaneous

miscarriage. Finally, the long-term effects of such immunization regimens are questioned in regard to the optimal source of donor leukocytes and the benefit-risk ratio against the potential problems associated with anaphylaxis, infection, and problems with prospective organ transplants in such individuals.

Recent evidence is also emerging concerning the possible role of sperm isoimmunization in causing problems with infertility and reproductive failure. A decrease in the miscarriage rate has been noted in individuals subsequently treated with prednisone (Jones, 1976; Mathur et al., 1981). The implications of these results need further study before clear-cut therapeutic guidelines are set.

Systemic lupus erythematosus (SLE) is an autoimmune disease that may be associated with a high rate of pregnancy wastage. Immune complexes formed by transplacental passage of maternal antibodies deposit themselves on trophoblast membrane and may be causative for the increased fetal wastage seen in this disease (Grennan et al., 1978). Patients in remission and without lupus nephritis have the best prognosis during pregnancy, although the spontaneous abortion rate is high—almost 30% in a well-controlled series (Estes and Larson, 1965). Part of the early fetal losses may be due to the high incidence of cardiovascular defects—specifically, complete heart block—in infants born of afflicted individuals (Chameides et al., 1983). The use of steroids to decrease the high miscarriage rate has not proved to be universally successful (Fraga et al., 1973; Hartikainen-Sorri and Kaila, 1980).

Furthermore, an association between a pre-lupus-type syndrome and chronic abortions may exist. In one such reported case the individual was asymptomatic but possessed a "lupus" anticoagulant in her plasma. The placenta of the aborted pregnancy showed fibrinoid necrosis and massive infarction. The plasma of this patient inhibited the formation of prostacycline by rat aortic rings. Since prostacycline is an important physiologic inhibitor of platelet aggregation and is a powerful vasodilator, it was hypothesized that placental infarction due to lack of sufficient amounts of prostacycline may have been the pathogenesis (DeWolf et al., 1982). Furthermore, in a recent prospective analysis of 155 couples with two or more consecutive pregnancy losses, 7.5% of the women had a positive antinuclear antibody (ANA) test result, whereas the expected rate was defined as 2%. The significance of this was unclear although the possible association of this with manifestation of lupus at a later date was speculated (Harger et al., 1983). Until the exact relationship between this lupus-like syndrome and spontaneous miscarriage is clarified, no specific therapy can be suggested.

Miscellaneous Factors

Abnormal maternal thyroid function has not been conclusively linked to an increased incidence of miscarriage. An indirect association with the presence of thyroid antibodies and Down's syndrome in younger mothers has been implicated; this may indirectly relate to the slight increase in spontaneous losses seen in hypothyroidism (Fralkow, 1967). Maternal diabetes has shown no direct cause-and-effect relationship with the incidence of first-trimester miscarriages (Crane and Wahl, 1981). However, when compared with a control population a recent study correlating abnormally high levels of glycosylated hemoglobin levels (Hb A_{1c}) showed a higher rate of spontaneous miscarriage (Wright et al., 1983). The implication is that with poorer diabetic control the possible incidence of miscarriage is greater reinforcing the need for strict diabetic control even prior to a contemplated pregnancy.

The effect of alcohol is an especially vibrant issue in today's society, with many recent studies showing direct susceptibility of the early embryo to the effects of alcohol. Cigarette smoking and/or alcohol consumption in excess both increase the rate of spontaneous miscarriages. No increase in the detection of anomalies on abortal specimens has been detected in women who conceive within six months after discontinuation of an oral contraceptive.

Recently a rat-embryo culture system was described showing the toxic effects of D-mannose on the growth and development of early embryos. The hypothesis that emerged from this study was that "major congenital lesions may occur coincidentally with relative minor disturbances in glycolysis before oxidative maturation in the embryo unit." Perhaps this new model can be used to study and explain the possible role of a multiple of exogenous toxins such as Agent Orange, anesthetics, over-the-counter prescriptions, alcohol, and such exogenous factors as nutrition, all of which have been implicated in early miscarriage (Freinkel et al., 1984).

James, in his review of the efficacy of psychotherapy in women who experience recurrent fetal losses maintains that proper "supportive therapy" will produce the best prognosis (80% vs. 45%). However, these were not randomized double-blind studies from which one could conclude that psychotherapy offered a better result than an elaborate investigation of the causative factors in first-trimester miscarriage. Patients who have experienced a miscarriage require accessory support systems to help them cope. They should be counseled that their feeling of loss is real and be allowed to express their grief. With such reassurance, they can also better cope with the extensive evaluation of habitual miscarriage. An excellent book for both the physician and patient, which deals with methods of coping with pregnancy loss is *When Pregnancy Fails* by S. Borg and J. Lasker (Boston, Beacon Press, 1981).

PROGNOSIS

Two studies in the recent literature looking at etiologies for recurrent abortion and subsequent reproductive performance place this chapter in perspective. Tho et al. studied 100 couples from 1968 through 1977 and selected those with poor reproductive performance on the basis of (1) two or more histologically documented abortions, and (2) one or more abortions associated with a phenotypically abnormal child. Harger et al. studied 155 couples from 1977 through 1981 who had had at least two or more consecutive pregnancy losses, with at least three occurring in 106 women. Both studies found that chromosomal analysis and investigation for müllerian defects as anatomic causes for miscarriages gave the greatest yield.

In the first study a genetic etiology was found in 25% of the cases and this had the poorest prognosis. Müllerian anomalies were found in 15%, with an overall success rate of term pregnancy following surgical correction of 60%. The best prognosis was in the "endocrine" group found to have retarded endometrial development; this group represented 23%, with an overall success rate of 91% following hormonal supplementation.

In the latter study, 15.4% of the couples demonstrated chromosomal anomalies and in 27% there was a uterine morphologic abnormality in the female. The incidence of a positive finding did not increase with repetitive abortions following the second arguing in favor of starting an evaluation after the second miscarriage (Table 11–2). There was a high rate of positive ANA titers in asymptomatic females detected in this study. Also, a high rate of colonization with T-mycoplasma is reported although a significant number of these patients who remained culture positive post-treatment had successful pregnancies. The overall prognosis for subsequent livebirths

was good if the diagnostic evaluation was normal (77%) or abnormal (71%) (Table 11–3). A factor contributing to recurrent pregnancy loss was found in 68% of women with three or more losses and diagnostic studies that gave the highest yield were tubogram, peripheral lymphocyte karyotypes, and cervical cultures for T mycoplasma.

Both of these studies present an encouraging prognosis for deciphering the diagnostic dilemma of recurrent abortion and for reassuring patients as to possible outcome.

MANAGEMENT OF PATIENT

Patients who present with a history of spontaneous miscarriage in either the first or second trimester should have a careful history taken (e.g., diabetes, lupus, etc.) and a complete physical examination (e.g., palpation of a bicornuate uterus, myoma, etc.). Note should be made of the phenotype (if developed) and/or genotype (if specimen was karyotyped) of the abortal specimen. Couples who have had two or more spontaneous miscarriages are appropriate for diagnostic evaluation. Care should be taken to instruct the couple to preserve the fetal specimen as carefully as possible if a subsequent miscarriage ensues. The clinician should send the fetal specimen for karyotypic analysis.

If the latter is abnormal it may be a random

TABLE 11–2.—ABNORMAL LABORATORY TEST RESULTS ASSOCIATED
WITH RECURRENT PREGNANCY LOSSES*

	NO. OF PREGNANCY LOSSES			
	≥ 4	3	2	TOTAL
TEST	NO. (%)	NO. (%)	NO. (%)	NO. (%)
Karyotype	5/88 (5.7)	12/112 (10.7)	4/72 (5.6)	21/272 (7.7)
Hysterosalpingogram	8/30 (27)	11/45 (24)	11/37 (30)	30/112 (27)
Thyroid function	0/30	2/52 (3.9)	0/37	2/119 (1.7)
Antinuclear antibody	1/32 (3.1)	5/51 (10)	3/37 (8.1)	9/120 (7.5)
Cervical culture				
Mycoplasma hominis	7/40 (18)	8/61 (13)	7/46 (15)	22/147 (15)
Ureaplasma urealyticum	22/40 (55)	27/61 (44)	22/46 (48)	71/147 (48)

*Abnormal test result/total number of tests performed. The chance that a given diagnostic test will be abnormal does not increase linearly with an increasing number of pregnancy losses. (Adapted from Harger J.H., et al.: *Obstet. Gynecol.* 62:574–581, 1983.)

TABLE 11–3.—RELATIONSHIP BETWEEN APPARENT CAUSE OF PREGNANCY
LOSSES AND PROGNOSIS OF SUBSEQUENT PREGNANCIES

ABNORMALITY	NO. OF NEXT PREGNANCIES	ABORTIONS	STILLBIRTHS	LIVE BIRTHS
Cytogenetic (total)	18 (100%)	4 (25%)	0	14 (78%)
Balanced translocation	8	2	0	6
X-chromosome mixoploidy	5	1	0	6
Pericentric inversion	3	1	0	2
Uterine (total)	15 (100%)	3 (20%)	2 (13%)	10 (67%)
Intrauterine synechiae	5	1	1	3
Subseptate or bicornuate	4	1	0	3
Other	6	1	1	4
Positive antinuclear antibody test	7 (100%)	3 (43%)	. . .	4 (57%)
Cervical culture positive for				
Ureaplasma urealyticum	40 (100%)	11 (27%)	0	29 (73%)
Successful therapy	19	6	0	13
Unsuccessful therapy	7	1	0	6
Not treated	14	4	0	10

*Adapted from Harger J.H., et al.: *Obstet. Gynecol.* 62:574–581, 1983.

event or it may be due to a translocation carrier state in either parent (most often the woman). These abnormalities may be detected by peripheral blood karyotypic analysis (with current banding techniques) on the husband and wife. If these are abnormal, appropriate advice may be given (as described previously). If normal, the couple may have other causes for repeated pregnancy loss or may be in the category of persons who suffer repeat trisomic abortuses although they are normal on chromosomal analysis.

If no definitive genetic defect is found an analysis of possible anatomic anomalies (e.g., septate uterus), infections (e.g., T mycoplasma), immunologic factors (e.g., history of lupus) should be investigated via the appropriate methods mentioned. In the absence of a possible genetic factor it is important that all these studies are done in their entirety in each individual. Genetic factors are the only proved cause of habitual miscarriage, and in the absence of such, all other factors have varying degrees of an association. The association of a uterine septum and the incidence of a spontaneous abortion is stronger, but even here the abnormality is at times first diagnosed at term delivery. Therefore, the next step in the evaluation of a couple with spontaneous miscarriage is to obtain a tubogram to look for an anatomic defect (and a hysteroscopy/laparoscopy when indicated), cultures for T mycoplasma, and a timed endometrial biopsy.

Despite the suggested association of positive ANA titers in asymptomatic patients, this study offers no direct benefit. Its association (in the absence of overt lupus erythematosus) with habitual miscarriage is speculative. By the same token, in the absence of overt disease, thyroid function tests and oral glucose tolerance testing are not beneficial. The analysis of histocompatibility at major HLA sites and sperm isoimmunity are areas of active unsettled investigation. Care should be taken in using such research tools in the current practical evaluation of habitual aborters.

In closing, it is worth mentioning several review articles dealing with the analysis of habitual miscarriage (Glass and Golbus, 1978; Fabricant et al., 1978; Simpson et al., 1982; Kamran, 1982; Stenchever, 1983; and Rock and Zacur, 1983). The reader is referred to these to widen his perspective of this controversial subject.

BIBLIOGRAPHY

Alberman E., Elliott M., Creasy M., et al.: Previous reproductive history in mothers presenting with spontaneous abortion. *Br. J. Obstet. Gynaecol.* 82:366–373, 1975.

Andrews W.C.: Luteal phase defects. *Fertil. Steril.* 32:501–509, 1979.

Barbieri R.L., Evans S., Kistner R.: Danazol in the treatment of endometriosis: Analysis of 100 cases with a four year followup. *Fertil. Steril.* 37:737–746, 1982.

Barbot J., Parent B., Dubuisson J.B.: Contact hysteroscopy: Another method of endoscopic examination of the endometrial cavity. *Am. J. Obstet. Gynecol.* 136:721–726, 1980.

Barnes A.B., Colton T., Gunderson J., et al.: Fertility and outcome of pregnancy in women exposed in utero to diethylstilbestrol. *N. Engl. J. Med.* 302:609–613, 1980.

Batzer F.R.: Hormonal evaluation of early pregnancy. *Fertil. Steril.* 34:1–13, 1980.

Beer A.E., Quebbeman J.F., Ayers J.W.T.: The immunobiology of abortion, in Shulman S., Dondero F., Nicotra M. (eds.): *Immunological Factors in Human Reproduction*, Serono Symposium no. 45. York, Academic Press, 1982.

Beer A.E., Quebbeman J.F., Ayers J.W.T., et al.: Major histocompatibility complex antigens, maternal and paternal immune responses, and chronic habitual abortion in humans. *Am. J. Obstet. Gynecol.* 141:987–999, 1981.

Boue J., Boue A.: Chromosomal analysis of two consecutive abortions in each of 43 females. *Hum. Genet.* 19:275–280, 1973.

Boue J., Boue A., Lazar P.: Retrospective and prospective epidemiological studies of 1,500 karyotyped spontaneous human abortions. *Teratology* 11–12:11–26, 1975.

Boue J.G., Boue A., Lazar P., et al.: Outcome of pregnancies following a spontaneous abortion with chromosomal anomalies. *Am. J. Obstet. Gynecol.* 116:806–812, 1973.

Buttram V.S.: Müllerian anomalies and their management. *Fertil. Steril.* 40:159–163, 1983.

Buttram N.C., Reeter R.C.: Uterine leimyomata: Etiology, symptomatology, and management. *Fertil. Steril.* 36:433–445, 1981.

Cadkin A.V., Sabbagha R.E.: Abnormal pregnancy, in *Diagnostic Ultrasound Applied to Obstetrics and Gynecology*. Hagerstown, Md, Harper & Row, pp. 149–164, chap. 14, 1980.

Carr B.R., MacDonald P.C., Simpson E.R.: The role of lipoproteins in the regulation of progesterone secretion by the human corpus luteum. *Fertil. Steril.* 38:303–311, 1982.

Caudle M.R., Rote N.S., Scott J.R., et al.: Histocompatibility in couples with recurrent spontaneous abortion and normal fertility. *Fertil. Steril.* 39:793–798, 1983.

Chameides L., Fruex R.C., Vetter V., et al.: Association of maternal systemic lupus erythematosus with congenital complete heart block. *N. Engl. J. Med.* 297:1204–1207, 197.

Charles D., Edwards W.E.: Infectious complications of cervical cerclage. *Am. J. Obstet. Gynecol.* 141:1065–1071, 1981.

Chartier M., Roger M., Barrat J., et al.: Measurement of plasma human chorionic gonadotropin (hCG) and β-hCG activities in the late luteal phase: Evidence of the occurrence of spontaneous menstrual abortions in infertile women. *Fertil. Steril.* 31:134–135, 1979.

Chez R.: Proceedings of the symposium, Progesterone, Progestins and Fetal Development. *Fertil. Steril.* 30:21–26, 1978.

Crane J.P., Wahl N.: The role of maternal diabetes in repetitive spontaneous abortion. *Fertil. Steril.* 36:477–479, 1981.

Daly D.C., Jaban N., Walters C., et al.: Hysteroscopic resection of the uterine septum in the presence of a septate cervix. *Fertil. Steril.* 39:560–563, 1983.

Damber M-G., vonSchoultz B., Solheim F., et al.: Prognostic value of the pregnancy zone protein during early pregnancy in spontaneous abortion. *Obstet. Gynecol.* 51:677–682, 1978.

DeWolf F., Carreras L.O., Moerman P., et al.: Decidual vasculopathy and extensive placental infarction in a patient with repeated thromboembolic accidents, recurrent fetal loss, and a lupus anticoagulant. *Am. J. Obstet. Gynecol.* 142:829–834, 1982.

DiZerega G.S., Hodgen G.D.: Luteal phase dysfunction infertility: A sequel to aberrant folliculogenesis. *Fertil. Steril.* 35:489–499, 1981.

Dmowski W.P., Cohen M.R.: Antigonadotropin (danazol) in treatment of endometriosis. *Am. J. Obstet. Gynecol.* 130:41, 1978.

Drake T.S., O'Brien W.F., Ramwell P.W., et al.: Peritoneal fluid thromboxane B2 and 6-keto prostaglandin $F_{1\alpha}$ in endometriosis. *Am. J. Obstet. Gynecol.* 140:401–404, 1981.

Driscoll S.G., Kundsin R.B., Horne H.W., et al.: Infections and first trimester losses: Possible role for mycoplasmas. *Fertil. Steril.* 20:1017–1019, 1969.

Edmonds D.K., Lindsay K.I., Miller J.F., et al.: Early embryonic mortality in women. *Fertil. Steril.* 38:447–453, 1982.

Elias S., LeBeau M., Simpson J.L., et al.: Chromosome analysis of ectopic human conceptuses. *Am. J. Obstet. Gynecol.* 141:698–703, 1981.

Elles R.G., Williamson R., Neazi M., et al.: Absence of maternal contamination of chorionic villi used for fetal-gene analyses. *N. Engl. J. Med.* 308:1433–1435, 1983.

Estes D., Larson D.L.: Systemic lupus erythematosus and pregnancy. *Clin. Obstet. Gynecol.* 8:307–321, 1965.

Fabricant J.D., Boue J., Boue A.: Genetic studies on spontaneous abortion. *Contemp. Ob/Gyn* 11:73–79, 1978.

Fitzsimmons J., Wapner R., Jackson L.: Repeated pregnancy loss. *Am. J. Med. Genet.* 16:7–13, 1983.

Fraga A., Mintz G., Orazco J.H., et al.: Systemic lupus erythematosus: Fertility, pregnancy, fetal wastage, and survival rate with treatment. A comparative study. *Arthritis Rheum.* 16:541, 1973.

Fralkow P.J.: Thyroid antibodies, Down's syndrome and maternal age. *Nature* 214:1253–1254, 1967.

Freedman J.M.: Genetic disease in the offspring of older fathers. *Obstet. Gynecol.* 57:745–749, 1981.

Freinkel N., Lewis N.J., Akazawa S., et al.: The honeybee syndrome: Implications of the teratogenicity of mannase on rat embryo cultures. *N. Engl. J. Med.* 310:223–230, 1984.

Friberg J.: Mycoplasmas and ureaplasmas in infertility and abortion. *Fertil. Steril.* 33:351–359, 1980.

Gerenier M., Drazancic A., Kuvacic I., et al.: HLA antigen studies in women with recurrent gestational disorders. *Fertil. Steril.* 31:401–404, 1979.

Glass R.H., Golbus M.S.: Habitual abortion. *Fertil. Steril.* 29:257–265, 1978.

Goldheizer J.W.: Double-blind trial of a progestin in habitual abortion. *J.A.M.A.* 188:651–654, 1964.

Green L.K., Harris R.E.: Uterine anomalies: Frequency of diagnosis and obstetric complications. *Obstet. Gynecol.* 47:427–429, 1976.

Grennan D.M., McCormick J.N., Wojtacha D., et al.: Immunological studies of the placenta in systemic lupus erythematosus. *Ann. Rheum. Dis.* 37:129–134, 1978.

Hammond M.G., Talbert L.M.: Clomiphene citrate therapy of the infertile woman with low luteal phase progesterone levels. *Obstet. Gynecol.* 59:275–279, 1982.

Harger J.H., Archer D.F., Marchese S.G., et al.: Etiology of recurrent pregnancy losses and outcome of subsequent pregnancies. *Obstet. Gynecol.* 62:574–581, 1983.

Harger J.H.: Comparison of success and morbidity in cervical cerclage procedures. *Obstet. Gynecol.* 56:543–548, 1980.

Harris M.J., Poland B.J., Dill F.J.: Triploidy in 40 human spontaneous abortuses: Assessment of phenotype in embryos. *Obstet. Gynecol.* 57:600–606, 1981.

Hartikainen-Sorri A., Kaila L.: Systemic lupus erythematosus and habitual abortion. *Br. J. Obstet. Gynaecol.* 87:729–731, 1980.

Hassold T.J.: A cytogenetic study of repeated spontaneous abortions. *Am. J. Hum. Genet.* 32:723–730, 1980.

Heinonen O.P., Slone D., Monson R.R., et al.: Cardiovascular birth defects and antenatal exposure to female sex hormones. *N. Engl. J. Med.* 296:67–70, 1977.

Heritage D.W., English S.C., Young R.B., et al.: Cytogenetics of recurrent abortions. *Fertil. Steril.* 29:414–417, 1978.

Herbst A.L., Hubby M.M., Azizi F., et al.: Reproductive and gynecologic surgical experience in diethylstilbestrol-exposed daughters. *Fertil. Steril.* 141:1019–1028, 1981.

Hertig A.T., Rock J., Adams E.C., et al.: Thirty-four fertilized human ova, good, bad, and indifferent, recovered from 210 women of known fertility. *Pediatrics* 23:202–211, 1959.

Hertz J.B., Mantoni M., Svenstrup B.: Threatened abortion studied by estradiol 17β in serum and ultrasound. *Obstet. Gynecol.* 55:324–328, 1980.

Honore L.H.: A significant association between spontaneous abortion and tubal ectopic pregnancy. *Fertil. Steril.* 32:401–402, 1979.

Horne H.W., Kundsin R.B., Kosasa T.S.: The role of *Mycloplasma* infection in human reproductive failure. *Fertil. Steril.* 25:380–388, 1974.

James W.H.: The problem of spontaneous abortion: X. The efficacy of psychotherapy. *Am. J. Obstet. Gynecol.* 85:38–40, 1963.

Jansen R.P.S.: Spontaneous abortion incidence in the treatment of infertility. *Am. J. Obstet. Gynecol.* 143:451–473, 1982.

Joaff R., Ballas S.: Traumatic hypoamenorrhea-amenorrhea (Asherman's syndrome). *Fertil. Steril.* 30:379–387, 1978.

Jones H.W., Acosta A., Andrews M.C., et al.: What is a pregnancy? A question for programs of in vitro fertilization. *Fertil. Steril.* 40:728–733, 1983.

Jones H.W.: Reproductive impairment and the malformed uterus. *Fertil. Steril.* 26:137–148, 1981.

Jones W.R.: Immunological aspects of infertility, in Scott J.S., Jones W.R. (eds.): *Immunology of Human Reproduction.* London, Academic Press, 1976, pp. 375–413.

Joshi S.G., Bank J.F., Henriques E.S., et al.: Serum levels of a progestagen-associated endometrial protein during the menstrual cycle and pregnancy. *J. Clin. Endocrinol. Metab.* 55:642–647, 1982.

Jovanovic L., Dawood M.Y., Landesman R., et al.: Hormone profile as a prognostic index of early abortion. *Am. J. Obstet. Gynecol.* 130:274–278, 1978.

Kamran S.M.: What causes habitual abortion? *Contemp. Ob/Gyn* 20:45–64, 1982.

Kaufman R.H., Adam E., Bender G., et al.: Upper genital tract changes and pregnancy outcome in offspring exposed in utero to diethylstilbestrol. *Am. J. Obstet. Gynecol.* 137:299–308, 1980.

Kaufman M.H.: Ethanol induced chromosomal anomalies at conception. *Nature* 302:258, 1983.

Keller D.W., Wiest W.G., Askin F.B., et al.: Pseudocorpus luteum insufficiency: A local defect of progesterone action on endometrial stroma. *Fertil. Steril.* 48:127–132, 1979.

Khudr G.: Cytogenetics of habitual abortion: A review. *Obstet. Gynecol. Surv.* 29:299–310, 1974.

Kim H.J., Ksu L.Y.F., Paduc S., et al.: Cytogenetics of fetal wastage. *N. Engl. J. Med.* 293:844–847, 1975.

Kistner R.W., Patton G.W.: Endoscopy, in Kistner R.W., Patton G.W. (eds.): *Atlas of Infertility Surgery.* Boston, Little Brown & Co., 1975, pp. 21–44, chap. 2.

Kistner R.W., Patton G.W.: Surgery of the uterus, in Kistner R.W., Patton G.W. (eds.): *Atlas of Infertility Surgery.* Boston, Little Brown & Co., 1975, pp. 65–93, chap. 5.

Kundsin R.B.: Mycoplasmas in genitourinary tract infection and reproductive failure. *Prog. Gynecol.* 5:275–282, 1970.

Kundsin R.B.: Personal communication, 1984.

Kundsin R.B., Driscoll S.G., Ming P.L.: Strain of *Mycoplasma* associated with human reproductive failure. *Science*, September 1967, pp. 1573–1574.

Lagrew D., Wilson E.A., Jawad J.: Determination of gestational age by serum concentrations of human chorionic gonadotropin. *Obstet. Gynecol.* 62:37–40, 1983.

Lopata A.: Concepts in human in vitro fertilization and embryo transfer. *Fertil. Steril.* 40:289–301, 1983.

McConnell H.D., Carr D.H.: Recent advances in the cytogenetic study of human spontaneous abortions. *Obstet. Gynecol.* 45(5):547–552, 1975.

McShane P., Reilly R.J., Schiff I.: Pregnancy outcomes following Tompkins metroplasty. *Fertil. Steril.* 40:190–194, 1983.

Madore C., Hawes W.E., Many F., et al.: A study of the effects of induced abortion on subsequent pregnancy outcome. *Am. J. Obstet. Gynecol.* 139:516–521, 1981.

March C.M.: Hysteroscopy: The womb revisited. *Fertil. Steril.* 39:455–457, 1983.

March C.M., Israel R.: Gestational outcome following hysteroscopic types of adhesions. *Fertil. Steril.* 36:455–459, 1981.

Marshall F.F., Beisel D.S.: The association of uterine and renal anomalies. *Obstet. Gynecol.* 51:559–562, 1978.

Masson G.W., Anthony F., Wilson M.S., et al.: Comparison of serum and urinary HCG levels with SP_1 and PAPP-A levels in patients with first trimester vaginal bleeding. *Obstet. Gynecol.* 61:223–226, 1983.

Mathur S., Baker E.R., Williamson H.O., et al.: Clinical significance of sperm antibodies in infertility. *Fertil. Steril.* 36:486–495, 1981.

Michels V.V., Medrano C., Venne V.L., et al.: Chromosome translocations in couples with multiple spontaneous abortions. *Am. J. Hum. Genet.* 34:507–513, 1982.

Mishell D.R., Thorneycroft D.H., Nagata Y., et al.: Serum gonadotropin and steroid patterns in early human gestation. *Am. J. Obstet. Gynecol.* 117:631–639, 1973.

Musich J.R., Behrman S.J.: Obstetric outcome before and after metroplasty in women with uterine anomalies. *Obstet. Gynecol.* 52:63–66, 1978.

Naylor A.F., Warburton D.: Sequential analysis of spontaneous abortion: II. Collaborative study data showing that gravidity determines a very substantial rise in risk. *Fertil. Steril.* 32:282–286, 1979.

Neuwirth R.S.: Hysteroscopic management of symptomatic submucus fibroids. *Obstet. Gynecol.* 62:509–511, 1983.

Nordlander C., Fuchs T., Hammarstrom L., et al.: Human leukocyte antigens group A in couples with unexplained infertility. *Fertil. Steril.* 40:60–65, 1983.

Noyes R.W., Hertig A., Rock J.: Dating the endometrial biopsy. *Fertil. Steril.* 1:3, 1950.

Oksenberg J.R., Persitz E., Amar A., et al.: Mixed lymphocyte reactivity nonresponsiveness in couples with multiple spontaneous abortions. *Fertil. Steril.* 39:525–530, 1983.

Poland B.J., Miller J.R., Jones D.C., et al.: Reproductive counseling in patients who have had a spontaneous abortion. *Am. J. Obstet. Gynecol.* 127:685–691, 1977.

Poland B., Yuen B.H.: Embryonic development in consecutive specimens from recurrent spontaneous abortion. *Am. J. Obstet. Gynecol.* 130:512–515, 1978.

Quagliarello J., Szlachter N., Nesselbaum J.S., et al.: Serum relaxin and human chorionic concentrations in spontaneous abortions. *Fertil. Steril.* 36:399–401, 1981.

Quagliarello J., Weiss G.: Clomiphene citrate in the management of infertility associated with shortened luteal phases. *Fertil. Steril.* 31:373–377, 1979.

Quinn P.A., Shewchuk A.B., Shuber J., et al.: Efficacy of antibiotic therapy in preventing spontaneous pregnancy loss among couples colonized with genital mycoplasmas. *Am. J. Obstet. Gynecol.* 45:239–244, 1983.

Rock J.A., Guzeck D.S., Sengos C., et al.: The conservative surgical treatment of endometriosis: Evaluation of pregnancy success with respect to the extent of the disease as categorized using contemporary classification systems. *Fertil. Steril.* 35:131–137, 1981.

Rock J.A., Jones H.A.: The clinical management of the double uterus. *Fertil. Steril.* 28:798–806, 1977.

Rock J.A., Zacur H.A.: The clinical management of repeated early pregnancy loss. *Fertil. Steril.* 39:123–140, 1983.

Rocklin R.E., Kitzmiller J.L., Carpenter C.B., et al.: Maternal-fetal relation—absence of an immunologic blocking factor from the serum of women with chronic abortions. *N. Engl. J. Med.* 295:1209–1213, 1976.

Rolfe B.E.: Detection of fetal wastage. *Fertil. Steril.* 37:655–660, 1982.

Rosenberg S.A., Luciano A.A., Riddick D.H.: The luteal phase defect: The relative frequency of, and encouraging response to, treatment with vaginal progesterone. *Fertil. Steril.* 34:17–20, 1980.

Sanfilippo J.S., Yussman M.A., Smith O.: Hysterosalpingography in the evaluation of infertility: A six year review. *Fertil. Steril.* 30:636–643, 1978.

St. Michel P., DiZerega G.S.: Hyperprolactinemia and luteal phase dysfunction infertility. *Obstet. Gynecol. Surv.* 38:248–254, 1983.

Saxena B.B., Landesman R.: Diagnosis and management of pregnancy by the radioreceptor assay of human chorionic gonadotropin. *Am. J. Obstet. Gynecol.* 131:97–107, 1978.

Schenker J.S., Margalioth E.J.: Intrauterine adhesions: An updated appraisal. *Fertil. Steril.* 37:593–610, 1982.

Schoenbaum S., Monson R.R., Stubblefield P.G., et al.: Outcome of delivery following an induced or spontaneous abortion. *Am. J. Obstet. Gynecol.* 136:19–24, 1980.

Schmidt G., Fowler W.C., Talbert L., et al.: Reproductive history of women exposed to diethylstilbestrol in utero. *Fertil. Steril.* 33:21–24, 1980.

Schweditsch M.O., Dubin N.H., Jones G.S., et al.: Hormonal considerations in early human pregnancy and blighted ovum syndrome. *Fertil. Steril.* 31:252–257, 1979.

Scott J.R.: Immunologic aspects of recurrent spontaneous abortion. *Fertil. Steril.* 38:301–302, 1982.

Seegar-Jones G., Maffezzoli R.D., Strott C.A., et al.: Pathophysiology of reproductive failure after clomiphene-induced ovulation. *Am. J. Obstet. Gynecol.* 108:847–867, 1970.

Semmens J.P.: Congenital anomalies of the female genital tract. *Obstet. Gynecol.* 19:328–350, 1962.

Siegler A.M.: Hysterosalpingography. *Fertil. Steril.* 40:139–158, 1983.

Simpson J.L., Elias S., Martin A.O.: Parental chromosomal rearrangements associated with repetitive abortions. *Fertil. Steril.* 36:584–590, 1981.

Simpson J.L.: Genes, chromosomes and reproductive failure. *Fertil. Steril.* 33:107–116, 1980.

Simpson J.L., Golbus M.S., Martin A.O., et al.: Spontaneous abortion and fetal wastage, in *Genetics in Obstetrics and Gynecology.* New York, Grune & Stratton, Inc., chap. 7, pp. 121–132, 1982.

Simpson J.L.: Repeated suboptimal pregnancy outcome. *Birth Defects* 17:113–142, 1981.

Singh D.N., Hara S., Foster H., et al.: Reproductive performance in women with sex chromosome mosaicism. *Obstet. Gynecol.* 55:608–611, 1980.

Smart Y.C., Roberts T.K., Clancy R.L., et al.: Early pregnancy factor: Its role in mammalian reproduction—research review. *Fertil. Steril.* 35:397–402, 1981.

Soules M.R., Hughes C.L., Askel S., et al.: The function of the corpus luteum of pregnancy and ovulatory dysfunction and luteal phase deficiency. *Fertil. Steril.* 36:31–40, 1981.

Spaepen M.S., Kundsin R.B., Horne H.W.: Tetracycline resistant T-strain mycoplasmas *(Ureaplasma urealyticum)* from patients with a history of reproductive failure. *Antimicrob. Agents Chemother.* 9:1012–1018, 1976.

Stein Z.: Early fetal loss. *Birth Defects* 17:95–111, 1981.

Stenchever M.A.: Habitual abortion. *Contemp. Ob./Gyn.* 22:162–174, 1983.

Stetten G., Rock J.A.: A paracentric chromosomal inversion associated with repeat pregnancy wastage. *Fertil. Steril.* 40:124–126, 1983.

Stillman R.J.: In utero exposure to diethylstilbestrol: Adverse effects on the reproductive tract and reproductive performance in male and female offspring. *Am. J. Obstet. Gynecol.* 142:905–921, 1982.

Stray-Pedersen B., Lorentzen-Styr A-M.: Uterine *Toxoplasma* infections and repeated abortions. *Am. J. Obstet. Gynecol.* 128:716–721, 1977.

Taylor C., Faulk W.P.: Prevention of recurrent abortion with leukocyte transfusion. *Lancet* 2:68–69, 1981.

Taylor P.J., Hamon J.E.: Hysteroscopy. *J. Reprod. Med.* 28:359–390, 1983.

Taylor-Robinson D., McCormack W.M.: The genital mycoplasmas. *N. Engl. J. Med.* 302:1003–1010, 1063–1067, 1980.

Tho S.P.J., Byrd J.R., McDonough P.G.: Chromosome polymorphism in 110 couples with reproductive failure and subsequent pregnancy outcome. *Fertil. Steril.* 38:688–693, 1982.

Tsuji K., Nakano R.: Chromosome studies of embryos from induced abortions in pregnant women age 35 and over. *Obstet. Gynecol.* 52:542–544, 1978.

Upadhyaya M., Hibbard B.M., Walker S.M.: The role of mycoplasmas in reproduction. *Fertil. Steril.* 39:814–818, 1983.

Vaitukaitis J.L., Braunstein G.D., Ross G.T.: A radioimmunoassay which specifically measures human chorionic gonadotropin in the presence of human luteinizing hormone. *Am. J. Obstet. Gynecol.* 113:751, 1972.

Valle R.F., Sciarra J.J.; Current status of hysteroscopy in gynecologic practice. *Fertil. Steril.* 32:619–632, 1979.

Verma R.S., Shah J.V., Dosik H.: Size of Y chromosome not associated with abortion risk. *Obstet. Gynecol.* 61:633–634, 1983.

Verp M.S., Rzeszotarski M.S., Martin A.O., et al.: Relationship between Y chromosome length and first trimester abortion. *Am. J. Obstet. Gynecol.* 45:433–438, 1983.

Verp M.S., Simpson J.L., Elias S., et al.: Heritable aspects of uterine anomalies: I. Three familial aggregates with müllerian fusion anomalies. *Fertil. Steril.* 40:80–90, 1983.

Warburton D., Fraser F.C.: On the probability that a woman who has had a spontaneous abortion will abort in subsequent pregnancies. *Br. J. Ostet. Gynaecol.* 68:784–787, 1961.

Warburton D., Fraser F.C.: Spontaneous abortion risks in man: Data from reproductive histories collected in a medical genetics unit. *Hum. Genet.* 16:1–25, 1964.

Wentz A.C.: Endometrial biopsy in the evaluation of infertility. *Fertil. Steril.* 33:121–124, 1980.

Wheeler J.M., Johnston B.M., Malinak L.R.: The relationship of endometriosis to spontaneous abortion. *Fertil. Steril.* 39:656–660, 1983.

Wright A.W., Pollack A., Nicholson H., et al.: Spontaneous abortion and diabetes mellitus. *Postgrad. Med. J.* 59:295–298, 1983.

CHAPTER TWELVE

The Management of Molar Pregnancy and Gestational Trophoblastic Tumors

DONALD PETER GOLDSTEIN, M.D.
ROSS S. BERKOWITZ, M.D.

GESTATIONAL TROPHOBLASTIC TUMORS (GTT) are one of the rare human malignancies that can be predictably cured even in the presence of widespread metastases (Goldstein and Berkowitz, 1982a; Bagshawe, 1976; Jones and Lewis, 1974). GTT include a spectrum of interrelated neoplasms, including invasive mole and choriocarcinoma, that have varying propensities for local invasion and distant spread. While GTT most commonly follow a hydatidiform mole, they may ensue after any gestational event, including ectopic and term pregnancy or spontaneous and therapeutic abortion. Important advances have been made in the diagnosis, management, and follow-up of molar pregnancy and GTT since the introduction of chemotherapy in 1956. This chapter will review these advances and discuss basic principles in the management of these conditions based on the experience accumulated at the New England Trophoblastic Disease Center (NETDC) between 1965 and the present.

HISTORICAL BACKGROUND

Li, Hertz, and Spencer inaugurated a new era in the treatment of GTT in 1956 when they reported the complete regression of metastatic choriocarcinoma in three women treated with methotrexate. Hertz and co-workers reviewed the initial five-year experience with chemotherapy for metastatic GTT at the National Cancer Institute in 1961 (Hertz et al., 1961). Methotrexate induced complete remission in 28 (47%) of 63 patients with metastatic disease. In 1961, Brewer and co-workers reported the survival of patients with choriocarcinoma at Northwestern University, Chicago (Brewer et al., 1961). Only six of 103 patients with metastatic choriocarcinoma were free of tumor at five years following their diagnosis. Brewer and associates also reviewed the five-year survival rates in patients with "nonmetastatic" choriocarcinoma treated by hysterectomy (Brewer et al., 1963). Only 29 (41.4%) of 70 patients with "localized" tumor survived despite prompt hysterectomy. Postoperatively, the remaining patients developed metastases and died from widespread dissemination. Surgical therapy alone, therefore, had limited ability to achieve cure in choriocarcinoma. Because of the dramatic success of chemotherapy in metastatic GTT, Hertz and co-workers then administered chemotherapy as primary treatment in nonmetastatic disease (Hertz et al., 1963). Chemotherapy effectively eliminated the need for hysterectomy in these patients and thereby enabled the preservation of fertility.

During the mid-1960s and early 1970s, it became increasingly apparent that certain patients with metastatic GTT were relatively resistant to single-agent chemotherapy and experienced a high mortality rate. Ross and coworkers observed that patients with high human chorionic gonadotropin (HCG) levels, prolonged delays in diagnosis, and brain or liver metastases were resistant to single-agent chemotherapy. Primary intensive combination chemotherapy was then employed in high-risk metastatic GTT and resulted in a substantial improvement in survival (Hammond et al., 1973).

The management of GTT has since been refined and guided by the experience from a growing number of regional centers in this country and abroad. Virtually all patients with nonmetastatic and low-risk metastatic GTT can now expect cure with chemotherapy (Goldstein and Berkowitz, 1982b). Patients with high-risk metastatic disease can expect an 80% survival rate with aggressive multimodality therapy. The experience in GTT thus represents one of the most dramatic triumphs of chemotherapy in the treatment of human malignancy (Table 12–1).

ANTECEDENT PREGNANCY

Figure 12–1 summarizes the interrelationships among the various types of pregnancies and GTT. Approximately 20% of all pregnancies terminate in spontaneous abortions and about one half of such abortuses are either pathologic or blighted ova. In two thirds of the abnormal pregnancies, the chorionic villi show early hydatidiform swelling. Hertig estimated that true hydatidiform mole occurs once in approximately 2,000 pregnancies in this country, an incidence of .05%. Molar pregnancy, however, is considerably more common in other regions of the world (Table 12–2).

Choriocarcinoma, usually metastatic, fol-

TABLE 12–1.—SUMMARY OF NETDC CLINICAL MATERIAL FROM JULY 1, 1965 TO JUNE 30, 1976

Total no. of patients admitted	865
Total no. of patients with a diagnosis, of molar pregnancy	624 (72%)
Uncomplicated	512 (82%)
Complicated	112 (18%)*
Total no. of patients with a diagnosis of GTT	241 (28%)†
Nonmetastatic	142 (59%)
Metastatic	99 (41%)
Remissions	227 (94%)
Deaths	14 (6%)

*Includes patients originally admitted with a diagnosis of molar pregnancy who subsequently developed a trophoblastic tumor.
†Includes patients who developed complications following evacuation of a molar pregnancy.

lows delivery in about 1:160,000 live births and in approximately 1:20 moles. The overall incidence of this highly malignant type of GTT is, therefore, 1:40,000 gestations. Most clinicians are well aware of the 15% to 20% risk of development of persistent GTT following molar pregnancy, but frequently overlook this complication when the antecedent pregnancy is nonmolar and somewhat remote in time. Patients in the latter group, in whom there is a delay in diagnosis, frequently present with late advanced GTT that is often resistant to conventional chemotherapy.

MORPHOLOGY

GTT develops in the placenta at the site of the cytotrophoblast and syncytiotrophoblast. Figure 12–2 illustrates the appearance of a normal chorionic villus with fetal vessels throughout the villous stroma and single layers of normal-appearing trophoblastic cells. According to Hertig and Mansell, hydatidiform mole develops when fetal vascularity is lost and the villi become hydropic from progressive accumulation of fluid within the connective tissue spaces of the chorionic villi, forming multiple, isolated grapelike cysts called *vesicles* (Fig 12–3). Microscopic examination of the villi demonstrates varying degrees of trophoblastic proliferation ranging from minimal

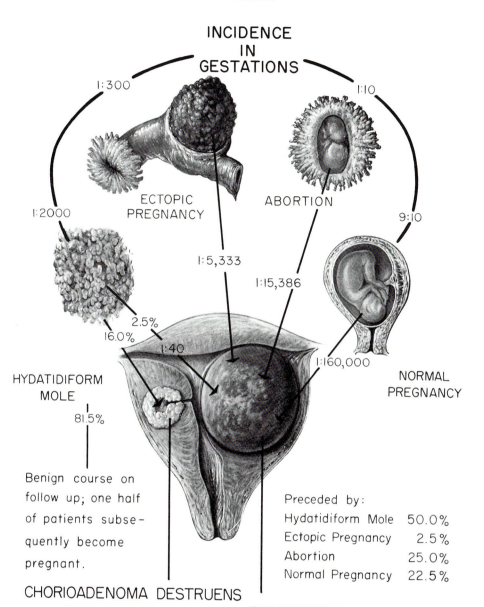

INCIDENCE
IN
GESTATIONS

1:300

1:10

ECTOPIC
PREGNANCY

ABORTION

1:2000

9:10

1:5,333

1:15,386

2.5%

16.0%

1:40

1:160,000

HYDATIDIFORM
MOLE

NORMAL
PREGNANCY

81.5%

Benign course on
follow up; one half
of patients subse-
quently become
pregnant.

Preceded by:
Hydatidiform Mole 50.0%
Ectopic Pregnancy 2.5%
Abortion 25.0%
Normal Pregnancy 22.5%

CHORIOADENOMA DESTRUENS

CHORIOCARCINOMA

Fig 12–1.—Schematic representation of the relation of various types of pregnancy to chorio-adenoma destruens (invasive mole) and chorio-carcinoma (true chorionepithelioma). Note that when pregnancies are followed by chorionic malignancy a hydatidiform mole can give rise to either variety of chorioma, although the other types of pregnancy appear to give rise only to chorio-carcinoma. The more pathologic or abnormal the pregnancy, the more likely it is to give rise to a true choriocarcinoma. The tendency of any one type of pregnancy to become malignant is indicated by the ratios or percentages on the interconnecting lines. (From Hertig A.T., Gore H.M.: Tumors of the female sex organs: part 2, Tumors of the vulva, vagina and uterus, sec. 9, fasc. 33, *Atlas of Tumor Pathology.* Washington, D.C., Armed Forces Institute of Pathology, 1960.)

TABLE 12–2.—Worldwide Incidence of Molar Pregnancy*

COUNTRY	INCIDENCE	AUTHOR
Taiwan (Formosa)	1:120	Wei & Ouyang (1963)
Philippines	1:173	Acosta-Sison (1959)
Mexico	1:200	Márquez-Monter et al. (1963)
India	1:160–1:400	Pai (1967)
Japan	1:232	Hasegawa (1957)
Hong Kong	1:242	Chun et al. (1964)
Russia	1:333	Karzavina (1949)
Israel	1:460	Brandes & Peretz (1965)
France	1:500	Brindeau et al. (1952)
Hong Kong	1:530	King (1956)
Guatemala	1:670	Aramliura (1958)
Australia	1:695	Beischer & Fortune (1968)
Australia	1:820	Coppleson (1958)
Chile	1:829	Cabrera (1946)
Great Britain (various)	1:835	Das (1938)
Great Britain (Belfast)	1:1,190	Stevenson et al. (1959)
Brazil	1:1,071	Fernandes & Marques (1957)
Holland	1:1,200	De Snoo (1946)
U.S.A.	1:1,000	Douglas (1959)
U.S.A.	1:1,349	Mueller & Lapp (1949)
U.S.A. (Boston)	1:2,062	Hertig & Sheldon (1947)
U.S.A.	1:2,500	Novak (1950)
U.S.A. (Chicago)	1:1,699 (deliveries) 1:2,093 (pregnancies)	Brewer & Gerbie (1967)
U.S.A. (Rhode Island)	1:1,450	Yen & MacMahon (1968)

*After Bagshawe K.D.: *Choriocarcinoma.* Baltimore, Williams & Wilkins Co., 1969, p. 32.

to marked hyperplasia with or without invasion, increased mitotic activity, and atypicality (Fig 12–4). Hertig and Sheldon have shown that the potential for a hydatidiform mole to manifest persistent GTT correlates well with its histologic appearance. Hydatidiform moles with marked trophoblastic hyperplasia and anaplasia have an increased risk of development of persistent GTT.

Choriocarcinoma also originates in the trophoblastic cells of the villus, but in contrast to hydatidiform mole is composed of sheets of malignant-appearing cytotrophoblast and syncytiotrophoblast. Choriocarcinoma is sufficiently undifferentiated to lose the ability to recapitulate the normal villous structure while retaining the ability to produce HCG. Grossly, choriocarcinoma may be localized in the uterus, where it appears red, granular, and hemorrhagic, either as a discrete nodule or as a tumor mass that fills the uterine cavity (Fig 12–5). Microscopically, choriocarcinoma

recapitulates the pattern exhibited by the 14-day implantation site, with the typical plexiform pattern of pure trophoblast and an admixture of blood clot and necrotic tissue (Fig 12–6).

Following molar evacuation, persistent GTT may have the histologic pattern of either hydatidiform mole or choriocarcinoma. However, after nonmolar gestations, persistent GTT exhibits only the histologic features of choriocarcinoma.

HYDATIDIFORM MOLE

Complete vs. Partial Hydatidiform Mole

Pathologic and Chromosomal Features

Hydatidiform mole may be categorized as either a complete (classical) mole or partial mole on the basis of gross morphologic and histopathologic features and karyotype (Table 12–3).

Complete moles have no identifiable em-

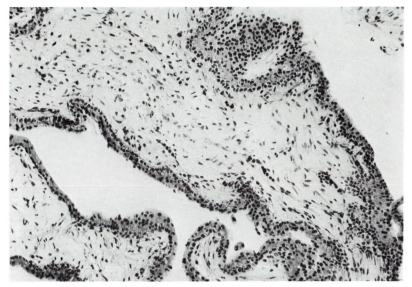

Fig 12–2.—Normal villus of early pregnancy showing fetal vessels throughout the stroma and single layers of normal-appearing cytotrophoblastic syncytiotrophoblastic tissue.

bryonic or fetal tissues. The chorionic villi have generalized hydatidiform swelling and are diffusely enveloped by atypical and hyperplastic trophoblast (Driscoll, 1981). Recent cytogenetic studies provide important information concerning the genesis of complete moles. Complete hydatidiform moles generally have a 46 XX karyotype and the molar chromosomes are derived entirely from paternal origin (Kajii and Ohama, 1977). Complete moles appear to arise from an ovum that has been fertilized by a haploid sperm, which then duplicates its own chromosomes after meiosis (Yamashita et al., 1979). The ovum nucleus may be either absent or inactivated. While most complete moles have a 46 XX chromosomal pattern, about 10% of complete moles have a 46 XY karyotype (Pattillo et al.,

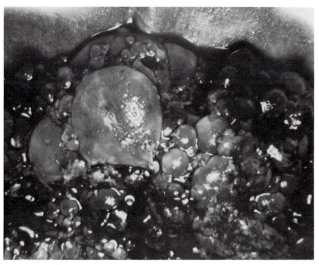

Fig 12–3.—Hydatidiform mole showing swollen, fluid-filled vesicles of varying sizes.

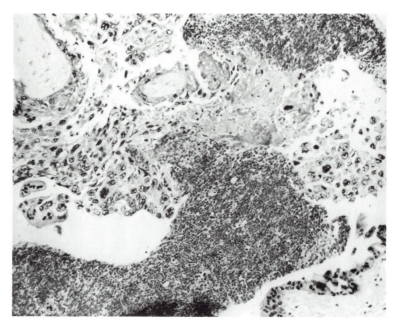

Fig 12–4.—Hydatidiform mole showing hyperplasia and anaplasia of epithelial elements. Note syncytial border of villus at lower right and "tissue-culture" growth of pure trophoblast in center.

1981). The molar chromosomes in the 46 XY complete mole also appear to be derived entirely from paternal origin (Surti et al., 1979). A 45 X complete mole has also been recently described (Berkowitz et al., 1982b). Complete hydatidiform mole therefore appears to be the morphologic expression of a variety of chromosomal patterns.

Partial hydatidiform moles are characterized by the following pathologic features: (1) variously sized chorionic villi with focal hydatidiform swelling and cavitation; (2) marked vil-

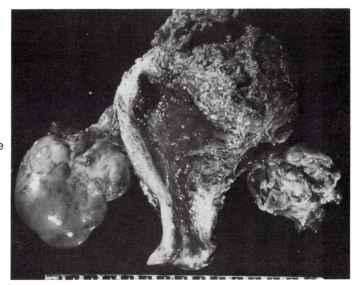

Fig 12–5.—Uterine choriocarcinoma with massive destruction of uterine wall.

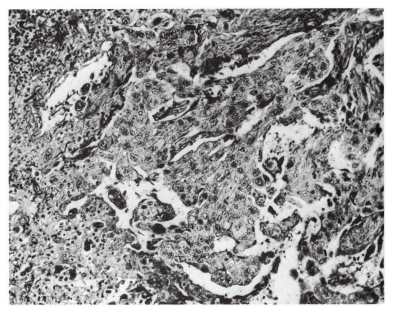

Fig 12–6.—Typical plexiform arrangement of trophoblastic cells in choriocarcinoma.

lous scalloping; (3) focal trophoblastic hyperplasia, with or without atypia; (4) prominent stromal trophoblastic inclusions; and (5) identifiable fetal or embryonic tissues (Szulman and Surti, 1978b). Partial moles generally have a triploid karyotype with the extra haploid set of chromosomes derived from either parent, but most often from the father (Szulman and Surti, 1978a). When fetuses are identified with partial moles, they generally have stigmata of triploidy, including growth retardation and multiple congenital anomalies.

Complete Hydatidiform Mole

Signs and Symptoms

Table 12–4 reviews the initial signs and symptoms of the first 306 patients with complete molar pregnancy managed at the

New England Trophoblastic Disease Center (NETDC) (Goldstein et al., 1981).

VAGINAL BLEEDING.—Vaginal bleeding is the most common symptom in patients with complete molar pregnancy (Curry et al., 1975) occurring in 97% of patients. Molar tissues may separate from the decidua and disrupt maternal vessels, thereby inducing bright-red vaginal bleeding. The endometrial cavity may be expanded by large volumes of retained blood. When the intrauterine clots undergo oxidation and liquefaction, "prune juice"–like fluid may leak into the vagina. Because the vaginal bleeding may be prolonged and considerable, half of the patients present with anemia (hemoglobin level, 10 gm/dl or less).

TABLE 12–3.—COMPLETE VS. PARTIAL HYDATIDIFORM MOLE

	COMPLETE MOLE	PARTIAL MOLE
Fetal or embryonic tissue	Absent	Present
Hydatidiform swelling of chorionic villi	Diffuse	Focal
Trophoblastic hyperplasia	Diffuse	Focal
Scalloping of chorionic villi	Absent	Present
Trophoblastic stromal inclusions	Absent	Present
Karyotype	46 XX; 46 XY	Triploid

TABLE 12–4.—CLINICAL SIGNS IN 306 PATIENTS
WITH COMPLETE HYDATIDIFORM MOLE
AT THE NETDC

SIGN	NO. (%) OF PATIENTS
Vaginal bleeding	297 (97)
Anemia	165 (54)
Excessive uterine enlargement	156 (51)
Toxemia of pregnancy	83 (27)
Hyperemesis gravidarum	80 (26)
Hyperthyroidism	21 (7)
Trophoblastic emboli	6 (2)

EXCESSIVE UTERINE SIZE.—The uterus is excessively enlarged in relation to the gestational age in 51% of patients with complete hydatidiform mole. The endometrial cavity may be expanded by both molar tissue and retained blood. Although the uterus may reach the xiphoid, there is no detectable fetal heartbeat. Excessive uterine size is generally associated with markedly elevated HCG levels because uterine enlargement partially results from exuberant trophoblastic proliferation. While excessive uterine size is one of the classic signs of complete molar pregnancy, it is important to remember that almost half of the patients with complete mole lack this clinical finding.

TOXEMIA.—At the time of presentation, preeclamptic toxemia is observed in 27% of patients with complete hydatidiform mole. Although preeclampsia is often associated with marked edema, hypertension, proteinuria and clonus, eclamptic convulsions rarely develop. Toxemia occurs almost exclusively in patients with excessive uterine enlargement and markedly elevated HCG levels. Curry et al. observed that 81% of their patients with molar pregnancy and toxemia had excessive uterine size. The diagnosis of hydatidiform mole should be considered in any woman in whom toxemia develops early in pregnancy.

HYPEREMESIS GRAVIDARUM.—Hyperemesis requiring antiemetic and/or intravenous therapy occurs in 26% of patients with complete hydatidiform mole. Infrequently, severe electrolyte disturbances may develop that require treatment with parenteral fluids. Hyperemesis develops primarily in patients with excessive uterine size and markedly elevated HCG levels. The cause of hyperemesis in these patients has not been explained.

HYPERTHYROIDISM.—Clinically evident hyperthyroidism is observed in 7% of patients with complete molar gestation at the time of diagnosis. These patients may present with tachycardia, warm skin, tremor, and thyroid enlargement. The diagnosis of hyperthyroidism is confirmed by detecting elevated serum levels of free thyroxine (T_4) and triiodothyronine (T_3). Laboratory evidence of hyperthyroidism may be commonly detected in patients with hydatidiform moles. Galton and associates measured thyroid function tests in 11 patients with molar pregnancy before and after molar evacuation. Before molar evacuation, all patients had elevated values for free T_4, thyroidal ^{131}I uptake, and protein-bound ^{131}I. The thyroid function test results rapidly returned to normal in all patients following molar evacuation.

If hyperthyroidism is detected, it is important to administer β-adrenergic blockers prior to induction of anesthesia for molar evacuation, since anesthesia or surgery may precipitate a "thyroid storm" in a patient with uncontrolled or inadequately treated hyperthyroidism. Thyroid storm may be manifested by hyperthermia, delirium, convulsion, coma, atrial fibrillation, or cardiovascular collapse. The administration of β-adrenergic blockers prevents or rapidly reverses many of the metabolic and cardiovascular complications of thyroid storm.

Some investigators have implicated HCG as the thyroid stimulator in hydatidiform mole (Kenimer et al., 1975; Nisula and Taliadouros, 1980). Positive correlations between serum HCG and serum total T_4 or total T_3 concentrations have been observed in some, but not all, studies. While HCG has thyrotropic activity in the mouse, in vitro experiments with

HCG have shown no thyrotropic activity with human thyroid membranes (Amir et al. 1980). Nagataki and co-workers also found no correlation between serum HCG and free T_4 levels in ten patients with molar pregnancy. The identity of the thyrotropic factor in hydatidiform mole has therefore not been clearly delineated. While some investigators have speculated about a separate chorionic thyrotropin, this entity has not yet been isolated.

Trophoblastic embolization.—Two percent of patients with complete hydatidiform mole develop trophoblastic embolization to the pulmonary vasculature, and present with the acute onset of chest pain, dyspnea, tachypnea, and tachycardia (Kohorn et al., 1978). Patients may experience severe respiratory distress in the recovery room after molar evacuation due to trophoblastic embolization. Auscultation of the chest usually reveals diffuse rales and chest roentgenogram may demonstrate bilateral pulmonary infiltrates (Fig 12–7). The electrocardiogram (ECG) may indicate right-sided heart strain due to an acute increase in pulmonary vascular resistance. The signs and symptoms of respiratory distress generally resolve within 72 hours with supportive care and supplemental oxygen.

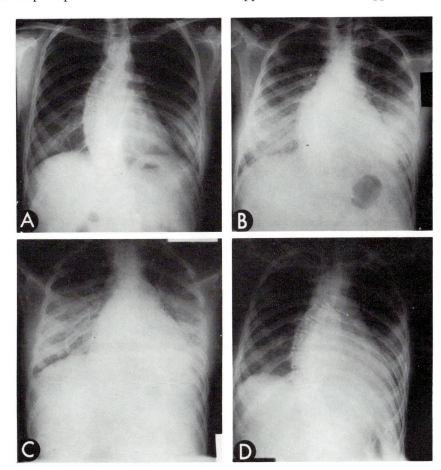

Fig 12–7.—Chest roentgenograms of patient in whom trophoblastic embolization developed immediately following suction evacuation of molar pregnancy. The condition generally runs its course in 72 to 96 hours, as shown by complete clearing of both lung fields **(D)**.

Anticoagulation is usually not indicated in the management of trophoblastic embolization, although digitalis may be indicated in severe cases.

THECA-LUTEIN OVARIAN CYSTS.—Prominent theca-lutein ovarian cysts (greater than 6 cm in diameter) develop in about half of patients with complete hydatidiform mole (Berkowitz and Goldstein, 1981a). The cysts contain amber-colored or serosanguineous fluid and are usually multilocular. Ovarian enlargement occurs almost exclusively in patients with markedly elevated HCG levels. The formation of theca-lutein cysts may also be related to increased serum levels of prolactin (Osathanondh et al., 1981). Theca-lutein cysts may be difficult to palpate on physical examination because the uterus may also be excessively enlarged. However, ultrasonography can accurately document their presence and size. Following molar evacuation, theca lutein cysts normally regress spontaneously within two to four months (Scheer and Goldstein, 1973.).

Since prominent theca-lutein cysts frequently cause symptoms of marked pelvic pressure or fullness, they may be decompressed by laparoscopic or transabdominal aspiration after molar evacuation to relieve symptoms of pelvic pressure and to reduce the risk of cystic torsion or rupture (Berkowitz et al., 1980b). If a patient with theca-lutein cysts manifests acute pelvic pain, laparoscopy should be performed to assess possible cystic torsion or rupture. Laparoscopic manipulation may successfully manage incomplete ovarian torsion or cystic rupture.

Partial Hydatidiform Mole

Presenting Signs and Symptoms

Between June 1967 and January 1982, diagnoses of partial hydatidiform mole were made in 33 patients at the NETDC. The presenting sign or symptom was vaginal bleeding in 23 patients (69.7%), absent fetal heartbeat in five patients (15.1%), excessive uterine size in three patients (9.1%), and preeclampsia in

two patients (6.1%). The uterine size was small for gestational dates in 16 patients (48.5%), appropriate in 13 patients (39.4%), and large for gestational dates in only four patients (12.1%). The presenting clinical diagnosis was threatened or incomplete abortion in ten patients (30.3%), missed abortion in 18 patients (54.6%), and hydatidiform mole in only five patients (15.1%). Preevacuation HCG levels were measured in 14 patients and exceeded 100,000 mIU/ml in only three. The three patients with HCG levels greater than 100,000 mIU/ml were the only ones in whom preeclampsia developed. Patients with partial hydatidiform mole usually do not have the clinical features that are characteristic of complete (classic) molar pregnancy. These patients generally present with the signs and symptoms of spontaneous or missed abortion, and the diagnosis of partial mole may only be made after histologic review of the curettage specimens (Szulman and Surti, 1982).

Diagnosis of Hydatidiform Mole

Human Chorionic Gonadotropin

Human chorionic gonadotropin is a predictable and constant secretory product of the trophoblastic cell (Goldstein, 1976). Like the other glycoprotein hormones luteinizing hormone [LH], follicle-stimulating hormone [FSH] and thyroid-stimulating hormone [TSH]), HCG is composed of two polypeptide chains (α and β) attached to a carbohydrate moiety. There is considerable cross-reactivity between HCG and LH because they share indistinguishable α-chains. The β-chain of the four glycoprotein hormones is biochemically unique and confers immunologic and biologic specificity. In 1972, Vaitukaitis and co-workers developed a highly sensitive and specific radioimmunoassay for HCG based on the immunologic properties of the β-subunit structure. The β-subunit radioimmunoassay is particularly useful in quantitating low levels of HCG to prevent interference from physiologic levels of LH.

Marked elevation of HCG levels has long been regarded as a valuable diagnostic sign of hydatidiform mole. The increased number of proliferating trophoblastic cells of a molar pregnancy may produce larger quantitites of HCG than seen at the corresponding gestational age in a normal single pregnancy (Fig 12–8). The HCG level in patients with a single pregnancy rarely exceeds 100,000 mIU/ml after the 12th week of gestation. In contrast, molar pregnancy may be associated with much higher HCG levels. However, in about half of the patients with molar gestations, the endometrial cavity is not excessively enlarged by trophoblastic proliferation. The HCG levels in these patients may actually be lower than the levels seen in normal pregnancies of the same gestational age. Therefore, the HCG level alone cannot conclusively establish or refute the diagnosis of hydatidiform mole. The clinician must also consider the possibility of a multiple gestation when a patient presents with markedly elevated HCG levels, excessive uterine enlargement, and vaginal bleeding.

Ultrasonography

Ultrasonography is a sensitive and reliable noninvasive technique for distinguishing a normal intrauterine gestation from a molar pregnancy. Because of the marked hydatidiform swelling of the chorionic villi, molar pregnancy produces a characteristic vesicular or "snowstorm" pattern on the ultrasonogram (Fig 12–9). If a normal pregnancy is present, the gestational sac should be visualized from the sixth to the tenth week of gestation and the fetal head should be identified after the 14th week of gestation. The following conditions may be confused with a hydatidiform mole during an ultrasound examination: (1) early pregnancy with coexisting uterine fibroids, (2) normal pregnancy in the tenth to 13th weeks of gestation, (3) tangential section of a normal placenta, (4) intrauterine clotted blood, and (5) missed abortion. However, ultrasonography is remarkably accurate in the diagnosis of hydatidiform mole when it is performed and interpreted by a skilled and experienced individual. Furthermore, unlike

amniography, ultrasonography does not expose the mother or her fetus to the potential hazards of ionizing radiation or invasive procedures.

Natural History of Hydatidiform Mole

Complete hydatidiform moles are well recognized to have a potential for developing local invasion or distant spread. Following molar evacuation, local uterine invasion occurs in 15% of patients and metastasis develops in 4% of patients (Goldstein et al., 1979).

We recently reviewed 858 patients with complete hydatidiform mole at the NETDC to identify factors that predispose to persistent GTT (Table 12–5). At the time of presentation, 41% of the patients had the following signs of marked trophoblastic proliferation: HCG level greater than 100,000 mIU/ml, uterine size larger than appropriate for gestational age, and theca-lutein cysts larger than 6 cm in diameter. After molar evacuation, 31.0% of these patients manifested local uterine invasion and metastases developed in 8.8%. The risk for persistent GTT is greatly reduced in the patients who did not present with signs of marked trophoblastic growth. Following molar evacuation, only 3.4% of these patients had local invasion and metastases developed in 0.6%. Therefore, patients with hydatidiform moles with markedly elevated HCG levels and excessive uterine size are at increased risk of having persistent GTT develop, and are categorized as high-risk patients.

An increased risk of postmolar GTT has also

TABLE 12–5.—SEQUELAE OF LOW-RISK AND HIGH-RISK COMPLETE HYDATIDIFORM MOLE

OUTCOME	NO. (%) OF PATIENTS*	
	LOW-RISK	HIGH-RISK
Normal involution	486/506 (96)	212/352 (60.2)
Persistent GTT		
Nonmetastatic	17/506 (3.4)	109/352 (31.0)
Metastatic	3/506 (0.6)	31/352 (8.8)
Total	506/858 (59)	352/858 (41)

*All patients managed by evacuation with no prophylactic chemotherapy.

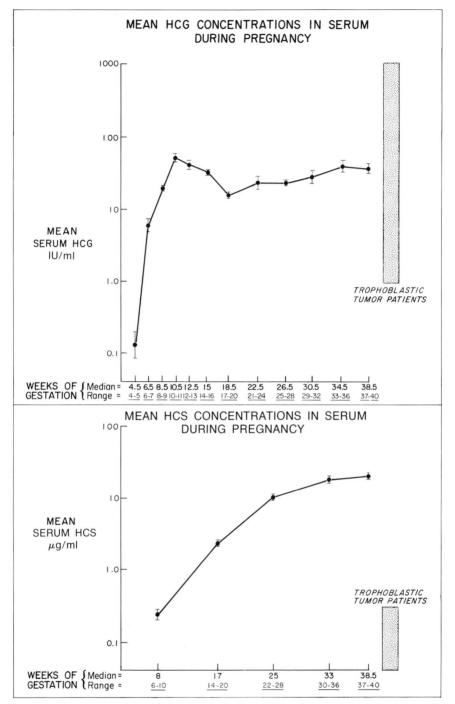

Fig 12–8.—Graphs showing the characteristic pattern of serum HCG and human chorionic somatomammotropin (HCS) levels in normal pregnancy. Also illustrated is the range of serum HCG and HCS values in a series of patients with trophoblastic disease (invasive mole and choriocarcinoma).

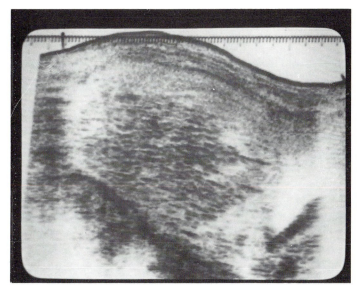

Fig 12–9.—Gray-scale ultra-sonogram of a molar pregnancy in situ. The uterus is completely filled with low-level echoes resembling normal placenta. In addition there are areas of irregular sonoluminescence due to hemorrhage. Circular echo patterns of the vesicles are shown.

been observed in women older than 40 years. Tow reported that 37% of women older than 40 years with molar pregnancy manifested persistent GTT. Hydatidiform moles in older women are frequently aneuploid, and this may be related to their increased potential for local invasion and metastasis (Tsuji et al., 1981).

Only one (3%) of our patients with partial mole developed persistent GTT with local uterine invasion and required chemotherapy to achieve remission (Berkowitz et al., 1979). Partial hydatidiform moles therefore appear to have a limited potential to develop post-molar tumor. This generally agrees with the experience reported by other investigators. To date, there have been no reported cases of choriocarcinoma following partial molar pregnancy.

Treatment

After diagnosis of a hydatidiform mole is made, the patient is carefully evaluated for the presence of associated medical complications, including preeclampsia, electrolyte imbalance, hyperthyroidism, and anemia. The patient's condition is first stabilized, and then a decision must be made concerning the most appropriate method of evacuation. Table 12–

TABLE 12–6.—TREATMENT PROTOCOL FOR HYDATIDIFORM MOLE (NETDC)

Preservation of fertility
  Low-risk patient
    Suction evacuation
    No prophylactic chemotherapy
  High-risk patient
    Suction evacuation
    Prophylactic chemotherapy
Sacrifice of fertility
  Low-risk patient
    Hysterectomy
    No prophylactic chemotherapy
  High-risk patient
    Hysterectomy
    Prophylactic chemotherapy
Follow-up
  HCG determinations weekly until normal for three consecutive weeks, then monthly until normal for six consecutive months
  Effective contraception during gonadotropin follow-up

6 reviews the protocol for managing patients with hydatidiform mole at the NETDC.

If the patient no longer desires to preserve fertility, hysterectomy may be performed with the mole in situ. The ovaries may be conserved at the time of surgery even though theca-lutein cysts are present. However, prominent ovarian cysts should be decompressed by puncture aspiration. Although hysterectomy eliminates the risks associated with local invasion, it does not preclude the possibility of distant spread.

Suction evacuation is the preferred method regardless of uterine size in patients who desire to preserve fertility (Goldstein and Berkowitz, 1982a). It is best to begin an oxytocin infusion in the operating room prior to the induction of anesthesia. The cervix should be gently dilated to accommodate a cannula size that is appropriate for the volume of molar tissue. A rigid 12-mm cannula is usually satisfactory, since this size permits rapid evacuation and involution of the uterus. As the cervix is being dilated, the surgeon frequently encounters an increased amount of uterine bleeding. However, active uterine bleeding should not deter the prompt completion of cervical dilation. If the uterus is larger than 14 weeks' size, one hand should be placed on top of the fundus and the uterus should be massaged to stimulate uterine contraction to reduce the risk of uterine perforation. When suction evacuation is thought to be complete, a sharp curettage using the large Reynolds curette should be performed to remove any residual molar tissue. The curettings from suction and sharp curettage are separately submitted for pathologic review.

After molar evacuation, pelvic examination should be performed to determine the presence of theca-lutein cysts, which may have been masked by the enlarged uterus. Since these cysts regress spontaneously, it is helpful to evaluate their size initially to establish a baseline for future comparison.

Abdominal hysterotomy for the evacuation of a molar pregnancy is an obsolete procedure and should be utilized only when the suction apparatus is unavailable or experience with its use is limited.

If the diagnosis of molar pregnancy is made at the time of spontaneous expulsion, suction evacuation should be carried out immediately. When the diagnosis of hydatidiform mole is unexpectedly made by the pathologist after routine curettage, no further curettage is necessary if the uterus is firm and involuted.

Prophylactic Chemotherapy

The use of prophylactic chemotherapy at the time of molar evacuation is controversial (Goldstein, 1974). The controversy concerns the wisdom of exposing all patients to potentially toxic treatment when only about 19% are at risk for developing persistent GTT.

Between July 1965 and June 1979 at the NETDC, 247 patients with complete molar pregnancy received dactinomycin (actinomycin D) prophylactically at the time of evacuation (Table 12–7). Local uterine invasion subsequently developed in only ten patients (4%) and no patient developed metastases. Furthermore, all ten patients who developed local invasion subsequently achieved remission after only one additional course of chemotherapy. Prophylactic chemotherapy therefore not only prevented metastases, but also reduced the incidence and morbidity of local uterine invasion. Prophylactic chemotherapy may be particularly useful in the management of high-risk complete molar pregnancy, especially when hormonal follow-up is unavailable or unreliable. Prophylactic chemotherapy should not be administered to patients with partial molar pregnancy because of their limited risk of developing persistent GTT.

Hormonal Follow-up

After molar evacuation, all patients must be followed-up fastidiously with quantitative

TABLE 12–7.—PROPHYLACTIC DACTINOMYCIN IN MOLAR PREGNANCY (NETDC, JULY 1965 THROUGH JUNE 1979)

	NO. (%) OF PATIENTS	
OUTCOME	DACTINOMYCIN*	NO DACTINOMYCIN†
Normal involution	237 (96)	698 (81.4)
Persistent GTT		
Nonmetastatic	10 (4)‡	126 (14.6)
Metastatic	0	34 (4)
Totals	247 (100)	858 (100)

*Suction evacuation (or hysterectomy) with prophylactic dactinomycin.
†Suction evacuation (or hysterectomy) without prophylactic dactinomycin.
‡Required only one course of single-agent chemotherapy to achieve remission.

HCG measurements to facilitate the early detection of persistent GTT. The necessity of careful hormonal follow-up cannot be overemphasized. Ideally, HCG should be measured using the β-subunit radioimmunoassay, which detects HCG specifically and quantitatively from high levels down to extinction. Patients are followed-up with weekly β-subunit levels until they are normal for three consecutive weeks and then monthly levels until they are normal for six consecutive months.

Patients are encouraged to use effective contraception during the entire interval of gonadotropin follow-up. We believe that intrauterine devices should not be inserted until the patient achieves a normal HCG level because of the potential risk of a foreign body in a subinvoluted uterus containing invasive tumor. If the patient does not want surgical sterilization, she is then confronted with the choice of using either oral contraceptives or barrier methods.

The incidence of postmolar GTT has been reported to be increased in patients who used oral contraceptives before gonadotropin remission (Stone et al., 1976). However, data from the NETDC indicate that oral contraceptives do not increase the risk of postmolar trophoblastic disease (Berkowitz et al., 1981c). Postmolar GTT developed in 14.3% of our patients using barrier methods and 18.9% of our patients using oral contraceptives ($P > .10$). The contraceptive method also did not influence the mean HCG regression time. We therefore believe that oral contraceptives may be safely prescribed after molar evacuation during the entire interval of gonadotropin follow-up.

GESTATIONAL TROPHOBLASTIC TUMORS

Natural History

Nonmetastatic Disease

Locally invasive GTT develops in 15% of patients following molar evacuation and infrequently after other gestations (Berkowitz et al., 1981a). These patients usually present with irregular vaginal bleeding, theca-lutein cysts, uterine subinvolution, or asymmetric enlargement and elevated HCG levels. The trophoblastic tumor may perforate through the myometrium, producing intraperitoneal bleeding, or erode into uterine vessels, causing vaginal hemorrhage. Bulky necrotic trophoblastic tumor may involve the uterine wall and serve as a nidus for sepsis. Patients with uterine infection may develop a purulent vaginal discharge and acute pelvic pain.

Metastatic Disease

Metastatic GTT occurs in 4% of patients after molar evacuation and infrequently following other pregnancies (Berkowitz and Goldstein, 1981). Metastatic GTT is usually associated with the presence of choriocarcinoma. Choriocarcinoma has a tendency for early vascular invasion with widespread dissemination. Because trophoblastic tumors are perfused by many fragile vessels, metastatic lesions are often hemorrhagic.

The pulmonary parenchyma is the most common site of metastasis (Table 12–8). At the time of presentation at the NETDC, 80% of patients with metastatic GTT have lung involvement. Patients with pulmonary metastases may have chest pain, cough, hemoptysis, dyspnea, or an asymptomatic lesion on chest roentgenogram. Respiratory symptoms may be protracted over many months or have an acute onset. GTT may produce four principal radiographic patterns in the lungs: (1) al-

TABLE 12–8.—COMMON
METASTATIC SITES AND
RELATIVE INCIDENCE

SITE	INCIDENCE (%)
Lungs	80
Vagina	30
Pelvis	20
Brain	10
Liver	10
Bowel, kidney, spleen	<5
Other	<5
Undetermined*	<5

*Persistent HCG titer following hysterectomy.

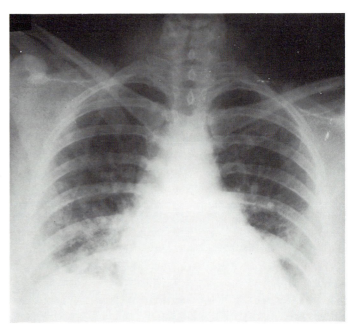

Fig 12–10.—Chest roentgenogram showing miliary-type metastases.

veolar or "snowstorm" pattern (Fig 12–10), (2) discrete rounded densities (Fig 12–11), (3) pleural effusion, and (4) embolic pattern resulting from pulmonary arterial occlusion (Sung et al., 1982; Libshitz et al., 1977; Bagshawe and Garnett, 1963). Because the respiratory symptoms and radiographic findings may be striking, the patient may be thought to have a primary pulmonary disease. Regrettably, the diagnosis of GTT may only be confirmed after a thoracotomy is performed.

Patients with GTT may develop pulmonary

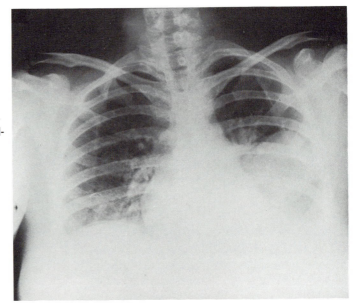

Fig 12–11.—Chest roentgenogram showing multiple tumor nodules of varying sizes in both lung fields.

hypertension secondary to pulmonary arterial occlusion by trophoblastic emboli. Hendrickse and associates examined 25 Nigerian patients with GTT and acute dyspnea and documented trophoblastic emboli in 15 patients. Progressive respiratory distress and pulmonary hypertension developed in four patients with recurrent trophoblastic emboli. Fortunately, pulmonary hypertension resolved in all four patients after they attained gonadotropin remission with chemotherapy. Bagshawe and Noble examined cardiopulmonary function in 52 patients with trophoblastic pulmonary involvement, and nine patients had significant pulmonary hypertension. Although patients with pulmonary hypertension may be extremely symptomatic, the chest roentgenogram may reveal only minimal changes.

Some patients with extensive pulmonary metastases have minimal or no gynecologic symptoms. The reproductive organs may be free of trophoblastic tumor in patients with widespread metastases. Pao-Chang and Shu-Chao performed postmortem examinations in 28 patients who died of GTT at the University of Hong Kong, and 27 patients had extensive pulmonary involvement. Nine (32%) of the patients had no detectable trophoblastic tumor in the uterus or other reproductive organs despite a thorough examination.

Vaginal metastases are present in 30% of patients with metastatic GTT. Vaginal lesions are generally highly vascular and may therefore appear reddened or violaceous. Vaginal metastases may occur in the fornices or suburethrally and cause irregular bleeding or a purulent discharge (Fig 12–12).

Liver metastases occur in 10% of patients with disseminated trophoblastic disease. Hepatic involvement is encountered almost exclusively in patients with extensive tumor burdens and prolonged delays in diagnosis. Patients may develop epigastric or right upper quadrant pain because metastases may stretch Glisson's capsule. Hemorrhagic lesions may cause hepatic rupture and exsanguinating intraperitoneal bleeding (Fig 12–13).

Trophoblastic tumor involves the brain in 10% of patients with metastatic GTT. Cerebral involvement is generally seen in patients

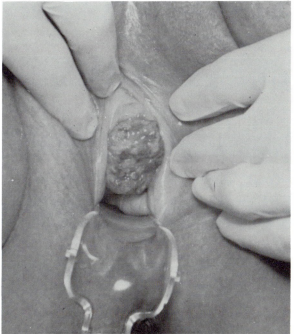

Fig 12–12.—Fungating suburethral metastasis of choriocarcinoma with necrosis and infection.

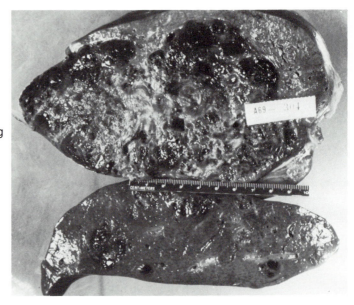

Fig 12–13.—Liver showing diffuse involvement with choriocarcinoma.

with late advanced disease. Most patients with brain metastases have concurrent pulmonary involvement. Because cerebral lesions may undergo spontaneous hemorrhage, patients may develop acute focal neurologic deficits (Fig 12–14).

Staging System

An anatomic staging system for GTT was adopted at a meeting of the International Society for the Study of Trophoblastic Neoplasms in October 1979 at the University of Hong Kong (Table 12–9). This staging system

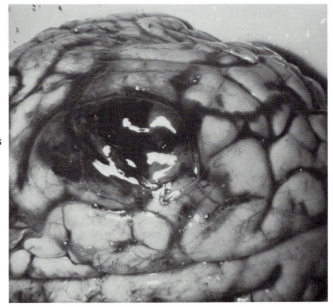

Fig 12–14.—Cerebral metastasis of choriocarcinoma with recent hemorrhage.

TABLE 12–9.—STAGING OF GESTATIONAL
TROPHOBLASTIC TUMORS

STAGE	
I	Confined to uterine corpus
II	Metastases to pelvis and vagina
III	Metastases to lung
IV	Distant metastases

will hopefully enable the objective comparison of data among various centers. Stage I includes all patients with persistently elevated HCG levels and tumor confined to the uterine corpus. Stage II comprises all patients with tumor outside of the uterus but localized to the vagina and/or pelvis. Stage III includes all patients with pulmonary metastases, with or without uterine, vaginal, or pelvic involvement. Precise morphologic diagnosis is not easily obtained in stage III without open thoracotomy. However, we do not advocate performing thoracotomy in these patients merely to obtain information concerning the histologic pattern. We therefore base our histologic diagnosis on the known morphology as determined by reviewing the previous pathologic findings, endometrial curettings, and antecedent pregnancy. Stage IV patients have far advanced disease with involvement of the brain, liver, kidneys, or gastrointestinal tract.

Patients with stage IV disease are in the highest-risk category because they are the most likely to be resistant to chemotherapy. Stage IV tumors generally have the histologic pattern of choriocarcinoma and more commonly follow a nonmolar pregnancy.

In addition to anatomic staging, it is useful to consider other variables to predict the likelihood of drug resistance and assist the clinician in the selection of an appropriate treatment protocol. A prognostic scoring system, based on one developed by Bagshawe, reliably predicts the potential for chemotherapy resistance (Table 12–10) (Bagshawe, 1976). When the prognostic score is 7 or greater, the patient is placed in a high-risk category and usually requires combination chemotherapy to achieve remission. In general, patients with stage I disease have a low-risk score and patients with stage IV disease have a high-risk score. Therefore, the distinction between low and high risk mainly applies to stages II and III GTT.

Diagnostic Evaluation

The optimal management of GTT requires a thorough evaluation of the extent of the disease process prior to the initiation of treatment. All patients with persistent GTT should undergo a careful pretreatment assessment,

TABLE 12–10.—PROGNOSTIC SCORE IN GTT

	0	1	2	3
Antecedent pregnancy	Hydatidiform mole	Nonmole abortion; ectopic	Term pregnancy	. . .
Interval between end of antecedent pregnancy and initial therapy (mo.)	<3	3–6	7–12	>12
HCG value at time of initial therapy (mIU/ml)	$<10^3$	10^3–10^4	10^4–10^5	$>10^5$
ABO blood group	. . .	. . .	B or AB	. . .
Largest tumor (cm)	<2	. . .	2–5	>5
Site of metastasis		Lung	GI tract; kidney; spleen	Brain; liver
No. of metastases identified	. . .	1–4	4–8	>8
Previous chemotherapy	. . .	. . .	Failed prophylactic chemotherapy	Failed therapeutic chemotherapy

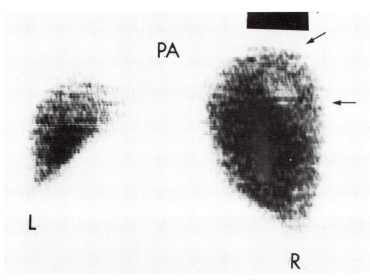

Fig 12–15.—Liver scan using technetium Tc 99m showing a single large metastasis of choriocarcinoma deep in the left lobe. Arrows indicate extent of lesion.

including a complete history and physical examination; HCG levels; hepatic, thyroid, and renal function tests; baseline levels of peripheral blood and platelet counts. The metastatic workup should include a chest roentgenogram, liver isotope scan (Fig 12–15), ultrasonography of the abdomen and pelvis, head computed tomographic (CT) scan (Fig 12–16) and, in some cases, selective angiography of

abdominal and pelvic organs (Fig 12–17). While the liver isotope scan may be useful for diagnosis, small, scattered lesions may be overlooked by this technique. Selective angiography may be more sensitive in detecting hepatic metastases but is associated with the potential risks of an invasive procedure. Our experience with both ultrasound and CT scan of the liver is limited, but it is hoped that

Fig 12–16.—Computed tomographic scan of large intracranial metastasis of choriocarcinoma showing filling defect.

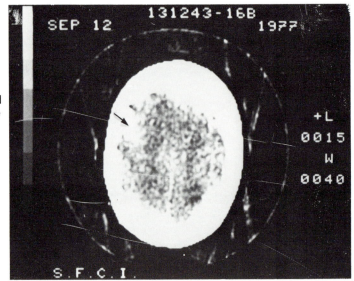

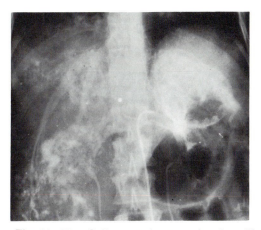

Fig 12–17.—Celiac arteriogram showing diffuse involvement of hepatic parenchyma by choriocarcinoma.

these techniques will be helpful in detecting hepatic lesions. The introduction of the head CT scan has facilitated the early detection of asymptomatic cerebral lesions. HCG levels are measured in the cerebrospinal fluid in patients with choriocarcinoma and/or metastatic disease to detect cerebral metastases. Stool guaiac tests should also be routinely performed in patients with persistent GTT. If the guaiac test is positive or the patient reports gastrointestinal symptoms, a full radiographic evaluation of the gastrointestinal tract should be undertaken.

Pretreatment Endometrial Curettage

We have recently evaluated the pathologic characteristics of pretreatment endometrial curettings as a predictor of response to chemotherapy in 37 patients with postmolar GTT (Berkowitz et al., 1980a). Pretreatment endometrial curettings demonstrated worsened trophoblastic histologic findings as compared with the antecedent hydatidiform mole in seven patients. Six (85.7%) of these patients with worsened trophoblastic histologic findings required multiple courses of chemotherapy to achieve remission. Patients with worsened trophoblastic histologic findings may represent part of the spectrum of trophoblastic neoplasms with a more virulent natural history. In contrast, no trophoblastic tumor

was present in the endometrial curettings in 20 patients. Nineteen of these patients attained complete HCG remission after only one course of chemotherapy. The only patient in this group who required several courses of chemotherapy had multiple pulmonary metastases. The pathologic findings from a pretreatment curettage may aid in the selection of patients who may be benefited by hysterectomy. If the pretreatment curettage reveals worsened trophoblastic histologic features, primary hysterectomy may be advised to potentially reduce the exposure to chemotherapy and its toxic effects.

Pelvic Ultrasonography

We have recently assessed the accuracy of ultrasonography in detecting trophoblastic uterine involvement in patients with persistent GTT. Pelvic ultrasonography was performed in 39 patients with persistent GTT as part of their pretreatment evaluation. During the same hospitalization, the patients also underwent laparoscopy and endometrial curettage (37 patients) or hysterectomy (two patients). Ultrasonography indicated trophoblastic uterine involvement in 20 patients (51.3%) and the sonographic interpretation was histologically confirmed in all 20 patients by endometrial curettage and/or hysterectomy. Among the 19 patients in whom the uterus appeared normal by ultrasound, endometrial curettings demonstrated only scanty fragments of trophoblastic tumor in six patients (31.6%). Pelvic angiography was performed in seven patients and consistently confirmed the ultrasound findings, including a solitary resistant uterine nodule in one patient. Pelvic ultrasonography therefore appears to be useful in detecting extensive trophoblastic uterine involvement and may also aid in identifying sites of resistant uterine tumor. Because ultrasonography can accurately and noninvasively detect extensive trophoblastic uterine tumor, it may aid in the selection of patients who will be benefited by hysterectomy. When the uterus has marked trophoblastic invasion, hysterectomy may substantially reduce the trophoblastic tumor burden. A reduction in the tumor burden may limit the exposure to chemotherapy that is necessary to induce gonadotropin remission (Hammond et al., 1980).

HCG in Cerebrospinal Fluid

Cerebral metastases may be associated with elevated levels of HCG in the cerebrospinal fluid (CSF). Bagshawe and Harland measured plasma-CSF ratios of HCG levels in 33 patients with trophoblastic cerebral involvement and the ratio was less than 60 in 29 of the patients. Cerebral metastases were first suggested in 13 of the patients by the level of HCG in the CSF.

To further understand the relationship between HCG levels in the blood and CSF, we measured serum-CSF ratios of HCG levels in 36 normal pregnant women and in six patients with choriocarcinoma (Berkowitz et al., 1981d). Levels of HCG in the CSF correlated well with those in the serum in both the first and third trimesters in normal pregnancy. However, the serum-CSF HCG ratio was less than 60 in one patient undergoing first-trimester abortion and in one patient with nonmetastatic choriocarcinoma. Furthermore, the serum-CSF HCG ratio exceeded 100 in two patients with documented trophoblastic cerebral metastases. Because rapid changes in the serum HCG levels may not be promptly reflected in the CSF, a single serum-CSF HCG ratio may be misleading. Unless supported by other clinical or radiographic data, a single serum-CSF HCG ratio is insufficient to diagnose trophoblastic cerebral metastases.

Management of Stage I GTT

Tables 12–11 and 12–12 review the NETDC protocol for the management of Stage I disease and the results of therapy. The selection of treatment is based primarily on the patient's desire to preserve fertility (Berkowitz et al., 1981a).

If the patient no longer wishes to preserve fertility, hysterectomy with adjuvant single-agent chemotherapy may be performed as primary treatment. Adjuvant chemotherapy is

TABLE 12–11.—TREATMENT PROTOCOL FOR STAGE I GTT (NETDC)

Initial
  Sequential methotrexate/dactinomycin
  or
  Hysterectomy with adjunctive chemotherapy
Resistant
  MAC* or
  Hysterectomy with adjunctive chemotherapy
  Local resection
  Pelvic infusion
Follow-up
  HCG measurement
    Weekly until normal 3 times
    Monthly until normal 12 times
Contraception
  12 consecutive mo. of normal HCG titers

*MAC indicates a combined regimen of methotrexate, dactinomycin (actinomycin D), and cyclophosphamide.

TABLE 12–12.—(NETDC, JULY 1965 THROUGH DECEMBER 1981) STAGE I GTT (CONFINED TO UTERINE CORPUS)

REMISSION THERAPY	NO. (%) OF PATIENTS	NO. (%) OF REMISSIONS
Initial	227 (96.2)	
Sequential methotrexate/dactinomycin		207 (91.2)
Hysterectomy		20 (8.8)
Resistant	9 (3.8)	
MAC*		4 (44.4)
Hysterectomy		2 (22.2)
Local uterine resection		2 (22.2)
Pelvic infusion		1 (11.2)
Totals	236 (100)	236 (100)

*MAC indicates a combined regimen of methotrexate, dactinomycin (actinomycin D), and cyclophosphamide.

administered for three reasons: (1) to reduce the likelihood of disseminating viable tumor cells at surgery, (2) to maintain a cytotoxic level of chemotherapy in the bloodstream and tissues in case viable tumor cells are disseminated at surgery, and (3) to treat any occult metastases that may be already present at the time of surgery (Lewis et al., 1966a). Chemotherapy may be safely administered at the time of hysterectomy without increasing the incidence of wound complications or sepsis (Lewis et al., 1966b). Hysterectomy is performed midway during the chemotherapeutic protocol. Twenty patients were treated by primary hysterectomy and adjuvant chemotherapy at the NETDC and all achieved complete remission with no additional therapy.

Single-agent chemotherapy is the preferred treatment in patients with stage I disease who desire to retain fertility. Primary single-agent chemotherapy was administered to 216 patients with stage I GTT and 207 patients (95.8%) achieved complete remission. The remaining nine resistant patients subsequently attained remission with either further chemotherapy or surgical intervention. When the patient desires to preserve fertility, we favor administration of combination chemotherapy in resistant stage I disease. If the patient's condition is resistant to both single-agent and combination chemotherapy and the patient wants to retain fertility, local uterine resection may be considered. When local resection is planned, a preoperative ultrasound and/or arteriogram may help to identify the site of the resistant tumor.

All patients with stage I, II, and III GTT are followed up with weekly HCG determinations until the results are normal for three consecutive weeks, and then monthly determinations until they are normal for 12 consecutive months. Patients are encouraged to use effective contraception during the entire interval of gonadotropin follow-up.

Management of Stage II GTT

The NETDC protocol for the management of stage II disease and the results of treatment are outlined in Tables 12–13 and 12–14. While low-risk patients are treated with primary single-agent chemotherapy, high-risk patients are managed with primary combination chemotherapy. Between July 1965 and December 1981, 25 patients with stage II disease were treated at the NETDC and all patients achieved remission. Single-agent chemotherapy induced complete remission in 15 (88.2%) of 17 low-risk patients. In contrast, only two of eight high-risk patients achieved remission with single-agent treatment.

Vaginal metastases may bleed profusely because they may be highly vascular and friable (Goldstein and Berkowitz, 1980). When bleeding is worrisome, bleeding may be controlled by packing the hemorrhagic lesion or performing wide local excision. The administration of one or two courses of chemotherapy may result in avascular planes around the vaginal tumor. Operative blood loss may also be reduced by excising the vaginal lesion with electrocautery. Infrequently, bilateral hypogastric artery ligation may be required to control hemorrhage from vaginal metastases.

TABLE 12–13.—TREATMENT PROTOCOL FOR STAGE II
GTT (NETDC)

Low-risk patients*	
Initial	Sequential methotrexate/dactinomycin
Resistant	MAC†
High-risk patients*	
Initial	MAC†
Resistant	CHAMOCA, VBP†
Follow-up	
HCG	Weekly until normal 3 times; monthly until
measurement	normal 12 times
Contraception	12 consecutive mo. of normal HCG levels

*Local resection optional.
†MAC indicates a combined regimen of methotrexate, dactinomycin (actinomycin D), and cyclophosphamide; CHAMOCA, the Bagshawe multiagent regimen; and VBP, vinblastine, bleomycin, and cisplatin (Platinol).

TABLE 12–14.—(NETDC, July 1965 Through December 1981) Stage II GTT (Metastases to Pelvis and Vagina)

REMISSION THERAPY	NO. (%) OF PATIENTS	NO. (%) OF REMISSIONS
Low-risk patients	17 (68)	
Initial		
Sequential methotrexate/dactinomycin		15 (88.2)
Local resection	3	
Resistant		
MAC*		2 (11.8)
Local resection	2	
High-risk patients	8 (32)	
Initial		
Sequential methotrexate/dactinomycin		2 (25.0)
MAC*		4 (50.0)
Local resection	2	
Resistant		
MAC*		1 (12.5)
CHAMOCA*		1 (12.5)
Local resection	1	
Total	25 (100)	25 (100.0)

*For explanation of chemotherapeutic regimens, see footnote for Table 12–13.

Management of Stage III GTT

The NETDC protocol for the treatment of stage III disease and the results of therapy are reviewed in Tables 12–15 and 12–16. Low-risk patients are treated with primary single-agent chemotherapy and high-risk patients are managed with combination drug treatment. Eighty patients with stage III disease were managed at the NETDC between July 1965 and December 1981 and all attained complete remission. Gonadotropin remission was induced with single-agent chemotherapy in 53 (91.4%) of 58 patients with low-risk dis-

ease and in 13 (59.1%) of 22 patients with high-risk disease. All patients, who were resistant to single-agent treatment, subsequently achieved remission with combination chemotherapy.

Thoracotomy has a limited role in the management of stage III GTT. However, if a patient has a persistent viable pulmonary metastasis despite intensive chemotherapy, thoracotomy may be performed to excise the resistant focus (Shirley et al., 1972; Edwards et al., 1975). An extensive metastatic workup should be performed prior to surgery to ex-

TABLE 12–15.—Treatment Protocol for Stage III GTT (NETDC)

Low-risk patients*	
Initial	Sequential methotrexate/dactinomycin
Resistant	MAC†
High-risk patients*	
Initial	MAC†
Resistant	CHAMOCA,† VBP†
Follow-up	
HCG measurements	Weekly until normal 3 times; monthly until normal 12 times
Contraception	12 consecutive mo. of normal HCG levels

*Local resection optional
†For explanation of chemotherapeutic regimens, see footnote for Table 12–13.

TABLE 12–16.—(NETDC, July 1965 Through December 1981) Stage III GTT (Metastases to Lung)

REMISSION THERAPY	NO. (%) OF PATIENTS	NO. (%) OF REMISSIONS
Low-risk patients	58 (72.5)	
Initial		
Sequential methotrexate/dactinomycin		53 (91.4)
Local resection	5	
Resistant		
MAC*		5 (8.6)
Local resection	3	
High-risk patients	22 (27.5)	
Initial		
Sequential methotrexate/dactinomycin		13 (59.1)
MAC*		6 (27.3)
Local resection	5	
Resistant		
MAC*		2 (9.1)
CHAMOCA*		1 (4.5)
Local resection	2	
Total	80 (100.0)	80 (100.0)

*For explanation of chemotherapeutic regimens, see footnote for Table 12–13.

clude other sites of persistent disease. Furthermore, it is important to note that fibrotic pulmonary nodules may persist for months on chest roentgenogram after complete gonadotropin remission is attained (Swett and Westcott, 1974).

Hysterectomy may be required in patients with metastatic GTT to control uterine hemorrhage or sepsis. Furthermore, in patients with extensive uterine tumor, hysterectomy may substantially reduce the trophoblastic tumor burden and thereby limit the need for multiple courses of chemotherapy (Hammond et al., 1980).

Management of Stage IV GTT

Tables 12–17 and 12–18 outline the NETDC protocol for the management of stage IV disease and the results of treatment. These patients are at greatest risk of developing rapidly progressive and unresponsive tumors despite aggressive therapy. All patients who have died from GTT at the NETDC have had stage IV disease.

TABLE 12–17.—Treatment Protocol for Stage IV GTT (NETDC)

Initial	
MAC†	
Brain	Whole-head irradiation (3,000 rads); craniotomy to manage complications
Liver	Resection to manage complication
Resistant*	
CHAMOCA†	
VBP†	
Hepatic arterial infusion	
Follow-up	
HCG measurements	Weekly until normal 3 times; monthly until normal 24 times
Contraception	24 consecutive mo. of normal HCG levels

*Local resection optional.
†For explanation of chemotherapeutic regimens, see footnote for Table 12–13.

TABLE 12–18.—(NETDC, JULY 1965 THROUGH DECEMBER 1981) STAGE IV GTT (DISTANT METASTASES)

REMISSION THERAPY*		NO. (%) OF REMISSIONS
Before 1975		
Initial		
Sequential methotrexate/dactinomycin	5	
Resistant		6/20 (30.0)
MAC†	1	
1975 or after		
Initial		
Sequential methotrexate/dactinomycin	2	
MAC†	2	
Resistant		10/14 (71.4)
High-dose methotrexate/dactinomycin	4	
MAC†	1	
CHAMOCA†	1	

*Radiotherapy and surgery utilized when indicated.
†For explanation of chemotherapeutic regimens, see footnote for Table 12–13.

All patients with stage IV disease should be treated with primary intensive combination chemotherapy and the selective use of radiation therapy and surgery (Surwit and Hammond, 1980). Before 1975, only six (30%) of 20 patients with stage IV disease at the NETDC attained complete remission. However, after 1975, ten (71.4%) of 14 patients with stage IV tumors achieved gonadotropin remission. This gratifying improvement in survival has resulted from the use of primary combination chemotherapy in conjunction with radiation and surgical treatment.

The management of hepatic metastases is particularly difficult and problematic. If a patient is resistant to systemic chemotherapy, hepatic arterial infusion of chemotherapy may induce complete remission in selected cases (Goldstein et al., 1967). Hepatic resection may also be required to control acute bleeding or to excise resistant tumor.

If cerebral metastases are detected, whole brain irradiation (3,000 rads in ten fractions) should be promptly instituted. The risk of spontaneous cerebral hemorrhage may be reduced by the concurrent use of combination chemotherapy and brain irradiation (Brace, 1968; Weed and Hammond, 1980). Brain irradiation may be both hemostatic and tumoricidal. Craniotomy should be performed to manage life-threatening complications with the hope that the patient will ultimately be cured with chemotherapy. Craniotomy may be required to provide acute decompression or to control bleeding. Hammond and co-workers reported performing craniotomy in six of their patients to control bleeding and three of these patients ultimately achieved complete remission (Hammond et al., 1980). Infrequently, cerebral metastases that are resistant to chemotherapy may be amenable to local resection. Fortunately, patients with cerebral metastases who achieve remission generally have no residual neurologic deficits.

Patients with stage IV disease are followed up with weekly HCG determinations until the results are normal for three consecutive weeks, and then monthly determinations until they are normal for 24 consecutive months. These patients require prolonged gonadotropin follow-up because they have an increased risk of late recurrence.

CHEMOTHERAPY

Single-Agent Chemotherapy

Selection of Single-Agent Chemotherapy

Single-agent chemotherapy with either dactinomycin (actinomycin D) or methotrexate has induced comparable and excellent remission rates in both nonmetastatic and metastatic GTT (Osathanondh et al., 1975). The selection of chemotherapeutic regimens should be influenced by the associated systemic toxic effects. An optimal regimen should maximize the response rate while minimizing the morbidity.

Bagshawe and Wilde first reported administering methotrexate with citrovorum factor in GTT to reduce systemic toxic effects. We have previously observed that methotrexate–citrovorum factor was both effective and safe in the management of GTT (Berkowitz and Goldstein, 1979; Berkowitz et al., 1982a). When compared with dactinomycin or methotrexate alone, methotrexate–citrovorum factor reduced the number of courses of chemotherapy required to attain complete gonadotropin remission. Furthermore, methotrexate–citrovorum factor caused less toxic response in the treatment of GTT than either dactinomycin or methotrexate alone.

We have recently evaluated the comparative toxic effects of dactinomycin, methotrexate alone, and methotrexate–citrovorum factor (Berkowitz et al., 1981b). Seventy-five patients with stage I GTT were selected at random from the files of our tumor registry. The patients' in-hospital records and follow-up data were carefully reviewed to assess the degree of hematologic, hepatic, and epithelial toxic effects that followed the first course of chemotherapy. While only one patient (4%) treated with methotrexate–citrovorum factor developed thrombocytopenia and/or granulocytopenia, myelosuppression was caused by methotrexate alone and by dactinomycin in 32% and 48% of the patients, respectively. Hepatotoxic effects only developed in patients treated with methotrexate alone (20%). Neither methotrexate alone nor methotrexate–citrovorum factor caused marked alopecia or generalized rash. In contrast, dactinomycin induced marked alopecia and generalized rash in 52% and 24% of the patients, respectively. Methotrexate–citrovorum factor is therefore the least toxic single-agent regimen available for the treatment of GTT.

Methotrexate–citrovorum factor has been the preferred single-agent regimen in the treatment of GTT at the NETDC since 1974 (Table 12–19). Between September 1974 and December 1981, 118 patients with GTT were treated with primary methotrexate–citrovorum factor therapy at the NETDC. Complete remission was induced with methotrexate–citrovorum factor in 104 patients (88.2%) and 85 (81.7%) of these patients required only one course of therapy to attain remission. Methotrexate–citrovorum factor induced remission in 96 (91.4%) of 105 patients with stage I GTT and in eight (61.5%) of 13 patients with low-risk stages II and III GTT. Resistance to methotrexate–citrovorum factor was more common in patients with choriocarcinoma, metastases, and with pretreatment HCG levels greater than 50,000 mIU/ml. Following therapy with methotrexate–citrovorum factor, thrombocytopenia, granulocytopenia, and hepatotoxic effects developed in only three (2.5%), eight (6.8%), and 15 (12.7%) patients, respectively. Methotrexate-citrovorum factor should be the preferred single-agent regimen in the management of GTT in patients with

TABLE 12–19.—METHOTREXATE AND CITROVORUM FACTOR PROTOCOL

DAY	TIME	THERAPY*
1	8 A.M.	CBC, platelet count, SGOT determination
	4 P.M.	Methotrexate, 1.0 mg/kg
2	4 P.M.	Citrovorum factor, 0.1 mg/kg
3	8 A.M.	CBC, platelet count, SGOT determination
	4 P.M.	Methotrexate, 1.0 mg/kg
4	4 P.M.	Citrovorum factor, 0.1 mg/kg
5	8 A.M.	CBC, platelet count, SGOT determination
	4 P.M.	Methotrexate, 1.0 mg/kg
6	4 P.M.	Citrovorum factor, 0.1 mg/kg
7	8 A.M.	CBC, platelet count, SGOT determination
	4 P.M.	Methotrexate, 1.0 mg/kg
8	4 P.M.	Citrovorum factor, 0.1 mg/kg

Follow-up tests: CBC, platelet count, and SGOT determination 3 times weekly for 2 weeks, then as needed.

Subsequent course(s)
  With response: repeat treatment at same dose
  Without response: add 0.5 mg of methotrexate and 0.05 mg of citrovorum factor to initial dose; if no response to latter, switch agent (all drugs are given intramuscularly)

*CBC indicates complete blood cell count; SGOT, serum glutamic oxaloacetic transaminase.

no preexisting liver disease. Methotrexate–citrovorum factor not only achieves an excellent therapeutic outcome with minimal toxic effects, but also effectively limits chemotherapy exposure.

Administration of Single-Agent Chemotherapy

The HCG level is measured weekly after each course of chemotherapy and the HCG regression curve serves as the primary basis for determining the need for additional treatment (Goldstein, 1972). After the first treatment, further chemotherapy is withheld as long as the HCG level is falling progressively. Additional single-agent chemotherapy is not administered at any predetermined or fixed time interval. A second course of chemotherapy is administered under the following conditions: (1) the HCG level stays at a plateau for more than three consecutive weeks or re-elevates, (2) the HCG level does not decline by one log within 18 days after completing the first treatment, (3) old metastases enlarge or recur, and (4) new lesions develop.

If a second course of methotrexate–citrovorum factor is required, the dosage of methotrexate is unaltered if the patient's response to the first treatment was adequate. An adequate response is defined as a fall in the HCG level by one log following a course of chemotherapy. When the response to the first treatment is inadequate, the dosage of methotrexate is increased 2 mg/kg in four divided doses. If the response to two consecutive courses of methotrexate–citrovorum factor is inadequate, the patient's condition is considered to be resistant to methotrexate and dactinomycin is promptly substituted (Table 12–20).

Combination Chemotherapy

The preferred combination drug regimen at the NETDC is the MAC III (triple therapy) protocol, which includes methotrexate–citrovorum factor, dactinomycin (actinomycin D), and cyclophosphamide (Table 12–21). The MAC III protocol has achieved satisfactory remission rates with acceptable toxic effects. If patients are resistant to MAC III, they are then treated with either a modified Bagshawe multiagent regimen or vinblastine, bleomycin, and cisplatin. Surwit and co-workers reported using a modified Bagshawe multiagent regimen in six patients whose conditions were resistant to triple therapy, and five patients achieved complete remission (Surwit et al., 1979). Vinblastine, bleomycin, and cisplatin also induced complete remission in two pa-

TABLE 12–20.—DACTINOMYCIN
(ACTINOMYCIN D) PROTOCOL

DAY	TIME	THERAPY*
1	8 A.M.	CBC, platelet count, SGOT determination
	8 P.M.	Dactinomycin, 12 μg/kg, IV
2	8 A.M.	CBC, platelet count, SGOT determination
	8 P.M.	Dactinomycin, 12 μg/kg, IV
3	8 A.M.	CBC, platelet count, SGOT determination
	8 P.M.	Dactinomycin, 12 μg/kg, IV
4	8 A.M.	CBC, platelet count, SGOT determination
	8 P.M.	Dactinomycin, 12 μg/kg, IV
5	8 A.M.	CBC, platelet count, SGOT determination
	8 P.M.	Dactinomycin, 12 μg/kg, IV

Follow-up tests: CBC, platelet count, and SGOT
  determination 3 times weekly for 2 weeks, then as needed
Subsequent course(s)
  With response: repeat treatment at same dose
  Without response: add 3 μg/kg of dactinomycin to initial
  dose

*CBC indicates complete blood cell count; SGOT, serum glutamic oxaloacetic transaminase; and IV, intravenously.

TABLE 12–21.–MAC III PROTOCOL

DAY	TIME	THERAPY*
1	8 A.M.	CBC, platelet count, SGOT determination
	8 P.M.	Methotrexate, 1.0 mg/kg, IM
		Dactinomycin, 12 µg/kg, IV
		Cyclophosphamide, 3 mg/kg, IV
2	8 A.M.	CBC, platelet count
	8 P.M.	Citrovorum factor, 0.1 mg/kg, IM
		Dactinomycin, 12 µg/kg, IV
		Cyclophosphamide, 3 mg/kg, IV
3	8 A.M.	CBC, platelet count, SGOT determination
	8 P.M.	Methotrexate, 1.0 mg/kg, IM
		Dactinomycin, 12 µg/kg, IV
		Cyclophosphamide, 3 mg/kg, IV
4	8 A.M.	CBC, platelet count
	8 P.M.	Citrovorum factor, 0.1 mg/kg, IM
		Dactinomycin, 12 µg/kg, IV
		Cyclophosphamide, 3 mg/kg, IV
5	8 A.M.	CBC, platelet count, SGOT determination
	8 P.M.	Methotrexate, 1.0 mg/kg, IM
		Dactinomycin, 12 µg/kg, IV
		Cyclophosphamide, 3 mg/kg, IV
6	8 P.M.	Citrovorum factor, 0.1 mg/kg, IM
7	8 A.M.	CBC, platelet count, SGOT determination
	8 P.M.	Methotrexate, 1.0 mg/kg, IM
8	8 P.M.	Citrovorum factor, 0.1 mg/kg, IM

Follow-up tests: CBC, platelet count, and SGOT determination 3 times weekly for 2 weeks, then as needed

*MAC III indicates triple therapy with methotrexate–citrovorum factor, dactinomycin (actinomycin D), and cyclophosphamide; CBC, complete blood cell count; SGOT, serum glutamic oxaloacetic transaminase; IM, intramuscularly; and IV, intravenously.

tients who were resistant to triple therapy (Schlaerth et al., 1980). Etoposide (VP-16-213), an epipodophyllin derivative, has been noted to have antitumor activity in GTT and may play a role in the development of newer combination regimens (Newlands and Bagshawe, 1980). The optimal combination drug protocol in GTT has not yet been defined. There has been no controlled study to objectively assess the comparative efficacies of the available drug regimens. A collaborative study among several institutions will be necessary to adequately evaluate the relative merits of the various combination drug protocols.

Patients who require combination chemotherapy must be treated intensively to attain remission. We administer combination chemotherapy every three weeks or as frequently as toxic effects permits until the patient achieves three consecutive normal HCG levels. After the patient attains normal HCG levels, at least one additional course of chemotherapy is administered to reduce the risk of recurrence.

SUBSEQUENT PREGNANCIES

Pregnancies After Molar Pregnancy

Patients with hydatidiform moles can anticipate normal reproduction in the future (Pastorfide and Goldstein, 1973). Between July 1965 and December 1978, 912 patients were managed at the NETDC for molar pregnancy. These patients had 783 subsequent pregnancies that resulted in 511 full-term live births (65.2%), 76 premature deliveries (9.7%), six ectopic pregnancies (0.8%), and four stillbirths (0.5%) (Table 12–22) (Berkowitz and Goldstein, 1981b). First-trimester sponta-

TABLE 12–22.—Subsequent
Pregnancies in Patients With
Hydatidiform Mole (NETDC, 1965
Through 1978)

OUTCOME	NO. (%)
Pregnancy	
Term delivery	511 (65.2)
Stillbirth	4
Premature delivery	76 (9.7)
Spontaneous abortion	
1st trimester	147 (18.7)
2nd trimester	10
Therapeutic abortion	20
Ectopic	6
Repeated mole	9*
Total pregnancies	783
Delivery	
Congenital malformations	30 (5.0)
Major obstetric complications	83 (14.0)
Total deliveries	591

*Four patients had three consecutive moles.

neous abortion occurred in 147 pregnancies (18.7%) and congenital malformations were detected in 30 infants (5%). Furthermore, there was no increase in perinatal morbidity or mortality.

However, when a patient has had a molar pregnancy, she is at increased risk of developing a trophoblastic tumor in subsequent conceptions (Federschneider et al., 1980). Nine (1:150) of our patients have had at least two consecutive molar gestations between July 1965 and December 1981. The later molar pregnancies are characterized by worsening histologic findings and increased risk of postmolar GTT. Patients with repetitive hydatidiform moles may also have a limited capacity to sustain a normal pregnancy. Only two of our patients have had a normal subsequent term pregnancy after two prior hydatidiform moles.

It therefore seems prudent to obtain ultrasonography in the first trimester of any subsequent pregnancy to confirm normal gestational development. Furthermore, the placenta or products of conception from subsequent pregnancies should undergo thorough pathologic review. An HCG measurement should also be obtained six weeks after

the completion of any future conception to exclude occult trophoblastic neoplasia.

Pregnancies After GTT

Data from the NETDC, National Cancer Institute, and Charing Cross Hospital, London, indicate that patients with GTT who are successfully treated with chemotherapy can expect normal reproduction in the future (Berkowitz and Goldstein, 1981b; Van Thiel et al., 1970; Walden and Bagshawe, 1976). Between July 1965 and December 1978, 186 patients were treated for stage I GTT at the NETDC. After achieving complete remission, these patients had 118 subsequent pregnancies that resulted in 77 full-term live births (65%), four premature deliveries (4%), three ectopic pregnancies (3%), and one stillbirth (1%) (Table 12–23). First-trimester spontaneous abortion occurred in 24 pregnancies (20%) and congenital anomalies were detected in only three infants (4%). The incidence of spontaneous abortion appears to be slightly increased in this population. However, these patients undergo meticulous clinical scrutiny and HCG monitoring and therefore their incidence of subsequent spontaneous abortion is most likely consistent with the general population. It is particularly reassuring that the frequency of congenital malformations is not increased because che-

TABLE 12–23.—Subsequent
Pregnancies in Patients With Stage
I GTT (NETDC, 1965 Through 1978)

OUTCOME	NO. (%)
Pregnancy	
Term delivery	77 (65)
Stillbirth	1
Premature delivery	4
Spontaneous abortion	
1st trimester	24 (20)
2nd trimester	3
Therapeutic abortion	5
Ectopic pregnancy	3
Repeat molar pregnancy	1
Total pregnancies	118
Delivery	
Congenital malformations	3 (4)
Major obstetric complications	7 (9)
Total deliveries	82

motherapeutic agents have a teratogenic and mutagenic potential.

THE ROLE OF THE REGIONAL TROPHOBLASTIC DISEASE CENTER

The question often arises regarding the optimal conditions under which patients should be treated. Brewer et al. (1971) compared the results of therapy of patients managed at a regional center (Northwestern University) to those of patients treated at the surrounding hospitals. Sixty-two (87%) of 71 patients with metastatic GTT survived when they were treated at the regional center. In contrast, only 29 (45%) of 65 patients with metastatic GTT survived when they were managed in neighboring hospitals.

The proper management of GTT is a time-consuming endeavor that requires a thorough understanding of the disease process. It therefore seems prudent to refer most patients to regional centers when centers are accessible. If referral is a genuine financial or social hardship for the patient, the local physician should obtain experienced consultation to guide therapy. However, we believe that all patients who require aggressive combination chemotherapy should be referred to regional centers regardless of possible personal hardships. These patients must not be deprived of the clinical experience, intensive therapy, and supportive measures that are available in regional centers. Patients with GTT deserve the full benefits of modern technology and treatment to maximize their opportunity for cure.

BIBLIOGRAPHY

Amir S.M., Sullivan R.C., Ingbar S.H.: In vitro response to crude and purified HCG in human thyroid membranes. *J. Clin. Endocrinol. Metab.* 51:51–58, 1980.

Bagshawe K.D.: Risks and prognostic factors in trophoblastic neoplasia. *Cancer* 38:1373–1385, 1976.

Bagshawe K.D., Garnett E.S.: Radiological changes in the lungs of patients with trophoblastic tumours. *Br. J. Radiol.* 36:673–679, 1963.

Bagshawe K.D., Harland S.: Immunodiagnosis and monitoring of gonadotropin-producing metastases in the central nervous system. *Cancer* 38:112–118, 1976.

Bagshawe K.D., Noble M.I.M.: Cardio-respiratory aspects of trophoblastic tumours. *Quart. J. Med.* 35:39–54, 1966.

Bagshawe K.D., Wilde C.E.: Infusion therapy for pelvic trophoblastic tumors. *Br. J. Obstet. Gynaecol.* 71:565–570, 1964.

Berkowitz R.S., Desai U., Goldstein D.P., et al.: Pretreatment curettage—a predictor of chemotherapy response in gestational trophoblastic neoplasia. *Gynecol. Oncol.* 10:39–43, 1980a.

Berkowitz R.S., Goldstein D.P.: Methotrexate with citrovorum factor rescue for nonmetastatic gestational trophoblastic neoplasms. *Obstet. Gynecol.* 54:725–728, 1979.

Berkowitz R.S., Goldstein D.P.: Pathogenesis of gestational trophoblastic neoplasms. *Pathobiol. Annu.* 11:391–411, 1981a.

Berkowitz R.S., Goldstein D.P.: Pregnancy outcome after molar gestation. *Contemp. Ob/Gyn* 18:69–77, 1981b.

Berkowitz R.S., Goldstein D.P., Bernstein M.R.: Laparoscopy in the management of gestational trophoblastic neoplasms. *J. Reprod. Med.* 24:261–264, 1980b.

Berkowitz R.S., Goldstein D.P., Bernstein M.R.: Management of nonmetastatic trophoblastic tumors. *J. Reprod. Med.* 26:219–222, 1981a.

Berkowitz R.S., Goldstein D.P., Bernstein M.R.: Methotrexate with citrovorum factor rescue as primary therapy for gestational trophoblastic disease. *Cancer* 50:2024–2027, 1982a.

Berkowitz R.S., Goldstein D.P., Jones M.A., et al.: Methotrexate with citrovorum factor rescue—reduced chemotherapy toxicity in the management of gestational trophoblastic neoplasms. *Cancer* 45:423–426, 1981b.

Berkowitz R.S., Goldstein D.P., Marean A.R., et al.: Proliferative sequelae after evacuation of partial hydatidiform mole. *Lancet* 2:804–805, 1979.

Berkowitz R.S., Goldstein D.P., Marean A.R., et al.: Oral contraceptives and postmolar trophoblastic disease. *Obstet. Gynecol.* 58:474–478, 1981c.

Berkowitz R.S., Osathanondh R., Goldstein D.P., et al.: Cerebrospinal fluid human chorionic gonadotropin levels in normal pregnancy and choriocarcinoma. *Surg. Gynecol. Obstet.* 153:687–689, 1981d.

Berkowitz R.S., Sandstrom M., Goldstein D.P., et

al.: 45, X complete hydatidiform mole. *Gynecol. Oncol.* 14:279–283, 1982b.

Brace K.C.: The role of irradiation in the treatment of metastatic trophoblastic disease. *Radiology* 91:540–544, 1968.

Brewer J.I., Eckman T.R., Dolkart R.E., et al.: Gestational trophoblastic disease—a comparative study of the results of therapy in patients with invasive mole and with choriocarcinoma. *Am. J. Obstet. Gynecol.* 109:335, 1971.

Brewer J.I., Rinehart J.J., Dunbar R.W.: Choriocarcinoma—a report of the five or more years' survival from the Albert Mathieu Chorionepithelioma Registry. *Am. J. Obstet. Gynecol.* 81:574–582, 1961.

Brewer J.I., Smith R.T., Pratt G.B.: Choriocarcinoma: Absolute five year survival rates of 122 patients treated by hysterectomy. *Am. J. Obstet. Gynecol.* 85:841–843, 1963.

Curry S.L., Hammond C.B., Tyrey L., et al.: Hydatidiform mole—diagnosis, management and long-term follow-up of 347 patients. *Am. J. Obstet. Gynecol.* 45:1–8, 1975.

Driscoll S.G.: Trophoblastic growths—morphologic aspects and taxonomy. *J. Reprod. Med.* 26:181–191, 1981.

Edwards J.L., Makey A.R., Bagshawe K.D.: The role of thoracotomy in the management of pulmonary metastases of gestational choriocarcinoma. *Clin. Oncol.* 1:329–339, 1975.

Federschneider J.M., Goldstein D.P., Berkowitz R.S., et al.: The natural history of recurrent molar pregnancy. *Obstet. Gynecol.* 55:457–459, 1980.

Galton V.A., Ingbar S.H., Jimenez-Fonseca J., et al.: Alterations in thyroid hormone economy in patients with hydatidiform mole. *J. Clin. Invest.* 50:1345–1354, 1971.

Goldstein D.P.: The chemotherapy of gestational trophoblastic disease: Principles of clinical management. *J.A.M.A.* 220:209–213, 1972.

Goldstein D.P.: Prevention of gestational trophoblastic disease by use of actinomycin-D in molar pregnancies. *Obstet. Gynecol.* 43:475–479, 1974.

Goldstein D.P.: Chorionic gonadotropin. *Cancer* 38:453–459, 1976.

Goldstein D.P., Berkowitz R.S.: Management of gestational trophoblastic neoplasms. *Curr. Probl. Obstet. Gynecol.* 3:1–42, 1980.

Goldstein D.P., Berkowitz R.S.: *Gestational Trophoblastic Neoplasms: Clinical Principles of Diagnosis and Management.* W.B. Saunders Co., Philadelphia, 1982a, pp. 1–301.

Goldstein D.P., Berkowitz R.S.: Nonmetastatic and low-risk metastatic gestational trophoblastic neoplasms. *Semin. Oncol.* 9:191–197, 1982b.

Goldstein D.P., Berkowitz R.S., Bernstein M.R.: Management of molar pregnancy. *J. Reprod. Med.* 26:208–212, 1981.

Goldstein D.P., Berkowitz R.S., Cohen S.M.: The current management of molar pregnancy. *Curr. Probl. Obstet. Gynecol.* 3:1–39, 1979.

Goldstein D.P., Couch N.P., Hall T.: Infusion therapy in the treatment of choriocarcinoma and related trophoblastic tumors. *Surg. Forum* 18:426–428, 1967.

Hammond C.B., Borchert L.G., Tyrey L., et al.: Treatment of metastatic trophoblastic disease: Good and poor prognosis. *Am. J. Obstet. Gynecol.* 115:451–457, 1973.

Hammond C.B., Weed J.C. Jr., Currie J.L.: The role of operation in the current therapy of gestational trophoblastic disease. *Am. J. Obstet. Gynecol.* 136:844–856, 1980.

Hendrickse J.P., Willis A.J.P., Evans K.T.: Acute dyspnoea with trophoblastic tumours. *Br. J. Obstet. Gynaecol.* 72:376–383, 1965.

Hertig A.T.: *Human Trophoblast.* Springfield, Ill., Charles C. Thomas Publisher, 1968.

Hertig A.T., Mansell H.: Tumors of the female sex organs, part 1: Hydatidiform mole and choriocarcinoma, sec. 9, fasc. 33, *Atlas of Tumor Pathology.* Washington, D.C., Armed Forces Institute of Pathology, 1956.

Hertig A.T., Sheldon W.H.: Hydatidiform mole: A pathologico-clinical correlation of 200 cases. *Am. J. Obstet. Gynecol.* 53:1, 1947.

Hertz R., Lewis J.L. Jr., Lipsett M.B.: Five years' experience with the chemotherapy of metastatic choriocarcinoma and related trophoblastic tumors in women. *Am. J. Obstet. Gynecol.* 82:631–640, 1961.

Hertz R., Ross G.T., Lipsett M.B.: Primary chemotherapy of nonmetastatic trophoblastic disease in women. *Am. J. Obstet. Gynecol.* 86:808–814, 1963.

Jones W.B., Lewis J.L. Jr.: Treatment of gestational trophoblastic disease. *Am. J. Obstet. Gynecol.* 120:14–20, 1974.

Kajii T., Ohama K.: Androgenetic origin of hydatidiform mole. *Nature* 268:633–634, 1977.

Kenimer J.G., Hershman J.M., Higgins H.P.: The thyrotropin in hydatidiform moles is human chorionic gonadotropin. *J. Clin. Endocrinol. Metab.* 40:482–487, 1975.

Kohorn E.I., McGinn R.C., Bernard J., et al.: Pulmonary embolization of trophoblastic tissue in molar pregnancy. *Obstet. Gynecol.* 51:16–20, 1978.

Lewis J. Jr., Gore H., Hertig A.T., et al.: Treatment of trophoblastic disease—with rationale for the use of adjunctive chemotherapy at the time of indicated operation. *Am. J. Obstet. Gynecol.* 96:710–718, 1966a.

Lewis J. Jr., Ketcham, A.S., Hertz R.: Surgical intervention during chemotherapy of gestational trophoblastic neoplasms. *Cancer* 19:1517–1522, 1966b.

Li M.C., Hertz R., Spencer D.B.: Effect of methotrexate therapy upon choriocarcinoma and chorioadenomas. *Proc. Soc. Exp. Biol. Med.* 93:361–366, 1956.

Libshitz H., Baber C.E., Hammond C.B.: The pulmonary metastases of choriocarcinoma. *Obstet. Gynecol.* 49:412–416, 1977.

Nagataki S., Mizuno M., Sakamoto S., et al.: Thyroid function in molar pregnancy. *J. Clin. Endocrinol. Metab.* 44:254–263, 1977.

Newlands E.S., Bagshawe K.D.: Anti-tumour activity of the epipodophyllin derivative VP-16-213 (etoposide:NSC-141540) in gestational choriocarcinoma. *Eur. J. Cancer* 16:401–405, 1980.

Nisula B.C., Taliadouros G.S.: Thyroid function in gestational trophoblastic neoplasia: Evidence that the thyrotropic activity of chorionic gonadotropin mediates the thyrotoxicosis of choriocarcinoma. *Am. J. Obstet. Gynecol.* 138:77–85, 1980.

Osathanondh R., Berkowitz R., deCholnoky C., et al.: Endocrine factor for theca-lutein cyst in gestational trophoblastic neoplasia. *Placenta* 3(suppl.):270–271, 1981.

Osathanondh R., Goldstein D.P., Pastorfide G.B.: Actinomycin D as the primary agent for gestational trophoblastic disease. *Cancer* 36:863–866, 1975.

Pao-Chang H., Shu-Chao P.: Chorionepithelioma: An analytical study of 28 necropsied cases, with special reference to the possibility of spontaneous regression. *J. Pathol. Bacteriol.* 72:95–104, 1956.

Pastorfide G.B., Goldstein D.P.: Pregnancy with hydatidiform mole. *Obstet. Gynecol.* 42:67–70, 1973.

Pattillo R.A., Sasaki S., Katayama K.P., et al.: Genesis of 46, XY hydatidiform mole. *Am. J. Obstet. Gynecol.* 141:104–105, 1981.

Ross G.T., Goldstein D.P., Hertz R., et al.: Sequential use of methotrexate and actinomycin D in the treatment of metastatic choriocarcinoma and related trophoblastic disease in women. *Am. J. Obstet. Gynecol.* 93:223–229, 1965.

Scheer K.I,., Goldstein D.P.: Use of ultrasonography to follow regression of theca-lutein cysts. *Radiology* 108:673–674, 1973.

Schlaerth J.B., Morrow C.P., DePetrillo A.D.: Sustained remission of choriocarcinoma with cis-platinum, vinblastine and bleomycin after failure of conventional combination drug therapy. *Am. J. Obstet. Gynecol.* 136:983–985, 1980.

Shirley R.L., Goldstein D.P., Collins J.J. Jr.: The role of thoracotomy in the management of patients with chest metastases from gestational trophoblastic disease. *J. Thorac. Cardiovasc. Surg.* 63:545–550, 1972.

Stone M., Dent J., Kardana A., et al.: Relationship of oral contraception to development of trophoblastic tumour after evacuation of a hydatidiform mole. *Br. J. Obstet. Gynaecol.* 83:913–916, 1976.

Sung H.C., Wu P.C., Hu M.H., et al.: Roentgenologic manifestations of pulmonary metastases in choriocarcinoma and invasive mole. *Am. J. Obstet. Gynecol.* 142:89–97, 1982.

Surti U., Szulman A.E., O'Brien S.: Complete (classic) hydatidiform mole with 46, XY karyotype of paternal origin. *Hum. Genet.* 51:153–155, 1979.

Surwit E.A., Hammond C.B.: Treatment of metastatic trophoblastic disease with poor prognosis. *Obstet. Gynecol.* 55:565–570, 1980.

Surwit E.A., Suciu T.N., Schmidt H.J., et al.: A new combination regimen for resistant trophoblastic disease. *Gynecol. Oncol.* 8:110–118, 1979.

Swett H.A., Westcott J.L.: Residual nonmalignant pulmonary nodules in choriocarcinoma. *Chest* 65:560–562, 1974.

Szulman A.E., Surti U.: The syndromes of hydatidiform mole: I. Cytogenetic and morphologic correlations. *Am. J. Obstet. Gynecol.* 131:665–771, 1978a.

Szulman A.E., Surti U.: The syndromes of hydatidiform mole: II. Morphologic evolution of the complete and partial mole. *Am. J. Obstet. Gynecol.* 132:20–27, 1978b.

Szulman A.E., Surti U.: The clinicopathologic profile of the partial hydatidiform mole. *Obstet. Gynecol.* 59:597–602, 1982.

Tow W.S.H.: The influence of the primary treatment of hydatidiform mole on its subsequent course. *Br. J. Obstet. Gynaecol.* 73:545–552, 1966.

Tsuji K., Yagi S., Nakano R.: Increased risk of malignant transformation of hydatidiform moles in older gravidas: A cytogenetic study. *Obstet. Gynecol.* 58:351–355, 1981.

VanThiel D.H., Ross G.T., Lipsett M.B.: Pregnancies after chemotherapy of trophoblastic neoplasms. *Science* 169:1326–1327, 1970.

Walden P.A.M., Bagshawe K.D.: Reproductive performance of women successfully treated for gestational trophoblastic tumors. *Am. J. Obstet. Gynecol.* 125:1108–1114, 1976.

Weed J.C. Jr., Hammond C.B.: Cerebral metastatic choriocarcinoma: Intensive therapy and prognosis. *Obstet. Gynecol.* 55:89–94, 1980.

Yamashita K., Wake N., Araki T., et al.: Human lymphocyte antigen expression in hydatidiform mole: Androgenesis following fertilization by a haploid sperm. *Am. J. Obstet. Gynecol.* 135:597–600, 1979.

CHAPTER THIRTEEN

Endocrine Disorders

VERONICA A. RAVNIKAR, M.D.

ENDOCRINE PROBLEMS in the female center on disorders of absent or infrequent menses, galactorrhea, and/or hirsutism (with possible virilization). Etiologies for these disordered symptoms are varied. They are best compartmentalized into problems with hypothalamic, pituitary, uterine, ovarian, and/or adrenal functioning. Discussion in this chapter will be divided into two major categories: endocrinologic problems that upset normal pubertal development and factors that occur after puberty to upset normal menstrual functioning.

Important advances in diagnosis and treatment of endocrinologic problems in the female have occurred with the availability of radioimmunoassays of the glycoprotein and steroid hormones. Furthermore, the isolation and synthesis of the hypothalamic decapeptide luteinizing hormone–releasing hormone (LH-RH) (also known as gonadotropin-releasing hormone [GnRH]) has been extremely significant in defining the pulse generator characteristics of the hypothalamic-pituitary axis. The 1978 Nobel Prize was shared by Dr. Rosyln Yallow for her work on radioimmunoassays and by Drs. Roger Guillemin and Andrew Schally. The latter two were honored for their work in isolation, sequencing, and synthesis of the decapeptide LH-RH (Porter et al.).

Luteinizing hormone–releasing hormone has become both a probe and a treatment in certain hormonal disorders. Finally, the long-term effects of disordered menstruation have been broadened with studies showing the specific skeletal changes (osteoporosis) caused by hypoestrogenemia. The diagnostic and therapeutic option and directives in female gynecologic endocrinology has truly blossomed in the last two decades.

PUBERTY

The prerequisites for the development of normal reproductive function in the female are: (1) normal ovaries capable of secreting steroids (estrogen and progesterone) in response to pituitary gonadotropins (LH and follicle-stimulating hormone [FSH]); (2) normal hypothalamus capable of responding to elevated levels of steroids by appropriate pulsatile secretion of LH-RH; (3) a normal pituitary that is sensitive to LH-RH and estrogen (or progesterone) and contains a pool of releasable LH large enough to provide an LH surge. There are many current reviews by major researchers in the field that both document the interrelationships of the hypothalamic-pituitary-ovarian cycle in the normal state (Porter et al., 1980; Yen, 1977). Furthermore, the studies in rhesus monkeys that have undergone oophorectomy document the profound changes that occur when the amplitude and/or the frequency of LH-RH pulses are changed (Knobil, 1981). The harmony of the menstrual cycle is a product of an elaborate pubertal process in which the hypothalamic-pituitary-ovarian axis develops concomitant to noted physical changes in the female. It is after the completion of the pubertal process that an individual is fully mature and able to reproduce. Physical changes were documented by Marshall and Tanner (Fig 13–1) and are the secondary sexual characteristics. There are average ages for the growth-spurt completion, thelarche (breast development), adrenarche (hair development), and menarche (onset of the first menstrual cycle). The onset of the pubertal event in each individual is variable and influenced profoundly by genetic and environmental factors (chronic disease and nutrition). In fact, the average onset of puberty in the United States is between ages 8 and 13 years. It is earlier than the average worldwide because of better nutrition. Also, since there is wide variation between the age at the onset of puberty among individuals (8 to 18 years), bone age correlates best with pubertal age. Special charts are therefore available to correlate specific so-

matic findings of puberty with appropriate bone age (Greulich and Pyle, 1959). Therefore, when evaluating an individual with delayed or advanced puberty, it is more important to match the bone age with other somatic pubertal changes.

To understand the hormone changes during puberty, it is worthwhile to review the changes in LH/FSH secretion from the time in utero to puberty (Grumbach et al., 1974; Conte et al., 1980; Sklar et al., 1980). It is now speculated that gonadarche and adrenarche are separate events. Puberty is felt to be controlled by an "LH-RH sensitivity threshold" in the hypothalamus that decreases with increased maturity of the hypothalamic-pituitary axis. Therefore, the central nervous system (CNS) appears to control the onset of puberty and, thus, the secretion of steroid hormones. However, after normal pubertal development has been accomplished, the hypothalamic-pituitary axis becomes sub-

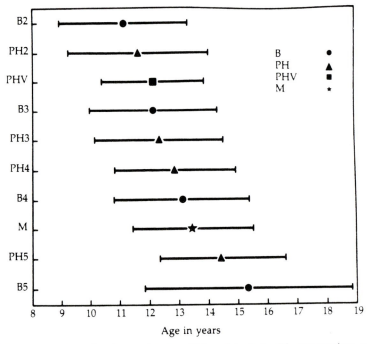

Fig 13–1.—Mean age at each stage of puberty. The center of each symbol represents the mean; the length of the symbol is equivalent to 2 SD on each side of the mean. B indicates breast; PH, pubic hair; M, menarche; and PHV, peak height velocity. (Adapted from Marshall W.A., Tanner J.M.: *Arch. Dis. Child.* 44:291, 1969.)

servient to the positive and negative feedback signals from the ovary. The pituitary control of adrenarche is not completely understood. Adrenarche causes pubic and axillary hair growth. It precedes the growth spurt by two years and involves an acceleration in size of the zona reticularis. There is subsequent increased secretion of androgens (dehydro-epiandrosterone [DHEA] and its sulfated form [DHEA-S] and androstenedione).

At midgestation, LH and FSH secretion by the fetus reach their highest levels and then decrease to low or undetectable levels to puberty. Therefore, the levels of circulating LH and FSH are low. But after the clearance of the maternal steroids from the placenta, there is decreased inhibition. Therefore, there is a temporary increase in LH and FSH to about 2 to 4 years of age. However, pituitary secretion of gonadotrope decreases again from about ages 4 to 11 years. This is felt to be due to the development of an intrinsic CNS inhibitory mechanism that suppresses pulsatile LH-RH release. This in turn is also more sensitive to the "gonadostat"—the feedback effect of prevailing steroids. Chronologically, the onset of puberty is thus heralded by a decrease in the CNS inhibitory restraint and a decrease in the negative feedback effect. There is then an increase in LH-RH secretion and pituitary responsiveness.

This responsiveness is demonstrated by the LH response to exogenous LH-RH administration. Prepubertal children show a minimal response to LH-RH, secreting a small but significant LH peak. Pubertal children and adults have a much greater LH response to LH-RH administration. This increase in pituitary reserve and secretion of LH is the hallmark of puberty and it is elicited prior to any physical evidence of secondary sexual development. Another maturational change seen in puberty is sleep-associated pulsatile LH secretion (Boyar et al., 1972).

The final phase of the maturational changes that take place is the development of cyclic release of LH due to the positive feedback of estradiol. This elicits the midcycle surge in gonadotropins seen after puberty in the normal female menstrual cycle. A typical cyclic adult pattern, however, is not achieved until luteal progesterone concentrations are adequate (greater than 10 ng/ml) (Lemarchand-Beraud, 1982).

Concomitant with these changes are also differences in adrenocortical functioning with an increase in adrenal androgen (adrenarche) (DHEA-S). Adrenal maturation, however, is a separate event. In agonadal children, a decrease in basal gonadotropins also occurs at ages 4 to 11 years, attesting to the isolated importance of a maturing CNS inhibitory influence during this period. Children with Addison's disease show the same pattern of gonadotropin secretion as that seen in normal and agonadal children and have a normal pubertal growth spurt. Premature adrenarche (before 8 years) is not consonant with premature gonadarche. Adrenarche also occurs in patients with both hypergonadotropic and hypogonadotropic hypogonadism (not hypopituitarism) (Grumbach, 1980).

Finally, in the prepubertal rhesus monkey, menstrual cycles can be initiated by infusions of GnRH for six minutes once every hour (Wildt et al., 1980). When the regimen is discontinued, the animals promptly revert to an immature state. All of this then leads us to the principle that the time frame between infancy and the onset of puberty is a state of "functional GnRH inactivity," which is terminated by mature pulsatile GnRH secretion.

"Minimum weight" is another criterion that appears to control normal menstrual function. About 4.5 kg of fat is gained from menarche to age 18 years. At age 18 years, mean fat is 16.0 ± 3 kg, 28% of the mean body weight of 57.1 ± 0.6 kg. This increase in fatness then reflects a decrease of 55.1 ± 0.2 oz of total water/body weight at menarche to 52.1 ± 0.2% at age 18 years. Losses of weight of 10% to 15% of body weight affect the menstrual cycle. Therefore, a relative degree of fatness plays a role in determining sexual maturation (Frisch, 1974, 1980; Sherman et al., 1981).

Abnormalities of the pubertal process involve isosexual or heterosexual precocity or delayed puberty. There also may be variations on the pubertal process with premature thelarche and premature adrenarche occurring in isolated form.

PRECOCIOUS PUBERTY

Puberty is considered precocious if secondary sexual characteristics occur prior to 8 years of age. This occurs in the general population in an incidence between 1/5,000 to 1/10,000. The female-to-male ratio is between 4:1 and 8:1. This is usually accompanied by accelerated linear growth (advanced bone age). Precocity may be due to constitutional or organic causes. The majority of patients with isosexual precocious puberty are of a constitutional or idiopathic form (85% of females) and it may be familial. It is, however, vital to distinguish these patients from those who have precocity based on lesions of the brain, ovary, or adrenal glands. Therefore, sexual precocity may be due to central or CNS causes (includes constitutional) or extrapituitary causes (ovarian tumors, adrenal tumors).

Central nervous tissue lesions and inflammatory processes such as hydrocephalus, meningitis, and brain abscesses can accelerate maturation. Central nervous tissue tumors such as gliomas, pinealomas, teratomas, and hypothalamic hamartomas (of tuber cinerum) may be involved. A much higher proportion of boys than girls will have tumors as a cause of precocity. Computed tomographic techniques reveal CNS lesions that may have been missed in the past. Therefore, the incidence of true idiopathic precocity may be lower. Ovarian tumors such as granulosa or theca cells of the ovary can cause precocity due to excess estrogen secretion. Virilization in females with accelerated adrenarche can be due to adrenal adenomas, carcinomas, arrhenoblastomas, or gonadoblastomas or congenital adrenal hyperplasia.

The most common cause of isosexual precocity is "constitutional." This is premature initiation of the normal physiologic and endocrinologic processes of adolescence. Breast development, appearance of pubic and axillary hair, and menstruation occur at a chronological age 2.5 SD below the mean for the onset of gonadal development (by age 8 years). The inciting factors are unknown.

Uterine bleeding in constitutional sexual precocity has been reported in infants as young as three months. Most patients are in the group aged 5 to 8 years. When premature menarche occurs during infancy, the bleeding may be the first abnormality noted. Premature breast development is not always associated with constitutional precocity. Some may ovulate and have moliminal symptoms.

The secretion of estrogen by the prematurely stimulated ovary results in an acceleration of linear growth and an advancement of bone age. X-rays of the carpal bones as well as the epiphyses of the knees and elbows will show advancement of bone age. Girls aged 8 or 9 years with constitutional sexual precocity usually are taller for their age group. However, because of premature epiphyseal closure, their adult height is usually below average. In addition, they may show rather excessive feminine hip contour and fat deposition in the buttocks. This appearance occasionally may be emphasized by the relative shortness of the lower extremities compared with the torso.

The diagnostic criteria in premature menstruation of constitutional etiology are: (1) gradual development and growth of pubic hair followed by uterine bleeding with moliminal symptoms if ovulation has occurred; (2) initial acceleration of linear growth and x-ray evidence of advanced bone age; (3) a computed axial tomographic (CAT) scan of the sella turcica that is normal; (4) elevated levels of urinary estrogens and detectable levels of urinary gonadotropins with normal serum DHEA-S and urinary 17-ketosteroids and 17-hydroxysteroids; (5) levels of serum LH and FSH above prepubertal levels but not usually as high as adult levels; (6) cornified cells on vaginal smears.

Kupperman and Epstein have pointed out the value of a therapeutic test with progestational steroids in differentiating idiopathic sexual precocity from that due to estrogenic secretion from a granulosa cell ovarian tumor. The vaginal smear in constitutional precocity shows midzone changes (estrogenic) or secretory (progestational) changes. The vaginal smear in a patient with a granulosa cell tumor will show only proliferative, cornified cells, since ovulation does not occur (shift to left). Exogenous progestins such as norethindrone, norethynodrel, or medroxyprogesterone acetate given to those with constitutional sexual precocity will suppress gonadal secretion. There will be a diminution of estrogen secretion and the vaginal smear will appear atrophic (basal cells). Since progestins will not inhibit estrogens secreted autonomously from the ovary, the vaginal pattern in these cases will show an atypical secretory pattern.

The treatment of patients with constitutional sexual precocity is predicated on the attempt to delay premature closure of the epiphysis. Treatment in this area has been revolutionized by the development of GnRH agonists. However, to date, GnRH agonists are not routinely available. It is still worthwhile to review older modalities of treatment.

The past treatment of choice has been Depo-Provera in doses of 200 to 300 mg given intramuscularly (IM) every 14 days (Hahn et al., 1964). This suppresses the pituitary gonadotropins and reduces the secretion of steroids from the gonads. A diminution in breast size is noted, together with diminished estrogenic activity in the vaginal smear. Amenorrhea follows. The bone age of the patient is followed and when adequate height is reached, the treatment is discontinued. However, Depo-Provera has been somewhat disappointing in that normal skeletal maturation has not consistently been achieved. The long-term effects on adrenal and menstrual function are also unknown.

Phenothiazine derivatives (chlorpromazine) can also suppress gonadal function by suppressing FSH and LH secretion (possibly due to hyperprolactinemia) (Sulman, 1959; Liv et al., 1965). The usual dose of chlorpromazine is 2.5 mg, four times a day. Abnormal electroencephalographic (EEG) patterns seen at times in patients with constitutional precocious puberty are reversed with chlorpromazine. Cyproterone acetate, an antiandrogen, not available in the United States, and danazol (17α-ethinyltestosterone) has also been used.

With the institution of LH-RH analogue (D-Trp^6-Pro^9-NEt-LHRH) therapy, new treatment has been instituted for precocity, which is very effective. The effects of LH-RH analogues are also completely reversible. Since normal hypothalamic-pituitary function is pulsatile, giving a long-acting LH-RH analogue desensitizes the pituitary LH-RH receptors. Gonadotropin release is inhibited and pubertal changes are interrupted. A recent report (Mansfield et al., 1983) documented its effect in nine girls with central precocious puberty who were treated with daily subcutaneous injections of LH-RH$_\alpha$ of 4 to 8 μg/kg of body weight. The doses were adjusted until plasma estradiol levels and maturation indices were suppressed to prepubertal levels. This did not interfere with established adrenarche, but did in those who were preadrenarcheal. The selective, reversible effects on gonadarche were: (1) regression of secondary sexual characteristics; (2) cessation of menses; (3) decrease of growth velocity and slowing of skeletal maturation, which lead to an increase in adult height; and (4) return of age-appropriate behavior. The latter is a very beneficial psychologic effect. Children with precocious puberty have excessive activity and emotional lability, which cause behavioral problems. To date, this treatment is still available only at the National Institute of Child Health and Human Development (NICHD) in Bethesda, Md, or through Dr. William F. Crowley, Jr., at the Massachusetts General Hospital in Boston.

Premature menses may also be due to organic causes both central (CNS) or peripheral (ovarian, adrenal).

Destructive lesions of the posterior hypothalamus cause premature pubescence. Most likely, this is due to the lack of the normal inhibitory influence by the hypothalamus. The pituitary subsequently releases high levels of gonadotropins. Computerized axial tomography of the skull has aided diagnosis of rare CNS tumors such as hamartomas of the tuber cinerum. The latter is benign, rarely damages the hypothalamus itself, and usually is asymptomatic (Loop, 1964). Pinealomas can also cause precocity.

Inflammation and scarring of the hypothalamus may lead to irritation and premature discharge of pulses to the anterior pituitary. Therefore, postencephalatic states, meningitis, and cranial trauma may precipitate precocious development. Treatment, again, would be the same as for the constitutional type.

Congenital lesions of the brain may also accelerate puberty. Notable amongst these is McCune-Albright syndrome identified by the triad of precocious puberty, large cafe-au-lait spots, and polyostotic fibrous dysplasia (Albright et al., 1937; Benedict, 1962). The latter are identifiable as disseminated cystic bone lesions with loss of bone trabecular architecture. The skin and skeletal features occur together unilaterally. Pathologic fractures in the areas of fibrous dysplasia may first call attention to the disorder. The base of the skull is also involved, and optic compression may occur. It has been suggested that this is actually precocious pseudopuberty, since ovulation rarely occurs. This occurs subsequently at the time of normal pubescence, and fertility is not impaired. The treatment again would center on delaying accelerated growth.

Some other CNS related lesions that may cause precocious puberty are gliomas associated with neurofibromatosis, and isolated LH-producing tumors (Rosenfeld et al., 1980). Other miscellaneous causes of precocious puberty include juvenile hypothyroidism. In such, precocious menstruation, breast enlargement, and galactorrhea may occur in the absence of pubic hair and growth accelera-

tion. This may be due to an increase in thyroid-stimulating hormone (TSH) along with LH and FSH. Administration of thyroid supplements reverses the situation (Van Wyk and Grumbach, 1960). Finally, exogenous steroid hormones may cause precocity.

The isosexual type of precocious pseudopuberty is more often due to estrogen-producing tumors of the ovary. Although these lesions are quite rare, they are usually assumed to be the cause of precocious bleeding in most young females. Pedowitz et al. reviewed the literature in 1955 and were able to find precocious pseudopuberty in only 85 patients. Sixty-five of these had granulosa-theca cell tumors; three, dysgerminomas; 12, teratomas; and five were reported as "follicular cysts." Thus, it should be remembered that only about 5% of granulosa cell tumors and only 1% of thecomas occur before puberty. Pedowitz and associates reported two cases of precocious pseudopuberty, one in a 14-month-old infant with a thecoma and one in a 10-year-old girl with a granulosa cell tumor. A recent report documented that in a 3½-year-old girl with isosexual precocious puberty, the hyperestrogenism caused by the granulosa cell tumor was due to the secretion of 17β-estradiol de novo by the tumor (Madden and MacDonald, 1978).

The youngest reported case of precocious puberty due to an ovarian tumor was in an infant, 14 weeks of age. Premature bleeding was most commonly seen in the granulosa-theca cell group, 56 patients having this symptom. In 74 patients of the total 85, vaginal bleeding was part of the symptomatology (Figs 13–2 and 13–3).

Endocrine assays may be of extreme value in differential diagnosis. As previously mentioned, hormone levels corresponding to those of normal adults (cyclic estrogen-progesterone and normal gonadotropins) suggest true precocious puberty. Increased levels of estrogen with absence of cyclic variation strongly suggest a granulosa-theca cell tumor. Solid teratomas and dysgerminomas that contain chorionic elements may be associated

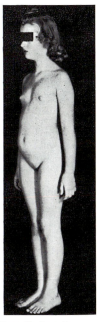

Fig 13–2.—Constitutional sexual precocity in a 7-year-old girl who had just noted menarche. Vaginal smear showed evidence of estrogen stimulation. Height was above normal and bone age was 9 years. Level of 17-ketosteroids was 3 mg/24 hours and gonadotropins, 8 mouse uterine units (muu)/ 24 hours. (From Lloyd C.W.: The ovaries, in Williams R.H. [ed.]: *Textbook of Endocrinology,* ed. 3. Philadelphia, W.B. Saunders Co., 1962.)

with elevated levels of gonadotropins in urine, occasionally sufficient to give positive results in a test for pregnancy. The estrogen production by the theca cells of the granulosa-theca cell tumors is undoubtedly responsible for the premature menses, breast enlargement, increased bone age, and acceleration of linear growth. In the vaginal smear there is a high percentage of cornified cells but without evidence of progesterone activity. The levels of gonadotropins and 17-ketosteroids in patients with feminizing granulosa-theca cell tumors are normal.

The diagnosis of an ovarian neoplasm as a cause of precocious pseudopuberty may be aided by the abdominal and rectovaginal examinations. Of the 85 patients in the study of Pedowitz and associates, 76 were found to

have an abdominal mass and 65 a pelvic mass. In addition, 21 of these patients complained of pain and 12 had ascites.

Premature uterine bleeding may be one of the symptoms in solid teratoma of the ovary, and, indeed, it was a presenting complaint in ten of 12 cases reported by Pedowitz and associates. These tumors contained chorionic elements that secrete gonadotropic hormone. Therefore, the contralateral ovary may be stimulated by the chorionic gonadotropin to produce sufficient estrogen for endometrial proliferation and subsequent vaginal bleeding. Assays of chorionic gonadotropins in urine in patients with teratomas will frequently show elevated values. Chorionic tissue was identified in eight of the 12 teratomas reported in the literature. The sexual precocity associated with lesions of this type is not accompanied by ovulation and therefore the vaginal smear will show evidence of estrogen effect only and the basal body temperatures will be monophasic. Another diagnostic point is the absence of axillary hair in prepubescent females with ovarian teratomas. Thus, the finding of premature bleeding with sexual precocity, breast development, absent axillary hair, and high urinary gonadotropin levels (which may give a positive pregnancy test result) is indicative of a solid teratoma of the ovary, particularly if a pelvic mass is palpable.

The mortality rate in patients with embryonic solid teratoma is about 100%. Despite the high degree of malignancy, complete hysterectomy and bilateral salpingo-oophorectomy should be performed. Neither methotrexate nor other chemotherapeutic agents have been of value in nongestational chorionic tumors.

Precocious puberty due to dysgerminomas has also been associated with elevated gonadotropin levels in urine. In the usual type of dysgerminoma occurring in the adult female, specific elaboration of chorionic gonadotropin has been described in only one patient. Occasionally granulosa-theca cell elements may be found in a dysgerminoma which, because of the elevated levels of estrogen secretion,

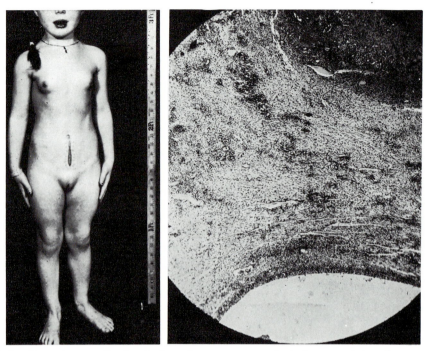

Fig 13–3.—Sexual precocity due to hypothalamic lesion in 3½-year-old girl with vaginal bleeding. Bone age was 4 years, the sella turcica normal. Gonadotropin excretion was 16 muu/24 hours; 17-ketosteroids, 2 mg/24 hours; and estrogens in urine, 20 μg/24 hours. An EEG showed changes localizing the lesion in the hypothalamus; the pneumoencephalogram excluded tumor. Therapy with medroxyprogesterone resulted in complete disappearance of precocious maturation. The midline scar was due to unwarranted exploration after the first episode of bleeding. Photomicrograph at right shows active ovarian stroma and a cystic graafian follicle obtained at biopsy at the time of laparotomy. (From Lloyd C.W.: The ovaries, in Williams R.H. [ed.]: *Textbook of Endocrinology,* ed. 3. Philadelphia, W.B. Saunders Co., 1962.)

may cause sexual precocity and uterine bleeding.

The removal of the ovarian neoplasm usually results in a rapid fall of the previously elevated levels of gonadotropin and estrogen. Reappearance of such hormonal entities, prior to the menarche, suggests a recurrence of the original tumor or the possibility of distant metastases.

Since in more than 90% of patients, precocious puberty will be found to be of constitutional or idiopathic type, exploratory laparotomy for patients with sexual precocity is not warranted unless ovarian enlargement can be identified. Ovarian neoplasms that show surface or peritoneal extension and are nonencapsulated are preferably treated by complete hysterectomy and bilateral salpingo-oophorectomy. In the case of a neoplasm of relatively low malignancy, such as an encapsulated granulosa-theca cell tumor, unilateral salpingo-oophorectomy is the treatment of choice. Most patients having the latter lesion were living and well without evidence of disease from three to five years following surgery in the series of Pedowitz and associates.

The treatment of encapsulated dysgerminomas has usually, in the past, been conservative because of the belief that this neoplasm was relatively benign. Evidence, however, by Pedowitz and co-workers indicates a five-year mortality rate of 73% with a tendency toward early recurrence. In addition, involvement of the contralateral ovary has been reported in about 35% of patients. In view of this high mortality rate and the bilaterality of the lesion, complete extirpation of the pelvic organs seems warranted.

A unilateral cystic ovary has been described in several patients with premature menarche and other signs of premature pubescence. Such lesions may result from pituitary gonadotropic stimulation associated either with lesions of the hypothalamus or with true constitutional sexual precocity. In several instances, however, removal of the ovarian cyst was followed by regression of the signs of sexual precocity. Removal of such a cyst is adequate therapy; the ovary should be preserved.

Although adrenocortical hyperfunction may result in the development of axillary and pubic hair, vaginal bleeding is rare. The development of adrenal hyperplasia, adenoma or malignancy in fact usually delays the onset of normal menstruation in prepubescent females. The differential diagnosis should not be difficult because, even in the presence of vaginal bleeding, breast development is unusual but clitoral enlargement is common. Careful physical examination together with a determination of urinary 17-ketosteroid concentrations will suffice to differentiate the site of hormone production. The level of 17-ketosteroids in urine is elevated (usually greater than 30 mg/24 hr), the degree depending on whether adrenal hyperplasia, adenoma, or neoplasm is present. The case of late-onset congenital adrenal hyperplasia will be discussed later in the chapter in the area of menstrual disorders and hirsutism. Dexamethasone suppression tests may be used to differentiate between congenital adrenal hyperplasia and adrenal tumors. The latter is not suppressed with exogenous steroids.

Workup of Precocious Puberty

The first crucial steps in an initial evaluation of precocious puberty are careful history taking (rule out exogenous steroid administration, history of encephalitis, cerebral trauma) and meticulous physical examination. Blood pressure, accelerated development of the-

larche, pubarche, gonadarche, and growth spurt are noted. Skin changes and any cafe-au-lait spots are documented. Pelvic and abdominal examination may indicate presence of an ovarian or adrenal mass, which is further confirmed by ultrasound scanning. Bone x-rays document accelerated linear growth and epiphyseal closure (and also exclude fibrous dysplasia). A skull x-ray or CAT scan rules out intracranial pathologic lesions. Chemical precocity is indicated by adolescent levels of FSH, LH, and 17β-estradiol. Thyroid function tests exclude hypothyroidism. Elevated urinary 17-ketosteroids excretion points to either possible late-onset congenital adrenal hyperplasia or an adrenal neoplasm (especially if documented by scan). In the latter condition, suppression does not occur with a dexamethasone suppression test, whereas suppression does occur in congenital adrenal hyperplasia. Increased urinary human chorionic gonadotropin (HCG) may indicate a rare trophoblastic tumor. Exogenous LH-RH administration can be used to discriminate between extrapituitary causes of precocity (ovarian tumors) and central causes. The latter will have a pubertal LH response after such stimulation whereas the former will not. Finally, if the use of exogenous steroids, CNS disease, hypothyroidism, late-onset congenital adrenal hyperplasia, McCune-Albright syndrome, and adrenal or ovarian masses are excluded, then idiopathic isosexual precocious puberty is the most likely diagnosis.

DELAYED MENARCHE

The term *delayed menarche* indicates the absence of menses in females by age 18 years. This may be classified into three groups: constitutional delay, hypogonadotrophic hypogonadism, and hypergonadotrophic hypogonadism.

The majority of patients with delayed adolescent development manifest no demonstrable organic pathologic conditions. The developmental retardation in these individuals represents a normal variation in endocrine function that will usually be rectified by time alone. For this reason, a most perplexing problem is *when* to commence a diagnostic program. The answer lies in the individualization of each case, taking into account the history, findings of physical examination, and the emotional attitudes of the patient and her family. The practice of initiating therapy to promote sexual development, however, is to be deplored unless adequate diagnostic studies have been undertaken.

The endocrine defect in delayed adolescent development and delayed menarche is the lack of proper estrogenic stimulation necessary for maturation of the accessory sex organs and initiation of uterine bleeding. The secretion of estrogen is dependent on the elaboration of gonadotropin hormones from the adenohypophysis. The secretion of gonadotropins may be diminished or entirely lacking. In these individuals, for reasons unknown, it is assumed that both FSH and LH are held in abeyance.

Malnutrition due to starvation or chronic wasting diseases may be contributory. Similarly, emotional or psychosomatic factors are known causes of secondary amenorrhea and may act to delay the onset of the puberty. Imbalances of other endocrine organs, such as the thyroid or adrenal glands, may also delay adolescent development and the menarche.

Clinical evaluation of the patients manifesting delayed adolescent development should begin with a complete and thorough history and physical examination. Careful scrutiny of the accessory sex organs and the genitalia is mandatory. The internal genitalia may be examined rectally; negligible mental trauma and physical discomfort ensue if the examiner is reassuring and careful. Bone x-rays document bone age. Neurologic and ophthalmologic examinations are indicated if suspicious signs or symptoms such as headaches, scotomata, or diplopia are manifested.

The importance of a thorough rectovaginal examination is emphasized by the fact that delayed menarche may on occasion be due to a congenital mechanical obstruction in the vagina or cervix. Most commonly this is an imperforate hymen, and rectal examination reveals accumulated menstrual discharge in the vagina. Normal menses will immediately follow incision into the hymen and relief of the obstruction.

Assay of gonadotropins will distinguish between pituitary and ovarian failure. An elevated serum gonadotropin titer suggests ovarian failure (hypergonadotropic hypogonadism). Diminished titers focus attention on pituitary dysfunction (hypogonadotrophic hypogonadism). Plasma FSH levels appear to be the single most reliable assay for the presence or absence of ovarian failure (Goldenberg et al., 1973). Estrogens measured in urine or blood are in the range of the prepubertal or postmenopausal female. Yet the function of the endometrium is not altered, since uterine bleeding may be induced by the administration of estrogens alone or estrogens followed by progesterone.

As previously stated, the majority of patients with delayed adolescent development manifest no discernible pathologic condition. The prognosis for normal sexual development and reproductive function is excellent. In the absence of proved lesions or hormonal deficiencies, the use of endocrine preparations is deemed inadvisable. Reassurance, explanation, and passage of time constitute the desired therapeutic regimen. Systemic abnormalities such as obesity, cachexia, infection, and diabetes should be appropriately treated. Adequate psychiatric therapy, if indicated, should be initiated.

Hypogonadotrophic Hypogonadism

The causes for hypogonadotrophic hypogonadism are isolated gonadotropin deficiency, congenital defects associated with gonadotropin insufficiency, CNS tumors, chronic disease (diabetes mellitus), and malnutrition (anorexia nervosa).

Isolated LH or FSH deficiency has been documented (Rabin et al., 1972; Hashimoto et al., 1972). Whether these isolated deficiencies of either hormone are due to hypothalamic or pituitary malfunction is unknown.

Certain congenital defects are associated

with gonadotropin deficiency. These are Kallmann's, Prader-Willi and Laurence-Moon-Biedl syndromes.

The association of congenital absence of the sense of smell and congenital hypogonadotropic hypogonadism is known as Kallmann's syndrome. This can occur in men and women and is associated with complete lack of secondary sexual characteristics. Other associated developmental anomalies are unilateral or bilateral hypoplasia of olfactory bulbs, multiple facial anomalies (cleft palate and lip), right aortic arches, color blindness, renal agenesis, neurosensory deafness, and insulin-dependent diabetes mellitus. This syndrome is associated with low FSH and LH secretion and low gonadal steroid secretion. Patients with this syndrome respond to exogenous LH-RH with varying levels of LH and FSH secretion and to exogenous gonadotropins with ovulation. They do not respond to clomiphene citrate (Clomid) (which requires normal pituitary functioning). Therefore, the condition is an isolated pituitary deficiency of LH and FSH secretion. Inheritance is considered to be autosomal recessive with variable expression (Lieblich et al., 1982; White et al., 1983).

Pulsatile LH-RH administration has again served as a probe and treatment for such individuals. When pulses of LH-RH (0.025 µg/kg) are given intravenously every two hours for five days, there is a changing pattern of gonadotropin (LH, FSH) secretion similar to that found in puberty. In females, the initial FSH response to LH-RH is rapid and then declines after three days. Plasma estradiol levels rise to adult follicular levels after day 2 of treatment. Luteinizing hormone responses to continued LH-RH treatment are initially low, but then increase with further treatment. A standard LH-RH test (2.5 µg/kg) given at the end of persistent pulsatile secretion showed an increase in LH secretion and a decrease in FSH, similar to that found in pubertal maturation (Valk et al., 1980). Finally, a successful ovulatory response to repetitive subcutaneous LH-RH pulses (25 ng/kg) at two hourly intervals for 27 days, produce a normal menstrual cycle. This is documented by a biphasic temperature response, anatomic changes in ovary consistent with ovulation and a normal pattern of gonadotropin and gonadal steroid concentration (Crowley and McArthur, 1980).

Therefore, these patients may today undergo ovulation-induction therapy with pulsatile LH-RH therapy. The use of exogenous pulsatile LH-RH via pump in establishing normal puberty is also being researched successfully. However, to date, the latter is not routinely available. Therefore, after cranial tumors have been excluded, maturation of accessory sex organs can be achieved with hormonal preparations (Premarin, Estinyl) once linear growth has ceased. This is lifetime supplementation and should continue until the menopause. Medroxyprogesterone acetate (Provera) therapy should be added for its sparing effects on the uterus. A typical replacement schedule is Premarin, 0.625 mg days 1 to 25 of each month, followed by Provera, 10 mg on days 15 to 25.

Prader-Willi syndrome is inherited as an autosomal recessive trait. It is associated with childhood-onset obesity, mental retardation, and hypogonadism. Laurence-Moon-Biedl syndrome is another autosomal recessive trait associated with obesity. It is additionally associated with genital atrophy, mental retardation, skull deformities, retinitis pigmentosa, polydactyly, and syndactyly.

Central nervous system tumors that may be associated with hypogonadotrophic hypogonadism are craniopharyngioma, histiocytosis X, and gliomas. Radiation therapy can also destroy hypothalamic pituitary functioning.

Craniopharyngiomas occur in 5% to 10% of all intracranial tumors and the majority of children are 7 to 12 years of age. The major clinical manifestations are that of hypothalamic dysfunction with disruption of the pubertal process, increased intracranial pressure, visual defects, and diabetes insipidus. Radiographically, the majority of these present as enlargement of the sella turcica with diffuse calcified flecks in the sella or suprasellar regions. Nonspecific signs of increased intracranial pressure may also be present, such as separation of the suture lines on plain radiographs.

Histiocytosis X is a histiocytic hyperplasia involving systemic proliferation of the cellular elements of the reticuloendothelial system. The nonlipid reticuloendotheliosis involves inflammatory histiocytic proliferation with, at times, formation of granulomatous lesions. Hand-Schüller-Christian disease is the type presenting as exophthalmos, membranous bone defects, and diabetes insipidus. Granulomatous lesions pressing on the pituitary can cause problems with hypothalamic-pituitary function. Hypothalamus gliomas and other tumors such as teratomas or dermoids, depending on their bulk and compressive effects, can cause sexual infantilism. Radiation therapy of tumors can cause residual hypothalamic dysfunction (Chutorian, 1972; Einhorn, 1972).

Finally, although hypothyroidism and chronic hydrocephalus can be associated with precocity, they can also cause delayed sexual development (Phansey et al., 1984).

Chronic diseases and malnutrition can also disrupt the pubertal process. Among these are weight loss, malnutrition, cystic fibrosis, regional enteritis, rheumatoid arthritis, sickle cell disease, diabetes mellitus, and renal failure.

Prominent among these causes for delayed puberty are anorexia nervosa and childhood athleticism.

Anorexia nervosa (pubertal starvation amenorrhea) is associated with an extremely distorted attitude toward eating and body image. This is combined with an excess of weight loss of greater than 25%, combined with amenorrhea, bradycardia, overactivity, bulimia (gorging and vomiting), and growth of lanugo body hair. Since this disorder occurs primarily in adolescent girls, it is considered as one of the causes of delayed pubertal development. However, its onset can occur in any female before the age of 25 years and therefore may be associated with secondary amenorrhea. Also, starting during puberty, it may subse-

quently manifest itself with a fluctuating course of exacerbations and remissions. Whether or not this dysfunction is another expression of endogenous depression is controversial. In fact, it is difficult to determine whether or not the metabolic (low blood pressure, low pulse rate) and neuroendocrinologic (decreased excretion of gonadotropins, decreased estrogen levels) abnormalities in anorexia are a cause or a result of the syndrome. Plasma levels of norepinephrine and urinary excretion of 3-methoxy-4-hydroxyphenylglycol (MHPG) are low in anorectic patients and recover after weight loss. This derangement of catecholamine metabolism can explain the hypothalamic dysfunction (norepinephrine stimulates LH release) and disordered cardiovascular response. Depressed patients, however, also have decreased urinary MHPG levels (Gross et al., 1979).

Anorectics with profound weight loss are hypogonadotropic and have a prepubertal response to bolus LH-RH injection (2.5 µg/kg of body weight) and do not have LH peaks during the day or sleep. Subsequent pulsatile LH-RH administration (0.025 to 0.05 µg/kg) initially increases FSH release, followed by a decline. This is followed with a rise in LH and peripheral estradiol secretion (Marshall and Kelch, 1979). Cortisol metabolism is also altered with mean plasma cortisol concentrations elevated with normal circadian rhythm. Cortisol half-life is prolonged, cortisol production is normal or increased and the metabolic clearance rates of cortisol are reduced. Thyroid function is generally normal except for low triiodothyronine (T_3) levels and elevated reverse T_3 levels (Boyar et al., 1977). With the administration of naloxone (produces opiate-receptor blockage in hypothalamus), anorectics whose amenorrhea precedes the weight loss have an elevation of LH and an elevation of β-endorphin–like substances. Serum ACTH and cortisol levels, however, remain unaltered (Baranowska et al., 1984). This may mean that there is an excess of exogenous opiates in the hypothalamus. The treatment of anorectics is predicated on a team effort combining psychiatric care along with parental involvement in the group therapy. It is one of the extreme examples of the metabolic adaptations to starvation and of the importance of critical body weight to the sustenance of reproductive functioning.

Professional athletes and dancers who begin vigorous training prior to adolescence delay menarche and have a higher percentage of amenorrhea. Runners especially have a higher incidence of amenorrhea, which appears to correlate with the number of miles run (Warren, 1980; Sanborn et al., 1982). Whether or not the hypogonadotropism is induced by the increased levels of β-endorphin or prolactin is debatable (Dixon et al., 1984; Howlett et al., 1984; Boyden et al., 1982). We already know that a critical body weight is important for normal adolescent development. Professional competitors and performers are notably lower in weight. The loss of bone mineral that appears to be correlated with the hypoestrogenic state has initiated the controversy of giving hormonal supplements to amenorrheic individuals along with calcium carbonate. The bone loss especially in the trabecular type of spinal bone seems to be similar to the physiologic menopausal loss that is abated with estrogen supplementation (Drinkwater et al., 1984; Heaney et al., 1978).

Hypergonadotrophic Hypogonadism

The next category of patients with delayed pubertal development are those with primary gonadal failure—hypergonadotrophic hypogonadism. The condition in the majority of these is due to chromosomal abnormalities such as gonadal dysgenesis and its variants. However, anything else that may destroy the ovary, such as autoimmune ovarian failure or radiation-induced ovarian failure, can cause hypogonadism.

Gonadal dysgenesis (Turner's syndrome) is responsible for about 40% of cases of failure of menarche. Thirty-eight percent of Turner's patients remain undiagnosed until puberty. Gonadal dysgenesis may occur with a normal chromosomal complement (46 XX, 46 XY) in 38%. If a Y chromosome is present, extirpation of the gonads is mandatory, since there is a high rate of malignant transformation (Simpson, 1976). In gonadal dysgenesis, the gonad is replaced by a fibrous streak with dense fibrous stroma and absent oocytes. These patients have normal external and internal genitalia. However, secondary sex characteristics do not develop. Some of Turner's stigmata include: (1) height lower than normal (average, 141 ± 0.62 cm); and (2) webbing of the neck; (3) low nuchal hairline; (4) shield-shaped chest; and (5) cardiovascular, skeletal, and auditory abnormalities. Moreover, chromosomal variants may have some different somatic presentation. In 45 X/45 XX patterns, 12% menstruate. Deletions of the short arm of the X chromosome usually result in normal stature and therefore 46 X isochromosome Xq have normal stature. It is recommended that amenorrheic individuals with gonadal dysgenesis are given hormonal therapy, to be initiated after the maximal adult height has been reached.

The study of the gonadotropin dynamics in patients with gonadal dysgenesis are interesting. Patients with Turner's syndrome display a negative correlation between mean 24-hour LH and FSH secretion and total body fat and percentage body fat indices. This is of interest since it again supports body fat factor in controlling gonadotropin secretion, despite the absence of gonadal steroids (Boyar et al., 1981). In these agonadal patients, LH-RH–induced LH and FSH responses are within the normal range for prepubertal patients 6 to 10 years of age, but then change after age 11 years with elevation of FSH and LH—the hallmarks of agonadal patients (Ross et al., 1983). Estrogen infusions in such patients (aged 12 to 35 years) abolish the pulsatile release of LH and, to a lesser extent, FSH (Yen et al., 1972).

The remaining causes for gonadal failure will be discussed further in the section dealing with primary and secondary amenorrhea.

MALE PSEUDOHERMAPHRODITISM

Testicular feminization or male pseudoher-maphroditism may be complete or incom-plete. It involves 46 XY individuals who have bilateral testes, female external genitalia, and a blindly ending vagina or no müllerian deriv-atives. Therefore, they are phenotypic fe-males but genetic males. Thelarche is normal but there is an absence of pubic and axillary hair. The initial presentation may actually be that of primary amenorrhea or an inguinal hernia (testes). The gene responsible may be an X-linked recessive or male limited autoso-mal dominant. Some may have clitoromegaly and are thus considered to represent an in-complete form of the syndrome. Their gonads require extirpation due to their malignant po-tential. This syndrome may be caused by de-ficient or defective cytoplasmic androgen re-ceptors (Simpson, 1976). Plasma testosterone levels are normal for males with elevated lev-els of LH but with normal FSH levels (Naf-tolin et al., 1983).

Müllerian aplasia refers to absent vagina and all or almost all of the uterus; this is the most frequent cause of vaginal agenesis. Vag-inal atresia may occur along with the presence of a normal uterus. Winter's syndrome is an autosomal recessive trait in which vaginal atresia is associated with middle ear anoma-lies and renal agenesis. Müllerian aplasia leads to absence of the uterine corpus, uter-ine cervix, and upper portion of the vagina. If a rudimentary uterus is present, then the term Rokitansky-Küster-Hauser syndrome is used. Renal anomalies (vertebral anomalies) are frequently associated with müllerian apla-sia. Müllerian aplasia has to be differentiated from testicular feminization; this is done by karyotypic analysis and determination of plasma testosterone levels (Simpson, 1982).

An incomplete type of male pseudoher-maphroditism (pseudovaginal perineoscrotal hypospadias) is an autosomal recessive trait. It is associated with ambiguous pseudofemale genitalia in genetic males. This results from deficient production of dihydrotestosterone due to a 5α-reductase deficiency (Simpson, 1976). These genetic males, depending on the degree of abnormality, are generally raised as females but show signs of masculinization at puberty.

Female pseudohermaphroditism results from androgen excess due to adrenal enzyme deficiencies inherited as an autosomal reces-sive trait. These are 21-hydroxylase, 11β-hy-droxylase, and 3β-hydroxysteroid dehydroge-nase deficiencies. These will be discussed un-der the heading "Menstrual Disorders," since they cause hirsutism, amenorrhea, and, rarely, problems with lack of pubertal development.

McDonough's group reported 252 patients with abnormalities of delayed pubertal devel-opment. Forty-three percent of these had ovar-ian failure and most of these were due to sex chromosome abnormalities. Fourteen percent had physiologic or constitutional delay of pu-berty. Another 15% had congenital absence of vagina or uterus (Reindollar et al., 1981).

The differential diagnosis, therefore, of pa-tients with delayed puberty involves a careful history taking (especially of the pubertal mile-stones of female relatives) and of nutritional or systemic medical problems. Physical ex-amination should include: height, weight, as-sessment for Turner's stigmata, Tanner stag-ing of breasts and pubic hair, evaluation of genital defects, and neurologic evaluation of the sense of smell. If levels of gonadotropins are elevated, then karyotyping is in order and may lead to the diagnosis of gonadal dysgen-esis or male pseudohermaphroditism. If levels of gonadotropins are low, then an olfactory check will indicate Kallmann's syndrome. A skull roentgenogram or CAT scan will rule out a tumor, and LH-RH testing may be in order to rule out hypopituitarism.

MENSTRUAL DISORDERS

This text section will deal with issues of pri-mary and secondary amenorrhea, and oligo-menorrhea.

The designation *primary amenorrhea* de-notes menarche that has not occurred by age

18 years. In the previous section, we have dealt with the hypogonadotropic and hypergonadotropic states that cause this syndrome in combination with delayed puberty. Primary amenorrhea is associated with normal pubertal development in vaginal or müllerian aplasia. Patients who have complete androgen insensitivity may also have normal thelarche, but do not have normal hair development and are amenorrheic. In deciphering the cause of primary amenorrhea, it is worthwhile to look at the patient's secondary sex characteristics. If there is good sexual development, then testicular feminization, müllerian agenesis, vaginal atresia, and polycystic ovarian disease, are

possibilities. If there is poor or little sexual development, then gonadal dysgenesis, anorexia nervosa, or prepubertal athleticism are possibilities.

A recent review crystallized the diagnostic technique of evaluating patients with primary amenorrhea (Maschak et al., 1981). In this study, 62 patients with primary amenorrhea were analyzed under the major subdivisions of breast development: present or absent (Fig 13–4). This concise and complete analysis again showed that the majority of patients with primary amenorrhea will have hypogonadotropic hypogonadism or gonadal dysgenesis. The second and third categories are fur-

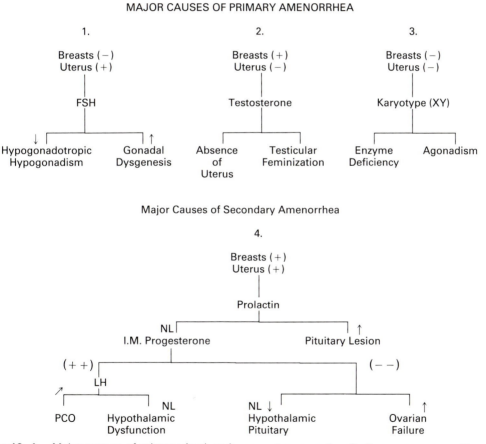

Fig 13–4.—Major causes of primary *(top)* and secondary *(bottom)* amenorrhea. Plus signs indicate normal development; minus signs, abnormal development. NL indicates normal; double plus sign, positive finding or response; and double minus sign, negative finding or response. For description of categories 1 through 4, see text. (Modified from Maschak C.A., et al.: *Obstet. Gynecol.* 57:715–720, 1981.)

ther discriminated by plasma testosterone levels. The fourth category, which includes patients with normal breast and uterine development is discriminated by prolactin levels, which rule out a pituitary tumor. If the patient is normoprolactinemic, then a progesterone intramuscular challenge test discerns estrogen status. If the latter is adequate, withdrawal bleeding occurs, and further LH measurements discriminate between patients with polycystic ovarian disease syndrome and hypothalamic dysfunction. If the progesterone withdrawal test is negative, then further FSH level testing rules out ovarian failure. This final diagnostic category is not primarily associated with primary amenorrhea, but rather with secondary amenorrhea. It will be discussed further. The systemic approach these authors offer, however, is very valuable in the diagnostic evaluation of primary amenorrhea.

Secondary amenorrhea denotes loss of menses for more than a six-month period in a woman who has had previously normal cycles. Oligomenorrhea denotes irregular but consistent periods occurring at intervals of two to five months. Chronic anovulation usually accompanies secondary amenorrhea or oligomenorrhea. The most common causes for secondary amenorrhea or oligoamenorrhea are (1) hypothalamic dysfunction; (2) hyperprolactinemia; and (3) excess androgen production.

In this section, hypothalamic dysfunction will be briefly reviewed, since it has already been mentioned as one of the etiologies for hypogonadotropic hypogonadism resulting in disordered puberty. Anorexia nervosa and/or excessive weight loss, malnutrition, stress, sustained systemic illness, and certain levels of exercise activity are all possible causes for such. This diagnosis is reached through exclusion, since pituitary, ovarian, and adrenal dysfunction must first be eliminated. Most patients with hypothalamic amenorrhea have normal puberty. With the onset of amenorrhea, gonadotropins and estrogen levels decrease. Depending on the length of their disorders and whether or not they have secondary amenorrhea, they may be nor-

moestrogenic or hypoestrogenic. Physical examination also serves as a bioassay of estrogen status, since well-cornified, rugated vaginal epithelium denotes normal estrogen status. Poorly cornified vaginal epithelium with scant cervical mucus denotes a low-estrogen state. The progesterone challenge test (100 ng of progesterone in oil) produces withdrawal bleeding if there is a normal estrogen state.

The three important factors to exclude are pregnancy, a pituitary tumor, or premature menopause. This is done by β-subunit HCG precluding pregnancy; LH, FSH, and prolactin level assays and a CAT scan of the pituitary, if necessary, exclude hyperprolactinemia or hypergonadotropism. Other pathologic processes are therefore ruled out and hypothalamic amenorrhea is indicated. Patients should be encouraged to gain weight or decrease exercise activity if these are thought to be causative factors. Hormonal supplementation should be suggested to prevent osteoporosis. If such patients desire pregnancy, then ovulation induction with Clomid, Pergonal, and, more recently, pulsatile LH-RH therapy is suggested.

Hyperprolactinemia is associated with variable findings of amenorrhea, oligomenorrhea, or galactorrhea. About 30% to 45% of persons with secondary amenorrhea will have galactorrhea, and when both of these symptoms are present, 75% to 90% will have hyperprolactinemia. Anywhere between 15% and 40% of patients with amenorrhea will have hyperprolactinemia. Finally, the triad of amenorrhea, galactorrhea, and hyperprolactinemia is associated with pituitary adenomas in more than 50% of cases. If a patient has chronic anovulation syndrome alone, then the incidence of hyperprolactinemia is lower (Coulam et al., 1982).

Prolactin is a protein hormone composed of 198 amino acids. It is produced by the acidophilic cells in the lateral wing of the pituitary gland. Recently, it has also been discovered in decidual cells of the human uterus during the late secretory phase of the menstrual cycle (Riddick and Kusmick, 1977).

Prolactin levels rise when the pituitary

stalk is sectioned, and therefore it is felt to be under chronic inhibition by a pituitary inhibitory factor. Dopamine, a biogenic amine, is produced in tuberoinfundibular neurons that terminate on portal vessels, and dopamine receptors have been found in the anterior pituitary gland (Quigley et al., 1980). Prolactin secretion is also mediated by norepinephrine, serotonin, acetylcholine, opiate, and histamine-containing neurons. Prolactin concentrations are normally lower in men and prepubertal and menopausal females, probably due to effects of estrogen on prolactin secretion. Hyperprolactinemia is normal during pregnancy and immediately post partum. Pharmacologic causes of hyperprolactinemia are thyroid-releasing hormone (TRF) administration, estrogen therapy, use of dopamine-receptor blocking agents (phenothiazines, metochloropropramide, sulpride, pimozide), catechol-depleting agents (reserpine, α-methyldopa), imipramine, and amphetamines (Frantz, 1978; Barbieri and Ryan, 1983).

Pathologic causes of hyperprolactinemia are prolactin-secreting pituitary tumors, pituitary stalk compression or section, hypothyroidism, acromegaly, renal failure, and ectopic production (bronchogenic cancer and hypernephroma). The detrimental effect of high prolactin levels is possibly an inhibitory effect on follicular steroidogenesis and/or an inhibition of gonadotropin secretion by blockage of LH-RH pulses. Both LH and FSH pulses are suppressed, LH more so than FSH, so that the FSH-LH ratio is somewhat equal or higher.

Therefore, all patients with amenorrhea and/or galactorrhea should be evaluated for hyperprolactinemia. If this is detected, then a CAT scan, with contrast, of the sella determines the presence of and extent of a pituitary adenoma. Tumors that are greater than 1 cm in diameter are termed *macroadenomas*, whereas those less than 1 cm are termed *microadenomas*. The debate continues whether transphenoidal microsurgery for microadenoma removal or pharmacologic intervention with bromocriptine (a dopamine agonist) is better (Barbieri and Ryan, 1983).

The most dangerous sequela of macroadenoma is extension of the suprasellar region, and subsequent compression of the optic chiasm, which can cause visual defects. The deleterious effects of these tumors are a result of local expansion and compression: removal of a macroadenoma surgically does not offer a good chance for resolving the hyperprolactinemia, but is done of necessity to prevent local expansion. Proton-beam radiation therapy, either as primary therapy or as an adjunct when the tumor has not been completely removed, is another possible therapy. However, a major side effect is the insidious development of panhypopituitarism. Management of a hyperprolactinemia depends on whether a tumor is or is not detected by CAT scan. If no tumor is detected, then treatment with bromocriptine is in order. Treatment of hyperprolactinemia is necessary in women who are not desirous of pregnancy, since bone loss occurs in hyperprolactinemia (Kliblanski et al., 1980). If a tumor is present (either microadenoma or macroadenoma), then patients may be offered either surgery or chemotherapy. Resolution of the hyperprolactinemia may not occur after treatment of macroadenomas, in which case postsurgical treatment with bromocriptine (Parlodel) may still be required. Patients with such a disorder, no matter the therapeutic course, should have periodic prolactin level checks every six months. Computed axial tomographic scans should be repeated at appropriate yearly intervals. Patients who achieve pregnancy with this disorder generally do well in pregnancy.

Patients must be monitored for signs of extrasellar expansion (headache, visual field loss) (Magyar and Marshall, 1978). Furthermore, there is no definite indication that birth control pills cause prolactinomas, although women with irregular menses before taking oral contraceptives still appear to have a higher incidence (Shy et al., 1983).

Excess androgen production involves a variety of syndromes and is accompanied by varying levels of hirsutism and/or virilization and secondary amenorrhea or oligomenorrhea. It incorporates a spectrum of disorders identified loosely as polycystic ovarian disease syndrome. Parts of the spectrum, although of extremely low incidence, have been identified. These are the adult-onset adrenal hyperplasia and the complex associated with hyperandrogenism, insulin resistance, and acanthosis nigricans (HAIR-AN syndrome) (Barbieri and Ryan, 1983).

The ovaries of these individuals are typically enlarged or normal sized, with a smooth hard capsule. On cross-section, there are many tiny subcapsular cysts and an increase in stroma density.

The pathophysiology of the polycystic ovary is heterogeneous, with biochemical and clinical variability. Therefore, the finding of polycystic ovaries is felt to be a sign and not a diagnosis. In this syndrome, there is no basic lack of secretion from either the pituitary or the ovary. However, the normal cyclicity of secretion of these hormones is aberrant, with chronic, elevated levels of LH and a subsequent LH:FSH ratio that is elevated. The pituitary is also extremely sensitive to exogenous LH-RH and immunoreactive (IR)–LH-RH levels are elevated (Goldzieher, 1981; Ravnikar et al., 1983). Evidence indicates increased inhibin concentrations in the follicles of these patients, which could explain the selective decrease in FSH levels. Serum androstenedione and testosterone are also elevated or are at upper levels of normal in patients with polycystic ovary–type syndrome. Plasma estrone levels are also elevated or at upper limits of normal and sex hormone–binding globulin is lower (Goldzieher, 1981).

Detailed study of the excess of androgenic hormones produced by these individuals has resulted in some important findings. It has been found that even though the absolute concentrations of these hormones may be within the normal range, testosterone's metabolic clearance rate (liters per 24 hours), (which is the ratio at which a hormone is irreversibly removed from the circulation over its total concentration in the plasma), and its production rate (micrograms per 24 hours) are significantly higher than normal. This in turn decreases sex hormone–binding globulin lev-

els and releases more testosterone into the periphery. Although testosterone is the most potent androgen, androstenedione is the principal ovarian androgen, and a significant amount is peripherally converted into testosterone. It is the free, unbound testosterone levels that are most important when the source of hyperandrogenism is the ovary (Goldzieher, 1981; Coney, 1984). The production rate of androstenedione is also elevated. Both testosterone and androstenedione are suppressed in these individuals by administration of exogenous estrogens and, therefore, most of the testosterone and androstenedione is thought to come from the ovary. Dehydroepiandrosterone (DHEA) is the principal adrenal androgen and dehydroepiandrosterone sulfate (DHEA-S) is the principal conjugated form. This androgen is suppressed by exogenous steroids (dexamethasone); therefore, this androgen is felt to come primarily from the adrenal. Using this concept, suppression tests are performed.

First, an individual is administered 1 mg of dexamethasone at 11 P.M. and a specimen for serum cortisol determination is drawn at 8 A.M. If it is above the normal laboratory value (more than 20 μg/dl), then the further workup is carried out for hypercortisolism due to Cushing's disease. Following these, the patient is subjected to a full five-day course of dexamethasone, 2 mg/day. Plasma levels of testosterone, DHEA, DHEA-S, and androstenedione are measured. This suppression test will generally decrease DHEA-S levels, since these primarily emanate from the adrenal. After this, oral contraceptives (such as Demulen) are administered for one month and an androgen profile is again checked. This again will suppress testosterone and androstenedione, since these are mainly ovarian products. In practice, however, these tests have actually been hampered by their nonselective nature in suppressing just one target organ and, therefore, in determining the exact source for the hyperandrogenism. This is complicated by the fact that testosterone production also occurs in the adrenal, and there is a minimal DHEA-S production from the ovary. It is still worthwhile to perform these, however, to rule out nonsuppression of these androgens, which would indicate a tumor.

In our laboratory the normal levels for reproductive-age women for these androgenic hormones are: testosterone, 0.3 to 0.75 ng/ml; free testosterone, 1.1% to 2.4% of total testosterone; and dehydroepiandrosterone sulfate, 0.8 to 3.4 μg/ml. Levels of testosterone greater than 2.5 to 2.0 ng/ml or DHEA-S levels greater than 0.7 μg/ml prompt an evaluation for an androgen-secreting tumor with CT scan and possible laparotomy.

When women with hyperandrogenism are evaluated, plasma free testosterone levels (determined from obtaining a ratio between total testosterone and sex-hormone–binding globulin (SHBG) or by equilibrium dialysis) are elevated in 80% of patients and is the most frequently elevated parameter (Coney, 1984). Total plasma testosterone is elevated in only 40% of patients; DHEA-S levels are elevated in 60%. Levels of DHEA-S vary inversely with a patient's weight, whereas plasma free testosterone levels are higher in obese women due to SHBG suppression (Wild et al., 1983).

Long-acting LH-RH analogue therapy has been used recently to attempt to decipher the source of the hyperandrogenism (Chang et al., 1983). When patients with polycystic ovarian syndrome are compared with normal subjects after administration of LH-RH analogue, the patients with polycystic ovarian syndrome had the following findings: LH levels rose but pulse amplitude decreased, FSH levels remained the same, plasma estradiol levels dropped to menopausal levels, and testosterone and androstenedione levels decreased. It had no demonstrable effect on the adrenal hormones cortisol, DHEA, or DHEA-S. This probe again determined that the exclusive source of testosterone and androstenedione in most patients with polycystic ovarian syndrome is ovarian and not adrenal in origin.

A precise etiology of polycystic ovarian disease is available only in a minority of patients. Hyperthecosis, dermoid tumors, and androgen-producing tumors are responsible for only a minority of cases. Therefore, a basic hypothetical etiology appears to be responsible for the majority of cases. The postulated defects in this syndrome are a central dopamine deficiency creating an increase in LH-RH output and/or increased inhibin levels due to ineffective follicular maturation. The hyperandrogenism may either be the precursor or the result of the disorder (either due to abnormal hypopituitary signals or abnormal follicular maturation). Some suggest that the genesis of polycystic ovarian syndrome is due to an exaggerated adrenarche resulting from an excess of a yet unidentified adrenal factor at puberty. Recently, pubertal patients with polycystic ovarian syndrome have been found not to have normal sleep-associated LH pulsations (Zumoff et al., 1983). Some patients with hyperandrogenism may have abnormal increases in certain precursor adrenal hormone levels prior to cortisol production after exogenous ACTH administration (Gibson et al., 1980). This has spurred interest about whether some patients with polycystic ovarian syndrome may have incomplete forms of congenital adrenal hyperplasia.

Classically, the most common form of congenital adrenal hyperplasia is a 21-hydroxylase deficiency. The usual clinical presentation is of a girl with abnormal genitalia (either clitoromegaly or hypospadias) and advanced adrenarche. The laboratory parameters indicate elevation of 17-hydroxyprogesterone levels and urinary pregnanetriol levels. An 11β-hydroxylase deficiency presents with the same clinical features, except that these patients also exhibit hypertension. They have increased serum compound S levels and high urinary secretion of tetrahydrocortisone. A 3β-hydroxysteroid dehydrogenase deficiency is associated with the inability to convert pregnenolone to progesterone; DHEA levels may be elevated and these patients, again, may present in adrenal insufficiency. A 17-hydroxylase deficiency includes a concomitant complete block in steroid synthesis. Males have ambiguous genitalia, present as phenotypic females, and may be seeking medical attention for primary amenorrhea. The laboratory parameters show a low secretion of 17-ketosteroids and 17-hydroxyprogesterone in the urine and a high level of progesterone, deoxycorticosterone acetate, and corticosterone, thereby causing hypertension. And finally, an 18-hydroxysteroid dehydrogenase deficiency presents as an inability to synthesize aldosterone, but there is no cortisol deficiency. A description of the therapy for all forms of congenital adrenal hyperplasia is too complex to delineate here. However, it is important to monitor for adrenal insufficiency in these patients and to control excess androgen production adequately by administration of long-acting exogenous adrenal steroids.

We now recognize that phenotypically normal adult women may present with hirsutism and menstrual irregularities. Their hyperandrogenism appears to be best suppressed with exogenous glucocorticoids. This is known as the adult-onset form of congenital adrenal hyperplasia, mainly due to an incomplete 21-hydroxylase deficiency. A number of patients with this condition have polycystic ovaries.

Congenital adrenal hyperplasia is inherited as an autosomal recessive trait and the gene responsible for the 21-hydroxylase deficiency is closely linked to the HLA-B locus on chromosome 6. Obligate heterozygotes (parents of such individuals) have greater 17-hydroxyprogesterone levels and a greater absolute rate of rise of 17-hydroxyprogesterone—after an ACTH challenge in comparison to controls. Patients with adult-onset congenital adrenal hyperplasia, however, have an increase in 17-hydroxyprogesterone levels after ACTH that is very dramatic and much greater than that in obligate heterozygotes. This led to the hypothesis that there are several alleles of the genotype at the 21 hydroxylase locus. Finally, another group of patients whose disorder has been labeled as cryptic congenital adrenal hyperplasia have been identified also. They are phenotypically normal (no amenorrhea and no

hirsutism) but chemically abnormal. Their baseline 17-hydroxyprogesterone levels are elevated and their levels of 17-hydroxyprogesterone after ACTH stimulation are elevated above levels of those with obligate heterozygosity for congenital adrenal hyperplasia, but are lower than those of patients with congenital adrenal hyperplasia (Rosenwaks et al., 1979; Chrousos et al., 1982; Levine et al., 1981; Kohn et al., 1982; New et al., 1983). There may also be the possibility of reduced 3β-hydroxysteroid dehydrogenase activity in some women with polycystic ovaries (Lobo and Goebelsmann, 1981).

Finally, recent investigative work is uncovering the effects of hyperinsulinism on ovarian steroidogenesis (Barbieri and Ryan, 1983). In normal-weight patients with polycystic ovarian syndrome who are hyperandrogenic, there is a significantly higher basal level of IR-insulin and an elevated response of insulin to a glucose challenge (Barbieri et al., 1984; Burghen et al., 1980; Chang et al., 1983; Shoupe et al., 1983). Therefore, individuals with polycystic ovarian syndrome have a significant amount of insulin resistance. The true significance of its effect both on ovarian steroidogenesis and on health, has yet to be determined.

Patients with hypothalamic amenorrhea should be counseled as to the possible causes of their dysfunction. Patients suffering from effects of excessive dietary restriction, specifically anorectics, and bulemics, should receive appropriate psychiatric referral. The care of such individuals is founded on a multidisciplinary approach. There is no long-term effect on the uterus and ovaries in such individuals. This is important, since many worry that they will not be able to carry a child if they have had prolonged amenorrhea due to exercise or anorexia. However, they should be made aware of the long-term skeletal effects producing osteoporosis and resulting from prolonged amenorrhea. Adequate diet, reasonable exercise, and exogenous calcium supplementation help decrease premature onset of osteoporosis.

If amenorrhea or oligomenorrhea are due to hyperprolactinemia, then a careful evaluation of pituitary sellar contents is mandatory. If a large pituitary adenoma exists, then it is best removed transphenoidally by an experienced neurosurgeon. The incidence of recurrent hyperprolactinemia is great, and patients should be made aware of this. If there is a microadenoma or if no tumor is visible on sellar CAT scan, then medical therapy with bromocriptine (Parlodel) is indicated. Therapy should be initiated at the lowest level possible and titrated against serum prolactin levels until the latter are brought into the normal range. Rarely is a dose of Parlodel of 7.5 mg/day or greater necessary to bring the serum prolactin level down to the normal range. Yearly CAT scans should be performed to rule out suprasellar enlargement of the pituitary. I treat all hyperprolactinemic patients, even if they are not interested in fertility, since there is an association between osteoporosis and hypoestrogenemia due to elevated prolactin levels.

Patients with diagnoses of polycystic ovarian syndrome should have intermittent withdrawal of menses with a progestin because of the high incidence of endometrial hyperplasia in this disorder (Coulam et al., 1983).

Patients who desire fertility and who have disorders of oligoovulation or anovulation have a decent success rate with ovulation-induction therapy. Treatment with bromocriptine (Parlodel), a dopamine agonist, is very successful in inducing ovulation in patients with hyperprolactinemia. Successful pregnancy occurs in more than 80% of such patients (Hammond, 1984). Clomiphene citrate, which works as an antiestrogen at estrogen receptor sites in the hypothalamus, is most successful in patients who do not have an estrogen deficiency. Therefore, patients with hypothalamic amenorrhea with normal estrogen status, or patients with polycystic ovarian disease have the highest chance of success. Overall, such patients have an 85.2% chance of ovulating and 42.8% of conceiving (Gysler et al., 1982). The discrepancy between these two rates may be due to the antiestrogen effects of Clomid on cervical mucus, which produces inhospitable mucus and an inadequate secretory lining in the uterus. When Clomid therapy fails, treatment with Pergonal (FSH, LH) may be in order. Patients who are hypoestrogenemic and hypogonadotropic respond best to this therapy. Pergonal therapy needs careful monitoring, with plasma estradiol measurements and ultrasound scanning of the follicles to reduce the chance of hyperstimulation (Oelsner et al., 1978; Schwartz et al., 1980). The chance of success with such therapy depends on the type of patient treated, but approaches 60% to 70%.

Clomid and Pergonal therapy both have a high incidence of hyperstimulation and multiple pregnancy (9% to 20%, depending on the series). The use of LH-RH therapy for induction of ovulation has again revolutionized therapy in this area. Low-dose pulses of LH-RH are administered either subcutaneously or intravenously (Mason et al., 1984; Miller et al., 1983; Hurley et al., 1984). With such therapy, the selection of follicles for ovulation is much more orderly; therefore, the dangers of hyperstimulation are lessened, as are the chances of multiple pregnancies.

CONCLUSION

In this chapter the normal changes in the pubertal process and the causes of dysfunction involving either delayed or precocious maturation have been reviewed. The major causes of amenorrhea and oligoamenorrhea in patients beyond puberty have also been discussed. A careful analysis based on the patient's age, history, and findings on physical examination are the key elements in determining the etiology of abnormal reproductive function. Advances in pharmacologic techniques have improved our ability to treat such patients, the most prominent among these being LH-RH therapy.

BIBLIOGRAPHY

Albright F., et al.: Syndrome characterized by osteitis fibrosa disseminata, areas of pigmentation and endocrine dysfunction with precocious puberty in females. *N. Engl. J. Med.* 216:727, 1937.

Baranowska B., Rozbicka G., Jeske W., et al.: The role of endogenous opiates in the mechanism of inhibited luteinizing hormone (LH) secretion in women with anorexia nervosa: The effect of naloxone on LH, follicle-stimulating hormone prolactin, and β-endorphin secretion. *J. Clin. Endocrinol. Metab.* 59:412–416, 1984.

Barbieri R.L., Makris A., Ryan K.J.: Insulin stimulates androgen accumulation in incubations of human ovarian stroma and theca. *Obstet. Gynecol.* 64(suppl.):73, 1984.

Barbieri R.L., Ryan K.J.; Bromocriptine: Endocrine pharmacology and therapeutic applications. *Fertil. Steril.* 39:727–741, 1983.

Barbieri R.L., Ryan K.J.: Hyperandrogenism, insulin resistance, and acanthosis nigricans syndrome: A common endocrinopathy with distinct pathophysiologic features. *Am. J. Obstet. Gynecol.* 147:90, 1983.

Benedict P.H.: Endocrine features of Albright's syndrome (fibrous dysplasia of bone). *Metabolism* 11:30, 1962.

Boyar R., Finkelstein J., Roffwarg H., et al.: Synchronization of augmented luteinizing hormone secretion with sleep during puberty. *N. Engl. J. Med.* 287:582–586, 1972.

Boyar R.M., Hellman L.D., Roffwarg H., et al.: Cortisol secretion and metabolism in anorexia nervosa. *N. Engl. J. Med.* 296:190–193, 1977.

Boyar R.M., Ramsey B.S., Chipman J., et al.: Regulation of gonadotropin secretion in Turner's syndrome. *N. Engl. J. Med.* 298:1328–1331, 1981.

Boyden T.W., Pamenter R.W., Grosso D., et al.: Prolactin responses, menstrual cycles, and body composition of women runners. *J. Clin. Endocrinol. Metab.* 54:711–714, 1982.

Buchanan G.C., Tredway D.R., Pittard J.C., et al.: Gonadotropin secretion and hypothyroidism. *Obstet. Gynecol.* 50:392–396, 1977.

Burghen G.A., Givens J.R., Kitabchi A.E.: Correlation of hyperandrogenism with hyperinsulinism in polycystic ovarian disease. *J. Clin. Endocrinol. Metab.* 50:113, 1980.

Chang R.J., Laufer L.R., Meedrum D.R., et al.: Steroid secretion in polycystic suppression by long acting gonadotropin releasing agonist. *J. Clin. Endocrinol. Metab.* 56:897, 1983.

Chang R.J., Nakamura R.M., Judd H.L., et al.: Insulin resistance in nonobese patients with polycystic ovarian disease. *J. Clin. Endocrinol. Metab.* 57:356, 1983.

Chrousos G.P., Loriaux L., Mann D.L., et al.: Late-onset 21-hydroxylase deficiency mimicking idiopathic hirsutism or polycystic ovarian disease. *Ann. Intern. Med.* 96:143–148, 1982.

Coney P.-J.: Polycystic ovarian disease: Current concepts of pathophysiology and therapy. *Fertil. Steril.* 42:667, 1984.

Chutorian A.M.: Tumors of the central nervous system, in Barnett, Einhorn A. (eds.): *Pediatrics.* New York, Appleton-Century-Crofts, 1972.

Conte F.A., Grumbach M.M., Kaplan S.L., et al.: Correlation of luteinizing hormone and follicle-stimulating hormone release from infancy to 19 years with the changing pattern of gonadotropin secretion in agonadal patients: Relation to the restraint of puberty. *J. Clin. Endocrinol. Metab.* 50:163, 1980.

Coulam C.B., Annegers J.F., Kranz J.S.: Chronic anovulation syndrome and associated neoplasia. *Obstet. Gynecol.* 61:403–407, 1983.

Coulam C.B., Annegers J.F., Kranz J.S.: The association between pituitary adenomas and chronic anovulation syndrome. *Am. J. Obstet. Gynecol.* 143:319–324, 1982.

Crowley W.F. Jr., McArthur J.W.: Simulation of the normal menstrual cycle in Kallmann's syndrome by pulsatile administration of luteinizing hormone-releasing hormone (LHRH). *J. Clin. Endocrinol. Metab.* 51:173–175, 1980.

Dixon G., Eurman P., Stern B.E., et al.: Hypothalamic function in amenorrheic runners. *Fertil. Steril.* 42:377–383, 1984.

Drinkwater B.L., Nilson K., Chestnut C.H. III, et al.: Bone mineral content of amenorrheic and eumenorrheic athletes. *N. Engl. J. Med.* 311:277–281, 1984.

Einhorn A.: The reticuloendotheliosis and sarcoidosis, in Barnett, Einhorn A. (eds.): *Pediatrics.* New York: Appleton-Century-Crofts, 1972.

Frantz A.G.: Physiology in medicine: Prolactin. *N. Engl. J. Med.* 298:201–207, 1978.

Frisch R.E.: A method of prediction of age of menarche from height and weight at ages 9 through 13 years. *Pediatrics* 53:384–390, 1974.

Frisch R.E.: Critical weight at menarche, initiation of the adolescent growth spurt, and control of puberty, in Grumbach M.M., Grave G.D., Mayer F.E. (eds.): *Control of the Onset of Puberty.* New York, John Wiley & Sons, 1974, pp. 403–423.

Frisch R.E.: Pubertal adipose tissue: Is it necessary for normal sexual maturation? Evidence from the rat and human female. *Fed. Proc.* 39:2395–2400, 1980.

Frisch R.E., McArthur J.W.: Menstrual cycles: Fatness as a determinant of minimum weight for height necessary for their maintenance or onset. *Science* 185:949–951, 1974.

Gibson M., Lackritz R., Schiff I., et al.: Abnormal adrenal responses to adrenocorticotropic hormone in hyperandrogenic women. *Fertil. Steril.* 33:43, 1980.

Goldenberg R.L., Grodin J.M., Rodbard D., et al.: Gonadotropins in women with amenorrhea: The use of plasma follicle-stimulating hormone to differentiate women with and without ovarian follicles. *Am. J. Obstet. Gynecol.* 116:1003–1112, 1973.

Goldzieher J.W.: Polycystic ovarian disease. *Fertil. Steril.* 35:371, 1981.

Greulich W.W., Pyle S.I.: *Radiographic Atlas of Skeletal Development of the Hand and Wrist*, ed. 2. Stanford, Calif., Stanford University Press, 1959.

Gross H.A., Lake C.R., Ebert M.H., et al.: Catecholamine metabolism in primary anorexia nervosa. *J. Clin. Endocrinol. Metab.* 49:805–809, 1979.

Grumbach M.M.: The neuroendocrinology of puberty. *Hosp. Pract.*, March 1980, pp. 51–60.

Grumbach M.M., Roth J.C., Kaplan S.L., et al.: Hypothalamic pituitary regulation of puberty in man: Evidence and concepts derived from clinical research, in Grumbach M.M., Grave G.D., Mayer F.E. (eds.): *Control of the Onset of Puberty.* New York, John Wiley & Sons, 1974, pp. 115–166.

Gysler M., March C.M., Mishell D.R. Jr., et al.: A decade's experience with an individualized clomiphene treatment regimen including its effect on the postcoital test. *Fertil. Steril.* 37:161–173, 1982.

Hahn H.B. Jr., Hayles A.B., Albert A.: Medroxyprogesterone and constitutional precocious puberty. *Mayo Clin. Proc.* 39:182, 1964.

Hammond C.B.: Bromocriptine mesylate in hyperprolactinemic infertility: A review. *Adv. Ther.* 1:285–298, 1984.

Hashimoto T., Miyai K., Izumi K., et al.: Isolated gonadotropin deficiency with response to luteinizing hormone-releasing hormone. *N. Engl. J. Med.* 287:1059–1062, 1972.

Heaney R., Ricker R., Saville P.: Menopausal changes in CA^{++} performance. *J. Clin. Med.* 92:953–963, 1978.

Howlett T.A., Tomlin S., Ngahfoong L., et al.: Release of β-endorphin and met-enkephalin during exercise in normal women: Response to training. *Br. Med. J.* 1:1950–1952, 1984.

Hurley D.M., Brian R., Outch K., et al.: Induction of ovulation and fertility in amenorrheic women by pulsatile low-dose gonadotropin-releasing hormone. *N. Engl. J. Med.* 310:1069–1074, 1984.

Kliblanski A., Neer R.M., Beitins I.Z., et al.: Decreased bone density in hyperprolactinemic women. *N. Engl. J. Med.* 303:1511–1514, 1980.

Knobil E.: Patterns of hypophysiotropic signals and gonadotropin secretion in the Rhesus monkey. *Biol. Reprod.* 24:44–49, 1981.

Kohn B., Levine L.S., Pollack M.S., et al.: Late-onset steroid 21-hydroxylase deficiency: A variant of classical congenital adrenal hyperplasia. *J. Clin. Endocrinol. Metab.* 55:817, 1982.

Kupperman H.S., Epstein J.A.: Medroxyprogesterone acetate in the treatment of constitutional sexual precocity. *J. Clin. Endocrinol. Metab.* 22:456, 1962.

Lemarchand-Beraud T., Zufferey M.-H., Reymond M., et al.: Maturation of the hypothalamo-pituitary-ovarian axis in adolescent girls. *J. Clin. Endocrinol. Metab.* 54:241–246, 1982.

Levine L.S., Dupont B., Lorenzen F., et al.: Genetic and hormonal characterization of cryptic 21-hydroxylase deficiency. *J. Clin. Endocrinol. Metab.* 53:1192, 1981.

Lieblich J.M., Rogol A.D., White B.J., et al.: Syndrome of anosmia with hypogonadotropic hypogonadism (Kallmann syndrome): Clinical and laboratory studies in 23 cases. *Am. J. Med.* 73:506, 1982.

Liu N., Grumbach M.M., de Napoli R.A., et al.: Prevalence of electroencephalographic abnormalities in idiopathic precocious puberty and premature pubarche: Bearing on pathogenesis and neuroendocrine regulation of puberty. *J. Clin. Endocrinol. Metab.* 25:1296, 1965.

Lobo R.A., Goebelsmann U.: Evidence for reduced 3β-ol-hydroxysteroid dehydrogenase activity in some hirsute women thought to have polycystic ovary syndrome. *J. Clin. Endocrinol. Metab.* 53:394, 1981.

Loop J.W.: Precocious puberty-pneumoencephalography demonstrating a harmartoma in the absence of cerebral symptoms. *N. Engl. J. Med.* 271:409, 1964.

McArthur J.W., Johnson L., Hourihan J., et al.: Endocrine studies during the refeeding of young women with nutritional amenorrhea and infertility. *Mayo Clin. Proc.* 51:607–616, 1976.

Madden J.D., MacDonald P.C.: Origin of estrogen in isosexual precocious pseudopuberty due to a granulosa-theca cell tumor. *Obstet. Gynecol.* 51:210–220, 1978.

Magyar D.M., Marshall J.R.: Pituitary tumors and pregnancy. *Am. J. Obstet. Gynecol.* 132:739, 1978.

Mansfield M.J., Beardsworth D.E., Loughlin J.S.,

et al.: Long-term treatment of central precocious puberty with a long-acting analogue of luteinizing hormone-releasing hormone. *N. Engl. J. Med.* 309:1286–1290, 1983.

Marshall J.C., Kelch R.P.: Low dose pulsatile gonadotropin-releasing hormone in anorexia nervosa: A model of human pubertal development. *J. Clin. Endocrinol. Metab.* 49:712–718, 1979.

Mashchak C.A., Kletzky O.A., Davajan V., et al.: Clinical and laboratory evaluation of patients with primary amenorrhea. *Obstet. Gynecol.* 57:715–720, 1981.

Marshall W.A., Tanner J.M.: Variation in pattern of pubertal changes in girls. *Arch. Dis. Child.* 44:291, 1969.

Mason P., Adams J., Morris D.V., et al.: Induction of ovulation of pulsatile luteinising hormone release hormone. *Br. Med. J.* 288:181–185, 1984.

Mecklenburg R.S., Loriaux D.L., Thompson R.H., et al.: Hypothalamic dysfunction in patients with anorexia nervosa. *Medicine* 53:147–157, 1974.

Miller D.S., Reid R.R., Cetel N.S., et al.: Pulsatile administration of low-dose gonadotropin-releasing hormone. *J.A.M.A.* 250:2937–2941, 1983.

Naftolin F., Pujol-Amat P., Corker C.S., et al.: Gonadotropins and gonadal steroids in androgen insensitivity (testicular feminization) syndrome: Effects of castration and sex steroid administration. *Am. J. Obstet. Gynecol.* 147:491–496, 1983.

New M.I., Lorenzen F., Lerner A.J., et al.: Genotyping steroid 21-hydroxylase deficiency: Hormonal reference data. *J. Clin. Endocrinol. Metab.* 57:320, 1983.

Oelsner G., Serr D.M., Mashiach S., et al.: The study of induction of ovulation with menotropins: Analysis of results in 1897 treatment cycles. *Fertil. Steril.* 30:538–543, 1978.

Pedowitz P., Felmus L.B., Mackles A.: Precocious pseudopuberty due to ovarian tumors. *Obstet. Gynecol. Surv.* 10:633, 1955.

Phansey S.A., Holtz G.L., Tsai C.C., et al.: Chronic hydrocephalus and primary amenorrhea with partial deficiency of gonadotropin-releasing factor. *Fertil. Steril.* 42:137–139, 1984.

Porter J.C., Nansel D.D., Gudelsky G.A., et al.: Neuroendocrine control of gonadotropin secretion. *Fed. Proc.* 39:2896–2901, 1980.

Quigley M.E., Judd S.J., Gilliland G.B., et al.: Functional studies of dopamine control of prolactin secretion in normal women with hyperprolactinemic pituitary microadenoma. *J. Clin. Endocrinol. Metab.* 50:994–998, 1980.

Rabin D., Spitz I., Bercovici B., et al.: Isolated deficiency of follicle-stimulating hormone. *N. Engl. J. Med.* 287:1313, 1972.

Ravnikar V.A., Elkind-Hirsch K., Schiff I., et al.: Peripheral immunoreactive-LHRH concentrations in polycystic ovarian disease, abstract no. 268. Presented at the 30th annual meeting of the Society for Gynecologic Investigation, Washington, D.C., 1983.

Reindollar R.H., Byrd J.R., McDonough P.G.: Delayed sexual development: A study of 252 patients. *Am. J. Obstet. Gynecol.* 140:371–380, 1981.

Riddick D.R., Kusmick W.R.: Decidua: A possible source of amniotic fluid prolactin. *Am. J. Obstet. Gynecol.* 127:187, 1977.

Rosenfeld R.G., Reitz R.E., King A.B., et al.: Familial precocious puberty associated with isolated elevation of luteinizing hormone. *N. Engl. J. Med.* 303:859–862, 1980.

Rosenwaks Z., Lee P.A., Jones G.S., et al.: An attenuated form of congenital virilizing adrenal hyperplasia. *J. Clin. Endocrinol. Metab.* 49:335, 1979.

Ross J.R., Loriaux D.L., Cutler G.D. Jr.: Developmental changes in neuroendocrine regulation of gonadotropin secretion in gonadal dysgenesis. *J. Clin. Endocrinol. Metab.* 57:288–293, 1983.

Sanborn C.F., Martin B.J., Wagner W.W. Jr.: Is athletic amenorrhea specific to runners? *Am. J. Obstet. Gynecol.* 143:859, 1982.

Schwartz M., Jewelewicz R., Dyrenfurth I., et al.: The use of human menopausal and chorionic gonadotropins for induction of ovulation. *Am. J. Obstet. Gynecol.* 138:801–807, 1980.

Sherman B., Wallace R., Bean J., et al.: Relationship of body weight to menarcheal and menopausal age: Implications for breast cancer risk. *J. Clin. Endocrinol. Metab.* 52:488–493, 1981.

Shoupe D., Kumar D.D., Lobo R.A.: Insulin resistance in polycystic ovary syndrome. *Am. J. Obstet. Gynecol.* 147:588, 1983.

Shy K.K., McTiernan A.M., Daling J.R., et al.: Oral contraceptive use and the occurrence of pituitary prolactinoma. *J.A.M.A.* 249:2204–2207, 1983.

Simpson J.L.: Common gynecologic disorders, in Golbus M., Martin A.O., Sarto G. (eds.): *Genetics in Obstetrics and Gynecology.* New York, Grune & Stratton, Inc., 1982, pp. 144–150.

Simpson J.L.: *Disorders of Sexual Differentiation: Etiology and Clinical Delineation.* New York, Academic Press, 1976, pp. 259–302, 371–388.

Simpson J.L.: Male pseudohermaphroditism, in Simpson J.L. (ed.): *Disorders of Sexual Differentiation: Etiology and Clinical Delineation.* New York, Academic Press, 1976, pp. 183–224.

Sklar C.A., Kaplan S.L., Grumbach M.M.: Evidence for dissociation between adrenarche and gonadarche: Studies in patients with idiopathic precocious puberty, gonadal dysgenesis, isolated gonadotropin deficiency, and constitutionally delayed growth and adolescence. *J. Clin. Endocrinol. Metab.* 51:548–556, 1980.

Sulman F.G.: The mechanism of the push and pull principle: II. Endocrine effects of hypothalamus depressants of the phenothiazine group. *Arch. Int. Pharmacodyn. Ther.* 118:298, 1959.

Valk T.W., Corley K.P., Kelch R.P., et al.: Hypogonadotropic hypogonadism: Hormonal responses to low dose pulsatile administration of gonadotropin-releasing hormone. *J. Clin. Endocrinol. Metab.* 51:730–738, 1980.

Vande Wiele R.I.: Anorexia nervosa and the hypothalamus. *Hosp. Pract.*, December 1977, pp. 45–51.

Van Wyk J.J., Grumbach M.M.: Syndrome of precocious menstruation and galactorrhea in juvenile hypothyroidism: An example of hormonal overlap in pituitary feedback. *J. Pediatr.* 57:416, 1960.

Walsh B.T., Katz J.L., Levin J., et al.: The production rate of cortisol declines during recovery from anorexia nervosa. *J. Clin. Endocrinol. Metab.* 53:203, 1981.

Warren M.P.: The effects of exercise on pubertal progression and reproductive function in girls. *J. Clin. Endocrinol. Metab.* 51:1150–1156, 1980.

White B.J., Rogol A.D., Brown K.S., et al.: The syndrome of anosmia with hypogonadotropic hypogonadism: A genetic study of 18 new families and a review. *Am. J. Med. Genet.* 15:417–435, 1983.

Wild R.A., Umstot E.W., Andersen R.N., et al.: Androgen parameters and their correlation with body weight in 138 women thought to have hyperandrogenism. *Am. J. Obstet. Gynecol.* 146:602, 1983.

Wildt L., Marshall G., Knobil E.: Experimental induction of puberty in the infantile female Rhesus monkey. *Science* 207:1373–1375, 1980.

Yen S.S.C.: Regulation of the hypothalamic-pituitary-ovarian axis in women. *J. Reprod. Fertil.* 51:181–191, 1977.

Yen S.S.C., Tsai C.C., Vandenberg G., et al.: Gonadotropin dynamics in patients with gonadal dysgenesis: A model for the study of gonadotropin regulation. *J. Clin. Endocrinol. Metab.* 35:897–904, 1972.

Zumoff B., Freeman R., Coupey S., et al.: A chronobiologic abnormality in luteinizing hormone secretion in teenage girls with the polycystic-ovary syndrome. *N. Engl. J. Med.* 309:1206–1209, 1983.

CHAPTER FOURTEEN

Steroid Therapy

ROBERT BARBIERI, M.D.

DURING THE PAST TWO DECADES scientific advances in the understanding of steroid structure and function have resulted in a dramatic increase in the number of therapeutic steroid agents available to the gynecologist. Optimal clinical applications of these agents requires a thorough understanding of both steroid structure and the biology of steroid synthesis and action. These concepts are reviewed in this chapter.

BIOLOGIC CONSIDERATIONS

Steroid Structure

The cyclopentanophenanthrene ring system is the basic carbon skeleton for all steroid compounds. This ring system consists of one ring of five carbon atoms (cyclopentane) and three rings, each composed of six carbon atoms (phenanthrene) (Fig 14–1). The rings are designated A, B, C, and D. The numbering of the carbon atoms in the ring system is important and should be memorized. Since the ring system is relatively planar, stereoisomers do occur and need to be distinguished. Atoms or molecules above the plane of the carbon ring system are designated "β" and those below the plane are designated "α."

There are three physiologically important steroid nuclei: estrane (18 carbon atoms), androstane (19 carbon atoms), and pregnane (21 carbon atoms) (Fig 14–1). All the important gonadal steroids are derivatives of these three steroid nuclei. Specific suffixes and symbols are used to indicate changes in these basic structures. For example, when the C-4, C-5 carbon bond is unsaturated, and a double bond is present, the suffix "ene" replaces the "ane" ending. If a keto ($=O$) group is substituted for two hydrogens, the suffix "one" is used together with the number of the carbon to which it is attached. The 4-ene-3-one grouping is present in many biologically active steroids (testosterone, progesterone, cortisol). If a hydroxy (OH) group is substituted for a hydrogen the suffix "ol" is used.

In Figure 14–2 the structural formula for progesterone is shown. Progesterone is a derivative of the C-21 compound, pregnane. Since there is a double bond in ring A, the term pregnane is changed to pregnene. The position of the double bond (between carbon atoms 4 and 5) is designated as "Δ^4." Two ketone groups are present, one on the carbon 3 and another on the carbon 20 atom; thus 3,20-dione (meaning two ketone groups). Therefore, the systematic name for progesterone is Δ^4-pregnene-3,20-dione. Figure 14–2 also shows the structure and systematic name for 17-hydroxyprogesterone. Note that the –OH group at the C-17 position is below the plane of the carbon ring and is therefore designated 17-α-ol.

Biochemistry of Steroid Biosynthesis

The quantitatively important sources of steroid production are the ovaries, the testes, and the adrenals. Each of these glands makes hormones that are unique to that gland. For example, the ovary secretes large amounts of

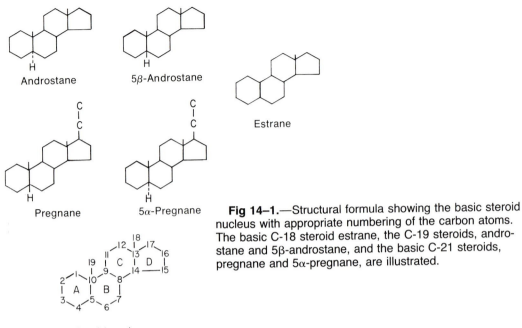

Androstane 5β-Androstane

Estrane

Pregnane 5α-Pregnane

Fig 14–1.—Structural formula showing the basic steroid nucleus with appropriate numbering of the carbon atoms. The basic C-18 steroid estrane, the C-19 steroids, androstane and 5β-androstane, and the basic C-21 steroids, pregnane and 5α-pregnane, are illustrated.

Sterid nucleus
(Cyclopentanophenanthrene)

estradiol. The testis secretes large amounts of testosterone. The adrenal gland is responsible for the production of cortisol and aldosterone. In addition to these unique steroid products, each gland can produce some common "core" steroids: progesterone, 17-hydroxyprogesterone, and androstenedione (Fig 14–3). These "core" steroids are the important precursors for the production of all gonadal steroids, glucocorticoids and mineralocorticoids. Discussion of the biosynthesis of these core steroids follows.

Cholesterol is the parent steroid from which all the gonadal steroids, glucocorticoids, and mineralocorticoids are derived. Classical concepts of steroidogenesis state that the steroid producing glands, such as the ovary, synthesize cholesterol from acetate and then utilize the cholesterol to produce progestins, estrogens, and androgens. However, recent evidence suggests that plasma cholesterol is the precursor for adrenal and ovarian steroid hormones. In the circulation, cholesterol is carried in lipoprotein packages, which consist of a core of apolar cholesterol and cholesterol esters surrounded by a shell of amphiteric phospholipids and apoproteins. The low-density lipoproteins (LDL) and the high-density lipoproteins (HDL) contain most of the cholesterol present in the circulation. The adrenal and ovarian cells responsible for steroidogenesis have membrane receptors for

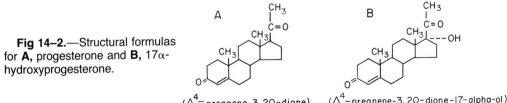

Fig 14–2.—Structural formulas for **A**, progesterone and **B**, 17α-hydroxyprogesterone.

(Δ^4– pregnene-3, 20-dione)   (Δ^4–pregnene-3, 20-dione-17-alpha-ol)

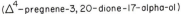

The Core Reactions

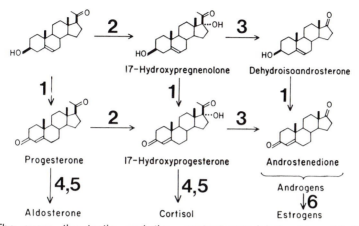

Fig 14–3.—The ovary, the testis, and the adrenal produce six common "core" steroids. The core δ^5 steroids are pregnenolone, 17α-hydroxy-pregnenolone, and dehydroepiandrosterone. The core δ^4 steroids are progesterone, 17α-hydroxy-progesterone, and androstenedione. The core steroids are the important precursors for the production of all gonadal steroids, glucocorticoids, and mineralocorticoids. Progesterone is an important gonadal steroid, and is the precursor for all mineralocorticoids. 17α-Hydroxyprogesterone is the precursor for all glucocorticoids. Androstenedione is the precursor for the androgens and estrogens. Enzyme no. 1 is 3β-hydroxyster-oid-dehydrogenase-isomerase; enzyme no. 2, 17α-hydroxylase; enzyme no. 3; 17,20-lyase; enzyme no. 4, 21-hydroxylase; enzyme no. 5, 11β-hydroxylase; and enzyme no. 6; aromatase.

the LDL lipoprotein package. The circulating LDL binds to these receptors and becomes incorporated into the cell by a process of endocytosis. The cholesterol from the LDL is released for utilization by the cell by the action of lysosomal enzymes.

Once cholesterol is released from the lipoprotein package it must be transported to the mitochondria where it binds to the cholesterol cleavage enzyme and is metabolized to pregnenolone (Fig 14–4). Pregnenolone is then metabolized to the other "core steroids" (progesterone, 17-hydroxyprogesterone, and androstenedione) by three enzyme systems (Fig 14–3). In turn, progesterone can be secreted, or metabolized, to the important mineralocorticoid, aldosterone. 17-Hydroxyprogesterone can be secreted, or metabolized, to the important glucocorticoid, cortisol. Androstenedione can be secreted, or metabolized, to the gonadal steroids, testosterone and estradiol (Fig 14–5).

There are only three types of reactions that all steroids can undergo: (1) removal or addition of hydrogen such as in the conversion of pregnenolone to progesterone (3β-hydroxysteroid dehydrogenase, (2) hydroxylations (addition of –OH) such as occurs in the conversion of progesterone to 17-hydroxyprogesterone (17-hydroxylase), and (3) conjugation reactions such as sulfo- and glucuro-conjugates.

The sequential conversion of cholesterol (C-26) to progesterone (C-21), to androstenedione (C-19), and, finally, to estradiol (C-18) requires the sequential removal of different carbon side chains. These cleavage reactions are accomplished by multiple hydroxylations of neighboring carbon bonds. This produces a highly unstable intermediate compound, which reaches a lower-energy state by separation of the carbon side chain from the parent steroid nucleus. For example, in the conversion of cholesterol to pregnenolone, multiple hydroxylations occur at the C-20, C-22 carbon bond leading to a breakdown of

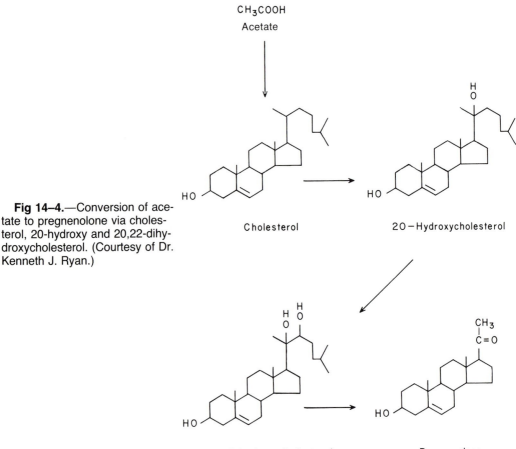

CH₃COOH
Acetate

Cholesterol

20−Hydroxycholesterol

20, 22-Dihydroxycholesterol

Pregnenolone

Fig 14–4.—Conversion of acetate to pregnenolone via cholesterol, 20-hydroxy and 20,22-dihydroxycholesterol. (Courtesy of Dr. Kenneth J. Ryan.)

the parent compound to pregnenolone and the isocaproic aldehyde side chain (Fig 14–4). The following enzymes involve cleavage of carbon side chains from the parent molecule: cholesterol cleavage enzyme, 17,20-lyase, and aromatase (Figs 14–3 to 14–5).

Steroid hormones are produced in the gonads and adrenals and secreted in the circulation. In the circulation, steroids are transported to peripheral tissues where further chemical transformations can occur. In the liver, multiple hydroxylation, hydration, and conjugation reactions occur leading to loss of steroid activity. However, in some peripheral tissues, potent steroid agonists can be locally produced from weak precursors. For example, the weak androgen, androstenedione,

can be converted in fat tissue to the important estrogen, estrone, by the enzyme aromatase. This *peripheral conversion* is of utmost importance in such disease states as polycystic ovarian disease and endometrial hyperplasia.

Another important peripheral conversion is that of androstenedione into the potent androgen testosterone. In women, 50% to 70% of circulating testosterone arises from the peripheral conversions of androstenedione derived from the ovary and adrenal.

Functional Anatomy of Ovarian Steroidogenesis

The ovary is composed of a large number of follicles surrounded by the ovarian stroma. The stroma is composed of spindle-shaped, fi-

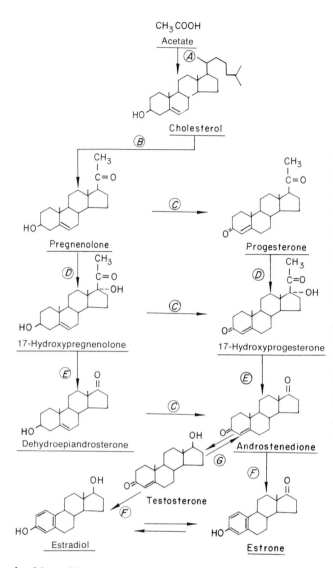

Fig 14–5.—Possible metabolic pathways for the ovarian biogenesis of estrogens. Letters above arrows denote the following metabolic pathways and the enzyme systems involved: **A,** formation of the sterol nucleus; **B,** cleavage of cholesterol side chain with formation of C-21 steroid; **C,** isomerase reaction with changing of double bond from C-5 to C-4, and dehydrogenation at C-3: 3β-ol dehydrogenases; **D,** 17 α-hydroxylation, i.e., introduction of hydroxy radical in α position on C-17; **E,** cleavage of side chain, converting C-21 to C-19 steroids; **F,** aromatization, i.e., introduction of double bonds into *ring A* with conversion of C-19 to C-18 steroids; **G,** 17β-ol dehydrogenase reactions (reversible), i.e., conversion of hydroxy radical in β position on C-17 to ketone group, or vice versa. (From Smith O.W., Ryan K.J.: *Am. J. Obstet. Gynecol.* 84:141, 1962.)

broblasticlike elements with the capacity to differentiate into steroidogenically active theca cells. *The follicle is the functional unit of the ovary.* The follicle is a sphere consisting of four parts: an outer wall of concentrically arranged cells (the theca), an inner wall of cuboidally shaped cells (the granulosa), an oocyte, and a central cavity containing follicular fluid.

Follicular development can be conceptually divided into four stages: (1) primordial, (2) preantral, (3) antral, and (4) preovulatory (Fig 14–6). The primordial follicle consists of an oocyte arrested in the diplotene stage of meiotic prophase surrounded by a single layer of granulosa cells. The primordial follicle progresses to the preantral stage with the multilayer proliferation of the granulosa cells, an enlargement of the oocyte, and the transformation of the neighboring stroma into theca cells. In the antral follicle, fluid that has accumulated in the intercellular spaces of the granulosa cells coalesces to form a cavity. During the transformation from the preantral to the antral follicle, the theca cells and the granulosa cells continue to increase in num-

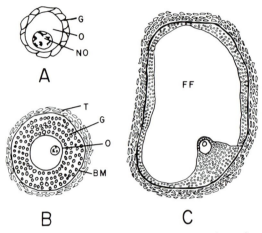

Fig 14–6.—A, schematic representation of a primordial follicle. **B,** schematic representation of a preantral follicle. **C,** schematic representation of an antral follicle. G indicates granulosa cells; O, oocyte; NO, nucleus of oocyte; BM, basement membrane; and FF, follicular fluid.

ber. In the preovulatory follicle the oocyte resumes meiosis and approaches the completion of its reduction division. The luteinizing hormone (LH) surge causes luteinization of the theca and granulosa cell layers, thereby preparing these cells for progesterone production.

The follicle consists of *two steroidogenically active cellular compartments*, each with a specific role. The theca cells (outer shell of follicle) contain LH receptors but not follicle-stimulating hormone (FSH) receptors. The human theca makes large amounts of androstenedione and smaller amounts of testosterone and estradiol. Since the theca is vascularized, it secretes these three steroids into the circulation. The theca is separated from the avascular granulosa cells by a basement membrane. The androstenedione from the theca diffuses across the basement membrane of the granulosa cells where it is aromatized to estradiol. The granulosa cell aromatase (androgen → estrogen) enzyme system is stimulated by FSH. Isolated theca cells and isolated granulosa cells make very little estradiol. When these two cellular components are recombined, large amounts of estrogen are made.

TABLE 14–1.—STEROID PRODUCTS OF THE THECA, GRANULOSA, AND STROMAL CELLS

CELL TYPE	STIMULATING HORMONE	STEROID PRODUCT
Theca cells	LH	Androstenedione
Granulosa cells	FSH	Estradiol
Stromal cells	LH	Androstenedione
Corpus luteum	LH (FSH)	Progesterone

This synergism of thecal androgen production stimulated by LH, and granulosa cell aromatase stimulated by FSH is termed the *two-cell theory of ovarian estrogen production* (Table 14–1).

A healthy follicle grows extremely rapidly. A primordial follicle (10^2 granulosa cells) can be transformed into a preovulatory follicle (10^8 granulosa cells) within 14 days. However 99% of all follicles fail to successfully make the transition from primordial follicles to preovulatory follicles. Recent evidence suggests that follicular atresia is produced by a high intrafollicular ratio of androgens to estrogens. Follicular health, as measured by the ability of the follicle to grow, and the presence of a healthy oocyte is correlated with high intrafollicular concentrations of estradiol and FSH. These observations have led to the hypothesis that the *intrafollicular microenvironment determines the health and growth potential of each follicle*. Since the granulosa cells, oocyte, and follicular fluid are surrounded by a basement membrane and are in an avascular environment, each follicle can develop a unique microenvironment. Therefore, in large measure, *it is the events within the follicle that determine if it will grow or become atretic*.

Steroid Receptors

A basic tenet of endocrinology is that *all hormones exert their effects* at the target tissue *by first interacting with receptors* specific for that hormone. The hormone-receptor complex is then able to produce specific changes in cell function. In general, all steroid hormone-receptor complexes exert their effects on target cells by altering *gene tran-*

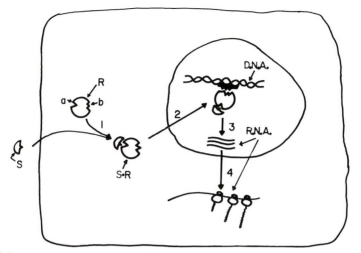

Fig 14–7.—Schematic representation of the important steps required for steroid action. *Step 1:* Binding of steroid to receptor. *Step 2:* Steroid-receptor complex undergoes an activation step *(transformation)* and then *translocates* to the nucleus. *Step 3: Transcription* of DNA into RNA. *Step 4: Translation* of RNA into new protein. S indicates steroid; R, receptor; a, steroid binding site; b, chromatin- or DNA-binding site; SR, steroid-receptor complex.

scription. Figure 14–7 summarizes this process. The first step in steroid action is steroid binding to the hormone receptor. This step can be quantitatively characterized by Scatchard analysis, which determines both the affinity constant for hormone-receptor interaction and the number of receptor sites present. After hormone binding, the receptor undergoes some type of enzymatic or conformational change called *transformation.* Transformation of the steroid-receptor complex is followed by the second step: *translocation* to the nucleus and binding to DNA. The third step is increased *transcription* of DNA into messenger RNA (mRNA). Each steroid hormone induces the specific transcription of a characteristic set of genes. The mRNA is processed and exits the nucleus to the cytoplasm where it is *translated* into new proteins.

An important concept is that some steroids are hormone *antagonists.* For example, the antiestrogen clomiphene can bind to the estrogen receptor; but the clomiphene-estrogen receptor complex does not stimulate a pattern of new protein formation characteristic of estrogen agonists. In fact, clomiphene treatment prevents the cell from responding to later estrogen stimulation. The therapeutic value of steroid antagonists is obvious, and a discussion of these compounds follows.

In general, naturally occurring steroid hormones bind with high affinity and high specificity to one hormone receptor type. For example, estradiol binds with high affinity and specificity to the estradiol receptor; but it does not bind well to progesterone, testosterone, or glucocorticoid receptors. Unfortunately, some synthetic steroids bind to multiple receptor types. Norethindrone, a major component of many oral contraceptives, binds to both progesterone and androgen receptors. This multiplicity of receptor binding complicates the interpretation of the effects of these synthetic steroids.

Principles of Steroid Pharmacology

Administration of a steroid to a patient results in a complex process of absorption, metabolism, transformation, and receptor interaction, which often makes it difficult to predict the ultimate results of drug therapy. The clinician should appreciate the enormous complexity of steroid absorption, metabolism, and action in order to optimally utilize these agents. Some important areas of concern are discussed in the following paragraphs.

For many steroids, *route of administration* determines the ultimate pattern of circulating parent compound and metabolites. For example, the administration of estradiol by mouth results in the appearance of large amounts of estrone in the circulation. This is due to the oxidation of estradiol at the 17 position by gut and liver enzymes. However, administration of estradiol via the vaginal mucosa or other cutaneous routes results in the appearance of large amounts of estradiol in the circulation and small amounts of estrone. This occurs because the skin contains very little of the enzyme, 17β-hydroxysteroid dehydrogenase, which converts estradiol to estrone.

Many steroids can be *metabolized to highly active products within steroid target tissues*. In some cases inactive steroids are metabolized to active steroids. In other cases steroids of one class (e.g., androgens) are metabolized to steroids of another class (e.g., estrogens). For example, estrone sulfate, which is a major component of conjugated estrogens, is an inactive estrogen. However, it can be metabolized in the endometrium to the potent estrogen, estradiol. The differential presence of key steroid-metabolizing enzymes in various target tissues may result in one tissue responding exuberantly to the administered "prehormone" while another tissue is unresponsive. An example of the metabolism of one class of active steroid (progestin or androgen) to another class of active steroid (estrogen) may occur with a major component of the combined oral contraceptive, norethindrone. Norethindrone, a potent progestin and a weak androgen, can be metabolized to ethinyl estradiol by the human aromatase enzyme system.

A major problem encountered when using synthetic steroids is that the same steroid can bind to *multiple classes of steroid receptor*. For example, norethindrone can bind to both the progesterone and the androgen receptor systems. Danazol can bind to androgen, progesterone, and glucocorticoid receptors. The binding of one steroid to multiple classes of receptor results in a complex pattern of hormone action.

Occasionally gynecologists use steroid hormone preparations that contain multiple active ingredients. These heterogeneous agents can produce a complex pattern of hormonal effects. For example, a preparation of conjugated estrogens (Premarin) contains sulfate esters of estrone, equilin, 17α-dihydroequilin, 17α-estradiol, equilenin, and 17α-dihydroequilenin. Each of these compounds has a slightly different pattern of absorption and metabolism, which can result in complex effects.

THERAPEUTIC USES

Estrogen Therapy

Virtually every body organ contains cells that have intracellular estrogen receptors and exhibit specific cellular responses to estrogen stimulation. The ubiquitous actions of estrogen on reproductive and nonreproductive tissues makes it important for the gynecologist prescribing these drugs to appreciate the full range and complexity of their actions.

HYPOTHALAMUS AND PITUITARY.—Estrogens lower LH and FSH secretion. FSH secretion is especially sensitive to the negative feedback effects of estrogen. Paradoxically, the administration of high doses of estrogen to women with normal cycles in the follicular phase can cause an increase in LH secretion (positive feedback effect of estrogen). High-dose estrogen therapy can also increase prolactin secretion. The vasomotor flush associated with hypoestrogenic states is probably an event mediated by the hypothalamus. The physiology of the vasomotor flush is discussed in Chapter 15.

VAGINA AND VULVA.—Hypoestrogenism results in the loss of the subcutaneous fat, vascularity, and elasticity of the labia minora and majora. The vagina develops increased blood flow and increased "superficial cells" in response to estrogen stimulation.

UTERUS.—Hypoestrogenism results in inadequate cervical mucus production. Endocervical glands, the endometrium, and the myometrium atrophy in a hypoestrogenic environment. Leiomyomata uteri are notoriously sensitive to estrogen stimulation and can grow to a massize size in response to high-dose estrogen therapy.

FALLOPIAN TUBE.—The epithelium of the oviduct is markedly changed as a result of estrogen stimulation. In response to estrogen, epithelial height increases with growth and prominence of the ciliated cells as well as enlargement of the secretory cells.

BREASTS.—The use of estrogenic substances in both male and female subjects has provided abundant evidence to confirm the stimulative effects of the mammary epithelium of animals. Use of exogenous estrogens induces mammary epithelial growth in human female castrates. Bilateral oophorectomy and the natural menopause will result in a decrease in breast size. In menopausal women, estrogen replacement often does not completely reverse the breast atrophy. This may be due to a decreased sensitivity of this end-organ to estrogen stimulation.

URETHRA AND BLADDER.—Hypoestrogenism produces atrophy of the squamous epithelium of the outer urethra and the transitional epithelium of the inner urethra and bladder.

BONE.—Hypoestrogenism produces a reduction of bone mass per unit volume of bone (osteoporosis).

LIVER.—Estrogen increases the production of a large number of circulating binding globulins including sex-hormone–binding globulin, thyroid-binding globulin, and corticosteroid-binding globulin. Hypoestrogenism results in a decrease in these liver proteins.

Estrogen administration can result in a broad range of adverse effects. The most serious of these adverse effects are deep venous thrombosis, pulmonary embolism, coronary artery thromboemboli, and cerebrovascular accidents (see Chapters 15 and 16). Other adverse effects include nausea, vomiting, jaun-

dice, chloasma, headache, and migraine. Most of these adverse effects are dose related.

A major area of continuing controversy is whether exogenously administered estrogens cause cancer. It is likely that the administration of high doses of exogenous estrogens to postmenopausal women does increase the risk of development of endometrial cancer. The relative risk is estimated to be in the range of 2 to 7. In general, the estrogen-induced endometrial cancers are stage I and of a low histologic grade. It is likely that the administration of a synthetic progestin for ten to 14 days per month will decrease the risk of development of endometrial cancer in patients taking replacement estrogens. Preliminary reports suggest that breast cancer may be linked to postmenopausal estrogen use. However the reported relative risk is in the range of 1.5 to 2.0. The administration of a synthetic progestin for ten to 14 days per month appears to decrease the risk of breast cancer development.

There are numerous estrogens available for therapeutic use (Table 14–2). For simplicity of discussion these can be divided into two groups: (1) naturally occurring estrogens and (2) synthetic estrogens. The naturally occurring estrogens available for oral use include estradiol, estrone, and estrone sulfate (Fig 14–8). The major synthetic estrogens available for oral use include: ethinyl estradiol and mestranol (the 3-methyl ether of ethinyl estradiol). As noted previously, when considering estrogen therapy, dose and route of administration are important considerations.

Exogenous estrogens are used for three main indications: (1) as contraceptive agents (see Chapter 16), (2) as replacement therapy for hypoestrogenic patients (see Chapter 15), and (3) for a variety of other gynecologic disorders (menorrhagia, endometriosis, Asherman's syndrome, and cervical mucus abnormalities) (Tables 14–3 and 14–4).

Hypoestrogenic patients are at risk for a variety of problems: osteoporosis, genitourinary tract atrophy, and accelerated cardiovascular disease. At greatest risk for these complications are patients who have never had ade-

TABLE 14–2.—ESTROGEN PREPARATIONS CURRENTLY AVAILABLE
FOR THERAPEUTIC USE

ESTROGEN	ROUTE OF ADMINISTRATION	TYPICAL DOSES AVAILABLE (MG)
Estradiol (Estrace)	Oral	1.0; 2.0
Estrone sulfate (Ogen)	Oral	0.625; 1.25; 2.5
Conjugated estrogens (Premarin)	Oral	0.3; 0.625; 1.25
	Intravenous	2.5
Estradiol valerate	Intramuscular	20.0
Ethinyl estradiol (Estinyl)	Oral	0.02; 0.05; 0.5

TABLE 14–3.—STANDARD REGIMEN FOR REPLACEMENT
OF ESTROGEN

	DOSE (MG)	DAYS OF MONTH
Conjugated estrogens	0.625	1 to 31
Medroxyprogesterone acetate (Provera Tablets)	10	18 to 31

TABLE 14–4.—BIOASSAYS FOR ESTROGENS, PROGESTINS,
AND ANDROGENS

STEROID	BIOASSAY
Estradiol	Cornification of vaginal epithelium in castrated rodents (Allen and Doisy)
Progesterone	Induction of secretory changes in the endometrium of castrated, immature, estrogen-primed rabbits (Clauberg assay)
Testosterone	Induction of growth in secondary sexual glands and muscles (prostate, seminal vesicles, and levator ani)

quate ovarian follicular function (Turner's syndrome) and those with early loss of follicular function (premature menopause, early castration). Patients who experience menopause at a normal age are at less risk for these complications. However, with the continuing rapid increase in life expectancy, women are living a progressively increasing proportion of their lives in a hypoestrogenic state. This trend may eventually produce a larger increase in the complications of hypoestrogenism.

A standard regimen for estrogen administration in a hypoestrogenic woman would include conjugated estrogens (0.625 mg daily) and medroxyprogesterone acetate (10 mg for days 18 to 30 each month). If necessary, higher doses of conjugated estrogens (1.25 mg) can be used. Replacement regimens containing less than ten days of progesterone therapy are associated with a high risk of development of endometrial hyperplasia and, possibly, carcinoma. Ethinyl estradiol can also be used as replacement therapy. In general, doses of approximately 0.005 to 0.010 mg of ethinyl estradiol have a biologic potency equivalent to 0.625 mg of conjugated estrogens.

The use of a combined estrogen-progester-

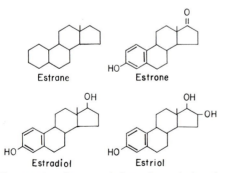

Fig 14–8.—Structural formulas of the three naturally occurring estrogens, together with the basic steroid nucleus, estrane.

one replacement regimen will result in continued menses for the majority of patients until at least age 65 years. After age 65 years the endometrium appears to become refractory to continued sequential estrogen and progesterone therapy and fewer women will continue to experience menses. Recent studies have demonstrated that estrogen can be replaced via topical application to the skin or via vaginal application. Further research will be required to demonstrate the clinical practicability of these regimens.

Estrogens can be used as the sole agent for the treatment of dysfunctional uterine bleeding. In general, however, combinations of estrogen and progestogens are used for the treatment of menometrorrhagia. Severe menorrhagia unresponsive to the oral administration of combined estrogen-progestogens can often be controlled by the administration of intravenous conjugated estrogens (25 mg intravenous bolus).

In patients with Asherman's syndrome, conjugated estrogens in doses of 1.25 to 2.5 mg/day are often used to stimulate endometrial proliferation. In infertile patients with inadequate cervical mucus, conjugated estrogens (0.625 to 1.25 mg/day) can be used in an attempt to increase mucus quantity and quality. The use of estrogens in the treatment of endometriosis is reviewed in Chapter 9.

Antiestrogen Therapy

Clomiphene and tamoxifen are the two most widely used antiestrogens (Fig 14–9). The stereochemical structures of clomiphene and tamoxifen are similar to estradiol. Clomiphene is extensively employed in the induction of ovulation (Chapter 10). Clomiphene blocks the suppressive effects of estradiol on pituitary secretion of FSH. The administration of clomiphene results in an increase in circulating FSH, thereby stimulating the growth of a cohort of follicles. Tamoxifen is

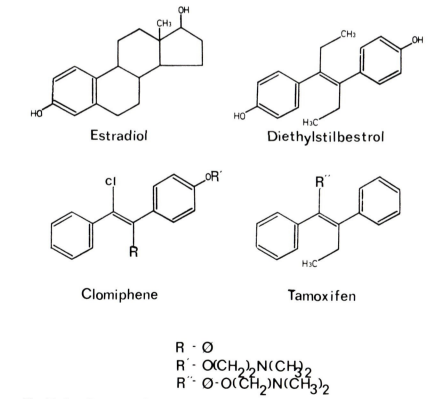

$$R \cdot \varnothing$$
$$R' \cdot O(CH_2)_2N(CH_3)_2$$
$$R'' \cdot \varnothing \text{-} O(CH_2)N(CH_3)_2$$

Fig 14–9.—Structure of estradiol, diethylstilbestrol, clomiphene, and tamoxifen. Note the similarities in the structure of these compounds.

TABLE 14–5.—USE OF C-21 PROGESTINS IN THE TREATMENT OF A VARIETY OF BENIGN GYNECOLOGIC DISEASES

DISEASE	RECOMMENDED STEROID	DOSE PER DAY (MG)	LENGTH OF THERAPY (DAYS)
Induction of withdrawal bleeding	Medroxyprogesterone acetate	10	5
Menorrhagia of dysfunctional uterine bleeding	Medroxyprogesterone acetate	20	10 to 14
Menopause	Medroxyprogesterone acetate	20	Continuous (if used as a single agent)
Inadequate luteal phase	Progesterone vaginal suppositories	75 (in divided doses)	14
Premenstrual syndrome	Progesterone vaginal suppositories	75 (in divided doses)	7 to 10

widely used in the treatment of breast carcinoma. Many breast carcinomas are dependent on estrogen for continued growth. The administration of the antiestrogen, tamoxifen, produces objective tumor regression in many of these tumors.

Progestational Therapy

Progesterone has a wide spectrum of biologic activities (Table 14–5). In general, the biologic actions of progesterone cannot be fully expressed unless the tissue is first exposed to estrogen. In all likelihood this is due to the fact that in most reproductive tissues progesterone receptors (required for progesterone action) are induced by estrogens. Another general rule is that in the müllerian-derived structures, estrogens are concerned with growth and progesterone with differentiation.

Progesterone has the physiological task of facilitating nidation of the fertilized ovum and nourishing the ensuing pregnancy. To accomplish this goal, progesterone has actions on multiple reproductive tissues. These actions include (1) secretory changes in the endometrium, (2) decidua formation at the site of nidation, and (3) reduction in myometrial contractility. Other actions of progesterone include inhibition of gonadotropins, effects on the cervical mucus, differentiation of the mammary glands, and modulatory effects on hypothalamic temperature regulation.

Three classes of progestational agents are available for therapeutic use: (1) natural progesterone, (2) C-21 synthetic progestins (medroxyprogesterone acetate), and (3) C-19 synthetic progestins (norethindrone, norethindrone acetate, and norgestrel). Progesterone has little biologic effect if given orally because it is rapidly metabolized to inactive products by intestinal and hepatic enzymes. However, when progesterone is administered by vaginal suppositories it is biologically active. The C-21 synthetic progestins (medroxyprogesterone acetate and megestrol acetate) have a spectrum of activity similar to that of progesterone. These compounds are orally active because synthetic substitutions at C-6 and C-21 prevent intestinal and hepatic metabolism. The C-19 synthetic progestins (norethindrone) bind to progesterone *and* androgen receptors and therefore have a spectrum of activity quite different than that of progesterone. The synthetic C-19 progestins are discussed in detail in Chapter 16.

Many investigators have reported that the C-21 progestins are of value in the treatment of patients with habitual abortion, premature labor, and idiopathic infertility. In general, these studies were not well controlled. To date there is no convincing evidence that progestin therapy is of value in these conditions.

An extremely controversial subject is the potential teratogenic and carcinogenic effects of certain synthetic progestins. For example, medroxyprogesterone acetate has been reported to induce breast neoplasms in beagle dogs and endometrial cancer in monkeys. The relevance of these observations to humans is unclear. Some investigators have suggested that the administration of synthetic progestins to pregnant women can induce urogenital abnormalities in their male offspring. These reports require that the gynecologist carefully evaluate the pros and cons of treating a pregnant woman with synthetic progestins.

Antiprogestational Agents

Antiprogestational agents would have obvious therapeutic value in the medical termination of an early, unwanted pregnancy, and in the treatment of endometriosis. The synthetic antiprogestational compound gestrinone (R-2323) has been demonstrated to be effective in the treatment of endometriosis. The synthetic antiprogestational agent RU-486 has been demonstrated to be effective in terminating early unwanted pregnancies. Both agents are still undergoing experimental trials and are not available for use in the United States.

Androgen Therapy

Androgens are classically described as agents that either induce growth or maintain functional competency in male secondary sexual glands (prostate, seminal vesicles, etc.). Like the estrogens and the progestins, the androgens can have effects on both reproductive and nonreproductive tissues. Androgens have important effects on the following reproductive tissues: hypothalamus-pituitary (lowers LH and FSH levels), endometrium (induces atrophy), breast (induces atrophy), and ovary (causes disordered folliculogenesis). Androgens also have major effects on nonreproductive tissues such as the skin (increases hair growth and sebum production), muscles (increases hypertrophy and hyperplasia), and bone (inhibits the bone loss of a hypoestrogenic state).

The administration of androgenic substances to women results in the common side effects of weight gain (increased muscle mass and fluid retention), amenorrhea (decreased LH and FSH, disordered folliculogenesis, endometrial atrophy), acne, oily skin, hirsutism, deepening of the voice, male-pattern baldness, and clitoromegaly. These side effects have severely limited the use of androgens in the treatment of gynecologic disorders.

The only synthetic androgen in widespread clinical use is danazol. The use of danazol in the treatment of endometriosis is discussed in detail in Chapter 9. Danazol in doses of 50 to 200 mg/day has also been shown to be of value in the treatment of fibrocystic breast disease. At these doses of danazol, many women will continue to ovulate. Since danazol is teratogenic to the developing female embryo, the physician must be sure that the patient does not become pregnant while taking danazol.

Antiandrogen Therapy

Cyproterone acetate (Fig 14–10) is the only antiandrogen in wide clinical use. This compound binds to the androgen receptor but prevents the synthesis of proteins normally induced by androgen agonists such as testosterone. Cyproterone acetate is especially effective in the treatment of hirsutism. A gradual reduction in unwanted androgen-dependent hair will occur over the first year of therapy. Cyproterone acetate is in clinical use in Europe and Canada, but is unavailable in the United States.

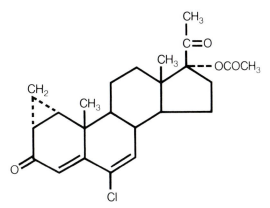

Fig 14–10.—The chemical structure of cyproterone acetate.

BIBLIOGRAPHY

Baird D.T., Horton R., Longcope C., et al.: Steroid prehormones. *Perspect. Biol. Med.* 3:384, 1968.

Barbieri R.L., Lee H., Ryan K.J.: Danazol binding to rat androgen, glucocorticoid, progesterone and estrogen receptors: Correlation with biological activity. *Fertil. Steril.* 31:182, 1979.

Barbieri R.L., Petro Z., Canick J.A., et al.: Aromatization of norethindrone to ethinyl estradiol by human placental microsomes. *J. Clin. Endocrinol. Metab.* 57:299, 1983.

Chen L., O'Malley B.W.: Mechanism of action of the sex steroid hormones. *N. Engl. J. Med.* 294:1322, 1976.

DeVore G.R., Owens O., Kase N.: Use of intravenous Premarin in the treatment of dysfunctional uterine bleeding—a double-blind randomized control study. *Obstet. Gynecol.* 59:285, 1982.

Dorrington J.H., Armstrong D.T.: Effects of FSH on gonadal functions. *Recent Prog. Horm. Res.* 35:301, 1979.

Downs K.A., Gibson M.: Clomiphene citrate therapy for luteal phase defect. *Fertil. Steril.* 39:34, 1983.

Fritz M.A., Sperott L.: The endocrinology of the menstrual cycle: The interaction of folliculogenesis and neuroendocrine mechanisms. *Fertil. Steril.* 38:509, 1982.

Gambrell R.D.: The menopause: Risks and benefits of estrogen-progestogen replacement therapy. *Fertil. Steril.* 37:457, 1982.

Gambrell R.D., Bagnell C.A., Greenblatt R.B.: Role of estrogens and progesterone in the etiology and prevention of endometrial cancer: A review. *Am. J. Obstet. Gynecol.* 146:696, 1983.

Grody W.W., Schrader W.T., O'Malley B.W.: Activation, transformation and subunit structure of steroid hormone receptors. *Endocr. Rev.* 3:141, 1982.

Healy D.M., Baulieu E.E., Hodgen G.D.: Induction of menstruation by an antiprogesterone steroid RU486 in primates. *Fertil. Steril.* 40:253, 1983.

Hodgen G.D.: The dominant ovarian follicle. *Fertil. Steril.* 38:281, 1982.

Lindsay R., Aitken J.M., Anderson J.: Long term prevention of osteoporosis by estrogen. *Lancet* 1:1038, 1976.

Lyon F.A.: The development of adenocarcinoma in young women receiving long-term sequential oral contraception. *Am. J. Obstet. Gynecol.* 123:299, 1975.

MacDonald P.C., Rombaut R.P., Siiteri P.K.: Plasma precursors of estrogen: I. Extent of conversion of plasma androstenedione to esterone in normal males and nonpregnant normal, castrate and adrenalectomized females. *J. Clin. Endocrinol. Metab.* 27:1103, 1967.

Mikhail G.: Hormone secretion by the human ovary. *Gynecol. Invest.* 1:5, 1970.

Nissen E.D., Kent F.D., Nissen S.E., et al.: Association of liver tumors with oral contraceptives. *Obstet. Gynecol.* 48:49, 1976.

Nora J.J., Nora A.H.: Birth defects and oral contraceptives. *Lancet* 1:941, 1973.

Richards J.S.: Hormonal control of ovarian follicular development: A 1978 perspective. *Recent Prog. Horm. Res.* 35:343, 1979.

Ryan K.J., Petro Z.: Steroid biosynthesis by human ovarian granulosa and theca cells. *J. Clin. Endocrinol. Metab.* 26:46, 1966.

Ryan K.J., Smith O.W.: Biogenesis of steroid hormones in the human ovary. *Recent Prog. Horm. Res.* 21:367, 1965.

Vermeulen A., Storia T., Verdonck L.: The apparent free testosterone concentration as an index of androgenicity. *J. Clin. Endocrinol. Metab.* 33:759, 1971.

Wentz A.C.: Progesterone therapy of the inadequate luteal phase. *Curr. Probl. Obstet. Gynecol.* 6(4):1, 1982.

CHAPTER FIFTEEN

Menopause

ISAAC SCHIFF, M.D.

MENOPAUSE describes the permanent cessation of menses, which in the United States usually happens in women at a mean age of 50 years. The condition constitutes but one part of the climacteric, during which period women undergo endocrine, somatic, and psychological changes. The changes are related both to aging and to estrogen depletion, but it is nearly impossible to quantify the respective effects of each. This notwithstanding, the present chapter focuses on the consequences of declining estrogen production in postmenopausal women and on the possible beneficial value of replacement therapy.

AGING OF THE OVARY

Unlike testicular function, which declines rather gradually over time, ovarian function fails quite abruptly and dramatically. It is misleading to think, however, that the ovary has not been aging at all until this time; in actuality it has begun to age even before birth. For example, at 20 weeks' gestation as many as 7 million oogonia are present; in the succeeding weeks there occurs a precipitous drop in this number, so that at birth only approximately 600,000 are present. Following birth the number of oocytes continues to decline even before the onset of puberty (Schiff and Wilson, 1978).

It is rather interesting that a precise timetable of ovarian follicular depletion seemingly exists. Exactly why millions of fetal ovarian follicles should progressively decrease in number over the years and cease their activity altogether toward the end of the fifth decade of female life remains a mystery, which is no doubt related to the still poorly understood general aging process.

ENDOCRINE CHANGES

With the decline in the number of ovarian follicles, the steroid production of the ovaries decreases as well since the ovary is both an endocrine organ and a reproductive organ. The predominant estrogen produced by the ovary is estradiol, and it is the diminished values of that hormone that signal menopause. Postmenopausal women, however, are not totally lacking estrogens. Estrogen production at low levels does continue, the source now being the androgens—specifically, androstenedione, which comes predominantly from the adrenal gland and in part from the ovarian stroma; these androgens are converted into estrone by the peripheral tissues such as fat, liver, and kidneys (MacDonald et al., 1978). Estrone, however, is a weaker estrogen than estradiol, and many menopausal women therefore develop symptoms of estrogen insufficiency. By the same token, in women whose bodies carry considerable fat, more of the adrenal androgens that are produced are converted to estrogens; consequently, such women suffer less from estrogen-deficiency conditions, such as osteoporosis. With regard to the sure diagnosis of menopause, it cannot reliably be made by simply measuring plasma estrogen levels; there is too great an overlap of ranges of the lower estrogen levels in premenopausal women during menstruation and the levels in postmenopausal women. For assurance that menopause has indeed begun, one can make use of the well-known endocrinologic principle that organ failure relates to a decline in the hormone levels of the stimulating organ. Thus, to diagnose ovarian failure, plasma follicle-stimulating hormone (FSH) and luteinizing hormone (LH) might be obtained; if the FSH and LH levels are greater than 50 mIU/ml it is fairly certain that organ function is compromised (Schiff, 1980).

In the following section, the various conditions associated with menopause are discussed.

GENITAL ATROPHY

Vulva

The changes that occur in the female vulva at around age 50 years are usually more related to the general aging process than to estrogen loss specifically. On physical examination of the organ, one perceives decreased subcutaneous fat and elastic tissue, increased wrinkling, and sparser and coarser pubic hair; the labia majora are shrunk more than the labia minora, and the relative proportions of the prepubertal female are thus reestablished. The Bartholin glands are found to be less efficient for purposes of lubrication. Clinically, the vulva may be found to have become pruritic and a source of irritation.

Vagina

With a decreasing estrogen supply the glycogen in the epithelial cells of the vagina diminishes, and an increased pH results. The changed constitution leads to an inhibition in the growth of lactobacilli, and, consequently, other contaminating organisms may flourish. The latter flora include a mixture of streptococci, staphylococci, and diphtheroid and coliform organisms, which may be responsible for the bouts of vaginal discharge and infection that may afflict women at this time. Al-

though it is tempting to use antibiotics to treat these conditions, estrogens serve better by getting to the source of the problem. In addition, the vaginal mucosa may demonstrate a flattening of the papillae, resulting in a disappearance of the rugae; the vagina will thus appear smoother and thinner. All of these changes explain, in large part, the frequent complaints by postmenopausal women of dyspareunia, burning, and occasionally bleeding (from breaks in the epithelium of the vaginal mucosa).

Other menopausal changes in the vagina include the general coloring, which turns from red to pale pink. If the vagina becomes irritated due to atrophy, inflammation may turn it deep red again. The vaginal walls become smooth and the orifice narrows due to a loss of elastic tissue; in fact, in extreme cases the vagina may actually become stenosed.

Urethra

It is known that the urethra has the same biological origin as the vagina—essentially the embryonic urogenital sinus. Thus, as the vagina undergoes atrophy, so may the urethra. Affected women may complain of dysuria and frequency. Again, the addition of antibiotics will provide temporary relief; the prescription of low-dose estrogens will attack the symptoms at their source (Smith, 1972; Smith et al., 1970).

Uterus and Tubes

The postmenopausal uterus tends to be small and firm. Because of estrogen depletion fibroids tend to regress. The vascularity is reduced, a feature that can be easily observed at the time of a hysterectomy. There is an inward migration of the squamocolumnar junction, which makes it more difficult to diagnose cervical cancer. As for the fallopian tubes, the fimbria begin to show deciliation and decreased secretion (Gaddum-Rosse et al., 1975).

SEXUAL FUNCTION

Although older women experience a decrease in both the intensity and duration of

sexual response, they are nevertheless capable of having an active sex life—as a growing number of them do (Masters and Johnson, 1966). For these women, sex remains an important part of the postmenopausal years; indeed, it usually seems that the more frequent their sexual activity, the better their capacity for a satisfactory response. Complaints of dryness may still be common, frequently due to some degree of atrophy; in this case, estrogen is a beneficial treatment. However, even the administration of estrogens locally results in their systemic absorption (see the discussion on estrogen replacement later on in this chapter).

VASOMOTOR FLUSHES

There are two predominant and indisputable symptoms of menopause: genital atrophy and vasomotor flushes (Rybo and Westerberg, 1971). As regards to flushes, it is estimated that about 60% to 70% of menopausal women will experience them at one time or another. In 10% to 20% of cases, the flushing will be so severe that some form of therapy will be indicated.

Vasomotor flushes occur very irregularly, with no apparent rhyme or reason to their onset (i.e., no precipitating event). They do, however, seem to occur more frequently at night than in the daytime. When they do occur, they may do so as infrequently as once or twice a day or as often as once or twice an hour or more. In the past, the only evidence for the existence of flushes came from the testimony of the women experiencing them; now temperature monitoring devices provide objective confirmation of the phenomenon.

Despite the unpredictability of their occurrence, flushes do have some characteristic associations. For example, a "hot flash"—a kind of anxiety—almost always precedes the flush and is subjectively experienced by the woman as a premonition that she is about to develop a flush. The flush itself is characterized by a reddening of the face and an elevation of body temperature. The women experiencing a flush has the feeling that the flush lasts only a

few minutes, but monitoring the temperature of the skin surface of the metacarpal indicates that the temperature may stay raised as long as 20 to 30 minutes (Tataryn et al., 1979). After the temperature falls, the woman may suffer a sweating episode in which the body cools off. It is the recurrent episodes of flash followed by flush and sweating that constitute the entire vasomotor flush syndrome. The description alone is sufficient to suggest how disturbing flushes can be to some of the women who experience them.

The chemistry of vasomotor flushing, as has been noted, is not clear. Of the theories put forward, perhaps the most plausible is that the flush is triggered by the *decline in*, rather than the absolute value of, estrogen levels. For example, it has been shown independently by Tataryn et al. and by Casper et al. that gonadotropin, or LH, levels surge during vasomotor flushes. But the LH surge is not the cause of the vasomotor flush, as it is known that injections of gonadotropins do not produce a flush. Moreover, women who have undergone hypophysectomy and who consequently do not produce appreciable amounts of FSH or LH in their systems will experience vasomotor flushes (Meldrum et al., 1981). But the measurement of LH–releasing hormone (LH-RH) in peripheral blood may demonstrate a connection (Fig 15–1). It has been demonstrated that rises are accompanied by spikes in plasma LH-RH levels. Furthermore, it is thought that the plasma LH-RH level presumably reflects central secretion of LH-RH. It is also known, for example, that the injection of LH-RH into the hypothalamus of rats causes a decrease in core temperature and an increase in peripheral temperature; the increase in the latter temperature amounts to a flush. Thus, the source of vasomotor flushes may be elevation of hypothalamic LH-RH (Ravnikar et al., 1984).

One of the major concerns for identifying the etiology of a flush is to come up with a form of therapy. It has been known for a long time that estrogens are clearly a palliative. On the other hand, it has been known that placebo is also remarkably effective—in the

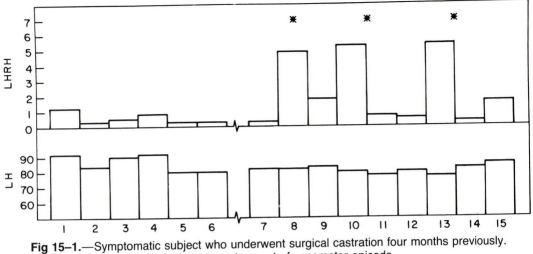

Fig 15–1.—Symptomatic subject who underwent surgical castration four months previously. Asterisk represents onset of vasomotor episode.

short term. A prospective double-blind randomized crossover study done by Coope showed that estrogens will relieve flushes much more significantly than placebo, and that when women initially receiving estrogens cross over to placebo, the flushes return dramatically. The results show that estrogens, though effective, still do not produce a permanent cure. On the other hand, the women initially receiving placebo who crossed over to estrogen therapy experienced even further relief of their symptoms. Women for whom estrogen replacement therapy is prescribed should, therefore, be told that flushing may return on cessation of treatment.

Although estrogens work, there is often a risk of serious side effects and complications for the women taking them (see the discussion following). Thus, other forms of therapy have been assayed. For example, depo-medroxyprogesterone acetate appears to be effective (Bullock et al., 1975), but the side effects of the drug include irregular vaginal bleeding and suppression of adrenal function. Because an intramuscular injection may persist as long as six months, oral medroxyprogesterone acetate would seem to be a better remedy (Ortiz et al., 1977). In a double-blind crossover study using medroxyprogesterone acetate, 20 mg, it was found that women re-

ceiving the drug experienced a 74% decline in vasomotor flushes in the last four weeks of a three-month trial, and that crossover to placebo produced an immediate worsening of symptoms (Fig 15–2) (Schiff et al., 1980). By contrast women who started on placebo experienced a significant decline (26%) in symptoms during the latter part of their treatment, and then a further decline of 35% after being placed on drug. Medroxyprogesterone acetate given orally also may involve disagreeable side effects: a woman may have symptoms usually associated with the premenstrual phase and may feel bloated, and a small weight gain is not uncommon. Nevertheless, the drug remains a quite effective one, as a follow-up study in which vasomotor flushes were measured objectively confirmed this (Albrecht et al., 1981). Once again, in the second study placebo was found to be effective—this time objectively—but not as effective as drug (Fig 15–3).

Because of the LH and LH-RH surges during a flush, it would be logical to suppose that neurotransmitters or drugs affecting neurotransmitters could alter flush frequency. Clonidine, a catecholamine that stimulates postsynaptic α-adrenergic receptors, would seem to be such a drug, and indeed a dose of

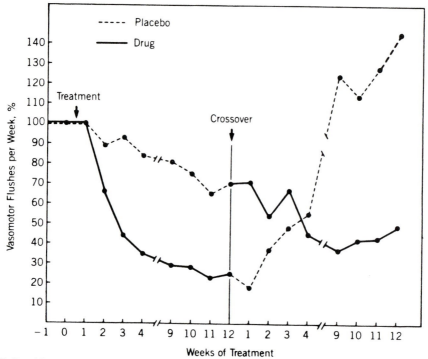

Fig 15–2.—Mean number of vasomotor flushes as a percentage change from pretreatment (week −1 to 0). Change of treatment regimen (crossover) occurred at 12 weeks. Weeks 5 to 8, unassociated with major variability, are not included. (From Schiff I., Tulchinsky D., Cramer D., et al.: *J.A.M.A.* 244:1443, 1980.)

0.4 mg/day of the substance reduces flushing by close to 50% (Laufer et al., 1982). Norepinephrine, also a catecholamine, causes release of LH-RH, and some of the hypothalamic neurons containing LH-RH are in close proximity to the temperature control center in the hypothalamus. Thus, catecholamines may ultimately provide the link between the LH-RH levels, LH levels, and vasomotor flushes. At the present time, however, estrogen replacement therapy remains clearly the most efficacious treatment.

OSTEOPOROSIS

Osteoporosis, defined by a reduction in the mass of structural bone per unit volume, is a significant disease of older women. About 20% of all women suffer a hip fracture by the time they reach age 90 years, brought on, in four cases out of five, by osteoporosis; 16% of

women die within three months of the accident due to postfracture complications (Heaney, 1976). Furthermore, about 25% of all white women over age 60 years suffer spinal compression fractures, which produce a reduction in height. (In 1980 there were more than 14,000,000 women in the United States older than 65 years.) Osteoporosis is not only associated with an increase in hip fractures, but also of fractures of the radius. In fact, there is a dramatic increase in such fractures among postmenopausal women, but not among older men. Again, with osteoporosis, the decline in estrogen levels among postmenopausal women seems to be the cause. Men, who have a higher bone density than women to begin with, experience a very small steroid loss after age 50 years, while women experience a rapid decline in estrogen production. It is also known that oophorectomy is followed by a rise in plasma calcium level,

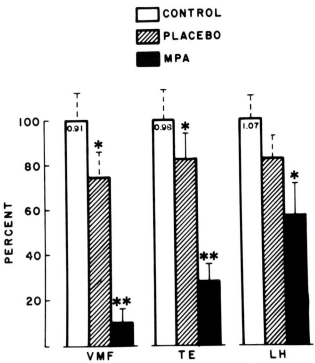

Fig 15–3.—The number at the top of each open bar indicates the number of observations per hour of the association between the various phenomena during the control period (no medications). The associations between these phenomena during administration of placebo (hatched bars) and medroxyprogesterone acetate (solid bars) are expressed as percentages of the control period. One asterisk indicates *P* <.05 when compared to control values; two asterisks, *P* >.05 when compared to both control and placebo values; *VMF,* vasomotor flushes that the patients subjectively report; and *TE,* temperature elevations that the patients report. (From Albrecht B.H., Schiff I., Tulchinsky D., et al.: *Am. J. Obstet. Gynecol.* 139:631, 1981.)

which suggests that a decline in estrogens leads to increased calcium resorption from the bone (Gallagher et al., 1974). Conversely, the intake of estrogen by postmenopausal women causes a decline in plasma and urinary calcium levels and, thus, an inhibition of bony resorption (Lindsay and Herrington, 1983).

Reifenstein and Albright were among the first physicians to prescribe estrogens for the prevention of osteoporosis; women who took the drug were later found to have lost less bone than women who did not. A later prospective double-blind study performed by Lindsay and co-workers and carried out over a five-year period clearly demonstrated that mestranol decreased bone loss; in fact, therapy even led to a slight increase in bone density during the first three years of treatment. Placebo, on the other hand, had no effect. They showed in a follow-up study that if the estrogen therapy is terminated, bone loss begins again at a very high rate, so that three years after the cessation of treatment, women who had previously taken estrogens showed the same bone densities as those who had not taken any for eight years.

What is more important to assess is whether the estrogens that attenuate osteoporosis result in a decreased incidence of fractures. Weiss et al. performed a case-control study and found that the risk of fractures related to osteoporosis were 50% to 60% lower in women who had used estrogens for six years or longer. Similarly, in a study by Pag-

inini-Hill et al. the risk ratio for fractures with oral estrogens taken in excess of 60 months was 0.42, with the risk being even smaller among drug-taking oophorectomized women. It was further found that the risk decreased significantly with duration but not with size of dose; thus, one does not have to use massive amounts of estrogens to control osteoporosis—doses of conjugated estrogens of 0.625 mg/day suffice.

Other means of managing osteoporosis and the attendant fracture risk include calcium and vitamin D treatment. Of great interest is the finding by Riggs et al. that sodium fluoride, a potent stimulator of bone formation that can increase the mass of the axial skeleton, is also effective; in fact, sodium fluoride plus calcium seems more effective than calcium alone. The drawbacks to fluoride treatment include widespread side effects: 38% of those treated with the substance suffered rheumatic symptoms such as joint pain or swelling, and gastrointestinal tract symptoms such as nausea and vomiting, and some, as a

consequence, had to discontinue therapy (Fig 15–4).

The most accurate method to diagnose osteoporosis is the bone biopsy, but the procedure is invasive and clearly not routinely indicated. A simple test available to most physicians is a lateral roentgenogram of the spine, which will also give evidence of any spinal compression fractures. An instrument that is now available in many centers is the bone densitometer, which measures bone density by means of photon absorptiometry. A radiation source such as I 125 emits photons; the instrument counter then gives a visual image of the amount of radiation passing through the peripheral bones, and, thus, a measure of bone quantity. A drawback is that the machine can only be used on the forearm or the hand; it cannot be used on the spine. Dual absorptiometry can be used for the spine. The very accurate quantitated computed tomographic (CT) scan can also be directed to the vertebral spine, and what it shows is that in general mineral loss is greater

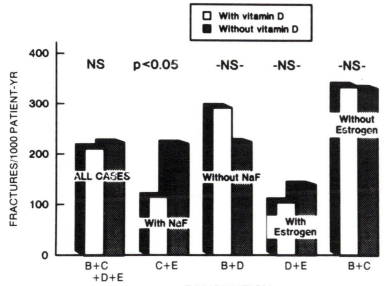

Fig 15–4.—Comparison of fracture rates after various combinations of therapy with and without vitamin D. Except in the groups receiving sodium fluoride, in whom the addition of vitamin D marginally reduced the incidence of fractures, no significant (NS) effect of vitamin D could be demonstrated. (From Riggs B.L., Seeman E., Hodgson S.F., et al.: *N. Engl. J. Med.* 306:446, 1982.)

in the spinal trabecular bone than in the forearm or hand (Genant et al., 1982). However, the CT scan is not a widely available piece of equipment that can be routinely used.

An important concomitant factor in the management of osteoporosis in older women is the ability to identify the women at risk. Thin, slender, white women who smoke are at greatest risk; obese women, whose fat tissue serves as a source for the increased peripheral conversion of adrenal androgens to estrogens, are at least risk. Once a woman at risk is identified she may be followed routinely by either photon absorptometry or CT scan. When bone density falls significantly, an appropriate therapy should be considered.

CARDIOVASCULAR SYSTEM

The increased incidence of coronary artery disease that aging women suffer was first thought to be related to the changes occurring at menopause; if one looks at the curves describing the ratio of male-to-female deaths due to coronary heart disease against age, one may indeed conclude that such is the case (Furman, 1971). The ratio of male deaths to female deaths among 35-year-old white coronary parents who were previously healthy is about 8:1. The ratio falls dramatically after age 50 years, and by the ninth decade of life it becomes 1:1. (The divergent values of the ratio, which indicate a sex difference, are not as great among nonwhites or among whites with diabetes or hypertensive disorders.) Thus, it was thought that menopause was implicated in heart disease and that estrogens were a preventative. But when one considers the absolute mortality figures for women and men separately, rather than ratios, one finds that the curve for women has a steady slope as it passes through the age of menopause. (In fact, it is the men's curve that changes greatly—accelerating at first and then tending to decelerate after age 50 years or so; it is now thought that perhaps the high-risk coronary males die off earlier.) Even though this information comes from data gathered in the 1950s, when many more men than women smoked and many more men than women worked outside the home, it has been found to be consistent in the 1970s (Fig 15–5). Nevertheless, the flawed analysis led in the 1950s and 1960s to the widespread prescription of estrogens in the hopes of controlling coronary artery disease. But the results of the Coronary Drug Project, a double-blind study carried out over an 18-month period at 53 separate medical centers and involving men ages 30 to 65 years who had suffered a previous myocardial infarction, showed that the men given conjugated estrogens, 5 mg, suffered about twice the number of nonfatal myocardial infarcts, three times the number of pulmonary emboli, and $1^1/_2$ times the number of deaths as the men given placebo. The men given conjugated estrogens, 2.5 mg, showed no increased attack or death rate. The Coronary Drug Project thus laid to rest the notion that estrogens are beneficial to patients with heart disease, at least in the case of men.

With regard to women, the Boston Collaborative Drug Study showed in two multipurpose surveys of patients hospitalized for nonfatal myocardial infarctions that there was no evidence of a statistically significant association between the use of estrogens and myocardial infarctions among women aged 40 to 75 years (Rosenberg et al., 1976). More recently retrospective studies have demonstrated a protective effect of estrogens in that the risk ratio of myocardial infarctions of estrogen users was 0.43 compared with controls (Ross et al., 1981). However, there may have been a selection process in that healthy women may be given hormones, and physicians may avoid giving them to women at risk. We have to await results of prospective studies. If estrogens are confirmed to have this beneficial effect on heart disease, they could have a very dramatic effect on life expectancy.

By contrast, convincing evidence exists that the cardiovascular system of younger women

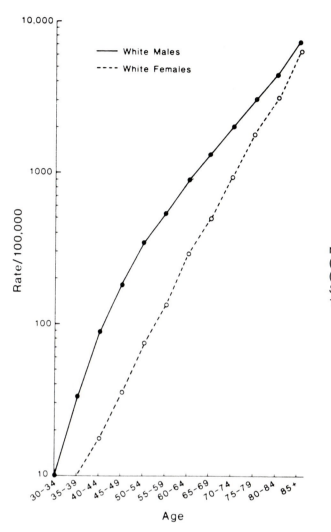

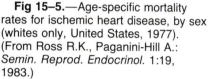

Fig 15–5.—Age-specific mortality rates for ischemic heart disease, by sex (whites only, United States, 1977). (From Ross R.K., Paganini-Hill A.: *Semin. Reprod. Endocrinol.* 1:19, 1983.)

is adversely affected by estrogen deprivation at an early age. For example, a study of the autopsy records of a number of women who had been castrated before age 40 years showed a greater incidence of coronary artery disease than women castrated between ages 40 to 50 years (Ryan, 1976). Other recent studies suggest, however, that hysterectomy alone with preservation of ovarian function also results in an increased incidence of coronary disease (Rosenberg et al., 1981; Gordon et al., 1978).

A possible connection between estrogens and cardiovascular disease may be seen in the effect of estrogens on serum lipids. Cholesterol levels are generally higher in young men than in young women. In men, the levels peak sometime around age 40 to 45 years; in women the levels appear to peak at a later age. However, the addition of estrogens does not restore the premenopausal lipid pattern. Nevertheless, the addition of estrogens does bring about an increase in high-density lipoproteins, which are significant in that they are elevated in persons who exercise and are thought to be responsible for their decreased infarction risk (Ross and Paganini-Hill, 1983; Notelovitz et al., 1983). This could explain the finding of a decreased life expectancy for all cause mortality in women who are not given estrogens (Bush et al., 1983).

PSYCHOLOGY

The effect of estrogens on the emotional state of postmenopausal women presents a controversial subject. For one thing, there is no good standard methodology in the testing protocols for what are ultimately subjective variables. Another matter is that truly reliable, objective control groups do not really exist. Thus the large-scale epidemiologic studies seem to suggest that depression, insomnia, irritability, and cognitive functioning do not correlate with the menopause, while the intervention trials that have been done seem to suggest otherwise.

A double-blind crossover study performed by Campbell comparing conjugated estrogens, 1.25 mg, with placebo used a graphic scale to measure a subject's emotional state. The results showed that the women who suffered severe vasomotor symptoms before the experiment began evinced, on estrogen intake, significant improvement in vasomotor flushes, urinary frequency, vaginal dryness, insomnia, headaches, irritability, and some other emotional variables such as memory, anxiety, and worry. On the other hand, the women who were not suffering from flushes showed improvement only in memory, anxiety, and worry. Thus, many of the emotional improvements due to estrogen intake may be solely the consequence of a dominolike effect set off by the attenuation of the flushes. In a year-long study (also done by Campbell) on women with less severe vasomotor flushes, the estrogens produced significant relief only for hot flushes, urinary frequency, vaginal dryness, and insomnia.

If estrogens do affect emotional state, it must be because of some biochemical interaction in the brain. Klaiber et al. have suggested that estrogens work by effecting a reduction in monoamine oxidase activity, which is normally increased in depressed patients; given in high doses to such patients, the hormones do seem to function as a monoamine oxidase inhibitor. A number of other studies have looked at the effect of estrogens on cognitive function, but the results are contradictory and inconclusive. Most investigators think, however, that any improvement in cognitive function is probably related to the improvement in emotional state, and that the latter comes about most likely because of the diminished flushes.

As mentioned previously, epidemiologic studies show very little correlation between menopause and insomnia. Yet, the experience of many physicians is that a connection exists: their menopausal patients make recurrent complaints of insomnia. Thompson and Oswald, in a double-blind parallel study using estrone sulfate and placebo, recorded patients' electroencephalographic (EEG) patterns and found that the estrogens, while not affecting total sleep time, did improve rapid eye movement (REM) sleep. Schiff et al. performed a double-blind crossover study with conjugated estrogens, 0.625 mg, and found that the women receiving drug evidenced fewer flushes, a shorter time between "lights out" and sleep onset (i.e., "sleep latency"), more REM sleep, and a greater percentage of REM sleep than the same women receiving placebo (Table 15–1). In addition, it was found that sleep latency tended to decrease most in the patients ranked highest in psychological well-adjustment by the attendant physician and nurse (Schiff et al., 1979; Regestein et al., 1981). A possible interpretation of the results is that fewer flushes means better sleep—the "insomnia" having been the consequence of frequent nighttime flushes. Thus, in the case of a menopausal woman experiencing severe vasomotor flushes and insomnia, estrogens will probably remedy both symptoms (Erlik et al., 1981). But if a woman's insomnia is related to other causes, such as fam-

TABLE 15–1.—EFFECTS OF PLACEBO AND
ESTROGEN TREATMENT ON VARIOUS SLEEP
FACTORS IN 27 PATIENTS*

	PLACEBO	DRUG
Sleep latency, min†	19.1 ± 6.1	12.2 ± 8.6
Total sleep time, min	426.2 ± 55.6	438.3 ± 43.2
Total REM sleep, min‡	70.4 ± 9.7	95.4 ± 14.8
REM time, %†	16.5 ± 1.1	21.7 ± 2.1
Awake time, %	13.7 ± 2.2	10.4 ± 1.9
Sleep stage, % of time		
I	10.2 ± 1.3	10.9 ± 1.7
II	40.3 ± 2.1	38.3 ± 2.1
III	11.0 ± 1.0	10.4 ± 1.2
IV	83.0 ± 1.3	8.3 ± 1.1

*All values given as mean ± SEM. (From Schiff I., et al.: *J.A.M.A.* 242:2405, 1979.)
†$P < .05$.
‡$P < .005$.

ily difficulties or deep-rooted psychological problems, the benefit of drug therapy would be doubtful.

COMPLICATIONS OF ESTROGEN REPLACEMENT THERAPY

Estrogens are known to be associated with various side effects, risks, and complications, including some forms of cancer. To take one clear example, the Boston Collaborative Drug Surveillance Program revealed a 2.5-fold increase of surgically confirmed gallbladder disease with the use of estrogens by postmenopausal women. But it is the suspected relationship of estrogen to cancer—e.g., endometrial and breast cancer—that is of most concern.

Endometrial Cancer

Since 1975, a number of published case-control studies have shown an increased risk of development of endometrial cancer among women taking estrogens (Smith et al., 1975; Ziel et al., 1975; Hulka et al., 1980; Antunes et al., 1979). The risk tends to be dose- and duration-related, i.e., it increases with the size and prolongation of prescription. Part of

the reason that it has been relatively easy to study the connection between estrogens and endometrial cancer is that there is a short latency period between the use of the drug and the onset of the disease; some studies have shown the period to be as short as six months, others have shown it to be as long as two years. It appears also that once the drug is discontinued the increased risk over normal tends to disappear (in fact, after six months the relative risk returns to unity), and so at least the long-term aftereffects are nil. Moreover, estrogens tend to be associated with low-grade cancers, namely, stage IA histological grade 1, and not with the more advanced and lethal tumors. Although endometrial cancer meets all the pathologic criteria of a true cancer, women who contract the disease after taking estrogens do not suffer a higher mortality rate than women free of the condition (Fig 15–6) (Chu et al., 1982).

The reason that estrogens cause cancer in menopausal women but not, obviously, in premenopausal women may very well have to do with the presence in the functioning ovary of progesterone, the hormone implicated in menstrual bleeding. Progesterone added to an estrogen regimen produces some unwanted withdrawal bleeding, but it also arrests the development of cystic and adenomatous hyperplasia, the precursor of endometrial cancer. A large-scale study carried out at the Wilford Hall Air Force Base in Texas (Gambrell, 1982) and a study done in England (Whitehead et al., 1982) confirm the significantly decreased incidence of hyperplasia and of endometrial cancer when progestins are included (at least for ten days a month) in an estrogen program. Theoretically the progesterone is effective because it converts estrogen in the form of estradiol to a less potent estrogen (namely, estrone), and it also causes a decrease in mitosis of the cells and in estrogen receptors. What progesterone achieves, therefore, is more stable endometrial growth (Table 15–2).

Past studies have shown that sequential

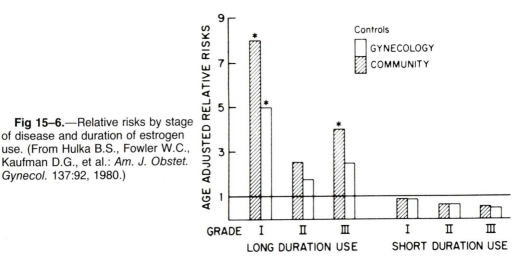

Fig 15–6.—Relative risks by stage of disease and duration of estrogen use. (From Hulka B.S., Fowler W.C., Kaufman D.G., et al.: *Am. J. Obstet. Gynecol.* 137:92, 1980.)

*Relative risks significantly different from 1, p<.05

oral contraceptives, which contain progestins and pharmacologic doses of estrogens, were associated with endometrial cancer. The reason that the regimen of estrogens along with progestin prescribed for postmenopausal women does not produce the same risk is probably because of the smaller estrogen doses involved.

Breast Cancer

Breast cancer, clearly a more serious concern, has a higher mortality rate among postmenopausal women than any other cancer. Whether or not added estrogens increase that rate is a subject of controversy: some studies have shown the effect and others have not. Hoover et al. found a twofold increased risk

of contracting breast cancer with ten years of use of estrogens. Ross et al. found a 2.5-fold increased risk of the disease among postmenopausal women whose ovaries were intact and who had taken 1.25 mg of conjugated estrogens for three years or more. This was not seen in women taking estrogens whose ovaries were removed. More recently, Hulka et al. found no increased risk either, except in the cases in which the estrogens were administered by injection and in which the women came from families with a strong history of breast cancer. All in all, it is difficult to interpret the conflicting data. For one thing, breast cancer seems to have a longer latency period than endometrial cancer, and, thus, the decline in risk after discontinuation of

TABLE 15–2.—INCIDENCE OF ENDOMETRIAL CANCER AT WILFORD HALL USAF MEDICAL CENTER BY THERAPY GROUP, 1975 TO 1979*

	PATIENT-YEARS OF OBSERVATION	NO. OF PATIENTS WITH CANCER	INCIDENCE PER 100,000 WOMEN
Estrogen-progestin users	7,063	5	70.8
Estrogen users	2,302	10	434.4
Estrogen vaginal cream users	1,318	1	75.9
Progestin or androgen users	761	0	. . .
Untreated women	2,477	6	242.2
Total	13,921	22	158.0

*From Gambrell R.D. Jr.: *J. Reprod. Med.* 27(suppl.):531, 1982.

drug may not provide a sufficient safeguard against the disease. At a minimum, and until further information becomes available, caution should be exercised in prescribing the drug—i.e., administration by injection should be avoided and no drug should be prescribed for women with a strong family history. Concern over complications should be shared with drug takers.

Progestins added to the estrogens may, again, lessen the breast cancer risk; some preliminary data from Gambrell seem to suggest this result (Fig 15–7). But one should recall that progestins are not without their side effects and complications—e.g., withdrawal bleeding every month, bloating and constant premenstrual symptoms, weight gain, and lowered high-density lipoprotein levels. Neither have the long-term effects of the drug on the cardiovascular system been fully worked out. Other studies have suggested that progestins may increase the risk of breast tumors in beagle dogs; although it is generally accepted that beagle dogs are not a good model for studying breast tumors and the risk has not been confirmed in humans, the information should be noted.

Other risks of estrogen replacement therapy are described in Chapter 16 in the section on oral contraceptives.

ROUTES OF ADMINISTRATION OF ESTROGEN

At one time it was thought that if estrogens were administered vaginally they would not be absorbed systemically, but such is not the case. In fact, estrogens applied locally are absorbed immediately into the plasma, bypassing the liver; prescribed this way, they may be neither bound nor altered to a weaker form, and, thus, may end up being more potent.

Such would be the case, for example, with estradiol. Estradiol is the predominant estrogen of younger women, and it would seem to make sense to prescribe this form of drug to postmenopausal women. However, it has

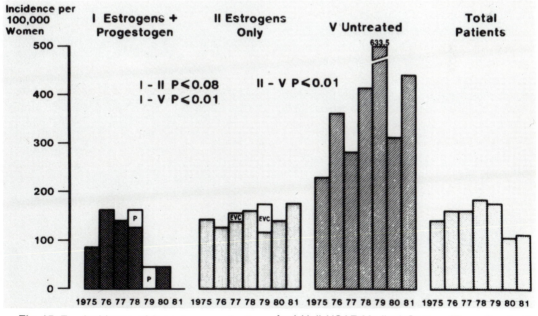

Fig 15–7.—Incidence of breast cancer in the various treatment groups compared with untreated women from 1975 through 1981 at Wilford Hall USAF Medical Center. (From Gambrell R.D. Jr.: *Semin. Reprod. Endocrinol.* 1:27, 1983.)

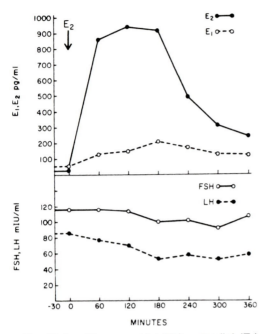

Fig 15–8.—Plasma estriol (E_1), estradiol (E_2), LH, and FSH concentrations before and after the vaginal administration of 0.5 mg of micronized E_2. (From Schiff I., Tulchinsky D., Ryan K.J.: *Fertil. Steril.* 28:1063, 1977.)

been shown that estradiol taken by mouth is converted to estrone. Estradiol placed in the vagina is absorbed systemically and remains estradiol (Fig 15–8) (Schiff et al., 1977).

It used to be thought that estriol was a much safer form of estrogen than the others; this is because women who have had children and have thus presumably been exposed to high levels of estriol experience a decreased incidence of breast and endometrial cancer. It has since been shown that estriol clearly supports breast cancer growth in vitro. At this time there is no evidence that estriol is any safer than any other form of estrogen. When estriol is taken orally most of it becomes conjugated and thus has very little biologic activity (Schiff et al., 1978); estriol taken vaginally remains an active substance (Schiff et al., 1980).

The most widely prescribed estrogen in this country is a conjugated estrogen (trade name, Premarin), which is obtained from the

urine of pregnant mares. There is no evidence that Premarin is any safer or any more dangerous than other forms of estrogen, for, ultimately, all of the estrogens work at the level of the receptor. Size of dose and route of administration are matters to be concerned with.

When estrogens bypass the liver they will cause a decreased production of some of the binding globulins that are normally present when estrogens are taken orally. There would be a reduction in renin substrate and, thus, less risk for hypertension (Campbell and Whitehead, 1982). The long-term health significance of these effects is not clear.

MONITORING THE PATIENT DURING MENOPAUSE

The woman given estrogens ought to be seen by her physician twice a year. At these times, the physician should monitor the patient for height, weight, and blood pressure, and should also carry out a complete interval history and physical examination. The patient ought already to have been familiarized with the possible warning signs for the development of endometrial hyperplasia or cancer, such as irregular bleeding; she ought to be performing regular breast self-examinations as well. Because the estrogens and progesterone may alter the lipid profile of some women it is a good idea for a lipid profile to be drawn a few months after the start of therapy. An endometrial biopsy may also be in order—despite the protection provided by the progestins—if only to reassure patient and physician that all is going well.

SUMMARY

Postmenopausal women continue to produce estrogens that are derived by the peripheral conversion in fat of adrenal and ovarian androgens. Thus, to diagnose menopause one has to demonstrate elevated plasma FSH and LH levels, rather than a simple plasma estrogen level.

There are two predominant complaints that

menopausal women describe: (1) vasomotor flushes and (2) genital atrophy. The etiology of vasomotor flushes has not been definitively elucidated, but it appears to be related to estrogen depletion. The rapid estrogen loss that occurs either with natural menopause as a result of depletion of follicles or as a result of surgical castration probably has a resultant effect on neurotransmitters such that there is an elevation of LH-RH in the hypothalamus. This elevation most likely causes LH surges, which often accompany the vasomotor flushes. Flushes can be measured objectively by noting the associated peripheral elevation of temperature. Subjectively, a flash usually forewarns a woman of the flush to follow. Flushes are very disturbing to women who experience them, and, certainly, therapy is warranted for those who desire it. Effective therapy includes estrogens, progestin, and α-adrenergic agonists. One ought to keep in mind that placebo can be efficacious, and any new drug should be compared with placebo. As for genital atrophy, it is now well understood that sexuality remains an important aspect of the life of older women, and here again estrogens are an effective—indeed the only effective—therapy. Although estrogens can be prescribed only locally, they will nevertheless be absorbed systemically.

Osteoporosis is associated with high morbidity and mortality among postmenopausal women. Every effort should be made to identify women most at risk for the condition; thin, slender, white women who smoke are at greatest risk. Objective monitoring of bone density can be performed with the aid of photon absorptiometry, lateral roentgenogram of the spine, or CT scan of the spine. Estrogens prescribed for osteoporosis ought to be started within a few years of the menopause, because that is when the loss of bone is greatest. Other therapies for osteoporosis include administration of calcium in the area of 1.2 gm/day, sodium fluoride in a dose of 30 to 40 mg/day, and exercise. Sodium fluoride ought only be prescribed by a specialist in bone endocrinology, for the undesirable side effects

are rather high. Finally, just as one measures blood pressure to determine efficacy of antihypertensive medications, one should always keep ongoing records of bone density.

As for heart disease, there is no evidence of a sudden acceleration in myocardial infarct incidence after the menopause. Women who undergo premature menopause are found to be more at risk for heart disease. It is not known whether added estrogen can reverse the heart disease risk of women who have undergone castration prior to age 40 years; one suspects, nevertheless, that there exists a beneficial effect. As for older women, it is known that estrogens in low doses do not increase their risk of suffering atherosclerotic heart disease. Some retrospective studies have indeed shown a decreased risk, but those studies were not properly randomized—e.g., a woman at risk for heart disease is not usually given estrogens by her physician.

Estrogens have a beneficial effect on the sleep behavior of women suffering hot flashes. Some prospective studies have shown that estrogens have a positive effect on cognitive thinking as well as on mood. Again, one has to interpret the results rather carefully, since in many situations the beneficial effect may be ultimately due to the reduction in vasomotor flushes, which may produce a domino-like effect on the other factors.

The risks associated with estrogen replacement therapy that are of most concern include those for endometrial cancer and breast cancer. Endometrial cancer has been clearly connected to the use of estrogen. A short latency period exists between the onset of therapy and the development of the disease; and stopping the drug eliminates the higher relative risk within a half year or so. Although endometrial cancer has a high morbidity, an estrogen-induced increased mortality has not been demonstrated. Moreover, a progestin added for at least ten days each month to the estrogen regime reduces the cancer risk to a lower rate than the no therapy figure. As for breast cancer, although the data are still inconclusive, long-term use of estrogen in high doses seems to be detrimental. The hoped-for beneficial effect of added progestins has not yet been studied.

Women receiving estrogen replacement therapy should be seen twice a year. A lipid profile should be obtained for women with a family history of heart disease. Blood pressure ought also to be checked. An endometrial biopsy should be performed a minimum of once a year, and if endometrial hyperplasia is demonstrated, the hormones ought to be stopped. Women taking an estrogen plus a progestin should undergo an endometrial biopsy about once every two years. If bleeding develops, the biopsy ought to be performed immediately.

The regimen currently most frequently prescribed is conjugated estrogens, 0.625 mg from the first to the 25th day of each month, and added progestin, such as medroxyprogesterone acetate, 10 mg from the 15th to the 25th day of the month. More than 90% of women with uterus in situ will experience some form of withdrawal bleeding during the last few days of the month.

At present, no conclusive data exist that suggest either that all women ought to be given hormones or that no women at all ought to be given hormones. The most reasonable procedure to follow would seem to be to review the foreseeable benefits and risks of hormone replacement therapy with each individual patient, and to have the patient participate in the decision of whether or not to pursue treatment. If the patient elects to be treated, then careful follow-up monitoring is maintained so that all of the benefits can be obtained from hormone replacement therapy while minimizing any risks or side effects.

BIBLIOGRAPHY

Albrecht B.H., Schiff I., Tulchinsky D., et al.: Objective evidence that placebo and oral medroxyprogesterone acetate therapy diminish menopausal vasomotor flushes. *Am. J. Obstet. Gynecol.* 139:631–635, 1981.

Antunes C.M.F., Stolley P.D., Rosenshein N.B., et al.: Endometrial cancer and estrogen use. *N. Engl. J. Med.* 300:9–13, 1974.

Boston Collaborative Drug Surveillance Program: Surgically confirmed gallbladder disease, venous thromboembolism, and breast tumors in relation to postmenopausal estrogen therapy. *N. Engl. J. Med.* 190:15, 1974.

Bullock J.L., Massey F.M., Gambrell R.D. Jr.: Use of medroxyprogesterone acetate to prevent menopausal symptoms. *Obstet. Gynecol.* 46:165, 1975.

Bush T.L., Cowman L.D., Barrett-Connor E., et al.: Estrogen use and all-cause mortality. Preliminary results from the lipid research clinics—program follow-up study. *J.A.M.A.* 249:903–906, 1983.

Campbell S.: Double blind psychometric studies on the effects of natural estrogens on postmenopausal women, in Campbell S. (ed.): *The Management of Menopause and Postmenopausal Years.* University Park Press, Baltimore, 1976, pp. 149–158.

Campbell S., Whitehead M.I.: Potency and hepato-cellular effects of oestrogens after oral, percutaneous, and subcutaneous administration, in VanKeep P.A., Utian W.H., Vermeulen A. (eds.): *The Controversial Climacteric.* MPT Press Ltd., Boston, 1982, pp. 103–125.

Casper R.F., Yen S.S.C., Wilkes M.M.: Menopausal flushes: A neuroendocrine link with pulsatile luteinizing hormone secretion. *Science* 205:823–825, 1979.

Chu J., Schweid A.I., Weiss N.S.: Survival among women with endometrial cancer: A comparison of estrogen users and nonusers. *Am. J. Obstet. Gynecol.* 143:569–572, 1982.

Coope J.: Double blind cross-over study of estrogen replacement therapy, in Campbell S. (ed.): *The Management of the Menopause and Postmenopausal Years.* University Park Press, Baltimore, 1976, pp. 159–168.

The Coronary Drug Project Research Group: The Coronary Drug Project: Initial findings leading to modifications of its research protocol. *J.A.M.A.* 214:1303, 1970.

Erlik Y., Tataryn I., Meldrum D., et al.: Association of waking episodes with menopausal hot flushes. *J.A.M.A.* 245:1741, 1981.

Furman R.H.: Coronary heart disease and the menopause, in Ryan K.J., Gibson D.C. (eds.): *Menopause and Aging.* U.S. Department of Health, Education and Welfare publication no. 73-319, 39, 1971.

Gallagher J.C., Nordin B.E.C.: Calcium metabolism and the menopause, in Curry A.S., Hewitt J.V. (eds.). *Biochemistry of Women: Clinical*

Concepts. CRC Press, Cleveland, 1974, pp. 145–175.

Genant H.K., Cann C.E., Ettinger B., et al.: Quantitative computed tomography of vertebral spongiosa: A sensitive method for detecting early bone loss after oophorectomy. *Ann. Intern. Med.* 97:699–705, 1982.

Gordon T., Kannel W.B., Hjortland M.C., et al.: Menopause and coronary heart disease: The Framingham Study. *Ann. Intern. Med.* 89:157–161, 1978.

Heaney R.P.: Estrogens and postmenopausal osteoporosis. *Clin. Obstet. Gynecol.* 19:791, 1976.

Herrmann H.W., Beach R.C.: The psychotropic properties of estrogens. *Pharmacopsychiatria* 11:164, 1978.

Hoover R., Gray L.A., Cole P., et al.: Menopausal estrogens and breast cancer. *N. Engl. J. Med.* 295:401, 1976.

Hulka B.S., Chambless L.E., Deubner D.C., et al.: Breast cancer and estrogen replacement therapy. *Am. J. Obstet. Gynecol.* 143:638, 1982.

Hulka B.S., Kaufman D.G., Fowler W.C. Jr., et al.: Predominance of early endometrial cancers after long-term estrogen use. *J.A.M.A.* 244: 2419–2422, 1980.

Gaddum-Rosse P., Rumery R.E., Blandan R.J., et al.: Studies on the mucosa of postmenopausal oviducts: Surface appearance, ciliary activity, and the effect of estrogen treatment. *Fertil. Steril.* 26:951–969, 1975.

Gambrell R.D. Jr.: Clinical use of progestins in the menopausal patient. *J. Reprod. Med.* 27 (suppl.):531–538, 1982.

Klaiber E.L., Broverman D.M., Vogel W., et al.: The use of steroids in depression, in Itil T.M., Laudahn G., Herrmann W.M. (eds.): *The Psychotropic Effects of Hormones.* Spectrum Publication Inc., New York, 1976.

Laufer L.R., Erlik Y., Meldrum D.R., et al.: Effect of clonidine on hot flashes in postmenopausal women. *Obstet. Gynecol.* 60:583–586, 1982.

Lindsay R., Herrington B.S.: Estrogens and osteoporosis. *Semin. Reprod. Endocrinol.* 1:55–67, 1983.

Lindsay R., Aitken J.M., Anderson J.B., et al.: Long-term prevention of postmenopausal osteoporosis by oestrogen. *Lancet* 1:1038, 1976.

Lindsay R., MacLean A., Kraszewski A., et al.: Bone response to termination of oestrogen treatment. *Lancet* 1:1325, 1978.

MacDonald P.C., Edman C.D., Hemsell D.L., et al.: Effect of obesity on conversion of plasma androstenedione to estrone in postmenopausal women with and without endometrial cancer. *Am. J. Obstet. Gynecol.* 130:448–455, 1978.

Masters W.H., Johnson V.E.: *Human Sexual Response.* Boston, Little Brown & Co., 1966.

Meldrum D.R., Erlik Y., Lu K.K.H., et al.: Objectively recorded hot flushes in patients with pituitary insufficiency. *J. Clin. Endocrinol. Metab.* 52:684–687, 1981.

Notelovitz M., Gudat J.C., Ware M.D., et al.: Lipids and lipoproteins in women after oophorectomy and the response to oestrogen therapy. *Br. J. Obstet. Gynecol.* 90:171–177, 1983.

Ortiz A., Hiroi M., Stanczyk F.Z., et al.: Serum medroxyprogesterone acetate (MPA) concentrations and ovarian function following intramuscular injection of depo-MPA. *J. Clin. Endocrinol. Metab.* 44:32, 1977.

Paganini-Hill A., Ross R.K., Gerkins V.R., et al.: Menopausal estrogen therapy and hip fractures. *Ann. Intern. Med.* 95:28–31, 1981.

Ravnikar V., Elkind-Hirsch K., Schiff I., et al.: Vasomotor flushes and the release of luteinizing hormone–releasing hormone in postmenopausal women. *Fertil. Steril.* 41:881–887, 1984.

Regestein Q.R., Schiff I., Tulchinsky D., et al.: Relationships among estrogen-induced psychological changes in hypogonadal women. *Psychosom. Med.* 43:147–155, 1981.

Reifenstein E.C. Jr., Albright, F.: The metabolic effects of steroid hormones in osteoporosis. *J. Clin. Invest.* 26:24, 1947.

Riggs B.L., Seeman E., Hodgson S.F., et al.: Effect of the fluoride/calcium regimen on vertebral fracture occurrence in postmenopausal osteoporosis. *N. Engl. J. Med.* 306:446–450, 1982.

Rosenberg L., Armstrong B., Phil D., et al.: Myocardial infarction and estrogen therapy in postmenopausal women. *N. Engl. J. Med.* 294:1256, 1976.

Rosenberg L., Hennekens C.H., Rosner B., et al.: Early menopause and the risk of myocardial infarction. *Am. J. Obstet. Gynecol.* 139:47–51, 1981.

Ross R.K., Paganini-Hill A.: Estrogen replacement therapy and coronary heart disease. *Semin. Reprod. Endocrinol.* 1:19–25, 1983.

Ross R.K., Mack T.M., Paganini-Hill A., et al.: Menopausal oestrogen therapy and protection from death from ischaemic heart disease. *Lancet* 1:858–860, 1981.

Ross R.K., Paganini-Hill A., Gerkins V.R., et al.: A case-control study of menopausal estrogen therapy and breast cancer. *J.A.M.A.* 243:1635, 1980.

Ryan K.J.: Estrogens and atherosclerosis. *Clin. Obstet. Gynecol.* 19:805, 1976.

Rybo G., Westerberg H.: Symptoms in the postmenopause—a population study. *Acta Obstet. Gynecol. Scand.* 50 (suppl. 9):25, 1971.

Schiff I.: The effects of conjugated estrogens on gonadotropins. *Fertil. Steril.* 33:333–334, 1980.

Schiff I., Wilson E.: Clinical aspects of aging of the female reproductive system, in Schneider E.L. (ed.): *Aging: 4. The Aging Reproductive System.* Raven Press, New York, 1978, pp. 9–28.

Schiff I, Regestein Q., Tulchinsky D., et al.: Effects of estrogens on sleep and psychological state of the hypogonadal woman. *J.A.M.A.* 242:2405–2407, 1979.

Schiff I., Tulchinsky D., Ryan K.J.: Vaginal absorption of estrone and estradiol-17β. *Fertil. Steril.* 28:1063–1066, 1977.

Schiff I., Tulchinsky D., Cramer D., et al.: Oral medroxyprogesterone treatment of postmenopausal symptoms. *J.A.M.A.* 244:1443–1445, 1980.

Schiff I., Tulchinsky D., Ryan K.J., et al.: Plasma estriol and its conjugates following oral and vaginal administration of estriol to postmenopausal women: Correlations with gonadotropin levels. *Am. J. Obstet. Gynecol.* 138:1137–1141, 1980.

Schiff I., Wentworth B., Koos B., et al.: Effect of estriol administration on the hypogonadal woman. *Fertil. Steril.* 30:278–282, 1978.

Smith D.C., Prentice R., Thompson D.J., et al.: Association of exogenous estrogens and endometrial carcinoma. *N. Engl. J. Med.* 293:1164, 1975.

Smith P.: Age changes in the female urethra. *Br. J. Urol.* 44:667, 1972.

Smith P., Roberts M., Slade N.: Urinary symptoms following hysterectomy. *Br. J. Urol.* 42:3, 1970.

Tataryn I.V., Lomax P., Meldrum D.R., et al.: Objective techniques for the assessment of postmenopausal hot flashes. *Obstet. Gynecol.* 57:340–344, 1981.

Tataryn I.V., Meldrum D.R., Lu K.H., et al.: LH, FSH and skin temperature during the menopausal hot flash. *J. Clin. Endocrinol. Metab.* 49:152–154, 1979.

Thomson J., Oswald I.: Effect of oestrogen on the sleep, mood, and anxiety of menopausal women. *Br. Med. J.* 2:1317, 1977.

Weiss N.S., Ure C.L., Ballard J.H., et al.: Decreased risk of fractures of the hip and lower forearm with postmenopausal use of estrogen. *N. Engl. J. Med.* 303:1195, 1980.

Whitehead M.I., Townsend P.T., Pryse-Davies J., et al.: Effects of various types and dosages of progestogens on the postmenopausal endometrium. *J. Reprod. Med.* 27(suppl.):539–548, 1982.

Williams A.R., Weiss N.S., Ure C.L., et al.: Effect of weight, smoking, and estrogen use on the risk of hip and forearm fractures in postmenopausal women. *Obstet. Gynecol.* 60:695–698, 1982.

Ziel H.K., Finkle W.D.: Increased risk of endometrial carcinoma among users of conjugated estrogens. *N. Engl. J. Med.* 293:1167, 1975.

CHAPTER SIXTEEN

Conception Control: Contraception, Sterilization, and Pregnancy Termination

PHILLIP G. STUBBLEFIELD, M.D.

THE WIVES OF North African desert tribesmen mixed gunpowder solution and foam from a camel's mouth and drank the potion. Egyptian women inserted pessaries made from crocodile dung into the vagina, or used tampons made from lint soaked in fermented acacia juice. The Chinese fried quicksilver in oil and drank it, or swallowed 14 live tadpoles three days after menstruation. Greek women of the second century made vaginal plugs of wool soaked in sour oil, honey, cedar gum, pomegranate, and fig pulp. These and similar practices were described in an account of contraceptive practices written by Soranos, a Greek physician living in Rome. He was quoted by scholars for the next 1,500 years (Himes, 1963). In the Middle Ages, potions were prepared from willow leaves, iron rust or slag, clay, and the kidney of a mule. European brides of the 17th century were instructed to sit on their fingers while riding in their coaches or to place roasted walnuts in the bosom, one for every barren year desired.

These are but a few of the more picturesque methods of "contraception" used in efforts to achieve family planning. Obviously, preventing pregnancy was as much a concern to the ancients as to modern men and women. A number of reasonably effective means for contraception have been known for a long time: the condom since the 16th century, the cervical cap since the early 19th century, the diaphragm and vaginal spermicides since the late 19th century, and intrauterine devices (IUDs) since early in the present century. The only truly new method is the use of female sex steroids to prevent pregnancy. During the 1960s the oral contraceptives (OCs) and the modern versions of the IUD largely supplanted the older, less effective methods in America. However, by the mid-1970s the rare but serious complications of these methods were appreciated and many couples turned back to the diaphragm or condom, or to surgical sterilization. A 1976 survey of the contraceptive practice of several thousand American couples is summarized in Table 16–1. Quite appropriately, contraceptive choice varied with age. Oral contraceptives were still first choice among women aged 29 years or younger, condoms were the second choice, while diaphragms and IUDs were about equal in popularity. For couples aged 30 years or over, surgical sterilization was the leading method of fertility control (Forrest and Henshaw, 1983). We suspect that 1983 data, soon to be analyzed will show less use of OCs and far greater use of the diaphragm. The availability of legal abortion since 1973 has meant that couples could bal-

583

TABLE 16–1.—PERCENTAGE DISTRIBUTION OF U.S. WOMEN AGED
15 TO 44 YEARS EXPOSED TO RISK OF UNINTENDED PREGNANCY,
BY CONTRACEPTIVE METHOD CURRENTLY USED, ACCORDING
TO AGE GROUP*

		AGE GROUP (YR)					
METHOD	TOTAL	15–19	20–24	25–29	30–34	35–39	40–44
Sterilization	32	†	6	25	43	62	61
Tubal	19	†	4	15	25	36	35
Vasectomy	13	†	2	10	17	26	26
Pill	27	44	50	34	17	8	5
IUD	6	3	6	8	9	6	4
Condom	12	21	13	12	12	8	11
Spermicides	4	7	3	3	4	3	5
Diaphragm	5	1	7	7	7	3	3
Withdrawal	3	5	3	3	2	2	2
Rhythm	2	†	1	1	1	3	2
Other	†	2	†	†	1	†	†
None	8	18	11	6	5	6	8
Total	100	100	100	100	100	100	100

*From Forrest J.D., Henshaw S.K.: *Fam. Plann. Perspect.* 15:157–166,
1983.
†Less than 0.5%.

ance the risk of pregnancy with less-effective
methods against the side effects and complications from the pill or IUDs.

As a background to the discussion of specific methods of contraception we will first address two concerns common to all methods:
effectiveness and safety.

EFFECTIVENESS

Four factors determine the effectiveness of
a contraceptive method: the user's fecundability, frequency of intercourse, the care with
which the method is used, and the biological
effectiveness of the method. Fecundability,
the probability of pregnancy when no contraception is used, is strongly influenced by age.
Girls are relatively less fecundable immediately after menarche because of the frequent
occurrence of anovulatory cycles; however,
their fecundability improves to reach a peak
in the late teens and early 20s and then declines steadily thereafter. The more frequently a couple has intercourse, the greater
the probability of conception. Proper use of
the contraceptive method is critical, and is
also strongly influenced by personal factors
such as age, race, education, socioeconomic

status, and religion, and by experience with a
particular contraceptive method. Thus it is
not surprising that the group most often using
legal abortion in the United States is composed of women 18 to 25 years old. A multi-
variate analysis of a large U.S. data set, the
1973 and 1976 National Surveys of Family
Growth, found that four factors accounted for
most of the difference in contraceptive failure
between different subgroups of our population: contraceptive method, intent (to delay a
later desired pregnancy or to prevent preg-

TABLE 16–2.—PERCENTAGE OF
WOMEN WHO EXPERIENCE
CONTRACEPTIVE FAILURE WITHIN
THE FIRST YEAR OF CONTRACEPTIVE
USE, BY METHOD, STANDARDIZED
BY INTENTION, INCOME, AND AGE
(JULY 1, 1970 TO JAN. 1, 1976)

METHOD	PERCENT
Pill	2.4
IUD	4.6
Condom	9.6
Spermicides	17.9
Diaphragm	18.6
Rhythm	23.7
Other	11.9

*From Schirm A.L., et al.: *Fam.
Plann. Perspect.* 14:68–75, 1982.

nancy altogether), age of the user, and family income (Schirm et al.). United States pregnancy rates for the different methods after standardization for these factors is given in Table 16–2.

The actual biological effectiveness of a method cannot be measured independent of the other factors, but can be estimated from large prospective studies with close medical supervision to insure that the couples are really using the method. Pregnancy rates with different methods as actually observed in a sample of 17,000 English couples are given in Table 16–3. As can be seen, the age of the woman was a major determinant of pregnancy rate. Still lower pregnancy rates have been obtained in some large studies, for example, 1 per 100 per year with the diaphragm in a large sample of young women from New York City reported by Lane and colleagues (1976). However, large population-based samples in the United States show much higher pregnancy rates, indicating that couples receiving only routine health care may experience more frequent contraceptive failure (Table 16–2). The difference between the best results and the usual results have to do with failure to use the method, and the differences are greater for methods that require a great deal of care (such as the oral contraceptive and the diaphragm) than for the IUD, which requires much less on the part of the user. Which pregnancy rates should be quoted in advising a patient: those from Table 16–2 or 16–3? The fairest approach is to give both rates as a range of what might be expected.

SAFETY

The alternatives to sexual abstinence are contraception and pregnancy. Estimates of the risk in using a contraceptive method must therefore include two components: health risk from complications of the contraceptive *and* the health risk from pregnancy, should the method fail. Both risks vary with the method, but also with the user. Age is a most important factor. Younger people have more contraceptive failures, but are less likely to die from complications of contraception or from pregnancy. A computer simulation of risks of death associated with different choices for fertility control, first performed by Tietze and Lewit, has been recently updated by Ory (Table 16–4). These calculations show that for women younger than 35 years, any contracep-

TABLE 16–3.—PREGNANCY RATES PER 100 WOMEN-YEARS FOR DIFFERENT METHODS OF CONTRACEPTION, BY AGE OF THE USER AND BY DURATION OF USE (OXFORD FAMILY PLANNING ASSOCIATION STUDY; N = 17,000)*

	DURATION			
	AGED 25–34 YR		AGED ≥35 YR	
METHOD	≤2 YR	≥4 YR	≤2 YR	≥4 YR
Oral contraceptive with 0.05 mg estrogen	0.25	0.09	0.17	0.10
Oral contraceptive with <0.05 mg estrogen	0.38	. . .	0.23	. . .
Progestin-only minipill	2.5	. . .	0.5	. . .
Diaphragm	5.5	2.3	2.8	0.8
Condom	6.0	3.6	2.9	0.7
Lippes loop C	2.4	2.0	1.1	0.6
Lippes loop D	2.3	2.3	1.8	0.4
Saf-T-Coil	2.3	1.4	1.6	0.5
Cu-7 IUD	3.1	. . .	0.6	. . .
Female sterilization	0.45	0.0	0.08	0.09
Male sterilization	0.08	0.0	0.0	0.03

*(From Vessey M., et al.: *Lancet* 1:841–843, 1982.)

TABLE 16–4.—CUMULATIVE RISK OF MORTALITY PER 100,000 NONSTERILE WOMEN, BY FERTILITY CONTROL METHOD, ACCORDING TO AGE GROUP*†

	AGE GROUP (YR)							
REGIMEN	15–19	20–24	25–29	30–34	35–39	40–44	15–44	15–34
None	35	37	46	74	129	141	462	192
Abortion	3	6	7	10	9	6	41	26
Pill/nonsmoker	3	3	5	10	70	160	251	21
Pill/smoker	12	18	34	68	257	588	977	132
IUD	6	6	6	7	10	10	45	25
Condom	6	8	4	1	2	2	23	19
Diaphragm	10	6	6	6	11	14	53	28
Condom plus abortion	<1	<1	<1	<1	<1	<1	1	1
Rhythm	12	8	8	8	14	18	68	36

*Assumes that sexual activity begins at age 15 years, then multiplies annual risk by 5.
†(From Ory H.W.: *Fam. Plann. Perspect.* 15:57–63, 1983.)

tive method is safer than no method. However, because of a risk for heart attack and stroke with OCs, which increases with age, and is dramatically increased by smoking cigarettes, use of OCs is ill advised beyond age 35 years for smokers and age 40 years for nonsmokers. At any age, the safest method is diaphragm or condom backed by early, legal abortion should the method fail. This is because there is no method-related risk of death from condom or diaphragm use, and the risk of death from early abortion in the United States is only 1 per 100,000 abortions. Ory has also calculated the cumulative risk of reproduction: risk of contraception used to delay pregnancy until a stated age, then risk of bearing one child, plus the risk of a subsequent surgical sterilization by tubal ligation (Table 16–5). At any age, the major component of risk is not from contraception, but from the pregnancies, and this risk increases rapidly with maternal age. Specific methods of contraception, their mechanism of action, advantages, disadvantages, and use in clinical practice are discussed herein. By making judicious choices at different ages, maximal benefit for least risk can be obtained. Thus, a woman might choose to use the pill when she is young because she needs the excellent protection from pregnancy that it affords, is at

TABLE 16–5.—CUMULATIVE MORTALITY RISK PER 100,000 WOMEN USING VARIOUS FERTILITY CONTROL METHODS, BEARING ONE CHILD, AND UNDERGOING TUBAL STERILIZATION, BY FERTILITY CONTROL METHOD, ACCORDING TO AGE AT FIRST BIRTH*

METHOD OF FERTILITY CONTROL	AGE AT FIRST BIRTH (YR)				
	20	25	30	35	40
Abortion	19	27	45	82	126
Pill/nonsmoker	19	25	42	79	185
Pill/smoker	28	49	94	190	482
IUD	22	31	49	83	127
Condom	26	33	52	86	113
Diaphragm/spermicide	26	35	52	86	132
Condom plus abortion	16	20	32	59	94
Rhythm	28	39	58	94	144
Mortality risk from bearing the one wanted child	12	15	27	54	89

*(From Ory H.W.: *Fam. Plann. Perspect.* 15:57–63, 1983.)

low risk for serious complications from pill use, and will extract maximal protection against future gynecologic cancer. She might use any of the other methods to space the births of her children during her late 20s and early 30s, and then either she or her husband obtain surgical sterilization when the family is completed.

CONDOMS

During the 16th century, the Italian anatomist Fallopius, for whom the fallopian tubes are named, devised a linen sheath for the penis, an effective forerunner of the condom. Madame de Sevigne, in a letter to her daughter in 1671, called the condom an "armor against enjoyment and a spider web against danger." Casanova (1725–1798), in his *Memoirs,* indicated he used condoms both to prevent venereal disease and pregnancy. He was not a fan, however: "I do not care to shut myself up in a piece of dead skin in order to prove I am perfectly alive." The English referred to condoms as "French letters," but on the continent they were thought to be of English origin. Casanova wrote of "preservatives the English have invented to put the fair sex under shelter from all fear" (Himes, 1963, p. 195). Condoms were used extensively in brothels during the 18th century. Some condoms of that period were recently discovered in a locked box in an English country home. Made around 1790 of animal intestine, they were of excellent quality (Peel, 1963). Condoms have been made in large quantities since the vulcanization of rubber was developed in the middle of the 19th century.

As used today, the condom is a covering for the penis and is usually made of rubber, although condoms made from animal intestine are still sold, and are preferred by some for being better at transmitting sensation. The condom captures and holds the seminal fluid, thus preventing its deposition in the vagina. The condom has the proved advantage, shared with other barriers, of reducing risk for sexually transmitted diseases and cervical cancer.

Objections to the condom include the possibiity that it may rupture and allow sperm to enter the vagina, that putting it on just prior to penetration interferes with spontaneity, and, most important, that the condom reduces sensation for both partners. We suspect that the latter problem contributes greatly to nonuse and much more to unwanted pregnancies than does the very occasional rupture of a condom. Indeed, until recently, most U.S. condoms were thicker, stronger, and less able to transmit sensation than necessary. Thinner condoms are made and sold in Japan and are the leading method of contraception in that country. Recently, condoms lubricated with a spermicide to improve efficacy are being sold in the United States.

COITUS INTERRUPTUS

Coitus interruptus is perhaps the oldest of the effective contraceptive methods. It is mentioned in the Bible when, in Genesis 38:7–10, Onan is cursed for "spilling his seed." Withdrawal of the penis just prior to ejaculation takes a great deal of willpower, and neither the man nor his partner know until the last minute whether he will be able to do so. Another concern is that the pre-ejaculatory excretion of urethral fluids with sexual excitement may occasionally contain live sperm that could produce conception even without vaginal ejaculation. The penis must be completely withdrawn both from the vagina and from the external genitalia, as pregnancy has occurred from ejaculation on the female external genitalia without penetration. Other alterations of sexual behavior to prevent conception are oral-genital lovemaking and anal intercourse. Anal intercourse is common in some parts of the world as a means of preserving technical virginity as well as avoiding pregnancy.

RHYTHM METHOD

The rhythm method consists of periodic abstinence in an attempt to avoid intercourse during the time that the woman may be ovulating. Two versions of the rhythm method are presently taught: the ovulation method and the symptothermal method. The ovulation method attempts to make use of the fact that many women can note the increased mucus made by the cervical glands in the days prior to ovulation just by feeling at the vaginal opening with their fingers. Sexual abstinence is practiced from the first day the mucus is noted until four days after the "peak" day when maximal mucus is noted. With the symptothermal method, the first day of abstinence is predicted by subtracting 21 from the length of the shortest menstrual cycle in the preceding six months, or the first day mucus is detected, whichever comes first. The end of the fertile period is predicted by use of basal body temperature. The woman takes her temperature every morning and resumes intercourse three days after the thermal shift, the rise in body temperature that signals that the corpus luteum is producing progesterone, and, hence, that ovulation has occurred. Sadly, despite claims by advocates of near-perfect results, formal trials of the rhythm methods have been disappointing. In the study of Wade et al., the symptothermal method was best, with pregnancy rates of 9.4 per 100 woman-years, while the pregnancy rate with the ovulation method was very high (24.8 per 100 woman-years). Even a week's abstinence around the time of actual ovulation is no insurance against fertilization, for sperm may survive several days in the female genital tract. Pregnancies have been observed to occur after a single coitus seven days prior to apparent ovulation indicated by basal body temperature. Use of the rhythm method has been reported to increase fetal risk. Avoidance of intercourse at midcycle means that when conception does occur, it is likely to involve either old sperm or old ova. Guerrero and colleagues have shown that such conceptions more often lead to spontaneous abortion than do conceptions from midcycle intercourse, and others have linked rhythm failures to a higher than usual rate of fetal malformations (Guerrero and Rojas, 1975).

LACTATION

Ovulation is suppressed for a variable period of time in women who are nursing their infants. The duration of the antiovulatory effect is variable, but is very strongly influenced by the frequency and duration of nursing. Women who do not nurse will have a menstrual period from one to three months after birth, but women who nurse for 18 months experience amenorrhea until eight to 13 months after birth. Ovulation and menstruation eventually return even among women who continue to lactate, and the onset of ovulation in an individual woman cannot be predicted. An additional method of contraception should be used as soon as other foods are started to supplement lactation because the infant will nurse less and ovulation will occur (McCann et al., 1981).

VAGINAL CONTRACEPTION

Vaginal spermicides are preparations combining a spermicidal chemical with a base of cream, jelly, aerosol foam, foaming tablet, or suppository. Suppositories made of quinine in cocoa butter were made and sold in England in the last century and continued in use until recently. The active ingredient of modern preparations is a surface active chemical that immobilizes sperm, usually nonoxynol 9 or octoxynol. The best results, 5 pregnancies per 100 woman-years, are usually obtained by aerosol foam–based spermicides, probably because they disperse instantly to fill the vagina, while melting suppositories may melt incompletely and fail to cover the cervical os with spermicide.

The possible hazards of the spermicidal chemicals has been of great concern in recent years even though the most-used spermicide, nonoxynol 9 is not absorbed from the human vagina (Malyk, 1983). In 1981 Jick and colleagues reported that major malformations were increased among infants born after failure of spermicides. Several much larger studies have found no such hazard (Shapiro et al.,

1982). In the article by Linn and colleagues, from Boston, the rate of major malformations among offspring of nonusers of contraception was 3.6% in a sample of 12,440 women interviewed just after delivery. The rates of major malformation among offspring of 703 diaphragm users and 199 foam users who reported contraceptive failure were 2.0%. Oral contraceptive failure was associated with a 1.8% rate of malformation among 223 births studied, and the offspring of those 752 using other methods (condoms, withdrawal, rhythm or IUD) had a malformation rate of 3.7% (Linn et al., 1983). As a general rule, when small studies report a finding not confirmed in larger, better-controlled studies, one should believe the larger studies; hence, nonoxynol 9 and related compounds may be presumed safe at present. Abortion of a desired pregnancy should not be advised solely on the basis of failure of spermicidal contraception.

VAGINAL BARRIERS

The vaginal diaphragm that is widely used in the United States is but one of four types of rubber vaginal barriers that existed at the beginning of the 20th century. All are still made and sold in England (Fig 16–1). Both cervical caps and vaginal diaphragms were used in the United States through the 1950s, but only the diaphragm continued in production, probably because it was easier to fit, insert, and remove. The cervical cap was rediscovered by American women who went to England, and has been reintroduced into the United States, largely through the efforts of feminist womens' health centers.

The vaginal barriers deserve serious attention. When used consistently they can be highly effective. They are safe and they offer noncontraceptive benefits. Women who use diaphragms or condoms are less likely than nonusers to develop pelvic inflammatory disease (Kelaghan et al., 1982). They also offer some protection against cervical cancer. Harris et al., reported the relative risk of severe dysplasia among users of condoms or diaphragms to be 0.4 at five to nine years of use and only 0.2 when the barriers had been used for ten years or more (1980).

Diaphragm

The diaphragm consists of a circular metal spring covered with fine latex rubber. There are several types as determined by the spring rim: coil, flat, or arcing. Coil-spring and flat-spring diaphragms become a flat oval when compressed for insertion. Arching diaphragms form an arc, or half moon, when compressed and, in our experience, are the easiest to insert correctly. Diaphragms are made in diameters that increase by 5-mm increments from 50 to 90 mm. Most women can be fitted with one in the middle range, from 65 to 75 mm. Too large a diaphragm will produce discomfort and even vaginal ulcerations; however, the actual effect of diaphragm size or type on pregnancy rates is unknown. The practitioner must not only fit the diaphragm for the patient, but must instruct her in its insertion, and verify by examination that she

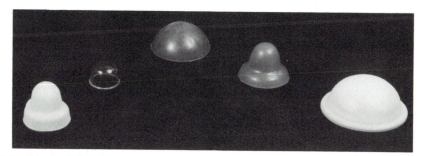

Fig 16–1.—Vaginal barriers *(left to right):* Prentiff cavity rim cervical cap, plastic cap, vault cap, vimule, and vaginal diaphragm. (Courtesy of Dr. Stubblefield.)

can insert it correctly to cover the cervix and upper vagina. In present times, the diaphragm is always used in combination with a spermicide; however, the contribution of the spermicide to pregnancy prevention seems never to have been determined. Customarily a teaspoon or so of water-soluble spermicidal jelly or cream is placed inside the diaphragm prior to use. If intercourse will be repeated, addition spermicidal jelly should be inserted into the vagina without removing the diaphragm. The diaphragm is left in place at least six hours after intercourse, then removed, washed, dried, and put away until needed again. It should never be dusted with talc, as the practice of dusting the female genitals with talc has been associated with ovarian cancer.

The Cervical Cap

As there is no present U.S. manufacturer, cervical caps are imported from England, and must be prescribed by a physician registered as an investigator and following a protocol approved by the Food and Drug Administration. The cap is much smaller than the diaphragm, ranging in external diameter from 22 to 35 mm, has no metal rim, and covers only the cervix. While it is harder to fit the cap and instruction in its use takes more time, women who have already learned to use the vaginal diaphragm readily learn to use the cap. The advantage of the cap over the diaphragm is that it can be left in place several days and hence is more convenient. Formerly, caps were left in place for the entire interval between the menses. Caps are used with spermicide, but again, the contribution of the spermicide to the efficacy is not known. A recent trial with the Prentiff cap by Koch in Boston found a pregnancy rate of 8 per 100 among his first 400 patients (Koch, 1982).

HAZARDS OF THE DIAPHRAGM.—Diaphragm use appears to somewhat increase the risk for bladder infections, probably because it rests under the urethra and may hinder clearing of the bacteriuria that inevitably results from vaginal intercourse. Prolonged wearing of the diaphragm to allow for multiple acts of intercourse may be especially likely to produce cystitis. As of early 1984, 18 cases of toxic shock have been linked to diaphragm use (*M.M.W.R.*, 1984). Whether this represents causation or only accidental association is unclear, as a formal epidemiologic study comparing toxic shock cases with controls found no increased risk from diaphragm use (Davis et al., 1980).

The cervical cap, while it is worn for several days at a time, does not compress the urethra, and has not been associated with cystitis.

Sponge and Spermicide

One of the more useful of the ancient methods of contraception was the natural sea sponge, dipped in salt water and inserted into the vagina as a barrier. A new version combines medical grade urethane sponge with the spermicide, nonoxynol 9 (Fig 16–2). The new sponge (trade name, Today), is left in place for up to 24 hours, and contains sufficient spermicide for multiple acts of intercourse. It is sold without a prescription and at a modest price, and thus offers a female equivalent of

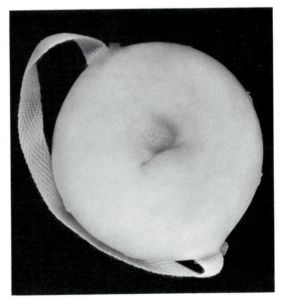

Fig 16–2.—The Today contraceptive sponge. (Courtesy of Dr. Stubblefield.)

the condom in availability and convenience. In the U.S. trials, the pregnancy rate was 10 per 100 women-years, which was as good as the diaphragm in the same trials, but much less effective than the one to three per 100 women-years obtained in other diaphragm trials. By early 1984, four cases of toxic shock had occurred among sponge users, an estimated attack rate of 10 per 100,000 users per year (*M.M.W.R.*, 1984). Whether this association implies causation is not yet clear.

INTRAUTERINE DEVICES

The first IUDs were made by Ota in Japan and Graffenberg in Germany more than 50 years ago, but widespread use awaited the development of the modern, flexible plastic devices. Of all the models devised, the Lippes loop designed by Dr. Jack Lippes of Buffalo, N.Y., in the 1960s remains the standard against which others are judged. Present plastic IUDs are stretched into a straight rod for insertion through the cervical canal without need for dilation, and then resume their original loop, spiral, or "T" shape when released into the uterine cavity.

Mechanism of Action

The mechanism of action of IUDs is still not entirely clear. Our current concept is that IUDs provoke a low-grade inflammatory response in the endometrium that results in formation of a sort of "biological foam," which contains strands of fibrin, phagocytic cells, and proteolytic enzymes released from these cells into the uterine cavity. Copper IUDs continuously release a small amount of the metal, producing a still greater inflammatory response. All IUDs stimulate the formation of prostaglandins within the uterus, consistent with both smooth-muscle contraction and inflammation. Scanning electron microscopic studies of the endometrium in IUD-wearing women show alterations in the surface morphology of cells, especially of the microvilli of ciliated cells (El Badrawi et al., 1981). There are major alterations in the composition of proteins within the uterine cavity, and new

proteins and proteinase inhibitors are found in washings from the uterus (Umapathysivam and Jones, 1980). The altered intrauterine environment interferes with implantation of the fertilized ova, but also interferes with sperm passage through the uterus, and, hence, reduces the chance of fertilization. A laparoscopic study was successful about half the time in obtaining sperm in washings from the fallopian tubes of control women at midcycle, while among women wearing IUDs there were no sperm in the tubal washings (Habashi et al., 1980). Women who wear IUDs are *less* likely to experience an ectopic pregnancy than nonusers of contraception, but should pregnancy occur in an IUD wearer, it will be ectopic in about 5% of cases. This is because the fallopian tubes are less well protected against pregnancy than is the uterus.

The huge clinical trial reported by Tietze and Lewit (1970) established that larger versions of the same IUD (Lippes loop C or D) have lower pregnancy rates and lower rates of expulsion, but more removals for pain and bleeding than do smaller versions of the same devices (Lippes loop A or B). This observation and the discovery by Zipper that certain metal wires inhibit fertility when placed inside the uterus led to the development of the small IUD wrapped with copper wire, the copper T* and Cu-7 (Tatum, 1982). Another approach to improving the efficacy of a small IUD was the development of the progesterone-releasing T-shaped IUD (Progestasert). Both of these medicated IUDs have lower pregnancy rates than the unmedicated "T" devices, but are not consistently superior to the older Lippes loop C or D. Intrauterine devices presently sold in the United States are pictured in Figure 16–3.

The great advantage of the IUD is that it requires only a simple office visit for insertion of the device, to provide for several years of convenient contraception. The main difficulty with IUDs is not the pregnancy rate of 2 to 4 per 100 woman-years, or the expulsion rate of

---

*Tatum-T is the U.S. trademark for the copper T 200.

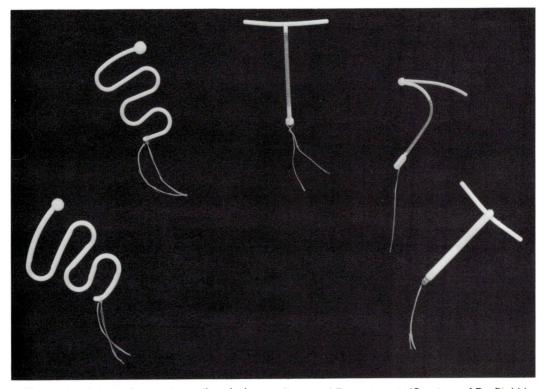

Fig 16–3.—Intrauterine contraceptive devices presently sold in the United States *(left to right):* Lippes loop D, Lippes loop B, copper T 200, Cu-7, and Progestasert. (Courtesy of Dr. Stubblefield.)

3 to 15 per 100 women-years, but rather the continuing problem of removal for medical reasons: excessive menstrual bleeding or pain. Rates for medical removal range from 5 to 20 per 100 women-years. In general, the IUD is better suited for older women who have had some pregnancies than for younger women who have not. Younger women have higher pregnancy rates, more expulsions, and more removals for medical reasons. For this reason and because of concerns about serious infection and later fertility, many physicians will not insert IUDs in nulliparous women.

IUDs and Infection

Modern plastic IUDs were at first perceived as a near perfect contraceptive and rapidly became of great importance in family planning programs worldwide. Initial enthusiasm was soon tempered because of prob-

lems with bleeding and pain; a syndrome of chronic progressive endometritis in IUD wearers was recognized (Burnhill, 1972). Intrauterine contraception suffered a serious setback when, in the early 1970s, it was appreciated that IUDs could be associated with death from infection if pregnancy occurred. Though one particular IUD, the Dalkon Shield figured importantly in initial reports of sepsis, other IUDs were also implicated and strong associations between IUD use and pelvic inflammatory disease (PID) in nonpregnant women was found. Laboratory studies revealed that the multifilament tail of the Dalkon Shield could act as a wick, pulling bacteria from the vagina into the uterus, and the device was withdrawn from the market. More recently, good epidemiologic studies of PID have established the precise relation between different types of IUDs and PID. A recent U.S. study found the relative risk for PID among IUD users compared with non-users of contraception to be 8.3 for the Dalkon Shield, 2.2 for the Progestasert, 1.9 for the Cu-7, 1.3 for the Saf-T-Coil, and 1.2 for the Lippes loop (*M.M.W.R.*, 1983). Mishell and colleagues (1966) demonstrated that bacteria were introduced into the uterine cavity with insertion, but found that the uterus soon sterilized itself. More recently, Sparks and colleagues (1981) found bacteria in the uterus after insertion of IUDs with tails, but none when tailless versions of the same devices had been inserted. Early IUDs had no tails, but tails were added to the plastic devices to facilitate insertion and removal and to allow early detection if expulsion had occurred. Risk of infection from modern IUDs with monofilament tails clearly is much less than seen with the wicklike tail of the Dalkon Shield, but perhaps future work should again evaluate whether the tail is needed at all.

Clinical Management of IUDs

Contraindications to IUD use include pregnancy, history of PID, undiagnosed genital bleeding, uterine anomalies (although a woman with separate uterine cavities might wear two IUDs) and fibroid tumors of more than small size. Intrauterine devices have usually been inserted just after menstruation, but White and colleagues' large study (1980) found competing risks depending on the timing of insertion in the menstrual cycle: more expulsions with postmenstrual insertion, more removals for pain and bleeding but fewer expulsions with later insertions. Actual insertion is preceded by a pelvic examination to determine uterine size and position. The cervix is then exposed with a speculum, grasped with a tenaculum, and gently pulled downward to straighten the angle between cervical canal and uterine cavity; then the IUD, previously loaded into its inserter, is gently introduced through the canal and the inserter is withdrawn. Failure to use a tenaculum increases risk of perforation. Syncope from bradycardia associated with manipula-

tions of the cervix is common, especially in women of low parity, and many physicians offer paracervical block with local anesthesia or premedicate the patient with atropine. Of the IUDs available in the United States, the copper devices are preferable to the small Lippes loops, A nd B, and hence would be selected for young women or women of low parity. Women who have had a child can tolerate the C or D Lippes loop, and patient and physician are free to choose between these and the copper devices. The Progestasert has not been popular because of its expense and the need for annual replacement, but does offer the prospect of reduced, rather than increased, menstrual flow.

Intrauterine devices are readily inserted immediately after an abortion. The safety of this treatment has been amply demonstrated (Rosenfield and Castadot, 1974). Insertion soon after childbirth is especially desired in the third world countries, but expulsion of present devices is frequent after postpartum insertion. The worst time for IUD insertions is probably the conventional six weeks or so after childbirth. By this time, the cervical canal has closed down, but the uterus is still soft, and risk of perforation is increased.

Perforation of IUDs through the uterine wall generally only occurs at insertion, though it usually is not recognized until pregnancy occurs, infection develops, or the IUD string disappears as the partially perforated IUD is pulled upward through the uterine wall by uterine contractions. An exception to this is the downward migration of "T" or "7"-shaped devices, which have at times eroded through the posterior wall of the cervix into the vagina. Suspected perforation is managed by removing the IUD. When, as is usually the case, mere traction on the strings is not sufficient, laparoscopy is indicated.

Lost IUD

Whenever the IUD strings cannot be found · on examination, the cervical canal should be gently probed to find them. If this maneuver is not successful, ultrasound is performed to identify the location of the IUD as either inside the uterus or inside the pelvic cavity. A simple roentgenogram will also suffice, but it is necessary to first mark the location of the uterine cavity, either by inserting another IUD of a different shape, placing a uterine sound, or injecting contrast material as for a hysterosalpingogram. If the location of the device is intrauterine, it can be left in place or removed by dilation and curettage with hysteroscopy, depending on the circumstances.

Duration of Use

Annual rates of pregnancy, expulsions, and medical removals *decrease* with each year of use (Tietze and Lewit, 1970), and most of the risk of PID is in the first few months after insertion (Burkman, 1981). Hence, a woman who has had no problem with her IUD by year 4, for example, is very unlikely to experience problems in the subsequent year. Current recommendations are to replace the copper T 200 and Cu-7 at three-year intervals. However, large studies have shown the T 200 still effective after five and six years, with fewer pregnancies or expulsions in the sixth year than in the fifth (Zipper et al., 1972).

The supply of progesterone in the Progestasert becomes exhausted after one year, and it must be replaced. The life span of plastic devices such as the Lippes loop is not known, but many women have worn them for a decade or longer. Lippes and Zielezny reported ten-year statistics for loops C and D. The ten-year cumulative pregnancy rate was only 5 per 100, and 32% of the original group were still wearing their IUDs after ten years (Lippes and Zielezny, 1975). The probability of colonization of the cervical canal with *Actinomyces* increases with duration of use, and this organism has occasionally been associated with PID. Diagnosis of *Actinomyces* infection by cervical cytologic examination yields false-positive results, but until it is clear that colonization is not harmful, we prefer to look for this organism in long-term wearers of IUDs and to remove the IUD when *Actinomyces* is found. If *Actinomyces* is not present, and the wearer has no pelvic pain or excessive bleeding and wishes to continue intrauterine contraception, we see no reason that she not continue until menopause.

Management of IUDs in Pregnancy

If the IUD strings are visible, the IUD should be removed as soon as pregnancy is detected. There is a twofold increased risk of spontaneous abortion following removal, but the prospect for later septic abortion, premature rupture of the membranes, and premature birth is much greater if the device is left in than when it is removed or expelled (Tatum et al., 1976). Where the strings are not visible, an ultrasound examination should localize the IUD and determine whether an unnoticed expulsion has occurred. If the IUD is present, an informed decision should be made by the patient, with an awareness of the risks of all options, whether to continue the pregnancy or elect termination. She must be aware of the risks of septic abortion, including death (particularly if the device has a multifilament tail), should the pregnancy continue with the device in place. If the patient elects to continue the pregnancy she must be closely observed. She should be advised to report all abnormal symptoms, such as flulike syndrome, fever, abdominal cramping and pain, or bleeding, because symptoms may be insidious. Death has been known to occur within 72 hours of onset of symptoms. At the earliest sign of sepsis, high-dose antibiotic therapy effective against aerobic and anaerobic organisms should be started and the uterus promptly evacuated. If PID is suspected in the nonpregnant patient the IUD should be removed and adequate antibiotic therapy begun immediately.

IUDs and Fertility

Intrauterine devices somewhat increase the wearers risk for PID, and PID increases the risk for subsequent infertility and ectopic pregnancy. Nonetheless, the large Oxford Study found that women gave birth just as promptly after IUD removal as they did after discontinuing use of the diaphragm (Vessey et al., 1976).

New IUDs

The copper T, Cu-7 and Progestasert are considered second-generation IUDs. Third-generation IUDs, already available in Europe and Canada, offer still greater improvement, and for the first time, randomized clinical trials show some of these to be superior to the Lippes loop. The copper T 380A, which has sleeves of copper on its arms instead of copper wire, had a total four-year pregnancy rate of only 1.9% in one large trial and thus is close to oral contraceptives in effectiveness (Sivin and Tatum, 1981). The Nova T, another version of the familiar copper T had a three-year cumulative pregnancy rate of only 1.9%, compared with 5.0% for the copper T-200, the device sold in the United States (Nigren et al., 1981). The Progestasert releases small amounts of natural progesterone, sufficient to produce endometrial atrophy and good contraception, but not enough to block ovulation. Experimental devices releasing the very potent progestin, norgestrel, can block ovulation (Nilsson et al., 1980).

HORMONAL CONTRACEPTION

In 1940, Sturgis and Albright reported that injections of estrogen blocked ovulation in women; however, the implications of this discovery for contraception awaited the synthesis of the orally active progestins in the 1950s (Rock et al., 1956). The progestins (progesteronelike hormones) that were first used contained trace amounts of estrogen as a by-product of synthesis. These compounds were highly effective in producing amenorrhea and preventing conception. The pure progestins that were produced subsequently also prevented conception, but produced an unacceptable bleeding pattern with irregular spotting and staining. The estrogen was added back intentionally, and the modern combined oral contraceptive (OC) resulted. Still, these compounds would have remained curiosities in search of medical uses had it not been for the determined efforts of the family-planning pioneer, Margaret Sanger, who recognized the enormous potential of hormonal contraception to free women from the slavery of unplanned and/or unwanted reproduction. She convinced the scientists to proceed with large-scale human trials and raised the funds to support the trials from private charity. The pill was so successful that by 1980, 50 million women were using it worldwide.

The estrogen in combination OCs is either ethinyl estradiol, or its methyl ester, mestranol. Steroid hormones must be bound by a cytosol receptor and carried into the nucleus of the cell in order to have an effect. Human estrogen receptors have little affinity for mestranol, and it must be converted to ethinyl estradiol by the liver before it can have an effect. In animal assays, ethinyl estradiol is somewhat more potent than mestranol, but in doses presently used for hormonal contraception the two appear equivalent in humans (Goldzieher et al., 1978).

The progestins used in OCs in the United States are pictured in Figure 16–4. Progestins can be divided into two or three groups based on their chemical structure. The 19-nor steroids are called estrane progestins and are structurally most similar to androgen. The other major group is the 17-acetoxy progestins, called pregnane progestins because of their structural similarity to progesterone. The pregnane progestins are bound by progesterone receptors. However, of the 19-nor compounds, only norethindrone and norgestrel have high affinity for progesterone receptors. The other 19-nor compounds are converted to norethindrone (Rozenbaum, 1982). Norgestrel is considerably different from the other 19-nor compounds in biological effect and in structure, and is described as a gonane progestin. The progestins differ in their progestational potency, in their estrogenic activity, their androgenic activity and their glucocorticoid activity. Most of the 19-nor

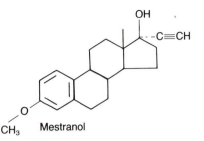

Ethinyl estradiol

Mestranol

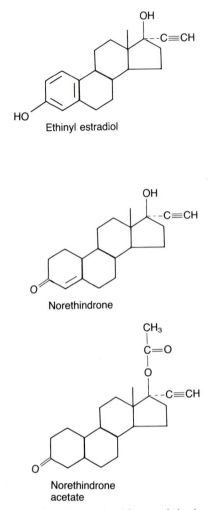

Norethindrone

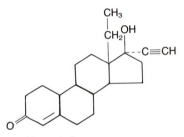

Norgestrel

Norethindrone
acetate

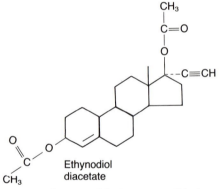

Ethynodiol
diacetate

Fig 16–4.—Synthetic steroids used in low-dose oral contraceptives sold in the United States today. Estrogens: ethinyl estradiol and mestranol. Progestins: norethindrone, norethindrone acetate, norgestrel, and ethynodiol diacetate.

progestins will bind to androgen receptors. Norethindrone has mild androgenic activity while norethynodrel has none, and indeed has some estrogenic activity. Norgestrel has much greater progestational and androgenic potency than the others. It exists as two stereoisomers. Only levonorgestrel is biologically active.

Mechanism of Action

Combination OCs suppress ovulation. The first OCs contained much higher doses of hor-mones than necessary for this purpose. A daily dose of 10 mg of the progestin noreth-indrone will block ovulation, as will 80 μg of ethinyl estradiol or mestranol (Goldzieher, 1982). Modern OCs contain much less hor-mone, as for example, 1 mg of norethindrone combined with only 35 μg of ethinyl estra-diol, yet are still able to prevent ovulation be-cause of the effect of the two hormones taken together, an example of synergism. Oral con-traceptives diminish the ability of the pitu-itary gland to synthesize gonadotropins when stimulated by gonadotropin-releasing hormone (GNRH) (Dericks-Tan et al., 1983). The result is very low levels of follicle-stimulating hormone (FSH) and luteinizing hormone (LH), hence, no stimulation of the ovaries and no ovulation. Women taking OCs do exhibit occasional surges of FSH and LH, but these are rarely sufficient to produce follicular maturation and ovulation. Examination at surgery of the ovaries of women taking combined OCs shows them to be small, inactive, and without any recent corpora lutea. As noted, progestins taken by themselves in high enough doses will also block ovulation. The effect of these preparations on gonadotropins is different. Follicle-stimulating hormone and LH are only moderately suppressed; there is some ovarian follicular activity with production of estradiol, but ovarian estrogen surges are not answered by pituitary release of the large amount of LH needed for ovulation. It is as if the progestins blocked the positive-feedback response of estrogens on the hypothalamus and pituitary (Goldzieher, 1982). In addition to blocking ovulation, combination OCs prevent conception by producing scant, dry cervical mucus, and an atrophic uterine lining. These same effects are produced by low doses of progestins without estrogen, the so-called minipills. Preparations containing for example, 0.35 mg of norethindrone per day, do not block ovulation and are thought to inhibit fertility because of the effects on cervical mucus, endometrium, and perhaps on tubal motility or corpus luteum function.

Presently, combination OCs containing only 30 to 35 μg of ethinyl estradiol combined with a low dose of one of the 19-nor progestins (see Table 16–2) are favored in the United States. The preparation containing 50 μg of estrogen are slightly more effective, but use-effectiveness pregnancy rates with all the combination OCs in the 30- to 50-μg dose range are well below 1 per 100 women-years. The progestin-only minipills have significantly higher pregnancy rates, 2 to 3 per 100 women-years, and are comparable to IUDs in use effectiveness (see Table 16–2). As we shall see, higher-dose progestin regimens have pregnancy rates comparable to those of the combined OCs.

Risks of Hormonal Contraception

By 1967, case reports of venous thrombosis, pulmonary embolism, and stroke among women taking combination OCs began to appear, and by the early 1970s several large studies confirmed these hazards of OC use (Royal College of General Practitioners, 1977; Vessey et al., 1976; Ramcharan et al., 1981). The relation of OC use to heart attack was at first unclear, but by 1975 a definite connection was demonstrated by Mann and Inman and the risk found to increase substantially with age. Subsequent reanalysis of the Mann and Inman data by Jain found that most of the risk for heart attack was among pill users who were also cigarette smokers (Jain, 1976). The influence of age and cigarette smoking on risk of death from vascular disease (primarily heart attack and stroke) is given in Table 16–6. Risk is significant for smokers after age 40 years, and is detectable even at age 35 years. There is apparent risk of death for nonsmokers from pill use as well; however, the risk is small, and even in this huge sample the risk ratios for nonsmokers were not statistically significant at any age. Risk of vascular disease in women is strongly influenced by other personal factors such as obesity, hypertension, high blood cholesterol levels, and nondrinking of alcohol (Table 16–7). Surprisingly, pill use by itself was not related to heart attack risk in the American Walnut Creek Study reported in Table 16–7, in contradistinction to the British data, but was related to risk for venous thrombosis, pulmonary embolism, and stroke. Duration of use has not been important in determining risk in the British studies (Layde et al., 1981). However, past users have been found to have some persistent risk (Slone et al., 1981).

The blood type of the user may affect risk of thrombosis from OC use. Women with blood type A or AB are more likely to suffer

TABLE 16–6.—MORTALITY RATES PER 100,000 WOMEN-YEARS, NUMBER OF DEATHS FROM CIRCULATORY DISEASES, AND RELATIVE RISK, BY AGE GROUPS AND SMOKING STATUS*†

| AGE GROUP (YR) AND SMOKING STATUS | DEATHS FROM CIRCULATORY DISEASE | | | | RELATIVE RISK (95% CONFIDENCE LIMITS) |
| | EVER-USERS | | CONTROLS | | |
	RATE	NO.	RATE	NO.	
15–25					
Nonsmokers	0.0	0	0.0	0	. . .
Smokers	10.5	1	0.0	0	
25–34					
Nonsmokers	4.4	2	2.7	1	1.6 (0.2–17.4)
Smokers	14.2	6	4.2	1	3.4 (0.5–24.6)
35–44					
Nonsmokers	21.5	7	6.4	2	3.3 (0.8–14.7)
Smokers	63.4	18	15.2	3	4.2 (1.4–12.8)
≥45					
Nonsmokers	52.4	4	11.4	1	4.6 (0.6–33.6)
Smokers	206.7	17	27.9	2	7.4 (2.1–25.7)

*Royal College of General Practitioners Study, 1968 to 1979 (N = 46,000 women).
†(From Layde P.M., et al.: *Lancet* 1:541–542, 1981.

TABLE 16–7.—RELATIVE RISK OF VASCULAR DISEASE BY VARIOUS FACTORS (WALNUT CREEK STUDY)*

FACTOR	MI†	SUBARACHNOID HEMORRHAGE	OTHER STROKE	IDIOPATHIC VENOUS THROMBOSIS
Smoking	2.9‡	5.7‡	4.8‡	3.9‡
Current OC use	0.8	6.5‡	0.7	7.6‡
Current OC use matched for smoking	0.8	6.5‡	0.6	6.7‡
Smoking and current OC use	2.8	21.9‡	2.0	6.1‡
Past use of OCs§	0.8	5.3‡	1.2	0.3
History of hypertension	4.1‡	1.9	2.4	NA†
Obesity	3.2‡	0.7	1.0	0.5
Gallbladder disease	6.6‡	3.6	0.6	3.0
Hypercholesterolemia	4.0‡	1.2	2.8	0.0
Nondrinker	3.1‡	0.4	0.8	1.0
Current noncontraceptive estrogen use	1.2	1.6	0.9	0.7

*(From Petitti D.B., et al.: *J.A.M.A.* 242:1150–1154, 1979. Copyright 1979, American Medical Association.)
†MI indicates myocardial infarction; NA, not applicable. Obesity is defined as 15% above height and age-specific cohort mean.
‡*P*<.01 by chi-square analysis.
§Excludes current users.

thrombosis while taking OCs than are women of blood type O (Jick et al., 1969).

Choice of OC also influences risk. There is growing evidence that deaths from vascular disease are fewer with the 30- to 35-μg estrogen preparations than with the 50-μg pills that were standard until recently, and these have already been shown to be safer than the older preparations containing 80 to 100 μg of estrogen (Meade et al., 1980). The relation of the precise hormonal composition of the pill to risk of illness has excited lengthy debate.

Norgestrel has marked antiestrogenic effects at the dose usually used in low-dose combination OCs. At first the antiestrogenic potency of norgestrel was thought to be an advantage, as low-dose formulations containing norgestrel could be shown to reverse estrogen-induced changes in many plasma proteins and it was thought that this might reduce complications. More recently, the appreciation that norgestrel reduces blood levels of high-density lipoprotein (HDL) has led to the opposite conclusion, that norgestrel-containing OCs might be less desirable because lowered levels of HDL in other contexts appear to be associated with increased risk of heart attack (Bradley et al., 1978). These concerns are only theoretical at this point, and are not borne out by any actual demonstration of increased risk. Indeed, the facts seem otherwise. As noted by Kay (1980), the Royal College of General Practitioners reported no cases of arterial disease with use of low-dose norgestrel OCs in 184,000 woman-months of use.

Table 16–8 can be used to estimate the maximal risk that would be expected for individual women of different ages from taking OCs. We say maximal, because selection of 30- to 35-μg pills and administration of pills only to women who have no other risk factors should result in marked reduction in vascular disease.

Oral contraceptives with 50 to 80 μg of estrogen increase circulating clotting factors such as factor VII, and depress anticoagulant factors such as antithrombin III; however, the 30- and 35-μg estrogen pills have minimal, if any measurable effect on these factors. Oral contraceptives may alter the aggregability of platelets and affect the blood vessel wall. However, present means for measuring these effects give equivocal results (Mammen, 1982). At higher doses, estrogens increase circulating levels of cholesterol and triglycerides, but also increase levels of HDL, a beneficial effect. At the same dose of estrogen, pills containing higher doses of progestin are more apt to produce vascular disease than those with low doses of progestin (Meade et al., 1980). This effect may have to do with the lowering of circulating HDL levels. Women taking OCs must produce more insulin in response to a given amount of glucose and some manifest a diabetic glucose tolerance test result. Blood pressure increases slightly while on the pill, and a small percent of users will

TABLE 16–8.—SERUM HIGH-DENSITY LIPOPROTEIN CHOLESTEROL CONCENTRATION, ACCORDING TO ORAL CONTRACEPTIVE FORMULATION*

			ADJUSTED CONCENTRATION OF HDL (MG/DL)		
GROUP	NO.	COMPOUND (MG)	MEAN ± SE	DIFFERENCE FROM NONUSER LEVEL	P†
1	137	Mestranol (0.05), norethindrone (1.0)	60.1 ± 1.3	0.1	NS‡
2	140	Mestranol (0.08), norethindrone (1.0)	62.8 ± 1.3	2.8	<.05
3	37	Mestranol (0.10), norethindrone (2.0)	61.4 ± 2.5	1.4	NS
4	21	Ethinyl estradiol (0.05), norethindrone acetate (1.0)	60.8 ± 3.3	0.8	NS
5	21	Ethinyl estradiol (0.05), norethindrone acetate (2.5)	50.3 ± 3.3	−9.7	<.01
6	64	Ethinyl estradiol (0.05), norgestrel (0.3)	50.4 ± 1.9	−9.6	<.001
7	15	Ethinyl estradiol (0.02), norgestrel (0.3)	55.2 ± 3.9	−4.8	NS
8	71	Mestranol (0.10), ethynodiol diacetate (1.0)	65.0 ± 1.8	5.0	<.01
9	15	Ethinyl estradiol (0.05), ethynodiol diacetate (1.0)	66.2 ± 3.9	6.2	NS
10	22	Mestranol (0.10), norethynodrel (2.5)	73.1 ± 4.0	13.1	<.001

*(From Bradley D.D., et al.: N. Engl. J. Med. 299:17–20, 1978. Reprinted by permission.)
†Probability that adjusted mean differs from nonuser mean.
‡NS indicates not significant.

become clinically hypertensive, with the percent increasing with each year of use. Both the alteration in glucose metabolism and the effects on blood pressure seem related more to the progestin than to the estrogen, and are less with the preparations with the least potency.

OCs and Other Illnesses

Extensive knowledge as to the effects of contraception on health has been provided by long-term prospective studies such as that begun in 1967 at Oxford. Rates of hospital referral among the 17,032 women in this study were published in 1976. Women using the pill were compared to IUD wearers and diaphragm users. Pill use was associated with more referrals for cerebrovascular disease, venous thrombosis and embolism, and gallbladder disease, for example (Vessey et al., 1976). Intrauterine device wearers were more apt to develop anemia, salpingitis, and PID.

The contraceptive benefits of OCs are obvious. There are other immediate benefits: reduction in dysmenorrhea, reduction in the amount of bleeding, and increased regularity of the menstrual cycle are some. The Oxford study found that OC users experienced *reduced* referrals for benign breast lesions, menstrual disorder, ovarian cysts, and malignant neoplasms than did the diaphragm group (Vessey et al., 1976). Other noncontraceptive benefits are now well demonstrated. It is not surprising that ovulation suppression with OCs prevents some ovarian retention cysts that would otherwise require surgery, but in addition it is now known that prolonged use of OCs reduces the woman's risk of developing later ovarian cancer and also reduces the risk for cancer of the endometrium (Centers for Disease Control [CDC] and Steroid Hormone Study, 1983a and 1983b). The CDC has estimated that 1,700 deaths from ovarian cancer and 2,000 deaths from endometrial cancer are *prevented* each year because of OC use by American women.

The same CDC study found no increased risk from breast cancer, and in fact a weak protective effect was found for women who first used the pill more than 15 years earlier or who had used the pill for more than 11 years (CDC and Steroid Hormone Study, 1983c). Use of OCs does increase the risk for adenomas of the liver, a potentially life-threatening complication. Fortunately, these tumors are exceedingly rare, even among long-term pill users.

The relation between OC use and cancer of the uterine cervix continues to be controversial. The diaphragm and other barriers are known to reduce the risk for cervical neoplasia, presumably because they reduce transmission of herpes, condyloma virus, or some other sexually transmitted causative agent. Pill use is frequently associated with increased rates for cervical neoplasia, but expert scrutiny of these studies leads to the observation that none of the studies adequately controls for other possibly causative factors; most important, age at first intercourse and number of sexual partners (Swann and Petitti, 1982). The Oxford study recently found pill users to develop cervical dysplasias and cancer at a more rapid rate than a control group of IUD wearers, but as they did not adjust their data for differences in age at first intercourse or cigarette smoking among the two groups, the controversy continues (Vessey et al., 1983).

Oral Contraceptives and Infection

Oral contraceptives do appear to increase the prevalence of yeast infections of the vagina. Formerly it was thought that they increased the severity of gonorrheal infection, but it is now clearly demonstrated that OC use *reduces* the chance of developing PID *by 50%* (Burkeman, 1981).

Do OCs cause more good than harm? While most assume that oral contraceptives do increase risk for heart attack, thrombotic and hemorrhagic stroke, and venous thrombosis and embolism, the amount of risk attributable to the present low-dose OCs used by women who have no other known risk factor is so low as to be difficult to determine, even at this point, after many years of investigation. Because of the lives eventually spared from ovarian and endometrial cancer, Ory has calculated that pill use among nonsmokers prior to age 35 years and smokers prior to age 30 years produces a net benefit (Table 16–9).

Clinical Management of Oral Contraception

Much has been written about selecting the right OC for the individual patient. Most such plans have been based on inferences poorly based in fact. Clinical judgments should be based on randomized, blinded trials of different preparations. Two such trials exist (Goldzieher et al., 1971; Ravenholt et al., 1978). The Goldzieher study was of higher-estrogen pills, but is still relevant because of its demonstration that side effects such as nausea, which is supposedly pill related, were also experienced during control cycles when the women were taking placebo OCs. All women in the study used vaginal contraceptives as well as the different pills. The Ravenholt study compared three 50-μg estrogen preparations on a blinded, crossover basis so that each woman reported detailed information on the three different pills: ethinyl estradiol, 0.050 mg, with d,1-norgestrel, 0.5 mg (Ovral); mestranol, 0.050 mg, with norethindrone, 1.0 mg (Norinyl 1 + 50 or Orthonovum 1/50); and ethinyl estradiol, 0.050, with norethindrone acetate, 1.0 mg (Norlestrin 1/50). Vaginal bleeding was least among cycles with the norgestrel-containing OC, while 10% or so experienced breakthrough bleeding from days 10 to 22 in the first three months while receiving the other two pills. Nausea was more frequent with the norgestrel preparation, while breast pain was most frequent while taking the norethindrone preparation. Most other symptoms studied were not consistently different among the three pills.

New OC users should begin with a 30- to 35-μg estrogen preparation. We feel that 80- to 100-μg preparations have no use for contraception. The practitioner should select one of the preparations containing 30 to 35 μg of ethinyl estradiol as first choice (Table 16–10). Norgestrel-containing preparations have been very popular because they appear to give a lower incidence of breakthrough bleeding and spotting than the other low-dose preparations. The norgestrel preparations are billed as having the lowest dose of progestin, but this ignores the much greater potency of norgestrel when compared to norethindrone and the other 19-nor progestins. Pike and Henderson (1983) related breast cancer risk among young women to early use of high-progestin OCs, a finding not confirmed by other, larger trials. And as mentioned previously, these preparations lower blood levels of HDL, a theoretical disadvantage. Since the lower-progestin pills work as well for most users, we would, at the present moment, reserve the norgestrel preparations for women who have persistent breakthrough bleeding while taking the other pills. The latest development in oral contraception are the biphasic and triphasic pills. These provide a very low dose of the steroids in the first part of the cy-

TABLE 16–9.—CUMULATIVE NUMBER OF DEATHS CAUSED OR AVERTED PER 100,000 WOMEN USING OCs UNTIL THE STATED AGE, THEN HAVING TWO WANTED CHILDREN FOLLOWED BY TUBAL STERILIZATION, UNITED STATES*

	SMOKERS		NONSMOKERS	
AGE (YR)	DEATHS CAUSED	DEATHS AVERTED	DEATHS CAUSED	DEATHS AVERTED
25	65	110	41	110
30	121	108	68	108
35	244	106	133	106

(*From Ory H.W.: *Fam. Plann. Perspect.* 15:57–63, 1983.)

TABLE 16–10.—U.S. ORAL CONTRACEPTIVES CONTAINING 0.050 MG OF ESTROGEN OR LESS*

TRADE NAME†	PROGESTIN AND DOSE (MG)	ESTROGEN AND DOSE (MG)
Formulations containing 0.050 mg of estrogen		
Ovral	d,1-Norgestrel, 0.5	Ethinyl estradiol, 0.050
Norlestrin 1/50	Norethindrone acetate, 1.0	Ethinyl estradiol, 0.050
Demulen 1/50	Ethynodiol diacetate, 1.0	Ethinyl estradiol, 0.050
Ovcon-50	Norethindrone, 1.0	Ethinyl estradiol, 0.050
Ortho-Novum 1/50		
Norinyl 1 + 50	Norethindrone, 1.0	Mestranol, 0.050
Formulations containing 0.030 to 0.035 mg of estrogen		
Lo/Ovral	d,1-Norgestrel, 0.3	Ethinyl estradiol, 0.035
Nordette	d-Norgestrel, 0.15	Ethinyl estradiol, 0.035
Norlestrin 2.5/50	Norethindrone acetate, 2.5	Ethinyl estradiol, 0.050
Loestrin 1.5/30, Norlestrin 1.5/30	Norethindrone acetate, 1.5	Ethinyl estradiol, 0.030
Demulen 1/35	Ethynodiol diacetate, 1.0	Ethinyl estradiol, 0.035
Ortho-Novum 1/35, Norinyl 1.35	Norethindrone, 1.0	Ethinyl estradiol, 0.035
Modicon, Brevicon	Norethindrone, 0.5	Ethinyl estradiol, 0.035
Ovcon-35	Norethindrone, 0.4	Ethinyl estradiol, 0.035
Loestrin 1/20	Norethindrone acetate, 1.0	Ethinyl estradiol, 0.020
Biphasic formulations‡		
Ortho-Novum 10/11	First 10 days:	
	Norethindrone, 0.5	Ethinyl estradiol, 0.035
	Next 11 days:	
	Norethindrone, 1.0	Ethinyl estradiol, 0.035
Triphasic formulations‡		
Trinorinyl	First 7 days:	
	Norethindrone, 0.5	Ethinyl estradiol, 0.035
	Next 9 days:	
	Norethindrone, 1.0	Ethinyl estradiol, 0.035
	Next 5 days:	
	Norethindrone, 0.5	Ethinyl estradiol, 0.035
Ortho-Novum 7/7/7	First 7 days:	
	Norethindrone, 0.5	Ethinyl estradiol, 0.035
	Next 7 days:	
	Norethindrone, 0.75	Ethinyl estradiol, 0.035
	Next 7 days:	
	Norethindrone, 1.0	Ethinyl estradiol, 0.035
Triphasil	First 6 days:	
	d-Norgestrel, 0.050	Ethinyl estradiol, 0.030
	Next 5 days:	
	d-Norgestrel, 0.075	Ethinyl estradiol, 0.040
	Next 10 days:	
	d-Norgestrel, 0.125	Ethinyl estradiol, 0.030
Progestin only, minipill		
Ovrette	d,1-Norgestrel, 0.075	
Micronor, Nor-Q.D.	Norethindrone, 0.35	

*Listed in order of progestin potency within groups of similar estrogen doses.
†For purposes of identification only.
‡Most formulations are also available as 28-day preparations containing placebos for the last seven days of the cycle.

cle with increasing dose thereafter. The total hormone dose for the 21 days of administration is thus considerably reduced, which should reduce side effects, yet the progressive increase in dose as the cycle progresses prevents the increase in breakthrough bleed-ing that is usually found as the dose is reduced.

Bleeding or spotting in between menstrual periods is a common problem of oral contraceptives that is more bothersome with the low-dose preparations. Increasing the dose of either the estrogen, the progestin, or both, reduces breakthrough bleeding but increases side effects and risk. Therefore one should make every effort to manage the bleeding without increasing the dose. This is accomplished by reassuring the patient that breakthrough bleeding is expected, especially during the first three pill cycles, and by using additional estrogen only temporarily as suggested by Speroff (1982): 20 μg of ethinyl estradiol for seven days whenever breakthrough bleeding is persistent. Amenorrhea is another problem of low-dose pills. Provided pregnancy is ruled out by serum human chorionic gonadotropin (HCG) assay, the problem is invariably one of transient endometrial atrophy. The OCs have turned off the woman's own production of estrogen and progesterone, and the synthetic steroids provided in the pill have produced so little growth of the endometrium that there is nothing to be shed; this accounts for the absence of the usual withdrawal bleeding during the week without medication. Some women will accept this pattern and may continue taking the same low-dose pill, but most will request change to a 50-μg estrogen preparation.

Headaches developing in women taking OCs are a worrisome symptom. Women who have suffered a stroke while taking OCs report several weeks of severe headache before the stroke occurred. Although most women who have headaches while on OCs will not have a stroke, we advise the discontinuation of pill use for this symptom.

Pregnancy and the Pill

Some authors have reported an increase in spontaneous abortions when pregnancy occurs with the OCs, and masculinization of the external genitalia of a female fetus has been reported from the older high-dose preparations. However, recent studies have found no increase in malformations among infants born to women following pill use, including those who have experienced contraceptive failure (Linn et al., 1983).

Fertility after OC Use

Initially there were concerns that some women might never resume spontaneous menstruation and, hence, would be infertile after OC use. Our current concept is that while there is a delay of a few months in return to ovulatory cycles after discontinuing the pill, there is no permanent sterility. Women with amenorrhea for more than six months after stopping the pill deserve a full evaluation, as a substantial proportion of this group will eventually be diagnosed as having prolactin-producing pituitary tumors. Women who had regular cycles prior to pill use and used the pill only for contraception have very low rates for developing such tumors. It is the women who were given OCs because of menstrual irregularity who more often have subsequent development of pituitary tumors, and presumably the slow-growing tumor was already present and producing menstrual irregularity before the OCs were given (Shy et al., 1983).

Sexuality and Oral Contraceptives

Occasionally, women taking OCs will complain of reduced sexual interest. The effect of OCs on sexuality has been difficult to determine. However, a sensitive study by Adams and colleagues (1978) recorded all episodes of female-initiated sexual behavior throughout the menstrual cycle and noted an increase at the time of ovulation, which was abolished in women who were taking OCs.

OTHER MEANS FOR HORMONAL CONTRACEPTION

We have already discussed the minipills, those containing only a very low dose of progestin and no estrogen. These have higher pregnancy rates than combination pills, frequently produce bothersome irregular bleeding, and, in most studies, only 50% of the subjects will continue taking the minipills beyond one year of use. Nonetheless, they do work well for the other 50%, and are an alternative for those who want to avoid estrogens.

High-dose progestins are more effective. The most successful of those presently available is injectable medroxyprogesterone acetate (Depo-Provera). Given as a 150-mg injection every three months, Depo-Provera produces amenorrhea and contraception as effective as the combination pill. Depo-Provera produces weight gain and a diabetic shift in the glucose tolerance test, but is otherwise very well tolerated. Several months to a year may be required for return to fertility after the last injection, but permanent sterility does not result. Unfortunately, studies of progestins in dogs revealed that Depo-Provera and the related progesterone-like 17-acetoxy progestins, such as chlormadinone, produce breast tumors. The 19-nor progestins, such as norethindrone, do not do this, but we now understand that this is because the dog's progesterone receptors, unlike those in humans, will not bind to the 19-nor progestins. This does not mean that norethindrone is safer than medroxyprogesterone acetate, but rather that the dog is a poor test animal for predicting human toxic effects from these agents. No serious human illness has been reported from use of Depo-Provera, and it probably is safer than the combination OCs, but although FDA-approved for other purposes in the United States, it is not approved for contraception (Liskin, 1983).

Vaginal Rings

Silastic rings worn in the vagina will release steroid hormones that are absorbed at a constant rate, allowing contraception with blood levels of the steroids well below the peak levels that are seen with OCs. Rings containing levonorgestrel and natural estradiol will suppress ovulation and, in international trials, have been quite successful (Roy and Mishell, 1983).

Norplant

Another, very important approach to hormonal contraception is the sustained release of steroids from polydimethylsiloxane (Silastic) reservoirs. The Norplant systems consists of six Silastic rods implanted beneath the skin through a large needle. These release norgestrel at a constant low rate, sufficient to block ovulation in most cycles, and provide continuous contraception for as long as five years. In the international trials supervised by the Population Council, now exceeding 2,500 woman-years of use, the pregnancy rate has been only 0.3 per 100 woman-years, better than any IUD and comparable to the combination OC (Sivin et al., 1983). The system is soon to be licensed in Finland, its country of manufacture.

HORMONAL CONTRACEPTION FOR MEN

The same negative feedback of sex steroids that can block ovulation in women will also suppress spermatogenesis in men; however, a truly practical method for hormonal contraception has not yet been developed. The validity of the principle was demonstrated some years ago by Briggs and Briggs (1974). They treated a group of men with 20 μg of ethinyl estradiol combined with 10 mg of the androgen methyltestosterone, taken twice a day. After 12 weeks of therapy, the sperm counts were 0. Another approach has been the use of androgens alone, as for example, testosterone enanthate injected every ten days (Steinburger, 1980).

POSTCOITAL CONTRACEPTION

Implantation of the fertilized ovum is thought to occur on the sixth day after fertilization. This interval provides an opportunity to prevent pregnancy even after fertilization. The first successful postcoital method was developed by Morris and Van Waaganen (1973) who used high doses of estrogens. Diethylstilbestrol, 25 mg twice a day for five days, has been the most used, but any other estrogen in comparable doses will work. Several possible mechanisms for the antifertility effect of postcoital estrogens have been proposed: altered tubal motility, a change in the endometrium that would inhibit implantation, and interference with corpus luteum function mediated by prostaglandin. The high-dose estrogen regimen produces significant nausea and vomiting, and antiemetics must be prescribed as well. Estrogens in early pregnancy may produce vaginal abnormalities and vaginal cancer in female offspring, so a woman who experiences pregnancy in spite of postcoital estrogen should be allowed to terminate the pregnancy if she desires.

The progestin norgestrel also works as a postcoital contraceptive. In a large trial women took 0.4 mg of levonorgestrel after each act of intercourse as their only contraceptive. The pregnancy rate was only 1.7 per 100 woman-years, but cycle disturbances were frequent (Kesseru et al., 1973). The same progestin, combined with estrogen in the oral contraceptive Ovral also is effective, and is available in the United States. As studied by Yuzpe and Smith (1982), the woman takes two Ovral tablets within 72 hours after intercourse, and then two more tablets 12 hours later. The pregnancy rate is about 5%, and the side effects are minimal.

A third postcoital option is insertion of a copper IUD. This was first studied by Lippes, who found no pregnancies when the copper T was inserted within 72 hours of intercourse. A subsequent article reported 191 patients treated in this fashion, with only one pregnancy occurring (Black et al., 1980). Still another option is early abortion by minisuction (see following sections) after early diagnosis of pregnancy. In our practice, the Ovral method is the one most used.

STERILIZATION

The great popularity of surgical sterilization in the United States has to do with the strong desire of individuals to control their own fertility, their appropriate concern about the safety and effectiveness of present contraceptive methods, and, most important, the availability of safe and reasonably easy surgical techniques. The major advances in recent years have been in the development of two sterilization procedures for women: laparoscopy and minilaparotomy.

Laparoscopy

The peritoneal cavity was first visualized through a tube inserted via a small incision early in this century. However, this technique had no practical application until modern fiberoptics made possible the easy illumination of the abdominal cavity. Laparoscopy was perfected in Germany during the 1960s and began to be widely available in the United States in the early 1970s. Instruments for laparoscopy are pictured in Figure 16–5. The surgical technique is as follows: The surgeon grasps the abdominal wall and elevates it, then inserts a needle through the lower margin of the umbilicus into the abdominal cavity to produce a pneumoperitoneum with either carbon dioxide or nitrous oxide gas. A small transverse incision is then made at the lower margin of the umbilicus and a sharp trocar is thrust into the cavity. The laparoscope is then inserted through the trocar sleeve, and connected to a light source via a fiberoptic cable. Some laparoscopes have an additional channel to allow insertion of a probe for surgical manipulations (single-puncture technique), but more commonly, a second puncture of the abdominal wall is made in the lower midline just above the pubic symphysis (two-puncture technique). The operating probe is inserted through the second trocar sleeve, and then, under direct vision through the laparoscope, the fallopian tubes are grasped.

In present practice, any of three techniques are used to produce sterilization via the laparoscope: electrical coagulation, application of a small Silastic rubber band (Fallope Ring), or application of a plastic and metal clip (Hulka clip). The Fallope Ring is placed around a loop of the fallopian tube so as to produce necrosis of that loop. When laparoscopy sterilization was first introduced, electrical coagulation was accomplished using high-voltage sources and unipolar technique where the patient is connected to a ground plate. However, this procedure occasionally produced electrical burns of the intestine, a potentially life-threatening complication. Modern elec-

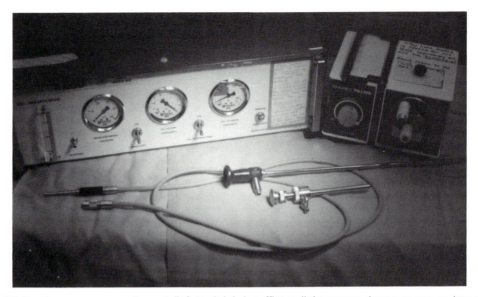

Fig 16–5.—Laparoscopy equipment *(left to right):* Insufflator, light source, laparoscope and trocars, fiberoptic cable. (Courtesy of Dr. Stubblefield.)

trosurgery units develop radiofrequency current at low voltage and are electronically isolated from ground, much reducing the incidence of injury to intestine or other structures inside the abdomen. A further very important development was the perfection of the bipolar forcep, which limits flow of electric current to the area between the two branches of the probe (Rioux and Cloutier, 1974) (Fig 16–6). Both Fallope Ring and Hulka Clip techniques allow tubal occlusion without the use of electric current. In practice, the electric and nonelectric techniques each have advantages and disadvantages. The mechanical devices completely prevent risk of electrical injury, but the Fallope Ring produces considerable postoperative pain and neither can be used if the tubes are thickened from previous salpingitis. On the other hand, salpingitis as a complication of the surgery, although quite rare, occurs more often after electrical coagulation than after the Fallope Ring procedure. Pregnancy after tubal sterilization occurs approximately once in 400 cases, and is somewhat less likely after electrocoagulation; however, about half of such pregnancies are ectopic. When pregnancy oc-

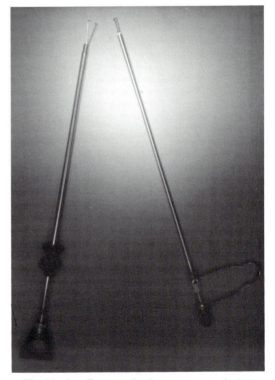

Fig 16–6.—Forceps for laparoscopy tubal sterilization: bipolar electrocoagulator *(left),* Fallope Ring applicator *(right).* (Courtesy of Dr. Stubblefield.)

curs after failure of Fallope Ring sterilization, it will more often be intrauterine (McCann and Kessel, 1976). Reversal of sterilization is more successful after mechanical occlusion than after electrocoagulation, as the latter method destroys much more of the tube, leaving less for the reconstructive surgeon to work with. Laparoscopy sterilization is usually performed in the hospital under general anesthesia, but can be done under local anesthesia with intravenous sedation, and is readily accomplished without overnight hospitalization.

Open Laparoscopy

Standard laparoscopy carries with it a small but definite risk of injury to major blood vessels with insertion of the sharp trocar. With the alternative technique called *open laparoscopy*, developed by Hasson, neither needle nor sharp trocar is used, but rather the peritoneal cavity is opened directly through an incision at the lower edge of the umbilicus. A special funnel-shaped sleeve, the Hasson cannula, is then inserted and the laparoscope introduced through this (Hasson, 1982).

Minilaparotomy

Minilaparotomy refers to use of a very small abdominal incision, just sufficient for the surgeon to operate directly on the tubes. Sterilization immediately after childbirth (postpartum sterilization) has been practiced for years, utilizing a small incision and taking advantage of the fact that immediately after birth the tubes and uterus are situated in the abdominal cavity rather than deep in the pelvis in their usual location. Interval sterilization (at any time other than post partum) would require a large incision, sufficient for the surgeon to insert his or her hand into the pelvis. To accomplish interval sterilization with a small incision requires use of a probe placed within the uterus to elevate it under the incision so that the surgeon can reach the tubes. Interval minilaparotomy sterilization was developed by Uchida in Japan (1975), and, more recently, further developed and popularized for out of hospital use by Osa-

thanondh of Thailand (1974). After making a small suprapubic incision, the surgeon may apply a Fallope ring or Hulka clip, but more commonly will surgically remove a loop of the tube after ligating the base of the loop with absorbable suture material (Pomeroy technique). Minilaparotomy can be accomplished on an outpatient basis under local anesthesia if the patient is slender, as is often the case in underdeveloped countries. In the United States it will usually require overnight hospitalization. The great advantage of minilaparotomy is that only simple surgical instruments and local anesthesia are required and the training of the surgeon is much easier. The sophisticated instrumentation for laparoscopy is expensive, requires maintenance, and is more appropriate for developed countries where specialists can be thoroughly trained in its use.

In the United States, tubal sterilization has been reasonably safe. There were 4 deaths per 100,000 procedures in the interval 1977 to 1981, well below the risk of one pregnancy. Tubal sterilization could be made still safer. Almost half of the deaths were from complications of general anesthesia, usually related to the use of mask ventilation (Peterson et al., 1983). If general anesthesia will be used for laparoscopy, endotracheal intubation is mandatory because the pneumoperitoneum increases the risk of aspiration.

Late Sequelae of Tubal Sterilization

Increased menstrual irregularity and pain have been linked to tubal sterilization for more than 30 years. The problem is that many women develop these symptoms even though they have not had tubal surgery. Neil and colleagues studied three groups of women: those sterilized by laparoscopy with tubal coagulation, those sterilized by open laparotomy with Pomeroy ligation, and those whose husbands had had vasectomy (Neil et al., 1975). They found the most menstrual symptoms in the first group, fewer in the second group, and least among the wives of vasectomized men. A larger study found no menstrual function changes, provided women discontinuing oral contraceptives and IUDs were excluded (Kwak et al., 1980). Important information is provided by the Collaborative Review of Sterilization (CREST) of the Centers for Disease Control (DeStefano, Huezo, Peterson et al., 1983). Interviews were conducted of 2,546 women before tubal sterilization and 2 years after. On the average, cycle length decreased by a very small amount, 0.03 days. Fewer women reported irregular cycles after sterilization than before. The reported amount of menstrual bleeding did not increase. Women having bipolar electrocoagulation or Silastic band sterilization more often reported *decreased* menstrual pain at the two-year interview, but women who had unipolar sterilization, the technique reported in the article by Neil et al., cited previously, had *increased* pain subsequently. This makes some sense, as there is more tissue destruction with the unipolar electrocautery. Bioplar cautery, the newer of the two techniques is also safer, and the older unipolar method should be discontinued.

Reversing Tubal Sterilization

Reanastomosis of the tubes after sterilization is possible, but a lengthy and expensive microsurgical procedure is required and success, defined as subsequent intrauterine pregnancy, can be expected only in 60% or so of cases. Clinical trials presently in progress may provide an alternative approach to sterilization that offers the prospect of easy reversibility. Silastic rubber is injected into the tubes via the uterine cavity using a hysteroscope, a small telescope that allows visualization of the uterine cavity and the tubal ostia through the cervical canal from the vagina. The Silastic cures in place at body temperature to form tubal plugs that prevent conception, but that can be removed without surgery. Preliminary results are encouraging (Reed and Erb, 1980).

Male Sterilization

Vasectomy, excision of a portion of the vas deferens, provides permanent sterilization for men much more easily that do any of the techniques performed for women. Vasectomy is readily accomplished with local anesthesia in an office setting. Though men frequently worry that vasectomy will decrease their sexual performance, this concern has been proved groundless (Liskin, Pile, and Quillin, 1983). Studies in vasectomized monkeys revealed the rapid development of significant atherosclerosis, raising the specter that vasectomized men might suffer from increased heart attacks. Fortunately, several large-scale human studies have found no connection between vasectomy and vascular disease (Walker et al., 1981; Goldacre et al., 1983). Vasectomy must be regarded as a permanent means of sterilization; however, in about half of cases, modern techniques of microsurgery will reverse the procedure and allow subsequent fertility.

PREGNANCY TERMINATION

With so many effective means of contraception available, why is abortion necessary? Contraceptive failure is part of the answer, for as we have seen, the existing methods are used by our population fail more often than most realize (Table 16–3). Another aspect is fear of side effects and complications of contraception. The Ory calculations cited in Table 16–4 show that condom or diaphragm backed up by legal abortion is the safest contraceptive approach. Quite appropriately, many couples are influenced by such considerations. However, equally important is failure to use contraception. Our most fertile age group, ages 18 to 25 years, is also the group that uses contraception the least (Table 16–1). Poor education about sexuality certainly accounts for part of this, but risk taking, whether conscious or unconscious, also plays a role in contraceptive failure. Contraception is preventive medicine, while abortion is employed after the fact, when the individual knows she has a problem. Finally, the issue of availability is very important. Societies control access to contraception. The oral contraceptive is not available at all in some developed countries, and all contraceptives are in short supply in the Third World. In our own country, minors are frequently unable to obtain contraceptive services and pay the price of unwanted pregnancies. Abortion, on the other hand, is available in all societies; the only differences have to do with whether the abortions are legal and safe, or illegal, dangerous, and expensive.

Abortion has been practiced since ancient times. Greek and Roman records describe instruments that clearly were curets meant for scraping the uterine cavity. The technique of uterine aspiration, or vacuum curettage, is more recent. It seems to have been first described in its present form by the Chinese in 1958 (Wu, 1958). In the United States, approximately 1,500,000 abortions are performed each year and the national ratio of abortions to live births is 325:1,000. Married women rarely choose abortion in the United States. Their abortion ratio is 100:1,000. Unmarried women and adolescents, not surprisingly, have high abortion ratios: 1,600:1,000 for unmarried women and 2,000:1,000 for adolescents (CDC, 1979).

The risk of death from legal abortion in the United States has been remarkably low and, overall, is much less than the risk of death from continued pregnancy (Table 16–11). However, risk increases with gestational age and may exceed the risk of continuing the pregnancy for abortions performed at or after 16 menstrual weeks. Fortunately, 92% of our abortions are performed in the first trimester, when abortion is safest.

First-Trimester Abortion

Because it is safer and less traumatic, uterine aspiration has replaced the older technique of dilation and sharp curettage (D&C). Since many gynecologic training programs still fail to teach abortion techniques, the procedure for a first-trimester uterine aspiration will be described in detail. The reader is also referred to the monographs by Burnhill and Levin (1975), and Hern's *Abortion Practice* (1984). Bimanual examination is performed to note uterine size and position (anterior or posterior). Next, the cervix is exposed with a speculum. Short specula such as the Moore modification of the Graves bivalve are preferred (Fig 16–7). The cervix is infiltrated at the 12 o'clock position with 2 ml of 1% chloroprocaine or lidocaine with epinephrine 1:200,000. Then the cervix is grasped with a single-toothed tenaculum placed vertically with one branch inside the cervical canal to avoid tearing. Next, 9 ml of the lidocaine is injected just beneath the vaginal mucosa at the 4 o'clock position on the cervix and a similar injection is made at the 8 o'clock position.

TABLE 16–11.—DEATH-TO-CASE RATE FOR LEGAL ABORTIONS BY WEEKS OF GESTATION, UNITED STATES, 1972 TO 1980*

GESTATION (WK)	NO. OF DEATHS[†]	NO. OF ABORTIONS[‡]	RATE[§]	RELATIVE RISK[‖]
>8	19	4,073,472	0.5	1.0
9–10	31	2,382,516	1.3	2.6
11–12	25	1,197,915	2.1	4.2
13–15	20	419,767	4.8	9.6
16–20	55	430,907	12.8	25.6
>21	14	91,343	15.3	30.6
Total	164	8,595,920	1.9	

*From *Abortion Surveillance, 1979–1980.* Atlanta, Centers for Disease Control, 1983.
[†]Excludes deaths from ectopic pregnancy.
[‡]Based on distribution of 6,108,658 abortions (71.1%).
[§]Deaths per 100,000 abortions.
[‖]Based on index rate of less than 8 menstrual weeks' gestation of 0.5 deaths per 100,000 abortions.

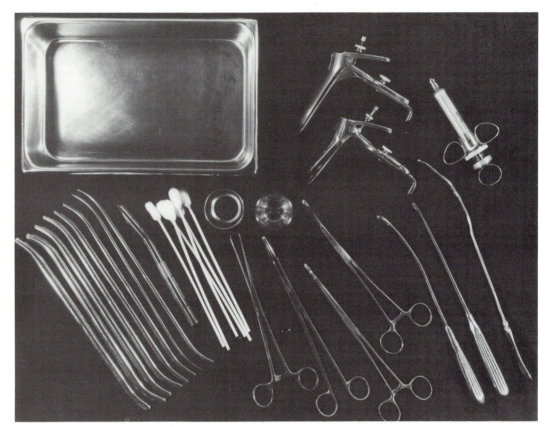

Fig 16–7.—Instrument kit for vacuum curettage abortion *(left to right):* sterile tray, Graves' speculum, Moore speculum, control syringe, uterine sound, no. 1 curettee, no. 3 curette, curved Foerrester forcep, straight Foerrester forcep, Moore ovum forcep, single-tooth tenaculum, medicine glasses, cotton swabs, plastic vacurette, Pratt cervical dilators. (From Stubblefield P.G.: Surgical techniques for first trimester abortion, in Sciarra J.J., Zatuchni G.I., Daly M.J. (eds.): *Gynecology and Obstetrics.* Hagerstown, Md., Harper & Row, 1982, vol. 6, chap. 57. Used with permission.)

This accomplishes a paracervical block. A uterine sound is very gently inserted, and depth and direction of the cavity are noted. Cervical dilation is then gradually accomplished using tapered dilators such as the Pratt, Hawkins-Ambler, or the Denniston dilators. We especially favor the latter as they are blunt at the end, but then taper gently, and being made of durable plastic are somewhat flexible. Slow, gentle dilation is essential. Dilation is the most perilous step in abortion, as this is when most perforations occur.

General anesthesia is avoided if at all possible. General anesthesia increases the risk of perforation, major visceral injury, hemorrhage, and death from abortion, and increases the possibility that hysterectomy will have to be performed, probably because it prevents the patient from signaling by her pain response that the surgeon is pushing too hard with an instrument (Peterson, 1979; Grimes et al., 1976).

Dilatation should be just sufficient to allow insertion of a vacuum cannula of the appropriate size for that gestation, usually of external diameter 1 to 2 mm less than the estimated gestational age in menstrual weeks. Abortions before eight weeks' gestation are

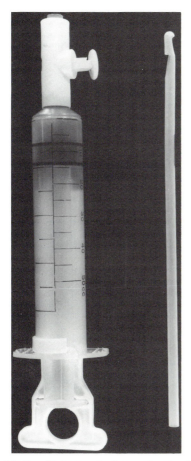

Fig 16–8.—Instruments for early abortion: 6-mm Karman cannula and modified 50-ml plastic syringe. (Courtesy of International Projects Assistance, Chapel Hill, N.C.)

accomplished with the 6-mm Karman cannula. For these early abortions, the modified 50-cc plastic syringe is a sufficient vacuum source (Fig 16–8). At eights weeks and beyond, electric vacuum pumps usually are used. An excellent hand-powered pump sufficient for procedures through the end of the first trimester is available at modest cost.*

After dilatation, the vacuum cannula is gently inserted into the uterine cavity and rotated several times to begin aspiration. The operator then begins an in-and-out motion

_____
*International Projects Assistance Services, 123 W. Franklin St., Chapel Hill, NC 27514.

while continuing to rotate the cannula. On the "out" stroke the cannula tip should be pulled back to the region just above the internal os, thus allowing the lower uterine segment to act as a funnel, linearizing the uterine content for entry into the cannula. When using the flexible Karman cannula, care must be taken not to rotate on the "in" stroke when the cannula is pressed against the uterine fundus, as this will break off the cannula tip. When the uterus is empty, there is increased resistance to motion of the cannula, and a grating feeling of the cannula scraping over the uterine lining is noted. A sharp curet is used to confirm that all tissue is removed. The curet is used not to scrape, but rather, as one would use a finger, to explore. Finally, the vacuum curet is gently reintroduced for a final check.

Immediately following the procedure, the surgeon must perform a fresh examination of the aspirated tissue to confirm that a pregnancy was removed, that all fetal parts are accounted for, and that there is no molar pregnancy. The fresh examination is best accomplished by washing the aspirated tissue in a strainer and then floating it in water in a clear plastic dish over a source of backlighting (Fig 16–9). If the gestational sac cannot be clearly identified, the uterus should be carefully reexplored to rule out continued pregnancy. If no gestational tissue is identified, the patient may have an ectopic pregnancy, but, alternatively, she may have had a false-positive pregnancy test result, have had an unrecognized early spontaneous abortion, or have a continued gestation in a normal or malformed uterus. She requires evaluation with a serum assay specific for human chorionic gonadotropin (β-HCG), pelvic ultrasound, and then diagnostic laparoscopy if the problem cannot otherwise be resolved.

LAMINARIA TENTS FOR DILATION.—This ancient device, the dried stem of a seaweed, was used in American obstetrics in the last century, and was reintroduced from Japan when abortion became legal in Hawaii (Hale

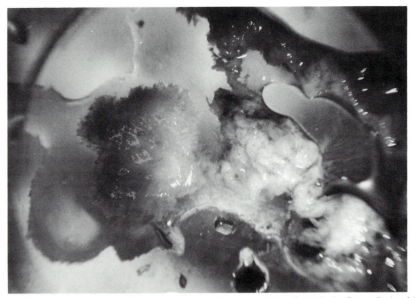

Fig 16–9.—Tissue specimen: 6-week pregnancy, as seen without magnification. The conceptus is on the left. To the right is the decidual lining of the uterus. (From Stubblefield P.G.: Surgical techniques for first trimester abortion, in Sciarra J.J., Zatuchni G.I., Daly M.J. (eds.): *Gynecology and Obstetrics.* Hagerstown, Md. Harper & Row, 1982, vol. 6, chap. 57. Used with permission.)

and Pion, 1972). *Laminaria* take up water and swell, producing gradual, atraumatic dilation of the cervix (Figs 16–10 and 16–11). Modest dilatation is accomplished in a few hours, but quite significant dilatation is produced when the tents are left in place overnight. Their use before first-trimester abortion reduces the risk for cervical injury or perforation. A large study found no increase in rates of infection when *Laminaria* were used (Schulz et al., 1983). A new synthetic alternative, Lamicel, consists of polyethylene sponge, impregnated with magnesium sulfate and compressed into a rod. The Lamicel extracts water from the cervix, producing softening and some dilatation more rapidly than do natural *Laminaria* tents. Yet another alternative for cervical dilatation may soon be provided. Synthetic analogues of the E prostaglandins produce considerable cervical softening and some dilatation with minimal side effects; however, at the moment their use is investigational.

Use of prophylactic antibiotics with abortion continues to be controversial. None have equaled the large study of Hodgson et al. (1975), which found considerable benefit from prophylactic tetracycline. However, Sonne-Holmes' group found the benefit to be limited to those women who had a history of previous pelvic infection (1981).

MANAGEMENT OF ABORTION COMPLICATIONS.—Pain, bleeding, and low-grade fever are the most common complications after first-trimester abortion. Although these symptoms may well respond to oral ergot preparations and a broad-spectrum antibiotic, routine reevacuation under local anesthesia quickly solves the problem, and will usually yield retained tissue or blood clots (Table 16–12).

From early experience with legal abortion came the first reports of a previously undescribed phenomenon: the acute hematometra or "redo syndrome." After abortion, the uterus fills with small clots and becomes overdistended, producing a dramatic increase in the patients' discomfort. Diagnosis is made by the demonstration of a tense, tender, en-

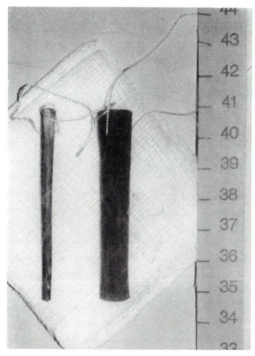

Fig 16–10.—Tents of *Laminaria japonicum.* Dry tent *(left)* as it would be just prior to insertion. Wet tent *(right)* as it would be after several hours exposure to water. (Courtesy of Mildred Hanson, M.D.)

TABLE 16–12.—FINDINGS OF REPEATED UTERINE EVACUATION IN 53 CONSECUTIVE PATIENTS PRESENTING WITH PAIN, BLEEDING, AND LOW-GRADE FEVER AFTER FIRST-TRIMESTER ABORTION*

FINDING	NO. OF PATIENTS
Retained tissue	24
Scant fragments of gestational tissue or decidua	4
Clot and gestational tissue mixture	10
Blood clot only (hematometra)	9
Continued pregnancy (intact gestational sac)	6
Total	53

*From Stubblefield P.G.: *Curr. Probl. Obstet. Gynecol.* 2:1–44, 1978.

The most feared immediate complication of abortion is perforation. The incidence in good hands is 1 or 2 per 1,000 first-trimester abortions. In our experience, perforation at abortion is most often at the junction of cervix and lower uterine segment, giving rise to either of two clinical syndromes depending on the precise location of the perforation (Berek and Stubblefield, 1979). A lateral perforation of the upper cervix into the broad ligament may lacerate the ascending branches of the uterine artery, producing immediate external hemorrhage as well as a broad ligament hematoma (Fig 16–12). These perforations are usually recognized at the time of abortion and necessitate the patient's immediate transfer to a hospital for laparoscopy. At laparoscopy in a young person there may be little sign of

larged uterus and by the response to the proper treatment: immediate reevacuation by vacuum curettage. The incidence of the syndrome is reduced if ergot or oxytocin is used during the abortion (Sands et al., 1976).

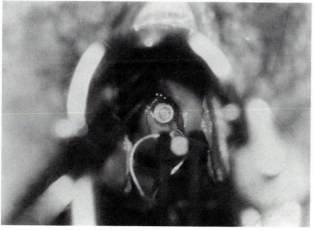

Fig 16–11.—Placing *Laminaria* tents into the cervical canal, as seen through a vaginal speculum. Tenaculum is on upper lip of cervix; one tent has been placed and a second is being inserted alongside the first. (Courtesy of Mildred Hanson, M.D.)

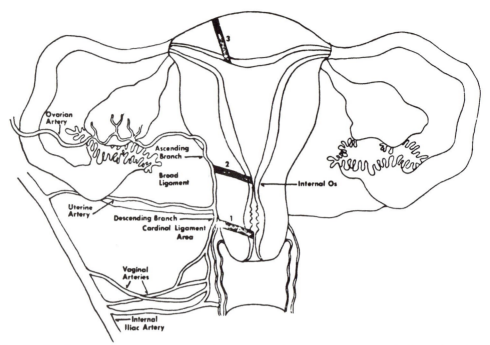

Fig 16–12.—Possible sites of uterine perforation at abortion; **1,** low cervical perforation with laceration of descending branches of uterine artery; **2,** perforation at junction of cervix and lower uterine segment with laceration of ascending branch of uterine artery; **3,** fundal perforation. (From Berek J.S., Stubblefield P.G.: *Am. J. Obstet. Gynecol.* 135:181–184, 1979. Used with permission.)

trauma, because spasm of the lacerated artery limits the size of the hematoma. It may be necessary to guide a probe from below, up through the perforation, and visualize the tip of the probe within the broad ligament in order to make the diagnosis. Management requires laparotomy, development of the bladder flap downward, as with cesarean section, opening of the broad ligament on the affected side, and positive identification of the ureter, followed by ligation of the severed uterine artery branches and suturing of the perforation. Hysterectomy should not be required.

Lateral perforations of the lower cervix cause lacerations of the descending branches of the uterine artery, within the dense substance of the cardinal ligaments. Perforations here produce only external bleeding. There is no internal bleeding and only minimal pain. Diagnosis is difficult, as bleeding will stop from vascular spasm; the patient may be sent home, only to experience recurrence of bleeding. Deaths have been reported from these perforations and the diagnosis must always be suspected when the postabortion patient has repeated hemorrhages and there is no tissue found in the uterus at reevacuation. Inflation of the balloon of a urinary catheter within the cervical canal will stop the hemorrhage and allow preparation of the patient for the necessary laparotomy. Lower perforations have usually been managed by hysterectomy, but Freiman (1979) has described a case where he was able the expose the cardinal ligaments and ligate the bleeding vessels. Selective radiologic arterial embolization might also be attempted. Midline perforations and fundal perforations may often be managed without laparotomy, but it is our preference to perform laparoscopy to determine the extent of injury and rule out injury to the intestine or urinary tract.

Significant postabortal infection is uncommon after legal abortion, occurring at a rate of 1 to 2 per 1,000 cases (Wulff and Freiman, 1977), but can rapidly endanger future fertility, and become life threatening. High-dose broad spectrum intravenous antibiotics are required, and prompt reevacuation of the uterus should be performed if physical examination gives any suggestion of retained tissue. The older practice of delay of a day or two for antibiotic treatment before curettage is to be strongly condemned. If retained tissue is suspected, the patient's condition should be rapidly stabilized with intravenous fluids and antibiotics, and curettage performed within a few hours at most.

Occasionally, agglutination of the cervical canal occurs following first-trimester abortion, producing a syndrome of amenorrhea with severe pain at the time of the expected menstruation. Treatment is gentle probing of the cervical canal, which opens the canal and permits egress of the trapped menstrual blood (Hakim-Elahi, 1976).

Midtrimester Abortion

Table 16–11 makes it quite clear that abortion is safer the earlier it is performed. Presently, 92% of U.S. abortions are performed in the first trimester, when abortion is safest (CDC, 1983). Women who seek abortion in the midtrimester are more commonly young, ambivalent, have had prenatal diagnosis of a fetal defect, or are seriously ill themselves. Presently there are several techniques for midtrimester abortion. Making a choice among them usually depends on gestational age and the experience of the surgeon. In 1973, when abortion became legal throughout the United States, it was widely taught that curettage procedures should never be performed after 12 menstrual weeks. The best alternative was amnioinfusion of hypertonic saline and this was difficult to do before 16 weeks. Women who requested abortion at 13 to 15 weeks' gestation were made to wait until 16 weeks for this reason. The error of this thinking became apparent in 1972 when Tietze reported that curettage procedures at 13 to 14 weeks were safer than saline infusion done subsequently. The significance of this finding for practice was not appreciated for years. Several articles by individual practitioners in England and subsequently in the United States described midtrimester curettage techniques and presented excellent results, but were also largely ignored (Bierer and Steiner, 1971; Slome, 1972; Finks, 1973; Peterson, 1979; Hanson, 1978). However, medical opinion changed rapidly following the publication by the CDC of a series of articles documenting the much greater safety of mid-

TABLE 16–13.—DEATH-TO-CASE RATE* AND DEATHS (IN PARENTHESES) FOR LEGAL ABORTIONS BY TYPE OF PROCEDURE AND WEEKS OF GESTATION, UNITED STATES, 1972 TO 1980†

TYPE OF PROCEDURE	GESTATION (WK)						TOTAL
	≤8	9–10	11–12	13–15	16–20	≥21	
Currettage	0.4(18)	1.2(29)	2.1(24)	0.0(0)	0.0(0)	0.0(0)	0.9(71)
Dilation and evacuation	0.0(0)	0.0(0)	0.0(0)	3.6(10)	10.7(9)	15.0(2)	5.5(21)
Instillation	0.0(0)	0.0(0)	0.0(0)	6.1(5)	13.0(41)	15.4(10)	10.6(56)
Saline	0.0(0)	0.0(0)	0.0(0)	1.9(1)	16.2(34)	15.1(7)	12.6(42)
Prostaglandin and other‡	0.0(0)	0.0(0)	0.0(0)	14.1(4)	6.6(7)	16.0(3)	7.1(14)
Hysterotomy/hysterectomy	0.0(0)	51.4(2)	35.3(1)	65.6(3)	64.6(3)	135.0(1)	44.6(10)
Total§	0.5(19)	1.3(31)	2.2(25)	5.4(20)	13.6(55)	17.7(14)	1.9(164)

*Deaths per 100,000 abortions, excluding deaths associated with ectopic pregnancy.
†From *Abortion Surveillance, 1979–1980.* Atlanta, Centers for Disease Control, 1983.
‡Denominators for rates include abortions reported as "other" type of procedure (1% of all abortions with procedure known).
§Includes four deaths for which type of procedure was classified as "other" and two for which type of procedure was unknown.

trimester dilation and evacuation techniques (D&E) over all other methods (Grimes et al., 1977). By 1980, D&E had become the most used method for abortion prior to 21 menstrual weeks. At 21 weeks and beyond, amnioinfusion was favored. Centers for Disease Control data on risk of death from abortion by the different procedures in the United States is reproduced in Table 16–13. The much greater risk attendant to hysterotomy or hysterectomy compared with that of the other means of abortion is readily apparent in these statistics.

DILATION AND EVACUATION.—D&E is demonstrably the best alternative in the early midtrimester. The other option is systemic administration of prostaglandins and according to Robins and Surrago, D&E is safer and more effective (1982). The several variations of the D&E technique have been reviewed elsewhere (Stubblefield, 1980). An excellent monograph on the subject was published by Hern in 1984. We follow the technique as described by Hanson (1978), except that we use a large-bore vacuum cannula system. Multiple *Laminaria japonica* tents* are inserted into the cervical canal the afternoon prior to the procedure, and the patient is then allowed to go home. The following morning, the *Laminaria* tents are removed, paracervical block is established, and intravenous sedation is accomplished with diazepam, 5 mg, and fentanyl, 0.05 to 0.10 mg. A 16-mm vacuum cannula system is used in combination with heavy ovum forceps to evacuate the uterus (Stubblefield et al., 1978). This procedure has been performed safely and in large numbers on our teaching service for several years (Altman et al., 1981).

The gynecologist wishing to learn D&E techniques is at a disadvantage, as few residency programs teach the procedure. Most learn by observing a skilled practitioner and then by beginning to perform the procedures only in the early midtrimester, and progressing to later gestations as skill increases.

As gestational age advances, uterine evacuation by D&E technique becomes progressively more difficult. The greater reliance on amnioinfusion techniques after 20 weeks reflects this difficulty. We suspect that after 15 weeks, D&E is best reserved for those surgeons who will regularly perform the procedure and thus maintain their skills. We strongly suggest use of *Laminaria* tents, and avoidance of general anesthesia to reduce the risk of perforation.

Dilation and evacuation in the late midtrimester is much facilitated by use of multiple insertions of *Laminaria* tents over two days' time, as advocated by Hern (1981), to achieve wide dilatations of the cervical canal. The addition of vasopressin to the solution of local anesthetic injected into the cervix is said to markedly reduce bleeding during the procedure and is advised for the more advanced gestations (Glick, 1980). One should use a dilute solution, 10 units in 60 ml to avoid hypertension. Vasopressin is contraindicated for women with hypertension or heart disease. The best results for abortion after 20 weeks are those reported by Hern for his outpatient procedure, which combines multiple sets of *Laminaria* tents, followed by amnioinfusion of urea, then extraction of fetus and placenta under paracervical block after labor has begun (Hern, 1981).

Use of ultrasound prior to the procedure is recommended so that the gynecologist does not undertake procedures beyond his or her level of competence. We believe ultrasound to be mandatory prior to all procedures at or after 20 weeks. Use of real-time ultrasound during the procedure has been advised by Darney (1981) and unquestionably offers great advantage for late midtrimester D&E.

MIDTRIMESTER ABORTION BY LABOR INDUCTION.—The standard for labor induction for midtrimester abortion has been amnioinfusion of hypertonic saline. Use of major surgery for

---

*Purchased from MediSpec Inc., 3483 Golden Gate Way, P.O. Box 53, Lafayette, CA 94549, or British Marketing Enterprise, Ltd., 589 First St., West Sonoma, CA 95476.

midtrimester abortion, hysterotomy and hysterectomy, was early recognized in this country as having unacceptably high rates of morbidity and mortality. With development of the D&E technique, the main use of the labor-induction methods is for late midtrimester abortion, the time when transient fetal survival is of great concern. Hypertonic saline and urea produce fetal death in utero, while prostaglandins do not predictably do this. Hypertonic saline, unfortunately, can be fatal if injected intravenously; it produces a chemical coagulopathy in all, which can be very serious in some, and is being replaced by newer methods. The most favored alternative at present is the combination of urea and low-dose prostaglandin $F_{2\alpha}$ by amnioinfusion (Burkman et al., 1978). The prostaglandins by themselves are effective abortifacients, but those presently available are associated with significant vomiting, diarrhea, and, in the case of E-series prostaglandins, fever.

Labor-induction methods share common problems of failed abortion, hemorrhage, and infection that may require immediate operative intervention. Presently available prostaglandins, given by intramuscular injection or vaginal suppository offer an important alternative. Incomplete abortion with later bleeding is a frequent problem. We have demonstrated that routine curettage done under local anesthesia after fetal abortion markedly reduces later complications (Stubblefield, 1978). If high-dose oxytocin is added to augment abortion induced by other means, the patient is at risk for cervical lacerations and uterine rupture.

SEQUELAE OF INDUCED ABORTION.—Older medical literature from Europe reported that women who had undergone induced abortions more often suffered later reproductive complications: sterility, spontaneous abortion, incompetent cervix, low-birth–weight infants, and premature infants. While most of these reports were allegations unsubstantiated by data, the technique for abortion usually used, dilation and sharp curettage under general anesthesia, may well have produced injury. Our group found no adverse effect of a single induced abortion except for some increased first-trimester bleeding in the next pregnancy; but that women who had two more induced abortions were found to be at greater risk for later spontaneous abortion (Levin et al., 1982). In our studies, it initially appeared that women reporting two or more prior induced abortions had a number of reproductive complications in the next pregnancy, but appropriate statistical control with logistic regression analysis found multiple abortions to be associated only with first-trimester bleeding, abnormal presentations, and premature rupture of the membranes, but not with low birth weight, prematurity, or perinatal loss (Linn et al., 1983). As expertly reviewed by Hogue and colleagues (1982), the recent U.S. studies have found no significant sequelae for later reproduction, provided appropriate scientific methodology is followed with controls for other adverse factors. Lack of adverse effect on later pregnancies may well be because of the safety of the prevalent means for abortion in the United States: early vacuum curettage under local anesthesia. We continue to be concerned that midtrimester D&E, if performed with forcible dilation, may damage the cervix and may later produce incompetent cervix or prematurity (Hogue and Peterson, 1984). We have demonstrated that by two weeks following *Laminaria* dilation for D&E, the cervix closes down to an internal diameter smaller than that prior to the abortion, and feel strongly that gradual dilation by *Laminaria* tents should always be used for midtrimester procedures (Stubblefield et al., 1982).

BIBLIOGRAPHY

Adams D.B., Gold A.R., Burt A.D.: Rise in female initiated sexual activity at ovulation and its suppression by oral contraceptives. *N. Engl. J. Med.* 299:1145–1150, 1978.

Altman A., Stubblefield P.G., Parker K., et al.: Midtrimester abortion by *Laminaria* and evacuation (L&E) on a teaching service: A review of 789 cases. *Adv. Plann. Parent.* 16:1–6, 1981.

Berek J.S., Stubblefield P.G.: Anatomical and clinical correlations of uterine perforations. *Am. J. Obstet. Gynecol.* 135:181–184, 1979.

Bierer I., Steiner V.: Termination of pregnancy in the second trimester with the aid of *Laminaria* tents. *Med. Gynecol. Sociol.* 6:9–10, 1971.

Black T.R., Goldstuck N.D., Spence A.: Post-coital intrauterine device insertion—a further evaluation. *Contraception* 22:653–658, 1980.

Bradley D.D., Wingerd J., Petitti D.B., et al.: Serum high density lipoprotein cholesterol in women using oral contraceptives, estrogens and progestins. *N. Engl. J. Med.* 299:17–20, 1978.

Briggs M.H., Briggs M.: Oral contraceptives for men. *Nature* 252:585–586, 1974.

Burkeman R.T., Atienza M., King T.M., et al.: Intra-amniotic urea as a midtrimester abortifacient: Clinical results and serum and urinary changes. *Am. J. Obstet. Gynecol.* 121:7–16, 1975.

Burkman R.T., and the Womens' Health Study: Association between intrauterine devices and pelvic inflammatory disease. *Obstet. Gynecol.* 57:269–276, 1981.

Burnhill M.S.: Syndrome of progressive endometritis associated with intrauterine contraceptive devices. *Adv. Plann. Parent.* 8:144–150, 1972.

Burnhill M.S., Levin H.: *Preterm Physician's Manual: Standard Medical Procedures,* ed. 3. Franconia, N.H., Preterm Institute, 1975.

Centers for Disease Control: *Abortion Surveillance 1977.* Atlanta, Centers for Disease Control, September 1979.

Centers for Disease Control: *Abortion Surveillance 1979–1980.* Atlanta, Centers for Disease Control, May 1983.

Centers for Disease Control Cancer and Steroid Hormone Study: Oral contraceptive use and the risk of ovarian cancer. *J.A.M.A.* 249:1596–1599, 1983.

Centers for Disease Control Cancer and Steroid Hormone Study: Oral contraceptive use and the risk of endometrial cancer. *J.A.M.A.* 249:1600–1604, 1983.

Centers for Disease Control Cancer and Steroid Hormone Study: Long-term oral contraceptive use and the risk of breast cancer. *J.A.M.A.* 249:1591–1604, 1983.

Clarkson T.B., Alexander N.J.: Long-term vasectomy: Effect on the occurrence and extent of atherosclerosis in Rhesus monkeys. *J. Clin. Invest.* 65:15–25, 1980.

Counsel carefully about sponge, toxic shock, CDC advises. *Contraceptive Technology Update* 5:29–32, 1984.

Darney P.D.: Midtrimester abortion under ultrasound guidance. Postgraduate course, National Abortion Federation, Tampa, Fla., Jan. 31, 1983.

Davis J.P., Chesney J., Wand P.J., et al.: Toxic shock syndrome: Epidemiologic features, recurrence, risk factors and prevention. *N. Engl. J. Med.* 303:1429–1435, 1980.

Dericks-Tan J.S.E., Kock P., Taubert H.D.: Synthesis and release of gonadotropins: Effect of an oral contraceptive. *Obstet. Gynecol.* 62:687–690, 1983.

DeStefano F., Greenspan J.R., Dicker R.C., et al.: Complications of interval laparoscopic tubal sterilization. *Obstet. Gynecol.* 61:153–158, 1983.

DeStefano F., Huezo C., Peterson H.B., et al.: Menstrual changes after tubal sterilization. *Obstet. Gynecol.* 62:673–681, 1983.

El Badrawi H.H., Hafez E.S., Barnhart M.I., et al.: Ultrastructural changes in human endometrium with copper and nonmedicated IUD's in utero. *Fertil. Steril.* 36:41–49, 1981.

Forrest J.D., Henshaw S.K.: What U.S. women think and do about contraception. *Fam. Plann. Perspect.* 15:157–166, 1983.

Finks A.I.: Midtrimester abortion. *Lancet* 1:263–264, 1973.

Freiman M.: Personal communication, 1980.

Glick E.: Personal communication, Oct. 4, 1980.

Goldacre M.J., Holford T.R., Vessey M.P.: Cardiovascular disease and vasectomy. *N. Engl. J. Med.* 308:805–808, 1983.

Goldzieher J.W.: Estrogens in oral contraceptives: Historical perspectives. *Johns Hopkins Med. J.* 150:165–169, 1982.

Goldzieher J.W., De La Pena A., Chenault C.B., et al.: Comparative studies of the ethinyl estrogens used in oral contraceptives: II. Anteovulatory potency. *Am. J. Obstet. Gynecol.* 122:625–636, 1975.

Goldzieher J.W., Moses L.E., Averkin E., et al.: A placebo controlled double blind crossover investigation of the side effects attributed to oral contraceptives. *Fertil. Steril.* 22:609–623, 1971.

Grimes D.A., Cates W.: Deaths from paracervical anesthesia used for first trimester abortion, 1972–1975. *N. Engl. J. Med.* 295:1397–1399, 1976.

Grimes D.A., Schulz K.F., Cates W. Jr., et al.: Midtrimester abortion by dilatation and evacuation: A safe and practical alternative. *N. Engl. J. Med.* 296:1141–1145, 1977.

Guerrero R., Rojas O.I.: Spontaneous abortion and aging of human ova and spermatozoa. *N. Engl. J. Med.* 293:573, 1975.

Grimes D.A., Schulz K.R., Cates W. Jr., et al.: Local vs. general anesthesia: Which is safer for performing suction curettage abortions? *Am. J. Obstet. Gynecol.* 135:1030–1035, 1979.

Habashi M., Sahwi S., Gawish S., et al.: Effect of Lippes loop on sperm recovery from human fallopian tubes. *Contraception* 22:549–555, 1980.

Hakim-Elahi E.: Postabortal amenorrhea due to cervical stenosis. *Obstet. Gynecol.* 48:723–724, 1976.

Hale R.W., Pion R.J.: *Laminaria:* An underutilized clinical adjunct. *Clin. Obstet. Gynecol.* 15:829–850, 1972.

Hanson M.S.: D&E midtrimester abortion preceded by *Laminaria*. Presented at the 16th annual meeting of the Association of Planned Parenthood Physicians, San Diego, Calif., Oct. 26, 1978.

Harris R.W.C., Brinton L.A., Cowdell R.H., et al.: Characteristics of women with dysplasia or carcinoma in situ of the cervix uteri. *Br. J. Cancer* 42:359–369, 1980.

Hasson H.M.: Open laparoscopy, in Zatuchni G.I., Daly M.J., Sciarra J.J. (eds.): *Gynecology and Obstetrics.* Philadelphia, Harper & Row, 1982, vol. 6, chap. 44, pp. 1–8.

Hern W.M.: Outpatient second trimester D&E abortion through 24 menstrual weeks gestation. *Adv. Plann. Parent.* 16:7–11, 1981.

Hern W.M.: *Abortion Practice.* Philadelphia, J.B. Lippincott Co., 1984.

Himes N.E.: *Medical History of Contraception.* New York, Gamut Press, 1963.

Hodgson J.E., Major B., Portman K., et al.: Prophylactic use of tetracycline for first trimester abortions. *Obstet. Gynecol.* 45:574–578, 1975.

Hogue C.J.R., Peterson W.F.: Outcome of pregnancy following midtrimester abortion by dilatation and evacuation. Presented at the National Abortion Federation Risk Management Seminar, Sept. 16, 1984, Atlanta.

Hogue C.J.R., Cates W. Jr., Tietze C.: The effects of induced abortion on subsequent reproduction. *Epidemiol. Rev.* 4:66–94, 1982.

Jain A.K.: Cigarette smoking, use of oral contraceptives, and myocardial infarction. *Am. J. Obstet. Gynecol.* 126:243–259, 1976.

Jick H., Walker A.M., Rothman K.J., et al.: Vaginal spermicides and congenital disorders. *J.A.M.A.* 245:1329–1332, 1981.

Jick H., Westerholm E., Vessey M.P., et al.: Venous thromboembolic disease and ABO blood type. *Lancet* 1:539–542, 1969.

Kafrissen M.E., Schulz K.R., Grimes D.A., et al.: A comparison of intra-amniotic instillation of hyperosmolar urea and prostaglandin $F_{2\alpha}$ vs dilatation and evacuation for midtrimester abortion. *J.A.M.A.* 251:916–919, 1984.

Kay C.R.: The happiness pill. *J. R. Coll. Gen. Pract.* 30:8–10, 1980.

Kelaghan J., Rubin G.L., Ory H.W., et al.: Barrier-method contraceptives and pelvic inflammatory disease. *J.A.M.A.* 248:184–187, 1982.

Kesseru E., Larrenaga A., Parada J.: Postcoital contraception with d-norgestrel. *Contraception* 7:367–369, 1973.

Koch J.P.: The Prentiff contraceptive cervical cap: A contemporary study of its clinical safety and effectiveness. *Contraception* 25:135–159, 1982.

Kwak H.M., Chi I.C., Gardner S.D., et al.: Menstrual pattern changes in laparoscopic sterilization patients whose last pregnancy was terminated by therapeutic abortion. *J. Reprod. Med.* 25:67–71, 1980.

Lane M.E., Arceo R., Sobrero A.: Successful use of the diaphragm and jelly by a young population: Report of a clinical study. *Fam. Plann. Perspect.* 8:81–86, 1976.

Layde P.M., Beral V., Kay C.R.: Further analysis of mortality in oral contraceptive users. *Lancet* 1:541–542, 1981.

Levin A.A., Schoenbaum S.C., Monson R.R., et al.: The association of induced abortion with subsequent pregnancy loss. *J.A.M.A.* 243:2495–2499, 1980.

Linn S., Schoenbaum S.C., Monson R.R., et al.: The relationship between induced abortion and outcome of subsequent pregnancies. *Am. J. Obstet. Gynecol.* 146:136–140, 1983.

Linn S., Schoenbaum S.C., Monson R.R., et al.: Lack of association between contraceptive usage and congenital malformation in offspring. *Am. J. Obstet. Gynecol.* 147:923–928, 1983.

Lippes J., Malik T., Tatum H.J.: The postcoital copper-T. *Adv. Plann. Parent.* 11:24–29, 1976.

Lippes J., Zielezny M.: The loop decade. *Mt. Sinai Med. J.* 4:353–356, 1975.

Liskin L.S.: Long-acting progestins–promise and prospects. *Popul. Rep. K* 11:17–55, 1983.

Liskin L.S., Pile J.M., Quillin W.F.: Vasectomy—safe and simple. *Popul. Rep.* 11:62–99, 1983.

Malyk B.: *Nonoxynol-9: Evaluation of Vaginal Absorption in Humans.* Raritan, N.J., Ortho-Pharmaceutical Corp., 1983.

Mammen E.F.: Oral contraceptives and blood coagulation: A critical review. *Am. J. Obstet. Gynecol.* 142:781–790, 1982.

Mann J.I., Inman W.G.W.: Oral contraceptives and death from myocardial infarction. *Br. Med. J.* 2:245–248, 1975.

McCann M.R., Liskin L.S., Piotrow P.T., et al.: Breast-feeding, fertility and family planning. *Popul. Rep. J*, no. 24, Nov./Dec. 1981.

McCann M.F., Kessel E.: International experience with laparoscopic sterilization: Follow up of 8,500 women. Presented at the 14th annual scientific meeting, Association of Planned Parenthood Physicians, Miami Beach, Nov. 10–12, 1976.

Meade T.W., Greenberg G., Thompson S.G.: Progestogens and cardiovascular reactions associated with oral contraceptives and a comparison of the safety of 50 and 30 mcg oestrogen preparations. *Br. Med. J.* 1:1157–1161, 1980.

Mishell D.R. Jr., Bell J.H., Good R.G., et al.: The intrauterine device: A bacteriologic study of the endometrial cavity. *Am. J. Obstet. Gynecol.* 96:119, 1966.

Leads from M.M.W.R. *J.A.M.A.* 251:1015–1016, 1984.

Morris J.M., Van Waaganen G.: Interception: The use of postovulatory estrogens to prevent implantation. *Am. J. Obstet. Gynecol.* 115:101–106, 1973.

Neil J.R., Hammond G.T., Nobel A.D., et al.: Late complications of sterilization by laparoscopy and tubal ligation: A controlled study. *Lancet* 2:669–671, 1975.

Nilsson C.G., Lahteenmaki P., Luukkainen T.: Patterns of ovulation and bleeding with a low levonorgestrel releasing intrauterine device. *Contraception* 21:155–164, 1980.

Nygren K., Nielsen N., Pyorala T., et al.: Intrauterine contraception with Nova T and Copper T-200 during three years. *Contraception* 24:529–542, 1981.

Ory H.W., and the Womens' Health Study: Ectopic pregnancy and intrauterine contraceptive devices: New perspectives. *Obstet. Gynecol.* 57:137–140, 1981.

Ory H.W.: Mortality associated with fertility and fertility control: 1983. *Fam. Plann. Perspect.* 15:57–63, 1983.

Osathanondh V.: Suprapubic mini-laboratory, uterine elevation technique: Simple, inexpensive and out-patient procedure for interval female sterilization. *Contraception* 10:251–262, 1974.

Peel J.: Manufacture and retailing of contraceptives in England. *Popul. Stud.* 17:113–125, 1963.

Peterson W.: Dilatation and evacuation: Patient evaluation and surgical techniques, in Zatuchni G.I., Sciarra J.J., Spiedel J.J. (eds.): *Pregnancy Termination: Procedures, Safety, and New Developments.* Hagerstown, Md., Harper & Row, 1979, pp. 184–191.

Peterson H.B., DeStefano F., Rubin G.L., et al.: Deaths attributable to tubal sterilization in the United States, 1977–1981. *Am. J. Obstet. Gynecol.* 146:131–136, 1983.

Petitti D.B., Wingerd J., Pellegrin F.A., et al.: Risk of vascular disease in women: smoking, oral contraceptives, noncontraceptive estrogens, and other factors. *J.A.M.A.* 242:1150–1154, 1979.

Ramcharan S., Pellegrin R.R., Hsu J.P.: The Walnut Creek Contraceptive Drug Study. National Institutes of Health publication no. 81-564, vol. 3, 1981.

Ravenholt R.T., Kessell E., Speidel J.J.: Comparison of the side effects of three oral contraceptives: A double blind cross-over study of Ovral, Norinyl and Norlestrin. *Adv. Plann. Parent.* 12:222–239, 1978.

Reed T.P., Erb R.A.: Tubal occlusion with silicone rubber: An update. *J. Reprod. Med.* 25:25–28, 1980.

Rioux J.E., Cloutier D.: A new bipolar instrument for laparoscopic tubal sterilization. *Am. J. Obstet. Gynecol.* 119:737, 1974.

Robins J., Surrago E.J.: Early midtrimester pregnancy termination: A comparison of dilatation and evacuation and intravaginal prostaglandin $F_{2\alpha}$. *J. Reprod. Med.* 27:415–419, 1982.

Rock J., Pincus G., Garcia C.R.: Effects of certain 19-nor steroids on the normal human menstrual cycle. *Science* 124:891–893, 1956.

Rosenfield A.J., Castadot R.G.: Early postpartum and immediate postabortion IUD insertion. *Am. J. Obstet. Gynecol.* 118:1104–1114, 1974.

Roy S., Mishell D.R.: Current status of research and development of vaginal contraceptive rings as a fertility control method in the female. *Res. Frontiers Fertil. Regulation* 2:1–10, 1983.

Royal College of General Practitioners: *Oral Contraceptives and Health.* London, Pitman Corp., 1974.

Royal College of General Practitioners' Oral Contraception Study. Incidence of arterial disease among oral contraceptive users. *J. R. Coll. Gen. Pract.* 33:75–82, 1983.

Rozenbaum H.: Relationships between chemical structure and biological properties of progestogens. *Am. J. Obstet. Gynecol.* 142:719–724, 1982.

Sands R.X., Burnhill M.S., Hakim-Elahi E.: Postabortal uterine atony. *Obstet. Gynecol.* 43:595–598, 1974.

Schulz K.F., Grimes D.A., Cates W. Jr.: Measures to prevent cervical injury during suction curettage abortion. *Lancet* 1:1182–1184, 1983.

Schirm A.L., Trussell J., Menken J., et al.: Contraceptive failure in the United States: The impact of social, economic and demographic factors. *Fam. Plann. Perspect.* 14:68–75, 1982.

Shapiro S., Slone D., Heinonen O., et al.: Birth defects and vaginal spermicides. *J.A.M.A.* 247:2381–2384, 1982.

Shy K.K., McTiernan A.M., Daling J.R., et al.: Oral contraceptive use and the occurrence of pituitary prolactinoma. *J.A.M.A.* 249:2204–2207, 1983.

Sivin I., Tatum H.J.: Four years of experience with the TCU 380A intrauterine contraceptive device. *Fertil. Steril.* 36:159–163, 1981.

Sivin I., Diaz S., Holma P.: A four year clinical

study of Norplant implants. *Stud. Fam. Plann.* 14:184–191, 1983.

Slome J.: Termination of pregnancy. *Lancet* 2:881, 1972.

Slone D., Shapiro S., Kaufman D.W., et al.: Risk of myocardial infarction in relation to current and discontinued use of oral contraceptives. *N. Engl. J. Med.* 305:420–424, 1981.

Sonne-Holmes S., Heisterberg L., Hebjorn S., et al.: Prophylactic antibiotics in first trimester abortion: A clinical controlled trial. *Am. J. Obstet. Gynecol.* 139:693–696, 1981.

Sparks R.A., Purrier B.G., Watt P.J., et al.: Bacteriological colonization of the intrauterine contraceptive device. *Br. Med. J.* 282:1189–1191, 1981.

Speroff L.: The formulation of oral contraceptives: Does the amount of estrogen make any clinical difference? *Johns Hopkins Med. J.* 150:170–175, 1982.

Steinberger E.: Current status of research on hormonal contraception in the male. *Res. Frontiers Fertil. Regulation* 1:1–12, 1980.

Stubblefield P.G.: Current technology for abortion. *Curr. Probl. Obstet. Gynecol.* 2:1–44, 1978.

Stubblefield P.G.: Midtrimester abortion by curettage procedures: An overview, in Hodgson J.E. (ed.): *Abortion and Sterilization: Medical and Social Aspects*. London, Academic Press, New York, Grune & Stratton, 1981, pp. 277–296.

Stubblefield P.G., Albrecht B.H., Koos B., et al.: A randomized study of 12-mm vs 15.9-mm vacuum cannulas in midtrimester abortion by *Laminaria* and vacuum curettage. *Fertil. Steril.* 29:512–517, 1978.

Stubblefield P.G., Altman A.M., Goldstein S.P.: Randomized trial of one versus two days of *Laminaria* treatment prior to late midtrimester abortion by uterine evacuation: A pilot study. *Am. J. Obstet. Gynecol.* 143:481–482, 1982.

Sturgis S.H., Albright F.: The mechanism of estrin therapy in the relief of dysmenorrhea. *Endocrinology* 26:68–72, 1940.

Swann S.H., Petitti D.B.: A review of problems of bias and confounding in epidemiologic studies of cervical neoplasia and oral contraceptive use. *Am. J. Epidemiol.* 115:10–18, 1982.

Tatum H.J., Connell-Tatum E.B.: Barrier contraception: A comprehensive overview. *Fertil. Steril.* 36:1–12, 1981.

Tatum H.J., Schmidt F.H., Jain A.K.: Management and outcome of pregnancies associated with a copper-T intrauterine contraceptive device. *Am. J. Obstet. Gynecol.* 126:869–877, 1976.

Tatum H.J.: Medicated intrauterine devices, in

Sciarra J.J., Zatuchni G.I., Daly M.J. (eds.): *Gynecology and Obstetrics: Fertility Regulation, Psychosomatic Problems, and Human Sexuality*. Philadelphia, Harper & Row, 1982, vol. 6, chapter 29.

Tietze C., Lewit S.: Evaluation of intrauterine devices: Ninth progress report of the Cooperative Statistical Program. *Stud. Fam. Plann.* 1:1–40, 1970.

Toxic shock syndrome and the vaginal contraceptive sponge. *M.M.W.R.* 32:221–222, 1983.

Uchida H.: Uchida tubal sterilization. *Am. J. Obstet. Gynecol.* 121:153–159, 1975.

Umapathysivam K., Jones W.R.: Effects of contraceptive agents on the biochemical and protein composition of human endometrium. *Contraception* 22:425–440, 1980.

Vessey M., Doll R., Peto R., et al.: A long term follow up study of women using different methods of contraception—an interim report. *J. Bios. Sci.* 8:373–420, 1974.

Vessey M., Lawless M., Yeates D.: Efficacy of different contraceptive methods. *Lancet* 1:841–843, 1982.

Vessey M., McPherson K., Lawless M., et al.: Neoplasia of the cervix uteri and contraception: A possible adverse effect of the pill. *Lancet* 2:930–934, 1983.

Wade M.E., McCarthy P., Abernathy J.R., et al.: A randomized prospective study of the use effectiveness of two methods of natural family planning: An interim report. *Am. J. Obstet. Gynecol.* 134:628–631, 1979.

Walker A.M., Jick H., Hunter J.R., et al.: Vasectomy and non-fatal myocardial infarction. *Lancet* 1:13–15, 1981.

White M.K., Ory H.W., Rooks J.B., et al.: Intrauterine device termination rates and the menstrual cycle day of insertion. *Obstet. Gynecol.* 55:220–224, 1980.

Wu Y.T.: Suction in artificial abortion: 300 cases (Chinese). *Chin. J. Obstet. Gynecol.* 6:447–449, 1958.

Wulff G., Freiman M.: Elective abortion: complications seen in a freestanding clinic. *Obstet. Gynecol.* 49:351, 1977.

Yuzpe A.A., Smith R.: Use of hormonal steroids for pregnancy interception, in Sciarra J.J., Zatuchni G.I., Daly M.J. (eds.): *Gynecology and Obstetrics: Fertility Regulation, Psychosomatic Problems, and Human Sexuality*. Philadelphia, Harper & Row, 1982, vol. 6, chap. 26.

Yuzpe A.A., Lancee W.J.: Ethinylestradiol and *dl*-norgestrel as a postcoital contraceptive. *Fertil. Steril.* 28:932–936, 1977.

Zipper J., Medel M., Goldsmith A., et al.: Six year continuation rates for Cu-T 200 users. *J. Reprod. Med.* 18:95–97, 1977.

CHAPTER SEVENTEEN

Medical Genetics

WAYNE A. MILLER, M.D.
RICHARD W. ERBE, M.D.

GENETIC PROBLEMS are frequently encountered initially by the gynecologist as primary physician to women. During routine prenatal evaluation the gynecologist may become aware of specific risk factors, such as advanced maternal age or a family history of serious genetic disorder. Patients frequently pose questions about the risks and nature of genetic and nongenetic birth defects. Subsequently the obstetrician is often the first to observe the presence of a serious congenital defect in the child, necessitating proper diagnosis, management, and interpretation to the parents. Thus the gynecologist must be familiar both with the fundamental principles of medical genetics and with those disorders of greatest relevance to maternal-fetal health and reproductive function.

This chapter addresses basic aspects of medical genetics, examples of genetic disorders that may present primarily with gynecologic complaints, and a genetically oriented approach to certain major gynecologic problems. For a more extensive treatment of the subjects presented in this chapter or for topics beyond the scope of this chapter, the reader is referred to Vogel and Motulsky (1979), Sutton (1980), and Simpson et al. (1982).

This work was supported in part by research grant no. HD06356 from the National Institute of Child Health and Human Development, DHEW, and by USPHS training grant 5 T01 GM02249.

BASIC PRINCIPLES

Mendel in the 1860s formulated many basic concepts of inheritance on which we depend today, but his work received little attention until it was rediscovered in the first decade of this century. At that time Garrod (Harris, 1963) proposed the term "inborn errors of metabolism" to unify his observations on alkaptonuria, albinism, cystinuria, and pentosuria, the four inherited disorders that he had studied in detail. The first identification of a molecular basis for a human genetic disease was in 1949 when Pauling noted the abnormal electrophoretic mobility of sickle hemoglobin. In 1957 Ingram showed that this altered mobility resulted from a changed amino acid sequence in the hemoglobin molecule. The deciphering of the genetic code, begun by Nirenberg in 1961, led to the recognition that the altered amino acid sequence of hemoglobin S resulted from a point mutation in the gene for the globin β-chain. The first specific enzyme defect in an inborn error of metabolism was identified in 1952 when Cori and Cori showed that glucose-6-phosphatase activity was deficient in glycogen storage disease, type II. The first mammalian gene, mouse globin, was cloned in 1977 (Tilghman et al., 1977) and the first restriction fragment length polymorphism (RFLP) was identified in 1978 (Wyman and White, 1978).

Chromosomes were described in the 1870s,

but not until 1956 was it determined that the normal diploid number of chromosomes in the human *karyotype,* or chromosome complement, is 46. The specific etiologic basis of a human chromosome disorder was first identified in 1959 when Lejeune demonstrated the presence of an extra number 21 chromosome in a child with Down's syndrome. The 46 chromosomes normally present occur in pairs, one member of the pair having been inherited from each parent. Twenty-two pairs are homologous and are designated the *autosomes.* The 23rd pair constitutes the *sex chromosomes,* the X and the Y. Although the chromosomes are always present in the nucleus of the cell, it is only immediately prior to cell division, i.e., at metaphase, that they condense and assume their characteristic form. At metaphase, each chromosome has already divided, the two sister chromatids thus produced remaining attached at the centromere, resulting in the familiar x-shaped appearance (not to be confused with the X chromosome). As shown schematically in Figure 17–1 the chromosome pairs are classified into seven groups, designated A through G, primarily on the basis of length and the position of the centromere (Bergsma et al., 1972). Figure 17–2 shows karyotypes of a normal female (A) and a normal male (B) stained by what was, until the early 1970s, the standard method. With this staining, normal chromosomes could be classified into groups without difficulty, but some of the pairs of homologues could not be distinguished. Furthermore, structurally abnormal chromosomes often could not be precisely characterized. Some useful additional information could be provided through the use of laborious special techniques, such as differential labeling of the chromosomes with tritiated thymidine followed by autoradiography.

In 1970 Caspersson and associates demonstrated that exposure of chromosomes to certain fluorescent compounds such as quinacrine hydrochloride or quinacrine mustard resulted in the appearance of bands, designated *Q-bands,* by which each chromosome pair as well as the X and the Y could be distinguished. Subsequently, several alternative banding techniques have been introduced, yielding different banding patterns and greater detail about certain specific chromosomal regions. In Figure 17–3 the chromosomes were first exposed to a dilute solution of trypsin and then to Giemsa stain to give characteristic

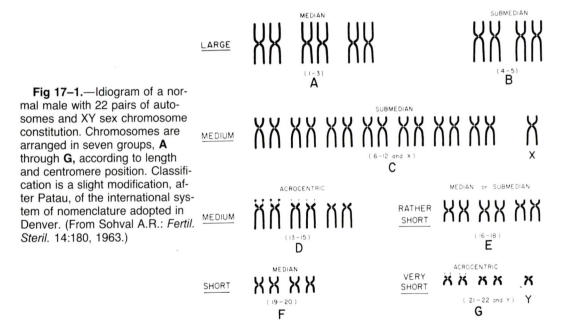

Fig 17–1.—Idiogram of a normal male with 22 pairs of autosomes and XY sex chromosome constitution. Chromosomes are arranged in seven groups, **A** through **G,** according to length and centromere position. Classification is a slight modification, after Patau, of the international system of nomenclature adopted in Denver. (From Sohval A.R.: *Fertil. Steril.* 14:180, 1963.)

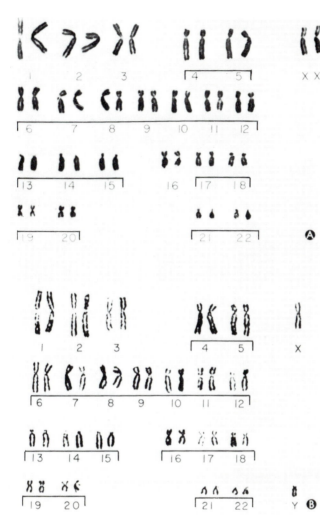

Fig 17–2.—**A,** normal female karyotype, and **B,** normal male karyotype stained with Giemsa. (From Hirschhorn K., Cooper L.C.: *Am. J. Med.* 31:442, 1961.) The chromosome pairs whose numbers are enclosed by *solid lines* cannot be distinguished using this staining technique.

G-bands. The locations and intensities of the G-bands are quite similar to those of the Q bands except for four chromosome segments. In contrast to the fluorescent banding, however, G-banding technique gives permanent preparations and requires no special microscopy equipment for observing the bands— hence its widespread use. So-called *minor variants,* structural variations with no apparent functional significance, occur frequently, making it possible in many instances to distinguish the maternally derived from the paternally derived member within each pair of homologues (Miller et al., 1973; Hoehn, 1975).

By convention, the karyotype is described by noting first the total number of chromosomes, followed by a designation of the sex chromosomes present, followed in turn by the description of any abnormality or variant (Bergsma et al., 1972). A normal female karyotype is designated 46 XX and a normal male is 46 XY. A patient with Turner's syndrome (see the section on Turner's syndrome) might have a 45 X karyotype, while Klinefelter's syndrome is associated with 47 XXY. Additional chromosomes are indicated by a plus sign (+) followed by the identity of the extra chromosome. For example, a male with trisomy 21 Down's syndrome is designated 47

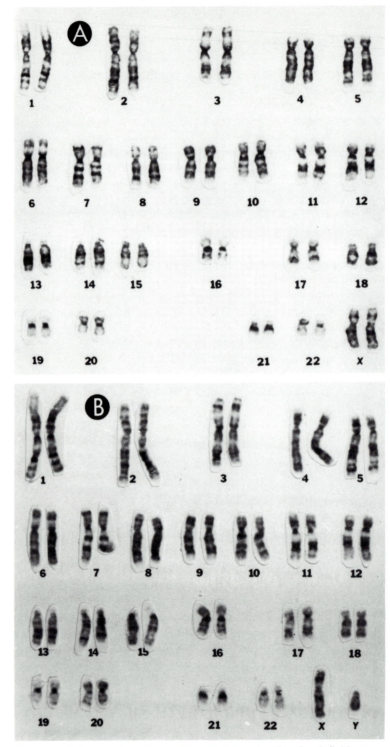

Fig 17–3.—A, normal female karyotype; **B,** normal male karyotype stained to reveal G-bands. The characteristic patterns of light and dark bands allow for definitive recognition of each chromosome pair.

XY +21. When a plus sign follows the number of a specific chromosome it indicates the presence of additional material on that chromosome as, e.g., in 46 XY 14+. The *short arm* of a chromosome is designated *p*, while the long arm is *q*. An addition is designated +; a deletion is −. Thus the karyotype of a male with the *cri du chat* syndrome, which is due to a deletion of the short arm of chromosome 5, is represented 46 XY 5p−. Translocations of part or all of one chromosome to another have a complex, but specific, terminology and are discussed further in the section "Meiosis."

The genotype or genetic constitution of an individual is encoded in the deoxyribonucleic acid (DNA) of the chromosomes (Watson, 1976; Stent, 1971). There are four nucleotide bases that make up each of the two strands of the DNA double helix. These nucleotide bases will pair only with a single complementary base on the opposite strand of the helix. When cell division occurs and the genetic material is duplicated, the two strands of DNA separate and two complementary daughter strands are formed by the *replication* enzymes, adenine opposite thymine and guanine opposite cytosine. The information encoded in the gene is used to form a strand of ribonucleic acid (RNA) by the process designated *transcription*. The sequence of DNA bases is transcribed by the precise pairing of specific complementary RNA bases to the DNA template. The messenger RNA strand in turn interacts with ribosomes, transfer RNA and various proteins in a process called *translation*, leading to the production of specific amino acid sequences. Not only the zygote, but each cell in the human body is thought to contain the entire genome (or genetic constitution), although the processes of differentiation allow the expression of certain portions of this genome in some cells and its repression in others, thus providing for specific cell types.

Recently developed recombinant DNA technologies hold great promise for medical genetics and have already produced much excitement. These technologies will be useful for diagnosis (especially prenatally) and for detecting carriers, as well as for fundamental studies of normal and pathologic gene action, and ultimately for gene therapy. Recombinant DNA studies rely on many concepts and techniques, only a few of which can be summarized here. More detailed reviews are available (Miller, 1981; Antonarakis et al., 1982). Most relevant to our presentation are the uses of recombinant DNA technologies in genetic diagnosis. These involve two basic approaches that will be described in some detail. The first approach is indirect and uses a nearby DNA marker not involved in causing the particular disorder to detect the presence of a disease-related gene or genes. Most often this linked, noncausal marker consists of what is called a restriction fragment length polymorphism (RFLP). In the second approach, the presence of the mutant gene is detected directly. Both approaches depend on the use of gene probes, restriction endonucleases, and gel electrophoresis. The DNA present in the nucleus of each cell in the body normally contains all of the genes of the individual. This DNA can be extracted from any convenient cell, such as a leukocyte or amniotic fluid cell. A consistent pattern of regular DNA fragments can be produced by incubation of this DNA with enzymes called *restriction endonucleases*, which cleave DNA at sequence-specific sites consisting of four, five, six, or seven DNA bases, the number and sequence depending on the specific restriction endonuclease used. The DNA restriction fragments can then be resolved by electrophoresis in agarose gels, which separate the fragments according to their lengths as shown in Figure 17–4. Although all of the genes of the individual are present somewhere in this display of fragments, identifying the location of any particular gene requires the addition of what is called a probe, a specially prepared segment of DNA containing the sequence of the gene being sought. Such probes are usually prepared from radioactively labeled precursors using various techniques to retrieve specific

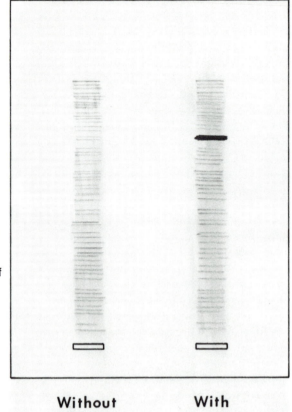

Fig 17–4.—Separation of restriction fragments by gel electrophoresis with and without gene-specific probe. Following digestion into fragments using a DNA sequence-specific restriction endonuclease, electrophoresis is used to separate the fragments according to their molecular lengths. Without hybridization with a gene-specific probe it is not possible to distinguish the fragment bearing the gene of interest. After hybridization with a specific probe, however, the fragment containing the gene of interest is readily identified, usually by autoradiography.

Without Probe

With Probe

gene sequences from either messenger RNA or directly from DNA. After electrophoresis, the radioactive probe is added, its complementary DNA sequence causes it to hybridize with the fragment containing the gene of interest, and the location of this fragment and gene can be identified by autoradiography as shown in Figure 17–4.

As noted previously, restriction endonucleases cleave the DNA at specific sequences. The fragment of DNA thus generated is that which normally connects two such sequence-specific cleavage sites. If one or more DNA bases within a cleavage site is changed by mutation, the restriction endonuclease no longer cleaves at that site, so the fragment of DNA containing that sequence is longer than it was before the mutation. We all carry a rather large number of mutations that change poten-

tial cleavage sites but do not seem to cause disease. In many cases the mutations have occurred in DNA sequences that do not normally code for proteins. These mutationally altered sequences found in individuals are inherited by progeny in a direct line of descent. Since these changes are relatively frequent in populations and are heritable, they are called *restriction fragment length polymorphisms* (RFLPs). The first application of recombinant DNA technology to the diagnosis of human genetic disease occurred in 1978 when Kan and Dozy (1978) developed a prenatal diagnostic test for sickle cell anemia using RFLPs. Their test took advantage of the concept of linkage, the fact that two markers that are close together on the same chromosome will assort nonrandomly, either both or neither being transmitted to the offspring of an individual. Kan and Dozy cleaved the DNA prior to electrophoresis using the restriction endonuclease Hpa I, which cleaves DNA at the sequence GTTAAC. After separating the fragments by electrophoresis and applying the radioactive globin-gene probe to locate the fragment containing the β-globin gene, the investigators found that the length of the DNA fragment on which the β-globin gene was located differed for the different β-globin genotypes. In individuals in their test group who had normal hemoglobin A, the β-globin gene was present on a fragment that was either 7.6 kilobases (kb) (i.e., 7,600 DNA bases) or 7.0 kb long, while the β-globin gene in persons with hemoglobin S was located on a 13.0-kb fragment. The β-globin gene probe did not react differently to the β^A-gene than to the β^S-gene; it was not sensitive to the change in a single DNA base in the rather large globin gene. Diagnosis was made possible by the presence of a second, linked mutation, which altered a nearby DNA sequence so that the Hpa I restriction endonuclease no longer cleaved at the nearby site, thus making the β^S-globin gene part of a longer fragment defined by the next adjacent Hpa I cleavage site (Fig 17–5). Taking advantage of this linked RFLP, the β-globin genotype of any individual could be deduced from the analysis of DNA in leukocytes, amniotic fluid cells, or any other nucleated cells. After incubation with Hpa I, electrophoresis of DNA from an individual with sickle cell trait and hemoglobin AS would have one band at 7.0/7.6 kb and a second band at 13.0 kb. In contrast, an individual with sickle cell anemia and hemoglobin SS would have a single band at 13.0 kb. This approach was successfully applied by Kan and Dozy to the prenatal diagnosis of a fetus at risk for sickle cell anemia and the correctness of the diagnosis, which in this case was sickle cell trait, was confirmed in the child following her birth. An important point is that analysis of DNA from amniotic fluid cells, which usually do not express the globin gene, correctly predicted the hemoglobin genotype for the adult hemoglobin that would not become the major hemoglobin until much later in gestation.

Although the prenatal diagnosis of sickle cell anemia was the first to be accomplished using RFLPs, other molecular diagnostic procedures have been developed for β-thalassemia, hemophilia B, phenylketonuria, analbuminemia, and, most recently, Huntington's disease (Giannelli et al., 1984; Camerino et al., 1984; Woo et al., 1983; Murray et al., 1983; Gusella et al., 1983). The techniques that use RFLPs are like all linkage analyses; they are essentially familial diagnoses and generally require the availability for analysis of samples from at least several family members. A single at-risk patient or fetus is insufficient for the application of this type of analysis.

The usefulness of the second approach, the direct detection of a mutant, disease-producing gene is also illustrated by sickle cell anemia. The direct detection of this disorder re-

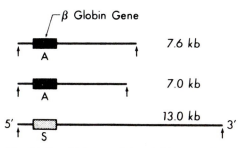

Fig 17–5.—Linkage of the globin gene to a restriction site polymorphism. *Hpa* I restriction endonuclease cleavage sites, indicated by *arrows*, to the left of the β-globin gene are constant, but those to the right differ depending on the specific globin gene present. These sites are closer in the case of the β^A-globin gene, so that the total length of the restriction fragment bearing the β^A-gene is either 7.6 kilobases (kb) or 7.0 kb in length. The mutation that produced the β^S-gene, however, is linked to a mutation that eliminated the nearest *Hpa* I cleavage site to the right, resulting in a longer fragment that is 13.0 kb in length. Thus, the differences in the length of the restriction fragment bearing the β^S-globin gene can be used to deduce the globin genotype of the individual whose DNA is being analyzed. (From Kan Y.W., Dozy A.M.: *Proc. Natl. Acad. Sci. U.S.A.* 75:5631–5635, 1978.)

cently became possible through the use of the restriction endonuclease Mst II, which cleaves at the CCTNAGG sequence present in the β^A-gene but not at the mutant sequence present in the β^S-gene. This direct analysis requires a DNA sample from only one individual or a single fetus at risk. Other types of direct DNA analysis are possible for α_1-antitrypsin deficiency and in cases where one or more genes have been deleted from the DNA such as in α-thalassemia (Kidd et al., 1983; Kidd et al., 1984; Wong et al., 1978).

In view of the rapid pace of advances in recombinant DNA technology, the list of serious genetic disorders diagnosable through linkage analysis using RFLPs or directly is likely to grow rapidly in the coming years.

It is important to distinguish between two fundamentally different cell types. *Germ cells* are the gonadal cells that, through the process of meiosis, form the gametes. The genetic information carried by the germ cells can thus be transmitted to subsequent generations of individuals. *Somatic cells* make up the remainder of the body, replicate by mitosis, and transmit their genetic information to their somatic cell progeny, but not between generations of whole individuals. Each cell has an ordered sequence of events in its life designated the *cell cycle*, shown in Figure 17–6. When two daughter cells are formed, each enters into a specific stage called the G_1 pe-

riod or first gap. During this time the chromosomes are present in the diploid number (2n) and are dispersed in the nucleus. The next stage of the cell cycle is the S period, which is defined as the time of DNA synthesis and duplication. At the end of this period the chromosome complement is doubled and the cell contains 4n chromosomes, twice the diploid number. The stage from the end of the S period to the initiation of mitosis is designated the G_2 period or second gap. These three stages of the cell cycle are collectively called *interphase*. The final phase of the cell cycle is *mitosis* in somatic cells, while in germ cells during gametogenesis the final phase is *meiosis*. Each of these can be divided into prophase, metaphase, anaphase, and telophase (Swanson et al., 1967; Hamerton, 1971).

Meiosis

Meiosis is the process by which the chromosome constitution of cells destined to become gametes is reduced from the diploid number of 46, or 2n, to the haploid number of 23, or n. To accomplish this, these cells divide twice while replicating their chromosomes only once, as diagrammed in Figure 17–7. In the first meiotic division, or meiosis I, the dispersed interphase chromatin first condenses. In step *a*, it becomes apparent that the chromosomes have already replicated in the previous S phase, yielding the 4n num-

Fig 17–6.—The cell cycle. Newly formed daughter cells enter into the G_1 period or first gap. At this stage, the chromosome number is diploid or 2n. The S period begins with initiation of DNA synthesis and ends when DNA replication is complete, bringing the chromosome complement to 4n. The G_2 period ends with the initiation of mitosis. The four stages of mitosis are prophase *(p)*, metaphase *(m)*, anaphase *(a)*, and telophase *(t)*.

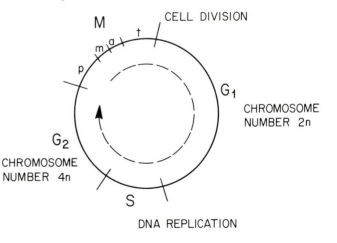

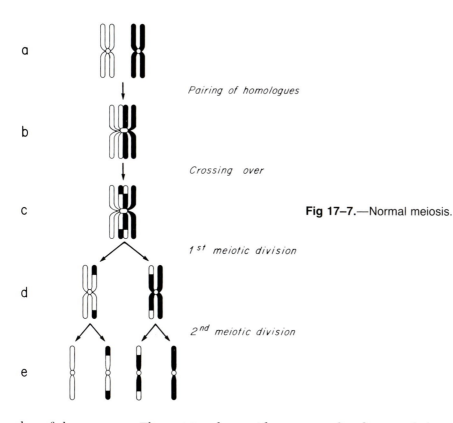

a

Pairing of homologues

b

Crossing over

c   **Fig 17–7.**—Normal meiosis.

1st meiotic division

d

2nd meiotic division

e

ber of chromosomes. These *sister chromatids,* each of which is half of the replicated chromosome, next separate everywhere along their length except at the centromere. In step *b*, a feature unique to meiosis, homologous chromosomes attract each other and, by the process known as *synapsis,* pair lengthwise at the equatorial region of the nucleus. At this stage, homologous segments of the maternal and paternal chromosomes are exchanged in a process called *crossing over,* step *c*. Longer chromosomes generally exhibit more crossing over, but it occurs even in the small chromosomes. Crossing over is a normal process that increases the range of genetic diversity beyond the combinations produced by the random assortment of homologous chromosomes. At the time of cell division in meiosis I, the homologous paired chromosomes separate and move toward opposite poles of the nucleus in the process called *disjunction,* step *d*. As a result of this disjunction and because the

maternal and paternal chromosomes were arranged in parallel, but at random, on the meiotic spindle, the products of the first meiotic division are two cells, each of which contains one member—maternal or paternal—of each of the 23 pairs of chromosomes. Generally about half of the chromosomes in each gametocyte will be of maternal origin and half of paternal origin. Since the maternal and paternal chromosomes have been separated by the first meiotic division, this is referred to as a *reduction division.* It will be recalled, however, that chromosomal replication to the 4n state occurred prior to the beginning of meiosis I and hence this reduction division still leaves the progeny cells with the 2n or diploid number of chromosomes. These paired chromatids that have remained joined at the centromere are identical except in those regions where crossing over has occurred with a chromatid of the homologous chromosome (McDermott, 1975).

Chromosome replication does not occur following meiosis I, and the gametogenic cells enter meiosis II with the 2n chromosome number. Meiosis II has been likened to a mitotic division because the chromatids align in the equatorial region, the spindle forms, the centromeres divide and one member of each chromatid pair moves to the opposite pole of the cell. Meiosis II differs from mitosis in that the progeny cells are haploid, with the n number of chromosomes, step *e*.

While these features of meiosis apply to both males and females, oogenesis and spermatogenesis differ in important respects. Oogenesis begins early in the embryonic ovary. The primary oocytes form during early fetal development and reach the late prophase of meiosis I by the fifth month of intrauterine life. The process of meiosis is arrested at what is termed the dictyotene stage of the meiosis I prophase. The meiotic processes resume 12 to 50 years later, after puberty, and only if that oocyte is to be activated in preparation for ovulation. This delay has been cited as a possible basis for certain of the chromosome anomalies shown to be due more often to errors in maternal than in paternal gametogenesis. When oogenesis resumes at metaphase in meiosis I, cell division results in two cells of very different sizes. The cell containing half of the chromosome complement but very little cytoplasm becomes the first polar body. The second meiotic division begins after the so-called pronucleus of the sperm has entered the large cell. Meiosis II in the oocyte is also highly asymmetric, yielding a small second polar body and an ovum that is nearly as large as the original primary oocyte. The male and female haploid pronuclei then unite to form the *zygote.*

Although development of testes proceeds much earlier in the embryo (Mittwoch, 1976), spermatogenesis is not initiated until puberty. In response to hormonal stimulation, primary spermatocytes are formed continuously by mitotic division and complete the first and second meiotic divisions. Each primary spermatocyte thus gives rise to four haploid sperm cells of equal size.

Nondisjunction, the failure of separation of paired chromosomes at metaphase—occurring during meiosis—leads to the formation of an aneuploid gamete, as shown in Figure 17–8. Instead of being diploid, the gamete will have an extra chromosome or will lack one chromosome. If these gametes are fertilized by normal gametes, the resulting zygote will be trisomic or monosomic, respectively. Monosomic cells can also be formed by *anaphase lag,* a process in which the migration of a chromosome is delayed, resulting in its exclusion from both daughter nuclei. Monosomies for the autosomes are lethal, whereas trisomies of many of the autosomes, while deleterious, are observed in live-born infants. Monosomy for the X chromosome results in Turner's syndrome, while monosomy with a Y chromosome but no X chromosome has not been observed. Trisomy of the X chromosome occurs and is associated with few, if any, serious abnormalities. By definition, trisomy refers to the presence of three homologous chromosomes and, since the X and Y are not homologous, XXY and XYY individuals are classified simply as having sex chromosome aneuploidy. Since the homologous chromosomes and the sex chromosomes normally separate in meiosis I, while the sister chromatids separate in meiosis II, the consequences of nondisjunction at these steps will differ. Nondisjunction in meiosis I results in a gamete with an extra homologous autosome or, in the case of the sex chromosomes in the male, both an X and a Y. If nondisjunction occurs in meiosis II, however, the extra chromosome in the gamete will be a sister chromatid. Thus, for example, XYY must result from a second meiotic division nondisjunction in the male parent, while XXY could result from nondisjunction in meiosis I of the male or in either meiosis I or meiosis II of the female parent. Occasionally nondisjunction occurs during both meiotic divisions, resulting in more complex aneuploidies, although sur-

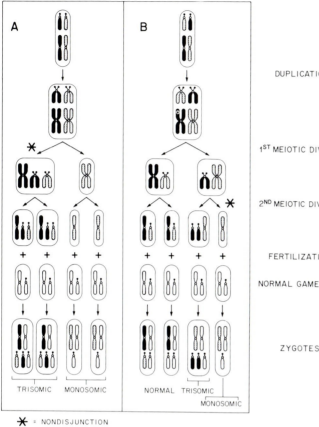

DUPLICATION

1ˢᵀ MEIOTIC DIVISION

2ᴺᴰ MEIOTIC DIVISION

FERTILIZATION

NORMAL GAMETES

ZYGOTES

✱ = NONDISJUNCTION

Fig 17–8.—A, nondisjunction at first meiotic division, resulting in abnormal gametes having an extra homologous chromosome; and **B,** nondisjunction at second meiotic division, resulting in abnormal gametes having an extra sister chromosome.

vival is limited to those involving the sex chromosomes.

Nondisjunction can also occur during mitosis and may result in *mosaicism* or the presence of two or more lines of cells differing in their genetic constitution but which have originated from single cells. Thus mitotic nondisjunction early in embryonic life would be expected to yield two daughter cells, one trisomic and the other monosomic. If an autosome were involved, the monosomic cell would be inviable while the progeny of the trisomic cell would coexist with the remaining diploid cells. For example, mitotic nondisjunction involving chromosome 21 could result in an individual with a 46 XY/47 XY +21 mosaicism.

Abnormalities in transfer of genetic information can also occur during meiosis if chromosomes are abnormal as the result of translocation. Chromosomes may become fragmented during either meiosis or mitosis and the fragments may become joined to other chromosomes or fragments of chromosomes in a process called *translocation.* As shown in Figure 17–9, if breaks occur in two chromosomes and the chromosomal material is simply exchanged, the translocation is said to be *reciprocal.* When the breakage and rejoining occur at the centromeres of the two chromosomes, the translocation is classified as the *centric fusion* or *Robertsonian* type. Translocations in which the sites of breakage and rejoining are not at the centromere are designated *non-Robertsonian.* Centric fusion translocations are far more common and usually involve the D and G group chromosomes, which have satellites, apparently because of

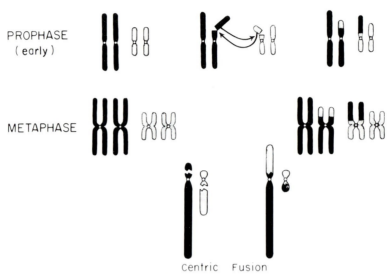

PROPHASE (early)

METAPHASE

Centric Fusion

Fig 17–9.—Mechanisms of translocation, *Top,* reciprocal translocation involving the exchange of parts of nonhomologous chromosomes early in prophase. *Center,* reciprocal translocation altering the structure of the individual chromosomes and the composition of the two pairs of homologous chromosomes at metaphase. *Bottom,* the mechanism of centric fusion, a special type of translocation involving acrocentric chromosomes. Breakage at or near the centromere occurs in both chromosomes. Of the two newly produced chromosomes, one is necessarily a minute fragment that is usually lost in a subsequent cell division. (From Sohval A.R.: *Am. J. Med.* 31:397, 1961.)

the tendency of these chromosomes to be in close physical proximity ("satellite association") during mitotic metaphase. Translocations are designated with the symbol *t* followed in parentheses by a designation of the chromosomes involved. For example, a translocation of the long arm of a chromosome 21 to the long arm of chromosome 14 is designated t(14q21q). If a sex chromosome is involved, it is listed first, e.g., t(X;2). Otherwise the chromosome having the lower number is specified first.

A reciprocal translocation with exchange of nonhomologous segments results in a rearrangement, but there is no loss of genetic material. The two new chromosomes will function well in mitotic division if each possesses a single centromere, although the minute chromosome produced in a centric fusion of acrocentric chromosomes is usually lost during subsequent divisions (see Fig 17–9). The individual with such a translocation is almost always phenotypically normal and is designated a *balanced translocation carrier*. Problems arise during meiosis when the homologous chromosome segments, rearranged by translocation, pair and then segregate in all possible combinations. As shown in Figures 17–10 and 17–11, the translocation carriers can form gametes having different chromosome contents, depending on the segregation patterns of segments and centromeres. A normal gamete can be produced and will result in a normal individual producing normal gametes and who therefore has no increased risk of a chromosome abnormality in his or her offspring. Nevertheless, four of the gametes are unbalanced. In the case of reciprocal translocations these contain two copies of a segment of one chromosome and lack a segment of another chromosome. In the case of centric fusion they are either missing an entire chromosome or have an extra chromosome. Fertilization with a normal gamete will contribute an additional complete haploid set of chromosomes and hence the zygotes will

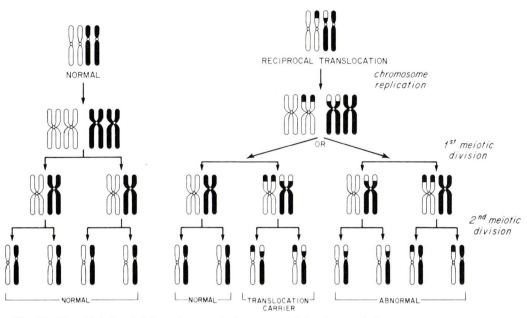

Fig 17–10.—Meiotic division of normal chromosomes and of chromosomes with reciprocal translocation. Shown here are two of the four possible abnormal chromosome complements resulting from random segregation of reciprocally translocated chromosomes.

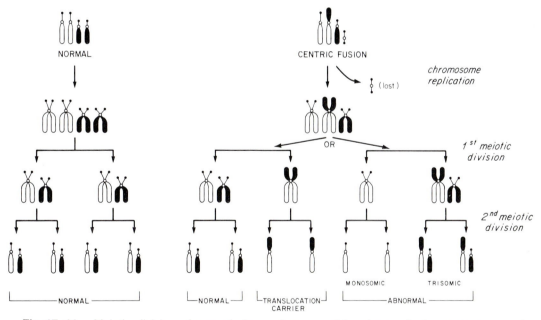

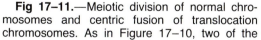

Fig 17–11.—Meiotic division of normal chromosomes and centric fusion of translocation chromosomes. As in Figure 17–10, two of the four possible abnormal chromosome complements are illustrated.

be chromosomally abnormal. Two of the possible gametes are balanced, containing a normal complement of structurally rearranged genetic information and, on fertilization, will produce an individual who is phenotypically normal. This individual, however, is a balanced translocation carrier and will also produce both chromosomally normal and abnormal gametes.

Mitosis

With fertilization, the resulting zygote enters the mitotic cell cycle. During interphase, which includes G_1, S, and G_2 are previously noted, the chromosomes are dispersed within the nucleus and, with two exceptions, cannot be visualized. These exceptions are the Barr body, which, as discussed in detail in the following section, is an inactivated and condensed X chromosome, and the Y *body*, a brightly fluorescent spot in the nuclei of male cells treated with quinacrine. Mitosis proper begins with prophase during which the chromosomes begin to condense and appear thin and threadlike. The chromosomes contract, revealing their distinctive morphologic features, and the sister chromatids become apparent, reflecting the fact that they have already replicated in the previous S period. In metaphase, the nuclear membrane disappears, the spindle appears, and the chromosomes align themselves along the midplane region of the cell. This alignment in mitosis occurs with individual chromosomes, in contrast to the alignment of paired homologues that is characteristic of the first meiotic division. In anaphase, the centromeres separate and the chromosomes migrate to opposite poles of the cell. Telophase begins when these chromosomes have reached the poles and begin to lose their distinct shapes. Formation of two new nuclear membranes and cell division complete telophase. Mitotic division thereafter occurs repetitively and, with rare exceptions, transmits the complete genome of the zygote to each successive progeny cell. The processes of differentiation result in selective expression and nonexpression of parts of the genome that determine specific cellular characteristics, including morphology, metabolic properties, and capacity to replicate.

Nondisjunction can occur during mitosis in a manner similar to that described for nondisjunction during meiosis II and results in monosomic and trisomic cells. Anaphase lag can occur in mitosis, producing a normal and a monosomic cell line. Depending on the stage of development during which the nondisjunction or anaphase lag occurs, some fraction of the cells in the body will contain aneuploid chromosome complements. An individual with different cellular genotypes that originated from a single cell is termed *mosaic* or *mixoploid*. In general, the earlier that the abnormal division occurs during development, the greater the proportion of aneuploid cells. There appear to be influences, however, that select against or for survival of certain cell lines. Hence, the final proportions of chromosomally normal and abnormal cells in a mosaic allow only a crude estimate of the timing of the nondisjunction or anaphase lag. The importance of mosaicism is that the expression of the abnormal complement may be modified by the normal cell line, producing individuals whose phenotype is intermediate between the normal and the full disease state.

The Single-Active-X Hypothesis

The *single-active-X or Lyon hypothesis* (Fig 17–12) is essential for understanding both normal X-chromosome function and certain sex chromosome disorders. Proposed in 1961 by Lyon and by several others simultaneously, this principle states that in females, at an early stage of embryonic development, one of the two normal X chromosomes is functionally inactivated in all somatic cells. This inactivation is irreversible and applies to all functions except replication of that X chromosome. Whether it is the maternal or paternal X chromosome that is inactivated in a given cell is both random and mutually exclusive; that is, the identity of the inactivated X

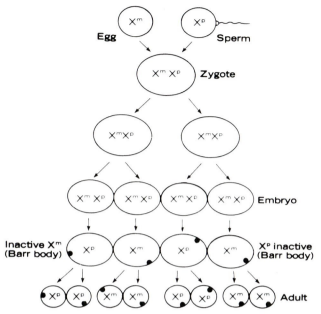

Fig 17–12.—Diagrammatic representation of X chromosome inactivation. (Reprinted by permission from Fralkow P.J.: *N. Engl. J. Med.* 291:26, 1974.)

chromosome (maternal or paternal) does not affect, nor is it affected by, the identity of the inactivated X chromosome in any other cell (Lyon, 1972, 1974). During interphase the inactive X is visible as a densely stained area adjacent to the nuclear membrane and is called the *nuclear chromatin* or *Barr body* (Fig 17–13). The maximal number of Barr bodies is one less than the number of X chromosomes present. Thus a normal male and a female with Turner's syndrome (45 X) have no Barr bodies. A normal female and a male with Klinefelter's syndrome (47 XXY) have one Barr body, while a triple-X (47 XXX) female has two Barr bodies. Sex chromatin status is usually evaluated by means of a buccal smear in which epithelial cells are scraped from the inner cheek and their DNA stained. A hundred or more cells are examined and their Barr body count tabulated to give the percentage that show Barr bodies. In normal females at least 20% of buccal epithelial cells contain Barr bodies, while in normal males the cells showing clumped nuclear chromatin that meets the criteria for a Barr body are, at most, 1% to 2%. For diagnostic purposes a person having 5% or more cells with Barr bodies is *chromatin positive*. A person with no Barr bodies is *chromatin negative*.

Normal males have only a single X chromosome, namely, that which was inherited from the mother, and the genes on this X chromosome are expressed. Normal females, however, have two X chromosomes, one of which was inherited from each parent. As shown in Figure 17–12, during development one or the other X chromosome is inactivated in each somatic cell. On the average, in the adult female there will be about equal numbers of cells with active maternally and paternally derived X chromosomes. The inactivation, however, occurs early in embryonic life, apparently at about day 16, when there are a relatively small number of primordial somatic cells destined for certain tissues and functions. Thus there is a finite probability that a deficiency encoded on one X chromosome will be expressed because of disproportional inactivation of the X with the normal gene. Correspondingly, some female carriers of X-linked recessive disorders cannot be detected by tests of function because of disproportionate inactivation of the X chromosome with the abnormal gene. Since X inactivation does not

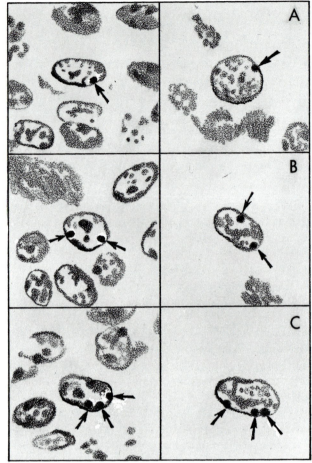

Fig 17–13.—Barr bodies in nuclei of cells from human skin *(left)* and buccal mucosa *(right).* **A,** XX normal female. **B,** XXXY male with mental deficiency. **C,** XXXXY eunuch with micro-orchism and mental deficiency.

occur in oocytes, this will not affect the inheritance of the X chromosome.

SEXUAL DIFFERENTIATION

Normal sexual development depends on the normal function of genes both on the X chromosomes and on the autosomes, as well as, in the case of males, on the Y chromosome. It has long been recognized that the presence of a Y chromosome leads to male development. Furthermore, since the features of Turner's syndrome have been observed in individuals with one X chromosome and an isochromosome resulting from centric fusion of the long arms of the Y[46,Xi(Yq)] it seems likely that the short arm of the Y chromosome contains the gene(s) that determine male sex. The observation in highly inbred strains of mice that females reject skin grafts from males led to the identification of the *H-Y antigen,* a Y-linked plasma membrane transplantation antigen that has been highly conserved during mammalian evolution. A second and related, but not identical, antigen is called serologically detectable male (SDM) antigen. Several assays for H-Y type antigens have been developed, but each has its limitations. H-Y antigen has been claimed by some to be the testis-determining substance that directs the initial steps leading to differentiation of the bipotential embryonic gonad as a testis. The presence of a testis nearly always signals the presence of H-Y antigen, but the presence of H-Y antigen may or may not be accompanied by testis development. Recent data, however, from clinical and laboratory studies in humans and mice indicate that neither H-Y transplantation antigen nor the SDM antigen is the primary cause of male gonadal determination (Silvers et al., 1982).

According to the current model, the presence of a Y chromosome, or at least Yp, induces the bipotential embryonic gonad to differentiate into a testis. Once male gonadal sex has been determined, histologic as well as biochemical differentiation begins. A nonsteroidal substance secreted locally causes regression of the müllerian ducts. Androgens are produced by the fetal testis but their uptake into cell cytoplasm and nucleus is dependent on the normal function of a specific androgen receptor that is encoded by the X chromosome and is present in probably all cells of both normal males and females. This androgen receptor is either completely absent or markedly defective (Amrhein et al., 1976) in complete testicular feminization, an X-linked recessive disorder (Meyer et al., 1975) analogous to the *Tfm* mutation well characterized in the mouse (Lyon and Hawkes, 1970). The clinical features of this and other relevant disorders of sexual development are described in a later section.

In normal males the synthesis of androgen stimulates development of the wolffian duct system. Even with a normal testis and wolffian system, proper differentiation of the male external genitalia requires the presence of the enzyme steroid 5α-reductase (Imperato-McGinley and Peterson, 1976). This enzyme converts testosterone to dihydrotestosterone, is present normally in cells throughout the body and is encoded by a locus on an autosomal chromosome. Deficiency of 5α-reductase results in a distinctive form of male pseudohermaphroditism characterized by ambiguous genitalia, a distinctly male puberty, and the absence of gynecomastia (Griffin and Wilson, 1980).

In the absence of the testis-determining factor, the bipotential gonad differentiates into an ovary, although normal ovarian development requires the presence of a second X chromosome. In the absence of androgen, the primitive wolffian system involutes and the external genitalia become female. The müllerian system differentiates independent of the ovary, showing equally good development if no gonad is present.

When only a single X chromosome is present, as is the case in 45 X Turner's syndrome, the external genitalia and müllerian duct system are normal in the newborn but ovarian development has been interrupted at a primitive stage. The resulting streak gonad is responsible for the sterility, primary amenorrhea, and failure to develop secondary sexual characteristics that are seen in these patients.

The exposure of a genetic female fetus to high levels of androgens, either from maternal sources or in a fetus having a masculinizing type of adrenogenital syndrome, results in female pseudohermaphroditism with varying degrees of virilization of the external genitalia but normal müllerian structures and ovaries, and absent wolffian structures.

Characterization of normal and abnormal sexual development thus requires information regarding the genetic sex, the gonadal sex, and the phenotypic sex of individuals. Normal sexual development depends on the functions of gene loci on both the autosomes and sex chromosomes, as well as on a hormonally normal intrauterine environment. More extensive reviews can be found in Simpson, 1976, and Saenger, 1984.

GENETIC DISORDERS

Genetic disorders can be classified into three major groups: (1) chromosome disorders, (2) mendelian or single gene disorders, and (3) multifactorial disorders.

Chromosome Disorders

Chromosome disorders result from abnormalities in the number or makeup of chromosomes that can be visualized with the microscope. The most common are aneuploid conditions, such as trisomies and monosomies, and chromosome rearrangements that result in deletions or additions of recognizable amounts of chromosome substance. Less often there are more complex defects, such as the formation of *ring chromosomes* in which the normally free ends are joined, or *isochromosomes* made up of two short arms or two long arms joined at a centromere, or *dicentric* chromosomes having two centromeres. Any of these abnormalities can be present in all cells or as a mosaic in which two or occasionally more chromosomally distinct cell lines are present. The specific disorders involving individual autosomal chromosomes differ from the sex chromosome disorders in both frequency and severity. For both autosome and sex chromosome disorders, the frequencies of conception differ markedly from those at birth, since many are lethal in utero. As a group, however, chromosome disorders are recognized clinically by the malformations that they produce. In some individuals with major chromosome abnormalities detected in screening consecutive newborns there are no accompanying physical features that would indicate the presence of the chromosome abnormality. The physician must consider obtaining a karyotype analysis in instances of unexplained fetal or neonatal demise, particularly when dysmorphic features are present, or when development is retarded as manifested by small size, failure to thrive, or microcephaly. Many of the major chromosome abnormalities that are compatible with survival produce some degree of mental retardation.

Most of these disorders occur as sporadic cases, arising from an error in gametogenesis in one or the other parent. While many are potentially heritable in classic mendelian patterns, few are actually transmitted, because of the frequently reduced fertility resulting from decreased survival, physical abnormalities of both functional and cosmetic importance, mental retardation, or actual sterility. Thus, in most instances risks of recurrence are calculated not according to mendelian principles but, instead, on a strictly empirical basis.

Hence, it is essential that the physician be familiar with the incidence and recurrence risks for each specific chromosome disorder encountered.

Autosomal disorders are present in about 1 per 256 live births (Hook and Hamerton, 1977). The most common type of autosomal abnormality results from nondisjunction in meiosis or, less often, in an early mitotic division. Such nondisjunction usually produces trisomic and/or monosomic cell lines. Although such nondisjunctional events are often lethal in utero (see the section "Spontaneous Abortion"), certain trisomies account for a substantial proportion of congenital malformations. The frequency of autosomal trisomies in live-born infants is 1 per 704 (Hook and Hamerton, 1977).

Structural rearrangements are the most common of the autosomal abnormalities in live-born children, occurring at the rate of 1 per 403. The majority of these, 1 per 515 live births, are present as balanced translocations, thereby providing a complete chromosome complement and producing no phenotypic abnormality. Unbalanced translocations with an abnormal chromosome complement and an observable disorder, however, are present in 1 per 1,852 live births (Hook and Hamerton, 1977).

Considering the fact that there are only two sex chromosomes while there are 44 autosomes, the incidence of sex chromosome disorders in live births (1 per 478) seems inordinately high. This is understandable in terms of differential survival. The defects produced by the sex chromosome abnormalities are less lethal and, in general, less damaging. Only monosomy Y (45 Y) appears to be incompatible with life. While XO conceptions exhibit a high rate of fetal wastage, some 45 X individuals survive to birth and beyond.

Single Gene Disorders

Single gene defects result from submicroscopic changes in individual genes. Usually these changes involve only a single nucleotide base in the DNA and occasionally several bases are deleted or inserted, but the changes are small relative to those in the chromosome disorders. The mode of inheritance depends upon whether the mutant gene is located on an autosome or a sex chromosome, and upon whether it is dominant or recessive. The manifestations of a mutant gene on the X chromosome differ in males and females. If the mutant gene is on an autosome, it is present in males and females with equal frequency. A disorder is said to be *dominant* when it is manifest as a disease in the heterozygote, i.e., an individual having a normal gene on one chromosome and a mutant alternative form, or *allele*, of this gene on the other chromosome of the pair. *Recessive* disorders are those that are expressed only when they are unopposed by a normal gene, i.e., when both alleles specify a disorder in the case of the paired autosomal loci and in males whose single X chromosome bears a mutant gene. To date, 3,368 mendelian phenotypes have been described (McKusick, 1983). Of these, 1,827 are autosomal dominant, 1,298 are autosomal recessive, and 243 are X-linked—almost all X-linked recessive. A complete family history is an essential part of the diagnostic evaluation and can be recorded in a pedigree using the symbols shown in Figure 17–14.

Autosomal dominant disorders often present a pattern of an affected parent having one or more affected children, as shown in Figure 17–15. The characteristics of autosomal dominant inheritance are (1) generation-to-generation transmission without intervening unaffected individuals, (2) equal frequency in males and females, (3) an average of 50% of the offspring of an affected parent having the disorder, (4) transmission from either sex to either sex, and (5) no recurrence of the disorder in the offspring of individuals who have an affected parent but did not themselves inherit the gene. The role of spontaneous mutation is readily apparent since it results in the occurrence of autosomal dominant disorders in families in which there are no other similarly affected individuals. Such a new mutation presumably was present in one of the parental gametes and therefore is present in all cells of the affected offspring. As a result, the offspring manifests the disorder and, since the abnormal gene is present in the gonads as well, this affected individual can transmit the gene to his or her offspring

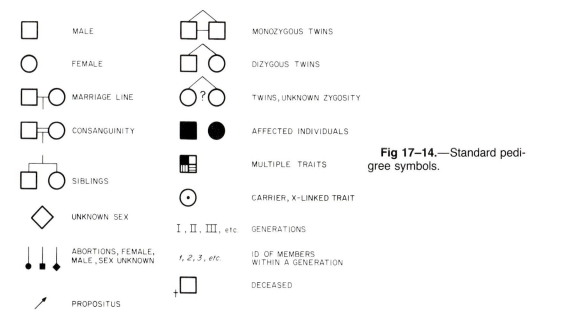

Fig 17–14.—Standard pedigree symbols.

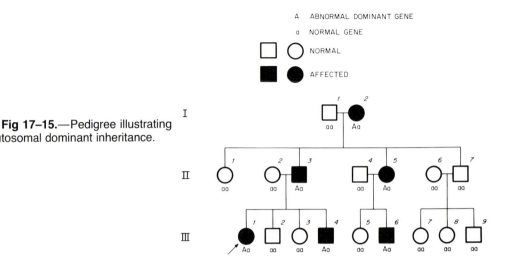

Fig 17–15.—Pedigree illustrating autosomal dominant inheritance.

in characteristic autosomal dominant pattern. With very few exceptions there are no specific laboratory abnormalities in the autosomal dominant disorders and hence the diagnosis relies heavily on clinical features, which often vary. The range of severity with which the characteristic features are manifest is termed *expressivity*. Some specific disorders show great variability of expressivity, while in others the variations between affected individuals in the same family and even between affected individuals in different families are quite small. Occasionally an autosomal dominant disorder will appear to skip a generation, producing characteristic abnormalities in, for example, an individual and one of his or her grandparents but not in either parent. In this case the gene is said to be *nonpenetrant* and the disorder to show *incomplete penetrance*. When complete examinations are carried out, however, the so-called unaffected parent frequently shows milder but definite evidence of the disorder. Incomplete penetrance is probably less common than is often supposed. Although the terms expressivity and penetrance are introduced here in conjunction with autosomal dominant disorders, they are entirely general concepts referring to alterations in the expression of the genome not only for any type of genetic disorder but for normal traits as well.

Autosomal recessive disorders occur when mutant disease-producing alleles are present at a locus on both chromosomes of the pair. Figure 17–16 shows a pedigree in which the affected child is the product of a first-cousin marriage. *Consanguinity*, or relatedness by blood, increases the probability that, when an abnormal autosomal recessive gene is present, a child will inherit one such gene from both parents and thus be an affected *homozygote*. The rarer an autosomal recessive gene for a disorder is, the greater will be the proportion of cases that are the products of consanguineous matings. In order to produce a disorder, the mutant alleles need not be identical, as they are in the homozygote, but they must both be abnormal. Thus, for example, an individual with hemoglobin SS disease (sickle cell anemia) is homozygous, having a β^S gene at the globin β-chain locus on each member of the chromosome pair, whereas a person with hemoglobin SC disease has a β^S gene on one chromosome and a β^C gene on the other. Yet both have red blood cell sickling disorders. An individual with paired abnormal, but nonidentical, alleles at a locus is termed a *genetic compound*.

The characteristics of autosomal recessive inheritance are (1) pedigrees in which unaffected parents give birth to one or more affected offspring, (2) equal frequency in males

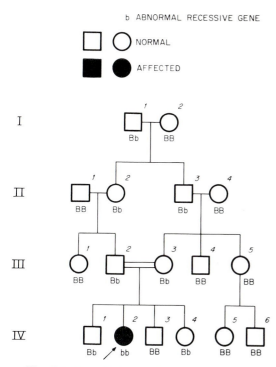

Fig 17–16.—Pedigree illustrating autosomal recessive inheritance. The double lines connecting individuals III-2 and III-3 indicate consanguinity, here a first-cousin mating.

and females, (3) an average of 25% of the offspring of carrier couples having the disorder, and (4) the presence of the carrier state in all offspring of couples in which one person is affected and the other is homozygous normal. Specific biochemical defects have been identified in a number of autosomal recessive disorders so that precise laboratory diagnosis is often possible. In many of these disorders the carriers can also be identified by direct testing. New mutations producing abnormal autosomal recessive alleles certainly occur, but in practice this is rarely observed. Such a fresh mutation, occurring at a frequency of perhaps 1 per 10,000 genes per generation, would almost always occur in an individual who was previously normal, and would thus produce only the carrier state. In turn, the carrier state would probably go unrecognized,

since it seldom has any substantial effect on the health of the carrier. The birth of a child having an autosomal recessive disorder to parents in whom specific tests have shown that one but not the other is a carrier requires—after rigorous exclusion of laboratory error—that a distinction be made between nonpaternity, nonmaternity, and a new mutation.

For genes on the X chromosome, dominant and recessive patterns must again be distinguished, although nearly all the described X-linked disorders are recessive. The *sine qua non* of either type of X-linked inheritance is the absence of male-to-male transmission, i.e., affected males do not transmit the disorder to any of their sons. This is readily understandable since, when a male transmits his X chromosome via the sperm, the conception will be female. In contrast, to produce a son, the father must transmit his Y chromosome. Male relatives having X-linked disorders are always related to one another through an intervening female. Figure 17–17 shows the pedigree pattern of an X-linked dominant disorder, such as hypophosphatemic rickets or ornithine carbamoyltransferase deficiency. The characteristics of X-linked dominant inheritance are as

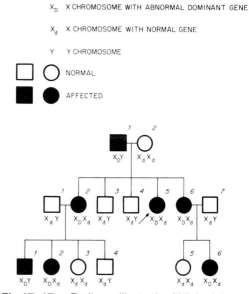

Fig 17–17.—Pedigree illustrating X-linked dominant inheritance.

follows: (1) male-to-male transmission is absent; (2) twice as many females are affected as males; (3) all female offspring of an affected male are themselves affected; (4) on the average, 50% of both male and female offspring of an affected female are themselves affected; and (5) the manifest severity of the disorder is greater in males than in females, since the latter have a normal gene on their second X chromosome and this appears to ameliorate the abnormalities.

Correspondingly, since the male has only a single X chromosome, X-linked recessive disorders will be expressed in males who are said to be *hemizygous* for the X chromosome, while females will be carriers but will not (except in rare instances) manifest the signs and symptoms of the disorder. A typical pedigree is shown in Figure 17–18. The characteristics of X-linked recessive inheritance are as follows: (1) male-to-male transmission is absent;

(2) there is a marked preponderance of affected males; (3) of the offspring of a carrier female, an average of 50% of the sons will be affected and 50% of the daughters will be carriers; (4) all of the daughters of an affected male will be carriers; and (5) the disorder does not recur in the progeny of unaffected sons or noncarrier daughters. Occasionally females manifesting X-linked recessive disorders are encountered and in most instances are found by family studies to be either (*a*) heterozygous but affected presumably because of disproportionate Lyon-type inactivation of the X chromosome with the normal gene or (*b*) homozygous, the father being affected and the mother a carrier of the disorder. Less often such an affected "female" will actually be 45 X or 46 XY with testicular feminization (see "Single Gene Defects") and thus be hemizygous for the X chromosome.

The occurrence of new mutations is readily

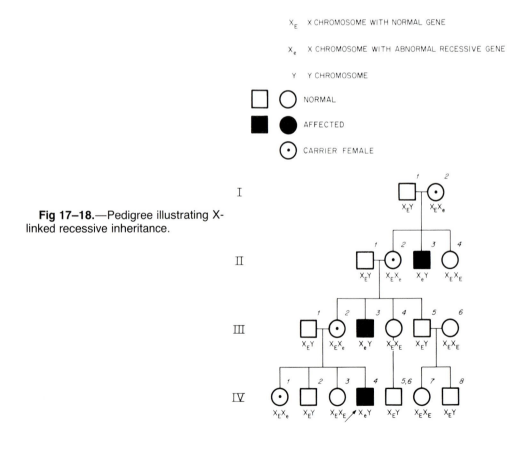

Fig 17–18.—Pedigree illustrating X-linked recessive inheritance.

apparent in the X-linked disorders as, e.g., in Duchenne-type muscular dystrophy. In this, the most severe type of muscular dystrophy, affected males show muscle weakness by about age 5 years, require a wheelchair or similar aids by their teens, and die by their early 20s. Since affected males never reproduce and, hence, never transmit the gene for Duchenne dystrophy, one might expect this disorder to decrease in frequency over the years and eventually disappear. Instead its frequency is thought to be nearly constant, with the genes that are lost each generation through the early death of affected males being replaced through mutation. The locus for Duchenne-type muscular dystrophy is on the X chromosome since the disorder follows an X-linked recessive pattern, and the mutation rate at that locus is about 1 per 10,000 per generation. This mutation rate applies to the Duchenne locus wherever the X chromosome is found and, since females have two X chromosomes and males have one, this new mutation is twice as likely to occur in females as in males. In this way the female becomes a heterozygous carrier of the gene for Duchenne-type muscular dystrophy and may have abnormally elevated levels of the muscle enzymes such as creatine phosphokinase or certain other laboratory abnormalities but will not have clinical manifestations. As noted in Figure 17–18, each of her sons has a 50% risk of being affected, while each of her daughters has a 50% risk of being a carrier.

When the diagnosis of Duchenne-type muscular dystrophy is established in a boy whose family history is negative, a new mutation is likely to be the basis. Accordingly, the chances that the mother is a carrier through new mutation are two thirds, while there is a one-third chance that the new mutation occurred in the affected son. Laboratory tests may or may not help in deciding whether the mother is a carrier. The birth of a second affected son means that the mother is surely a carrier since the alternative explanation, that of males affected through two separate mutations, would have a probability

of $(1/10,000)^2$ or $1/100,000,000$! It is in this and similar types of rather complex situations that a consultation with a medical geneticist can be particularly helpful.

Multifactorial Disorders

The group of multifactorial disorders encompasses a large number of quite heterogeneous abnormalities in which multiple genetic loci of smaller individual effects and environmental influences act together to produce defects. These disorders are sometimes referred to as *polygenic*, but, while reflecting the multiplicity of gene loci involved, this term overlooks the great importance of environmental factors. The characteristics of multifactorial inheritance include (1) the simulation of mendelian pedigree patterns in individual families but a complex, nonmendelian pattern for the disorder when many affected families are compared; (2) a recurrence risk that is generally about 5%; (3) altered sex ratio (i.e., more males affected than females or vice versa); (4) increased recurrence rate with increased severity of the disorder; (5) a further increase in the recurrence rate with each affected offspring; (6) increased risk of occurrence in the offspring of an affected individual of the less likely sex (e.g., there are three times as many males with pyloric stenosis as females; the risk of pyloric stenosis in offspring of a parent with pyloric stenosis is much greater if the affected parent is female rather than male); and (7) the presence of the disease in microforms (i.e., states in which one or more of the characteristic manifestations of the disorder are present but their expression is less severe). Examples of multifactorial disorders include anencephaly, meningomyelocele, cleft lip (alone or with cleft palate), pyloric stenosis, congenital dislocation of the hip, and various forms of congenital heart disease. The occurrence and recurrence risks are derived from empirical data about each specific disorder (Fraser and Hunter, 1975; Nora and Nora, 1976; Holmes et al., 1976) and a knowledge of the principles of multifactorial inheritance (Carter, 1968; Fraser, 1970).

GENETIC DISORDERS
IN GYNECOLOGY

Abnormalities of Sexual Differentiation

Sex Chromosome Abnormalities

TURNER'S SYNDROME.—Most often the Turner phenotype is associated with a 45 X chromosome constitution. Turner's syndrome occurs with a frequency of 1 per 2,500 live "female" births. The severity of this disorder is reflected in the fact that only about 1 in 64 conceptions that have a 45 X chromosome complement result in live births, the remainder being aborted spontaneously or stillborn. The diagnosis may be suspected at birth on the basis of small size and the presence of congenital lymphedema, which is usually transient but with slower disappearance of puffiness over the dorsal aspects of the toes and fingers. About 20% of patients have congenital cardiovascular malformations, the most frequent (about 70%) of which is coarctation of the aorta. Many patients are not diagnosed until later, often at puberty (Fig 17–19), based on the findings of short stature (the height rarely exceeding 5 feet), primary amenorrhea, infantile but female genitalia, a shield-shaped chest with widely spaced nipples, hypoplastic nails, and signs of estrogen deficiency. About half of the patients also show webbing of the posterolateral aspect of the neck, a short fourth metacarpal, and excessive numbers of pigmented cutaneous nevi. Intelligence is usually normal, mental retardation being present in about 10% of the cases. Urinary gonadotropin levels are markedly elevated. The ovaries consist of white streaks of gonadal tissue with absence or marked hypoplasia of germinal elements, and the patients are infertile (Smith, 1976). Most of the patients will have a 45 X karyotype and be chromatin negative by buccal smear. About 30% of patients with Turner's syndrome stigmata, however, will be mosaics, most often 45 X/46 XX. These individuals are often chromatin positive. In general, the smaller the proportion of 45 X cells, the fewer

the abnormalities. The karyotype of peripheral blood lymphocytes, however, may not always reflect precisely the proportions of normal and abnormal cells elsewhere. It has been postulated that some of the patients with Turner's syndrome who have been reported to be fertile are in fact X/XX mosaics who lack 46 XX cells in the karyotyped peripheral blood lymphocytes and the buccal epithelium. Mosaics with 45 X/46 XY are also seen, and these individuals may be masculinized to varying degrees. Dysgenetic gonads that contain a cell line with a Y chromosome are predisposed to gonadal malignancy, particularly gonadoblastoma (Scully, 1970a). Thus, when a cell line containing Y chromosome is identified in such a mosaic individual, prophylactic surgical removal of these dysgenetic gonads should be considered. Gonadal extirpation is not indicated for 45 X or 45 X/46 XX patients. These individuals can derive great psychological and social benefits from treatment with estrogens to promote the development of secondary sexual characteristics.

Other patients with features of Turner's syndrome have one normal X chromosome but are missing a portion of the second X chromosome, which has become abnormal by any of several possible mechanisms (Fig 17–20). Deletions resulting in the loss of parts of the X chromosome short arm, termed Xp, or long arm, Xq, produce phenotypic changes (Wyss et al., 1982). Patients with terminal Xp deletions have somatic traits characteristic of Turner's syndrome, whereas gonadal function is generally preserved. More extensive Xp deletions, extending to the proximal portion of band p11, are associated in most cases with a complete Turner's syndrome phenotype, including gonadal dysgenesis. With regard to the long arm, a large deletion of Xq, with the breakpoint at or proximal to band q21, produces gonadal dysgenesis with primary amenorrhea and, in half the cases, somatic Turner's syndrome features. A terminal deletion of Xq, with the breakpoint distal to q22, is generally associated with pure gonadal dysgenesis. In

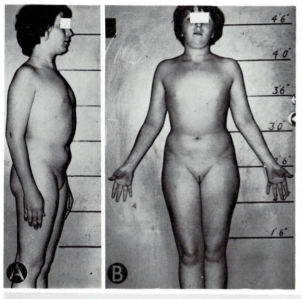

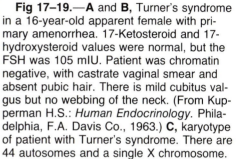

Fig 17–19.—A and **B,** Turner's syndrome in a 16-year-old apparent female with primary amenorrhea. 17-Ketosteroid and 17-hydroxysteroid values were normal, but the FSH was 105 mIU. Patient was chromatin negative, with castrate vaginal smear and absent pubic hair. There is mild cubitus valgus but no webbing of the neck. (From Kupperman H.S.: *Human Endocrinology.* Philadelphia, F.A. Davis Co., 1963.) **C,** karyotype of patient with Turner's syndrome. There are 44 autosomes and a single X chromosome.

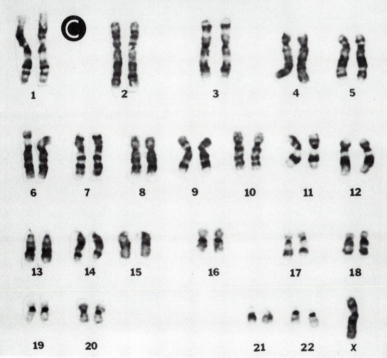

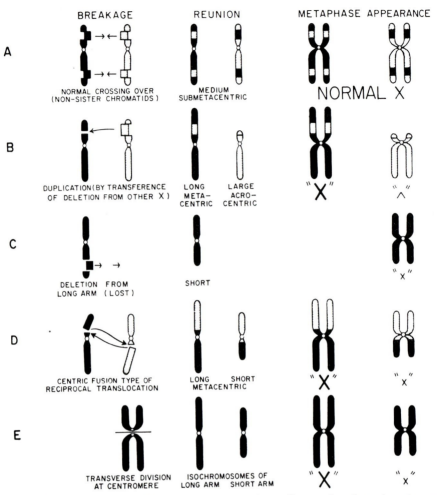

Fig 17–20.—Mechanisms of translocation producing structural abnormalities of X chromosome through improper reunion after breakage. Abnormally large metacentric X chromosomes are designated "**X**." Small Xs are represented as "x" or "^," depending on location of centromere. Black chromosome is derived from one parent, light from the other. (From Sohval A.R.: *Fertil. Steril.* 14:180, 1963.)

these cases, in contrast to those with more extensive deletions, secondary amenorrhea is particularly characteristic.

These deletions can arise through nonreciprocal translocation or the formation of isochromosomes in which two X chromosomes break at the centromere and rejoin incorrectly, with the short arms or the long arms fused to one another. In both cases, the imbalance arises when one of the two rearranged chromosomes is subsequently lost, usually during meiosis (Lindsten, 1963; Böök et al., 1973; Yanagisawa and Yokoyama, 1975). Some or all of the features of Turner's syndrome are produced when a translocation involving the X chromosome and an autosome results in the loss of critical portions of the X chromosome (Dorus et al., 1979). Structural abnormalities of the X chromosome may produce a corresponding alteration in the Barr bodies. In general when one X chromosome is normal and the other is structurally abnormal, it is the latter that is inactivated to form the Barr body, in marked contrast to the random choice for inactivation when two normal X chromosomes are present. Thus, a patient with an X deletion may show an unusually small Barr body, while one with additions to the X or with an isochromosome X may show large Barr bodies. These or any other abnormalities suspected from the results of a buccal smear must be confirmed by a complete karyotypic analysis (Polani et al., 1970).

Females with a 47 XXX chromosome constitution have been identified with a frequency of 1 per 1,100 live female births. These females appear normal at birth. Some later exhibit mild mental retardation, delayed neuromuscular maturation, learning and language disorders (Robinson et al., 1983), menstrual disturbances, and/or infertility (Puck et al., 1983).

Sex chromosome aneuploidies with still larger numbers of X chromosomes (48 XXXX; 49 XXXXX; etc.) are seen but are progressively more rare with increasing numbers of X chromosomes. The frequency of mental retardation increases with the degree of aneuploidy, but other features are quite variable. Usually sexual development is normal and these individuals are fertile. While buccal smears show increased numbers of Barr bodies—the maximal number being one less than the total number of X chromosomes—only a small percentage of cells will show the maximal number, the remainder showing fewer. As before, while the smear is an appropriate screening test, a full karyotype is required if a chromosome abnormality is suspected (Gerald, 1976).

KLINEFELTER'S SYNDROME.—Klinefelter syndrome is characterized by small, firm testes, azoospermia, gynecomastia, and elevated concentrations of plasma and urinary gonadotropins. The clinical phenotype is usually associated with a 47 XXY karyotype and occurs with a frequency of 1 per 900 live "male" births, but at much higher frequencies of approximately 1 per 50 stillborn males and 1 per 10 azoospermic adult males, thus being the most prevalent of the major sex chromo-

some disorders and the most frequent disorder of sexual differentiation. Studies of chromosome markers have shown that in about 60% of these individuals the nondisjunction that led to the presence of the extra sex chromosome occurred in the maternal gametes, while in 40% of the cases the nondisjunction was paternal. Affected males usually appear normal until puberty, at which time they develop eunuchoid body proportions, gynecomastia, and sparse facial and body hair (Fig 17–21). Height may be increased, with the lower extremities being relatively long. Lower-than-average intelligence is common and may account for the behavioral abnormalities that are frequently described (Walzer and Gerald, 1975). At puberty the testes remain small, rarely being larger than 2 cm in greatest diameter, and produce neither sperm nor adequate amounts of testosterone. The testes are characterized by hyalinized and fibrotic seminiferous tubules, hypoplastic interstitial cells, and absent spermatogenesis. Levels of urinary gonadotropins are increased. A buccal smear for screening will be chromatin positive, and karyotype will usually show a 47 XXY chromosome constitution. Some individuals with the stigmata of Klinefelter's syndrome are found to be mosaics for XXY/XY, or to have other karyotypic abnormalities such as 48 XXYY; 48 XXXY; etc. Therapy with testosterone can produce virilization but does not affect the sterility.

Nondisjunction of the Y chromosomes at the paternal second meiotic division results in 47 XYY. The frequency of XYY is about 1 per 1,000 male births. The phenotypic manifestations, particularly regarding behavior, have been the subject of much public and scientific controversy. Increased height is a frequent feature, intelligence may be decreased, and nodulocystic acne at adolescence may be severe (Philip et al., 1976). These individuals are fully masculinized and fertile. Interestingly, there have been no reported instances of XYY in father and son, indicating that the risk of transmission is very low. Whether there is any increase in the frequencies

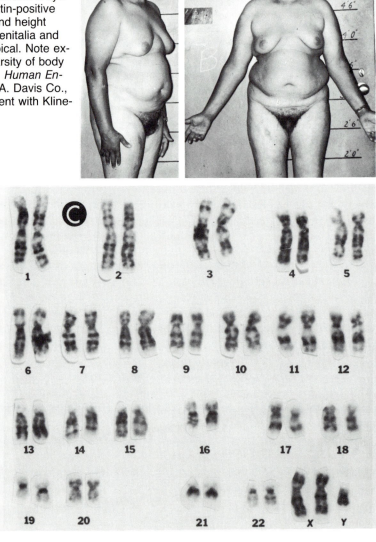

Fig 17–21.—A and **B,** Klinefelter's syndrome in 33-year-old chromatin-positive patient. Weight was 213 lb and height 67½ in. The small external genitalia and female fat distribution are typical. Note extreme gynecomastia and sparsity of body hair. (From Kupperman H.S.: *Human Endocrinology*. Philadelphia, F.A. Davis Co., 1963.) **C,** karyotype of a patient with Klinefelter's syndrome, 47 XXY.

of aggressive and criminal behavior is presently unresolved but a recent study by Witken et al. (1976) of a large group of Danish males has shown that criminal behavior is no more frequent in XYY males than in other males having comparable reductions in intelligence.

Single Gene Defects

The single gene disorders discussed in this section are inherited in simple mendelian autosomal recessive patterns, with the exception of testicular feminization, which is inherited in an X-linked recessive pattern.

Familial gonadal dysgenesis, XX type, is a

rare autosomal recessive disorder in which streak gonads are present in phenotypic females who have a 46 XX karyotype and usually lack the somatic stigmata of Turner's syndrome (Simpson et al., 1971; Perez-Ballester et al., 1970). Estrogens are deficient and gonadotropins are elevated. There have also been a few reports of gonadal dysgenesis in phenotypic females with a 46 XY karyotype. Some of these have been familial in a pattern compatible with either X-linked recessive inheritance or autosomal dominant inheritance with expression only in males (Espiner et al., 1970; Chemke et al., 1970). Although the specific defects in these disorders are not known, they may prove to be developmental abnormalities in which the basic lesion is in the gonad and the associated abnormalities are secondary to hypogonadism.

5α-*Reductase deficiency* is a recently recognized form of male pseudohermaphroditism that is inherited in an autosomal recessive pattern. This is an inborn error of steroid metabolism involving deficient conversion of testosterone to 5α-dihydrotestosterone. At birth only the external genitalia of affected males are abnormal. The phallus is small and the urethra opens on the perineum as part of a urogenital sinus. In most instances the urogenital sinus consists of an anterior urethral orifice with a blind vaginal pouch posteriorly. The scrotum is cleft and the testes, which are otherwise normal, may be in the inguinal canals, the abdomen, or labioscrotal folds. These clinical abnormalities led to the designation "pseudovaginal perineoscrotal hypospadias" prior to the recognition of the enzyme defect. Many of these children have been reared as females, with the error in sex assignment recognized only at puberty when masculinization occurs (Opitz et al., 1972; Imperato-McGinley et al., 1974; Imperato-McGinley and Peterson, 1976). The penis enlarges to adult proportions, the cleft scrotum elongates, the testes enlarge, muscle mass increases, the voice deepens, and body hair growth follows a male pattern. In addition to

a distinctly male puberty, the absence of gynecomastia is an important feature that distinguishes this disorder from other forms of male pseudohermaphroditism. Clearly it is exceedingly important to be aware of this disorder to avoid serious errors resulting from inappropriate management and incorrect sex assignment. The diagnosis should be suspected in any child with the genital ambiguities just noted and a male karyotype, and can be established by identification in cultured skin fibroblasts of decreased conversion of testosterone to 5α-dihydrotestosterone. This decrease is due to deficiency of the enzyme steroid 5α-reductase. Androgen receptors that are normally present in all cells can bind both testosterone and dihydrotestosterone, but the affinity of the receptor for dihydrotestosterone is much greater. During fetal development and childhood the circulating levels of testosterone are normally low and the 5α-reductase deficiency in affected individuals interferes with its conversion to the more potent androgen, dihydrotestosterone, resulting in incomplete masculinization. This is overcome at puberty when testosterone increases to normal pubertal levels and sufficiently large amounts of testosterone, the weaker androgenic compound, enter the cells to produce essentially normal virilization. Parents carrying a gene for this autosomal recessive disorder show normal sexual development but in most instances measurement of the appropriate urinary steroid indicates intermediate degrees of metabolic abnormality (Imperato-McGinley and Peterson, 1976).

Testicular feminization includes one or more X-linked recessive disorders that produce a striking type of male pseudohermaphroditism. The external genitalia are female as are the postpubertal secondary sex characteristics, except for the sparse or absent pubic and axillary hair (Fig 17–22). Internally, the urogenital sinus ends blindly, müllerian and wolffian structures are usually absent. The gonads consist of testes that have differentiated normally but show histologic changes result-

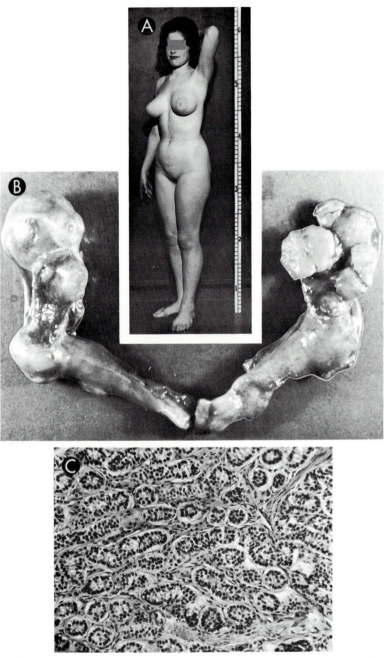

Fig 17–22.—Testicular feminization. **A,** 18-year-old apparent female with primary amenorrhea, minimal sexual hair, large breasts and areolae but small nipples. FSH concentration before surgery: over 13, less than 52 mIU; 17-ketosteroids, 21 mg/24 hours; 17-ketogenic steroids, 5.5 mg/24 hours; pregnanetriol, 1.2 mg/24 hours. **B,** gonads and rudimentary uterine structures removed from patient in **A.** Note nodular appearance of the gonad. **C,** photomicrograph of gonad. Immature testicular tubules are lined principally by primitive germ cells with some Sertoli's cells present. There is a marked resemblance to the fetal testis. (From Morris J.M., Mahesh V.B.: *Am. J. Obstet. Gynecol.* 87:731, 1963.)

ing from the effects of cryptorchidism. Plasma androgen levels are in the normal male range. Serum LH is increased, while the FSH level is usually normal (Kelch et al., 1972; Judd et al., 1972).

The syndrome of complete testicular feminization was in the past erroneously attributed to 5α-reductase deficiency. More recent studies on the basic defect have shown that in some families the affected siblings and individuals lack the cellular dihydrotestosterone-testosterone receptor and are therefore unable to initiate cytoplasmic effects and to transport androgen to its acceptor site in the nucleus where it normally interacts with chromatin to produce additional effects. This receptor-negative defect is analogous to that in the so-called *Tfm* mutation in the mouse (Lyon and Hawkes, 1970). There are, however, presumably steps beyond those presently identified, since clinically indistinguishable patients in other families have shown normal androgen binding as well as nuclear uptake and retention (Amrhein et al., 1976). For the receptor-negative form, the defect has been shown to be located on the X chromosome and inherited in an X-linked recessive pattern (Meyer et al., 1975). As with other instances where gonadal tissue containing a Y chromosome is located intra-abdominally, gonadal extirpation should be considered to avoid the possibility of gonadal malignancy, although the magnitude of the risk of malignancy is presently controversial.

A variety of male pseudohermaphrodites have been described with what has been called *incomplete testicular feminization* which has been attributed to lesser degrees of androgen insensitivity. No specific defects have been identified to explain the clinical findings. In general these individuals manifest some phallic enlargement, partial labioscrotal fusion, incomplete development of female secondary sexual characteristics at puberty, and pubertal hirsutism or even frank virilization.

In female pseudohermaphroditism, the karyotype is 46 XX, and the ovaries and mül-

lerian structures are normally developed but the external genitalia are virilized to some degree. *Congenital virilizing adrenal hyperplasia* is the commonest cause of female pseudohermaphroditism. In this group of autosomal, recessively inherited disorders, deficiencies of individual or, in rare instances, coupled adrenal enzymes interrupt normal steroid biosynthesis and decrease cortisol production (Fig 17–23). As a result, the anterior pituitary is derepressed and produces increased amounts of ACTH, leading morphologically to adrenal hyperplasia and biochemically to overproduction of other adrenal steroids, many of which are either themselves androgenic or become androgenic after conversion in nonadrenal tissues. In approximately half of the patients, the site of the specific block interferes with the production of cortisol, corticosterone, and aldosterone, leading to a sodium-losing state that is often life-threatening.

At birth, clinical features in females include some degree of clitoromegaly, labial fusion, and persistence of the urogenital sinus, and, depending on the specific enzyme defect, dehydration, and hypotension. Immediate therapy for affected newborns includes the replacement of the deficient steroid products and correction of the electrolyte and fluid imbalances. The clinical features beyond the newborn period and the appropriate management depend on the specific deficiency and its severity. This information is clearly important in the diagnosis and management of such patients, and the reader is referred to Liddle (1974) for further details. Because these disorders can produce genital ambiguities in both genetic males and females, accurate sex assignment by karyotype analysis is essential prior to undertaking surgical or sex-hormone therapy.

Other Endocrine Disorders

Familial isolated gonadotropin deficiency results in hypogonadism in both males and females because of deficiency of both follicle-stimulating hormone (FSH) and luteinizing hormone (LH). The levels of the other pitu-

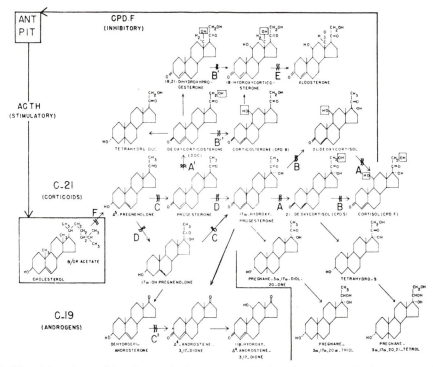

Fig 17–23.—Adrenal steroid pathways indicating sites of specific enzyme deficiencies: *A,* 21-hydroxylase; *B,* 11-hydroxylase; *C,* 3β-ol-dehydrogenase; *D,* 17-hydroxylase; *E,* 18-hydroxysteroid dehydrogenase; *F,* desmolase. (Courtesy of John F. Crigler, Jr., M.D., Harvard Medical School.)

itary hormones are normal. No associated somatic abnormalities have been described. Inheritance is in an autosomal recessive pattern (Ewer, 1968; Spitz et al., 1974).

The *Stein-Leventhal syndrome* is inherited in an autosomal dominant pattern with different manifestations in males and females, and variable expressivity among members of each sex. The clinical features in females consist of oligomenorrhea, hirsutism, and polycystic ovaries, frequently with secondary amenorrhea and infertility. Males suspected of having inherited the gene occasionally manifest hirsutism. Laboratory abnormalities consist of elevated androstenedione and luteinizing hormone levels in affected females (Givens et al., 1971).

Müllerian Tract Anomalies

Congenital absence of the vagina has been described in a large number of patients, although its exact frequency is uncertain. Based on the analysis of over 500 cases, Ross and Van de Wiele (1974) estimated that congenital absence of the vagina is second only to gonadal dysgenesis as a cause of primary amenorrhea. Absent vagina, however, can occur in association with several other types of malformations, as an isolated abnormality or as part of several malformation syndromes (Buchta et al., 1973; Bryan et al., 1959). Most cases are thought to be sporadic, i.e., to be the only ones in their respective families to be affected. In many instances, however, the relatives have not been examined for specific müllerian tract, renal, skeletal, and other abnormalities. Hence the ascertainment is incomplete, particularly in regard to more mildly affected individuals, and systems of classifications at present are necessarily only approximate, with many exceptions to be anticipated.

The Rokitansky-Küster-Hauser syndrome consists of congenital absence of the vagina and a rudimentary uterus composed of bicornuate muscular cords without or, less often, with a lumen. The ovaries, fallopian tubes, and associated ligaments are normal, as are the female secondary sexual characteristics, body proportions, endocrine functions, and karyotype. Autosomal recessive inheritance with the characteristic expression in females has been observed in some families. In many published reports the term *Rokitansky-Küster-Hauser syndrome* has been applied to patients having some of these features in association with various renal and skeletal abnormalities (Griffin et al., 1976). It seems likely that several and perhaps many different disorders are present within this broad spectrum, but their individual characteristics have not yet been resolved.

Some patients have been described with müllerian tract malformations associated with the *Klippel-Feil anomaly*, involving varying degrees of vertebral fusion, most often in the cervical spine. Some of these patients also manifest deafness. No simple pattern of inheritance has been identified.

Absent vagina is to be distinguished from *transverse vaginal septum* or *hydrometrocolpos*. In this autosomal, recessively inherited disorder a thick transverse membrane prevents the discharge of cervical secretions and menses. The remainder of the reproductive system is normal. Surgical removal of the septum allows full reproductive and sexual function.

Ovarian Tumors

Benign cystic teratomas (or dermoid cysts) of the ovary are, by definition, composed of tissues that have differentiated from all three germ layers: the ectoderm, mesoderm, and endoderm. It has been known for years that these ovarian teratomas have a 46 XX chromosome constitution. Although theoretically these tumors could arise by any of four mechanisms during meiosis, recent studies have examined both the cytogenetic and biochemical features relating to individual chromosomes from several of the homologous pairs (Linder et al., 1975). Based on the findings that the ovarian teratomas were consistently homozygous for morphologic centromeric markers, but often heterozygous for biochemical markers located at a distance from the centromeres, it was possible to demonstrate that these tumors arise from single oocytes after the first meiotic division but prior to completion of the second meiotic division. Either the second polar body is not formed or it is formed but recombines its haploid chromosome complement with that of the haploid oocyte to produce a diploid cell. In either case this diploid cell then undergoes parthenogenic development into a benign cystic teratoma.

The *Peutz-Jeghers syndrome* is an autosomal dominant disorder consisting of multiple hamartomatous gastrointestinal polyps accompanied by abnormal melanotic pigmentation, most frequently in the buccal and perioral areas. About 5% of females with Peutz-Jeghers syndrome have primary tumors in one or both ovaries. Although various pathologic diagnoses have been assigned, Scully (1970b) has found that a substantial proportion of these show a highly distinctive architecture that he designates as a "sex cord tumor with annular tubules" and that appear to be a specific manifestation of the Peutz-Jeghers gene.

Autosomal Chromosome Disorders

Several autosomal chromosome disorders are encountered frequently enough by the gynecologists, either directly or through questions from patients, that they deserve mention.

Down's syndrome is the commonest of the autosomal disorders with an overall incidence of 1 per 800 live births. The clinical features include small size, hypotonia, microcephaly, characteristic facies, transverse palmar or simian creases, and cardiovascular malformations of which ventricular septal defect is most common. Karyotype analysis of patients indicates that in 95% of cases the abnormalities result from trisomy 21, the presence of a third 21 chromosome in addition to the normal dip-

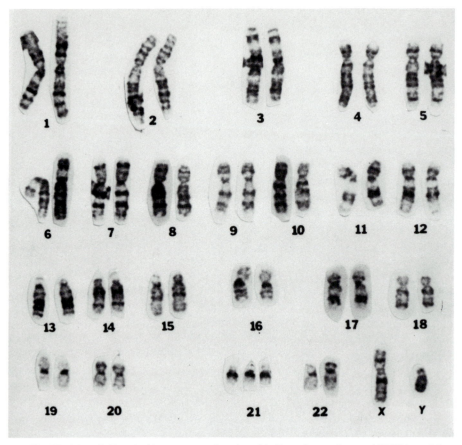

Fig 17–24.—G-Banded karyotype of male with Down's syndrome (47 XY + 21).

loid complement, as shown in Figure 17–24. About 2% of Down's syndrome patients are mosaics with both trisomy 21 and normal cell lines in blood and tissues. The remaining 3% of patients have translocation Down's syndrome of the D/G or G/G type. These individuals are abnormal because they possess three copies of part or all of the long arm of a 21 chromosome, which has been translocated to a D group (numbers 13 to 15 chromosome), to a 22 chromosome, or to another 21 chromosome. In the case of D/G translocations, about one third of patients have a parent—more often the mother—who is a balanced D/G translocation carrier. Theoretically, random segregation of chromosomes during gametogenesis would result in one third of the viable zygotes having Down's syndrome. In fact, the observed outcome is quite different, and varies with the sex of the carrier parent. The frequency of Down's syndrome of a female D/G translocation carrier is about 15%, while in offspring of a male translocation carrier the frequency is only about 3%. The unaffected offspring in both cases are equally divided between having normal chromosomes and being balanced translocation carriers.

While the overall incidence of Down's syndrome is 1 per 800 live births, the frequency of trisomy 21—95% of cases of Down's syndrome—increases from 1 per 2,300 live births for 20-year-old mothers to 1 per 40 live births at a maternal age of 45 years. This *maternal age effect*, the rise in frequency of meiotic nondisjunction with increasing maternal age, is seen not only in trisomy 21 but also in trisomy 18, trisomy 13, and Klinefelter's (47 XXY) syndrome. Despite this change in frequency, most children with these chromosome disorders are born to relatively young mothers because of the substantially greater total number of children born to the younger age group.

The *trisomy 18 syndrome* (47 XX or XY, +18), previously called Edward's syndrome, occurs in about 1 per 8,000 live births. It is characterized clinically by low birth weight, a clenched hand position, short sternum, and various other malformations. Affected females exceed males by a ratio of 3:1. Only about 10% of these patients survive the first year and these show a uniform degree of severe mental retardation.

The *trisomy 13 syndrome* (47 XX or XY, +13), previously called Patau's syndrome, occurs with a frequency of about 1 per 20,000 live births. Clinical features include malformations of eye, nose, lip, and forebrain; polydactyly; and defects of the skin and posterior scalp. About 20% of these individuals survive the first year and are severely retarded.

Miscellaneous Genetic Disorders With Female Reproductive Tract Anomalies

In addition to the conditions just described, many other genetic disorders that involve genital abnormalities are encountered primarily by the gynecologist. Further details regarding these disorders are available in Smith (1976) and McKusick (1983).

Ambiguous or malformed external genitalia are often found in Robinow's syndrome, trisomy 18 syndrome, and 18q syndrome and, less frequently, in de Lange's syndrome, fetal alcohol syndrome, and popliteal web syndrome.

Müllerian tract abnormalities, including bicornuate uterus and/or double vagina, are frequently reported in the cryptophthalmos syndrome, Johanson-Blizzard syndrome, and trisomy 13, and occasionally in Robert's syndrome and trisomy 18.

Hypogonadism is frequent in Down's syndrome, Prader-Willi syndrome, myotonic dystrophy, De Sanctis-Cacchione syndrome, and Laurence-Moon-Biedl syndrome, and occasionally in Noonan's syndrome, multiple lentigines syndrome, Albright's hereditary osteodystrophy, and Fanconi's anemia.

SPONTANEOUS ABORTION

Chromosome anomalies are present in a substantial proportion of abortuses. As reviewed by Carr (1971), most chromosomally abnormal conceptuses that are aborted spontaneously do so within the first trimester, 40% to 50% of such abortuses showing chromosome abnormalities. Most of these abnormalities are numerical, of which about 45% consist of trisomies, about 25% of polyploidy, and about 20% of 45 X. Retrospective and prospective karyotype analysis of 1,500 spontaneous abortions by Boue and Boue have yielded useful epidemiologic information. The presence of a chromosomal abnormality in a spontaneously aborted first conception was associated with a definite increase in the risk of some chromosome abnormality in a subsequent conception, but there was no consistency in the specific type of abnormality. In couples previously having only full-term deliveries, the occurrence of a chromosomally abnormal abortus was associated with a favorable prognosis for subsequent pregnancies, but a normal karyotype in the abortus signaled a higher (24% to 33%) risk of recurring abortion, postulated to reflect maternal causes such as incompetent cervix. The highest risk of recurring abortion (41.5%) was found in those couples who had already experienced one or more spontaneous abortions of a chromosomally abnormal fetus and where the mother was over 30 years of age. These authors found no effect of oral contraceptive use on the frequency of abortions or chromosome abnormalities. An increased frequency of chromosome abnormalities was observed after ovulation-inducing drugs and after occupational exposure of the fathers to radiation. There were no changes in fertility rate or in the frequency of congenital malformations in births following the abortions.

Bauld, Sutherland, and Bain (1974) conducted chromosome studies of consecutive stillbirths and neonatal deaths, compiling results of 153 cases during a one-year period. Chromosome abnormalities were found in 11 cases, giving a frequency of 7.2%. Most of the abnormalities were trisomies, of which trisomy 18 was most frequent. It should be noted that chromosome studies can often be carried out successfully if done hours or even several days after clinical death of the fetus, by using material from the spleen, lung, or sterile skin from which fibroblasts can be grown.

In these studies of spontaneous abortions and perinatal deaths, the vast majority of the chromosome abnormalities observed were of types that would be expected to arise de novo during parental gametogenesis rather than being transmitted from a parent who carries a chromosome abnormality. This distinction was addressed directly by Kim et al. (1975), who obtained karyotypes using the new banding techniques on a consecutive series of 50 couples who had more than two early abortions, stillbirths, live births, or a combination of the latter two, of infants with multiple congenital anomalies. Three women were found to be balanced reciprocal translocation carriers, but none of these translocations was detectable by chromosome analysis without banding. An additional woman was found to be a mosaic, and four parents—three females and one male—showed mitotic chromosome abnormalities. These authors estimated that between 6% and 16% of fetal wastage so defined results from parental chromosome abnormalities and that such couples could benefit from prenatal monitoring to detect chromosome abnormalities in future pregnancies. Such monitoring done in the second trimester would detect fetal chromosome abnormalities that had not resulted in spontaneous abortion but which would produce perinatal death or serious birth defects in surviving offspring.

PRENATAL DIAGNOSIS

Second trimester amniocentesis for prenatal diagnosis is both a safe and an important means for preventing the birth of children with various genetic disorders. The National Institute of Child Health and Human Development Collaborative Amniocentesis Registry Project found no increase in fetal loss when 1,040 pregnancies in which amniocentesis was performed were compared with 992 controls. Similarly, there were no major maternal complications in the study group. There have been reports of fetal injury resulting from the amniocentesis needle, but fortunately these instances are rare.

Amniocentesis should be performed between sixteen and eighteen weeks of gestation and should routinely be preceded or accompanied by ultrasound studies. Ultrasound imaging allows localization of the placenta, detection of multiple fetuses (which would confuse the interpretation of results of many studies), and assessment of gestational age by measurement of the biparietal diameter of the fetal head. Approximately 20 ml of amniotic fluid is withdrawn and, after separation by centrifugation with precautions to preserve sterility, the supernatant fluid is analyzed for α-fetoprotein content, and the cells are placed in culture for later chromosome analysis, biochemical studies, or molecular analyses.

The current indications for prenatal genetic diagnosis are generally considered to consist of the following: (1) maternal age of 35 years or greater; (2) history of a previous child with trisomy 21 (Down's syndrome); (3) pregnancy at risk for a mendelian disorder specifically diagnosable in utero; (4) presence of a balanced chromosome abnormality in either parent; (5) history of a previous child with anencephaly or meningomyelocele; and (6) elevated maternal serum α-fetoprotein concentration. When the fetus is at risk for having a severe X-linked recessive disorder—such as Duchenne-type muscular dystrophy or severe hemophilia A—that is not specifically diagnosable, amniocentesis for identification of male sex by karyotyping is another possible indication. At a maternal age of 35 years the risk of a chromosome abnormality is 1 per 200 live births and increases to 1 per 65 live births by age 40 years. The observed frequencies of chromosome abnormalities measured at 15 to 16 weeks of gestation have been higher than those found in newborn surveys. This apparent decrease in the frequencies of chromosome abnormalities between 15 and 16 weeks of gestation and birth has been attributed in part to the spontaneous abortion of some of these abnormal fetuses in the interim. The birth of a child with trisomy 21 appears to identify couples who are at higher risk for recurrence of this abnormality, although the reasons are not known. The risk of a second trisomy 21 for a woman less than age 35 years appears to be approximately 1% and is higher for older women, being about double the age-related occurrence risk. Although individuals differ in their perception of the importance of a 1% risk, in many instances the anxiety produced by the birth of the first affected child will prompt the couple to seek prenatal diagnosis. Analysis of the karyotype in cultured amniotic fluid cells will, of course, detect not only trisomy 21 but also any other major chromosome abnormality.

While the list of mendelian disorders specifically diagnosable in utero has increased steadily, it is still a minority of disorders that can be detected. Table 17–1 lists those disor-

TABLE 17–1.—INBORN ERRORS OF METABOLISM DIAGNOSABLE PRENATALLY

Lipidoses
  Cholesterol ester storage disease
  Fabry's disease
  Farber's disease
  Gaucher's disease, several forms
  G_{m1} gangliosidosis
    Type 1, generalized gangliosidosis
    Type 2, juvenile G_{m1} gangliosidosis
  G_{m2} gangliosidosis
    Tay-Sachs disease
    Sandhoff's disease
    AB variant
  Krabbe's disease
  Metachromatic leukodystrophy
  Multiple sulfatase deficiency
  Niemann-Pick disease
  Refsum's disease
  Wolman's disease
Mucopolysaccharidoses
  β-Glucuronidase deficiency
  Hurler's/Scheie's syndromes

Hunter's syndrome
I-cell disease
Morquio's syndrome
Maroteaux-Lamy syndrome
Sanfilippo's syndromes, A and B
Carbohydrate and glycoprotein metabolism disorders
  Aspartylglucosaminuria
  Fucosidosis
  Galactosemia
  Glucose-6-phosphate dehydrogenase deficiency
  Glucose phosphate isomerase deficiency
  Glycogenosis (glycogen storage disease) types II
    (Pompe's disease), III, and IV
  Mannosidosis
  Pyruvate decarboxylase deficiency
  "Pyruvate dehydrogenase complex" deficiency, several
    forms
Amino acid metabolism disorders
  Hyperphenylalaninemia due to dihydropteridine
    reductase deficiency
  Hyperprolinemia, type II
  Lysine metabolic errors
    Hyperlysinemia
    Saccharopinuria
  Sulfur pathway disorders
    Cystathionine synthase deficiency homocystinuria
    Sulfite oxidase deficiency
  Urea cycle disorders
    Argininosuccinicaciduria
    Citrullinemia
Organic acid metabolism disorders
  Glutaric aciduria
  Maple syrup urine disease, at least four forms
  Methylmalonic acidemia, three forms
  Propionic acidemia
Vitamin metabolism disorders
  5,10-Methylenetetrahydrofolate reductase deficiency
  Methylmalonic acidemia alone or with homocystinuria
Collagen disorders
  Ehlers-Danlos syndrome, types IV, V, and VIII
  Hydroxylysine deficient collagen disease
Miscellaneous disorders
  Acatalasia, several types
  Adenosine deaminase deficiency
  Chronic granulomatous disease
  Combined immunodeficiency due to adenosine
    deaminase or nucleoside phosphorylase deficiency
  Congenital adrenal hyperplasia due to 21-hydroxylase
    deficiency
  Cystinosis
  Hypercholesterolemia, familial—several forms
  Lesch-Nyhan syndrome
  Lysosomal acid phosphatase deficiency
  Menkes' disease
  Mucolipidosis
    Type II, I cell disease
    Type III, pseudo-Hurler polydystrophy
    Type IV
  Orotic aciduria, types I and II
  Porphyria
    Acute intermittent porphyria
    Congenital erythropoietic porphyria
    Protoporphyria
  Xeroderma pigmentosum

ders that have already been diagnosed prenatally, or in which the possibility of doing so is very likely, based on detection of the defect in cultured skin fibroblasts. In addition, several forms of β-thalassemia, sickle cell anemia, and hemophilia have been diagnosed experimentally by analysis of fetal erythrocytes. All of the disorders in Table 17–1 are inherited in autosomal recessive or X-linked recessive patterns except for acute intermittent porphyria and familial hypercholesterolemia which, along with myotonic dystrophy, are the only three autosomal dominant disorders of the more than 1,000 described that can be diagnosed in utero.

Anencephaly, encephalocele, meningomyelocele, and meningocele all appear to be part of a spectrum of neural tube disorders that manifest features of multifactorial inheritance. Couples who have given birth to a child with any of these disorders have a recurrence risk of about 2% for any of the disorders in this group. Thus, after the birth of an anencephalic child, the couple has about a 2% risk in the subsequent pregnancy of anencephaly, encephalocele, meningomyelocele, or meningocele. When the fetus is affected with any of these neural tube defects, the α-fetoprotein concentration will be elevated and this can be detected by analysis of the level in fluid obtained by amniocentesis. False-positive and false-negative results have been reported, and there are other fetal disorders that can elevate the α-fetoprotein concentrations. Acetylcholinesterase isozyme assay by electrophoresis provides a qualitative technique that has proved to be extremely useful in differentiating between the various causes of elevations in α-fetoprotein concentration (Haddow et al., 1983; Goldfine et al., 1983). Anencephaly is usually detected during the ultrasound examination prior to amniocentesis (Haddow and Miller, 1982).

Now that the safety of early second trimester amniocentesis has been established, and as diagnostic capabilities expand, the gynecologist can expect a steady increase in requests for information about prenatal diagnosis.

Recently there has been renewed interest in a technique first described by Hahnemann and Mohr (1968) and Kullander and Sandahl (1973). Chorionic villus biopsy (CVB) involves the transcervical sampling of placental tissue with guidance by ultrasound. Since it is performed between 8 and 11 weeks of gestation (amenorrhea) and the tissue can be analyzed directly without the need for culture, prenatal diagnosis can be performed much earlier in pregnancy and a result provided to the patient after a much shorter wait following the procedure, both of which are powerful advantages. To date, chorionic villi have been used for the cytogenetic, biochemical, and DNA analyses (Old and Ward, 1982; Simoni et al., 1983; Williamson et al., 1981). Since no amniotic fluid is obtained by this technique α-fetoprotein and acetylcholinesterase assays to screen for neural tube defects, omphalocoele, gastroschisis, and congenital nephrosis cannot be performed. If necessary, the tissue obtained can be established in culture and the volume of cells expanded beyond the amount provided by the initial biopsy sample. The 10 to 20 mg of chorionic villi regularly obtained provides a far greater amount of viable tissue than is obtained by amniocentesis and is sufficient for most biochemical assays and as a source of DNA for recombinant DNA techniques without the need for culture. For cytogenetic analyses, the relatively high mitotic rate of trophoblastic cells allow direct preparation of the sample for chromosome analysis.

The biopsy procedure itself requires both an experienced ultrasonographer and obstetrician-gynecologist. The ultrasonographer scans the uterus to determine the location of the placenta, the viability of the fetus by observing the fetal heart movements, and the gestation age by measuring crown-rump length. The obstetrician introduces the sampling instrument through the cervical canal, into the placenta, under direct ultrasound guidance, and takes the chorionic villus biopsy. The various instruments that have been used are of two basic types. One type includes direct visualization of the villi by means of a fiberoptic scope such as a fetoscope or contact hysteroscope, and biopsy under direct vision using the appropriate biopsy forceps or suction cannula (Gosden et al., 1982; Rodeck et al., 1983). The other type involves the use of a cannula and suction to obtain villi under ultrasound guidance (Ward et al., 1983). The advantages and disadvantage of the two types of approach seem comparable and user preference appears to be a major determinant of use.

Although the potential advantages of first-trimester prenatal diagnosis by means of chorionic villus biopsy appear to be enormous, the safety and accuracy of these diagnostic procedures have not been critically evaluated and, thus, chorionic villus biopsy cannot at present be regarded as an established method. Fetal risks are not clearly defined, although early studies suggest a fetal loss rate of approximately 5%. This rate is somewhat difficult to evaluate since data on spontaneous fetal loss rates after ultrasound proof of viability at 8 to 11 weeks' gestation are lacking. Since few pregnancies examined by these techniques have yet come to delivery, information is lacking regarding premature delivery, intrauterine growth retardation, third-trimester bleeding, rate of caesarean section, and fetal injury resulting from testing. Likewise, the maternal risks have yet to be evaluated. It is important to note that the frequency with which the procedure fails to result in a diagnosis and the accuracy of the diagnoses obtained are not known. Maternal cell contamination and unexplained chromosomal mosaicism and biochemical errors have been reported.

Chorionic villus biopsy cannot be considered at present as an alternative to amniocentesis at 16 to 18 weeks, the safety and accuracy of which are well established. Instead, chorionic villus biopsy should be reserved for those pregnancies that are known to be at high risk for genetic defects such as inborn errors of metabolism, X-linked disorders, and unbalanced chromosome translocation, so that the risk of the disorder is clearly higher than the likely risk of the new procedure. A scientifically valid, properly controlled study of first-trimester prenatal diagnosis is greatly needed.

GENETIC COUNSELING

As indicated at the onset, the gynecologist as primary physician to women is in a key position to assess the risk of, and to aid in preventing, serious genetic disorders in the patients' offspring.

The first step in genetic counseling is accurate and precise diagnosis; all that follows depends on this. In various instances this may be by history, by physical examination, or by review of medical records regarding the patient, affected relatives, or both. Since genetic heterogeneity is the rule, many common and rare disorders that superficially appear quite similar are fundamentally different with regard to recurrence risks, means of diagnosis, and management. For example, from the discussion of congenital absence of the vagina it will be recalled that this abnormality can be part of an autosomal recessive disorder with a 25% recurrence risk or it may be an isolated developmental anomaly with a negligible recurrence risk. The family history, and careful examination of the patient for associated anomalies, as well as complete examination of female relatives, may allow the physician to distinguish which of the possible etiologies applies in any given patient.

Once the diagnosis is established, the physician can provide information regarding the nature of the disorder, its mode of inheritance, the magnitude of the risk, the natural history of the disorder, and the prospects for treatment. Depending on the specific disorder in question and the potential burden that the family perceives would result from the birth of an affected child, the physician needs to discuss the relevant reproductive alternatives, including prenatal diagnosis, artificial insemination, and adoption of children. In addition to the informative aspects of counseling, the physician should also provide support for the emotional needs of the patient and often for those of the family as well.

It may also be advisable to consult a medical geneticist, not only for aid in diagnosis of rare disorders but also to make available additional educational and supportive resources.

BIBLIOGRAPHY

Amrhein J.A., Meyer W.J., Jones H.W., et al.: Androgen insensitivity in man: Evidence for genetic heterogeneity. *Proc. Natl. Acad. Sci. USA* 73:891, 1976.

Bardin C.W., Bullock L.P., Sherins R.J., et al.: Androgen metabolism and mechanisms of action in male pseudohermaphroditism: A study of testicular feminization. *Recent Prog. Horm. Res.* 29:65, 1973.

Bauld R., Sutherland, G.R., Bain A.D.: Chromosome studies in investigations of stillbirths and neonatal deaths. *Arch. Dis. Child.* 49:782, 1974.

Bergsma D., Hamerton J.L., Jacobs P.A., et al. (eds.): Paris Conference (1971): Standardization in human cytogenetics. *Birth Defects* 8(no. 7):2, 1972.

Böök J.A., Eilon B., Halbrecht I., et al.: Isochromosome Y (46,X,i(Yq)) and female phenotype. *Clin. Genet.* 4:410, 1973.

Boue J., Boue A.: Chromosomal analysis of two consecutive abortions in each of 13 women. *Hum. Genet.* 19:275, 1973.

Boue J., Boue A., Lazar P.: Retrospective and prospective epidemiological studies of 1500 karyotyped spontaneous human abortions. *Teratology* 12:11, 1975.

Bryan A.L., Nigro J.A., Counseller V.S.: 100 cases of congenital absence of the vagina. *Surg. Gynecol. Obstet.* 88:79, 1949.

Buchta R.M., Viseskul C., Gilbert E.F., et al.: Familial renal agenesis and hereditary renal adysplasia. *Eur. J. Pediatr.* 115:111, 1973.

Carr D.H.: Chromosomes and abortion. *Adv. Hum. Genet.* 2:201, 1971.

Camerino G., Grzeschik K.H., Jaye M., et al.: Regional localization on the human X chromosome and polymorphism of the coagulation factor IX gene (hemophilia B locus). *Proc. Natl. Acad. Sci. USA* 21:498, 1984.

Carter C.O.: Genetics of common disorders. *Br. Med. Bull.* 25:52, 1968.

Chemke J., Carmichel R., Stewart J.M., et al.: Familial XY gonadal dysgenesis. *J. Med. Genet.* 7:105, 1970.

De La Chapelle A., Tippett P.A., Wetterstrand G., et al.: Genetic evidence of X-Y interchange in a human XX male. *Nature* 307:170, 1984.

Dorus E., Amarose A.P., Tredway D.R., et al.: A reciprocal translocation (X;11) in a female with gonadal dysgenesis. *Clin. Genet.* 16:253, 1979.

Erbe R.W.: Prenatal diagnosis of inherited disease in Altman P.L., Katz D.D. (eds.): *Human Health and Disease*. Bethesda, Md., Federation of American Societies for Experimental Biology, 1977, p. 91.

Erickson R.P., Gondas B.: Alternative explanations of the differing behavior of ovarian and testicular teratomas. *Lancet* 1:410, 1976.

Espiner E.A., Veale A.M., Sands V.E., et al.: Familial syndrome of streak gonads and normal male karyotype in five phenotypic females. *N. Engl. J. Med.* 283:6, 1970.

Ewer R.W.: Familial monotropic pituitary gonadotropin insufficiency. *J. Clin. Endocrinol. Metab.* 28:783, 1968.

Ford E.H.R.: *Human Chromosomes*. New York, Academic Press, 1973.

Fraser F.C.: The genetics of cleft lip and cleft palate. *Am. J. Hum. Genet.* 22:336, 1970.

Fraser F.C., Hunter A.D.W.: Etiologic relations among categories of congenital heart malformations. *Am. J. Cardiol.* 36:793, 1975.

Gasser D.L., Silvers W.K.: Genetics and immunology of sex-linked antigens. *Adv. Immunol.* 15:215, 1972.

Gerald P.S.: Sex chromosome disorders. *N. Engl. J. Med.* 294:706, 1976.

Giannelli F., Choo K.H., Winship P.R., et al.: Characterisation and use of an intragenic polymorphic marker for detection of carriers of haemophilia B(factor IX deficiency). *Lancet* 1:239, 1984.

Givens J.R., Wiser W.L., Coleman S.A., et al.: Familial ovarian hyperthecosis: A study of two families. *Am. J. Obstet. Gynecol.* 110:959, 1971.

Goldfine C., Miller W.A., Haddow J.E.: Amniotic fluid gel cholinesterase densities ratios in fetal open defects of the neural tube and ventral wall. *Br. J. Obstet. Gynecol.* 90:238, 1983.

Gordan J.W., Ruddle F.H.: Mammalian gonadal determination and gametogenesis. *Science* 211:1265, 1981.

Gosden J.R., Mitchell A.R., Gosden C.M., et al.: Direct vision chorion biopsy and chromosome-specific DNA probes for determination of fetal sex in the first trimester. *Lancet* 2:1416, 1982.

Griffin J.E., Wilson J.D.: The syndromes of androgen resistance. *N. Engl. J. Med.* 302:198, 1980.

Griffin J.E., Edwards C., Maddin J.D., et al.: Congenital absence of the vagina. *Ann. Intern. Med.* 85:224, 1976.

Guellan G., Casanova M., Bishop C., et al.: Human XX males with Y single-copy DNA fragments. *Nature* 307:172, 1984.

Gusella J.F., Wexler N.S., Conneally P.M., et al.: A polymorphic DNA marker genetically linked to Huntington's disease. *Nature* 306:234, 1983.

Haddow J.E., Miller W.A.: Prenatal diagnosis of open neural tube defects. *Methods Cell Biol.* 26:67, 1982.

Haddow J.E., Morin M.E., Holman M.S., et al.: Acetylcholinesterase and fetal malformations: Modified qualitative technique for diagnosis of neural tube defects. *Clin. Chem.* 27:61, 1981.

Hahnemann N., Mohr J.: Genetic diagnosis in the embryo by means of biopsy from extraembryonic membrane. *Bull. Eur. Soc. Hum. Genet.* 2:23, 1968.

Hamerton J.L.: *Human Cytogenetics*, vol. 1 and 2. New York, Academic Press, 1971.

Hamerton J.L., Canning N., Ray M., et al.: A cytogenetic survey of 14,069 newborn infants: I. Incidence of chromosome abnormalities. *Clin. Genet.* 8:223, 1975.

Harris H.: *Garrod's Inborn Errors of Metabolism.* London, Oxford University Press, 1963.

Hoehn H.: Functional implications of differential chromosome banding. *Am. J. Hum. Genet.* 27:676, 1975.

Holmes L.B., Driscoll S.G., Atkins L.: Etiologic heterogeneity of neural tube defects. *N. Engl. J. Med.* 294:365, 1976.

Hook E.B., Hamerton J.L.: Frequency of chromosome abnormalities detected in consecutive newborns—differences between studies, in Hook E.B., Porter I.H. (eds.): *Population Cytogenetics: Studies in Newborns.* New York, Academic Press, 1977.

Hook E.B., Warburton D.: The distribution of chromosomal genotypes associated with Turner's syndrome: Livebirth prevalence rates and evidence for diminished fetal mortality and severity in genotypes associated with structural X abnormalities or mosaicism. *Hum. Genet.* 64:24, 1983.

Hsu L.Y., Shapiro L.R., Gertner M., et al.: Trisomy 22: A clinical entity. *J. Pediatr.* 79:12, 1971.

Imperato-McGinley J., Guerrero L., Gautier T., et al.: Steroid 5α-reductase deficiency in man: An inherited form of male pseudohermaphroditism. *Science* 186:1213, 1974.

Hsu L.Y., Peterson R.E.: Male pseudohermaphroditism: The complexities of male phenotypic development. *Am. J. Med.* 61:251, 1976.

Judd H.L., Hamilton C.R., Barlow J.J., et al.: Androgen and gonadotropin dynamics in testicular feminization syndrome. *J. Clin. Endocrinol. Metab.* 34:229, 1972.

Keenan B.S., Meyer W.J., Hadjian A.J., et al.: Syndrome of androgen insensitivity in man: Absence of 5α-dihydrotestosterone binding protein in skin fibroblasts. *J. Clin. Endocrinol. Metab.* 38:1143, 1974.

Kelch R.P., Jenner M.R., Weinstein R., et al.: Estradiol and testosterone secretion by human, simian, and canine testes, in males with hypogonadism and in male pseudohermaphrodites with the feminizing testes syndrome. *J. Clin. Invest.* 51:824, 1972.

Kidd V.J., Wallace R.B., Itakura K., et al.: α_1-Antitrypsin deficiency detection by direct analysis of the mutation in the gene. *Nature* 304:230, 1983.

Kidd V.J., Golbus M.S., Wallace R.B., et al.: Prenatal diagnosis of α_1-antitrypsin deficiency by direct analysis of the mutation site in the gene. *N. Engl. J. Med.* 310:639, 1984.

Kim H.J., Hsu L.Y.F., Paciuc S., et al.: Cytogenetics of fetal wastage. *N. Engl. J. Med.* 293:844, 1975.

Kullander S., Sandahl B.: Fetal chromosome analysis after transcervical placenta biopsies during early pregnancy. *Acta Obstet. Gynecol. Scand.* 52:355, 1973.

Liddle G.W.: The adrenal cortex, in Williams R.H. (ed.): *Textbook of Endocrinology*, ed. 5. Philadelphia, W.B. Saunders Co., 1974, pp. 233–282.

Linder D., Kaiser-McCraw B., Hecht F.: Parthenogenic origin of benign ovarian teratomas. *N. Engl. J. Med.* 292:63, 1975.

Lindsten J.: *The Nature and Origin of X Chromosome Aberrations in Turner's Syndrome: A Cytogenetical and Clinical Study of 57 Patients.* Stockholm, Almqvist and Wiksell, 1963.

Lyon M.F.: X chromosome inactivation and developmental patterns in mammals. *Biol. Rev.* 47:1, 1972.

Lyon M.F.: Mechanisms and evolutionary origin of variable X chromosome activity in mammals. *Proc. R. Soc. Lond. Biol.* 187:243, 1974.

Lyon M.F.: Hawkes S.G.: X-linked gene for testicular feminization in the mouse. *Nature* 227:1217, 1970.

McDermott A.: *Cytogenetics of Man and Other Animals—Outline Studies in Biology.* New York, John Wiley & Sons, 1975.

McKusick V.A.: *Mendelian Inheritance in Man: Catalogs of Autosomal Dominant, Autosomal Recessive and X-linked Phenotypes*, ed. 6. Baltimore, The Johns Hopkins University Press, 1983.

McKusick V.A., Bauer R.L., Koop C.E., et al.; Hydrometrocolpos as a simply inherited malformation. *J.A.M.A.* 189:813, 1964.

McKusick V.A., Weilbaecher R.G., Gragg G.W.: Recessive inheritance of a congenital malformation syndrome. *J.A.M.A.* 204:113, 1968.

Meyer W.J., Migeon B.R., Migeon C.J.: Locus on human X chromosome for dihydrotestosterone receptor and androgen insensitivity. *Proc. Natl. Acad. Sci. USA* 72:1469, 1975.

Miller O.J., Miller D.A., Warburton D.: Application of new staining techniques to the study of human chromosomes. *Prog. Med. Genet.* 9:1, 1973.

Milunsky A.: Prenatal diagnosis of genetic disorders. *N. Engl. J. Med.* 295:377, 1976.

Mittwoch U., Kirk D.: Superior growth of the right gonad in human foetuses. *Nature* 257:791, 1975.

Murray J.C., Demopulos C.M., Lawn R.M., et al.: Molecular genetics of human serum albumin: Restriction enzyme fragment length polymorphisms and analbuminemia. *Proc. Natl. Acad. Sci. USA* 80:5951, 1983.

Nora J.J., Nora A.H.: Recurrence risks in children having one parent with a congenital heart disease. *Circulation* 53:701, 1976.

Ohno S.: Major regulatory genes for mammalian sexual development. *Cell* 7:315, 1976.

Old J.M., Ward R.H.T., Petroum M., et al.: First trimester diagnosis for haemoglobinopathies: Three cases. *Lancet* 2:1413, 1982.

Opitz J.M., Simpson J.L., Sarto G.E., et al.: Pseudovaginal perineoscrotal hypospadias. *Clin. Genet.* 3:1, 1972.

Perez-Ballester B., Greenblatt R.B., Byrd J.R.: Familial gonadal dysgenesis. *Am. J. Obstet. Gynecol.* 107:1262, 1970.

Philip J., Lundsteen C., Owen D., et al.: The frequency of chromosome aberrations in tall men with special reference to 47,XYY + 47,XXY. *Am. J. Hum. Genet.* 28:404, 1976.

Polani P.E., Angell R., Giannelli F., et al.: Evidence that the Xg locus is inactivated in structurally abnormal X chromosomes. *Nature* 227:613, 1970.

Puck M.H., Bender B., Borelli J.B., et al.: Parents' adaptation to early diagnosis of sex chromosome anomalies. *Am. J. Med. Genet.* 16:71, 1983.

Rimoin D.L., Schimke R.N.: *Genetic Disorders of the Endocrine Glands.* St. Louis, C.V. Mosby Co., 1971.

Robinson A., Bender B., Borelli J., et al.: Sex chromosomal anomalies: Prospective studies in children. *Behav. Genet.* 13:321, 1983.

Rodeck C.H., Morsman J.M., Gosden C.M., et al.: The development of an improved technique for first trimester microsampling of chorion. *Br. J. Obstet. Gynecol.* 39:338, 1983.

Ross G.T., Van de Wiele R.L.: The ovaries, in Williams R.H. (ed.): *Textbook of Endocrinology,* ed. 5. Philadelphia, W.B. Saunders Co., 1974, pp. 368–422.

Saenger P.: Abnormal sex differentiation. *J. Pediatr.* 104:1–17, 1984.

Scully R.E.: Gonadoblastoma: A review of 74 cases. *Cancer* 24:1340, 1970a.

Scully R.E.: Sex cord tumor with annular tubules: A distinctive ovarian tumor of the Peutz-Jegher syndrome. *Cancer* 25:1107, 1970b.

Silvers W.K., Gasser D.L., Eicher E.M.: H-Y antigen, serologically detectable male antigen and sex determination. *Cell* 28:439, 1982.

Simpson J.L.: Repeated suboptimal pregnancy outcome. *Birth Defects* 17:113, 1981.

Simpson J.L.: *Disorders of Sexual Differentiation.* New York, Academic Press Inc., 1976.

Simpson J.L., Golbus M.S., Martin A.O., et al.: *Genetics in Obstetrics and Gynecology.* New York, Grune & Stratton, Inc., 1982.

Simpson J.L., Christakos A.C., Horwith M., et al.: Gonadal dysgenesis in individuals with apparently normal chromosome complements: Tabulation of cases and compilation of genetic data, in Bergsma D., McKusick V.A. (eds.): *The Clinical Delineation of Birth Defects,* vol. 10: *Endocrine System.* Baltimore, Williams & Wilkins Co., 1971.

Simoni G., Brambati B., Danesino C., et al.: Efficient direct chromosome analysis and enzyme determination from chorionic villi samples in the first trimester of pregnancy. *Hum. Genet.* 63:349, 1983.

Smith D.W.: *Recognizable Patterns of Human Malformations,* ed. 2. Philadelphia, W.B. Saunders Co., 1976.

Spitz I.M., Diamant Y., Rosen E., et al.: Isolated gonadotropin deficiency: A heterogeneous syndrome. *N. Engl. J. Med.* 290:10, 1974.

Stein Z.: Early fetal loss. *Birth defects* 17:95, 1981.

Stent G.S.: *Molecular Genetics.* San Francisco, W.H. Freeman and Co., 1971.

Sutton E.H.: *An Introduction to Human Genetics,* ed. 3. New York, Holt, Rinehart & Winston, 1980.

Swanson C.P., Merz T., Young W.J.: *Cytogenetics.* Englewood Cliffs, N.J., Prentice-Hall, Inc., 1967.

Tilghman S.M., Tiemeier D.C., Polsky F., et al.: Cloning segments of the mammalian genome: Bacteriophage containing mouse globin and surrounding gene sequences. *Proc. Natl. Acad. Sci. USA* 77:4406, 1977.

Vogel F., Motulsky A.G.: *Human Genetics: Problems and Approaches.* New York, Springer-Verlag, 1979.

Walzer S., Gerald P.S.: Social class and frequency of XYY + XXY. *Science* 190:1228, 1975.

Ward R.H.T., Modell B., Petro M., et al.: Method

of sampling chorionic villi in the first trimester of pregnancy under guidance of real-time ultrasound. *Br. Med. J.* 286:15423, 1983.

Watson J.D.: *Molecular Biology of the Gene*, ed. 3. New York, W.A. Benjamin Inc., 1976.

Williams R.H.: *Textbook of Endocrinology*, ed. 5. Philadelphia, W.B. Saunders Co., 1974.

Williamson R., Eskdale J., Coleman D.V., et al.: Direct gene analysis of chorionic villi: A possible technique for first trimester antenatal diagnosis of haemoglobinopathies. *Lancet* 2:1125, 1981.

Wilson J.D., George F.W., Griffin J.E.: The hormonal control of sexual development. *Science* 211:1278, 1981.

Witkin H.A., et al.: Criminality in XYY and XXY men. *Science* 193:547, 1976.

Wong M.B., Ma H.K., Todd D., et al.: Diagnosis of homozygous β-thalassemia in cultured amniotic-fluid fibroblasts. *N. Engl. J. Med.* 298:669, 1978.

Woo S.L.C., Lidsky A.S., Guttler F., et al.: Cloned human phenylalanine hydroxylase gene allows prenatal diagnosis and carrier detection of classical phenylketonuria. *Nature* 306:151, 1983.

Wyman A., White R.: A highly polymorphic locus in human DNA. *Proc. Natl. Acad. Sci. USA* 77:6754, 1980.

Wyss D., DeLozier C.D., Daniell J., et al.: Structural anomalies of the X chromosome: Personal observation and review of non-mosaic cases. *Clin. Genet.* 21:145, 1982.

Yanagisawa S., Yokoyama H.: Symptoms of Turner's syndrome and interstitial heterochromatin in i(Xq). *Clin. Genet.* 7:299, 1975.

CHAPTER EIGHTEEN

Gynecologic Infections

RUTH E. TUOMALA, M.D.

IN THIS CHAPTER, infectious diseases that affect the female genital tract will be discussed, with an emphasis on clinical diagnosis and management. The specific diseases that will be presented have been chosen on the basis of prevalence, importance of sequelae, or, in some cases, because they are considerations in the differential diagnosis of more common entities.

Infectious diseases that affect the upper genital tract are presented first. Next, infections of the lower genital tract, including infectious vaginitis and infections that produce lesions, will be considered. Finally, postoperative pelvic and wound infections are discussed.

PELVIC INFLAMMATORY DISEASE

Pelvic inflammatory disease (PID) is a disease of the upper genital tract that is characterized primarily by infection of the endosalpingeal cells lining the fallopian tubes. Infection may be confined to the tubes (salpingitis) or in addition involve the ovaries (salpingo-oophoritis). Infection may involve disruption and destruction of tubal architecture on a microscopic or obvious (gross) level. Marked inflammation resulting in the involvement of contiguous intraperitoneal structures in inflammatory processes and massive suppuration resulting in tubo-ovarian abscess formation can result in total destruction of normal architecture as well as functional impairment.

Pelvic inflammatory disease is a disease of sexually active, menstruating women. It is rare in premenarchal, postmenopausal, and celibate women, and when it does occur in these groups it is often secondary to spread from other foci of intra-abdominal sepsis such as ruptured appendiceal abscesses. The exact incidence of PID in the United States is unknown, although it is estimated to account for 250,000 annual hospitalizations, and 500,000 to 1 million new cases of PID are estimated to occur each year.

The majority of cases of PID are thought to be ascending infections, caused by microorganisms that ascend from the lower genital tract through the cervix, along the endometrium to the normally sterile tubes. Infection may also spread to the tubes and ovaries via the parametrium from cervical vessels and lymphatics. Pelvic inflammatory disease is a polymicrobial infection. Both organisms that are recognized to be sexually transmitted and organisms that are considered to be part of the normal, endogenous flora of the lower genital tract are participants in PID. Sexually transmitted organisms such as *Neisseria gonorrhoeae*, *Chlamydia trachomatis*, and *Mycoplasma hominis* may be found as sole pathogens in cases of PID or may be found along with other organisms. Current estimates are that in the United States, 25% to 80% of cases of PID involve the gonococcus. An exact role for *C. trachomatis* in PID in the United States is unknown, but *Chlamydia* may be an important pathogen in 10% to 20% of cases of PID.

Multiple species of aerobic and anaerobic bacteria normally found in the lower genital tract of asymptomatic women can be found at the site of upper genital tract infection both in the presence of and in the absence of sexually transmitted organisms. Pelvic inflammatory disease may be a pure aerobic, pure anaerobic, or mixed aerobic-anaerobic infection. In approximately two thirds of cases, anaerobes are involved. Aerobic endogenous bacteria that are associated with PID include the Enterobacteriaceae, particularly *Escherichia coli*, staphylococcal species, and streptococcal species, including the enterococci. Anaerobes that are associated with PID include peptococci, peptostreptococci, anaerobic streptococci, and *Bacteroides* species, including *B. fragilis* and *B. melaninogenicus*.

It is likely that key organisms are responsible for initial invasion of the upper genital tract and that other organisms can become involved in infection under altered conditions and structure of the upper genital tract. The exact microbial and host factors responsible for tissue invasion and infection are currently the subject of much ongoing research.

The exact organisms involved in a particular infection can be ascertained only by direct culture of the infected site. In pelvic inflammatory disease this involves culture of tubal exudate or cul-de-sac fluid performed at the time of laparoscopy or laparotomy. Cultures of the lower genital tract do not accurately reflect the organisms that are present in upper genital tract infection. Contamination of peritoneal fluid cultures obtained by culdocentesis by lower genital tract flora render these unacceptable specimens. The presumed microbiology of individual infections is largely an estimation based on usual organism involvement and to some extent, differential clinical presentation.

Diagnosis

The clinical diagnosis of PID is inexact. There are multiple potential symptoms and signs ascribable to PID as predicted by areas of inflammatory involvement. No symptoms or signs are pathognomic for PID.

Reports in which all clinical diagnoses of PID are confirmed by laparoscopy suggest that in one third of cases, the clinical diagnosis of PID is in error. Other conditions that may be diagnosed as PID include appendicitis, ectopic pregnancy, endometriosis, adhesions, and adnexal tumors, including ruptured or hemorrhagic functional ovarian cysts. In addition, some 10% to 15% of cases of PID initially are diagnosed as another process, such as those just listed.

For the majority of cases in which pelvic inflammatory disease is erroneously diagnosed, no pelvic pathologic features can be defined by laparoscopy. Without receiving treatment for PID, symptoms in these women resolve and long-term sequelae associated with PID do not ensue. A portion of disease in this group with normal visual findings may be infection confined to the lower genital tract, and a portion may involve disease of other organ systems.

The largest such laparoscopy series has been conducted on an ongoing basis by Weström and co-workers in Sweden. When these investigators compared the incidence of various symptoms and signs between women with PID and women with a laparoscopically normal pelvis, very few symptoms and signs were seen more frequently in the group of women with PID (Table 18–1). Although seen in a minority of cases, multiple signs and

TABLE 18–1.—SYMPTOMS AND SIGNS SEEN SIGNIFICANTLY MORE OFTEN IN PATIENTS WITH PID THAN IN THOSE WITH LAPAROSCOPICALLY NORMAL PELVIC FINDINGS*

	PID (%)	VISUALLY NORMAL (%)
Symptoms		
Fever and chills	41.0	20.0
Proctitis	6.9	2.7
Signs		
Adnexal tenderness	92.0	87.0
Palpable mass or swelling	49.4	24.5
Erythrocyte sedimentation rate >15 mm/hr	75.9	52.7
Abnormal discharge	63.2	40.2
Temperature >38 C	32.9	14.1

*From Jacobson L., Weström L.: *Am. J. Obstet. Gynecol.* 105:1088, 1969.

symptoms present in one person confer the greatest accuracy of clinical diagnosis.

Traditional laboratory studies do little to improve the accuracy of diagnosis of PID. The white blood cell (WBC) count is elevated both in women with PID and in normal women. The sedimentation rate is often elevated in women with PID and may be helpful in judging response to therapy, but is a nonspecific test, and the rate may also be elevated in a large number of normal women. Ultrasound and computed tomographic (CT) scanning may be of aid in detecting the presence of and following resolution of tubo-ovarian abscesses, but cannot accurately differentiate abscess formation from other causes of pelvic masses.

Virtually all women who have PID have WBCs present in lower genital tract discharge. If WBCs are not present in this discharge, the diagnosis of PID is unlikely. A Gram stain of this discharge that is positive for intracellular gram-negative diplococci supports but does not confirm a diagnosis of gonococcal PID, although a positive Gram stain can be helpful in determing therapy.

Normal cul-de-sac fluid contains 1,500 WBCs/cu mm. The great majority of cul-de-sac samples taken by culdocentesis from women with PID contain 15,000 to 30,000 WBCs/cu mm. Though not often helpful for culture, culdocentesis can be helpful in establishing a clinical diagnosis of PID.

When the differential diagnosis of pelvic pain is between PID and a surgical condition and in cases of nonresponse or recurrent clinical disease not associated with an obvious precipitating cause, diagnostic laparoscopy should be performed. Laparoscopic criteria for the diagnosis of PID are listed in Table 18–2.

To establish at least minimal criteria for the diagnosis of PID, and to better compare data between institutions, baseline criteria for a clinical diagnosis of PID have been proposed. These are listed in Table 18–3.

Approximately 5% of women with PID will have an associated syndrome of perihepatitis called the Fitz-Hugh–Curtis syndrome. This is an inflammatory, fibrinous perihepatitis associated with right upper quadrant pain and mildly deranged liver function tests. Eventual scarring results in the classic fibrous "violin-string" adhesions between the dome of the liver and the diaphragm. This process has been associated with both gonococcal and chlamydial PID.

Some risk factors for the occurrence of PID have been delineated and should be considered when taking a history from a woman who presents with pelvic pain. These risk factors include those related to sexual activity, age, and contraceptive practices.

A history of sexual activity is necessary to seriously consider the diagnosis of PID. Number of sexual partners and frequency of activity increase the risk of development of PID.

TABLE 18–2.—LAPAROSCOPIC CRITERIA
FOR ACUTE PID*

Minimum criteria
  Erythema of fallopian tubes
  Edema and swelling of fallopian tube
  Exudate from fimbria or on serosa of fallopian tube
Scoring
  Mild: minimum criteria, tubes freely movable and patent
  Moderate: more marked, tubes not freely movable, patency uncertain
  Severe: inflammatory mass

  *From Jacobson L.: *Am. J. Obstet. Gynecol.* 138:1006–1011, 1980.

TABLE 18–3.—CRITERIA FOR DIAGNOSIS
OF ACUTE PID*

Three of following are necessary:
  Lower abdominal pain and tenderness
  Rebound tenderness of lower abdomen
  Cervical motion tenderness
  Adnexal tenderness
In addition, at least *one* of following must be present:
  Fever ≥100.4 F
  Leukocytosis ≥10,500 WBCs/cu mm
  Inflammatory mass documented by pelvic examination and/or ultrasound
  Culdocentesis reveals WBCs and bacteria on stain of peritoneal fluid
  Gram-negative intracellular diplococci on Gram stain from cervix

  *From Hager W.D., et al.: *Obstet. Gynecol.* 61:113, 1983.

This risk is probably largely confined to women who are heterosexually active. Prior or concomitant documented sexually transmitted disease, including prior PID, and gonorrhea increase the risk of PID.

Age is an important risk factor for the occurrence of PID. Peak incidence of PID in the United States is the 15 to 24-year age group. After age 25 years, particularly after age 30 years, the incidence of PID declines markedly. It is unclear whether age-related risk is associated with sexual habits, the development of protective antibodies with age, or other factors.

Contraceptive practices influence the risk of pelvic inflammatory disease. Oral contraceptives and barrier methods both decrease the risk of pelvic inflammatory disease compared to use of no contraceptive method. The presence of an intrauterine device (IUD) increases the risk of PID 1.5 to 4.0 times that of women using no contraception. This risk is greatest for the Dalkon shield but is increased for all types of IUDs and does not appear to differ appreciably among all other types of IUDs. The risk of development of PID is most likely the greatest immediately after IUD insertion, but thereafter there is a risk of development of PID regardless of duration of IUD use, socioeconomic status, and parity. Nulliparous women may be at a greater risk for developing IUD associated PID than multiparous women, but this is controversial.

It was formerly thought that unilateral tubo-ovarian abscess formation was highly associated with IUD use and presumably occurred because of parametrial spread of infection secondary to erosion of the endometrium by the IUD. More recent studies have documented that approximately 60% of all tuboovarian abscesses are unilateral and that this percentage is constant regardless of whether an IUD is present or not.

All invasive gynecologic procedures are associated with a risk for upper genital tract infection. Such procedures include tubal lavage, hysterosalpingograms, endometrial biopsies, and dilation and curettages (D&Cs) done either for the purpose of diagnosis or therapeutic abortion. Such iatrogenic infection may be associated with either endogenous flora or sexually transmitted organisms. It is not clear whether prophylactic antibiotics prevent pelvic infections associated with gynecologic procedures or even which antibiotics would be appropriate in these varied settings.

There may be differences in the clinical presentation of PID depending on the primary pathogens involved. Gonococcal PID tends to present acutely within 48 hours of onset of symptoms with multiple symptoms and signs, including high fevers, peritoneal signs, and purulent vaginal discharge. It often presents as an initial episode of PID. Abscess formation is less frequent with gonococcal PID, and therapeutic response is usually prompt.

Nongonococcal PID is often recurrent disease, and presents with a more indolent course and less impressive symptoms and signs. Patients present after having symptoms for five to seven days and look less ill. Fever and peritoneal signs are less prominent, but sedimentation rates are more often elevated, abscess formation is more frequent, and response to therapy is less dramatic. Anaerobic organisms, particularly *Bacteroides fragilis* are of particular concern in multiple recurrences, in women over the age of 30 years, and when abscesses are present. The manifestations of PID associated with *Chlamydia trachomatis* may be the most subtle. Chronic, low-grade pelvic pain, irregular bleeding, elevated sedimentation rates, and a high percentage of tubal scarring may all be features of infection caused by this particular organism.

There are four well-documented long-term consequences of PID: disease recurrence, pelvic pain, infertility, and ectopic pregnancy. As previously mentioned, pelvic inflammatory disease is a recurrent disease, despite apparently adequate therapy. It remains to be seen whether aggressive attempts at elucidating the microbiology and treatment of sexual partners will appreciably decrease rates of recurrence of upper genital tract infections.

Approximately 20% of all women who have had documented PID will have some type of chronic pelvic pain. This may be sporadic or cyclic, or may be constant and debilitating. This sequela often eventuates in hysterectomy; PID and its sequelae are responsible for approximately 25% of abdominal hysterectomies performed in the United States each year.

Women who have had PID have an increased risk of infertility due to tubal obstruction. The risk of infertility is related to the number of episodes of infection, severity of episodes, and may also be associated with the infecting organism and adequacy of therapy (Table 18–4). If pregnancy is achieved after PID, there is an increased incidence of ectopic pregnancies. Pelvic inflammatory disease is thought to be the major factor in the increasing incidence of ectopic pregnancies in the United States.

Treatment

Although it is difficult to document, it is hoped that early, aggressive therapy of PID will decrease the incidence and severity of the long-term sequelae. To date there have been no good comparative trials that support a single therapeutic regimen as being most ef-

ficacious for the treatment of PID. Essential components of adequate therapy are frequent observation, thoughtful use of antibiotics, and contact tracing and treatment of sexual partners for the presence of gonorrhea and *Chlamydia*.

Suggested antibiotic treatment regimens as outlined by the Centers for Disease Control (CDC) are presented in Table 18–5. The efficacy and toxic effects of these regimens are untested, but the microbiologic rationale for their selection is sound.

Hospitalization for the treatment of PID with parenteral antibiotics under close observation is suggested for all patients with severe disease as defined by peritoneal signs or abscess formation. In addition, outpatients for whom the diagnosis is in doubt, who cannot take oral antibiotics for any reason, and in whom an initial course of oral therapy has failed should be hospitalized. An inability to maintain close observation as an outpatient may be another indication for hospitalization. In addition, suspected pregnancy is an indication for hospitalization. Pelvic inflammatory disease during pregnancy is quite rare; however when it does occur, it can be particularly virulent and requires close observation and aggressive antibiotic therapy.

Tubo-ovarian abscesses deserve a trial of medical therapy. The majority of abscesses less than 8 cm will respond to medical ther-

TABLE 18–4.—SUMMARY OF LONG-TERM SEQUELAE SEEN IN 415 CASES OF LAPAROSCOPICALLY DOCUMENTED PID AND IN 100 CONTROLS WITH LAPAROSCOPICALLY NORMAL PELVIC FINDINGS*

SEQUELAE	NORMAL PELVIS	PID
Chronic abdominal pain >6 months	5.0%	18.1%
Ectopic/intrauterine pregnancy	1/147	1/24
Involuntary infertility related to tubal factor	3.0%	17.3%

INFERTILITY RELATED EPISODES OF PID		INFERTILITY RELATED TO SEVERITY OF PID (FIRST EPISODE ONLY)	
NO. OF EPISODES	% INFERTILE	SEVERITY OF EPISODES	% INFERTILE
1	12.8	Mild	2.6
2	35.5	Moderate	13.1
3+	75.0	Severe	28.6

*From Weström L.: *Am. J. Obstet. Gynecol.* 121:707, 1975.

TABLE 18–5.—TREATMENT OF PID*

Inpatient therapy
    Doxycycline, 100 mg intravenously (IV) twice a day, plus cefoxitin, 2 gm IV four times a day, followed by doxycycline, 100 mg orally twice a day to complete ten to 14 days of therapy
    or
    Clindamycin, 600 mg IV four times a day plus gentamicin, 2 mg/kg IV followed by 1.5 mg/kg IV three times a day, followed by clindamycin 450 mg orally four times a day to complete ten to 14 days of therapy
    or
    Doxycycline, 100 mg IV twice a day plus metronidazole, 1 gm IV twice a day followed by both drugs at the same dosage orally to complete ten to 14 days of therapy
Ambulatory therapy
    Cefoxitin, 2 gm intramuscularly (IM) or amoxicillin, 2 gm orally, or ampicillin, 3.5 gm orally, or aqueous procaine penicillin G, 4.8 million units IM at two sites; preceded by probenecid, 1 gm orally, followed by doxycycline, 100 mg twice a day for ten to 14 days
    or
    Tetracycline hydrochloride, 500 mg orally for ten to 14 days

*Adapted from *M.M.W.R.* 31(suppl.):33–62, 1982.

apy on an acute basis. Ruptured tubo-ovarian abscesses, tubo-ovarian abscesses that do not respond to medical therapy within four to five days of institution of therapy, and abscesses that have responded acutely to therapy but that result in chronic pain require surgical extirpation. In cases of unilateral tubal ovarian abscess, unilateral adnexectomy with continued aggressive medical therapy is an accepted procedure. Well-localized, walled-off abscesses can occasionally be drained through colpotomy or rectal incisions. The major surgical therapy, however, of PID consists of total abdominal hysterectomy and bilateral salpingo-oophorectomy.

GONORRHEA

Gonorrhea is one of the most prevalent sexually transmitted diseases in the United States today. More than 1 to 1.5 million cases are reported each year. The peak age of occurrence of gonorrhea is less than 25 years of age, and gonorrhea is more common in urban populations and among lower socioeconomic status groups.

Gonorrhea may present as localized infection of the lower genital tract, as invasive infection of the upper genital tract, or as disseminated disease with systemic manifestations or it may be totally asymptomatic. The causative organism of gonorrhea is *Neisseria gonorrhoeae*, a gram-negative aerobic diplococcus that grows best in carbon dioxide and that is very sensitive to drying and extremes in temperature. The organism commonly infects columnar and transitional cells.

The majority of gonorrhea is transmitted through sexual activity. The incubation period is approximately three to five days in those cases in which symptoms are recognizable. In the female, *N. gonorrhoea* is harbored chiefly in the endocervix. It is also found in the urethra, rectum, and oropharynx, and occasionally may be found in one of these locations in the absence of cervical gonorrhea.

The manifestations of gonorrhea in women are most often subtle. Endocervical gonorrhea is associated with a purulent vaginal discharge, which may or may not be noticed as being abnormal. Occasionally irregular vaginal bleeding may also be noted. Urethral gonorrheal involvement of Skene's glands may be associated with symptoms of lower urinary tract infection, such as dysuria and frequency of urination. Rectal gonorrhea most often causes no symptoms. *Neisseria gonorrhoeae* that are present in the oropharynx may cause an acute pharyngitis; however, it is usually asymptomatic. Because colonization with *N. gonorrhoeae* in women produces either no symptoms or vague ones in 80% of cases, these women do not seek medical attention and form a major reservoir of disease transmission.

Lower genital tract gonorrhea can lead to infection of the Bartholin's glands and the formation of Bartholin's abscesses. Bartholin's abscesses associated with gonorrhea are most often unilateral, acutely suppurative, and painful. They may drain spontaneously or require incision and drainage; they occasionally resolve spontaneously.

Ten percent to 15% of women with endocervical gonorrhea will develop acute salpingitis. *Neisseria gonorrhoeae* can invade and infect the upper genital tract as a solitary pathogen or may be part of a polymicrobial infection. Some strains of *N. gonorrhoeae* are more pathogenic for the upper genital tract than others. A lipopolysaccharide toxin that is capable of damaging salpingeal cells and outer membrane pili that facilitate attachment of the gonococcus to host cells are two features of *N. gonorrhoeae* that are associated with pathogenicity for the upper genital tract. In addition, certain risk factors in the host that predispose to the occurrence of salpingitis have been defined as previously outlined. The exact organism and host factors that lead to invasion and infection of the upper genital tract by *N. gonorrhoeae* are incompletely understood. In the United States, estimates of the incidence of gonococcal salpingitis range from 25% to 80% of all cases of salpingitis.

Pharyngeal carriage of *N. gonorrhoeae* is most often asymptomatic. It can occasionally be associated with an acute, exudative pharyngitis. The etiology of pharyngeal gonorrhea is thought to be almost exclusively as a result of fellatio with an infected male. Although it is largely asymptomatic, pharyngeal gonorrhea is not thought to be very contagious or to be a major reservoir of disease transmission. It is, however, more resistant to therapy with the standard antimicrobial regimens. In addition, there may be a greater tendency for pharyngeal gonorrhea to disseminate, as the number of cases of disseminated gonococcal infection associated with pharyngeal gonorrhea appears to be disproportionately high.

The incidence of disseminated gonococcal infection (DGI) in all persons with gonorrhea is approximately 1% to 3%. Exact risk factors for the occurrence of DGI are unknown, although pregnancy may predispose to DGI. Twenty-eight percent to 42% of cases of DGI in some series have been in pregnant women.

Disseminated gonococcal infection usually presents in one of two distinct forms. It may present as a systemic illness associated with chills, fever, malaise, asymmetric polyarthralgias, and painful skin lesions. The fingers, toes, hands, wrists, and ankles are most frequently involved in what appears to be a tenosynovitis and, rarely, a frank, suppurative arthritis. Skin lesions classically appear as a slightly raised, erythematous base with a necrotic center, but may be petechial, papular, pustular, hemorrhagic, and, occasionally, bullous. These lesions are lightly scattered about the body, often on extremities. Up to 50% of acutely symptomatic patients with systemic DGI may have positive blood cultures.

The second common clinical syndrome of DGI is that of a septic, monoarticular arthritis. Knees are most frequently involved; elbow and ankle involvement are also seen. Joint effusion is exudative, often frankly purulent, with the gonococcus present by routine culture in approximately 50% of cases. Blood cultures are not positive.

Disseminated *N. gonorrhoeae* may also cause endocarditis, myocarditis, pericarditis, hepatitis, or meningitis.

Diagnosis

The diagnosis of gonorrhea is most accurately made by a culture of the organism on selective media, such as modified Thayer-Martin agar. The specimen should be plated directly on warmed media and incubated without delay to minimize false-negative results due to improper handling.

Obtaining specimens from multiple sites inceases the yield of culturing for suspected gonorrhea. The endocervix is the site most frequently positive in females, and should always be sampled. Cultures from the urethra, rectum, and pharynx may be positive even with negative cervical cultures, and should be performed when indicated by history, strong clinical suspicion of gonococcal disease, and in all cases of recurrent disease.

A Gram stain of cervical secretions may be

helpful in making a tentative diagnosis of gonorrhea in patients who are symptomatic or who have a history of contact with known gonorrhea. A Gram stain is considered to be positive if intracellular Gram negative diplococci are seen in a minimum of three polymorphonuclear leukocytes per high-power field. Approximately two thirds of women with endocervical gonorrhea will have suggestive Gram stains.

Treatment

Guidelines for treatment of gonorrhea are as outlined by current CDC recommendations (Table 18–6). The majority of *N. gonorrhoeae* organisms in the United States are sensitive to high-dose penicillin. Tetracycline is the treatment of choice in penicillin-allergic patients. When penicillin-resistant gonorrhea is suspected, therapy should be with either spectinomycin or cefoxitin.

Plasmid-mediated penicillinase or β-lactamase production by the gonococcus is responsible for penicillin resistance. First seen in the Far East and in West Africa, penicillinase-producing gonococci (PPNG) are recognized but not a major problem in most areas of the United States at this time. Because this is a concern, it is important to reculture all pertinent sites for gonorrhea three to seven days after therapy has been completed. If repeated cultures are positive, retreatment should be with a regimen as described for PPNG.

Most cases of positive gonorrhea cultures after therapy are due to reinfection from untreated sexual partners. It is now recognized that the prevalence of asymptomatic gonorrhea in males may be as high as 20% to 30%. Adequate contact tracing remains an integral part of adequate therapy for gonorrhea.

CHLAMYDIA

Chlamydia trachomatis is an obligate intracellular parasite of columnar and transitional epithelial cells whose role as a pathogen for the genital tract was first recognized to be as the causative agent of lymphogranuloma

TABLE 18–6.—TREATMENT OF GONORRHEA*

Uncomplicated anogenital or urethral infection
 Aqueous procaine penicillin G, 4.8 million units intramuscularly (IM) at two sites, preceded by probenecid, 1 gm orally
  or
 Tetracycline hydrochloride, 500 mg four times a day for seven days
  or
 Amoxicillin, 3.0 gm, or ampicillin, 3.5 gm, either given with probenecid, 1.0 gm orally
Pharyngeal infection
 Aqueous procaine penicillin G, 4.8 million units IM at two sites, preceded by probenecid, 1 gm orally
  or
 Tetracycline hydrochloride, 500 mg four times a day for seven days
Penicillinase-producing *Neisseria gonorrhoeae*
 Spectinomycin, 2 gm IM
  or
 Cefoxitin, 2 gm IM, preceded by probenecid, 1 gm orally
  or
 Cefotaxime, 1 gm IM
  or
 (For pharyngeal PPNG) trimethoprim-sulfamethoxazole, 80 mg-400 mg, nine tablets each day for five days
Disseminated gonococcal infection
 Aqueous crystalline penicillin G, 10 million units intravenously (IV) each day until improvement occurs, followed by amoxicillin or ampicillin, 500 mg orally four times a day to complete seven days of therapy
  or
 Amoxicillin, 3.0 gm, or ampicillin, 3.5 gm, orally, preceded by probenecid, 1 gm orally, followed by 500 mg of either amoxicillin or ampicillin orally four times a day for seven days
  or
 Tetracycline hydrochloride, 500 mg orally four times a day for seven days
  or
 Cefoxitin, 1 gm, or cefotaxime, 500 mg, IV four times a day for seven days
  or
 Erythromycin, 500 mg orally four times a day for seven days

*Adapted from *M.M.W.R.* 31(suppl.):33-62, 1982.

venereum (LGV). Non-LGV serotypes of *C. trachomatis* have now been associated with asymptomatic carriage in and a variety of infections of the female genital tract.

The overall prevalence of *C. trachomatis* in the female genital tract is 4% to 13%. It is a sexually transmitted organism, and more prevalent in the age group of those younger than 19 years, in nulliparas, and in oral contraceptive users. *Chlamydia* is frequently associated with gonorrhea; approximately 30% of the time it may be cultured from the genital tract after successful therapy for gonorrhea. It is recognized to be a major pathogen in cases of postgonococcal and nongonococcal urethritis in the male, and female partners of males with these syndromes are at high risk for chlamydial colonization and disease.

In addition to being a causative agent of pelvic inflammatory disease (PID), *C. trachomatis* has been associated with cervicitis and urethritis. The presence of *C. trachomatis* in the cervix has been associated with a distinct cervicitis characterized by a hypertrophic-appearing, often friable central eversion covered with purulent cervical mucus. Endocervical mucus will discolor the tip of a cotton-tipped applicator (positive "Q-tip" test) and microscopic examination will reveal the presence of WBCs. Antibiotic treatment for *Chlamydia* will result in reversion of these cervical changes to simple eversion without purulence.

The female urethral syndrome of dysuria, pyuria greater than 10 WBCs per high-power field, and negative bacterial culture has been associated with *C. trachomatis* in up to 50% of cases. Therapy with doxycycline will result in resolution of symptoms.

Chlamydia trachomatis has also been implicated as a cause of bartholinitis and late postpartum endometritis. It can also be transmitted to neonates at the time of birth through an infected maternal birth canal and in neonates is associated with a distinctive conjunctivitis and pneumonitis. *Chlamydia trachomatis* has recently been associated also with unexplained "silent" infertility due to tubal obstruction.

Diagnosis

The presence of *C. trachomatis* is determined most accurately by demonstrating the intracellular organism in tissue culture. Rapid immunofluorescent and histochemical staining techniques for the identification of chlamydial organisms have recently been introduced. These tests appear to be both sensitive and specific and can be expected to be more widely available and less expensive than the presently available culture techniques.

Invasive infection with *C. trachomatis* does produce an immunogenic response, and chlamydial antibodies are measurable using complement fixation, microimmunofluorescence and ELISA techniques. When a fourfold rise in IgG titer or the presence of specific IgM antibodies is documented, chlamydial disease may be diagnosed. The presence of pre-existing antibody, cross-reactivity of various serotypes of *Chlamydia* by serologic testing methods, and the lack of antibody response to some chlamydial infections and most chlamydial carriage limit the usefulness of chlamydial serologic analysis as a diagnostic tool.

Treatment

The drug of choice for the treatment of *Chlamydia* is tetracycline. The exact duration of therapy necessary to achieve cure is unknown. Tetracycline, 500 mg four times a day for seven to ten days is most likely adequate. Tetracycline, 250 mg four times a day for 21 days is also curative. *Chlamydia* are also sensitive to erythromycin and some sulfa drugs. Penicillins are not effective agents against *Chlamydia*. Although treatment to eliminate *Chlamydia* should be based on culture documentation, when such culture facilities are not available or culture is impractical, presumptive therapy may be instituted for suspected carriage or disease in a high-risk population.

Repeated cultures after therapy should be performed, at the earliest, three to four weeks after completion of antimicrobial therapy. All sexual partners must be referred for evaluation and treatment.

Actinomycosis

Infection by *Actinomyces israelii* is an infrequent cause of disease of the upper genital tract. *Actinomyces israelii* is a gram-positive, non–acid fast anaerobic bacterium with characteristic radially branching filamentous formation. It is most typically found in the oral cavity. Actinomycosis is a sporadic infection of soft tissues characterized by invasion of areas of trauma, with chronic, suppurative infection that results in tissue destruction, fibrosis, and the formation of draining sinuses. Active actinomycotic infection usually is polymicrobial, with other anaerobic organisms most frequently being involved.

Actinomycosis is a rare cause of indolent pelvic infection secondary to seeding of the upper genital tract from other intra-abdominal sources or hematogenous dissemination of *Actinomyces*. In addition, the occurrence of ascending pelvic actinomycosis has been described in the presence of an intrauterine device (IUD).

Colonization of the lower genital tract by *Actinomyces* is seen most frequently, though not exclusively, in IUD users. The prevalence of colonization increases with the duration of IUD use. A small percentage of women in whom colonization occurs will manifest upper genital tract infection associated with actinomycosis. This may be preceded by irregular patterns of vaginal bleeding, such as menorrhagia, metrorrhagia, and intermenstrual spotting, as well as by the development of mild, chronic pelvic discomfort. Often by the time of presentation of upper genital tract infection, the pelvic organs are massively indurated and fibrotic, with near total destruction of anatomy and adherence to surrounding structures. At this stage because of the minimal chance of restoration of structure and function by medical therapy and because of the occasional confusion in diagnosis with that of a malignant process, the outcome is frequently surgical removal of affected organs.

Diagnosis

The diagnosis of actinomycosis can be suspected by a suggestive Gram stain in association with nonstaining by acid-fast smear of tangled, filamentous structures. Histologic sections of actinomycotic infections show necrotic debris and inflammation associated with "sulfur granules," which are central organisms with branching filaments that stain yellow with a silver stain. Diagnosis can be confirmed by culture using appropriate anaerobic media and techniques.

The diagnosis of lower genital tract colonization by *Actinomyces* can be suspected by Papanicolaou smear. Aggregates of bacteria can have the appearance of actinomycotic filaments, and colonization suspected by Papanicolaou smear is confirmed using specific immunofluorescent staining techniques only 50% of the time. Such immunofluorescent staining is not widely available.

Treatment

When colonization is suspected by Papanicolaou smear, treatment with antibiotics has not been shown to effectively eliminate *Actinomyces* from the lower genital tract. Current recommendations are to remove IUDs in cases of suspected colonization and repeat Papanicolaou smears in a few months; if the smear is negative, the IUD may then be reinserted.

Actinomycosis is sensitive to penicillins, tetracycline, chloramphenicol, and clindamycin. Treatment of infection is with high-dose parenteral antibiotics, typically penicillin. The exact length of therapy necessary is not established, although the slow growth of these organisms and extensive involvement in cases of infection at other sites usually necessitate a minimum of six weeks of therapy. Treatment of actinomycotic pelvic infection should also include coverage for other organisms typically found in cases of upper genital tract infection, in particular, anaerobic organisms. Despite aggressive therapy, chances of surgical intervention are high.

GENITAL TRACT TUBERCULOSIS AS AN ETIOLOGIC AGENT FOR PELVIC INFLAMMATORY DISEASE

Tuberculosis is a rare cause of upper genital tract infection in developed countries. Today it most often presents in older women who were exposed to tuberculosis before the advent of effective chemoprophylaxis and in younger women who emigrate from countries where tuberculosis is endemic.

Genital tract tuberculosis is usually secondary to hematogenous spread from pulmonary or other non–genital tract foci. It can rarely spread to the genital tract from other intraperitoneal foci or from male sexual partners with tuberculous epididymitis.

The most frequent site of tuberculous involvement in the female genital tract is the fallopian tube. Central spread of infection will result in involvement of the uterus, cervix, and vagina and vulva, in order of decreasing frequency. Ovarian involvement in the tuberculous process varies from 5% to 30%.

Genital tract tuberculosis is an extremely indolent infection. Disease may not become manifest for more than ten years after initial seeding of the genital tract. Presenting symptoms may be those of unusual vaginal bleeding patterns, including altered menses, amenorrhea, and postmenopausal bleeding. Approximately 25% to 35% of women with pelvic tuberculosis may complain of vague, chronic lower abdominal or pelvic pain. The chief presenting complaint of young women with genital tract tuberculosis is infertility. Occasionally, women with genital tract tuberculosis can present with tuberculous peritonitis and ascites, although this is more frequently secondary to direct hemotogenous seeding of the peritoneum.

The diagnosis of genital tract tuberculosis may be suspected from past medical history, travel history, and a chest roentgenogram with evidence of healed pulmonary tuberculosis. Except for debilitated, systemically ill patients, a PPD skin test for tuberculosis will yield positive findings. Hysterosalpingogram may show characteristic changes suggestive of tuberculous infection including beading, sacculation, sinus formation, and the rigid "pipe-stem" pattern.

Diagnosis can be confirmed by histologic examination that reveals typical granulomas, or acid-fast stain and culture of surgical or endometrial biopsy specimens. Menstrual blood collected in a vaginal cup or cervical cap may also be submitted for culture.

The treatment of genital tract tuberculosis is primarily medical, with administration of two or three antituberculosis drugs over an 18 to 24-month period. Surgery is indicated if symptoms or physical examination suggest persistence or increase in disease despite adequate therapy or if culture or biopsy suggest resistant organisms. Surgical therapy most often consists of total abdominal hysterectomy and bilateral salpingo-oophorectomy.

GENITAL HERPES

Genital herpes is a sexually transmitted infection of increasing concern for sexually active women of all age groups, races, and socioeconomic status. Symptomatic genital herpes is the most frequent cause of painful lesions of the lower genital tract of women in the United States. Herpes infection of the lower genital tract has been associated with cervical cancer, although a causative role remains undefined. In addition, contact with genital herpes during passage through the birth canal has been associated with systemic neonatal infection, which carries major risks of serious morbidity and a high rate of mortality.

The exact prevalence of genital herpes infection is unknown, since not all people with active infections seek medical care. However, some consider that genital herpes may be one of the most frequent sexually transmitted diseases in the United States today.

Genital herpes is caused by the herpes simplex virus (HSV), a member of the DNA-containing Herpesviridae family. There are two major types of HSV, types 1 and 2 (HSV-1 and HSV-2), which are closely related and share some common antigens. While the majority of genital herpes lesions are caused by HSV-2 infections and HSV-1 primarily cause oral-labial lesions, it is clear that there is significant overlap. Approximately 85% to 90% of genital infections are caused by HSV-2, while the remainder are caused by HSV-1. This proportion varies, and up to 50% of genital lesions were found to be due to HSV-1 in a survey that took place in England.

Genital herpes is a recurrent infection. Periods of active infection are separated by periods of latency during which the inactive virus resides in the dorsal-root sacral ganglia. Under the stimulus of various endogenous and exogenous factors, the virus travels down the sensory nerve root to the lower genital area where virus replicates, outward manifestations of disease become apparent, and HSV can be identified by culture.

The lesions of genital herpes are typically painful lesions that begin as fluid-filled vesicles or papules, which progress to well-circumscribed, occasionally coalescent, shallow-based ulcers, and heal by reepithelialization of mucous membranes or by crusting over of epidermal surfaces. The clinical presentation and duration of active infection varies widely, and is dependent on virus type and on presentation as initial or recurrent disease.

Initial presentation of genital herpes infection occurs one to 45 days (mean, 5.8 days) after exposure to the virus. Manifestations of initial HSV infection are more severe and last longer than those of recurrent disease. Multiple painful, usually bilateral, lesions occur on the external genitalia. Symptoms tend to peak within eight to ten days and gradually decrease over the next week. Ulcers last four to 15 days, and the mean time from the onset of lesions to total healing is 20 to 21 days. Most often, local lesions are accompanied by bilateral, tender lymphadenopathy of the inguinal and, sometimes, femoral and iliac regions. When adenopathy of the deep inguinal nodes is present, it can be responsible for severe lower pelvic pain. Adenopathy appears somewhat after the onset of lesions and often takes longer to resolve, lasting beyond the period of the lesions themselves.

Local involvement includes urethritis in the majority of cases. Urination may be problematic either because of periurethral and vulvar edema or because of intense dysuria due to uretheral herpetic involvement.

Initial genital herpes infection involves the cervix in more than 80% of cases. Cervical involvement may be clinically apparent with friability of the cervix, ulcerative and occasionally necrotic lesions of the cervix, and a marked increase in cervical discharge. Both the exocervix and endocervix may be involved. In some cases, involvement of the cervix may not be clinically apparent, although virus can be cultured from the cervix.

Although HSV has been cultured from the fallopian tube, it is unclear how often the upper genital tract is involved during initial cases of genital herpes. At present, this is not felt to be a major clinical problem.

Coincident with initial symptomatic genital herpes infection, symptomatic pharyngitis has been reported to occur in approximately 10% of cases. The herpes simplex virus can be isolated from the pharynx of individuals with both symptomatic pharyngitis and from those without pharyngeal symptoms. Pharyngitis and pharyngeal viral shedding occur for genital infection with both HSV-1 and HSV-2.

Secondary spread of local lesions to other body sites occurs after the onset of lesions and before lesions have crusted over. Extragenital involvement is most often of sites below the waist such as the buttocks and upper legs; however, involvement of the fingers and eyes has also been reported. Secondary spread of lesions to extragenital sites is thought to be primarily due to autoinoculation.

In half to two thirds of cases of initial genital herpes infection, systemic symptoms are apparent. Fever, malaise, headache, and myalgias are common. Other systemic complications can include hepatitis, aseptic meningitis, and autonomic nervous system dysfunction.

Hepatitis exhibits a picture typical for hepatocellular necrosis, and presents after the onset of local genital lesions. This usually occurs within the first week of illness and is most often accompanied by other systemic symptoms.

Aseptic meningitis is seen much more frequently with HSV-2 than with HSV-1 infections. It has been reported to occur in up to 36% of initial genital herpes infections. The presentation is of headache, stiff neck, and photophobia, with or without fever. It is accompanied by a cerebrospinal fluid pleocytosis consisting largely of lymphocytes. Meningitis is self-limited, requires only supportive care, and resolves without permanent neurological sequelae. Encephalitis is rarely a complication of genital herpes infection.

Sacral autonomic nervous system dysfunction is a less common complication of inital genital herpes infection. Typical symptoms include decrease in sensation along the sacral nerve route distribution, inability to void due to bladder dysfunction, and constipation due to bowel dysfunction. Nerve dysfunction can be confirmed through electromyography; it may last up to six to eight weeks. Occasionally, sensory involvement may take the form of hypoesthesia in a radicular pattern. A presentation of self-limited transverse myelitis with paralysis has also been reported.

Recurrent genital herpes infection is typically less severe, of shorter duration, and less frequently involves systemic manifestations than initial disease. One to two days prior to the onset of recurrent lesions, prodromal symptoms may occur. This is typically described as a tingling sensation or hyperesthesia of the genital area where lesions will occur. The prodrome may also include a sacral dermatomal neuralgia with pain radiating to the buttocks and hips.

Recurrent genital lesions are fewer, smaller, and more often unilateral. Recurrent lesions may not have the typical ulcerative appearance, and may be more similar in appearance to a fissure or excoriation. Recurrences tend to occur in the same location and have the same appearance from episode to episode. Symptoms of recurrent lesions last four to eight days and the mean time to disappearance of recurrent lesions is nine to ten days. Both urethritis and cervicitis are less frequently seen with recurrent genital infection

than with initial infection. Tender local adenopathy may be present, but is usually less severe and of shorter duration. Systemic manifestations are uncommon.

The frequency of recurrent disease and the length of time between recurrences of active infection is highly variable. The average number of recurrences in women who have symptomatic recurrent genital herpes is five to eight per year. Recurrences may be precipitated by an obvious endogenous stimulus, such as cyclic hormonal variation or stress, or recurrent infection may be precipitated by exposure to HSV through sexual contact with an infected partner. It is unclear whether contact with exogenous virus precipitates recurrent infection or whether this is actually reinfection with a different viral strain. While it has been the general impression that frequency of recurrent disease decreases as time from initial infection increases, recent evidence suggests that the frequency of recurrent disease is independent of time. It is now apparent that the clinical presentation of genital herpes does not always follow classic patterns. Asymptomatic infection as defined by culture-positive viral shedding in the absence of symptoms or lesions has been documented to occur from both the cervix and the vulva. The prevalence of asymptomatic shedding is unknown, as is the frequency. It does appear that asymptomatic shedding is of brief duration, and lasts for an average of three to five days per episode.

Approximately 25% of initial genital herpes infections present in women who have preexisting antibody to HSV. These initial episodes tend to be less severe with fewer systemic manifestations, and are more typical of recurrent infection. Some of these mild initial episodes may actually be recurrent infection in a person with previous asymptomatic infection. In other cases, the presence of antibody to HSV-1 of oral-labial origin may serve to ameliorate the clinical expression of infection.

While initial presentation of genital herpes infection caused by HSV-1 cannot be distinguished from initial presentation of infection caused by HSV-2, HSV-1 is less likely to result in recurrent infection. Recurrences of infection after initial infection caused by HSV-1 are much less frequent and less severe. The reason for this type of specific difference in recurrence rates is unclear.

Diagnosis

The diagnosis of genital herpes is often suggested by characteristic clinical presentation and appearance of lesions. The most accurate diagnostic test to confirm clinical impression is virus isolation by tissue culture. The virus may be isolated from both vesicle fluid and the base of a wet ulcer. If vesicles are present, the vesicles should be unroofed and the fluid cultured directly. A single virus culture done of an appropriate lesion will identify live virus in 85% to 90% of cases. Less sensitive but helpful tests when viral cultures are not available rely on cytologic methods to identify changes in cells typically produced by the HSV. Scrapings of viral lesions may be gathered for a Papanicolaou smear or for Tzanck preparation. A Tzanck smear stained with either Wright's or Giemsa stain is positive if multinucleated giant cells are identified, as they may be in up to 50% of cases. Antibody testing is often of no value to the diagnosis of genital herpes infections. Forty percent to 60% of adults have antibodies to HSV-1, which represents past exposure to HSV-1 that may have resulted in clinically apparent infection or asymptomatic infection. Although it is possible to distinguish antibodies to HSV-2 from antibodies to HSV-1, there is an approximately 20% crossover that makes such identification inaccurate. In these cases, the existence of antibody to HSV at the onset of an initial genital herpes infection may preclude identification of this episode as either primary infection in a previously antibody-negative host or recurrent infection in a previously asymptomatic host. In addition, the presence of antibody to HSV at the onset of a herpes genital lesion may identify past exposure to this virus but not, however, help identify the etiology of active lesions. Occasionally, if there is no antibody to HSV present at the onset of a suspected primary genital herpes infection and antibody is documented to develop during the course of illness, antibody testing can be of some value.

Treatment

There is no therapy that effectively prevents recurrent genital herpes infection on a long-term basis. The currently available antiviral agent that holds the most promise for altering the course of genital herpes infection is acyclovir. Acyclovir is available in three forms. Topical application of acyclovir has been demonstrated to decrease the duration of symptoms and the length of viral shedding for initial disease. To be efficacious, topical therapy must be applied at onset of symptoms and must be applied frequently. Topical acyclovir is not effective in altering the course of recurrent genital herpes infection. Intravenous acyclovir effectively ameliorates the presentation of initial genital herpes infections and prevents recurrences in immunosuppressed individuals. In addition, intravenous acyclovir is used to treat disseminated herpetic infection in immunosuppressed individuals. The emergence of resistant herpes simplex virus to acyclovir has been documented with the use of intravenous acyclovir. Oral acyclovir has been demonstrated to significantly decrease recurrences of genital herpes in healthy adults when given on a long-term basis. Administration of oral acyclovir does not appear to alter the natural history of genital herpes infection, however, and recurrences of infection return to previous rates when therapy is discontinued. Of concern, the development of drug-resistant virus in patients receiving continual oral therapy has been demonstrated. The potential for drug resistance and long-term side effects of acyclovir therapy exist, and an exact role of oral acyclovir in the treatment of genital herpes remains undefined.

The mainstay of treatment of genital herpes infections remains care of local lesions and supportive care through any systemic illness.

Local measures to decrease superinfections of lesions and to increase comfort are encouraged. Use of an indwelling bladder catheter may be necessary in severe cases of herpes urethritis. Hospitalization for observation and supportive care during episodes of aseptic meningitis may be necessary. Finally, appropriate counseling must be provided to handle the emotional and informational needs of patients in whom genital herpes infection has been diagnosed.

SYPHILIS

Syphilis occurs when the causative organism, the spirochete *Treponema pallidum*, is inoculated into mucous membranes. This occurs most frequently during sexual activity. In the United States, approximately 20,000 new cases of syphilis are reported each year, predominantly in the 15 to 40-year-old age group.

Syphilis exists in well-described stages defined by both clinical presentation and time course.

The incubation period from contact to the onset of lesions of primary syphilis ranges from nine to 90 days, with an average time of three weeks. The lesion of primary syphilis is the chancre, a solitary, painless ulceration that forms at the site of inoculation. A chancre begins as a firm papule, and breaks down to become a well-demarcated ulcer with raised, rolled borders and a smooth, erythematous base. The average size of a chancre is 0.5 to 2.0 cm. Most frequently, these occur on the labia, posterior fourchette, cervix, or vagina, although pharyngeal and anal chancres also occur. Bilateral, firm, nontender regional adenopathy is common. Because chancres are not painful, they often go unnoticed and undetected. Spirochetes are found at the base of the ulcer, and chancres are infectious.

Nine to 90 days after chancre formation, or an average of six to 12 weeks after exposure, hematogenous dissemination of spirochetes occurs and the onset of symptoms of secondary syphilis takes place. The chancre of primary syphilis may still be present at this time. Secondary syphilis also has mucocutaneous manifestations, although systemic manifestations due to multiorgan involvement may be prominent. Macular, maculopapular, or primarily papular generalized skin eruptions are typical. Facial sparing and involvement of the palms and soles is classic. Pustular and discoid lesions as well as alopecia and mucous membrane patches are well-described variants of the mucocutaneous lesions of secondary syphilis. Another classic lesion of secondary syphilis is the condyloma lata, which is a confluence of raised, moist, flat condylomatous lesions occurring primarily in intertriginous areas. These lesions are also infectious.

Generalized, often tender, lymphadenopathy, fever, malaise, headache, sore throat, and arthralgias commonly present along with the skin lesions of secondary syphilis. Manifestations of involvement of other organ systems such as hepatitis and meningitis, also occur.

Following resolution of signs of secondary syphilis, this infection enters a latent period. Latent syphilis is classified as *early latent syphilis* for up to four years' duration. Syphilis of more than four years' duration is classified as *late latent syphilis*. During early latent syphilis of less than one year's duration, there can be a recurrence of symptoms of secondary syphilis. Otherwise, latent syphilis is asymptomatic and not infectious.

Manifestations of late syphilis are thought to be largely a result of endothelial damage and ongoing chronic inflammation. Five to 20 years or more after initial disease, the consequences of late syphilis present as single-system or multisystem involvement.

Benign, mucocutaneous late disease presents with painless, indolent, destructive lesions. The classic skin lesion of late syphilis is the solitary gumma, a progressive, granulomatous, necrotic ulcer, but lesions may also be nodular and multiple. Gummas and destructive lesions of late syphilis may also involve visceral organs, long bones, and joints.

Two other distinct forms of late syphilis are cardiovascular syphilis and neurosyphilis. Cardiovascular syphilis most prominently involves the aorta, resulting in aortic insufficiency and thoracic aortic aneurysms. Neurosyphilis may be asymptomatic, may present as acute meningitis, or may be responsible for gradual deterioration of intellectual and motor capacity.

Syphilis can be transmitted to the fetus at any stage of pregnancy, resulting in deformities, acute neonatal illness, and late manifestations of disease that have been described elsewhere. Congenital syphilis can be prevented or ameliorated by maternal treatment during pregnancy. For this reason, premarital and prenatal screening for syphilis are the rule.

Diagnosis

When an infectious lesion of syphilis such as a chancre is recognized, a dark-field examination should be performed on secretions from a cleaned lesion. If spirochetes are demonstrated, a diagnosis of syphilis may be made. False-negative results of dark-field examinations can occur, particularly when topical or systemic antimicrobial therapy suppresses the numbers of spirochetes.

The diagnosis of syphilis is most often made by serologic methods. Serologic tests for syphilis are of two types: the nontreponemal and the treponemal tests.

The nontreponemal tests most widely available are the VDRL slide tests and the rapid plasma reagin circle card test (RPR-CT). These tests detect the presence of cardiolipin, a nonspecific antigen produced during syphilitic infection. These tests are quantitative and serial titers may be used to judge therapeutic response. A positive result of a nontreponemal test is suggestive of, but not specific for, a diagnosis of syphilis. Positive nontreponemal tests for syphilis are also associated with a variety of conditions and disorders, including collagen-vascular diseases, lymphomas, drug abuse, sarcoidosis, and acute infections such as mononucleosis, *Mycoplasma* infections, and other febrile illnesses.

A definitive diagnosis of syphilis is made by testing for the presence of specific antitreponemal antibodies. The fluorescent treponemal antibody absorption test (FTA-ABS) is the treponemal test most widely used. This test will confirm a diagnosis of syphilis with a low false-positive rate of 1% to 2%. Once positive, an FTA-ABS result will remain positive despite successful therapy.

A serologic test for syphilis will be predictive of disease in about 75% of cases by the fourth week after exposure. By six weeks to three months, 99% to 100% of serologic tests will be positive. While a chancre may be present prior to seropositivity, secondary syphilis is almost always accompanied by a positive serologic test result. If a serologic test for syphilis remains negative three months after suspected exposure, the diagnosis of syphilis can be excluded.

When results of a screening serologic test for syphilis is positive the stage of disease is determined using historical guidelines. If presently asymptomatic and a result of a serologic test for syphilis (STS) performed within the preceding year was negative, early latent syphilis of less than one year's duration is diagnosed. If asymptomatic, and a result of an STS performed within the preceding four years was negative or the patient is younger than 30 years, early latent syphilis is diagnosed. If the patient is older than 30 years or a negative STS result within four years cannot be documented, late latent syphilis is diagnosed. If late latent syphilis is diagnosed, a lumbar puncture should be performed to rule out neurosyphilis, as neurosyphilis may be less responsive to standard therapy and requires close follow-up.

Treatment

Treatment of syphilis will abort acute disease and prevent progression of disease but will not alter permanent changes produced by tissue destruction. Primary therapy of syphilis is with benzathine penicillin. Penicillin-allergic patients are treated with tetracycline. The length of therapy is determined by the stage of disease (Table 18–7).

TABLE 18–7.–TREATMENT OF SYPHILIS*

Early syphilis (primary, secondary, or latent syphilis of less than one year's duration)
    Benzathine penicillin G, 2.4 million units, intramuscularly (IM) at a single session
    Penicillin-allergic patients:
        Tetracycline hydrochloride, 500 mg orally four times a day for 15 days
        or
        Erythromycin,† 500 mg orally four times a day for 15 days
Syphilis of more than one year's duration (except neurosyphilis)
    Benzathine penicillin G, 2.4 million units IM once a week for three successive weeks (7.2 million units total)
    Penicillin-allergic patients
        Tetracycline hydrochloride, 500 mg orally four times a day for 30 days
        or
        Erythromycin, 500 mg orally four times a day for 30 days
Neurosyphilis
    Aqueous crystalline penicillin G, 12 to 24 million units IV each day for ten days, followed by benzathine penicillin G, 2.4 million units IM once a week for three doses
    or
    Aqueous procaine penicillin G, 2.4 million units IM each day plus probenecid, 500 mg orally four times a day, both for ten days, followed by benzathine penicillin G, 2.4 million units IM weekly for three doses
    or
    Benzathine penicillin G, 2.4 million units IM once a week for three doses
    Penicillin-allergic patients
        Patients with histories of allergies to penicillin should have their allergy confirmed and managed in consultation with an expert

*Adapted from *M.M.W.R.* 31(suppl.):33–62, 1982.
†The efficacy of erythromycin has not been firmly established; therefore, complications and serologic follow-up should be assured.

After successful therapy, nontreponemal serologic test results will revert to negative in a large percentage of cases, depending on the duration of disease. Within two years, virtually all patients with secondary syphilis will have negative nontreponemal serologic tests. Within five years, approximately 45% of patients with latent syphilis will be seronegative. Titers should be followed after therapy until they stabilize or disappear. If titers increase, reinfection is presumed and retreatment indicated.

The Jarisch-Herxheimer reaction is a well-described phenomenon occurring in a variable number of patients treated for primary or secondary syphilis. Approximately 12 hours after therapy, skin lesions become more prominent, and pronounced systemic symptoms of fever, rigors, headache, myalgias, and arthralgias occur. This is presumed to be due to either release of treponemal toxins or to formation of circulating antigen-antibody complexes. Symptoms are self-limited, do not recur, and no specific therapy is indicated.

CHANCROID

Chancroid is a sexually transmitted disease caused by *Hemophilus ducreyi*, a short, thick, gram-negative bacillus that is a facultative anaerobe. Chancroid is characterized by painful genital ulcers and suppurative inguinal lymphadenopathy with a lack of systemic signs or symptoms.

After an incubation period of one to six days, the genital lesions of chancroid begin as small papules or vesicles, which become pustular and rupture, forming an ulcer within one to three days of their onset. Ulcers are not indurated, and have well-circumscribed but shaggy, overhanging margins. Surrounding the ulcer may be a rim of erythema. The base of the ulcer is covered with gray, adherent, sometimes necrotic, exudate, and it bleeds easily when the exudate is scraped off. Ulcers are painful and tender. Ulcers may be single, but are more often multiple. They vary in size from a few millimeters to 20 mm. Most often the labia, posterior fourchette, and the perianal region are involved, but the cervix and vagina may also be involved.

Regional lymph nodes are involved in more than 50% of cases. Bilateral involvement of inguinal nodes is common, although if genital lesions are unilateral, lymph node involvement will also be unilateral. Lymph nodes increase in size, suppurate, and become fluctuant, and overlying skin becomes thinned and necrotic, leading to spontaneous rupture and drainage. If lymph nodes are noted to be indurated and fluctuant, the lymph node may be aspirated and a large, chronic, draining sinus prevented.

Diagnosis

The diagnosis of chancroid can be made by scraping material from the edges of an ulcer or collecting material from a suppurating lymph node and culturing this on specific media. A Gram strain of this material reveals predominantly chaining gram-negative coccobacillary forms. *Hemophilus ducreyi* may be one of many bacterial species present in a lesion of chancroid; the diagnosis in these cases may be more difficult to document. The diagnosis of chancroid is often made by clinical presentation, and by excluding other causes of genital ulceration such as genital herpes, lymphogranuloma venereum and syphilis.

Treatment

If untreated, ulcers may persist, increase in size, and form more extensive, erosive lesions. Occasionally, local lesions may run a self-limited course. Treatment has classically consisted of administration of sulfa or tetracycline. There are increasing reports of sulfa resistance, however. Alternative therapy is administration of streptomycin and chloramphenicol. Treatment with either erythromycin or trimethoprim-sulfamethoxazole has also been reported to be beneficial. Treatment should be carried out for a minimum of one to three weeks, depending on the therapeutic response. Therapy should be continued for five to seven days after resolution of all lesions and symptoms.

At present, chancroid is most common in developing countries, particularly in the tropical and subtropical areas. It is not commonly reported in North America and Europe except for periodic, geographically isolated outbreaks.

LYMPHOGRANULOMA VENEREUM (LGV)

Lymphogranuloma venereum (LGV) is a sexually transmitted disease whose major clinical manifestations are due to infection of regional lymph nodes that drain sites of transient local genital infection. The causative organism of LGV is *Chlamydia trachomatis*, specifically immunotypes L1, L2, l3.

The transient mucosal or cutaneous lesion of LGV occurs at the site of inoculation four to 21 days after exposure. In females lesions are usually singular, although they may be multiple. They occur predominantly on the posterior vulva, urethral meatus, and medial labia, although the vagina and cervix may be involved. Lesions are small, vesicular, papular, or pustular lesions, less than 6 mm, which progress to small, shallow ulcers with irregular borders and an erythematous base. Ulcers are usually not painful and often not recognized. After a short period of time, local lesions heal spontaneously and after variable periods of latency, the symptoms of local lymphadenitis become manifest.

The symptoms of adenitis vary according to the lymph chains that are involved and the chronicity of infection. The immediate course of lymph node involvement entails a one- to four-week period during which multiple nodes become inflamed, suppurate, become fixated to overlying skin, and spontaneously rupture and drain. Chronic inflammation of involved lymphatics may lead to obstruction with retrograde edema and occasional ulceration. Involved tissue is often totally replaced by fibrosis and constriction with scarring. Repeated episodes of spontaneous rupture and drainage may lead to chronically draining sinuses, fistula formation, and scarring.

Initial LGV lesions of the anterior vulva and lower vagina drain into femoral and inguinal lymphatics, resulting in the "inguinal syndrome." Multiple nodes of both inguinal and femoral regions become firm, adherent to each other, and eventually form buboes, which are fluctuant and painful with skin fixation. If both the inguinal and femoral areas are involved, buboes are separated by the inguinal ligament forming the pathognomonic "groove sign." Involvement most often is unilateral. If fluctuant nodes are aspirated through normal skin, this can prevent spontaneous rupture with chronic sinus formation. Chronic inflammation of inguinal lymph nodes can lead to fibrous constriction of the inguinal area, often accompanied by draining sinuses. Hypertrophy and edema of vulvar lymphatic tissues can be marked. When this occurs it is called *esthiomene*, and is analogous to elephantiasis in the male. Overlying vulvar skin may ulcerate. Chronic inflammation in the vaginal and periurethral area can lead to stricture and fistula formation.

More often in the female, the perirectal and pelvic lymph nodes are involved, leading to "genitorectal" manifestations of LGV. This presents as a proctocolitis with bloody diarrhea and perianal discharge. Fibrosis of edematous mucosa eventually leads to stricture formation and rectovaginal fistulas are common.

As opposed to chancroid, systemic symptoms may be present at the time of presentation of LGV. Approximately 50% of patients will have fever, malaise, headache, and anorexia at the time of initial lymphadenitis

Diagnosis

The diagnosis of LGV is most frequently made by antibody testing. Complement fixation titers to *C. trachomatis* greater than or equal to 1:128 are suggestive of LGV. Antibody testing by microimmunoflourescence may show an increase in specific IgG titers, or the presence of specific IgM antibody. Chlamydial organisms may occasionally be isolated from the exudate of fluctuant or draining buboes. Histologic examination of involved nodes may show suggestive palisading aggregates of mononuclear cells surrounding granulomas or microabscesses, but may be fairly nonspecific and biopsy is not the primary mode of diagnosis.

Treatment

Treatment of LGV is usually with tetracycline given for at least two weeks after the remission of all systemic symptoms and local disease. Alternative therapies include sulfonamides and erythromycin.

Lymphogranuloma venereum is currently rare in North America and other industrialized countries. It is common in the tropical and semitropical areas, particularly in developing countries.

DONOVANOSIS (GRANULOMA INGUINALE)

Donovanosis, formerly termed *granuloma inguinale*, is a disease of the lower genital tract characterized by slowly progressive, hypertrophic ulceration with tissue destruction. Donovanosis is a sexually transmitted disease associated with the encapsulated gram-negative bacillus, *Calymmatobacterium granulomatis*.

The incubation period of donovanosis may be up to six months although it averages two to four months. The initial genital tract lesion is a painless, indurated, reddish-brown papule, which, over a course of days to weeks, erodes and ulcerates. Multiple lesions may coalesce and ulcerate. Ulcerations have well-defined borders and clean bases with exuberant granulation tissue. Lesions are fairly superficial, and spread by contact, autoinoculation, and lymphatic extension. Involved tissue undergoes repeated granulomatous proliferation, ulceration, and scarring with eventual extensive tissue destruction. Extension to the inguinal area is associated with subcutaneous induration, swelling, and eventual breakdown with "pseudobubo" formation. Lymph nodes may be slightly increased in size and occasionally tender, but they do not suppurate. Systemic signs are rare, and when they do occur are related to extensive disease with secondary infection.

Diagnosis

The diagnosis of donovanosis is established by demonstrating the presence of "Donovan bodies" in tissue preparations stained with Wright's or Giemsa stain. Donovan bodies are mononuclear cells containing large numbers of encapsulated bacilli. Scrapings of lesions, "crush" preparations of tissue, or biopsy samples taken from the edge of an ulcer all may reveal these characteristic formations.

Treatment

If untreated, lesions of donovanosis appear to undergo periods of spontaneous resolution or healing, with subsequent relapse of active disease. Active lesions resolve with antibiotic therapy and relapse less frequently. Occasionally prolonged courses of antibiotics need to be administered to prevent "recurrent" disease. The antibiotic of choice for treatment of donovanosis is doxycycline or tetracycline; erythromycin and ampicillin have also been demonstrated to be effective.

Donovanosis is currently rare in Europe and North America. It is most common in tropical and subtropical countries.

GENITAL WARTS

Genital warts are caused by the papillomavirus, a papovavirus structurally and probably antigenically related to the causative agent of common skin warts. Genital warts are sexually transmitted with an incubation period of approximately three months. There is a 60% transmission rate for genital warts, and infectivity may be affected by the number and the age of lesions. Genital warts of longer duration tend to be less infectious.

Genital warts are verrucose growths that typically appear as papillary, pink-to-white frondlike lesions. These lesions are superficial, and may be solitary or may coalesce into large cauliflowerlike masses. Any part of the vulva may be involved, but particularly the posterior fourchette. The perineum and perianal areas may be involved, as may be the vagina, cervix, and anal canal. For this reason, all patients with vulvar warts should have speculum examination performed and all patients with perianal warts should have a rectal examination and sometimes anoscopy should be performed. Warts that occur in the vagina and on the cervix usually appear as flat or papular lesions. Lesions are not usually painful, although they may be pruritic. When warts are exceptionally large they may be-

come necrotic and secondarily infected, with superficial bleeding, discharge, and fetid odor.

The growth of genital warts is stimulated by heat, moisture, and, probably, the number and age of lesions. In addition, some genital warts may grow remarkably during pregnancy, only to recede following the end of pregnancy. It is unclear whether this is related to hormonal factors or related to changes in local cellular immunity.

Diagnosis

The diagnosis of genital warts is suggested by a typical gross appearance and the exclusion of other processes by biopsy. Histologic features of genital warts include papillomatosis, acanthosis, and parakeratosis with vacuolization of epithelial cells.

Treatment

Genital warts are treated using either local cytotoxic agents or ablative therapy. Local application of 20% podophyllum in benzoin is an antimitotic agent that is incorporated into the wart and will cause sloughing of the tissue within three to four days after application. This treatment is slightly less effective for hyperkeratotic warts and may need to be repeated at weekly intervals for resolution of larger warts. Trichloroacetic acid and bichloroacetic acid may also be used.

Cryocautery, laser therapy, and electrocautery have all been used for ablative therapy with success. With cryocautery the lesions should be frozen to the base. Blistering and resolution of the lesion may take place with initial freezing or may require repeated freezings. Laser therapy and electrocautery both attempt to totally remove lesions at the time of initial therapy. Occasionally, the large size of warts necessitates surgical removal. Both electrocautery and surgical removal can be associated with significant blood loss, particularly during pregnancy.

Any associated vaginal infections should be treated concomitantly. The decrease in local moisture that results can be helpful in slowing down growth of lesions that are present. Occasionally, small lesions may resolve spontaneously with such symptomatic therapy. After initial disappearance or removal of lesions it is necessary to closely follow up patients and treat new or recurrent lesions promptly.

Condyloma acuminata has been associated with vulvar cancer and also with cervical koilocytotic atypia and dysplasia. It is not known whether this virus is simply a marker for malignancy or is capable of inducing malignant transformation. Women with a history of genital warts or women with persistent or atypical genital warts should be followed up for the possibility of dysplasia or malignancy, and biopsies of persistent or atypical lesions should be performed.

VAGINITIS

Vaginitis is characterized by abnormal discharge, vulvovaginal discomfort, or both abnormal discharge and discomfort. Many microorganisms, including those that have been associated with vaginitis, can be cultured from the vagina of totally asymptomatic women. Unless symptoms are present the diagnosis of vaginitis should not be made, and in the majority of cases treatment is not indicated.

An average of 4.7 to 6.7 organisms per person can be found on routine culturing of the vagina. Both aerobic and anaerobic bacteria are present. Organisms such as gram-negative enteric rods, *Staphylococcus* species, streptococci (including enterococci), anaerobic gram-positive cocci, and *Bacteroides* species, which are potential pathogens of the upper genital tract, are considered to be normal flora of the vagina. In addition, nonpathogens such as lactobacilli and diphtheroids are also frequently found. The normal pH of the vagina is 3.5 to 4.5. The pH of the vagina is influenced by the organic acid byproducts of metabolism, which are produced by the predominant species in the vaginal flora. Both vaginal pH and normal vaginal flora must be considered when diagnosing vaginitis. In addition, it is important to consider cervical mucus and normal vaginal

discharge when interpreting symptoms of vaginitis.

There are three types of infectious vaginitis currently recognized. These will be discussed in turn.

Candidiasis

The majority of candidiasis is caused by *Candida albicans*, an organism that can be found in the lower genital tract of 30% to 80% of women with minimal to no symptoms. A small number of fungal vaginal infections are caused by *C. glabrata*.

The hallmark of candidiasis is itching and irritation. Itching may be quite severe, and noticed either in the vaginal or vulvar area. Irritation may be associated with dysuria and dyspareunia. When discharge is present, it is commonly described as "cottage cheesy," or thick, white, and clumpy. Discharge is not always present with symptomatic candidiasis, however, and occasionally there may only be a thin watery discharge.

Symptoms of candidiasis frequently have their onset just prior to the menses. In addition, a number of precipitating factors for the occurrence of symptomatic candidiasis have been delineated. *Candida* species may frequently be found in the vagina and some of the precipitating factors for symptomatic candidiasis are those that foster overgrowth of the vagina by *Candida*. This may occur through depression of normal bacterial flora, depression of local cellular immunity, alterations in the metabolic and nutritional milieu of the vagina, and through unknown mechanisms. Precipitating factors for symptomatic candidiasis include the use of systemic antibiotics, immunosuppressive therapy, diabetes mellitus, pregnancy, stress, and, potentially, oral contraceptive agents.

Candidiasis often presents as apparent vulvitis or vulvovaginitis. Examination reveals well-demarcated erythema of the vulva with occasional satellite lesions surrounding the major rim of erythema. The vulva can be notably edematous. The vagina may also be edematous and erythematous, with erythema extending onto the squamous exocervix. It is not unusual for there to be excoriations and fissuring of the vulva and, occasionally, of the vagina. Even if discharge has not been described by the patient, an adherent clumpy white discharge may be found in the upper vagina. The pH of this discharge is most often less than 4.5. When a drop of the discharge is mixed with a drop of 10% potassium hydroxide, covered with a coverslip, and examined under the microscope, normal cellular elements will be lysed and the branching hyphae and bilobate buds of the *Candida* will be visible. In up to 25% of cases of symptomatic candidiasis, the potassium hydroxide wet preparation will be falsely negative. When candidiasis is suspected from the clinical presentation, diagnostic accuracy can be improved by use of the Gram stain or culture on specific media. Hyphae and buds are gram-positive; bilobate buds are slightly larger than WBCs. Solid media that can be used for specific *Candida* cultures include Nickerson's media and Sabouraud agar.

Initial treatment of candidiasis is with local vaginal antifungal preparations. Nystatin suppositories or cream can be used twice a day for 14 days. Miconazole and clotrimazole cream or suppositories are used once a day for seven days and have a slightly higher initial cure rate. It may be possible to use these preparations for shorter periods of time and achieve acceptable cure rates. Interest has developed in the use of boric acid, 600 to 650 mg in a gel capsule used daily for 14 days for the treatment of candidiasis. Initial results would indicate acceptable cure rates and the lack of compounding chemicals makes this an attractive therapeutic alternative in patients who develop a hypersensitivity reaction to other local anti-infective agents. The use of gentian violet–impregnated tampons is messy and occasionally irritating, but may prove useful in some patients.

Ketoconazole is a systemic oral antifungal agent that has been shown to be efficacious in the treatment of vulvovaginal candidiasis. It is not clear that this therapy is any more effective than local preparations. The exact duration of therapy to achieve highest cure rates is unknown; however, one- to two-week courses of therapy are probably effective in the majority of cases. With the use of more long-term ketoconazole, the most serious side effect is reversible but occasionally severe hepatotoxic reaction.

There are a number of approaches to recurrent candidiasis. Longer courses of therapy can be used. Since at least 10% of male sexual partners of women with candidiasis are found to have a candidal balanitis, it is reasonable to treat male sexual partners, particularly those who have displayed any symptoms. Gastrointestinal (GI) tract colonization by *Candida* is present in 50% of adults. For this reason, some advocate the simultaneous use of oral nystatin and local vaginal anti-infectives to decrease the GI tract colonization and prevent cross-contamination of the vagina by perirectal spread. The efficacy of this approach however remains unproved. Finally, it is occasionally necessary to remove all potential precipitating factors in order to achieve long-lasting cure.

Trichomoniasis

Trichomoniasis is caused by the flagellated parasite, *Trichomonas vaginalis*. Male partners of women with trichomoniasis may be found to harbor *Trichomonas*, and there is a high rate of reinfection of women whose male sexual partners are not treated concomitantly for *Trichomonas*; therefore, trichomoniasis is considered to be a sexually transmitted disease. It is often isolated along with other sexually transmitted organisms, in particular, *Neisseria gonorrhoeae*.

The incubation period for trichomoniasis is approximately 19 to 21 days. Symptoms often peak just after the menses. Classic symptoms of trichomoniasis include the presence of a copious, frothy discharge, along with symptoms of local pain and irritation. Dysuria, dyspareunia, and dull lower abdominal pain may be present. Occasionally, itching is the predominant local symptom.

Examination of the vulva and vagina is usually most remarkable for the presence of and appearance of discharge. On insertion of a speculum, copious discharge pools in the posterior blade. This discharge is most often homogeneous, ranges in color from white to greenish-yellow, and may be frothy. The pH of the discharge is greater than 6.0. A wet preparation made by mixing a drop of the discharge with a drop of normal saline, covered with a coverslip, and examination under the microscope at high, dry power will reveal motile trichomonads in the majority of cases of symptomatic trichomoniasis. These parasites are slightly larger than WBCs, ovoid, possess a central undulating membrane, and a terminal flagella. In addition, in the majority of cases of trichomoniasis, greater than 10 WBCs per high-power field will be found on wet preparation. Diagnostic accuracy in suspected cases with a negative wet preparation can be improved by culture in specific media such as Diamond media or Trichosel broth.

Occasionally, the cervix and upper vagina will have an appearance of raised, punctate erythema. This "strawberry" appearance is pathognomonic for trichomoniasis, but found in the minority of cases.

Trichomoniasis has been associated with cervical dysplasia, and may be a marker for cervical carcinoma. Although a causal relationship is doubtful, it may be reasonable for this reason, to treat even asymptomatic women who have *Trichomonas* present in the vagina.

The most effective therapy for trichomoniasis currently available in the United States is oral metronidazole. Two dosage regimens have been shown to be effective. Single high-dose therapy with 2 gm of metronidazole at once has been shown to effectively eradicate *Trichomonas* in 90% of cases. Occasionally, severe nausea and vomiting, particularly when taken in association with other medications, will preclude effective use of this dose schedule. Lower-dose longer-term therapy with 250 mg three times a day for seven to ten days may also be used. There is a high rate of reinfection of females if male sexual partners are not treated concomitantly; therefore, it is common practice for even asymptomatic male partners to be treated. When metronidazole cannot be used, intravaginal clotrimazole or boric acid may provide relief from symptoms and be curative in a small portion of cases.

Gardnerella-associated Vaginitis (Nonspecific Vaginitis)

Nonspecific vaginitis is an infection characterized by excessive discharge and odor. Although for many years the exact microbiologic etiology of this infection was unknown, it is now accepted that this infection is a result of synergistic activity between the aerobic *Gardnerella vaginalis* and vaginal anerobes to produce symptoms. *Gardnerella vaginalis* is commonly found as part of the vaginal flora in approximately a third of sexually active women. Without a critical concentration of vaginal anaerobic bacteria, this organism is not thought to be responsible for symptoms. The effect of anaerobic bacteria in acting with *G. vaginalis* to cause symptoms has been most convincingly shown using gas-liquid chromatography, on specimens from patients with symptomatic disease, which reveals organic-acid metabolites of anaerobes and disappearance of symptoms that correlated with the appearance of metabolites produced by *Lactobacillus* and streptococcal species.

The onset of odor and discharge associated with *Gardnerella*-associated vaginitis is evenly distributed throughout the menstrual cycle. Rarely is local discomfort a problem with this vaginitis. The diagnosis of *Gardnerella*-associated vaginitis is made with a high degree of certainty on examination of the patient and the discharge.

The discharge of *Gardnerella*-associated vaginitis is typically homogeneous, grayish-white to yellow-white, and somewhat adherent to the external vulva and the vaginal walls. Underlying edema or erythema of the vulva or vagina are not typical. The pH of this vaginal discharge is always greater than 4.5

and almost always greater than 5.0. When a drop of potassium hydroxide is added to a drop of discharge, an intense amine odor is elaborated, producing a positive "whiff test." The typical appearance of this discharge on normal saline wet preparation is of a paucity of WBCs and a predominance of "clue" cells. By Gram stain, clue cells can be identified as epithelial cells almost totally covered by small, gram-negative rods. There is a paucity of other organisms seen in the background. By wet preparation these cells are best identified by a stippled birefringence that so densely covers the epithelial cell that the normal borders and nuclei are obscured. Culture on specific media and the use of gas-liquid chromatography are rarely of benefit in a clinical setting.

The most effective treatment for *Gardnerella*-associated vaginitis that has been documented to date is metronidazole. This may be given as 500 mg twice a day or 250 mg three times a day for seven days. The single high-dose therapy used in *Trichomonas* is not believed to be effective for *Gardnerella*-associated vaginitis. Metronidazole is thought to be efficacious for curing this infection because of its effect on the vaginal anaerobes. When metronidazole is contraindicated, alternative therapy of ampicillin, 500 mg four times a day for seven days is effective in a smaller number of cases. The need to treat male sexual partners is controversial. Reinfection of women after treatment is common. Most would agree that in cases of recurrent *Gardnerella*-associated vaginitis, the male partner should also be treated. The use of intravaginal sulfa creams or acidifying agents in the treatment of this infection may be effective in some cases.

Other Causes of Vaginitis Symptoms

Excessive vaginal discharge may be a manifestation of cervicitis. Organisms associated with cervicitis include *T. vaginalis, N. gonorrhoeae, C. trachomatis,* and the herpes simplex virus. When diagnosed, these should be treated accordingly. In addition, excess vaginal discharge may be associated with cervical ectopy or eversion, with no apparent infectious etiology.

Discharge and odor is associated with the presence of foreign bodies in the vaginal vault. Although this is chiefly of concern in pediatric populations, forgotten tampons may be a source of discharge in any population.

In addition to vulvar dystrophies and dysplasias, vulvar discomfort may be due to hypersensitivity reactions. In particular, this should be considered in women who have received numerous courses of topical anti-infective therapy.

POSTOPERATIVE INFECTIONS

Virtually all major and minor surgical procedures during which there is some manipulation of the lower genital tract may result in localized postsurgical infection. The risk of operative site infection is most strongly correlated with contamination of the operative site by potential pathogens. Procedures that result in exposure of the upper genital tract, the intra-abdominal cavity, or of skin wounds to lower genital tract flora may result in significant postoperative infection.

In order to understand the microbiology of postoperative infection, it is necessary to discuss the microbiology of the lower genital tract. The vulva, vagina, and cervix of the lower genital tract are normally colonized with a wide variety of bacteria. The lower genital tract flora is polymicrobial, and includes both aerobic and anaerobic organisms. The exact composition of lower genital tract flora varies among individuals, and appears to be influenced by age, hormonal status, sexual experience, and possibly by immune status. Cell type may also affect flora, possibly because of differences in bacterial adherence to cell surfaces, and because of differences in cell turnover. Although it can clearly be demonstrated that the vulva, vagina, and cervix are colonized with similar species of organisms, the exact types and quantities of organisms present in each area may be distinct.

TABLE 18–8.—LOWER GENITAL
TRACT FLORA

ORGANISM	RANGE (%)	AVERAGE
Lactobacillus sp	10–97	75
Staphylococcus albus	5–75	50
Gardnerella vaginalis	8–40	30
Enterococcus	5–35	25
Streptococcus viridans	2–30	15
Group B *Streptococcus*	5–20	12
Escherichia coli	3–24	10
Staphylococcus aureus	1–12	5
Peptococcus	8–64	30
Peptostreptococcus	10–30	20
Bacteroides sp	5–35	20
B. fragilis	1–9	3
Fusobacterium	2–23	5

Bacteriologic surveys of lower genital tract flora have been performed on varied patient populations by several investigators. Table 18–8 depicts average prevalences of some bacteria that are commonly part of the endogenous genital tract flora.

The results of prevalence surveys of lower genital tract flora have been compared with infection site cultures. Some species of bacteria are frequently found at sites of infection and are classified as potential pathogens. Other organisms that are part of the normal lower genital tract flora do not commonly cause local or systemic infections and are considered to be of very low pathogenic potential. Certain bacterial species such as *Escherichia coli* and *Bacteriodes fragilis* appear to be underrepresented in the lower genital tract in comparison with their occurrence at the site of infections. This may represent a particular capability of organisms such as these to invade and cause infection. The presence of virulence factors in certain organisms may contribute to their pathogenicity; the presence of a polysaccharide capsular antigen that helps to resist phagocytosis and opsonization while enhancing tissue invasiveness is one such factor.

The pathogenic potential of the lower genital tract flora may also be determined by interactions between bacteria. There may be some organisms that are capable of initially invading tissue and causing an inflammatory reaction. Other organisms may be able to contribute to that inflammatory reaction and further the infectious process once initial tissue destruction has progressed and anaerobic conditions have been achieved. Therefore, the types and quantity of organisms present and the proportions of potential pathogens at an operative site may all be important determinants of postoperative infection.

The major aerobic pathogens of importance in postoperative infections are Enterobacteriaceae including *E. coli*, streptococci including *S. viridans* and enterococci, and staphylococci, in particular *S. aureus*. *Staphylococcus aureus* and streptococcal species may be found as sole pathogens at the site of wound infections and other organisms may be found as sole pathogens at the site of postoperative infection; however, most often these organisms are seen in combination with other aerobic or anaerobic organisms. The most numerous anaerobic pathogens are the anaerobic gram-positive cocci including anaerobic streptococci, peptococci, and peptostreptococci. *Bacteroides* species including *B. fragilis* and *B. melaninogenicus* are major anaerobic pathogens of wound and soft-tissue infection. *Clostridum perfringens* and other anaerobic bacteria are less prevalent but need to be considered as potential pathogens.

Cultures of the lower genital tract may not accurately reflect the organisms that are present at the site of postoperative infection. Unless material from postoperative abscesses or postoperative wound infections is obtained for culture, treatment of infections is most often based on knowledge of which species may be involved in infection. Aerobic organisms such as the streptococci and coliforms are of particular concern in acute illness. Anaerobes, in particular *Bacteroides* species, are of concern, particularly with abscess formation.

The risk of infection after hysterectomy ranges from 7% to 30%. After vaginal hysterectomy, major operative site infections are pelvic infections such as cuff cellulitis or pelvic abscess. After abdominal hysterectomy, there is the risk of both pelvic and major abdominal wound infection. Posthysterectomy pelvic cellulitis presents as fever and lower pelvic pain that occurs between two to five days after surgery. The vaginal cuff is often indurated, warm, and exquisitely painful. Postoperative pelvic abscesses of the vaginal cuff, pelvic floor and side walls, at the site of intra-abdominal blood collection, or in the adnexal structures usually present more than five days after hysterectomy or other intra-abdominal pelvic surgical procedures and may not become manifest until after discharge from the hospital. Pelvic cellulitis often responds to simple broad-spectrum antibiotic therapy, not including extensive coverage for *B. fragilis*. If there is a suggestion of early abscess formation, if response to initial therapy is not prompt, or if there is life-threatening or severe illness, antimicrobial coverage for gram-negative enteric bacilli, streptococci, anaerobic cocci, and *B. fragilis* must be provided. Blunt drainage of the vaginal cuff can be a helpful adjunct to antibiotic therapy; surgical management of postoperative abscesses must be considered when the response to antibiotic therapy is not prompt and complete.

Postoperative wound infections may present acutely with fever and incisional pain along with erythema, induration, warmth, and tenderness. The group A β-hemolytic *Streptococcus* cause wound infection and high fevers occurring within 24 to 48 hours of surgery, and wounds should always be inspected when fever occurs early in the postoperative period. A less immediate onset of wound infection is more typical, however. Often a wound infection is the cause of spiking, low-grade fevers, whose source does not become obvious until a collection of pus is discovered through spontaneous drainage or by wound exploration. More than 20% of wound infections become apparent after hospitalization. *Staphylococcus aureus* and other skin organisms are common causes of postoperative wound infections. After genital tract surgery, mixed flora may also cause wound infections. Because of the somewhat unique exposure to

mixed aerobic/anaerobic pathogens at the time of surgery, patients undergoing gynecologic surgery are at risk for development of a distinct but uncommon "synergistic" wound infection at the site of the abdominal wound. Synergistic wound infections occur when tissue planes are invaded by both aerobic and anaerobic organisms. It has been theorized that aerobic organisms cause initial tissue infection and damage and that anaerobic organisms then cause further tissue destruction in an atmosphere of decreased oxygen tension. Diabetes, debilitating disease, obesity, and prior radiation therapy are risk factors for the occurrence of synergistic infections.

Synergistic infections may be rapidly progressive with necrosis spreading along fascial lines or through the subcutaneous tissue in a matter of hours. This is termed *necrotizing fasciitis* or *cellulitis*. In such cases, fever and signs of systemic sepsis are almost always present. Examination of skin and subcutaneous tissue reveals necrotic eschar formation and underlying crepitance. Cross-table lateral x-ray may reveal a subcutaneous gas pattern. Necrotizing wound infection due to *C. perfringens* may also cause a similar picture.

In other cases, synergistic wound infections have a more insidious onset with lack of systemic signs. Physical pain is often intense, and by the time the characteristic skin changes of central necrosis with surrounding erythema of a violaceous hue become apparent, the subcutaneous tissue necrosis is more advanced than one would suspect from outward appearance. This type of infection is sometimes called progressive synergistic bacterial gangrene.

There are a number of combinations of flora that can cause synergistic wound infections. Original descriptions of these wound infections were of mixed aerobic staphylococcal and microaerophilic streptococcal infection. Combinations of *E. coli* and other gram-negative enteric bacilli or aerobic streptococci with anaerobic cocci and *Bacteroides* species can also be isolated from these types of wound infections. Antibiotic therapy in cases of suspected synergistic wound infections must provide broad-spectrum coverage for both aerobic and anaerobic organisms, and must also include coverage for clostridial infections. It is rare, however, that antimicrobial therapy alone will be curative. Most often, wide debridement of all affected tissues is necessary. In cases of rapidly progressive disease, prompt debridement may be lifesaving. At the time of surgery, the infected tissue appears to undermine the skin, and classically is described as appearing totally gray, stringy, and devitalized with a purulent and fetid or a "dishwater" discharge. All such devitalized tissue must be totally resected to the point of healthy-appearing, bleeding tissue. Healing should be by secondary intention. Fascial grafting with synthetic grafts may be necessary.

The risk of pelvic infection after vaginal hysterectomy and the risk of pelvic plus wound infection combined after abdominal hysterectomy is significantly reduced, but not eliminated, through the use perioperative antimicrobial prophylaxis. Parenteral antibiotics should be used for such prophylaxis, should be administered just prior to surgery, and

continued postoperatively for less than 24 hours. There is no benefit to the use of either extended preoperative or extended postoperative antibiotics for preventing infection. The usual type of antibiotics used for prophylaxis during hysterectomy are broad-spectrum first-generation antimicrobials, such as cefazolin. There does not appear to be any additional benefit in terms of further decrease in postoperative infection through the use of more expensive and toxic regimens that provide additional coverage for anaerobes and resistent gram negative enteric bacilli. In addition to expense and toxicity, the development of superinfection or infection by resistant organisms is a potential danger with use of more broad-spectrum antibiotic regimens.

The use of properly functioning, active intraperitoneal or subperitoneal drains does prevent some postoperative infection. It is not clear whether the use of such drains is as effective or is additive to the efficacy of perioperative antimicrobial prophylaxis. The efficacy of antimicrobial prophylaxis for other gynecologic surgical procedures such as adnexal surgery or infertility surgery has not been proved.

BIBLIOGRAPHY

Bartlett J.G., Moon N.E., Goldstein P.R., et al.: Cervical and vaginal bacterial flora: Ecological niches in the female lower genital tract. *Am. J. Obstet. Gynecol.* 130:658–661, 1978.

Bartlett J.G., Onderdonk A.B., Drude E., et al.: Quantitative bacteriology of the vaginal flora. *J. Infect. Dis.* 136:271–277, 1977.

Becker L.E.: Lymphogranuloma venereum. *Int. J. Dermatol.* 15:26–33, 1976.

Burkman R., Schlesselman S., McCaffrey L., et al.: The relationship of genital tract actinomycetes and the development of pelvic inflammatory disease. *Am. J. Obstet. Gynecol.* 143:585–589, 1982.

Burkman R.T., Women's Health Study: Association between intrauterine device and pelvic inflammatory disease. *Obstet. Gynecol.* 57:269–277, 1981.

Caplan L.R., Kleeman F.J., Berg S.: Urinary retention probably secondary to herpes genitalis. *N. Engl. J. Med.* 297:920–921, 1977.

Corey L., Adams H.G., Brown Z.A., et al.: Genital herpes simplex virus infections: Clinical manifestations course and complications. *Ann. Intern. Med.* 98:958–972, 1983.

Criteria for diagnosis and grading of salpingitis, editorial. *Obstet. Gynecol.* 61:113, 1983.

Dalaker K., Gjonnaess H., Kvile G., et al.: *Chlamydia trachomatis* as a cause of acute perihepatitis associated with pelvic inflammatory disease. *Br. J. Vener. Dis.* 57:41–43, 1981.

Daly J.W., King R., Monif G.R.G.: Progressive necrotizing wound infection in postirradiated patients. *Obstet. Gynecol.* 52(suppl.):5–8, 1978.

Douglas J.M., Critchlow C., Benedetti J., et al.: A double-blind study of oral acyclovir for suppression of recurrences of genital herpes simplex virus infection. *N. Engl. J. Med.* 310:1551–1556, 1984.

Edelman D.A., Berger G.S.: Contraceptive practice and tubo-ovarian abscess. *Am. J. Obstet. Gynecol.* 138:541–544, 1980.

Eschenbach D.A.: Vaginal infection. *Clin. Obstet. Gynecol.* 26:186–202, 1983.

Eschenbach D.A., Buchanan T.M., Pollock H.M., et al.: Polymicrobial etiology of acute pelvic inflammatory disease. *N. Engl. J. Med.* 293:166–171, 1975.

Eschenbach D.A., Harnisch J.P., Holmes K.K.: Pathogenesis of acute pelvic inflammatory disease: Role of contraceptive and other risk factors. *Am. J. Obstet. Gynecol.* 128:838–850, 1977.

Eschenbach D.A., Holmes K.K.: Acute pelvic inflammatory disease: Current concepts of pathogenesis, etiology and management. *Clin. Obstet. Gynecol.* 18:35–50, 1975.

Fiumara N.J.: Treatment of seropositive primary syphilis: An evaluation of 196 patients. *Sex. Transm. Dis.* 4:92–95, 1977.

Fiumara N.J.: Treatment of secondary syphilis: An evaluation of 204 patients. *Sex. Transm. Dis.* 4:96–99, 1977.

Fiumara N.J.: Reinfection primary, secondary, and latent syphilis: The serologic response after treatment. *Sex. Transm. Dis.* 7:111–115, 1980.

Fonts A.C., Kraus S.J.: *Trichomonas vaginalis:* Reevaluation of its clinical presentation and laboratory diagnosis. *J. Infect. Dis.* 141:137–143, 1980.

Galask R.P., Larsen B., Ohm M.J.; Vaginal flora and its role in disease entities. *Clin. Obstet. Gynecol.* 19:61–81, 1976.

Gardner H.L.: *Haemophilus vaginalis* vaginitis after 25 years. *Am. J. Obstet. Gynecol.* 137:385–391, 1980.

Gilstrap L.C., Herbert W.N.P., Cunningham E.G., et al.: Gonorrhea screening in male consorts of women with pelvic infection. *J.A.M.A.* 238:965–966, 1977.

Golde S.H., Israel R., Ledger W.J.: Unilateral tuboovarian abscess: A distinct entity. *Am. J. Obstet. Gynecol.* 127:807–812, 1977.

Hager W.D., Brown S.T., Kraus S.J., et al.: Metronidazole for vaginal trichomoniasis: Seven-day *v* single-dose regimens. *J.A.M.A.* 224:1219–1220, 1980.

Henry-Suchet J., Loffredo V.: Chlamydial and *Mycoplasma* genital infection in salpingits and tubal sterility. *Lancet* 1:539–543, 1980.

Holmes K.K., Counts G.W., Beaty H.N.: Disseminated gonococcal infection. *Ann. Intern. Med.* 74:979–993, 1971.

Holmes K.K., Mardh P.A.: *International Perspectives on Neglected Sexually Transmitted Diseases.* New York, Hemisphere Publishing Corporation, 1983, pp. 1–336.

Hunter C.A., Long K.R.: Vaginal and cervical pH in normal women and in patients with vaginitis. *Am. J. Obstet. Gynecol.* 75:872–874, 1958.

Jacobson L., Westrom L.: Objectivized diagnosis of acute pelvic inflammatory disease: Diagnostic and prognostic value of routine laparoscopy. *Am. J. Obstet. Gynecol.* 105:1088–1098, 1969.

Judson F.N., Allaman J., Dans P.E.: Treatment of gonorrhea: Comparison of penicillin G procaine, doxycycline, spectinomycin, and ampicillin. *J.A.M.A.* 230:705–708, 1974.

Kelaghan J., Rubin G.L., Ory H.W., et al.: Barrier-method contraceptives and pelvic inflammatory disease. *J.A.M.A.* 248:184–187, 1982.

Ketoconazole *(Nizoral):* A new antifungal agent. *Med. Lett. Drugs Ther.* 23:85–87, 1981.

Klein T.A., Richmond J.A., Mischell D.R. Jr.: Pelvis tuberculosis. *Obstet. Gynecol.* 48:99–105, 1976.

Larsen B., Galask R.P.: Vaginal microbial flora: Practical and theoretic relevance. *Obstet. Gynecol.* 55(suppl.):1005–1135, 1980.

Lee N.C., Rubin G.L., Ory H.W., et al.: Type of intrauterine device and the risk of pelvic inflammatory disease. *Obstet. Gynecol.* 62:1–6, 1983.

Lee T.J., Sparling F.: Syphilis: An algorithm. *J.A.M.A.* 242:1187–1189, 1979.

Lightfoot T.W., Gotschlich E.C.: Gonococcal disease. *Am. J. Med.* 56:347–356, 1974.

Linder J.G.E.M., Plantema F.H.F., Hoogkamp-Korstamje J.A.A.: Quantitative studies of the vaginal flora of healthy women and of obstetric and gynaecological patients. *J. Med. Microbiol.* 11:233–241, 1978.

Lynch P.J.: Sexually transmitted diseases: Granuloma inguinale, lymphogranuloma venereum, chancroid and infectious syphilis. *Clin. Obstet. Gynecol.* 31:1041–1052, 1978.

McCormack W.M. (ed.): *Diagnosis and Treatment of Sexually Transmitted Diseases.* Littleton, Mass, John Wright PSG Inc. 1983, pp. 1–260.

McLellan R., Spence M.R., Brockman M., et al.: The clinical diagnosis of trichomoniasis. *Obstet. Gynecol.* 60:30–34, 1982.

Mardh P.A., Ripa K.T., Svensson L., et al.: *Chlamydia trachomatis* infection in patients with acute salpingitis. *N. Engl. J. Med.* 296:1377–1379, 1977.

Mardh P.A., Weström L.: Adherence of bacteria to vaginal epithelial cells. *Infect. Immunol.* 13:661–666, 1976.

Mardh P.A., Weström L.: Tubal and cervical cultures in acute salpingitis with special reference to *Mycoplasma hominis* and T-strain mycoplasmas. *Br. J. Vener. Dis.* 46:179–186, 1970.

Mead P.B.: Cervical-vaginal flora of women with invasive cervical cancer. *Obstet. Gynecol.* 52:601–604, 1978.

Meisels A.: Dysplasia and carcinoma of the uterine cervix: IV. A correlated cytologic and histologic study with special emphasis on vaginal microbiology. *Acta Cytol.* 13:224–234, 1969.

Meleney F.L.: Bacterial synergism in disease processes. *Ann. Surg.* 94:961–981, 1931.

Meltzer R.M.: Necrotizing gasciitis and progressive bacterial synergistic gangrene of the vulva. *Obstet. Gynecol.* 61:757–760, 1980.

Miles M.R., Olsen L., Rogers A.: Recurrent vaginal candidiasis: Importance of an intestinal reservoir. *J.A.M.A.* 238:1836–1837, 1977.

Monif G.R.G.: *Infectious Diseases in Obstetrics and Gynecology.* New York, Harper & Row Publishers, 1982, pp. 1–671.

Müller-Schoop J.W., Wang S.P., Munzinger J., et al.: *Chlamydia trachomatis* as possible cause of peritonitis and perihepatitis in young women. *Br. Med. J.* 1:1022–1024, 1978.

Nahmias A.J., Roizman B.: Infection with herpes simplex viruses 1 and 2. *N. Engl. J. Med.* 289:667–674, 719–725, 781–789; 1973.

Oriel J.D.: Genital warts. *Sex. Transm. Dis.* 4:153–159, 1977.

Oriel J.D., Partridge B.M., Denny M.J., et al.: Genital yeast infections. *Br. Med. J.* 4:761–764, 1972.

Oriel J.D., Ridgway G.L.: *Genital Infection With Chlamydia trachomatis.* New York, Elsevier Biomedical, 1982, pp. 1–144.

Pheifer T.A., Forsyth P.S., Durfee M.A., et al.: Nonspecific vaginitis: role of *Haemophilus vaginalis* and treatment with metronidazole. *N. Engl. J. Med.* 298:1429–1434, 1978.

Polk B.F.: Antimicrobial prophylaxis to prevent mixed bacterial infection. *J. Antimicrob. Chemother.* 8:115–129, 1981.

Polk B.F. Shapiro M., Goldstein P., et al.: Randomised clinical trial of perioperative cefazolin in preventing infection after hysterectomy. *Lancet* 1:438–441, 1980.

Rein M.F.: Current therapy of vulvovaginitis. *Sex. Transm. Dis.* 8:316–370, 1981.

Rubin G.L., Ory H.W., Layde P.M.: Oral contraceptives and pelvic inflammatory disease. *Am. J. Obstet. Gynecol.* 114:630–635, 1982.

Rudolph A.H.: Examination of the cerebrospinal fluid in syphilis. *Cutis* 17:749–752, 1976.

Scaling S.T., Levinson C.J., Plavidal F., et al.: The correlation of pelvic ultrasound and laparoscopy in the diagnosis and management of gynecologic disorders. *J. Reprod. Med.* 21:53–58, 1978.

Schacter J.: Chlamydial infections. *N. Engl. J. Med.* 298:428–435, 490–495, 540–549; 1978.

Schiffer M.A., Elguezabel A., Sultana M., et al.: Actinomycosis infections associated with intrauterine contraceptive devices. *Obstet. Gynecol.* 45:67–71, 1975.

Scott W.C.: Pelvic abscess in association with intrauterine contraceptive devices. *Am. J. Obstet. Gynecol.* 131:149–156, 1978.

Sexually transmitted diseases treatment guidelines 1982. *M.M.W.R.* 31:33–62, 1982.

Spaulding L.B., Gelman S.R., Wood S.D., et al.: The role of ultrasonography in the management of endometritis/salpingitis/peritonitis. *Obstet. Gynecol.* 53:442–446, 1979.

Speigel C.A., Amsel R., Eschenbach D., et al.: Anaerobic bacteria in nonspecific vaginitis. *N. Engl. J. Med.* 303:601–607, 1980.

Stamm W.E., Wagner K.F., Amsel R., et al.: Causes of the acute urethral syndrome in women. *N. Engl. J. Med.* 303:409–415, 1980.

St. John R.K., Brown S.T.: International symposium on pelvic inflammatory disease. *Am. J. Obstet. Gynecol.* 138:845–1112, 1980.

Stone H.H., Martin J.D.: Synergistic necrotizing cellulitis. *Ann. Surg.* 175:702–711, 1972.

Straus S.E., Takiff H.E., Seidlin M., et al.: Suppression of frequently recurring genital herpes. *N. Engl. J. Med.* 310:1545–1550, 1984.

Sweet R.L., Mills J., Hadley K.W., et al.: Use of laparoscopy to determine the microbiologic etiology of acute salpingitis. *Am. J. Obstet. Gynecol.* 134:68–78, 1979.

Thompson S.E., Hager W.D., Wong K.H., et al.: The microbiology and therapy of acute pelvic inflammatory disease in hospitalized patients. *Am. J. Obstet. Gynecol.* 36:179–186, 1980.

Valicenti J.E., Pappas A.A., Graber C.D., et al.: Detection and prevalence of IUD-associated *actinomyces* colonization and related morbidity. *J.A.M.A.* 247:1149–1152, 1982.

Van Slyke K.K., Michel V.P., Rein M.F.: Treatment of vulvovaginal candidiasis with boric acid power. *Am. J. Obstet. Gynecol.* 141:145–148, 1981.

Weström L.: Effect of acute pelvic inflammatory disease on fertility. *Am. J. Obstet. Gynecol.* 121:707–713, 1975.

Wiesner P.J., Thompson S.E.: Gonococcal diseases. *D.M.* 26:1–44, 1980.

Wolner-Hanseen P., Mardh P.A., Svensson L., et al.: Laparoscopy in women with chlamydial infection and pelvic pain: A comparison of patients with and without salpingitis. *Obstet. Gynecol.* 61:299–303, 1983.

Index